EASY CODER

2008 EDITION

BY

PAUL K. TANAKA, M.D., C.P.C.

Published by
Unicor Medical, Inc.
4160 Carmichael Rd.
Montgomery, AL 36106
(334) 260-8150

ISBN-13: - 978-1-56781-216-9

Editing and Production:

In memory of Peter O. Tanaka

PREFACE

Unicor Medical, Inc. is the most innovative company in the field of medical coding. We have entirely reorganized the ICD-9 system in order to help produce fast, complete, and precise coding. Accurate ICD-9 coding not only helps to optimize reimbursement but also produces a savings in the amount of employee time and effort spent on the coding/reimbursement process. When used properly and in conjunction with all current coding and reimbursement guidelines, Easy Coder is an important investment in the future earnings of a practice or medical facility.

The purpose of Easy Coder is to help you: 1) find ICD-9 codes efficiently, 2) use multiple codes so that the complete nature of the encounter is fully described, and 3) ensure the specificity and accuracy of the codes selected so as to adequately justify the services involved, thereby optimizing reimbursements. Great care has been taken in this book to incorporate and follow Centers for Medicare and Medicaid Services (CMS) and the National Center for Health Statistics (NCHS) guidelines, as well as third party payor regulations.

The rules to survive in the new coding climate are very complex, and mistakes are common and are costly for all parties involved. Not only does the physician pay for coding errors, but patients also suffer unjustly when services are not covered. *Remember, you communicate with carriers through numbers.* You must fully and accurately describe patient encounters numerically. Easy Coder will help you do just that. And just as your office is committed to providing quality medical care for your patients, Unicor Medical, Inc. stresses a sincere corporate committment to assist you in every way possible.

DISCLAIMER

Unicor Medical's Easy Coder code book has been written for use with codes taken from the Federal Government. Information has been referenced from official CMS and NCHS material, and includes the same codes as those from Volumes 1 and 2, 2008, of the U.S. Department of Health and Human Services' official code books.

Unicor Medical, Inc. has made every reasonable effort to assure that the information contained in the Easy Coder is completely accurate. The ultimate responsibility for the correct assignment of diagnosis codes, however, falls upon the medical provider.

Unicor Medical, Inc. and its principals, employees, or staff neither explicitly nor implicitly warranty/guarantee that the contained codes, statements, or narratives are error-free. We disclaim any responsibility or liability if a dispute of payment based on codes from the book arises with any third party payor, nor do we bear any responsibility or liability as to any use of the book, either medically or otherwise.

Users of the book purchase the material without any warranty/guarantee of any kind, either expressed or implied, as to the fitness of the book for their use. Neither is any warranty/guarantee given for the consequences or results from Easy Coder's use.

THE UNICOR QUALITY GUARANTEE

We believe that your 2008 Easy Coder will be the fastest, easiest, and most accurate ICD-9 book you've ever used. You'll quickly become familiar with the innovative Easy Coder format when you read the *Introduction* on the following pages.

If you ever have a problem finding a code in Easy Coder, we'd be happy to help. Simply call us toll-free at 1-800-825-7421 between 8am and 5pm CST Monday through Friday. You'll speak with a member of our own coding staff who will quickly locate for you the code you need at no charge whatsoever.

Complimentary coding support is provided exclusively for ICD-9 coding and exclusively for users of Unicor Medical products. Coding support for 2008 Easy Coder users extends from October 1, 2007 through October 1, 2008.

Please use the following unique identification number when you call:

CODING AUTHORIZATION NUMBER
521-1

INTRODUCTION

ICD-9 CM coding is the process of assigning a numerical code to a written description of a diagnosis, problem, condition, etc. You should code all the documented current diagnoses, including underlying diseases and secondary diagnoses.

Easy Coder is designed to do much of the coding analysis for you by providing a format for the codes that is logical and simple, by incorporating many basic rules within the format of the book, and by providing "help text" windows throughout the book. It is important, though, to consistently stay up to date on all the numerous rules and guidelines that help define which codes are acceptable under which circumstances.

One of the most important rules to remember has to do with the sequencing of codes. Sequencing in ICD-9 coding is determined by the intensity and acuity of service, the inherent DRG value, and the "level of service." The procedure indicated on the claim must be commensurate with the diagnosis or diagnoses indicated, and appropriate secondary diagnoses must be filed.

Proper sequencing of the diagnosis codes is of utmost importance. Occasionally, however, the rules for proper sequencing may seem confusing. AHA coding and sequencing guidelines were derived from inpatient data and are not necessarily logical in all cases when they are adapted to the outpatient rules of coding. Although these coding guidelines are far from perfect, they, nevertheless, are the guidelines by which many carriers now pay or reject claims.

The main rule to remember is the "reason rule," which says that the reason for the patient visit (encounter) is coded first. The only exception to the reason rule applies in the following situation: After study, the physician's major work and effort is directed toward a certain diagnosis or procedure different from the one the patient originally came in for. Then the diagnosis that required the greater amount of effort should be coded first.

Now that you know how important it is to understand coding rules, and you are familiar with the important "reason rule," it's time to explain how Easy Coder makes following these rules easier and makes coding more efficient.

FINDING THE DIAGNOSIS

The traditional system of categories and exclusions does not exist in Easy Coder. Easy Coder is completely alphabetical. Some diagnoses have their own singular listing, while others are listed under a main boldface heading along with all the other types, kinds, states, conditions, or possible locations associated with that heading. For example, when you look up arthritis alphabetically, you'll find that arthritis is a main heading and that indented under it is a list of all the different types of arthritis.

The most important element is this: Whether it is a singular listing or part of a list under a main boldface heading, *each and every diagnosis is listed with its own correct code* at ultimate specificity. You will never find an exclusion in Easy Coder. Just look up the diagnosis alphabetically, and you'll find the exact code. There are three (3) ways that a diagnosis may be listed:

1. By the key word in the diagnosis

Most diagnoses are listed under a "key word." The key word is the most important or most descriptive word in the diagnosis. The key word is the word that gives you the most information about the diagnosis. It's usually a noun or a noun derivative.

Often you'll find that a key word for one diagnosis is also the key word for several other related or similar diagnoses. In this case, the key word is a main boldface heading, and it is followed by an indented listing of the various diagnoses, which usually convey particular types, states, or possible locations.

Once you determine the key word, look for that word alphabetically, just as if you were using a dictionary. Here are some examples of diagnoses and their key words:

biliary cirrhosis

Cirrhosis would be the key word in this example, since it tells you more about the diagnosis than biliary does. The word biliary describes what type of cirrhosis; it is secondary information.

Since the key word for this diagnosis is cirrhosis, you would find the diagnosis under the alphabetical listing for cirrhosis.

hiatal hernia

Hernia would be the key word for his diagnosis, since it gives the most important descriptive information. Hiatal, of course, describes the type of hernia.

2. By the anatomical site

The second way that a diagnosis may be listed is under the anatomical site. A diagnosis will typically be listed by anatomical site if it is surgical in nature, or if the condition or disorder involved is rather non-descriptive, such as "injury." Here are just a few examples of diagnoses that are listed this way:

progressive atrophy of the iris-- found alphabetically under iris
deviated nasal septum-- found alphabetically under septum
congenital absence of an arm-- found alphabetically under arm

Please note that it is not uncommon for a diagnosis to be listed by the anatomical site as well as by a key word or exactly as it was written in the documentation. In standard code books, diagnoses are listed only one way. *In Easy Coder, however, most diagnoses are listed several ways so that the need for multiple searches and cross referencing is practically eliminated.* For example, congestive heart failure can be found alphabetically under congestive and CHF. Laceration of the eyeball can be found alphabetically under laceration and ocular.

3. Exactly as it is written in the patient's record

Many diagnoses are listed exactly as they are written in the patient's record or chart from which you're coding. In other words, you'll simply look for the diagnosis alphabetically by the first word in its description, just as if you were using a dictionary. Here are just a few examples of diagnoses that are listed by the first word in the description:

spinal cord compression-- found alphabetically under spinal cord
hypertensive retinopathy-- found alphabetically under hypertensive
myocardial infarction--found alphabetically under myocardial

Note that *one word diagnoses* and *discrete diagnoses* are always found alphabetically under the first word of the diagnosis, exactly as they are written in the documentation. Again, here are just a few of the many possible examples:

intertrigo--found alphabetically under intertrigo
fructose intolerance-- found alphabetically under fructose
idiopathic hypertrophic subaortic stenosis-- found alphabetically under idiopathic

Also note that most diagnoses can be found not only under their exact medical name, but also under any common name, abbreviation, and acronym. For instance:

temporomandibular joint disorder--found alphabetically under temporomandibular, and under its common abbreviation, TMJ
hepatomegaly--found alphabetically under hepatomegaly and under its common name, liver enlargement

Remember, a diagnosis will always be listed alphabetically, either by the first word in the diagnosis (exactly as it's documented in the record), by a key word in the diagnosis, or by the anatomical site involved. A diagnosis may have its own singular one-line listing, or it may be part of a comprehensive listing under a main heading.

Main headings are words or phrases that are in **boldface** type and that are followed by a list of indented entries. A main heading may be the key word or the anatomical site for several various types, kinds, states, or locations of related or similar diagnoses. These specific diagnoses are given in an indented list immediately below the main heading. The indented entries are specific choices for the main heading. Note that the main headings have been set up for coding ease, not for classification of medical terms.

FINDING THE CODE

Easy Coder is organized to give you all the codes you need for every diagnosis in just one step. To the left of every diagnosis is a code. If the code is not at ultimate specificity already, a menu follows. If you need to use a second code in order to completely code for all additional diagnoses or underlying diseases, you'll find the second code provided for you to the right of the diagnosis, or you'll be reminded to select the appropriate additional code in cases where several codes could be applicable.

Following are descriptions of the symbols and formats used to ensure that you have all the digits and all the correctly sequenced codes needed to fully code the diagnosis. Note that all of the following symbols and formats may be used in conjunction with one another and more than one can appear at a time; apply all the necessary ones that appear for any diagnosis.

1. Menus

You will always be able to tell when a code is not at ultimate specificity because the code number will be in boldface type and there will be a pound sign (#) in the location where the fourth or fifth digit should be. There will be also be a "menu," a selection of choices, immediately following. You should choose the appropriate description from the menu and then append the corresponding digit to the base code in order to obtain ultimate specificity.

If the bold code number is 3 digits long and has one # sign next to it, the choice from the menu will take the diagnosis to its ultimate 4th digit specificity.

If the bold code number is 4 digits long and has one # sign next to it, the appropriate choice from the menu will take the diagnosis to its ultimate 5th digit specificity.

If the bold code number is 3 digits long and has two # signs next to it, two menus will follow, and the choices together will take the diagnosis to its 5th digit ultimate specificity.

Here's an example:

Dx= abdominal pain lower left quadrant

ABDOMEN, ABDOMINAL
789.0# Pain

4th Digit: 789.0
0. Unspecified site
1. Upper right quadrant
2. Upper left quadrant
3. Lower right quadrant
4. Lower left quadrant
5. Periumbilic
6. Epigastric.
7. Generalized
9. Other specified site (multiple)

To take the code for this diagnosis to ultimate specificity, you would select choice "4" from the 4th digit menu. The code for this diagnosis is 789.4 which is to ultimate specificity.

If the diagnosis were to another area of the abdomen you would choose the appropriate location and append that digit to the code.

Note: In a very few cases, you will see a single menu that contains both 4th and 5th digits. Some of the choices in the menu will have only a 4th digit; others will have a 4th and a 5th digit. Simply make the appropriate selection from the menu, and assign the corresponding digit or digits.

Here's an example:

BACTERIAL INFECTION

041.9 NOS
041.85 AEROBACTER AEROGENES
041.82 BACTEROIDES FRAGILIS
041.83 CLOSTRIDIUM PERFRINGENS
041.4 E COLI
041.81 EATON'S AGENT
041.3 FRIEDLANDER'S BACILLUS
041.84 GRAM-NEGATIVE ANAEROBES
041.85 GRAM-NEGATIVE BACTERIA NOS
041.5 H. INFLUENZAE
041.86 H. PYLORI (HELICOBACTER PYLORI)
041.3 KLEBSIELLA
041.85 MIMA POLYMORPHA
041.81 MYCOLPLASMA
041.81 PLEUROPNEUMONIA LIKE ORGANISMS
041.2 PNEUMOCOCCUS
041.6 PROTEUS (MIRABILIS) (MORGANII) (VULGARIS)
041.7 PSEUDOMONAS
041.85 SERRATIA (marcescens)
041.10 STAPHYLOCOCCUS UNSPECIFIED
041.11 STAPHYLOCOCCUS AUREUS
041.19 STAPHYLOCOCCUS OTHER
041.00 STREPTOCOCCUS
041.01 STREPTOCOCCUS GROUP A
041.02 STREPTOCOCCUS GROUP B
041.02 STREPTOCOCCUS GROUP C
041.04 STREPTOCOCCUS GROUP D
041.05 STREPTOCOCCUS GROUP G
041.09 STREPTOCOCCUS OTHER
041.89 OTHER SPECIFIED BACTERIA

The correct code for the organism E coli would be 041.4.

The correct code for the organism streptococcus, group D would be 041.04.

If there is only a 4th digit listed for your menu selection, then use just a 4th digit to take the code to ultimate specificity. If there are a 4th and a 5th digit listed, then append both digits to take the code to ultimate specificity.

2. "Use Additional Code(s)"

Sometimes more than one code is needed to correctly code a diagnosis. There are two conventions for referencing additional codes in Easy Coder. In the majority of cases, the additional code is listed in brackets to the right of the diagnosis. In some cases, when there are numerous codes that could be used as an additional code, and the selection of the correct additional code is dependent on what diagnoses were documented for the particular episode of care, a help box is provided reminding you to use the additional code that is correct for the encounter you are coding (if one is required). Remember, only code the diagnoses that are documented by the physician and that are relevant for that particular episode of care.

A. Additional Code in Brackets

Two codes

When a diagnosis requires a second code for an underlying disease or a secondary diagnosis, the appropriate second code may be listed in brackets to the right of the diagnosis. If both conditions inherent in the diagnosis are documented in the record, then the code in brackets is a mandatory part of correct coding for the particular diagnosis; it is not optional.

The relationship of the diagnosis to the codes is indicated by underlining. One code, either the code to the left of the diagnosis or the code in brackets to the right, will be underlined; also underlined will be part of the diagnosis description. *The code number that is underlined goes with the part of the diagnosis that is underlined. The code number that is not underlined goes with the part of the diagnosis that is not underlined.* Remember, though, underlining indicates correspondence only, not sequencing priority.

A code in a main heading

Easy Coder sometimes will list an additional code in brackets beside a main heading if that code may apply to all the diagnoses listed under that heading. The bracketed code, if used, would be sequenced after the primary code for the diagnosis.

Three codes

In some cases, a diagnosis requires two additional codes. In these cases, Easy Coder provides both of the additional codes to the right of the diagnosis. Both codes will be contained in brackets.

One of the three codes and one part of the diagnosis description will be underlined once. Another code and another part of the diagnosis description will be underlined twice. *The code with one underline goes with the part of the diagnosis with one underline. The code with two underlines goes with the part of the diagnosis with two underlines. Of course, the code that is not underlined goes with the part of the diagnosis that is not underlined.*

Sequencing

Any time Easy Coder gives you an additional code in brackets, it also puts the codes in order for sequencing. *Always sequence multiple codes from left to right.*

The code to the left of the diagnosis sequences first. The bracketed code immediately to the right of the diagnosis sequences second. If there are two bracketed codes located to the right of the diagnosis, the far-right code sequences third. The rule is easy: sequence left to right, regardless of which code is underlined, and regardless of which part of the diagnosis you actually looked up alphabetically. The work has already been done for you. Just sequence from left to right.

Here are some examples of additional codes in brackets. Remember, the underlining indicates the correspondence between the codes and the diagnosis. The sequencing is always done from left to right.

272.7 FABRY'S DISEASE CEREBRAL DEGENERATION [330.2]

The correct codes and sequencing for the above listing would be as follows:

272.7 Fabry's Disease
330.2 cerebral degeneration

DEMENTIA

985.8 DIALYSIS DUE TO ALUMINUM OVERLOAD [294.8] [E879.1]

The correct codes and sequencing for the above listing would be as follows:

985.8 Aluminum Overload
294.8 Dementia
E879.1 Dialysis

SPONDYLOSIS

WITH OSTEOPOROSIS [733.0#]

721.0 CERVICAL
721.1 CERVICAL WITH MYELOPATHY (CORD COMPRESSION)
721.3 LUMBAR

Remember that if the diagnosis did not include osteoporosis, you would have used only the codes 721.0 for the cervical spondylosis.

Remember that any time there is a # sign following a code, you need to append at least one more digit from the associated menu(s) in order to gain ultimate specificity. However, for the sake of space and clarity, the menus for the notated codes above have not been listed out in these examples.

B. Additional Code Reminder Box

For some diagnoses, coding guidelines suggest that an additional code be used to show the specific complication, manifestation, disease, etc., if one is documented. In most of these cases, there are numerous additional codes that may be applicable; the choice of which code is correct for the particular episode of care you are coding can only be determined by the documentation of the diagnoses seen during that episode.

In these cases, when there is not a specific code indicated in brackets, there will be a help text box nearby to remind you that you should use an appropriate additional code. As its name suggests, the additional code should be sequenced after the primary diagnosis, unless otherwise specified.

Here is an example of a help box reminding you to use an additional code:

USE AN ADDITIONAL CODE TO FURTHER SPECIFY THE COMPLICATION OF ANESTHESIA OR OTHER SEDATION.

ANESTHESIA COMPLICATING L & D

668.9# COMPLICATION NOS
668.1# CARDIAC COMPLICATIONS
668.2# CENTRAL NERVOUS SYSTEM COMPLICATIONS
668.0# PULMONARY COMPLICATIONS
668.8# OTHER SPECIFIED COMPLICATIONS

5th Digit: 668.0-9
0. EPISODE OF CARE NOS OR N/A
1. DELIVERED
2. DELIVERED POSTPARTUM COMPLICATION
3. ANTEPARTUM COMPLICATION
4. POSTPARTUM COMPLICATION

The 668 code identifies that there is a complication, but it does not identify the specific complication. To show exactly what the complication is, you need to use an additional code. Since there can be numerous conditions that are complications of anesthesia (such as hypoxia, hyperpyrexia, various types of cardiac dysrhythmia, etc.), you must select the additional code that specifies what the exact complication was for the specific episode of care you are coding. As the name suggests, the additional code is sequenced after the primary code (unless otherwise noted).

If your documentation indicates that the patient experienced hypoxia in reaction to the anesthesia given during delivery, the correct codes and sequencing would be as follows:

668.0# pulmonary complication / anesthesia complicating labor and delivery
799.02 hypoxia

MORPHOLOGY CODES

Morphology codes, or "M" codes, are an adaptation of the International Classification of Diseases of Oncology. Published by the World Health Organization, "M" codes indicate the histological origin and the behavior of neoplasms.

M-codes consist of five digits. Histological origin or cell-type is indicated by the first four digits, while the fifth digit indicates behavior.

The fifth digit indicates the following behaviors:

/0 benign
/1 uncertain whether benign or malignant, borderline malignancy
/2 carcinoma in situ
 intraepithelial
 non-infiltrating
 non-invasive
/3 malignant, primary site
/6 malignant, secondary site or metastatic
/9 malignant, uncertain whether primary or metastatic

The morphology codes given include a fifth digit for the assumed behavior based on the cell-type. However, the patient's records and documentation may indicate a different behavior and therefore prompt the use of a different fifth digit. For example, a Leydig Cell Tumor unspecified is generally assumed to be malignant and would be assigned a morphology code of M8650/3. But if the supporting documents for the case you are coding indicate that the tumor is benign, the appropriate behavior code would be /0 and the correct M-code would be M8650/0. Generally speaking, the documented description of the neoplasm should decide the appropriate morphology code where applicable.

The M code is listed in Easy Coder to the right of the diagnosis description.

When a morphological diagnosis contains two qualifying adjectives, and the adjectives correspond to different M-codes, use the higher number. Most likely, the higher number is a more specific description. For example, a papillary carcinoma has a morphology code of M8050/3, while a papillary serous carcinoma has a morphology code of M8460/3. For the correct code for papillary serous carcinoma, you would choose the higher of the two morphology numbers and select M8460/3.

Note that the fifth digit of /9 is inapplicable in the context of ICD-9, since all malignant neoplasms are presumed to be primary (/3) or secondary (/6) according to the information on the medical record.

E-CODES

An E-code is an ICD-9 code that provides supplementary information concerning the external cause of an injury. E-codes do not indicate the injury itself, but rather why the injury occurred. E-codes can be used to show the environmental events, circumstances, conditions, or nature of the condition, and they help provide to the carrier a more detailed analysis of what happened to the patient that resulted in the current condition. E-codes are also very important for reporting purposes.

E-codes can be used in conjunction with any other code from 001-999, but they can not be used alone and they can not be assigned as the principal diagnosis. The only E-codes that are mandatory nationwide are E-codes that indicate drugs that have caused adverse effects during therapeutic use. Several states, however, now require the use of any and all E-codes when applicable.

E-codes are listed in the back of Easy Coder. The section is divided into logical and easy-to-use categories. An E-code directory is provided at the beginning of the E-code section. The directory tells you on what page you'll find the various categories.

Following is an example of correctly using E-codes.

Scenario: A patient suffers a hip contusion after slipping on a wet spot on the floor and falling at the factory where he works.

After coding the contusion as 924.01, you're ready to find the correct E-codes. First, you'll turn to the E-code directory at the beginning of the E-code section and find the appropriate category which, in this case, would be "falls." When you turn to the page referenced in the directory, you'll then see three types of falls, one involving falls between two levels, one involving a fall on just one level, and one for fall unspecified. Since the scenario says the man slipped on the floor, only one level is involved.

FALLS FROM/INTO SAME LEVEL

E885.1	ROLLER SKATES OR INLINE SKATES
E885.9	SIDEWALK - MOVING
E885.2	SKATEBOARD
E885.3	SKIS
E885.9	SLIPPING ON ICE
E885.9	SLIPPING ON MUD
E885.9	SLIPPING ON OIL
E885.9	SLIPPING ON SLIPPERY SURFACE
E885.9	SLIPPING ON SNOW
E885.9	SLIPPING OR TRIPPING OTHER
E885.9	SLIPPING ON WET SURFACE
E885.4	SNOWBOARD
E886.0	SPORTS (COLLISION)
E885.9	STUMBLING OVER ANIMAL OR SMALL OBJECT
E885.9	TRIPPING OVER ANIMAL, CURB, RUG OR SMALL OBJECT
E886.9	OTHER AND UNSPECIFIED COLLISION

For the scenario above, you would choose code E885.9 from the types of falls listed. An injury code always sequences before an E-code, so you know that the 924.01 code comes first, followed by E885.9.

The correct sequenced codes for the above example are as follows:
924.01 hip contusion
E885.9 fall from/ into same level slipping, tripping, or stumbling

SUMMARY

All diagnoses are listed alphabetically. A diagnosis may be a singular one-line listing or part of an indented list of diagnoses under a main heading.

Find the diagnosis by looking alphabetically for the key word, the anatomical site, or the first word in the diagnosis description. Remember, the diagnosis may be listed under its exact medical name, common name, abbreviation, or acronym. If a proper name (such as Refsum's, Coat's, etc.) is in the description, the diagnosis is usually listed under the proper name.

The key word is usually a noun or a noun-based derivative. It is the most descriptive or most important word in the diagnosis description-- the word that gives the most information about the diagnosis.

Many diagnoses are listed at least two different ways to avoid cross-referencing and multiple searches.

If a code is followed by a # sign, choose the appropriate selection from the corresponding menu to take the code to ultimate specificity.

If an additional code is given in brackets, underlining indicates correspondence between the code and the diagnosis description only. It does not indicate sequencing. Sequence multiple codes from left to right.

SYMBOLS & FORMATS

The **"#"** sign indicates that the ICD-9 code is not to the ultimate specificity. The appropriate 4th or 5th digit menu will immediately follow the diagnoses.

The **"[ ]"** are used to enclose a supplementary code. If the diagnosis with which the code corresponds is documented in the patient's record, the supplemental code must be used. This code must be sequenced secondarily.

An underline **"__________"** under a code number and part of a diagnosis description means that that code and that part of the description correspond. Likewise, a double-underlined code corresponds with the double-underlined part of the diagnosis description.

The **"( )"** are used to enclose other words that can be used interchangeably in the diagnosis description, and for words used to make the meaning of the description clearer.

The **"0"** in place of a code indicates that the code(s) for that particular description is listed under a synonym. There will be a description telling you where to find the appropriate diagnosis. You may not select a diagnosis with a code of 0.

A

758.39 5Q DELETION CONSTITUTIONAL
238.73 5Q DELETION WITH HIGH GRADE MYELODYSPLASTIC SYNDROME
238.74 5Q DELETION WITH MYELODYSPLASTIC SYNDROME
238.74 5Q MINUS SYNDROME NOS
441.4 AAA (ABDOMINAL AORTIC ANEURYSM)
273.4 AAT DEFICIENCY (ALPHA-1 ANTITRYPSIN)
0 AB (ABORTION) SEE 'ABORTION'
781.99 ABAROGNOSIS

ABASIA/ASTASIA

307.9 NOS
781.3 Atactica (choreic) (paroxysmal trepident) (spastic) (trembling) (trepidans)
300.11 Hysterical

270.0 ABDERHALDEN-KAUFMANN-LIGNAC SYNDROME

ABDOMEN, ABDOMINAL

793.6 Abnormal (x-ray) (other test or study)
902.0 Aorta injury
908.4 Aorta injury late effect
787.3 Bloating
345.5# Convulsive, epileptic
5th digit: 345.5
0. Without mention of intractable epilepsy
1. With intractable epilepsy

787.3 Distention (gaseous)
746.87 Heart
868.00 Injury unspecified site
902.9 Injury blood vessel NOS
908.1 Injury late effect
868.09 Injury multiple or other specified site
868.10 Injury with open wound unspecified site
868.19 Injury with open wound multiple or other specified site
789.3# Mass
5th digit: 789.3
0. Unspecified site
1. Upper right quadrant
2. Upper left quadrant
3. Lower right quadrant
4. Lower left quadrant
5. Periumbilic
6. Epigastric
7. Generalized
9. Other specified site (multiple)

346.2# Migraine syndrome
5th digit: 346.2
0. Without mention intractable migraine
1. With intractable migraine

756.79 Muscle deficiency syndrome
959.12 Muscle injury
756.79 Obstipum

ABDOMEN, ABDOMINAL (continued)

789.0# Pain
5th digit: 789.0
0. Unspecified site
1. Upper right quadrant
2. Upper left quadrant
3. Lower right quadrant
4. Lower left quadrant
5. Periumbilic
6. Epigastric
7. Generalized
9. Other specified site (multiple)

0 Pregnancy see 'Ectopic Pregnancy (Ruptured) (Unruptured)'
728.84 Rectus diastasis
665.8# Rectus diastasis complicating pregnancy
5th digit: 665.8
0. Episode of care NOS or N/A
1. Delivered
2. Delivered with postpartum complication
3. Antepartum complication
4. Postpartum complication

756.79 Rectus diastasis congenital
789.4# Rigidity
739.9 Segmental or somatic dysfunction
789.3# Swelling
306.4 Symptom psychogenic
789.9 Symptom other
789.0# Syndrome acute
789.6# Tenderness
5th digit: 789.0, 3, 4, 6
0. Unspecified site
1. Upper right quadrant
2. Upper left quadrant
3. Lower right quadrant
4. Lower left quadrant
5. Periumbilic
6. Epigastric
7. Generalized
9. Other specified site (multiple)

756.70 Wall anomaly - NOS
756.71 Wall anomaly - prune belly syndrome
756.79 Wall anomaly - other
959.12 Wall injury
911.8 Wall injury other and NOS superficial
911.9 Wall Injury other and NOS superficial - infected

0 ABDOMINALGIA SEE 'ABDOMEN, ABDOMINAL', PAIN
277.31 ABDOMINALGIA PERIODIC
378.54 ABDUCENS NERVE DISORDER (ATROPHY) (PALSY)
951.3 ABDUCENS NERVE INJURY
277.39 ABERCROMBIE'S SYNDROME (AMYLOID DEGENERATION)
272.5 ABETALIPOPROTEINEMIA
790.91 ABG ABNORMAL
780.79 ABIONARCE
799.89 ABIOTROPHY
743.62 ABLEPHARON DEFORMITIES EYELID CONGENITAL

A

Abnormal tests, symptoms, signs, or ill-defined conditions may also be found under specific descriptions such as EKG, coma, chest, or x-ray.

ABNORMAL

787.5	Bowel sounds
786.7	Chest sounds
793.1	CXR
787.7	Feces
790.09	Findings anisocytosis
796.5	Findings antenatal screening
796.6	Findings neonatal screening
796.9	Findings other specified
781.2	Gait
781.0	Head movements
781.91	Height loss
374.43	Innervation syndrome eyelid
781.0	Involuntary movements
524.51	Jaw closure
781.0	Movements
786.7	Percussion chest
781.92	Posture
796.1	Reflex
786.4	Sputum (amount) (color) (odor)
792.1	Stool color
524.59	Swallowing (malocclusion)
783.1	Weight gain

783.21 Use an additional code to identify body mass index (BMI), if known. See 'Body Mass Index'.

783.21	Weight loss

ABNORMAL BODY FLUIDS OR SUBSTANCES

792.3	Amniotic fluid
792.0	Cerebrospinal
792.5	Cloudy (hemodialysis) (peritoneal) dialysis effluent
792.9	Peritoneal
792.9	Pleural
792.4	Saliva
795.2	Saliva in chromosomal analysis
792.2	Semen
792.2	Spermatozoa
786.4	Sputum (color) (amount) (odor)
792.1	Stool
792.9	Synovial
792.9	Vaginal
792.9	Other

ABNORMAL CULTURE

790.7	Blood
795.39	Microbiologic NEC
795.39	Nasal
0	Pap smear, cervix see 'Pap Smear'
795.39	Skin lesion NEC
792.0	Spinal fluid
795.39	Sputum
792.1	Stool
795.39	Throat
791.9	Urine
795.39	Wound
795.39	NEC

ABNORMAL FUNCTION STUDIES - BRAIN

794.00	Brain unspecified
794.01	Echoencephalogram
794.02	EEG (electroencephalography)
794.09	Other (scan)

ABNORMAL FUNCTION STUDIES - CARDIOPULMONARY

794.39	Ballistocardiogram
794.30	Cardiovascular unspecified
794.39	Cardiovascular other
794.31	ECG (electrocardiogram)
794.31	EKG (electrocardiogram)
794.2	Lung scan
794.39	Phonocardiogram
794.2	Pulmonary
794.39	Stress test
794.39	Vectorcardiogram

ABNORMAL FUNCTION STUDIES - NERVOUS SYSTEM

794.15	Auditory function studies
794.00	Central NOS
794.09	Central other specified
794.12	Electro-oculogram (EOG)
794.17	EMG (electromyogram)
794.11	ERG (electroretinogram)
794.10	Nerve stimulation unspecified
794.14	Oculomotor studies
794.19	Peripheral nerves other
794.11	Retinal
794.16	Vestibular function studies
794.13	Visually evoked potential

ABNORMAL FUNCTION STUDIES - OTHER

794.7	Basal metabolism
794.9	Bladder
794.9	Bone
794.4	Kidney
794.8	Liver
0	Liver function test see 'Abnormal Lab Test (Blood) Nonspecific', Liver
794.9	Pancreas
794.9	Placental
794.2	Pulmonary
794.4	Renal
794.9	Spleen
794.5	Thyroid
794.6	Other endocrine
794.9	Other

If there is a specific condition stated in the medical record, remember to code that condition (hypoglycemia, hyperkalemia, hyperlipidemia). Abnormal findings are to be used only when there is no definitive diagnosis.

ABNORMAL LAB TEST (BLOOD) NONSPECIFIC

790.99	NOS
790.99	Albumin globulin ratio
790.3	Alcohol level increased
795.79	Antibody NOS
790.91	Arterial blood gas or other exam of blood
790.7	Bacteremia any kind
790.92	Bleeding time prolonged
790.91	Blood gas level
790.6	Bun and creatine elevated

ABNORMAL LAB TEST (BLOOD) NONSPECIFIC (continued)

790.95 C-reactive protein elevated
275.40 Calcium
795.82 Cancer antigen 125 (CA 125)
795.81 Carcinoembryonic antigen (CEA)
790.6 Chemistries (except electrolytes)
272.9 Cholesterol (serum)
272.0 Cholesterol high
272.2 Cholesterol high with high triglycerides
790.5 Enzyme levels other
790.94 Euthyroid sick syndrome
790.29 Glucose (non-fasting)
790.29 Glucose elevated
790.21 Glucose elevated fasting
790.22 Glucose elevated tolerance test
790.21 Glucose fasting impaired (elevated)
790.09 Hematocrit
790.01 Hematocrit drop (precipitous)
795.79 Immunological other (immunoglobulins)
790.6 Lead
790.6 Liver function test (LFT)
790.5 Liver function test (LFT) – alkaline phosphatase
790.4 Liver function test (LFT) - aminotransferase
782.4 Liver function test (LFT) - bilirubin
790.5 Liver function test (LFT) – hepatic enzyme NEC
790.4 Liver function test (LFT) – lactate dehydrogenase
790.5 Other enzymes phosphatase amylase
276.8 Potassium deficiency
276.7 Potassium excess
790.93 PSA (elevated) prostatic specific antigen
790.09 RBC (red blood cells) volume morphology
790.1 SED rate elevated
790.29 Sugar abnormal
790.29 Sugar high NOS
790.21 Sugar high fasting
790.22 Sugar high tolerance test
251.2 Sugar low
796.0 Toxicology
790.4 Transaminase or LDH
272.1 Triglycerides high
272.2 Triglycerides high with high cholesterol
795.8# Tumor markers

5th digit: 795.8
1. Elevated carcinoembryonic antigen (CEA)
2. Elevated cancer antigen 125 (CA 125)
9. Other

790.6 Uric acid
790.8 Viremia any kind
288.60 White blood cell count elevated
288.69 White blood cell count elevated other
288.50 White blood cell count low
288.59 White blood cell count low other
288.9 White blood cell differential
288.9 White blood cell morphology
790.99 Other specified

ABNORMAL RADIOLOGICAL STUDY

793.#(#) Echogram
793.#(#) Thermography
793.#(#) Ultrasound
793.#(#) X ray

4th or 4th and 5th digit: 793
0. Skull and head
1. Lung field
2. Other intrathoracic
3. Biliary tract
4. Gastrointestinal tract
5. Genitourinary organs
6. Abdominal area including retroperitoneum
7. Musculoskeletal system
8#. Breast
80. Unspecified
81. Mammographic microcalcification
89. Other abnormal findings (calcification) (calculus)
9#. Other
91. Inconclusive due to excess body fat
99. Other abnormal findings (placenta)(skin)(subcutaneous)

When using code 793.91, Image test inconclusive due to excess body fat, use additional code to identify body mass index (BMI) which can be found at 'Body Mass Index'.

ABNORMAL URINALYSIS (NONSPECIFIC)

791.6 Acetonuria
791.0 Albuminuria
791.0 Bence Jones
791.4 Bilirubinuria
791.7 Cells, casts
791.1 Chyluria
791.9 Crystals
791.5 Glycosuria, glucose
791.2 Hemoglobinuria
791.6 Ketone acetone
791.6 Ketonuria
791.3 Myoglobinuria
791.0 Proteinuria
791.9 Pus in urine
796.0 Toxicology
791.9 Other

ABO INCOMPATIBILITY

773.1 Causing hemolytic disease (fetus) (newborn)
773.1 Fetus or newborn
999.6 Infusion or transfusion reaction
656.2# Maternal affecting management of mother

5th digit: 656.2
0. Episode of care NOS or N/A
1. Delivered
3. Antepartum complication

V26.35 ABORTER HABITUAL MALE PARTNER TESTING

646.3# ABORTER HABITUAL WITH CURRENT PREGNANCY

5th digit: 646.3
- **0. Episode of care NOS or N/A**
- **1. Delivered**
- **3. Antepartum complication**

629.81 ABORTER HABITUAL WITHOUT CURRENT PREGNANCY

> ***When an attempted termination of pregnancy results in a liveborn fetus, the appropriate code to assign is 644.21, early onset of delivery, with the appropriate code from V27.# outcome of delivery.***

> ***Code 639 should be assigned for all complications following abortion. Code 639 can not be assigned with codes from the categories 634-638, abortion by type.***

> ***Abortion is the removal or extraction of all or part of placenta or membrane with or without an identifiable fetus weighing less than 500 grams or over 22 weeks gestation. Use 644.21, early onset of delivery, premature labor with onset of delivery before 37 weeks gestation for reporting.***
>
> ***Spontaneous abortion occurs without instrumentation or chemical intervention (634.##).***
>
> ***Legally induced abortion is the therapeutic or elective termination of pregnancy (635.##).***
>
> ***Illegally induced abortion is preformed against provisions of state law or regulatory requirements. Use 636.# when a patient has abortion performed outside and is admitted to treat a complication or for completion.***
>
> ***Failed abortion is when the procedure fails and the woman is still pregnant (638.#).***

ABORTION

637.## Unspecified

638.# Failed attempted

636.## Induced - illegally

635.## Induced - legally

4th digit: 635, 636, 637, 638
- **0. With infection**
- **1. With delayed or excessive hemorrhage**
- **2. With damage to pelvic organs or tissue**
- **3. With renal failure**
- **4. With metabolic disorder**
- **5. With shock**
- **6. With embolism**
- **7. With other specified complications**
- **8. With unspecified complication**
- **9. Uncomplicated**

5th digit: 635, 636, 637
- **0. Unspecified**
- **1. Incomplete**
- **2. Complete**

ABORTION (continued)

632 Missed <22 weeks

632 Missed <22 weeks - with complication during treatment [639.#]

639.# Missed <22 weeks - with complication following treatment

4th digit: 639
- **0. Genital tract and pelvic infection**
- **1. Delayed or excessive hemorrhage**
- **2. Damage to pelvic organs and tissue**
- **3. Renal failure**
- **4. Metabolic disorders**
- **5. Shock**
- **6. Embolism**
- **8. Other specified complication**
- **9. Unspecified complication**

629.81 Recurrent or habitual without current pregnancy

639.0 Septic

639.0 Septic with shock

634.## Spontaneous <22 weeks

761.8 Spontaneous <22 weeks - affecting fetus or newborn

635.## Therapeutic

4th digit: 634, 635
- **0. With infection**
- **1. With delayed or excessive hemorrhage**
- **2. With damage to pelvic organs or tissue**
- **3. With renal failure**
- **4. With metabolic disorder**
- **5. With shock**
- **6. With embolism**
- **7. With other specified complications**
- **8. With unspecified complication**
- **9. Uncomplicated**

5th digit: 634, 635
- **0. Unspecified**
- **1. Incomplete**
- **2. Complete**

640.0# Threatened

5th digit: 640.0
- **0. Episode of care NOS or N/A**
- **1. Delivered**
- **3. Antepartum complication**

759.89 ABRACHIOCEPHALIA

759.89 ABRACHIOCEPHALUS

283.9 ABRAMI'S DISEASE (ACQUIRED HEMOLYTIC JAUNDICE)

> ***If abrasions are associated with an underlying injury, such as a fracture, code the underlying injury only. The abrasion is incidental to the injury.***

ABRASION

919.0 Site NOS

919.1 Site NOS infected

911.0 Abdominal wall

911.1 Abdominal wall infected

916.0 Ankle

916.1 Ankle infected

911.0 Anus

911.1 Anus infected

912.0 Arm upper

912.1 Arm upper infected

ABRASION (continued)

912.0 Axilla
912.1 Axilla infected
911.0 Back
911.1 Back infected
911.0 Breast
911.1 Breast infected
911.0 Buttock
911.1 Buttock infected
916.0 Calf
916.1 Calf infected
910.0 Cheek
910.1 Cheek infected
911.0 Chest wall
911.1 Chest wall infected
918.2 Conjunctival
918.1 Cornea
910.0 Ear
910.1 Ear infected
913.0 Elbow
913.1 Elbow infected
918.9 Eye
918.0 Eyelid and periocular area
910.0 Face
910.1 Face infected
915.0 Finger
915.1 Finger infected
911.0 Flank
911.1 Flank infected
917.0 Foot
917.1 Foot infected
913.0 Forearm
913.1 Forearm infected
911.0 Groin
911.1 Groin infected
910.0 Gum
910.1 Gum infected
914.0 Hand
914.1 Hand infected
917.0 Heel
917.1 Heel infected
916.0 Hip
916.1 Hip infected
911.0 Interscapular region
911.1 Interscapular region infected
916.0 Knee
916.1 Knee infected
911.0 Labia
911.1 Labia infected
906.2 Late effect - skin/subcutaneous tissue
916.0 Leg
916.1 Leg infected
910.0 Lip
910.1 Lip infected
919.0 Multiple
919.1 Multiple infected
910.0 Neck
910.1 Neck infected
910.0 Nose
910.1 Nose infected
911.0 Penis
911.1 Penis infected
911.0 Perineum
911.1 Perineum infected

ABRASION (continued)

910.0 Scalp
910.1 Scalp infected
912.0 Scapular region
912.1 Scapular region infected
911.0 Scrotum
911.1 Scrotum infected
912.0 Shoulder
912.1 Shoulder infected
911.0 Testis
911.1 Testis infected
916.0 Thigh
916.1 Thigh infected
910.0 Throat
910.1 Throat infected
915.0 Thumb
915.1 Thumb infected
917.0 Toe
917.1 Toe infected
911.0 Trunk
911.1 Trunk infected
911.0 Vagina
911.1 Vagina infected
911.0 Vulva
911.1 Vulva infected
913.0 Wrist
913.1 Wrist infected
919.0 Other sites
919.1 Other sites infected

0 ABRIKOSSOV'S TUMOR BENIGN SITE SPECIFIED SEE 'BENIGN NEOPLASM' CONNECTIVE TISSUE M9580/0

0 ABRIKOSSOV'S TUMOR MALIGNANT SITE SPECIFIED SEE 'CANCER', CONNECTIVE TISSUE, BY SITE M9580/3

641.2# ABRUPTIO PLACENTA
5th digit: 641.2
0. Episode of care NOS or N/A
1. Delivered
3. Antepartum complication

762.1 ABRUPTIO PLACENTAE AFFECTING FETUS OR NEWBORN

> ***When coding an infection, use an additional code, [041.#(#)], to identify the organism. See 'Bacterial Infection'.***

ABSCESS

682.9 Site NOS
567.22 Abdomen (abdominal cavity)
682.2 Abdominal wall
567.22 Abdominopelvic
474.9 Adenoid disease NOS
474.10 Adenoid with tonsil hypertrophy
255.8 Adrenal (capsule) (gland)
522.5 Alveolar (oral)
006.3 Amebic liver
566 Anal regions
682.6 Ankle
682.3 Antecubital space
540.1 Appendix with peritoneal abscess
611.0 Areola

ABSCESS (continued)

675.1# Areola due to pregnancy
5th digit: 675.1
0. Episode of care NOS or N/A
1. Delivered
2. Delivered with postpartum complication
3. Antepartum complication
4. Postpartum complication

682.3 Arm (any part except hand)
447.2 Artery (wall)
380.10 Auditory canal (external)
380.10 Auricle (ear)
380.10 Auricle (ear) staphylococcal [041.1#]
5th digit: 041.1
0. Unspecified
1. Aureus
9. Other

380.10 Auricle (ear) streptococcal [041.0#]
5th digit: 041.0
0. NOS
1. Group A
2. Group B
3. Group C
4. Group D (enterococcus)
5. Group G
9. Other strep

682.3 Axilla
682.2 Back (any part except buttock)
616.3 Bartholin's gland (nonobstetrical)
595.89 Bladder
006.8 Bladder amebic
730.2# Bone
730.0# Bone acute or subacute
730.1# Bone chronic (old)
5th digit: 730.0-2
0. Site NOS
1. Shoulder region
2. Upper arm (elbow) (humerus)
3. Forearm (radius) (wrist) (ulna)
4. Hand (carpal) (metacarpal) (fingers)
5. Pelvic region and thigh (hip) (buttock) (femur)
6. Lower leg (fibula) (knee) (patella) (tibia)
7. Ankle and/or foot (metatarsals) (toes) (tarsal)
8. Other (head) (neck) (rib) (skull) (trunk)
9. Multiple

324.0 Brain
006.5 Brain amebic
324.0 Brain cerebellar
324.0 Brain cystic
324.1 Brain intraspinal
324.0 Brain otogenic
013.3# Brain tuberculous
5th digit: 013.3
0. NOS
1. Lab not done
2. Lab pending
3. Microscopy positive (in sputum)
4. Culture positive - microscopy negative
5. Culture negative - microscopy positive
6. Culture and microscopy negative confirmed by other methods

ABSCESS (continued)

611.0 Breast
680.2 Breast carbuncle
675.1# Breast maternal due to pregnancy
5th digit: 675.1
0. Episode of care NOS or N/A
1. Delivered
2. Delivered with postpartum complication
3. Antepartum complication
4. Postpartum complication

614.3 Broad ligament acute
614.4 Broad ligament (chronic)
016.7# Broad ligament tuberculous
5th digit: 016.7
0. NOS
1. Lab not done
2. Lab pending
3. Microscopy positive (in sputum)
4. Culture positive - microscopy negative
5. Culture negative - microscopy positive
6. Culture and microscopy negative confirmed by other methods

519.19 Bronchus
528.3 Buccal cavity
597.0 Bulbourethral gland
727.89 Bursa
682.5 Buttock
372.20 Canthus

When coding an infection of an ostomy, use an additional code to specify the organism. See 'Bacterial Infection'.

569.61 Cecostomy with abscess of abdomen [682.2]
569.5 Cecum
540.1 Cecum with appendicitis
013.3# Cerebellar (cerebral) tuberculous
5th digit: 013.3
0. NOS
1. Lab not done
2. Lab pending
3. Microscopy positive (in sputum)
4. Culture positive - microscopy negative
5. Culture negative - microscopy positive
6. Culture and microscopy negative confirmed by other methods

324.0 Cerebellar (embolic)
324.0 Cerebral (embolic)
616.0 Cervix (stump) (uteri)
682.0 Cheek external
528.3 Cheek internal
682.2 Chest wall
682.0 Chin
363.00 Choroid
364.3 Ciliary body
569.5 Colon (wall)

When coding an infection of an ostomy, use an additional code to specify the organism. See 'Bacterial Infection'.

569.61 Colostomy with abscess of abdomen [682.2]
372.00 Conjunctiva

A

ABSCESS (continued)

682.9 Connective tissue NEC
370.55 Corneal
370.00 Corneal with ulceration
597.0 Cowper's gland
522.5 Dental
522.5 Dentoalveolar
681.9 Digit
380.10 Ear external auditory canal
380.11 Ear pinna
682.3 Elbow

> *When coding an infection of an ostomy, use an additional code to specify the organism. See 'Bacterial Infection'.*

569.61 Enterostomy with abscess of abdomen [682.2]
604.0 Epididymis
604.0 Epididymis E. coli [041.4]
604.0 Epididymis hemophilus influenza [041.5]
604.0 Epididymis klebsiella [041.3]
604.0 Epididymis pneumococcus [041.2]
604.0 Epididymis pneumoniae [041.89]
604.0 Epididymis proteus [041.6]
604.0 Epididymis pseudomonas [041.7]
604.0 Epididymis staphylococcal [**041.1#**]
5th digit: 041.1
0. Unspecified
1. Aureus
9. Other

604.0 Epididymis streptococcal [**041.0#**]
5th digit: 041.0
0. NOS
1. Group A
2. Group B
3. Group C
4. Group D (enterococcus)
5. Group G
9. Other strep

604.0 Epididymis other specified [**041.8#**]
5th digit: 041.8
1. Mycoplasma, Eaton's agent, PPLO
2. Bacteroides fragilis
3. Clostridium perfringens
4. Other anaerobes
5. Aerobacter aerogenes, mima polymorpha, serratia, (other gram-negative)
9. Other specified bacteria

324.0 Epidural (embolic) brain
324.1 Epidural (embolic) spinal
013.5# Epidural spinal cord tuberculous
5th digit: 013.5
0. NOS
1. Lab not done
2. Lab pending
3. Microscopy positive (in sputum)
4. Culture positive - microscopy negative
5. Culture negative - microscopy positive
6. Culture and microscopy negative confirmed by other methods

478.79 Epiglottis
530.86 Esophagostomy
530.19 Esophagus
380.10 External ear canal

ABSCESS (continued)

324.9 Extradural - NOS
324.0 Extradural - brain (embolic)
324.1 Extradural - spinal cord (embolic)
360.00 Eye
373.13 Eyelid
682.0 Face
614.2 Fallopian tube
728.89 Fascia
681.01 Felon
681.00 Finger
681.01 Finger felon
681.02 Fingernail
682.2 Flank
682.7 Foot (except toes)
682.3 Forearm
682.0 Forehead
575.0 Gallbladder (see also 'Cholecystitis', acute)

> *When coding an infection of an ostomy, use an additional code to specify the organism. See 'Bacterial Infection'.*

536.41 Gastrostomy with abscess of abdomen [682.2]
523.30 Gingival
682.5 Gluteal region
682.2 Groin
682.4 Hand (except fingers and thumb)
682.8 Head (except face)
429.89 Heart
682.7 Heel
682.6 Hip

> *When coding an infection of an ostomy, use an additional code to specify the organism. See 'Bacterial Infection'.*

569.61 Ileostomy with abscess of abdomen [682.2]
569.5 Ileum
540.1 Iliac fossa
682.2 Iliac region
683 Inguinal lymph gland or node
682.2 Inguinal region
540.1 Intestinal appendiceal
569.5 Intestinal nonappendiceal
997.4 Intestinal postoperative
560.81 Intestinal with obstruction adhesive
324.0 Intracranial (embolic)
326 Intracranial late effect
324.1 Intraspinal (spinal) (embolic)
364.3 Iris
566 Ischiorectal
526.4 Jaw (acute, chronic, suppurative)
682.0 Jaw skin

> *When coding an infection of an ostomy, use an additional code to specify the organism. See 'Bacterial Infection'.*

569.61 Jejunostomy with abscess of abdomen [682.2]
0 Joint see 'Arthritis Other Specified' pyogenic
590.2 Kidney
616.4 Labia (majus) (minus)

ABSCESS (continued)

375.30 Lacrimal (passages) (sac)
375.00 Lacrimal gland
373.31 Lacrimal system
478.79 Larynx
682.6 Leg (except foot)
528.5 Lip
597.0 Littre's gland
572.0 Liver
006.3 Liver amebic
513.0 Lung (multiple)
006.4 Lung amebic

When assigning code 449, use an additional code to identify the site of the embolism (433.0-433.9) (444.0-444.9). See 'Embolism', by site.

513.0 Lung with septic arterial embolism [449]
683 Lymph gland or node (acute)
0 Lymph gland see also 'Lymphadenitis'
0 Mammary gland submammary see 'Abscess' breast
383.00 Mastoid
383.01 Mastoid subperiosteal
513.1 Mediastinum
567.22 Mesenteric (suppurative peritonitis)
682.2 Mons pubis
528.3 Mouth
728.89 Muscle
567.31 Muscle psoas
681.9 Nail
478.19 Nasal septum
0 Nasal sinus see 'Sinusitis' chronic
478.29 Nasopharynx
682.1 Neck
675.0# Nipple maternal due to pregnancy

5th digit: 675.0
0. Episode of care NOS or N/A
1. Delivered
2. Delivered with postpartum complication
3. Antepartum complication
4. Postpartum complication

478.19 Nose (septum)
682.0 Nose external
478.19 Nose internal
567.22 Omentum
681.02 Onychia finger
681.11 Onychia toe
998.59 Operative wound
376.01 Orbit
324.0 Otogenic (embolic)
526.4 Palate - hard
528.3 Palate - soft
577.0 Pancreas
523.30 Paradontal (parodontal) (pericemental) (pericoronal) (peridental)
614.3 Parametric parametrium acute
614.4 Parametric parametrium chronic
478.22 Parapharyngeal
681.02 Paronychia finger
681.11 Paronychia toe
527.3 Parotid (duct) (gland)
528.3 Parotid region
682.2 Pectoral region

ABSCESS (continued)

614.4 Pelvic female (chronic)
614.3 Pelvic female acute
016.7# Pelvic female tuberculous
567.22 Pelvic male
016.5# Pelvic male tuberculous

5th digit: 016.5, 016.7
0. NOS
1. Lab not done
2. Lab pending
3. Microscopy positive (in sputum)
4. Culture positive - microscopy negative
5. Culture negative - microscopy positive
6. Culture and microscopy negative confirmed by other methods

567.22 Pelvirectal
607.2 Penis
566 Perianal
522.7 Periapical (tooth) with sinus
522.5 Periapical (tooth) without sinus
540.1 Periappendiceal
590.2 Perinephric
682.2 Perineum
523.31 Periodontal (parietal)
730.3# Periosteum

5th digit: 730.3
0. Site NOS
1. Shoulder region
2. Upper arm (elbow) (humerus)
3. Forearm (radius) (wrist) (ulna)
4. Hand (carpal) (metacarpal) (fingers)
5. Pelvic region and thigh (hip) (buttock) (femur)
6. Lower leg (fibula) (knee) (patella) (tibia)
7. Ankle and/or foot (metatarsals) (toes) (tarsals)
8. Other (head) (neck) (rib) (skull) (trunk) (vertebrae)
9. Multiple

566 Perirectal
590.2 Perirenal (tissue)
567.22 Peritoneum
998.59 Peritoneum postoperative
475 Peritonsillar
614.2 Peritubal
593.89 Periureteral
597.0 Periurethral
595.89 Perivesical
478.29 Pharynx
685.0 Pilonidal (cyst) (fistula) (sinus)
253.8 Pituitary
510.9 Pleura
510.0 Pleura with fistula
682.6 Popliteal
478.19 Postnasal
998.59 Postoperative

ABSCESS (continued)

614.4 Pouch of Douglas (chronic)
016.7# Pouch of Douglas tuberculous

5th digit: 016.7
- **0. NOS**
- **1. Lab not done**
- **2. Lab pending**
- **3. Microscopy positive (in sputum)**
- **4. Culture positive - microscopy negative**
- **5. Culture negative - microscopy positive**
- **6. Culture and microscopy negative confirmed by other methods**

682.6 Prepatellar
601.2 Prostate
567.31 Psoas muscle
511.0 Pulmonary
566 Rectal
566 Rectal submucosal
616.10 Rectovaginal
590.2 Renal and perinephric
363.00 Retina
376.01 Retrobulbar
567.22 Retrocecal
567.38 Retroperitoneal
998.59 Retroperitoneal postprocedural
478.24 Retropharyngeal
566 Retrorectal
527.3 Salivary gland
682.8 Scalp
355.0 Sciatic nerve
379.09 Scleral
017.2# Scrofulous
608.4 Scrotum (spermatic cord)
608.0 Seminal vesicle
478.19 Septum nasal
682.3 Shoulder
597.0 Skene's duct or gland
682.9 Skin NEC
608.4 Spermatic cord
013.5# Spinal cord tuberculous

5th Digit: 013.5, 017.2
- **0. NOS**
- **1. Lab not done**
- **2. Lab pending**
- **3. Microscopy positive (in sputum)**
- **4. Culture positive - microscopy negative**
- **5. Culture negative - microscopy positive**
- **6. Culture and microscopy negative confirmed by other methods**

289.59 Spleen
998.59 Stitch
324.9 Subarachnoid
324.0 Subarachnoid brain (cerebral)
567.22 Subdiaphragmatic

ABSCESS (continued)

324.9 Subdural - NOS
324.0 Subdural - brain (intracranial) (embolic)
324.1 Subdural - spinal cord (embolic)
013.3# Subdural - tuberculous brain
013.5# Subdural - tuberculous spinal cord

5th digit: 013.3, 5
- **0. NOS**
- **1. Lab not done**
- **2. Lab pending**
- **3. Microscopy positive (in sputum)**
- **4. Culture positive - microscopy negative**
- **5. Culture negative - microscopy positive**
- **6. Culture and microscopy negative confirmed by other methods**

567.22 Subhepatic
528.3 Sublingual
527.3 Sublingual gland
682.0 Submandibular
527.3 Submandibular gland
682.0 Submaxillary
527.3 Submaxillary gland
682.0 Submental (pyogenic)
527.3 Submental gland
566 Submucosal, rectum
567.22 Subphrenic
998.59 Subphrenic postoperative
682.2 Subscapular
681.9 Subungual
682.3 Supraclavicular (fossa)
566 Supralevator
682.0 Temple region
727.89 Tendon
604.0 Testis
604.0 Testis E. coli [041.4]
604.0 Testis hemophilus influenza [041.5]
604.0 Testis klebsiella [041.3]
604.0 Testis pneumococcus [041.2]
604.0 Testis pneumoniae [041.89]
604.0 Testis proteus [041.6]
604.0 Testis staphylococcal [**041.1#**]

5th digit: 041.1
- **0. Unspecified**
- **1. Aureus**
- **9. Other**

604.0 Testis streptococcal [**041.0#**]

5th digit: 041.0
- **0. NOS**
- **1. Group A**
- **2. Group B**
- **3. Group C**
- **4. Group D (enterococcus)**
- **5. Group G**
- **9. Other strep**

604.0 Testis other specified [**041.8#**]

5th digit: 041.8
- **1. Mycoplasma, Eaton's agent, PPLO**
- **2. Bacteroides fragilis**
- **3. Clostridium perfringens**
- **4. Other anaerobes**
- **5. Aerobacter aerogenes, mima polymorpha, serratia, (other gram-negative)**
- **9. Other specified bacteria**

A

ABSCESS (continued)

682.6 Thigh
510.9 Thorax
681.00 Thumb
254.1 Thymus
681.10 Toe
681.11 Toe onychia (paronychia)
681.11 Toenail
529.0 Tongue
522.5 Tooth/teeth (root)
523.30 Tooth/teeth (root) supporting structures NEC
478.9 Trachea

When coding an infection of an ostomy, use an additional code to specify the organism. See 'Bacterial Infection'.

<u>519.01</u> <u>Tracheostomy</u> with abscess of neck [682.1]
682.2 Trunk
<u>015.0#</u> <u>Tuberculous</u> [730.88]
5th digit: 015.0
0. NOS
1. Lab not done
2. Lab pending
3. Microscopy positive (in sputum)
4. Culture positive - microscopy negative
5. Culture negative - microscopy positive
6. Culture and microscopy negative confirmed by other methods

614.2 Tubo ovarian
614.6 Tubo ovarian with adhesions (postoperative) (postinfection)
608.4 Tunica vaginalis
682.2 Umbilicus
771.4 Umbilicus newborn
593.89 Ureter
597.0 Urethra
599.3 Urethral (caruncle)
615.9 Uterus - NOS
615.0 Uterus - acute
760.8 Uterus - affecting fetus or newborn
615.1 Uterus - chronic
670.0# Uterus - major maternal due to pregnancy (puerperal)
5th digit: 670.0
0. NOS
2. Delivered with postpartum complication
4. Postpartum complication

364.3 Uveitis
528.3 Uvula
616.10 Vaginal wall
616.10 Vaginorectal
608.4 Vas Deferens
360.04 Vitreous
478.5 Vocal cord
616.4 Vulva (nonobstetrical)
616.10 Vulvovaginal
616.3 Vulvovaginal gland
682.4 Wrist

0 ABSENCE SEE ANATOMICAL SITE
117.7 ABSIDIA INFECTION

304.6# ABSINTHE ADDICTION
5th digit: 304.6
0. NOS
1. Continuous
2. Episodic
3. In remission

0 ABSOLUTE NEUTROPHIL COUNT DECREASED (ANC) SEE 'NEUTROPENIA'

291.81 ABSTINENCE ALCOHOL SYNDROME
292.0 ABSTINENCE DRUG SYNDROME
202.5# ABT-LETTERER-SIWE SYNDROME (ACUTE HISTIOCYTOSIS X) M9722/3
5th digit: 202.5
0. Unspecified site, extranodal and solid organ sites
1. Lymph nodes of head, face, neck
2. Lymph nodes intrathoracic
3. Lymph nodes abdominal
4. Lymph nodes axilla and upper limb
5. Lymph nodes inguinal region and lower limb
6. Lymph nodes intrapelvic
7. Spleen
8. Lymph nodes multiple sites

799.89 ABULIA

When the cause of an injury is stated to be abuse, multiple codes should be assigned if applicable, to identify any associated injuries. Sequence in the following order:

1 . Type of abuse - child or adult (995.5, 995.8)

2. Type of injury

3. Nature of the abuse - see E-code directory 'Assault' (E904.0, E960-E966, E968)

4. Perpetrator of the abuse - see E-code directory 'Assault' (E967)

ABUSE

995.8# Adult (victim)
5th digit: 995.8
0. Maltreatment unspecified
1. Physical, battery
2. Emotional/psychological (deprivation)
3. Sexual
4. Neglect (nutritional), desertion
5. Other abuse and neglect, multiple forms

V62.83 Adult - counseling of perpetrator non-parental/non-spousal of physical/sexual abuse NEC
V61.12 Adult - counseling of perpetrator of spousal (partner) abuse
V61.11 Adult - counseling of victim of spousal (partner) abuse
V62.89 Adult - counseling of victim other specified abuse
995.84 Adult desertion
V71.81 Adult - evaluation (alleged)
V71.6 Adult - evaluation for battery (alleged)
V71.81 Adult - evaluation for neglect (alleged)
V71.5 Adult - evaluation for sexual (alleged)
V15.4# Adult history
5th digit: V15.4
1. Physical/sexual abuse, rape
2. Emotional abuse, neglect
9. Other psychological trauma

ABUSE (continued)

Substance abuse describes the practice of using drugs or alcohol to excess without reaching the state of physical dependence. Substance dependence is addiction. Dependence involves the loss of control, judgment and/or the ability to use in moderation. Dependence is marked by compulsive physical demands which are triggered by further ingestion.

V65.42 Alcohol counseling
303.9# Alcohol dependent
303.0# Alcohol dependent with acute intoxication
5th digit: 303.0, 9
0. NOS
1. Continuous
2. Episodic
3. In remission

V11.3 Alcohol history

When the cause of an injury is stated to be abuse, multiple codes should be assigned if applicable, to identify any associated injuries. Sequence in the following order:

1 . Type of abuse - child or adult (995.5, 995.8)

2. Type of injury

3. Nature of the abuse - see E-code directory 'Assault' (E904.0, E960-E966, E968)

4. Perpetrator of the abuse - see E-code directory 'Assault' (E967)

995.5# Child (victim)
5th digit: 995.5
0. Unspecified
1. Emotional/psychological (deprivation)
2. Neglect (nutritional), desertion
3. Sexual
4. Physical
5. Shaken infant syndrome
9. Other abuse and neglect, multiple forms

V62.83 Child - counseling of perpetrator non-parental of physical/sexual abuse NEC
V61.22 Child - counseling of perpetrator parental child abuse
V61.21 Child - counseling of victim
995.52 Child desertion
V71.81 Child - evaluation (alleged)
V71.6 Child - evaluation for battery (alleged)
V71.81 Child - evaluation for neglect (alleged)
V71.5 Child - evaluation for sexual (alleged)
V15.4# Child history
5th digit: V15.4
1. Physical/sexual abuse, rape
2. Emotional abuse, neglect
9. Other psychological trauma

ABUSE (continued)

304.## Drug - dependent (addiction)
4th digit: 304
0. Opioid
1. Sedative, hypnotic or anxiolytic
2. Cocaine
3. Cannabis
4. Amphetamine type
5. Hallucinogenic
6. Other specified
7. Mixed with opioid
8. Mixed
9. NOS

5th digit: 304
0. NOS
1. Continuous
2. Episodic
3. In remission

Substance abuse nondependent describes the practice of using drugs or alcohol to excess without reaching the state of physical dependence.

305.## Drug - nondependent (abuse)
4th digit: 305
0. Alcohol
2. Cannabis
3. Hallucinogen
4. Sedative, hypnotic or anxiolytic
5. Opioid
6. Cocaine
7. Amphetamine type
8. Antidepressant type
9. Mixed or other specified

5th digit: 305
0. NOS
1. Continuous
2. Episodic
3. In remission

V65.42 Drug counseling
V11.8 Drug history

***648.3# :** Code the specific maternal drug abuse or dependence with an additional code. See 'Abuse' drug.*

648.3# Drug maternal current (co-existent) in pregnancy
5th digit: 648.3
0. Episode of care unspecified or N/A
1. Delivered
2. Delivered with postpartum complication
3. Antepartum complication
4. Postpartum complication

655.5# Drug maternal in pregnancy with suspected damage to fetus
5th digit: 655.5
0. Episode of care unspecified or N/A
1. Delivered
3. Antepartum complication

V15.4# History (adult) (child)
5th digit: V15.4
1. Physical/sexual abuse, rape
2. Emotional abuse, neglect
9. Other psychological trauma

A

ABUSE (continued)

0 Substance see 'Abuse', drug
V65.42 Substance counseling
305.1 Tobacco (dependence)
V65.49 Tobacco use cessation counseling
V15.82 Tobacco use history

V62.3 ACADEMIC PROBLEM
313.83 ACADEMIC UNDERACHIEVEMENT DISORDER (EMOTIONAL DISTURBANCES OF CHILDHOOD OR ADOLESCENCE)

275.40 ACALCEROSIS
275.40 ACALCICOSIS
784.69 ACALCULIA NOS (AUDITORY) (VISUAL) (ORGANIC)

125.4 ACANTHOCHEILONEMA PERSTANS INFECTION
125.6 ACANTHOCHEILONEMA STREPTOCERCA INFECTION
530.89 ACANTHOSIS GLYCOGENIC ESOPHAGUS
701.2 ACANTHOSIS NIGRICANS ACQUIRED
759.89 ACARDIA

ACARIASIS

133.9 NOS
133.8 Demodex folliculorum
133.0 Scabies
133.8 Other specified

277.89 ACATALASEMIA
277.89 ACATALASIA
333.99 ACATHISIA DUE TO DRUGS

ACCESSORY

755.56 Carpal bone
752.19 Fallopian tube
755.01 Fingers
755.67 Foot bones
752.49 Hymen
748.69 Lobe of lung
756.82 Muscle anomalies other specified congenital
757.6 Nipple
752.0 Ovary congenital
755.00 Polydactyly, unspecified digits
756.2 Ribs
756.2 Ribs Cervical
755.02 Toes
744.1 Tragus congenital
753.4 Ureter
752.2 Uterus
756.19 Vertebra

ACCESSORY NERVE

352.4 Atrophy
352.4 Disorder
951.6 Injury
352.4 Neuritis

ACCOMMODATION

367.9 Disorder
367.89 Disorder drug induced or toxic
367.51 Paresis
367.53 Spasm

V62.4 ACCULTURATION PROBLEM

718.6# ACETABULUM UNSPECIFIED INTRAPELVIC PROTRUSION
5th digit: 718.6
0. Site NOS
5. Pelvic region and thigh (hip) (buttock) (femur)

736.39 ACETABULUM WANDERING
791.6 ACETONURIA
286.3 AC GLOBULIN DEFICIENCY
286.7 AC GLOBULIN DEFICIENCY ACQUIRED

530.0 ACHALASIA (OF CARDIA)
255.2 ACHARD-THIERS (ADRENOGENITAL) SYNDROME

ACHILLES

726.71 Tendinitis
727.81 Tendon contracture
845.09 Tendon laceration
892.2 Tendon laceration with open wound
727.67 Tendon rupture nontraumatic
845.09 Tendon rupture traumatic
892.2 Tendon rupture traumatic with open wound

536.0 ACHLORHYDRIA
756.4 ACHONDROPLASIA CONGENITAL

709.00 ACHROMA CUTIS
368.54 ACHROMATOPSIA
316 ACHROMATOPSIA PSYCHOGENIC [368.54]
536.3 ACHYLIA GASTRICA NEUROGENIC

656.8# ACID BASE BALANCE ABNORMAL AFFECTING MANAGEMENT OF MOTHER
5th digit: 656.8
0. Episode of care unspecified or N/A
1. Delivered
3. Antepartum complication

276.9 ACID BASE BALANCE DISORDER
276.4 ACID BASE BALANCE DISORDER MIXED (WITH HYPERCAPNIA)
536.8 ACID PEPTIC DISEASE
790.5 ACID PHOSPHATASE ABNORMAL BLOOD LEVEL
997.3 ACID PULMONARY ASPIRATION SYNDROME
668.0# ACID PULMONARY ASPIRATION SYNDROME - OBSTETRIC (MENDELSON'S)
5th digit: 668.0
0. Episode of care NOS or N/A
1. Delivered
2. Delivered with postpartum complication
3. Antepartum complication
4. Postpartum complication

ACIDEMIA

276.2 NOS
270.6 Arginosuccinic
656.3# Fetal affecting management of mother
5th digit: 656.3
0. Episode of care unspecified or N/A
1. Delivered
3. Antepartum complication

768.4 Fetal liveborn - onset unspecified
768.2 Fetal liveborn - onset before labor
768.3 Fetal liveborn - onset during labor and delivery
775.81 Newborn
270.7 Pipecolic

288.59 ACIDOCYTOPENIA, ACIDOPENIA

ACIDOPHIL

194.3 Carcinoma site NOS
0 Carcinoma site specified see 'Cancer', by site M8280/3
194.3 Basophil carcinoma (mixed) site NOS
0 Basophil carcinoma (mixed) site specified see 'Cancer', by site M8281/3

ACIDOSIS

276.2 NOS
656.8# Fetal affecting management of mother
5th digit: 656.8
0. Episode of care unspecified or N/A
1. Delivered
3. Antepartum complication
775.81 Fetal affecting newborn
250.1# Ketoacidosis
250.3# Ketoacidosis with coma
5th digit: 250.1, 3
0. Type II, adult-onset, non-insulin dependent (even if requiring insulin), or unspecified; controlled
1. Type I, juvenile-onset or insulin-dependent; controlled
2. Type II adult-onset, non-insulin dependent (even if requiring insulin); uncontrolled
3. Type I, juvenile-onset or insulin-dependent; uncontrolled
276.2 Lactic
276.2 Metabolic
775.81 Metabolic mixed with respiratory acidosis of newborn
775.7 Metabolic newborn late
775.81 Newborn
588.89 Renal tubular
276.2 Respiratory
276.4 Respiratory complicated by metabolic acidosis
775.81 Respiratory mixed with metabolic acidosis of newborn

ACIDURIA

791.9 NOS
270.6 Arginosuccinic
277.2 Beta-Aminoisobutyric (BAIB)
270.7 Glutaric type I
277.85 Glutaric type II (type IIA, IIB, IIC)
277.86 Glutaric type III
271.8 Glycolic
270.3 Methylmalonic
270.7 Methylmalonic with glycinemia
270.9 Organic
281.4 Orotic (congenital) (hereditary) (pyrimidine deficiency)

Carcinomas and neoplasms should be coded by site if possible. Code by cell type, "site NOS", only if a site is not specified in the diagnosis. Otherwise, refer to the appropriate category of neoplasm for a more specific code. See 'Cancer' 'Cancer Metastatic', 'Carcinoma In Situ', 'Neoplasm Uncertain Behavior', 'Neoplasm Unspecified Nature', or 'Benign Neoplasm'.

229.9 ACINAR CELL ADENOMA NOS
0 ACINAR CELL ADENOMA SITE SPECIFIED SEE 'BENIGN NEOPLASM', BY SITE M8550/0
199.1 ACINAR CELL CARCINOMA SITE NOS
0 ACINAR CELL CARCINOMA SITE SPECIFIED SEE 'CANCER', BY SITE M8550/3
238.9 ACINAR CELL TUMOR SITE NOS
0 ACINAR CELL TUMOR SITE SPECIFIED SEE 'NEOPLASM UNCERTAIN BEHAVIOR', BY SITE M8550/1
0 ACL (ANTERIOR CRUCIATE LIGAMENT) SEE 'ANTERIOR', CRUCIATE

ACNE

706.1 NOS
706.1 Conglobata
706.1 Conjunctiva
706.1 Cystic
695.3 Erythematosa
706.0 Frontalis
706.0 Necrotica
706.1 Neonatal
706.1 Pustular
695.3 Rosacea
692.72 Summer
706.0 Varioliformis
706.1 Vulgaris

993.2 ACOSTA'S DISEASE

ACOUSTIC

742.8 Nerve absence congenital
388.5 Nerve degeneration (atrophy)
388.5 Nerve disorder
388.5 Neuritis
094.86 Neuritis syphilitic
225.1 Neuroma
388.11 Trauma (ear) (explosive)

736.09 ACQUIRED DEFORMITY UPPER LIMB
736.89 ACQUIRED DEFORMITY ARM OR LEG OTHER NEC
0 ACQUIRED IMMUNE DEFICIENCY SYNDROME SEE 'AIDS'
781.99 ACRAGNOSIS
740.0 ACRANIA CONGENITAL
117.4 ACREMONIUM FALCIFORME INFECTION
781.99 ACROAGNOSIS
755.55 ACROCEPHALOSYNDACTYLY SYNDROME
756.0 ACROCEPHALY
701.9 ACROCHORDONS
443.89 ACROCYANOSIS
770.83 ACROCYANOSIS NEWBORN
0 ACROCYANOSIS NEWBORN MEANING TRANSIENT BLUE HANDS AND FEET – OMIT CODE

ACRODERMATITIS

686.8 NOS
701.8 Atrophicans chronica
696.1 Continua
686.8 Enteropathica
696.1 Perstans
696.1 Pustulosa continua

0 ACROHYPERHIDROSIS SEE 'HYPERHIDROSIS'
253.0 ACROMEGALY
443.82 ACROMELALGIA

A

ACROMIOCLAVICULAR

831.04 Dislocation closed
831.14 Dislocation open
739.7 Region segmental or somatic dysfunction
840.0 Separation (rupture) (tear) (laceration)
840.0 Strain (sprain) (avulsion) (hemarthrosis)

ACROPARESTHESIA

443.89 NOS
443.89 Simple (Schultze's type)
443.89 Vasomotor (Nothnagel's type)

300.29 ACROPHOBIA
710.1 ACROSCLEROSIS
710.1 ACROSCLEROSIS WITH LUNG INVOLVEMENT [517.2]
710.1 ACROSCLEROSIS WITH MYOPATHY [359.6]

ACTH

255.41 Insensitivity
255.3 Overproduction
255.3 Overproduction adrenal
253.1 Overproduction pituitary

ACTINIC

692.72 Cheilitis
692.82 Cheilitis chronic due to radiation
692.74 Cheilitis chronic NEC
692.89 Dermatitis
692.82 Dermatitis due to roentgen rays
692.70 Dermatitis solar (sun)
692.72 Dermatitis solar (sun) acute
692.74 Dermatitis solar (sun) chronic
692.82 Dermatitis other than sun
692.74 Elastosis
692.73 Granuloma due to solar radiation
370.24 Keratitis
702.0 Keratosis
702.0 Keratosis solar
692.75 Porokeratosis disseminated superficial (DSAP)
692.73 Reticuloid due to solar radiation

024 ACTINOBACILLUS MALLEI INFECTION

0 ACTINOMADURA SEE 'ACTINOMYCOSIS'
0 ACTINOMYCETALES SEE 'ACTINOMYCOSIS'

ACTINOMYCOSIS

039.9 Unspecified site
039.2 Abdominal
039.3 Cervicofacial
039.0 Cutaneous
039.3 Eyelid [373.5]
039.4 Madura foot
039.1 Pulmonary
039.1 Thoracic
039.8 Other specified sites

0 ACTINOMYCOTIC MYCETOMA SEE 'ACTINOMYCOSIS'
357.89 ACTINONEURITIS
286.3 ACTIVATING FACTOR (BLOOD) DEFICIENCY
780.99 ACTIVITY DECREASE FUNCTIONAL

789.0# ACUTE ABDOMINAL SYNDROME
5th digit: 789.0
0. Unspecified site
1. Upper right quadrant
2. Upper left quadrant
3. Lower right quadrant
4. Lower left quadrant
5. Periumbilic
6. Epigastric
7. Generalized
9. Other specified site (multiple)

282.62 ACUTE CHEST SYNDROME DUE TO SICKLE CELL DISEASE [517.3]
282.64 ACUTE CHEST SYNDROME DUE TO SICKLE CELL/Hb-C DISEASE [517.3]
282.42 ACUTE CHEST SYNDROME DUE TO SICKLE CELL THALASSEMIA [517.3]
282.69 ACUTE CHEST SYNDROME DUE TO SICKLE CELL DISEASE OTHER SPECIFIED [517.3]

415.0 ACUTE COR PULMONALE
411.1 ACUTE CORONARY SYNDROME
207.0# ACUTE ERYTHREMIC MYELOSIS M9840/3
5th digit: 207.0
0. Without mention of remission
1. With mention of remission

446.1 ACUTE FEBRILE MUCOCUTANEOUS LYMPH NODE SYNDROME (MCLS)
648.9# ACUTE FEBRILE MUCOCUTANEOUS LYMPH NODE SYNDROME (MCLS) MATERNAL CURRENT (CO-EXISTENT) IN PREGNANCY [446.1]
5th digit: 648.9
0. Episode of care NOS or N/A
1. Delivered
2. Delivered with postpartum complication
3. Antepartum complication
4. Postpartum complication

363.15 ACUTE POSTERIOR MULTIFOCAL PLACOID PIGMENT EPITHELIOPATHY
646.7# ACUTE YELLOW ATROPHY OF PREGNANCY (LIVER)
5th digit: 646.7
0. Episode of care NOS or N/A
1. Delivered
3. Antepartum complication

755.4 ADACTYLY LIMB NOS (CONGENITAL)
756.51 ADAIR-DIGHTON SYNDROME
170.# ADAMANTINOMA BONE AND ARTICULAR CARTILAGE M9310/0
4th digit: 170
0. Skull and face
1. Mandible
2. Vertebral column
3. Ribs, sternum, clavicle
4. Scapula, long bones of upper limb
5. Short bones of upper limb
6. Pelvic bones, sacrum, coccyx
7. Long bones of lower limb
8. Short bones of lower limb
9. Site NOS

426.9 ADAMS-STOKES (-MORGAGNI) SYNDROME (SYNCOPE WITH HEART BLOCK)

426.9 ADAMS-STOKES (SYNCOPE WITH HEART BLOCK) DISEASE

309.9 ADAPTATION REACTION NOS

ADD (ATTENTION DEFICIT DISORDER) - (ADULT) (CHILD)

314.00 NOS
314.00 Inattentive
314.01 With hyperactivity/impulsiveness
314.8 With other specified manifestations

> ***Substance dependence is addiction. Dependence involves the loss of control, judgment and/or ability to use in moderation. Dependence is marked by compulsive physical demands which are triggered by further ingestion.***

ADDICTION

303.0# Alcohol - acute episode
303.9# Alcohol - chronic

5th digit: 303.0, 9
0. NOS
1. Continuous
2. Episodic
3. In remission

304.## Drug

4th digit: 304
0. Opioid
1. Sedative, hypnotic or anxiolytic
2. Cocaine
3. Cannabis
4. Amphetamine type
5. Hallucinogenic
6. Other specified
7. Mixed with opioid
8. Mixed
9. NOS

5th digit: 304
0. NOS
1. Continuous
2. Episodic
3. In remission

ADDISON'S, ADDISONIAN

281.0 Anemia (pernicious)
255.41 Crisis (melanosis) (bronze)
255.41 Disease (primary adrenal insufficiency) NOS
255.41 Disease with myopathy [359.5]
701.0 Keloid
255.41 Melanoderma (melanosis) (adrenal) (cortical hypofunction)
255.41 Syndrome
017.6# Tuberculosis

5th digit: 017.6
0. Nos
1. Lab not done
2. Lab pending
3. Microscopy positive (in sputum)
4. Culture positive - microscopy negative
5. Culture negative - microscopy positive
6. Culture and microscopy negative confirmed by other methods

136.9 ADEM (ACUTE DISSEMINATED ENCEPHALOMYELITIS) – NOS AND INFECTIOUS [323.61]

323.81 ADEM (ACUTE DISSEMINATED ENCEPHALOMYELITIS) - NONINFECTIOUS

0 ADENITIS SEE 'LYMPHADENITIS'

> ***Carcinomas and neoplasms should be coded by site if possible. Code by cell type, "site NOS", only if a site is not specified in the diagnosis. Otherwise, refer to the appropriate category of neoplasm for a more specific code. See 'Cancer' 'Cancer Metastatic', 'Neoplasm Uncertain Behavior', 'Neoplasm Unspecified Nature', or 'Benign Neoplasm'.***

ADENOCARCINOMA

199.1 Site NOS
0 Site specified see 'Cancer', by site M8140/3
153.9 Adenomatous polyposis coli site NOS
0 Adenomatous polyposis coli site specified see 'Cancer', by site M8220/3
0 Alveolar site specified see 'Cancer', by site M8251/3
173.# Apocrine M8401/3
162.9 Bronchioloalveolar site NOS
0 Bronchioloalveolar site specified see 'Cancer', by site M8250/3
173.# Ceruminous M8420/3

4th digit: 173
0. Lip
1. Eyelid including canthus
2. Ear (auricle) auricular canal external (acoustic) or site unspecified
3. Unspecified parts of face, cheek external, chin, eyebrow, forehead, nose external, temple
4. Scalp and neck
5. Trunk, axilla, breast (or mastectomy site), buttock, groin, perianal skin, perineum, umbilicus
6. Upper limb including shoulder
7. Lower limb including hip
8. Other specified skin sites, contiguous or overlapping, undetermined point of origin

199.1 Clear cell site NOS
0 Clear cell site specified see 'Cancer', by site M8310/3
0 Endometrioid (borderline malignancy) site specified see 'Neoplasm Uncertain Behavior', by site M8381/1
183.0 Endometrioid (malignant) site NOS
0 Endometrioid (malignant) site specified see 'Cancer', by site M8381/3
220 Endometrioid site NOS
0 Endometrioid site specified see 'Benign Neoplasm', by site M8381/0
199.1 Follicular site NOS
0 Follicular site specified see 'Cancer', by site M8330/3
193 Follicular (trabecular type) site NOS
0 Follicular (trabecular type) site specified see 'Cancer', by site M8332/3
193 Follicular (well differentiated type) site NOS
0 Follicular (well differentiated type) site specified see 'Cancer', by site M8331/3

Carcinomas and neoplasms should be coded by site if possible. Code by cell type, "site NOS", only if a site is not specified in the diagnosis. Otherwise, refer to the appropriate category of neoplasm for a more specific code. See 'Cancer' 'Cancer Metastatic', 'Carcinoma In Situ', 'Neoplasm Uncertain Behavior', 'Neoplasm Unspecified Nature', or 'Benign Neoplasm'.

ADENOCARCINOMA (continued)

234.9 In situ site NOS
0 In situ site specified see 'Ca In Situ', by site M8140/2
151.9 Intestinal type site NOS
0 Intestinal type site specified see 'Cancer', by site M8144/3
157.9 Islet cell and exocrine (mixed) site NOS
0 Islet cell and exocrine (mixed) site specified see 'Cancer', by site M8154/3
199.1 Metastatic site NOS
0 Metastatic site specified see 'Cancer', by site, metastatic M8140/6
199.1 Mixed cell site NOS M8323/3
0 Mixed cell site specified see 'Cancer', by site M8323/3
199.1 Mucin producing site NOS
0 Mucin producing site specified see 'Cancer', by site M8481/3
199.1 Mucinous site NOS
0 Mucinous site specified see 'Cancer', by site M8480/3
199.1 Oxyphilic site NOS
0 Oxyphilic site specified see 'Cancer', by site M8290/3
199.1 Papillary site NOS
0 Papillary site specified see 'Cancer', by site M8260/3
193 Papillary and follicular site NOS
0 Papillary and follicular site specified see 'Cancer', by site M8340/3
233.0 Papillary noninfiltrating intraductal site NOS
0 Papillary noninfiltrating intraductal site specified see 'Carcinoma In Situ', by site M8503/2
199.1 Scirrhous site NOS
0 Scirrhous site specified see 'Cancer', by site M8141/3
199.1 Sebaceous site NOS
0 Sebaceous site specified see 'Cancer', by site M8400/3
199.1 Serous site NOS
0 Serous site specified see 'Cancer', by site M9014/3
199.1 Superficial spreading site NOS
0 Superficial spreading site specified see 'Cancer', by site M8143/3

Carcinomas and neoplasms should be coded by site if possible. Code by cell type, "site NOS", only if a site is not specified in the diagnosis. Otherwise, refer to the appropriate category of neoplasm for a more specific code. See 'Cancer' 'Cancer Metastatic', 'Carcinoma In Situ', 'Neoplasm Uncertain Behavior', 'Neoplasm Unspecified Nature', or 'Benign Neoplasm'.

ADENOCARCINOMA (continued)

173.# Sweat gland M8400/3
4th digit: 173
0. Lip
1. Eyelid including canthus
2. Ear (auricle) auricular canal external (acoustic)
3. Unspecified parts of face, cheek external, chin, eyebrow, forehead, nose external, temple
4. Scalp and neck
5. Trunk, axilla, breast (or mastectomy site), buttock, groin, perianal skin, perineum, umbilicus
6. Upper limb including shoulder
7. Lower limb including hip
8. Other specified skin sites, contiguous or overlapping, undetermined point of origin
9. Site NOS

199.1 Trabecular site NOS
0 Trabecular site specified see 'Cancer', by site M8190/3
199.1 Tubular site NOS
0 Tubular site specified see 'Cancer', by site M8262/3
199.1 Villous site NOS
0 Villous site specified see 'Cancer', by site M8262/3
194.1 Water clear cell site NOS
0 Water clear cell site specified see 'Cancer', by site M8322/3
199.1 With apocrine metaplasia site NOS
0 With apocrine metaplasia site specified see 'Cancer', by site M8573/3
199.1 With cartilaginous and osseous metaplasia site NOS
0 With cartilaginous and osseous metaplasia site specified see 'Cancer', by site M8571/3
194.3 With spindle cell metaplasia site NOS
0 With spindle cell metaplasia site specified see 'Cancer', by site M8572/3
199.1 With squamous metaplasia site NOS
0 With squamous metaplasia site specified see 'Cancer', by site M8570/3

ADENOFIBROMA

220 Site NOS
0 Site specified see 'Benign Neoplasm', by site
220 Clear cell site NOS M8313/0
0 Clear cell site specified see 'Benign Neoplasm', by site M8313/0
220 Endometroid M8313/0
236.2 Endometroid borderline malignancy M8381/1
183.0 Endometroid malignant M8381/3

ADENOFIBROMA (continued)

220 Mucinous site NOS M9015/0
0 Mucinous site specified see 'Benign Neoplasm', by site M8313/0

600.20 Prostate

> *See 'LUTS' or 'Lower Urinary Tract Symptoms' for the additional code to identify the specific lower urinary tract symptoms.*

600.21 Prostate with urinary obstruction, retention or other lower urinary tract symptoms (LUTS)

220 Serous site NOS
0 Serous site specified see 'Benign Neoplasm', by site

253.2 ADENOHYPOPHYSEAL

ADENOID

199.1 Cystic carcinoma site NOS
0 Cystic carcinoma site specified see 'Cancer', by site M8200/3
474.9 Disease
474.12 Hyperplasia (hypertrophy) (enlargement)
474.00 Hyperplasia (hypertrophy) (enlargement) with chronic tonsillitis
474.02 Hyperplasia (hypertrophy) (enlargement) with chronic tonsillitis and adenoiditis
474.10 Hyperplasia (hypertrophy) (enlargement) with tonsil hypertrophy (hyperplasia)
959.09 Injury
474.8 Tag
474.01 Tag infected
474.2 Vegetations

ADENOIDITIS

463 Acute
474.01 Chronic
474.02 Chronic with chronic tonsillitis
474.01 Chronic with hypertrophy (adenoid) (tonsillar)
474.02 Chronic with hypertrophy (adenoid) (tonsillar) with chronic tonsillitis

210.2 ADENOLYMPHOMA SITE NOS
0 ADENOLYMPHOMA SITE SPECIFIED SEE 'BENIGN NEOPLASM', BY SITE M8561/0

ADENOMA

229.9 Site NOS
0 Site specified see 'Benign Neoplasm', by site M8140/0

194.3 Acidophil basophil (mixed) site NOS
0 Acidophil basophil (mixed) site specified see 'Benign Neoplasm', by site M8281/0
227.3 Acidophil site NOS
0 Acidophil site specified see 'Benign Neoplasm', by site M8280/0

229.9 Acinar cell site NOS
0 Acinar cell site specified see 'Benign Neoplasm', by site M8550/3

ADENOMA (continued)

227.0 Adrenal cortical (clear cell type) site NOS M8401/0
0 Adrenal cortical (clear cell type) site specified see 'Benign Neoplasm', by site M8373/0
227.0 Adrenal cortical (compact cell type) site NOS
0 Adrenal cortical (compact cell type) site specified see 'Benign Neoplasm', by site M8371/0
227.0 Adrenal cortical (glomerulosa cell type) site NOS
0 Adrenal cortical (glomerulosa cell type) site specified see 'Benign Neoplasm', by site M8374/0
227.0 Adrenal cortical (heavily pigmented variant) site NOS
0 Adrenal cortical (heavily pigmented variant) site specified see 'Benign Neoplasm', by site M8372/0
227.0 Adrenal cortical (mixed cell type) site NOS
0 Adrenal cortical (mixed cell type) site specified see 'Benign Neoplasm' by type M8375/0
227.0 Adrenal cortical site NOS
0 Adrenal cortical site specified see 'Benign Neoplasm', by site M8370/0
227.0 Alveolar site NOS
0 Alveolar site specified see 'Benign Neoplasm', by site M8251/0

217 Apocrine breast soft tissue (connective or glandular tissue)

216.# Apocrine skin M8401/0

4th digit: 216

0. Lip
1. Eyelid including canthus
2. Ear external (auricle) (pinna)
3. Face (cheek) (nose)
4. Scalp, neck
5. Trunk, back, chest
6. Upper limb including shoulder
7. Lower limb including hip
8. Other specified sites
9. NOS

229.9 Basal cell site NOS
0 Basal cell site specified see 'Benign Neoplasm', by site M8147/0

227.3 Basophil site NOS
0 Basophil site specified see 'Benign Neoplasm', by site M8300/0

211.5 Bile duct site NOS
0 Bile duct site specified see 'Benign Neoplasm', by site M8160/0

235.7 Bronchial site NOS
0 Bronchial site specified see 'Neoplasm Uncertain Behavior', by site M8140/1

216.# Ceruminous

4th digit: 216

0. Lip
1. Eyelid including canthus
2. Ear external (auricle) (pinna)
3. Face (cheek) (nose)
4. Scalp, neck
5. Trunk, back, chest
6. Upper limb including shoulder
7. Lower limb including hip
8. Other specified sites
9. NOS

ADENOMA (continued)

227.1 Chief cell site NOS
0 Chief cell site specified see 'Benign Neoplasm', by site M8321/0

227.3 Chromophobe site NOS
0 Chromophobe site specified see 'Benign Neoplasm', by site M8270/0

229.9 Clear cell site NOS
0 Clear cell site specified see 'Benign Neoplasm', by site M8310/0

229.9 Embryonal site NOS
0 Embryonal site specified see 'Benign Neoplasm', by site M8191/0

237.4 Endocrine (multiple) site NOS
0 Endocrine (multiple) site specified see 'Neoplasm Uncertain Behavior', by site M8360/1

238.9 Endometrioid (borderline malignancy) site NOS
0 Endometrioid (borderline malignancy) site specified see 'Neoplasm Uncertain Behavior', by site M8380/1

229.9 Endometrioid Site NOS
0 Endometrioid Site Specified See 'Benign Neoplasm', by site M8380/0

226 Follicular site NOS
0 Follicular site specified see 'Benign Neoplasm', by site M8330/0

211.7 Islet cell site NOS
0 Islet cell site specified see 'Benign Neoplasm', by site M8150/0

211.5 Liver cell site NOS
0 Liver cell site specified see 'Benign Neoplasm', by site M8170/0

226 Macrofollicular site NOS
0 Macrofollicular site specified see 'Benign Neoplasm', by site M8334/0

226 Microfollicular site NOS
0 Microfollicular site specified see 'Benign Neoplasm', by site M8333/0

229.9 Mixed cell site NOS
0 Mixed cell site specified see 'Benign Neoplasm', by site M8323/0

229.9 Monomorphic site NOS
0 Monomorphic site specified see 'Benign Neoplasm', by site M8146/0

229.9 Mucinous site NOS
0 Mucinous site specified see 'Benign Neoplasm', by site M8480/0

226 Oxyphilic site NOS
0 Oxyphilic site specified see 'Benign Neoplasm', by site M8290/0

229.9 Papillary (intracystic) site NOS
0 Papillary (intracystic) site specified see 'Benign Neoplasm', by site M8504/0

229.9 Papillary site NOS
0 Papillary site specified see 'Benign Neoplasm', by site M8260/0

229.9 Pleomorphic site NOS
0 Pleomorphic site specified see 'Benign Neoplasm', by site M8940/0

ADENOMA (continued)

600.20 Prostate

> ***See 'LUTS' or 'Lower Urinary Tract Symptoms' for the additional code to identify the specific lower urinary tract symptoms.***

600.21 Prostate with urinary obstruction, retention or other lower urinary tract symptoms (LUTS)

216.# Sebaceous
216.# Skin appendage M8390/0
216.# Sweat gland M8400/0

4th digit: 216
- **0. Lip**
- **1. Eyelid including canthus**
- **2. Ear external (auricle) (pinna)**
- **3. Face (cheek) (nose)**
- **4. Scalp, neck**
- **5. Trunk, back, chest**
- **6. Upper limb including shoulder**
- **7. Lower limb including hip**
- **8. Other specified sites**
- **9. NOS**

229.9 Trabecular site NOS
0 Trabecular site specified see 'Benign Neoplasm', by site M8190/0

220 Tubular female site NOS
222.0 Tubular male site NOS
0 Tubular site specified see 'Benign Neoplasm', by site M8211/0

229.9 Tubulovillous site NOS
0 Tubulovillous site specified see 'Benign Neoplasm', by site M8263/0

238.9 Villous site NOS
0 Villous site specified see 'Neoplasm Uncertain Behavior', by site M8261/1

227.1 Water clear cell site NOS
0 Water clear cell site specified see 'Benign Neoplasm', by site M8322/0

229.9 ADENOMATOID TUMOR SITE NOS
0 ADENOMATOID TUMOR SITE SPECIFIED SEE 'BENIGN NEOPLASM', BY SITE M9054/0

153.9 ADENOMATOUS POLYPOSIS COLI SITE NOS
0 ADENOMATOUS POLYPOSIS COLI SITE SPECIFIED SEE 'BENIGN NEOPLASM', BY SITE M8220/0

229.9 ADENOMYOMA SITE NOS
0 ADENOMYOMA SITE SPECIFIED SEE 'BENIGN NEOPLASM', BY SITE M8932/0
600.20 ADENOMYOMA PROSTATE

> ***See 'LUTS' or 'Lower Urinary Tract Symptoms' for the additional code to identify the specific lower urinary tract symptoms.***

600.21 ADENOMYOMA PROSTATE WITH URINARY OBSTRUCTION, RETENTION OR LOWER URINARY TRACT SYMPTOMS

617.0 ADENOMYOSIS

785.6 ADENOPATHY (LYMPH GLANDS)
091.4 ADENOPATHY SYPHILIS SECONDARY
0 ADENOPATHY TUBERCULOUS SEE 'TUBERCULOSIS', LYMPH NODES

277.2 ADENOSINE DEAMINASE DEFICIENCY
199.1 ADENOSQUAMOUS CARCINOMA SITE NOS
0 ADENOSQUAMOUS CARCINOMA SITE SPECIFIED SEE 'CANCER', BY SITE M8560/3
0 ADENOTONSILITIS SEE 'TONSILITIS'
V01.79 ADENOVIRUS EXPOSURE
008.62 ADENOVIRUS GASTROENTERITIS
079.0 ADENOVIRUS INFECTION (INFECTING AGENT)
V56.31 ADEQUACY TESTING FOR HEMODIALYSIS
V56.32 ADEQUACY TESTING FOR PERITONEAL DIALYSIS

ADH (ANTIDIURETIC HORMONE) SECRETION

259.3 Ectopic
259.3 Inappropriate ectopic
253.6 Inappropriate neurohypophysical
253.6 Syndrome

ADHESION, ADHESIVE

568.0 Abdominal wall
762.8 Amnion to fetus affecting fetus or newborn
658.8# Amnion to fetus complicating childbirth
5th digit: 658.8
0. Episode of care NOS or N/A
1. Delivered
3. Antepartum complication

543.9 Appendix
0 Arachnoid see 'Adhesion, Adhesive', meningeal
381.89 Auditory tube
622.3 Band cervix
568.0 Band intestine (postoperative) (postinfection)
560.81 Band intestine obstructed (postoperative) (postinfection)
621.5 Band uterus
576.8 Bile duct (any)
596.8 Bladder (sphincter)
568.0 Bowel (postoperative) (postinfection)
560.81 Bowel obstructed (postoperative) (postinfection)
620.8 Broad ligament
726.0 Capsulitis shoulder
423.1 Cardiac
398.99 Cardiac rheumatic
568.0 Cecum (postoperative) (postinfection)
560.81 Cecum obstructed (postoperative) (postinfection)
622.3 Cervicovaginal
752.49 Cervicovaginal congenital
674.8# Cervicovaginal maternal due to pregnancy
5th digit: 674.8
0. Episode of care NOS or N/A
2. Delivered with postpartum complication
4. Postpartum complication

622.3 Cervicovaginal postpartal, old
622.3 Cervix (bands) (old laceration)
622.3 Cervix cicatrix (postpartum)
624.4 Clitoris
568.0 Colon (postoperative) (postinfection)
560.81 Colon obstructed (postoperative) (postinfection)
576.8 Common duct
743.63 Conjunctiva - congenital
372.63 Conjunctiva - extensive
372.62 Conjunctiva - localized

ADHESION, ADHESIVE (continued)

371.00 Cornea - NOS
371.03 Cornea - central
743.43 Cornea - congenital
743.42 Cornea - congenital interfering with vision
371.01 Cornea - minor
371.02 Cornea - peripheral
575.8 Cystic duct
568.0 Diaphragm (peritoneal)
560.81 Diaphragm obstructed (peritoneal) (postoperative) (postinfection)
568.0 Duodenum
560.81 Duodenum obstructed (postoperative) (postinfection)
385.10 Ear middle
385.19 Ear middle - drum head
385.11 Ear middle - drum head to incus
385.13 Ear middle - drum head to promontorium
385.12 Ear middle - drum head to stapes
385.19 Ear middle - other adhesions and combinations
608.89 Epididymis
478.79 Epiglottis
381.89 Eustachian tube
743.63 Eye - conjunctiva congenital
372.63 Eye - conjunctiva extensive
372.62 Eye - conjunctiva localized
371.00 Eye - cornea NOS
371.03 Eye - cornea central
743.43 Eye - cornea congenital
743.42 Eye - cornea congenital interfering with vision
371.01 Eye - cornea minor
371.02 Eye - cornea peripheral
360.89 Eye - globe
364.70 Eye - iris
996.79 Eye - iris to corneal graft
379.29 Eye - vitreous
374.46 Eyelid
997.99 Eyelid postoperative complication
V45.69 Eyelid surgically created (status)
755.11 Fingers congenital
575.8 Gallbladder
568.0 Gastrointestinal tract (postoperative)
560.81 Gastrointestinal tract obstructed (postoperative)
568.0 Ileocecal (postoperative) (postinfection)
560.81 Ileocecal obstructed (postoperative) (postinfection)
568.0 Ileum (postoperative) (postinfection)
560.81 Ileum obstructed (postoperative) (postinfection)
568.0 Intestine (postoperative) (postinfection)
560.81 Intestine obstructed (postoperative) (postinfection)
0 Intestine obstructed with hernia see 'Hernia', by site, incarcerated
0 Intestine obstructed with hernia gangrenous see 'Hernia', by site, gangrenous
0 Joint see 'Ankylosis'
593.89 Kidney
624.4 Labium (minus)
752.49 Labium (majus) (minus) congenital
572.8 Liver
511.0 Lung
519.3 Mediastinum
349.2 Meningeal (cerebral) (spinal)
742.4 Meningeal congenital cerebral
742.59 Meningeal congenital spinal
0 Meningeal tuberculosis see 'Tuberculosis', meninges
568.0 Mesenteric
568.0 Mesenteric postoperative (postinfection)
478.19 Nasal or intranasal

ADHESION, ADHESIVE (continued)

355.9 Nerve NEC
355.0 Nerve sciatic
378.60 Ocular muscle
568.0 Omentum
751.4 Omentum anomalous congenital
568.0 Omentum postoperative (postinfection)
385.10 Otitis
385.11 Otitis - drum head to incus
385.13 Otitis - drum head to promontorium
385.12 Otitis - drum head to stapes
385.19 Otitis - other adhesions and combinations
614.6 Ovary
614.6 Ovary postoperative (postinfection)
752.0 Ovary to cecum congenital
752.0 Ovary to kidney congenital
752.0 Ovary to omentum congenital
614.6 Parauterine
614.6 Parauterine postoperative (postinfection)
614.6 Parovarian
614.6 Parovarian postoperative (postinfection)
568.0 Pelvic peritoneal (postoperative) (postinfection)
648.9# Pelvic peritoneal complicating pregnancy, childbirth or puerperium

5th digit: 648.9
0. Episode of care NOS or N/A
1. Delivered
2. Delivered with postpartum complication
3. Antepartum complication
4. Postpartum complication

614.6 Pelvic peritoneal female (postoperative) (postinfection)
568.0 Pelvic peritoneal male
560.81 Pelvic peritoneal obstructed (postoperative) (postinfection)
568.0 Pelvic peritoneal postoperative
560.81 Pelvic peritoneal postoperative obstructed
752.69 Penis to scrotum (postinfectional) (postoperative) (congenital)
568.0 Periappendiceal (postoperative) (postinfection)
560.81 Periappendiceal obstructed (postoperative) (postinfection)
423.1 Pericardium
393 Pericardium rheumatic
017.9# Pericardium tuberculosus [420.0]

5th digit: 017.9
0. NOS
1. Lab not done
2. Lab pending
3. Microscopy positive (in sputum)
4. Culture positive - microscopy negative
5. Culture negative - microscopy positive
6. Culture and microscopy negative, confirmed by other methods

575.8 Pericholecystic
568.0 Perigastric (postoperative) (postinfection)
560.81 Perigastric obstructed (postoperative) (postinfection)
602.8 Periprostatic
568.0 Perirectal (postoperative) (postinfection)
560.81 Perirectal obstructed (postoperative) (postinfection)

ADHESION, ADHESIVE (continued)

751.4 Peritoneal - congenital
614.6 Peritoneal - female
568.0 Peritoneal - male
614.6 Peritoneal - pelvic, female
568.0 Peritoneal - pelvic, male
614.6 Peritoneal - postoperative, female
568.0 Peritoneal - postoperative, male
560.81 Peritoneal - postoperative obstructed
614.6 Peritoneal - to uterus
614.6 Peritoneal - to uterus postoperative (postinfection)
537.3 Peritoneal - with duodenal obstruction
560.81 Peritoneal - with intestinal obstruction
614.6 Peritubal
614.6 Peritubal postoperative (postinfection)
596.8 Perivesical
511.0 Pleura pleuritic
012.0# Pleural tuberculosis

5th digit: 012.0
0. NOS
1. Lab not done
2. Lab pending
3. Microscopy positive (in sputum)
4. Culture positive - microscopy negative
5. Culture negative - microscopy positive
6. Culture and microscopy negative confirmed by other methods

511.0 Pleuropericardial
624.4 Postpartal, old
605 Prepuce
511.0 Pulmonary
568.0 Pylorus (postoperative) (postinfection)
560.81 Pylorus obstructed (postoperative) (postinfection)
478.29 Rosenmuller's fossa
355.0 Sciatic nerve
608.89 Seminal vesicle
726.0 Shoulder (joint) (capsulitis)
726.2 Shoulder subscapular
608.89 Spermatic cord
752.89 Spermatic cord congenital
349.2 Spinal canal
355.9 Spinal nerve NEC
724.9 Spinal nerve root site NOS
723.4 Spinal nerve root cervical
724.4 Spinal nerve root lumbosacral
724.4 Spinal nerve root thoracic
568.0 Stomach (postoperative) (postinfection)
560.81 Stomach obstructed (postoperative) (postinfection)
726.90 Tendonitis site unspecified
726.0 Tendonitis shoulder
608.89 Testicle
755.13 Toes congenital
529.8 Tongue
750.12 Tongue congenital
519.19 Trachea
614.6 Tubo ovarian
614.6 Tubo ovarian postoperative (postinfection)
608.89 Tunica vaginalis
593.89 Ureter
598.2 Urethra postoperative

ADHESION, ADHESIVE (continued)

621.5 Uterus (intrauterine)
763.89 Uterus affecting fetus or newborn
654.4# Uterus complicating childbirth

5th digit: 654.4
0. Episode of care NOS or N/A
1. Delivered
2. Delivered with postpartum complication
3. Antepartum complication
4. Postpartum complication

614.6 Uterus to abdominal wall
623.2 Vagina (chronic) (postoperative) (postradiation)

0 ADHESIVE SEE 'ADHESION, ADHESIVE'
379.46 ADIE (-HOLMES) (PUPIL) SYNDROME
272.8 ADIPOSIS DOLORA
278.02 ADIPOSITY
278.1 ADIPOSITY LOCALIZED
278.02 ADIPOSITY WITH BODY MASS INDEX 25.0 AND ABOVE [**V85.#(#)**]

V85.#(#): These codes are for use in persons over 20 years old.

4th or 4th and 5th digit: V85
2#. 25-29
1. 25.0-25.9
2. 26.0-26.9
3. 27.0-27.9
4. 28.0-28.9
5. 29.0-29.9
3#. 30-39
0. 30.0-30.9
1. 31.0-31.9
2. 32.0-32.9
3. 33.0-33.9
4. 34.0-34.9
5. 35.0-35.9
6. 36.0-36.9
7. 37.0-37.9
8. 38.0-38.9
9. 39.0-39.9
4. 40 and over

253.8 ADIPOSOGENITAL DYSTROPHY
253.8 ADIPOSOGENITAL SYNDROME

ADJUSTMENT REACTION

309.9 NOS
309.23 Academic inhibition specified
309.29 Culture shock
309.1 Depressive reaction, prolonged
309.22 Emancipation disorder of adolescence and early adult life
309.0 Grief reaction
309.9 Juvenile
309.81 Posttraumatic
309.21 Separation anxiety

ADJUSTMENT REACTION (continued)

309.24 With anxiety
309.28 With anxiety and depressed mood mixed
309.4 With conduct and emotion disturbance
309.3 With conduct disturbance
309.0 With depressed mood
309.28 With mixed anxiety and depressed mood
309.4 With mixed conduct and emotion disturbance
309.82 With physical symptoms
309.83 With withdrawal
309.23 Work inhibition specified
309.89 Other

V68.9 ADMINISTRATIVE ENCOUNTER UNSPECIFIED PURPOSE
V68.81 ADMINISTRATIVE ENCOUNTER REFERRAL WITHOUT EXAM OR TREATMENT
V68.89 ADMINISTRATIVE ENCOUNTER OTHER SPECIFIED PURPOSE
379.8 ADNEXA DISORDER OTHER SPECIFIED (EYE)
V21.2 ADOLESCENCE
V61.29 ADOPTED CHILD PROBLEM
V68.89 ADOPTION - ENCOUNTER FOR ADMINISTRATIVE PURPOSES
V70.3 ADOPTION - MEDICAL EXAM

ADRENAL

759.1 Aberrant congenital
V45.79 Absence (gland) acquired
759.1 Absence (gland) congenital
759.1 Accessory congenital
255.3 Androgenic overactivity, acquired, benign
255.41 Atrophy (autoimmune) (capsule) (cortex) (gland) (with or without hypofunction)
255.41 Calcification (capsule) (gland)
194.0 Cortical carcinoma site NOS M8370/3
0 Cortical carcinoma site specified see 'Cancer', by site
255.41 Cortical crisis
255.41 Crisis (cortical)
255.8 Degeneration (capsule) (gland)
277.39 Degeneration lardaceous
255.41 Degeneration with hypofunction
255.9 Disorder NOS
255.2 Disorder adrenogenital
255.8 Disorder specified NEC
759.1 Ectopic gland congenital
255.8 Fibrosis gland (subcutaneous)
255.41 Function decrease
772.5 Hemorrhage perinatal
036.3 Hemorrhage syndrome
255.6 Hyperfunction medulloadrenal
255.3 Hyperfunction other (acquired) (benign) (cortical) (androgenic)
255.8 Hyperplasia
255.2 Hyperplasia congenital
255.0 Hyperplasia due to ACTH excess
255.2 Hyperplasia male with sexual precocity
255.41 Hypofunction (cortex) (gland)
255.41 Infarction
255.8 Inflammation

ADRENAL (continued)

868.01 Injury (traumatic)
868.11 Injury (traumatic) with open wound into cavity
908.1 Injury (traumatic) late effect
255.41 Insufficiency – NOS primary (gland) (acute) (chronic)
255.5 Insufficiency - medullary
036.3 Insufficiency - medullary meningococcal
017.6# Insufficiency - tuberculous

5th digit: 017.6
0. NOS
1. Lab not done
2. Lab pending
3. Microscopy positive (in sputum)
4. Culture positive - microscopy negative
5. Culture negative - microscopy positive
6. Culture and microscopy negative confirmed by other methods

255.41 Melanosis
255.41 Melasma
036.3 Meningococcic syndrome
359.21 Muscle myotonia
229.9 Rest tumor site NOS
0 Rest tumor site specified see 'Benign Neoplasm', by site M8671/0
255.41 Syndrome
255.8 Other specified disorder

259.3 ADRENALIN ECTOPIC SECRETION
255.41 ADRENOCORTICAL INSUFFICIENCY
255.3 ADRENOCORTICAL SYNDROME
0 ADRENOCORTICOTROPIC SEE 'ACTH'
255.41 ADRENOCORTICOTROPIN HORMONE (ACTH) INSENSITIVITY
255.2 ADRENOGENITAL DISORDERS
255.2 ADRENOGENITAL FEMINIZING SYNDROME
760.79 ADRENOGENITAL IATROGENIC SYNDROME AFFECTING FETUS OR NEWBORN
255.2 ADRENOGENITAL SYNDROME (ACQUIRED) (CONGENITAL)
255.2 ADRENOGENITAL VIRILISM SYNDROME (ACQUIRED) (CONGENITAL)
277.86 ADRENOLEUKODYSTROPHY (NEONATAL) (X-LINKED)
277.86 ADRENOMYELONEUROPATHY

When the cause of an injury is stated to be abuse, multiple codes should be assigned if applicable, to identify any associated injuries. Sequence in the following order:

1. Type of abuse - child or adult (995.5, 995.8)

2. Type of injury

3. Nature of the abuse - see E-code directory 'Assault' (E904.0, E960-E966, E968)

4. Perpetrator of the abuse - see E-code directory 'Assault' (E967)

ADULT

995.8# Abuse (victim)

5th digit: 995.8
0. Maltreatment unspecified
1. Physical, battery
2. Emotional/psychological (deprivation)
3. Sexual
4. Neglect (nutritional), desertion
5. Other abuse and neglect, multiple forms

V62.83 Abuse - counseling of perpetrator non-parental/non-spousal of physical/sexual abuse NEC
V61.12 Abuse - counseling of perpetrator of spousal (partner) abuse
V61.11 Abuse - counseling of victim of spousal (partner) abuse
V62.89 Abuse - counseling of victim of other specified abuse
995.84 Abuse desertion
V71.81 Abuse - evaluation (alleged)
V71.6 Abuse - evaluation for battery (alleged)
V71.81 Abuse - evaluation for neglect (alleged)
V71.5 Abuse - evaluation for sexual (alleged)
V15.4# Abuse history

5th digit: V15.4
1. Physical/sexual abuse, rape
2. Emotional abuse, neglect
9. Other psychological trauma

995.81 Maltreatment syndrome

ADULT RESPIRATORY DISTRESS SYNDROME

518.5 NOS
507.0 Associated with aspiration pneumonia
514 Associated with hypostatic pneumonia
518.81 Associated with respiratory failure - acute in other conditions
518.84 Associated with respiratory failure - acute and chronic in other conditions
518.83 Associated with respiratory failure - chronic in other conditions
518.5 Associated with shock
518.82 Associated with other conditions
518.5 Following trauma and surgery
518.5 Traumatic or postsurgical
518.82 Other specified

In ICD-9 terms, an adverse effect is a reaction to a substance properly administered, while a poisoning is a reaction to a substance improperly administered (accident, suicide attempt, or assault). Adverse effects are coded when the proper administration of a drug results in an adverse condition. Code the resultant condition first with an additional E-code from 'Drugs And Chemicals' index, 'Therapeutic' column (E930-E949).

ADVERSE EFFECT

995.20 Unspecified drug, medicinal, or biological substance (see also table of drugs and chemicals, therapeutic)
995.22 Anesthesia
995.21 Arthus phenomenon (reaction)
909.5 Drug (to correctly administered substance) late effect
994.8 Electric current (shock)
909.4 Electric current (shock) late effect
994.5 Exertion (excessive)
909.4 Exertion (excessive) late effect
994.4 Exposure (exhaustion)
909.4 Exposure (exhaustion) late effect
995.7 Food reaction NEC
995.7 Food reaction NEC with hives [708.0]
995.7 Food reaction NEC with wheezing [786.07]
994.2 Hunger
909.4 Hunger late effect
692.82 Infrared dermatitis
995.23 Insulin
995.20 Medication
692.82 Radiation dermatitis or eczema
692.82 Radioactive dermatitis
692.82 Radiotherapy dermatitis
255.8 Steroid [E932.0]
692.70 Sun dermatitis
692.82 Ultaviolet dermatitis
692.82 X-ray dermatitis
995.29 Other drug, medicinal, or biological substance (see also table of drugs and chemicals, therapeutic)

0 ADVICE SEE 'COUNSELING'
560.1 ADYNAMIC ILEUS
753.22 ADYNAMIC URETER
993.0 AERO OTITIS MEDIA
909.4 AERO OTITIS MEDIA LATE EFFECT
0 AEROBACTER AEROGENES SEE 'BACTERIAL INFECTION' OR SPECIFIED CONDITION
998.81 AERODERMECTASIA SURGICAL
993.3 AEROEMBOLISM
909.4 AEROEMBOLISM LATE EFFECT
306.4 AEROPHAGY CYCLICAL
993.1 AEROSINUSITIS
909.4 AEROSINUSITIS LATE EFFECT

AFFECTIVE

V11.1 Disorder - history
301.10 Personality disorder
296.90 Psychosis see also 'Mood Disorder'
296.99 Psychosis other see also 'Mood Disorder'
309.1 Seasonal disorder
292.84 Syndrome - organic drug induced
293.89 Syndrome - organic NEC

537.89 AFFERENT LOOP SYNDROME NEC

AFIBRINOGENEMIA

286.6 Acquired
641.3# Antepartum hemorrhage
5th digit: 641.3
0. Episode of care NOS or N/A
1. Delivered
3. Antepartum complication

639.1 Post abortion or ectopic/molar pregnancy
666.3# Postpartum
5th digit: 666.3
0. Episode of care NOS or N/A
2. Delivered with postpartum complication
4. Postpartum complication

115.1# AFRICAN HISTOPLASMOSIS
5th digit: 115.1
0. Unspecified
1. Meningitis
2. Retinitis
3. Pericarditis
4. Endocarditis
5. Pneumonia
9. Other

273.3 AFRICAN MACROGLOBULINEMIA SYNDROME
086.5 AFRICAN SLEEPING SICKNESS
082.1 AFRICAN TICK TYPHUS

Aftercare generally includes fitting and adjustments, checking, changing, cleansing, removal and replacement unless otherwise stated.

AFTERCARE

V58.9 NOS
V53.09 Auditory substitution device
V58.2 Blood transfusion
V53.02 Brain pacemaker (neuropacemaker)
V53.32 Cardiac defibrillator automatic implantable
V53.31 Cardiac pacemaker
V53.39 Cardiac device other specified
V56.1 Catheter - dialysis extracorporeal
V56.2 Catheter - dialysis peritoneal
V58.82 Catheter - nonvascular NEC
V53.6 Catheter - urinary
V58.81 Catheter - vascular
V53.01 Cerebral ventricular (communicating) shunt
V58.11 Chemotherapy session (adjunctive) (maintenance)
V53.1 Contact lenses
V53.90 Device NOS
V53.99 Device other
V58.49 Drain change or removal
V58.30 Dressing change - nonsurgical
V58.31 Dressing change - surgical
V58.83 Drug monitoring encounter - therapeutic
V58.83 Drug monitoring encounter - therapeutic with long term drug use [**V58.6#**]
5th digit: V58.6
1. Anticoagulants
2. Antibiotics
3. Antiplatelets/antithrombotics
4. Anti-inflammatories non-steroidal (NSAID)
5. Steroids
6. Aspirin
7. Insulin
9. Other

A

AFTERCARE (continued)

FRACTURE

V54.2# Pathological healing
V54.1# Traumatic healing
5th digit: V54.1-2
0. Arm
1. Arm upper
2. Arm lower
3. Hip
4. Leg
5. Leg upper
6. Leg lower
7. Vertebrae
9. Other (pelvis) (wrist) (ankle) (hand/foot) (fingers/toes)

AFTERCARE (continued)

V53.2 Hearing aid

Antibiotics, Coumadin, Digoxin, chemotherapy drugs, and any other drug with a risk of adverse reaction is considered to be a high-risk medication. Code V67.51 is used to identify patients that have completed high risk medication therapy.

HIGH RISK MEDICATION

V67.51 Completed therapy
V58.6# Current therapy (long term)
5th digit: V58.6
1. Anticoagulants
2. Antibiotics
3. Antiplatelets/antithrombotics
4. Anti-inflammatories non-steroidal (NSAID)
5. Steroids
6. Aspirin
7. Insulin
9. Other

V58.83 Drug monitoring encounter
V58.83 Drug monitoring encounter with long term drug use **[V58.6#]**
5th digit: V58.6
1. Anticoagulants
2. Antibiotics
3. Antiplatelets/antithrombotics
4. Anti-inflammatories non-steroidal (NSAID)
5. Steroids
6. Aspirin
7. Insulin
9. Other

AFTERCARE (continued)

V53.91 Insulin pump (fitting, adjustment, titration)
V65.46 Insulin pump training
V58.89 Medical NEC
V58.49 Myringotomy tube removal encounter
V53.02 Nervous system device - pacemaker
V53.09 Nervous system device - other
V53.02 Neuropacemaker (brain) (peripheral nerve) (spinal cord)
V58.30 Nonsurgical dressings
V58.5 Orthodontic
V53.4 Orthodontic device

AFTERCARE (continued)

ORTHOPEDIC

V54.9 Unspecified
V54.02 Adjustment/lengthening growth rod
V54.89 Amputation stump
V54.89 Change, checking or removal of an external device: (cast) (external fixation) (kirschner wire) (splint) (traction device)
V53.7 Fitting and adjustment of a device: (brace) (cast) (corset) (shoes)
V54.81 Joint replacement **[V43.6#]**
5th digit: V43.6
0. Site unspecified
1. Shoulder
2. Elbow
3. Wrist
4. Hip
5. Knee
6. Ankle
9. Other

V54.01 Removal (change) growth rod
V54.01 Removal (change) internal fixation device (fracture plate) (pin) (plates) (rod) (screws)
V54.09 Other internal fixation device
V54.89 Other NEC

OSTOMY

V55.9 NOS
V55.4 Cecostomy
V55.3 Colostomy
V55.5 Cystostomy
V55.4 Digestive other
V55.4 Enterostomy
V55.1 Gastrostomy
V55.2 Ileostomy
V55.4 Jejunostomy
V55.6 Nephrostomy
V55.0 Tracheostomy
V55.6 Ureterostomy
V55.6 Urethrostomy
V55.6 Urinary other
V55.8 Other specified site

AFTERCARE (continued)

V66.7 Palliative
V53.02 Peripheral nerve pacemaker (neuropacemaker)

Codes from this subcatagory should be used in conjunction with other aftercare codes to fully identify the reason for the aftercare encounter.

POSTOPERATIVE

V58.49 NOS
V58.78 Bone
V58.73 Circulatory system
V58.75 Digestive system
V58.49 Drain change or removal
V58.76 Genital organs
V58.76 Genitourinary system
V58.43 Injury
V54.81 Joint replacement
V58.78 Musculoskeletal
V58.42 Neoplasm
V58.72 Nervous system
V58.75 Oral cavity

AFTERCARE (continued)

POSTOPERATIVE (continued)

V58.44 Organ transplant [**V42.#(#)**]
4th or 4th and 5th digit: V42
0. Kidney
1. Heart
2. Heart valve
3. Skin
4. Bone
5. Cornea
6. Lung
7. Liver
8#. Other specified
81. Bone marrow
82. Peripheral stem cells
83. Pancreas
84. Intestine
89. Other specified
9. Unspecified

V58.74 Respiratory system
V58.71 Sense organs
V58.77 Skin
V26.22 Sterilization reversal
V58.77 Subcutaneous tissue
V58.75 Teeth
V58.43 Trauma
V58.76 Urinary system
V58.41 Wound closure planned
V58.49 Other specified

PROSTHESIS

V52.9 NOS
V52.0 Arm
V52.4 Breast
V52.3 Dental
V52.2 Eye
V52.1 Leg
V52.8 Other specified

AFTERCARE (continued)

V58.0 Radiotherapy
V53.09 Special senses device
V53.1 Spectacles
V53.02 Spinal cord pacemaker (neuropacemaker)
V58.32 Staple removal
V58.31 Surgical dressings
V58.32 Suture removal
V58.83 Therapeutic drug monitoring encounter
V58.81 Vascular catheter removal
V53.01 Ventricular shunt (cerebral) (communicating)
V53.09 Visual substitution device
V53.8 Wheelchair
V58.30 Wound dressing (packing) NOS or nonsurgical
V58.31 Wound dressing (packing) surgical
V58.89 Other specified

AFTER CATARACT

366.50 NOS
366.53 Obscuring vision
366.52 Other not obscuring vision

0 AGALACTIA SEE 'LACTATION' FAILURE

AGAMMAGLOBULINEMIA

279.00 NOS
279.2 Autosomal recessive
279.04 Bruton's type
279.2 Swiss-type
279.11 Thymic (hypoplasia) (dysplasia)
279.04 X-linked
279.2 X-linked recessive

751.3 AGANGLIONOSIS CONGENITAL

Elderly multigravida is a second or more pregnancy in a woman who will be 35 years of age or older at the expected date of delivery.

659.6# AGE ADVANCED MATERNAL COMPLICATING LABOR AND DELIVERY - ELDERLY MULTIGRAVIDA
5th digit: 659.6
0. Episode of care unspecified or N/A
1. Delivered
3. Antepartum complication

Elderly primigravida is a first pregnancy in a woman who will be 35 years of age or older at the expected date of delivery.

659.5# AGE ADVANCED MATERNAL COMPLICATING LABOR AND DELIVERY - ELDERLY PRIMIGRAVIDA
5th digit: 659.5
0. Episode of care unspecified or N/A
1. Delivered
3. Antepartum complication

Young maternal age is a pregnancy in a female who is less than 16 years old at the expected date of delivery.

659.8# AGE YOUNG MATERNAL COMPLICATING LABOR AND DELIVERY
5th digit: 659.8
0. Episode of care unspecified or N/A
1. Delivered
3. Antepartum complication

AGENESIS

742.8 Acoustic nerve
751.8 Digestive organ(s) or tract NOS (complete) (partial)
751.2 Digestive organ(s) or tract lower
750.8 Digestive organ(s) or tract upper
747.89 Ductus arteriosus
743.62 Eyelid
755.34 Femur NEC
755.37 Fibula NEC
755.29 Finger NEC
524.09 Jaw
524.09 Mandible
524.09 Maxilla
752.69 Penis
0 See also by anatomical site, absence congenital

312.0# AGGRESSIVE CONDUCT DISORDER (OUTBURST)
5th digit: 312.0
0. Unspecified
1. Mild
2. Moderate
3. Severe

301.3 AGGRESSIVE PERSONALITY DISORDER

A

307.9 AGITATION
308.2 AGITATION STATE, ACUTE REACTION TO STRESS
750.11 AGLOSSIA
784.69 AGNOSIA (AUDITORY) (VISUAL) (ORGANIC)
368.16 AGNOSIA VISUAL (PSYCHOPHYSICAL)
300.22 AGORAPHOBIA
300.21 AGORAPHOBIA WITH PANIC DISORDER (ATTACKS)
288.03 AGRANULOCYTIC ANGINA
288.09 AGRANULOCYTOPENIA

AGRANULOCYTOSIS

288.09 NOS
288.09 Chronic
288.01 Congenital
288.02 Cyclical
288.01 Genetic
288.01 Infantile
288.02 Periodic
288.09 Pernicious

784.69 AGRAPHIA (AUDITORY) (VISUAL) (ORGANIC)
742.2 AGYRIA CONGENITAL

253.1 AHUMADA-DEL CASTILLO SYNDROME (NONPUERPERAL GALACTORRHEA AND AMENORRHEA)

AIDS, ARC and symptomatic HIV infection are all reported with 042. This code should be sequenced as the principal diagnosis with an additional code for any manifestation. Exception: If the encounter is for an unrelated condition such as a trauma, sequence the trauma as the principal diagnosis, followed by the 042 code, and then the additional codes for any manifestations.

AIDS

042 NOS
042 NOS due to HIV II [079.53]
V65.44 Counseling
V01.79 Exposure
795.71 Inconclusive (nonspecific serologic evidence)
042 Like syndrome
647.6# Maternal current (co-existent) in pregnancy [042]
5th digit: 647.6
0. Episode of care NOS or N/A
1. Delivered
2. Delivered with postpartum complication
3. Antepartum complication
4. Postpartum complication

042 Related complex
042 Related complex due to HIV II [079.53]

136.0 AINHUM
0 AIR BLAST CONCUSSION SYNDROME SEE ANATOMICAL SITE, INJURY

AIR EMBOLISM

999.1 Following infusion perfusion or transfusion
673.0# Maternal due to pregnancy
5th digit: 673.0
0. Episode of care NOS or N/A
1. Delivered
2. Delivered with postpartum complication
3. Antepartum complication
4. Postpartum complication

958.0 Traumatic
908.6 Traumatic late effect

306.1 AIR HUNGER PSYCHOGENIC
993.9 AIR PRESSURE EFFECT
909.4 AIR PRESSURE LATE EFFECT
993.8 AIR PRESSURE OTHER SPECIFIED EFFECTS
994.6 AIR SICKNESS
909.4 AIR SICKNESS LATE EFFECT

AIRWAY

493.90 Disease reactive (see also 'Asthma')
519.8 Obstruction NEC
496 Obstruction chronic
519.11 Obstruction due to bronchospasm
934.9 Obstruction due to foreign body
506.9 Obstruction due to inhalation of fumes or vapors
478.75 Obstruction due to laryngospasm
495.9 Obstruction with allergic alveolitis NEC
0 Obstruction with asthma see 'Asthma'
494.# Obstruction with bronchiectasis
4th digit: 494
0. Without acute exacerbation
1. With acute exacerbation

0 Obstruction with bronchitis see 'Bronchitis', obstructive
492.8 Obstruction with emphysema NEC

081.2 AKAMUSHI DISEASE (SCRUB TYPHUS)
781.0 AKATHISIA
333.99 AKATHISIA DUE TO DRUGS
333.99 AKATHISIA NEUROLEPTIC INDUCED
291.1 AKS (ALCOHOLIC KORSAKOFF SYNDROME) SEE ALSO 'PSYCHOSIS ALCOHOLIC'
049.8 AKUREYRI DISEASE
759.89 ALAGILLE SYNDROME

ALALIA

784.3 Acquired
315.31 Developmental - expressive
315.32 Developmental - receptive mixed (expressive - receptive)

270.8 ALANINE METABOLISM DISORDERS
270.8 ALANINEMIA
050.1 ALASTRIM
791.9 ALBARRAN'S (COLIBACILLURIA) DISEASE
756.52 ALBERS-SCHONBERG'S SYNDROME
726.71 ALBERT'S DISEASE
270.2 ALBINISM
270.2 ALBINISM AMINO ACID METABOLISM AROMATIC DISTURBANCES
270.2 ALBINISM OCULAR

275.49 ALBRIGHT-MARTIN (-BANTAM) SYNDROME (PSEUDOHYPOPARATHYROIDISM)

756.59 ALBRIGHT-MCCUNE-STERNBERG SYNDROME (OSTEITIS FIBROSA DISSEMINATA)

756.59 ALBRIGHT STERNBERG SYNDROME

273.8 ALBUMIN ABSENCE (BLOOD)

790.99 ALBUMIN GLOBULIN RATIO ABNORMAL

791.0 ALBUMINURIA ABNORMAL FINDINGS

0 ALBUMINURIA MATERNAL COMPLICATING PREGNANCY WITH HYPERTENSION SEE 'PRE-ECLAMPSIA'

646.2# ALBUMINURIA MATERNAL COMPLICATING PREGNANCY WITHOUT MENTION OF HYPERTENSION

5th digit: 646.2
0. Episode of care unspecified or N/A
1. Delivered
2. Delivered with postpartum complication
3. Antepartum complication
4. Postpartum complication

> ***Substance abuse describes the practice of using drugs or alcohol to excess without reaching the state of physical dependence. Substance dependence is addiction. Dependence involves the loss of control, judgment and/or the ability to use in moderation. Dependence is marked by compulsive physical demands which are triggered by further ingestion.***

ALCOHOL

303.0# Abuse dependent - acute intoxication
303.9# Abuse dependent - in chronic alcoholism
305.0# Abuse nondependent

5th digit: 303.0, 9, 305.0
0. NOS
1. Continuous
2. Episodic
3. In remission

790.3 Blood level excessive (elevated)
V70.4 Blood test for alcohol
760.71 Fetal syndrome
760.71 Transmitted via placenta or breast milk affecting fetus or newborn

ALCOHOL INTOXICATION

303.0# Acute dependent
305.0# Acute nondependent

5th digit: 303.0, 305.0
0. NOS
1. Continuous
2. Episodic
3. In remission

291.4 Acute pathologic (idiosyncratic)

> ***Alcoholic (alcoholism induced) conditions require two codes, one for the alcoholic condition and one for the dependence. See 'Alcohol Abuse', (dependent). Sequencing depends on the reason for encounter. However, in the event of alcoholic psychoses, 291.#(#) should be sequenced first with the dependence code second.***

ALCOHOLIC (ALCOHOLISM INDUCED)

291.81 Abstinence symptoms or syndrome
291.1 Amnestic persisting syndrome
291.89 Anxiety

ALCOHOLIC (ALCOHOLISM INDUCED) (continued)

291.2 Brain syndrome (chronic)
425.5 Cardiomyopathy
303.9# Cerebellar ataxia [334.4]
303.9# Cerebral degeneration disease [331.7]

5th digit: 303.9
0. Unspecified
1. Continuous
2. Episodic
3. In remission

571.2 Cirrhosis of liver
291.5 Delusions
291.2 Dementia persisting
291.81 Deprivation symptoms or syndrome
345.## Epilepsy

4th digit: 345
0. Generalized nonconvulsive
1. Generalized convulsive
4. Partial, with impairment of consciousness
5. Partial, without impairment of consciousness
6. Infantile spasms
7. Epilepsia partialis continua
8. Other forms
9. Unspecified, NOS

5th digit: 345
0. Without mention of intractable epilepsy
1. With intractable epilepsy

345.3 Epilepsy grand mal status
345.2 Epilepsy petit mal status
571.2 Fatty liver
535.3# Gastritis

5th digit : 535.3
0. Without hemorrhage
1. With hemorrhage

291.3 Hallucinations
571.1 Hepatitis
291.1 Induced persisting amnestic disorder or syndrome
303.0# Intoxication acute

5th digit: 303.0
0. NOS
1. Continuous
2. Episodic
3. In remission

291.4 Intoxication pathological (idiosyncratic)
291.5 Jealousy
291.1 Korsakoff syndrome (AKS)
571.3 Liver damage
571.3 Liver disease
571.1 Liver disease acute
291.9 Mania NOS
0 Mental disorder see 'Psychosis Alcoholic'
291.89 Mood
357.5 Neuropathy
291.1 Neuropathy with psychosis
291.2 Organic brain syndrome
291.5 Paranoia (jealousy)
0 Psychosis see 'Psychosis Alcoholic'
V79.1 Screening
291.89 Sexual disorder
291.82 Sleep disorder

ALCOHOLIC (ALCOHOLISM INDUCED) (continued)

291.0 Withdrawal - delirium (tremens)
291.3 Withdrawal - hallucinosis (psychosis)
291.81 Withdrawal - symptoms or syndrome
760.71 Withdrawal - symptoms or syndrome affecting fetus or newborn

ALCOHOLISM

303.0# Acute
303.9# Chronic
5th digit: 303.0, 9
0. NOS
1. Continuous
2. Episodic
3. In remission

V61.41 Family problems
V11.3 History
655.4# Maternal with suspected damage to fetus
5th digit: 655.4
0. Episode of care NOS or N/A
1. Delivered
3. Antepartum complication

V79.1 Screening

571.3 ALD (ALCOHOLIC LIVER DISEASE)
571.1 ALD - ACUTE (ALCOHOLIC LIVER DISEASE)
288.2 ALDER'S (REILLY) SYNDROME (LEUKOCYTE GRANULATION ANOMALY)
271.2 ALDOLASE (HEREDITARY) DEFICIENCY

ALDOSTERONISM

255.10 NOS
255.13 Bartter's syndrome
255.10 Congenital
255.12 Conn's syndrome
255.11 Familial type I
255.11 Glucocorticoid-remediable
255.10 Hyperaldosteronism
255.10 Primary
255.14 Secondary other

237.2 ALDOSTERONOMA
279.12 ALDRICH (-WISKOTT) SYNDROME (ECZEMA-THROMBOCYTOPENIA)
085.1 ALEPPO BOIL
288.09 ALEUKIA CONGENITAL
284.9 ALEUKIA HEMORRHAGICA
284.89 ALEUKIA HEMORRHAGICA ACQUIRED (SECONDARY)
284.09 ALEUKIA HEMORRHAGICA CONGENITAL
315.01 ALEXIA DELAY IN DEVELOPMENT
784.61 ALEXIA WITH AGRAPHIA
733.7 ALGONEURODYSTROPHY
300.29 ALGOPHOBIA

202.1# ALIBERT-BAZIN SYNDROME (MYCOSIS FUNGOIDES) M9700/3
202.1# ALIBERT'S DISEASE (MYCOSIS FUNGOIDES) M9700/3
5th digit: 202.1
0. Unspecified site, extranodal and solid organ sites
1. Lymph nodes of head, face, neck
2. Lymph nodes intrathoracic
3. Lymph nodes abdominal
4. Lymph nodes axilla and upper limb
5. Lymph nodes inguinal region and lower limb
6. Lymph nodes intrapelvic
7. Spleen
8. Lymph nodes multiple sites

293.89 ALICE IN WONDERLAND SYNDROME

ALIMENTARY TRACT

751.8 Absence NOS (complete) (partial) (congenital)
V45.79 Absence acquired
751.5 Absence lower (complete) (partial) (congenital)
750.8 Absence upper (complete) (partial) (congenital)
751.8 Agenesis NOS (complete) (partial) (congenital)
751.2 Agenesis lower (complete) (partial) (congenital)
750.8 Agenesis upper (complete) (partial) (congenital)
751.5 Anomaly lower (complete) (partial) (congenital)
750.9 Anomaly upper unspecified (congenital)
750.8 Anomaly upper other specified (congenital)
751.8 Atresia (complete) (partial) (congenital)
751.2 Atresia lower (complete) (partial) (congenital)
750.8 Atresia upper (complete) (partial) (congenital)
0 Obstruction see 'Intestine, Intestinal', obstruction

790.5 ALKALINE PHOSPHATASE ABNORMAL BLOOD LEVEL
790.4 ALKALINE PHOSPHATASE ELEVATED

ALKALOSIS

276.3 NOS
276.3 Metabolic
276.3 Respiratory

270.2 ALKAPTONURIA AMINO ACID METABOLISM AROMATIC DISTURBANCES
270.2 ALKAPTONURIC OCHRONOSIS
620.6 ALLEN-MASTERS SYNDROME

ALLERGY, ALLERGIC

0 Anaphylactic shock see 'Anaphylaxis, Anaphylactic'
493.0# Asthma
5th digit: 493.0
0. NOS
1. With status asthmaticus
2. With (acute) exacerbation

518.6 Bronchopulmonary aspergillosis
558.3 Colitis
558.3 Colitis due to ingested foods **[V15.0#]**
5th digit: V15.0
1. Peanuts
2. Milk products
3. Eggs
4. Seafood
5. Other foods

372.14 Conjunctivitis (eczematous)

ALLERGY, ALLERGIC (continued)

477.8 Dandruff
525.66 Dental restorative material (existing)
0 Dermatitis see also 'Dermatitis' and 'Dermatitis Contact'
V07.1 Desensitization
558.3 Diarrhea
558.3 Diarrhea due to ingested foods **[V15.0#]**
5th digit: V15.0
1. Peanuts
2. Milk products
3. Eggs
4. Seafood
5. Other foods

V15.09 Diathesis
995.27 Drug correctly administered
360.19 Endophthalmitis
477.8 Epidermal (animal)
V19.6 Family history of allergy disorders
477.8 Feathers
691.8 Food - atopic dermatitis
692.5 Food - contact with skin
V65.3 Food - counseling and surveillance
693.1 Food - ingestion dermatitis
477.1 Food - rhinitis
535.4# Gastritis
5th digit: 535.4
0. Without hemorrhage
1. With hemorrhage

558.3 Gastroenteritis
558.3 Gastroenteritis due to ingested foods **[V15.0#]**
5th digit: V15.0
1. Peanuts
2. Milk products
3. Eggs
4. Seafood
5. Other foods

477.9 Hay fever
477.2 Hay fever – animal (cat) (dog) dander or hair
477.8 Hay fever – animal (cat) (dog) epidermal or feathers
477.8 Hay fever - dust (house) (stock)
477.0 Hay fever - pollens (grass) (grains) (ragweed) (trees)
493.0# Hay fever - with asthma
5th digit: 493.0
0. NOS
1. With status asthmaticus
2. With (acute) exacerbation

0 History see 'Allergy, Allergic History'
995.3 Hypersensitivity
364.04 Iridocyclitis
995.27 Medicine correctly administered
558.3 Milk protein
287.0 Purpura
995.3 Reaction
0 Reaction history see 'Allergy, Allergic History'
909.9 Reaction late effect
306.1 Reaction psychogenic - respiratory
995.27 Reaction NOS to correctly administered substance

ALLERGY, ALLERGIC (continued)

477.9 Rhinitis
477.2 Rhinitis – animal (cat) (dog) dander or hair
477.8 Rhinitis – animal (cat) (dog) epidermal or feathers
477.8 Rhinitis - dust (house) (stock)
477.1 Rhinitis - food
477.0 Rhinitis - pollens (grass) (grains) (ragweed) (trees)
493.0# Rhinitis - with asthma
5th digit: 493.0
0. NOS
1. With status asthmaticus
2. With (acute) exacerbation

999.5 Serum (prophylactic) (therapeutic)
995.0 Shock
V07.1 Shots
692.9 Skin reaction
V72.7 Testing
597.89 Urethritis
708.0 Urticaria

ALLERGY, ALLERGIC HISTORY

V15.09 Unspecified
V14.9 Unspecified medication
V14.6 Analgesic agent
V14.4 Anesthetic agent
V15.06 Bugs
V14.5 Codeine
V15.08 Contrast media used for x-rays
V15.09 Diathesis
V15.03 Eggs
V15.05 Food additives
V15.06 Insects (bites and stings)
V15.07 Latex
V15.02 Milk products
V14.5 Narcotic agent
V15.05 Nuts other than peanuts
V14.3 Other anti-infective agent
V14.1 Other antibiotic
V15.01 Peanuts
V14.0 Penicillin
V15.08 Radiographic dye
V15.04 Seafood ink (octopus) (squid)
V15.04 Shellfish
V15.06 Spiders (spider bite)
V14.2 Sulfonamides
V14.7 Vaccine
V15.05 Other specified food
V14.8 Other specified medicinal agents
V15.09 Other specified non-medicinal agents

117.6 ALLESCHERIA PETRIELLIDIUM BOYDII INFECTIONS

117.6 ALLESCHERIOSIS

757.1 ALLIGATOR BABY SYNDROME (ICHTHYOSIS CONGENITA)

701.1 ALLIGATOR SKIN DISEASE ACQUIRED

757.1 ALLIGATOR SKIN DISEASE CONGENITAL

116.1 ALMEIDA'S (BRAZILIAN BLASTOMYCOSIS)

A

ALOPECIA

704.00 NOS
704.01 Androgenetic
704.01 Areata
757.4 Congenital
316 Psychogenic [704.00]
091.82 Syphilitic
704.02 Telogen effluvium

330.8 ALPERS' DISEASE OR GRAY-MATTER DEGENERATION
273.4 ALPHA-1-ANTITRYPSIN DEFICIENCY
273.4 ALPHA-1-TRYPSIN INHIBITOR DEFICIENCY
255.2 ALPHA (17) (20) HYDROXYLASE DEFICIENCY
792.3 ALPHA FETOPROTEIN ABNORMAL FINDING IN AMNIOTIC FLUID
790.99 ALPHA FETOPROTEIN ABNORMAL FINDING IN BLOOD
V28.1 ALPHA FETOPROTEIN SCREENING BY AMNIOCENTESIS
271.8 ALPHA FUCOSIDASE DEFICIENCY
272.5 ALPHA LIPOPROTEIN DEFICIENCY
271.8 ALPHA MANNOSIDASE DEFICIENCY
993.2 ALPINE SICKNESS
909.4 ALPINE SICKNESS LATE EFFECT
759.89 ALPORT'S SYNDROME (HEREDITARY HEMATURIA-NEPHROPATHY-DEAFNESS)
335.20 ALS MOTOR NEURON DISEASE (BULBAR) (MIXED TYPE)
0 ALTE (APPARENT LIFE-THREATENING EVENT) CODE INDIVIDUAL SYMPTOM(S)

780.0# ALTERATION OF CONSCIOUSNESS
5th digit: 780.0
1. Coma
2. Transient awareness
3. Persistent vegetative state
9. Other (stupor, drowsiness, somnolence, semicoma, unconsciousness)

780.97 ALTERED MENTAL STATUS
780.93 ALTERED MENTAL STATUS - AMNESIA, MEMORY LOSS
118 ALTERNARIA INFECTION TO COMPROMISED HOST ONLY
993.2 ALTITUDE SICKNESS
909.4 ALTITUDE SICKNESS LATE EFFECT
435.9 ALVAREZ SYNDROME (TRANSIENT CEREBRAL ISCHEMIA)

ALVEOLAR

516.3 Capillary block syndrome
524.7# Dental anomaly
5th digit: 524.7
0. Unspecified (mandible) (maxilla)
1. Maxillary hyperplasia
2. Mandibular hyperplasia
3. Maxillary hypoplasia
4. Mandibular hypoplasia
5. Vertical displacement
6. Occlusal plane deviation
9. Other specified

524.75 Extrusion
959.09 Injury
526.5 Osteitis

ALVEOLAR (continued)

525.8 Process absence
750.26 Process absence congenital
525.2# Process atrophy (ridge)
5th digit: 525.2
0. Unspecified
1. Minimal of mandible
2. Moderate of mandible
3. Severe of mandible
4. Minimal of maxilla
5. Moderate of maxilla
6. Severe of maxilla

525.8 Process irregular
525.8 Ridge cleft
525.8 Ridge enlargement NOS
528.72 Ridge mucosa keratinization excessive
528.71 Ridge mucosa keratinization minimal
525.8 Ridge process anomaly

ALVEOLITIS

495.9 Allergic (extrinsic)
495.7 Allergic (extrinsic) - ventilation
495.8 Allergic (extrinsic) - specified type NEC
495.4 Due to aspergillus clavatus
495.6 Due to cryptostroma corticale
516.3 Fibrosing idiopathic (lung)
714.81 Fibrosing idiopathic (lung) - rheumatoid
526.5 Jaw
526.5 Sicca dolorosa

ALZHEIMERS

331.0 Dementia **[294.1#]**
331.0 Disease
331.0 Disease with dementia **[294.1#]**
331.0 Sclerosis
331.0 Sclerosis with dementia **[294.1#]**
5th digit: 294.1
0. Without behavioral disturbance or NOS
1. With behavioral disturbance

V15.81 AMA DISCHARGE (AGAINST MEDICAL ADVICE)
330.1 AMAUROTIC FAMILIAL IDIOCY

AMAUROSIS

369.00 NOS both eyes
362.34 Fugax
300.11 Hysterical
362.76 Leber's congenital
377.34 Tobacco
377.34 Toxic
0 Uremic see 'Uremia'

AMBLYOPIA

368.00 NOS
368.02 Deprivation induced
368.03 Refractive
368.01 Strabismic (suppressive)
377.34 Toxic

0 AMEBIASIS SEE 'AMEBIC, AMEBIASIS'

AMEBIC, AMEBIASIS

006.0 Acute infection
006.8 Ameboma
006.8 Appendicitis
006.8 Balanitis
006.5 Brain abscess (and liver) (and lung)

AMEBIC, AMEBIASIS (continued)

V02.2 Carrier
006.1 Chronic
006.6 Cutaneous
007.8 Due to organisms other than entamoeba histolytica
006.0 Dysentery acute
006.1 Dysentery chronic
006.3 Hepatic
006.9 Infection
136.2 Infection free-living specific
006.8 Infection other sites
006.3 Liver abscess
006.4 Lung abscess (and liver)
136.2 Meningoencephalitis (naegleria)
006.2 Nondysenteric colitis
006.6 Skin ulceration
006.6 Ulceration skin
006.8 Other sites

755.4 AMELIA
755.31 AMELIA LOWER LIMB
755.21 AMELIA UPPER LIMB ABSENCE CONGENITAL

AMELOBLASTOMA

213.# NOS (by site) M9310/0
170.# Malignant (by site) M9310/3
4th digit: 170, 213
0. Skull, face, upper jaw
1. Lower jaw NOS
2. Spine
3. Rib, sternum, clavicle
4. Long bones of upper limb, scapula
5. Short bones of upper limb
6. Pelvis, sacrum, coccyx
7. Long bones of lower limb
8. Short bones of lower limb
9. Site NOS

520.5 AMELOGENESIS IMPERFECTA
626.0 AMENORRHEA PRIMARY OR SECONDARY
256.8 AMENORRHEA HYPERHORMONAL [626.0]
066.1 AMERICAN MOUNTAIN TICK BORNE FEVER
0 AMI (ACUTE MYOCARDIAL INFARCTION) SEE 'MYOCARDIAL INFARCTION ACUTE'
270.9 AMINO ACID DEFICIENCY
270.9 AMINO ACID METABOLISM DISORDER
270.2 AMINO ACID METABOLISM DISORDER AROMATIC
775.89 AMINO ACID METABOLISM DISORDER NEONATAL TRANSITORY
270.8 AMINO ACID METABOLISM DISORDER OTHER
V09.4 AMINOGLYCOSIDES RESISTANT INFECTION (SEE DRUG RESISTANT MICROORGANISMS FOR COMPLETE LISTING)
270.6 AMMONIA METABOLISM DISORDER

AMNESIA

780.93 NOS
300.12 Dissociative
300.12 Hysterical
780.93 Retrograde
437.7 Transient global

AMNESTIC DISORDER

294.8 NOS
291.1 Alcohol-induced persisting
292.83 Drug induced persisting
294.0 In conditions classified elsewhere

AMNESTIC SYNDROME

294.0 NOS
291.1 Alcohol-induced persisting
292.83 Drug-induced persisting
294.0 Confabulatory
294.0 In conditions classified elsewhere
291.1 Korsakoff's
294.0 Persisting in conditions classified elsewhere
294.0 Posttraumatic

AMNIOCENTESIS

V28.1 Alphafetoprotein screening
V28.0 Chromosomal screening anomaly
762.1 Damaging placenta affecting fetus or newborn
V28.2 Other screening

AMNION, AMNIOTIC

762.9 Abnormality - NOS affecting fetus or newborn
762.8 Abnormality - other specified affecting fetus or newborn
762.8 Band affecting fetus or newborn
658.8# Band complicating pregnancy
5th digit: 658.8
0. Episode of care NOS or N/A
1. Delivered
3. Antepartum complication

792.3 Fluid abnormal
673.1# Fluid embolism maternal due to pregnancy
5th digit: 673.1
0. Episode of care NOS or N/A
1. Delivered
2. Delivered with postpartum complication
3. Antepartum complication
4. Postpartum complication

658.8# Fluid leakage
0 Infection (cavity) see 'Amnionitis'
658.9# Membrane or cavity problem
658.8# Nodosum
658.1# Sac rupture premature
5th digit: 658.1, 8-9
0. Episode of care NOS or N/A
1. Delivered
3. Antepartum complication

658.4# AMNIONITIS
5th digit: 658.4
0. Episode of care NOS or N/A
1. Delivered
3. Antepartum complication

762.7 AMNIONITIS AFFECTING FETUS OR NEWBORN
301.7 AMORAL PERSONALITY
292.89 AMOTIVATIONAL SYNDROME
305.7# AMPHETAMINE ABUSE (NONDEPENDENT)
304.4# AMPHETAMINE ADDICTION (DEPENDENT)
5th digit: 304.4, 305.7
0. NOS
1. Continuous
2. Episodic
3. In remission

530.89 AMPULLA ESOPHAGEAL
576.2 AMPULLA OF VATER OBSTRUCTION (OCCLUSION)
0 AMPULLA OF VATER OBSTRUCTION (OCCLUSION) WITH CALCULUS SEE 'CHOLEDOCHOLITHIASIS'
530.89 AMPULLA PHRENIC

A

A current complicated amputation is a traumatic amputation with delayed healing, treatment, foreign body, or infection.

AMPUTATION

0 Amputee (bilateral) (old) acquired see 'Amputation', status, by site

887.# Arm and/or hand traumatic
4th digit: 887
0. Below elbow unilateral
1. Below elbow unilateral complicated original admission
2. Above elbow unilateral
3. Above elbow unilateral complicated original admission
4. Level NOS unilateral
5. Level NOS unilateral complicated original admission
6. Bilateral (any level)
7. Bilateral (any level) complicated original admission

886.0 Finger traumatic
886.1 Finger traumatic - complicated original admission
896.0 Foot traumatic unilateral
896.1 Foot traumatic unilateral - complicated original admission
896.2 Foot traumatic bilateral
896.3 Foot traumatic bilateral - complicated original admission

997.62, Infection of an amputation stump, requires an additional code to identify the organism. See 'Bacterial Infection'.

997.62 Infection (late) (chronic) stump
0 Infection current traumatic amputation see 'Amputation', by site, traumatic complicated

905.9 Late effect (surgical) (traumatic)
997.6# Late effect stump
5th digit: 997.6
0. NOS
1. Neuroma of stump
2. Infection (chronic)
9. Other

897.# Leg traumatic
4th digit: 897
0. Unilateral below knee
1. Unilateral below knee complicated original admission
2. Unilateral above knee
3. Unilateral above knee complicated original admission
4. Unilateral level NOS
5. Unilateral level NOS complicated original admission
6. Bilateral any level
7. Bilateral any level complicated original admission

878.0 Penis traumatic
878.1 Penis traumatic - complicated original admission
353.6 Phantom limb syndrome
878.2 Scrotum and testes traumatic
878.3 Scrotum and testes traumatic - complicated original admission

AMPUTATION (continued)

V49.7# Status - lower limb
5th digit: V49.7
0. Unspecified level
1. Great toe
2. Other toe(s)
3. Foot
4. Ankle
5. Below knee
6. Above knee
7. Hip

V49.6# Status - upper limb
5th digit: V49.6
0. Unspecified level
1. Thumb
2. Other finger(s)
3. Hand
4. Wrist
5. Below elbow
6. Above elbow
7. Shoulder

V54.89 Stump aftercare
997.6# Stump complication
5th digit: 997.6
0. Unspecified
1. Neuroma
2. Infection (chronic)
9. Other

885.0 Thumb traumatic
885.1 Thumb traumatic - complicated original admission
895.0 Toe traumatic
895.1 Toe traumatic - complicated original admission
0 Traumatic see 'Open Wound', by site

740.0 AMYELENCEPHALUS CONGENITAL
742.59 AMYELIA CONGENITAL
474.8 AMYGDALOLITH

790.5 AMYLASE ABNORMAL LEVEL
790.4 AMYLASE ELEVATED
277.30 AMYLOID DISEASE OR DEGENERATION ANY SITE
277.39 AMYLOID INFILTRATE

AMYLOIDOSIS

277.30 NOS
277.39 Arthropathy [713.7]
277.39 Cardiomyopathy [425.7]
277.31 Glomerulonephritis [583.81]
277.39 Heart [425.7]
277.39 Hereditary cardiac [425.7]
277.31 Hereditary nephropathic [583.81]
277.39 Inherited systemic
277.39 Nephropathic [583.81]
277.31 Nephropathic hereditary [583.81]
277.39 Nephrotic Syndrome [581.81]
277.39 Neuropathic (portuguese) (swiss) [357.4]
277.39 Peripheral nerve (autonomic) [337.1]
277.39 Polyneuropathy [357.4]
277.39 Pulmonary [517.8]
277.39 Renal disease [583.81]
277.39 Secondary
277.39 With lung involvement [517.8]
277.39 With myopathy [359.6]
277.39 Other specified

A

271.0 AMYLOPECTINOSIS
275.1 AMYOSTATIC SYNDROME
728.2 AMYOTROPHIA
756.89 AMYOTROPHIA CONGENITA
353.5 AMYOTROPHIA NEURALGIC (NONDISCOGENIC)
335.20 AMYOTROPHIC LATERAL SCLEROSIS (SYNDROME)

AMYOTROPHY

005.1 Botulism [358.1]
250.6# Diabetic [353.1]
5th digit: 250.6
0. Type II, adult-onset, non-insulin dependent (even if requiring insulin), or unspecified; controlled
1. Type I juvenile-onset or insulin-dependent; controlled
2. Type II adult-onset, non-insulin dependent (even if requiring insulin); uncontrolled
3. Type I, juvenile-onset or insulin-dependent; uncontrolled

244.# Hypothyroid [358.1]
4th digit: 244
0. Postsurgical
1. Postablative (irradiation)
2. Iodine ingestion
3. PAS, phenylbut, resorcinol
8. Secondary NEC
9. NOS

353.5 Neuralgic
281.0 Pernicious anemia [358.1]
335.21 Spinal progressive
242.## Thyrotoxic [358.1]
4th digit: 242
0. Toxic diffuse goiter
1. Toxic uninodular goiter
2. Toxic multinodular goiter
3. Toxic nodular goiter unspecified
4. From ectopic thyroid nodule
8. Of other specified origin
9. Without goiter or other cause

5th digit: 242
0. Without storm
1. With storm

795.79 ANA POSITIVE (ANTINUCLEAR ANTIBODIES)
0 ANAEROBIC SEE 'SEPTICEMIA' OR SPECIFED CONDITION
282.3 ANAEROBIC GLYCOLYSIS WITH ANEMIA
770.88 ANAEROSIS OF NEWBORN
0 ANAL SEE 'ANUS, ANAL'
763.5 ANALGESICS OF L&D AFFECTING FETUS OR NEWBORN
301.4 ANANCASTIC PERSONALITY DISORDER

ANAPHYLAXIS - ANAPHYLACTIC

995.0 NOS
909.9 NOS late effect
995.0 Allergic shock
909.9 Allergic shock late effect
995.0 Due to drug (medicine) - correctly administered
909.9 Due to drug (medicine) - correctly administered late effect
977.9 Due to drug (medicine) - improperly administered
909.0 Due to drug (medicine) - improperly administered late effect

ANAPHYLAXIS – ANAPHYLACTIC (continued)

995.0 Due to nonmedical substance
909.9 Due to nonmedical substance late effect
977.9 Due to overdose
909.0 Due to overdose late effect
999.4 Due to serum (immunization)
909.3 Due to serum (immunization) late effect
287.0 Purpura
995.0 Reaction
909.9 Reaction late effect
995.0 Shock NOS
909.9 Shock NOS late effect
995.6# Shock due to food nonpoisonous
5th digit: 995.6
0. Unspecified food
1. Peanuts
2. Crustaceans
3. Fruits and vegetables
4. Tree nuts and seeds
5. Fish
6. Food additives
7. Milk products
8. Eggs
9. Other specified food

909.9 Shock due to food late effect
989.5 Shock due to sting or venom
909.1 Shock due to sting or venom late effect

199.1 ANAPLASTIC CARCINOMA SITE NOS
0 ANAPLASTIC CARCINOMA SITE SPECIFIED SEE 'CANCER', BY SITE M8021/3
782.3 ANASARCA
0 ANASARCA CARDIAC SEE 'HEART FAILURE'
752.62 ANASPADIAS CONGENITAL
747.60 ANASTOMOSIS ARTERIOVENOUS CONGENITAL NEC
997.4 ANASTOMOSIS COMPLICATION POSTSURGICAL - GASTROINTESTINAL
997.5 ANASTOMOSIS COMPLICATION POSTSURGICAL - URINARY
V45.3 ANASTOMOSIS GASTROINTESTINAL STATUS
534.## ANASTOMOTIC ULCER
4th digit: 534
0. Acute with hemorrhage
1. Acute with perforation
2. Acute with hemorrhage and perforation
3. Acute
4. Chronic or unspecified with hemorrhage
5. Chronic or unspecified with perforation
6. Chronic or unspecified with hemorrhage and perforation
7. Chronic
9. Unspecified as acute or chronic

5th digit: 534
0. Without obstruction
1. Obstructed

0 ANC (ABSOLUTE NEUTROPHIL COUNT) DECREASED SEE 'NEUTROPENIA'

A

ANCYLOSTOMA, ANCYLOSTOMIASIS

126.9 And necatoriasis
126.2 Braziliense infection
126.3 Ceylanicum infection
126.0 Duodenale infection
126.8 Infection other specified
126.1 Necator americanus

272.8 ANDERS (ADIPOSIS TUBEROSA SIMPLEX) DISEASE
271.0 ANDERSEN'S DISEASE (GLYCOGENOSIS IV)
272.7 ANDERSON'S DISEASE (ANGIOKERATOMA CORPORIS DIFFUSUM)
993.2 ANDES DISEASE
686.8 ANDREWS' DISEASE (PUSTULAR BACTERID)

Carcinomas and neoplasms should be coded by site if possible. Code by cell type, "site NOS", only if a site is not specified in the diagnosis. Otherwise, refer to the appropriate category of neoplasm for a more specific code. See 'Cancer' 'Cancer Metastatic', 'Carcinoma In Situ', 'Neoplasm Uncertain Behavior', 'Neoplasm Unspecified Nature', or 'Benign Neoplasm'.

ANDROBLASTOMA

236.2 Site NOS female
0 NOS female site specified see 'Neoplasm Uncertain Behavior', by site M8630/1
236.4 Site NOS male
0 NOS male site specified see 'Neoplasm Uncertain Behavior', by site M8630/1
220 Benign female site NOS
0 Benign female site specified see 'Benign Neoplasm', by site M8630/0
222.9 Benign male site NOS
0 Benign male site specified see 'Benign Neoplasm', by site M8630/0
183.0 Malignant female site NOS
0 Malignant female site specified see 'Cancer', by site M9310/3
186.9 Malignant male site NOS
0 Malignant male site specified see 'Cancer', by site M9310/3
0 Tubular (with lipid storage) female site specified see 'Benign Neoplasm', by site M8641/0
220 Tubular (with lipid storage) female site NOS
0 Tubular (with lipid storage) male site specified see 'Benign Neoplasm', by site M8641/0
222.0 Tubular (with lipid storage) male site NOS M8641/0

256.1 ANDROGEN HYPERSECRETION OVARIAN
259.5 ANDROGEN INSENSITIVITY (PARTIAL) SYNDROME (TESTICULAR FEMINIZATION)

When a patient is admitted and treated for anemia, and the treatment is directed only at that condition, the anemia would be the principal diagnosis, regardless of the underlying condition.

ANEMIA

285.9 NOS
282.2 6-Phosphogluconic dehydrogenase deficiency
280.9 Achlorhydric
281.8 Achrestic
281.0 Addison's (pernicious)
281.0 Addison-Biermer (pernicious)
288.09 Agranulocytic

ANEMIA (continued)

281.4 Amino acid deficiency
282.3 Anaerobic glycolysis disorder
284.#(#) Aplastic

4th or 4th and 5th digit: 284

0#.Constitutional

1. Red blood cell (Blackfan-Diamond) (congenital) (familial hypoplastic) (of infants) (primary) (pure)

9. Other (Fanconi's) (pancytopenia with malformations)

1. Pancytopenia

2. Myelophthisis (leukoerythroblastic) (myelophthisic)

8#.Other specified

1. Red blood cell (acquired) (adult) (secondary) (with thymoma)

9. Other specified (chronic systemic disease) (drugs) (infection) (radiation) (toxic) (paralytic)

9. NOS (aplastic) (aregenerative) (hypoplastic) (idiopathic) (nonregenerative) (medullary hypoplasia)

285.29 Aplastic chronic systemic disease
244.9 Aplastic myxedema
284.81 Aplastic red cell acquired (adult) (with thymoma)
284.01 Aplastic red cell congenital
284.01 Aplastic red cell pure
284.9 Aregenerative
284.01 Aregenerative congenital
280.9 Asiderotic
285.9 Atypical (primary)
282.2 Autohemolysis of selwyn and dacie (type I)
283.0 Autoimmune hemolytic
282.2 Baghdad spring
007.0 Balantidium coli
281.0 Biermer's (pernicious)
280.0 Blood loss NOS
285.1 Blood loss acute all types
998.11 Blood loss acute resulting from a procedure [285.1]
280.0 Blood loss chronic all types (iron deficiency)
998.11 Blood loss chronic resulting from a procedure [280.0]
238.72 Bomford-Rhoads
123.4 Bothriocephalus
126.9 Brickmakers see also 'Ancylostomiasis'
437.8 Cerebral
282.9 Childhood
280.9 Chlorotic
281.9 Chronic simple nutritional
284.01 Chronica congenita aregenerativa
283.0 Cold type (hemolytic) (symptomatic) (secondary)
281.0 Combined system disease NEC [336.2]
281.1 Combined system disease due to dietary deficiency [336.2]

CONGENITAL

284.01 Aplastic
776.5 Due to blood loss (fetal)
285.8 Dyshematopoietic
285.8 Dyserythropoietic
282.7 Heinz-body (Castles)
282.9 Hereditary hemolytic
281.0 Intrinsic factor deficiency (Castle's)
773.2 Isoimmunization

ANEMIA (continued)

CONGENITAL (continued)

282.2 Nonspherocytic type I
282.3 Nonspherocytic type II
281.0 Pernicious
282.0 Spherocytic

ANEMIA (continued)

282.49 Cooley's
0 Crescent see 'Sickle Cell'
281.0 Cytogenic
282.2 Dacie's (nonspherocytic) type I
282.3 Dacie's (nonspherocytic) type II
284.9 Davidson's

DEFICIENCY

281.9 NOS
282.3 2, 3 diphosphoglycurate mutase
282.3 2, 3 PG
282.2 6-PGD
282.2 6- Phosphogluronic dehydrogenase
281.4 Amino acid
281.3 B12 and folate
282.2 Enzyme, drug induced (hemolytic)
282.3 Enzyme deficiency NEC
282.2 Erythrocytic glutathione
281.2 Folate (dietary) (drug-induced)
281.2 Folic acid (dietary) (drug induced)
282.2 G-6-PD (erthrocytic) (glutathione)
282.2 GGS-R
282.2 Glucose-6-phosphate dehydrogenase (G-6-PD)
282.3 Glucose-phosphate isomerase
282.2 Glutathione peroxidase
282.2 Glutathione-reductase
282.3 Glyceraldehyde phosphate dehydrogenase
282.3 GPI
282.2 G SH
285.9 Hemoglobin
282.3 Hexokinase
280.9 Iron (FE)
280.8 Iron (FE) other specified
281.9 Nutritional NOS
280.9 Nutritional with poor iron absorption
281.8 Nutritional with specified deficiency NEC
280.1 Nutritional due to inadequate dietary iron intake
281.8 Nutritional other
282.2 Pentose phosphate pathway
282.3 PFK
282.3 Phosphofructo-aldolase
282.3 Phosphofructokinase
282.3 Phosphoglycerate kinase
282.3 PK
281.4 Protein
282.3 Pyruvate Kinase (PK)
V78.1 Screening unspecified
282.3 TPI
282.3 Triosephosphate isomerase
281.1 Vitamin B12 NEC
281.1 Vitamin B12 dietary
281.0 Vitamin B12 pernicious

ANEMIA (continued)

284.01 Diamond-Blackfan (congenital hypoplastic)
123.4 Dibothriocephalus
281.9 Dimorphic
281.8 Diphasic
032.89 Diphtheritic

ANEMIA (continued)

123.4 Diphyllobothrium
282.60 Drepanocytic see also 'Sickle Cell'
285.2# Due to chronic disease (illness)

5th digit: 285.2

1. End-stage renal disease (chronic kidney disease)
2. Neoplastic disease
9. Other NEC

283.9 Dyke-Young type (secondary) (symptomatic)
285.8 Dyserythropoietic (congenital) (types I, II, III)
285.8 Dyshemopoietic (congenital)
126.9 Egypt (see also 'Ancylostoma')
282.3 Embden Meyerhof pathway glycolysis defect
282.1 Elliptocytic see also 'Elliptocytosis'
0 Enzyme deficiency see 'Anemia', deficiency
126.9 Epidemic see also 'Ancylostoma'
285.21 EPO resistant
282.49 Erythroblastic familial
773.5 Erythroblastic late
285.21 Erythropoietin-resistant
285.9 Essential
281.9 Evans'
280.9 Faber's (achlorhydric anemia)
280.0 Factitious (self-induced blood letting)
284.09 Fanconi's (congenital pancytopenia)
282.49 Familial erythroblastic (microcytic)
284.01 Familial hypoplastic
282.49 Familial microcytic (erythroblastic)
V18.2 Family history
282.2 Favism
0 Fetus see 'Anemia', newborn or fetus
123.4 Fish tapeworm (D. Latum) infestation
282.2 Glutathione metabolism disorder
281.2 Goat's milk
288.09 Granulocytic
282.7 Heinz-body congenital
282.7 Hemoglobinopathy NOS
282.7 Hemoglobinopathy other

HEMOLYTIC

283.9 Acquired NOS
283.0 Acquired autoimmune (drug induced) (warm or cold type)
283.1# Acquired nonautoimmune

5th digit: 283.1

0. Unspecified
1. Hemolytic-uremic syndrome
9. Other non-autoimmune

283.2 Acquired with hemoglobinuria NEC
283.9 Acute
282.3 Acute due to enzyme deficiency
283.0 Autoimmune (acquired) (cold type) (idiopathic) (primary) (secondary) (symptomatic) (warm type)
282.9 Chronic
283.9 Chronic idiopathic
283.0 Cold type
282.0 Congenital spherocytic
282.3 Congenital nonspherocytic
283.0 Drug-induced
283.19 Due to cardiac condition
283.19 Due to prosthesis or shunt
283.19 Due to traumatic cardiac condition
283.19 Fragmentation (acquired)
282.9 Familial

A

ANEMIA (continued)

HEMOLYTIC (continued)

282.9 Hereditary NOS
282.1 Hereditary elliptocytotic (ovalocytosis) (congenital)
282.2 Hereditary G6PD (glutathione reductase) (enzyme deficiency) (drug induced) (glutathione-reductase) (favism)
282.7 Hereditary hemoglobinopathy NOS (HB-C) (HB-D) (HB- E) (fetal)
282.3 Hereditary hexokinase deficiency (PK) (TPI) (hexokinase) (nonspherocytotic type II)
0 Hereditary sickle cell see 'Sickle Cell'
282.0 Hereditary spherocytic (acholuric jaundice) (congenital) (Minkowski Chauffard syndrome) (spherocytosis)
0 Hereditary thalassemia sickle cell see 'Sickle Cell'
282.49 Hereditary thalassemia other and unspecified (Mediterranean) (Cooley's) (leptocytosis) (microdrepanocytosis)
282.8 Hereditary other specified (stomatocytosis)
283.9 Idiopathic (chronic)
283.19 Infectious (acquired)
283.0 Infectious autoimmune
283.19 Lederer's (acquired infectious hemolytic)
283.19 Mechanical (acquired)
283.19 Microangiopathic (acquired)
0 Newborn see 'Anemia', newborn or fetus
283.10 Non-autoimmune (acquired)
282.2 Nonspherocytic (hereditary) type I
282.3 Nonspherocytic (hereditary) type II
283.19 Secondary
283.0 Secondary autoimmune
282.7 Stransky regala type (HB-E)
283.19 Symptomatic
283.0 Symptomatic autoimmune
446.6 Thrombotic thrombocytopenic purpura
283.19 Toxic (acquired)
283.19 Traumatic cardiac
283.11 Uremic (adult) (child)
283.0 Warm type

ANEMIA (continued)

280.0 Hemorrhagic (chronic)
285.1 Hemorrhagic acute
285.8 Hempas
0 Herrick's see 'Sickle Cell'
282.2 Hexose monophosphate (HMP) shunt deficiency
282.49 High A2
126.9 Hookworm see also 'Ancylostoma'
280.9 Hypochromic (idiopathic) (microcytic) (normoblastic)
285.0 Hypochromic familial sex linked
285.0 Hypochromic pyridoxine-responsive
285.0 Hypochromic with iron loading
284.01 Hypoplasia congenital or familial
284.81 Hypoplasia red blood cells
284.9 Hypoplastic (idiopathic)
284.09 Hypoplastic of childhood
285.9 Idiopathic
280.9 Impaired absorption
285.9 Infantile
285.9 Infective
126.9 Intertropical see also 'Ancylostoma'

ANEMIA (continued)

280.# Iron deficiency
4th digit: 280
0. Due to chronic blood loss
1. Due to inadequate iron intake
8. Other specified (Patterson) (Plummer Vinson)
9. NOS (achlorhydric) (chlorotic)

285.1 Iron deficiency due to acute blood loss
280.8 Iron deficiency with sideropenic dysphagia
285.8 Jaksch's (pseudoleukemia infantum)
284.01 Joseph-Diamond-Blackfan (congenital hypoplastic)
280.9 Koilonychia
386.50 Labyrinth
283.19 Lederer's (acquired infectious hemolytic anemia)
282.49 Leptocytosis (hereditary)
284.2 Leukoerythroblastic
281.9 Macrocytic
281.2 Macrocytic nutritional
281.2 Macrocytic tropical
281.1 Malabsorption (familial) selective B12 with proteinuria
084.6 Malarial see also 'Malaria'
281.0 Malignant (progressive)
281.9 Malnutrition
084.6 Marsh see also 'Malaria'

Code the specific maternal anemia in addition to 648.2#. See 'Anemia'.

648.2# Maternal current (co-existent) in pregnancy
5th digit: 648.2
0. Episode of care unspecified or N/A
1. Delivered
2. Delivered with postpartum complication
3. Antepartum complication
4. Postpartum complication

282.49 Mediterranean (with hemoglobinopathy)
281.# Megaloblastic
4th digit: 281
2. Folate deficiency (congenital) (goat's milk) (nutritional megaloblastic)
3. Other (B12 with folate deficiency) (refractory)
9. NOS

281.9 Megaloblastic
281.2 Megaloblastic nutrition (of infancy)
281.3 Megaloblastic refractory
281.9 Megalocytic
283.19 Microangiopathic hemolytic
280.9 Microcytic (hypochromic)
282.49 Microcytic familial
282.49 Microdrepanocytosis
126.9 Miners'
285.8 Myelopathic
284.2 Myelophthisic (normocytic)
244.9 Myxedema
126.1 Necator americanus

ANEMIA (continued)

NEWBORN OR FETUS

773.2 Unspecified
773.1 ABO hemolytic disease
773.1 ABO due to maternal/fetal incompatibility
760.8 Affected by maternal anemia
776.5 Due to fetal blood loss
773.2 Due to isoimmunization - NOS
773.1 Due to isoimmunization - ABO
773.0 Due to isoimmunization - RH antibodies
773.0 Due to isoimmunization - RH (rhesus), anti-D (RH)
773.2 Due to isoimmunization - other specified
773.2 Erythroblastic
773.5 Late due to isoimmunization
776.5 Posthemorrhagic
776.6 Prematurity neonatal
773.0 RH due to maternal/fetal incompatibility

ANEMIA (continued)

284.9 Nonregenerative
285.9 Normocytic (not due to blood loss) (infectional)
284.2 Normocytic (normocytic)
281.9 Nutritional (deficiency)
280.1 Nutritional due to inadequate dietary iron intake
280.9 Nutritional due to poor iron absorption
281.2 Nutritional folate (of infancy)
281.2 Nutritional megaloblastic (of infancy)
282.9 Of childhood
281.4 Orotic aciduric (congenital) (hereditary)
289.89 Osteosclerotic
282.1 Ovalocytosis (hereditary)
084.6 Paludal
281.0 Pernicious (congenital)
281.0 Pernicious with combined subacute spinal cord degeneration [336.2]
281.0 Pernicious with myelopathy (cord compression) [336.3]
281.0 Pernicious with polyneuropathy [357.4]
285.9 Pleochromic
281.8 Pleochromic of sprue
285.8 Portal
280.0 Posthemorrhagic (chronic)
285.1 Posthemorrhagic acute
285.9 Postoperative NOS
998.11 Postoperative due to (acute) blood loss [285.1]
998.11 Postoperative due to chronic blood loss [280.0]
648.2# Postpartum

5th digit: 648.2

0. Episode of care NOS or N/A
1. Delivered
2. Delivered with postpartum complication
3. Antepartum complication
4. Postpartum complication

285.9 Pressure
285.9 Primary
285.9 Profound
285.9 Progressive
281.0 Progressive malignant
281.0 Progressive pernicious
285.8 Pseudoleukemica infantum
285.0 Pyridoxine responsive (hypochromic)
284.81 Red cell pure
284.01 Red cell congenital
238.72 Refractoria sideroblastica

ANEMIA (continued)

281.3 Refractory megaloblastic
238.72 Refractory (primary) (RA)
238.72 Refractory sideroblastic
280.9 Refractory sideropenic
238.73 Refractory with excess blasts – 1 (RAEB-1)
238.73 Refractory with excess blasts – 2 (RAEB-2)
238.72 Refractory with hemochromatosis
238.72 Refractory with ringed sideroblasts (RARS)
282.49 Rietti-Greppi-Micheli (thalassemia minor)
281.8 Scorbutic
285.9 Secondary
284.9 Semiplastic
285.9 Septic
0 Sickle cell see 'Sickle Cell'
282.60 Sickle cell NOS
282.5 Sickle cell trait
285.0 Sideroachrestic
285.0 Sideroblastic (acquired) (congenital) (drug-induced) (due to disease) (hereditary) (primary) (pyridoxine-responsive) (secondary) (sex-linked hypochromic) (vitamin B6 responsive)
238.72 Sideroblastic refractory
280.9 Sideropenic (refractory)
281.9 Simple chronic
282.0 Spherocytic (hereditary)
285.8 Splenic
272.7 Splenic familial (Gaucher's)
285.8 Splenomegalic
282.8 Stomatocytosis
095.8 Syphilitic
282.49 Target cell (oval)
0 Thalassemia sickle cell see 'Sickle Cell'
282.49 Thalassemia other and unspecified
287.5 Thrombocytopenia
284.89 Toxic (paralytic)
281.2 Tropical, macrocytic
017.9# Tuberculosis see also 'Tuberculosis'

5th digit: 017.9

0. Unspecified
1. Lab not done
2. Lab pending
3. Microscopy positive (in sputum)
4. Culture positive - microscopy negative
5. Culture negative - microscopy positive
6. Culture and microscopy negative confirmed by other methods

281.1 Vegan's
285.0 Vitamin B6 responsive
281.1 Vitamin B12 deficiency with spinal cord degeneration [336.2]
281.1 Vitamin B12 malabsorption with proteinuria
285.8 Von Jaksch's (pseudoleukemia infantum)
283.0 Warm type (hemolytic)
285.2# With chronic disease (illness)

5th digit: 285.2

1. End-stage renal disease (chronic kidney disease)
2. Neoplastic disease
9. Other NEC

280.9 Witts' (achlorhydric)
281.2 Zuelzer (Ogden) (nutritional megaloblastic)
285.8 Other specified type

A

740.# ANENCEPHALUS CONGENITAL
4th digit: 740
0. Anencephalus
1. Craniorachischisis
2. Iniencephaly

655.0# ANENCEPHALY FETALIS AFFECTING PREGNANCY MANAGEMENT
5th digit: 655.0
0. Episode of care NOS or N/A
1. Delivered
3. Antepartum complication

ANESTHESIA

995.22 Adverse effect of drug, medicinal and biological substance
995.22 Complication or reaction NEC
371.81 Eye
338.0 Hyperesthetic, thalamic
782.0 Skin
995.4 Shock (to correctly administered substance)
909.9 Shock (to correctly administered substance) late effect

668.##: Use an additional code to further specify the complication of anesthesia or other sedation.

ANESTHESIA COMPLICATING L & D

668.9# NOS
763.5 Affecting fetus or newborn
668.1# Cardiac
668.2# Central nervous system
668.0# Pulmonary
668.8# Other specified
5th Digit: 668.0-2, 8-9
0. Episode of care NOS or N/A
1. Delivered
2. Delivered with postpartum complication
3. Antepartum complication
4. Postpartum complication

701.3 ANETODERMA

ANEURYSM AORTIC

441.9 NOS
441.4 Abdominal
441.3 Abdominal ruptured
441.0# Dissecting (ruptured)
5th digit: 441.0
0. Unspecified site
1. Thoracic
2. Abdominal
3. Thoracoabdominal

647.0# Maternal - syphilitic current (co-existent) in pregnancy [093.0]
5th digit: 647.0
0. Episode of care NOS or N/A
1. Delivered
2. Delivered with postpartum complication
3. Antepartum complication
4. Postpartum complication

ANEURYSM AORTIC (continued)

648.9#: Use an additional code to identify the specific aortic aneurysm.

648.9# Maternal - vascular current (co-existent) in pregnancy
5th digit: 647.0
0. Episode of care NOS or N/A
1. Delivered
2. Delivered with postpartum complication
3. Antepartum complication
4. Postpartum complication

441.5 Ruptured site NOS
093.0 Syphilitic
441.2 Thoracic
441.1 Thoracic ruptured
441.7 Thoracoabdominal
441.6 Thoracoabdominal ruptured
0 Traumatic see 'Aorta, Aortic', injury

ANEURYSM ARTERIAL (CIRSOID) (FALSE) (VARICOSE) (RUPTURED)

442.9 Artery NOS
447.0 Arteriovenous acquired
0 Arteriovenous congenital see 'Aneurysm Congenital'
442.81 Carotid artery internal extracranial portion
0 Carotid artery internal intracranial portion see 'Aneurysm Cerebral'
442.84 Celiac artery
372.74 Conjunctival
442.3 Femoral artery
442.84 Gastroduodenal artery
442.84 Gastroepiploic artery
421.0 Heart valve (any) infective
442.84 Hepatic artery
442.2 Iliac artery
442.89 Innominate artery
442.3 Lower extremity

648.9#: Use an additional code to identify the specific arterial aneursym.

648.9# Maternal current (co-existent) in pregnancy
5th digit: 648.9
0. Episode of care NOS or N/A
1. Delivered
2. Delivered with postpartum complication
3. Antepartum complication
4. Postpartum complication

442.89 Mediastinal artery
442.84 Mesenteric artery
442.84 Pancreaticoduodenal artery
442.3 Popliteal artery
417.1 Pulmonary artery
442.1 Renal artery
442.89 Spinal artery
442.83 Splenic artery
442.82 Subclavian artery
442.84 Superior mesenteric artery
0 Traumatic see specific artery, injury
442.0 Upper extremity artery
442.84 Visceral artery

A

ANEURYSM CEREBRAL

437.3 Nonruptured NOS
437.3 Nonruptured carotid artery internal intracranial portion
0 Ruptured see 'Hemorrhage', by site
094.87 Ruptured syphilitic

ANEURYSM CONGENITAL

747.29 Aortic
747.6# Arteriovenous (peripheral)

5th digit: 747.6
- **0. Peripheral vascular unspecified site**
- **1. Gastrointestinal vessel**
- **2. Renal vessel**
- **3. Upper limb vessel**
- **4. Lower limb vessel**
- **9. Other specified site peripheral vascular**

747.89 Artery site NEC
747.81 Cerebral arteriovenous
747.89 Circulatory NEC
746.85 Coronary
746.85 Coronary artery
747.6# Peripheral
747.6# Peripheral artery

5th digit: 747.6
- **0. Peripheral vascular unspecified site**
- **1. Gastrointestinal vessel**
- **2. Renal vessel**
- **3. Upper limb vessel**
- **4. Lower limb vessel**
- **9. Other specified site peripheral vascular**

747.3 Pulmonary
747.3 Pulmonary arteriovenous
747.3 Pulmonary artery
747.62 Renal (peripheral vascular)
743.58 Retinal
743.58 Retinal artery
747.29 Sinus of valsalva
747.82 Spinal

ANEURYSM HEART

414.12 Coronary artery dissection
414.11 Coronary vessels
414.10 Mural
429.79 Postinfarction <8 wks. [**410.##**]

4th digit: 410
- **0. Anterior lateral**
- **1. Anterior**
- **2. Inferior lateral**
- **3. Inferior posterior**
- **4. Inferior other**
- **5. Lateral**
- **6. Posterior**
- **7. Subendocardial**
- **8. Other site**
- **9. Site NOS**

5th digit: 410
- **0. Episode of care unspecified**
- **1. Initial episode of care**
- **2. Subsequent episode of care**

429.79 Postinfarction >8 wks. [414.8]
414.10 Ventricular
414.10 Wall
414.19 Other

759.89 ANGELMAN SYNDROME
312.0# ANGER REACTION

5th digit: 312.0
- **0. Unspecified**
- **1. Mild**
- **2. Moderate**
- **3. Severe**

ANGIITIS

447.6 NOS
446.4 Allergic granulomatosis (lung)
446.20 Hypersensitivity
446.21 Hypersensitivity - Goodpasture's syndrome
446.29 Hypersensitivity - other specified

> ***648.9#: Use an additional code to identify the specific angiitis.***

648.9# Maternal current (co-existent) in pregnancy

5th digit: 648.9
- **0. Episode of NOS or N/A**
- **1. Delivered**
- **2. Delivered with postpartum complication**
- **3. Antepartum complication**
- **4. Postpartum complication**

446.0 Necrotizing

> ***All carriers do not regard cardiac angina, 413.9, with the same degree of medical urgency as preinfarction angina, 411.1. Code to the specificity documented.***

ANGINA CARDIAC

413.9 NOS
411.1 Accelerated
411.1 Crescendo
413.0 Decubitus
413.9 Effort
413.9 Exertional
411.1 Initial
413.0 Nocturnal
413.9 Pectoris
411.1 Preinfarction
413.1 Prinzmetal's
411.1 Progressive
306.2 Psychogenic
413.9 Stable
413.9 Syndrome (Heberden's)
411.1 Unstable
413.1 Variant

A

ANGINA CRURIS

443.9 NOS
440.2# Extremities arteries
440.2# Extremities arteries with chronic complete or total occlusion [440.4]
5th digit: 440.2
0. Unspecified
1. With intermittent claudication
2. With rest pain or rest pain and intermittent claudication
9. Other atherosclerosis extremities

> ***When coding atherosclerosis of the extremities use an additional code, if applicable, to identify chronic complete or total occlusion of the artery of the extremities (440.4).***

440.24 Extremities arteries with ischemic gangrene or ischemic gangrene and ulceration, or ulceration and intermittent claudication, rest pain [707.#(#)]
440.23 Extremities arteries with ulceration, or ulceration and intermittent claudication, rest pain [707.#(#)]
4th or 4th and 5th digit: 707
1#. Lower limb except decubitus
10. Unspecified
11. Thigh
12. Calf
13. Ankle
14. Heel and midfoot
15. Other parts of foot, toes
19. Other
8. Chronic of other specified site
9. Chronic site NOS

ANGINA INFECTIOUS

034.0 Erysipelatous
462 Erythematous
476.0 Exudative chronic
478.29 Faucium
462 Gangrenous
462 Malignant
034.0 Septic
034.0 Streptococcal

ANGINA MESENTERIC

557.1 Abdominal
557.1 Intestinal
557.1 Mesenteric

0 ANGIOBLASTOMA SITE SPECIFIED SEE 'NEOPLASM UNCERTAIN BEHAVIOR' M9161/1
0 ANGIOCHOLECYSTITIS SEE 'CHOLECYSTITIS', ACUTE

ANGIODYSPLASIA

569.84 Intestine
569.85 Intestine with hemorrhage
537.82 Stomach and duodenum
537.83 Stomach and duodenum with hemorrhage

995.1 ANGIOEDEMA (ALLERGIC) (TO CORRECTLY ADMINISTERED SUBSTANCE)
909.9 ANGIOEDEMA (ALLERGIC) (TO CORRECTLY ADMINISTERED SUBSTANCE) LATE EFFECT
277.6 ANGIOEDEMA HEREDITARY
210.7 ANGIOFIBROMA SITE NOS
0 ANGIOFIBROMA SITE SPECIFIED SEE 'BENIGN NEOPLASM' BY SITE M9160/0

286.4 ANGIOHEMOPHILIA (A) (B)
363.43 ANGIOID STREAKS CHOROID
216.# ANGIOKERATOMA M9141/0
4th digit: 216
0. Lip skin
1. Eyelid including canthus
2. Ear external (auricle) (pinna)
3. Face (cheek) (nose)
4. Scalp, neck
5. Trunk, back, chest
6. Upper limb including shoulder
7. Lower limb including hip
8. Other specified sites
9. Skin NOS

214.# ANGIOLIPOMA M8861/1
4th digit: 214
0. Skin and subcutaneous tissue of face
1. Skin and subcutaneous tissue other
2. Intrathoracic organs
3. Intra abdominal organs
4. Spermatic cord
8. Other specified sites
9. Unspecified site

238.1 ANGIOLIPOMA INFILTRATING SITE NOS
0 ANGIOLIPOMA INFILTRATING SITE SPECIFIED SEE 'NEOPLASM UNCERTAIN BEHAVIOR', BY SITE M8861/1

0 ANGIOMA SEE 'HEMANGIOMA'
709.1 ANGIOMA SERPIGINOSUM
757.32 ANGIOMATOSIS
083.8 ANGIOMATOSIS BACILLARY
228.09 ANGIOMATOSIS SYSTEMIC
223.0 ANGIOMYOLIPOMA SITE NOS
0 ANGIOMYOLIPOMA SITE SPECIFIED SEE 'BENIGN NEOPLASM', BY SITE M8860/0

171.# ANGIOMYOLIPOSARCOMA M8860/3
215.# ANGIOMYOMA M8894/0
171.# ANGIOMYOSARCOMA M8894/3
4th digit: 171, 215
0. Head, face, neck
2. Upper limb including shoulder
3. Lower limb including hip
4. Thorax
5. Abdomen (wall), gastric, gastrointestinal, intestine, stomach
6. Pelvis, buttock, groin, inguinal region, perineum
7. Trunk NOS, back NOS, flank NOS
8. Other specified sites
9. Site NOS

ANGIONEUROTIC EDEMA

995.1 NOS
909.9 NOS late effect
999.5 Due to serum
909.3 Due to serum late effect
995.1 Giant
909.9 Giant late effect
995.1 Quincke's
909.9 Quincke's late effect
995.1 Urticaria
909.9 Urticaria late effect

ANGIOPATHY

459.9	NOS
443.9	Peripheral NOS
250.7#	Peripheral diabetic [443.81]
443.89	Peripheral other specified
362.18	Retinalis (juvenilis)
362.10	Retinalis (juvenilis) background
250.5#	Retinalis (juvenilis) diabetic [362.01]

5th digit: 250.5, 7
- **0. Type II, adult-onset, non-insulin dependent (even if requiring insulin), or unspecified; controlled**
- **1. Type I, juvenile-onset or insulin-dependent; controlled**
- **2. Type II, adult-onset, non-insulin dependent (even if requiring insulin); uncontrolled**
- **3. Type I, juvenile-onset or insulin-dependent; uncontrolled**

362.29	Retinalis (juvenilis) proliferative
0	Retinalis (juvenilis) tuberculous see 'Tuberculosis', retinalis

443.9	ANGIOPLASTIC DISEASE
435.9	ANGIOPLASTIC DISEASE CEREBRAL
459.89	ANGIOPLASTIC DISEASE VEIN
V45.82	ANGIOPLASTY STATUS (PTCA)
128.8	ANGIOSTRONGYLUS CANTONENSIS INFECTION
159.1	ANGIOSARCOMA SPLEEN M9120/3
368.42	ANGIOSCOTOMA ENLARGED
524.2#	ANGLE'S DENTAL ARCH ANOMALY (MALOCCLUSION)

5th digit: 524.2
- **1. Class I**
- **2. Class II**
- **3. Class III**

780.99	ANHEDONIA
705.0	ANHIDROSIS
276.51	ANHYDRATION
276.51	ANHYDREMIA
0	ANIMAL BITE (SKIN SURFACE INTACT) SEE 'CONTUSION', BY SITE
0	ANIMAL BITE (SKIN SURFACE PENETRATED) SEE 'OPEN WOUND', BY SITE
743.45	ANIRIDIA CONGENITAL
127.1	ANISAKIASIS
127.1	ANISAKIS LARVA INFECTION
367.32	ANISEIKONIA
379.41	ANISOCORIA
743.46	ANISOCORIA CONGENITAL
790.09	ANISOCYTOSIS
367.31	ANISOMETROPIA

ANKLE

V49.74	Absence (acquired)
755.31	Absence congenital complete
755.32	Absence congenital partial
726.70	Bursitis
736.70	Deformity acquired
736.79	Deformity acquired specified
755.69	Deformity congenital
726.70	Enthesopathy

ANKLE (continued)

959.7	Injury
916.8	Injury other and NOS superficial
916.9	Injury other and NOS superficial infected
718.97	Joint calcification
718.97	Joint ligament relaxation
0	Joint ligament tear see 'Sprain'
0	Joint see also 'Joint'
718.17	Loose body (joint)
V54.81	Replacement aftercare [V43.66]
V43.66	Replacement status
845.00	Separation (rupture) (tear) (laceration)
845.00	Strain (avulsion) (hemathrosis)
726.70	Tendinitis

374.46	ANKYLOBLEPHARON
750.0	ANKYLOGLOSSIA SUPERIOR SYNDROME
720.0	ANKYLOSING SPONDYLITIS
721.6	ANKYLOSING VERTEBRAL HYPEROSTOSIS

ANKYLOSIS

385.22	Ear ossicles
385.21	Ear ossicles malleus
718.54	Finger
718.57	Foot
718.55	Hip
718.5#	Joint (fibrous) (osseous)

5th digit: 718.5
- **0. Site NOS**
- **1. Shoulder region**
- **2. Upper arm (elbow) (humerus)**
- **3. Forearm (radius) (wrist) (ulna)**
- **4. Hand (carpal) (metacarpal) (fingers)**
- **5. Pelvic region and thigh (hip) (buttock) (femur)**
- **6. Lower leg (fibula) (knee) (patella) (tibia)**
- **7. Ankle and/or foot (metatarsals) (toes) (tarsals)**
- **8. Other**
- **9. Multiple**

718.56	Knee
724.6	Lumbosacral (nonvertebral) (nondiscogenic)
385.21	Malleus
718.58	Neck
718.58	Rib
724.6	Sacroiliac (nonvertebral) (nondiscogenic)
724.6	Sacrum (nonvertebral) (nondiscogenic)
724.9	Spine (nonvertebral) (nondiscogenic)
718.57	Toes
521.6	Tooth

ANODONTIA

520.0	NOS
524.30	NOS with abnormal spacing
525.1#	Acquired

5th digit: 525.1
- **0. Unspecified**
- **1. Due to trauma**
- **2. Due to periodontal disease**
- **3. Due to caries**
- **9. Other**

524.30	Acquired causing malocclusion
0	ANOMALY, ANOMALOUS SEE BY SPECIFIED ANOMALY OR BY ANATOMICAL SITE
759.9	ANOMALY NOS CONGENITAL
759.7	ANOMALY MULTIPLE NOS CONGENITAL

A

757.5 ANONYCHIA CONGENITAL
V45.78 ANOPHTHALMOS ACQUIRED
743.00 ANOPHTHALMOS CONGENITAL
752.89 ANORCHIA
752.89 ANORCHISM (CONGENITAL)
783.0 ANOREXIA
307.1 ANOREXIA NERVOSA

ANOSMIA

781.1 NOS
478.9 Postinfectional
306.7 Psychogenic
951.8 Traumatic

780.99 ANOSOGNOSIA
756.50 ANOSTEOPLASIA
744.09 ANOTIA
628.0 ANOVULATORY CYCLE
799.02 ANOXEMIA
770.88 ANOXEMIA NEWBORN

ANOXIA, ANOXIC

799.02 NOS

BIRTH

768.9 Unspecified
768.6 Mild
768.6 Moderate
768.5 Severe
768.5 Severe with neurologic involvement

The codes for anoxia and anoxic brain damage during labor or at birth cannot be used alone. You must also code the cause of the anoxia or anoxic brain damage. Sequence the anoxia first and the cause second. Post-op anoxic brain damage does not require an additional code.

BRAIN DAMAGE

348.1 NOS
768.0 Causing fetal death - NOS or before onset of labor
768.1 Causing fetal death - during labor
997.01 Due to abortion
772.1# Due to hemorrhage intraventricular (perinatal)
5th digit: 772.1
0. Unspecified
1. Grade I (bleeding into germinal matrix)
2. Grade II (bleeding into ventricle)
3. Grade III (bleeding with enlargement of ventricle)
4. Grade IV (bleeding into cerebral cortex)

772.2 Due to subarachnoid hemorrhage perinatal cause
767.0 Due to subdural or cerebral hemorrhage
997.01 During or resulting from a procedure
639.8 Following abortion, ectopic or molar pregnancy
997.01 Post op

ANOXIA, ANOXIC (continued)

348.1 Cerebral
770.88 Cerebral newborn
997.01 Cerebral due to procedure
348.1 Encephalopathy
997.01 Encephalopathy due to a procedure

ANOXIA, ANOXIC (continued)

770.88 Fetal affecting newborn
993.2 High altitude
909.4 High altitude late effect

Fetal or newborn codes (760-779), sometimes require an additional code to further specify the cause of the condition, the infecting organism, or complicating diagnoses. Whenever appropriate, describe the patient's medical situation as clearly and concisely as possible using multiple codes.

INTRAUTERINE

768.9 Liveborn - NOS
768.4 Liveborn - onset NOS
768.2 Liveborn - onset before labor
768.3 Liveborn - onset during labor and delivery
768.0 Stillborn - death before onset of labor
768.1 Stillborn - death during labor

ANOXIA, ANOXIC (continued)

799.02 Pathological

989.5 ANT (FIRE ANT) BITE
995.0 ANT (FIRE ANT) BITE WITH ANAPHYLAXIS [989.5]
451.82 ANTECUBITAL VEIN PHLEBITIS

796.5 ANTENATAL SCREENING FINDINGS ABNORMAL
V28.9 ANTENATAL SCREENING OF MOTHER

ANTEPARTUM HEMORRHAGE

641.9# NOS
5th digit: 641.9
0. Episode of care NOS or N/A
1. Delivered
3. Antepartum complication

762.1 Affecting fetus or newborn
641.3# Associated with coagulation defects
641.8# Other
5th digit: 641.3, 8
0. Episode of care NOS or N/A
1. Delivered
3. Antepartum complication

ANTERIOR

360.34 Chamber flat (postinflammatory) (post op) (posttraumatic)
786.52 Chest wall syndrome
958.92 Compartment syndrome tibial
717.83 Cruciate ligament disruption (old)
717.9 Cruciate ligament relaxation
844.2 Cruciate ligament tear (strain) (rupture) - acute
335.9 Horn cell disease
335.8 Horn cell disease other
524.54 Occlusal guidance insufficient
433.8# Spinal artery syndrome
5th digit: 433.8
0. Without cerebral infarction
1. With cerebral infarction

721.1 Spinal artery compression syndrome
904.51 Tibial artery injury
908.3 Tibial artery injury late effect
958.92 Tibial (compartment) syndrome
904.52 Tibial vein injury
908.3 Tibial vein injury late effect

524.24 ANTERO-OCCLUSION

500 ANTHRACOSILICOSIS

500 ANTHRACOSIS

ANTHRAX

022.9 NOS
022.2 Colitis
795.31 Culture positive (nasal)
022.0 Cutaneous
V71.82 Evaluation for suspected exposure
V01.81 Exposure
022.2 Gastrointestinal
V71.82 Observation for suspected exposure
022.1 Pneumonia [484.5]
022.1 Pulmonary
022.1 Respiratory
022.3 Sepsis
022.8 Other specified manifestations

286.5 ANTI VIII A INCREASE

286.5 ANTI IX A INCREASE

286.5 ANTI X INCREASE

286.5 ANTI XI A INCREASE

V58.83 ANTI-INFLAMMATORIES NON-STEROIDAL DRUG MONITORING (NSAID) ENCOUNTER

V58.83 ANTI-INFLAMMATORIES NON-STEROIDAL DRUG MONITORING (NSAID) ENCOUNTER WITH LONG TERM USE [V58.64]

V67.51 ANTI-INFLAMMATORIES NON-STEROIDAL (NSAID) FOLLOW UP EXAM - COMPLETED THERAPY

V58.64 ANTI-INFLAMMATORIES NON-STEROIDAL (NSAID) FOLLOW UP EXAM - CURRENT THERAPY

611.0 ANTIBIOMA BREAST

V07.39 ANTIBIOTIC PROPHYLACTIC ADMINISTRATION

V58.83 ANTIBIOTICS DRUG MONITORING ENCOUNTER

V58.83 ANTIBIOTICS DRUG MONITORING ENCOUNTER WITH LONG TERM USE [V58.62]

V67.51 ANTIBIOTICS FOLLOW UP EXAM - COMPLETED THERAPY

V58.62 ANTIBIOTICS FOLLOW UP EXAM - CURRENT THERAPY

V09.1 ANTIBIOTICS (B-LACTAM) RESISTANT INFECTION (SEE DRUG RESISTANT MICROORGANISMS FOR COMPLETE LISTING)

760.74 ANTIBIOTICS TRANSMITTED VIA PLACENTA OR BREAST MILK AFFECTING FETUS OR NEWBORN

279.00 ANTIBODY DEFICIENCY SYNDROME (AGAMMAGLOBULINEMIC) (HYPOGAMMAGLOBULINEMIC)

279.04 ANTIBODY DEFICIENCY SYNDROME CONGENITAL

795.79 ANTIBODY TITER RAISED (ELEVATED)

795.79 ANTICARDIOLIPIN ANTIBODY SYNDROME

V58.83 ANTICOAGULANT DRUG MONITORING ENCOUNTER

V58.83 ANTICOAGULANT DRUG MONITORING ENCOUNTER WITH LONG TERM USE [V58.61]

V67.51 ANTICOAGULANT FOLLOW UP EXAM - COMPLETED THERAPY

V58.61 ANTICOAGULANT FOLLOW UP EXAM - CURRENT THERAPY

760.77 ANTICONVULSANTS TRANSMITTED VIA PLACENTA OR BREAST MILK AFFECTING FETUS OR NEWBORN

305.8# ANTIDEPRESSANT ABUSE (NONDEPENDENT)
5th digit: 305.8
0. NOS
1. Continuous
2. Episodic
3. In remission

0 ANTIDIURETIC HORMONE SEE ALSO 'ADH'

259.3 ANTIDIURETIC HORMONE SECRETION (ADH) ECTOPIC SECRETION

795.79 ANTIGEN ANTIBODY REACTION ABNORMAL

286.0 ANTIHEMOPHILIC FACTOR A DEFICIENCY

286.1 ANTIHEMOPHILIC FACTOR B DEFICIENCY

286.2 ANTIHEMOPHILIC FACTOR C DEFICIENCY

286.0 ANTIHEMOPHILIC GLOBULIN (AHG) DEFICIENCY

760.78 ANTIMETABOLIC AGENTS TRANSMITTED VIA PLACENTA OR BREAST MILK AFFECTING FETUS OR NEWBORN

758.39 ANTIMONGOLISM SYNDROME

0 ANTIMYCOBACTERIAL RESISTANT INFECTION SEE 'DRUG RESISTANCE'

795.79 ANTINUCLEAR ANTIBODIES RAISED (POSITIVE)

795.79 ANTIPHOSPHOLIPID ANTIBODY SYNDROME

V58.83 ANTIPLATELETS/ANTITHROMBOTIC DRUG MONITORING ENCOUNTER

V58.83 ANTIPLATELETS/ANTITHROMBOTIC DRUG MONITORING ENCOUNTER WITH LONG TERM USE [V58.63]

V67.51 ANTIPLATELETS/ANTITHROMBOTIC FOLLOW UP EXAM - COMPLETED THERAPY

V58.63 ANTIPLATELETS/ANTITHROMBOTIC FOLLOW UP EXAM - CURRENT THERAPY

301.7 ANTISOCIAL PERSONALITY DISORDER

289.81 ANTITHROMBIN III DEFICIENCY

286.5 ANTITHROMBINEMIA HEMORRHAGIC DISORDER DUE TO INTRINSIC CIRCULATING ANTICOAGULANTS

286.5 ANTITHROMBOPLASTINEMIA HEMORRHAGIC DISORDER DUE TO INTRINSIC CIRCULATING ANTICOAGULANTS

286.5 ANTITHROMBOPLASTINOGENEMIA HEMORRHAGIC DISORDER DUE TO INTRINSIC CIRCULATING ANTICOAGULANTS

V58.83 ANTITHROMBOTIC/ANTIPLATELETS DRUG MONITORING ENCOUNTER

V58.83 ANTITHROMBOTIC/ANTIPLATELETS DRUG MONITORING ENCOUNTER WITH LONG TERM USE [V58.63]

V67.51 ANTITHROMBOTIC/ANTIPLATELETS FOLLOW UP EXAM - COMPLETED THERAPY

V58.63 ANTITHROMBOTIC/ANTIPLATELETS FOLLOW UP EXAM - CURRENT THERAPY

273.4 ANTITRYPSIN DEFICIENCY

V07.2 ANTIVENIN ADMINISTRATION (PROPHYLACTIC)

307.9 ANTON BABINSKI SYNDROME (HEMIASOMATOGNOSIA)

473.0 ANTRITIS (CHRONIC)

473.0 ANTRITIS MAXILLA

461.0 ANTRITIS MAXILLA ACUTE

535.5# ANTRITIS STOMACH
5th digit: 535.5
0. Without hemorrhage
1. With hemorrhage

A

473.0 ANTRUM, ANTRA CLOUDY - MAXILLARY SINUS

ANURIA

788.5 NOS
997.5 Postoperative
997.5 Specified as due to procedure
958.5 Traumatic
908.6 Traumatic late effect
788.5 Unknown etiology

ANUS, ANAL

911.0 Abrasion
911.1 Abrasion infected
751.2 Absence (canal) (congenital)
569.49 Anusitis
751.2 Atresia congenital
911.2 Blister
911.3 Blister infected
099.52 Chlamydia trachomatis infection
569.49 Crypt
564.89 Contracture
787.99 Discharge NEC
569.49 Disease NEC
751.5 Duplication congenital
751.5 Ectopic congenital
565.0 Fissure
565.0 Fissure non-traumatic
565.0 Fissure non-traumatic with fecal incontinence [787.6]
863.89 Fissure traumatic
863.99 Fissure traumatic with open wound
565.1 Fistula (to skin)
751.5 Fistula congenital
911.6 Foreign body superficial
911.7 Foreign body superficial infected
751.2 Imperforate congenital
569.49 Infection
569.49 Inflammation
959.19 Injury
911.8 Injury superficial other and unspecified
911.9 Injury superficial other and unspecified infected
911.4 Insect bite
911.5 Insect bite infected
787.99 Mass
787.99 Neuralgia
569.49 Occlusion
751.2 Occlusion congenital
569.42 Pain
569.49 Papillae hypertrophy
211.4 Polyp - adenomatous
569.0 Polyp - nonadenomatous
569.1 Prolapse (canal) (sphincter)
751.5 Prolapse (canal) (sphincter) congenital
751.2 Septum congenital
564.6 Spasm
564.89 Sphincter dilatation
569.3 Sphincter hemorrhage
569.2 Sphincter stricture
569.2 Stenosis
751.2 Stenosis congenital
569.2 Stricture
751.2 Stricture congenital
911.6 Superficial FB
911.7 Superficial FB infected
787.99 Swelling

ANUS, ANAL (continued)

569.43 Tear nontraumatic, nonpuerperal (sphincter)
569.43 Tear nontraumatic, nonpuerperal (sphincter) with fecal incontinence [787.6]
564.89 Tightness
569.41 Ulcer

569.49 ANUSITIS

ANXIETY

291.89 Alcohol induced
300.4 Depression
300.00 Disorder
300.02 Disorder generalized
293.84 Disorder in conditions classified elsewhere
300.09 Disorder other specified
292.89 Drug induced
313.0 Fearfulness of childhood and adolescence
300.20 Hysteria
300.00 Neurosis

Organic anxiety syndrome, 293.84, is a transient organic psychosis secondary to a medical condition. Code the medical condition first followed by 293.84.

293.84 Organic syndrome
300.00 Reaction
309.21 Reaction separation
308.0 Reaction stress (acute)
309.21 Separation disorder
300.00 State
300.00 State nonsituational
300.00 Syndrome
293.84 Syndrome psychotic (organic) (transient)
309.24 With adjustment disorder
309.28 With adjustment disorder and depressed mood

305.4# ANXIOLYTIC ABUSE
304.1# ANXIOLYTIC ADDICTION (DEPENDENT)

5th digit: 304.1, 305.4
0. NOS
1. Continuous
2. Episodic
3. In remission

382.9 AOM (ACUTE OTITIS MEDIA)

AORTA, AORTIC

747.22 Absence congenital
746.89 Absence valve congenital
745.0 And pulmonary artery fusion congenital

ANEURYSM

441.9 NOS
441.4 Abdominal
441.3 Abdominal ruptured
747.29 Congenital
441.0# Dissecting (ruptured)

5th digit: 441.0
0. Unspecified site
1. Thoracic
2. Abdominal
3. Thoracoabdominal

AORTA, AORTIC (continued)

ANEURYSM (continued)

648.9#: Use an additional code to identify the aortic aneurysm.

648.9# Maternal current (co-existent) in pregnancy
5th digit: 648.9
0. Episode of care NOS or N/A
1. Delivered
2. Delivered with postpartum complication
3. Antepartum complication
4. Postpartum complication

441.5 Ruptured site NOS
093.0 Syphilitic
441.2 Thoracic
441.1 Thoracic ruptured
441.7 Thoracoabdominal
441.6 Thoracoabdominal ruptured
0 Traumatic see 'Aorta, Aortic', injury

AORTA, AORTIC (continued)

747.20 Anomaly congenital
747.22 Aplasia congenital

ARCH

747.21 Anomalies congenital
747.11 Atresia (congenital)
747.21 Double congenital
747.10 Hypoplasia congenital
747.11 Interruption congenital
747.21 Persistent convolutions
747.21 Persistent right
446.7 Syndrome

AORTA, AORTIC (continued)

440.0 Arteriosclerosis (degeneration) (deformans)
747.22 Atresia (congenital)
746.7 Atresia (congenital) with hypoplasia of ascending aorta and defective development of left ventricle (with mitral valve atresia)
996.1 Balloon complication (mechanical)
444.0 Bifurcation (occlusion) syndrome
237.3 Body tumor site NOS
0 Body tumor site specified see 'Neoplasm Uncertain Behavior', by site M8691/1
440.0 Calcification (arteritis)
747.10 Coarctation (preductal) (postductal) congenital
747.21 Dextraposition congenital
745.11 Dextratransposition congenital
093.0 Dilatation syphilitic
747.29 Dilation congenital
447.9 Disease
093.89 Disease syphilitic
441.0# Dissecting
5th digit: 441.0
0. Unspecified site
1. Thoracic
2. Abdominal
3. Thoracoabdominal

996.1 Graft complication (mechanical)
424.1 Incompetence see also 'Aortic Insufficiency'
902.0 Injury abdominal
908.4 Injury late effect
901.0 Injury thoracic

AORTA, AORTIC (continued)

INSUFFICIENCY

424.1 NOS
421.0 Bacterial (acute) (chronic)
746.4 Congenital
395.1 Rheumatic
396.3 With mitral insufficiency
396.3 With mitral insufficiency rheumatic
396.1 With mitral stenosis
396.1 With mitral stenosis rheumatic
093.22 With mitral stenosis syphilitic
396.8 With other valve multiple involvement, stenosis/insufficiency (rheumatic)

AORTA, AORTIC (continued)

902.0 Laceration abdominal traumatic (rupture) (hematoma) (avulsion) (aneurysm)
901.0 Laceration thoracic traumatic (rupture) (hematoma) (avulsion) (aneurysm)
747.21 Malposition congenital
424.1 Obstruction or occlusion see also 'Aorta, Aortic (Valve) Stenosis'
424.1 Regurgitation see also 'Aortic Insufficiency'
747.21 Ring (atresia) syndrome (congenital)
745.0 Septal defect congenital

STENOSIS

424.1 NOS
396.0 Atypical
421.0 Bacterial acute
421.0 Bacterial chronic
746.3 Congenital
746.7 Congenital in hypoplastic left heart
746.81 Congenital subaortic
747.22 Congenital supravalvular
425.1 Hypertrophic subaortic - idiopathic
395.0 Rheumatic
395.2 Rheumatic with insufficiency
093.22 Syphilitic
424.1 With insufficiency
421.0 With insufficiency bacterial (acute) (chronic)
093.22 With insufficiency syphilitic
396.2 With mitral insufficiency
396.2 With mitral insufficiency rheumatic
093.22 With mitral insufficiency syphilitic
396.0 With mitral stenosis
396.0 With mitral stenosis rheumatic
093.22 With mitral stenosis syphilitic
396.8 With other valve multiple involvement, stenosis/insufficiency (rheumatic)

AORTA, AORTIC (continued)

747.22 Stricture congenital
745.11 Transposition congenital
746.89 Valve atresia (congenital)
746.4 Valve bicuspid congenital
395.9 Valve disease rheumatic
424.1 Valve disorder
747.21 Vascular ring congenital

AORTITIS

447.6 NOS
447.6 Calcific
093.1 Luetic
391.1 Rheumatic acute
093.1 Syphilitic
090.5 Syphilitic congenital

0 AORTOCORONARY BYPASS GRAFT COMPLICATION SEE 'COMPLICATION'
V45.81 AORTOCORONARY BYPASS STATUS
444.0 AORTOILIAC EMBOLISM (OBSTRUCTION) (OCCLUSION) (INFARCTION) (THROMBOSIS)
745.0 AORTOPULMONARY DEFECT (COMMON TRUNCUS) (COMMUNICATION ABNORMAL) CONGENITAL

APEPSIA

536.8 NOS
536.0 Achlorhydric
306.4 Psychogenic

255.2 APERT-GALLAIS SYNDROME (ADRENOGENITAL)
524.20 APERTOGNATHIA
755.55 APERT'S SYNDROME (ACROCEPHALOSYNDACTYLY)
787.20 APHAGIA
307.1 APHAGIA PSYCHOGENIC

APHAKIA

379.31 Aphakia
743.35 Congenital
379.31 Postsurgical
V45.61 Status post cataract extraction

APHASIA

784.3 Unspecified
784.69 Apraxia-alexia syndrome
315.31 Developmental expressive
315.32 Developmental receptive mixed (expressive - receptive)
438.11 Late effect cerebrovascular disease
784.3 Unknown etiology

784.41 APHONIA
784.49 APHONIA CLERICORUM

APHTHAE, APHTHOUS

074.0 Angina
078.4 Aphthae epizootic
529.0 Cachectic
078.4 Epizootic
078.4 Fever
528.2 Oral
528.2 Stomatitis
528.2 Ulcer (oral) (recurrent)
616.50 Ulcer genital organ(s) female

429.83 APICAL BALLOONING SYNDROME

APNEA, APNEIC (SPELLS)

786.03 NOS
306.1 Psychogenic
770.81 Newborn (essential) (primary)
770.82 Newborn obstructive
770.81 Newborn sleep
770.82 Newborn other
770.82 Obstructive newborn
770.82 Obstructive perinatal period
770.81 Perinatal period
770.82 Perinatal period obstructive

APNEA, APNEIC (SPELLS) (continued)

780.57 Sleep unspecified

327.27: Code first the underlying condition

327.27 Sleep central in conditions classifiable elsewhere
327.21 Sleep central primary
770.81 Sleep newborn
327.23 Sleep obstructive (adult) (child)
327.20 Sleep organic NOS
327.29 Sleep organic other
780.53 Sleep with hypersomnia unspecified
780.51 Sleep with hyposomnia unspecified
780.51 Sleep with insomnia unspecified
780.57 Sleep with sleep disturbance

077.4 APOLLO CONJUNCTIVITIS
726.90 APONEUROSIS DISEASE

APOPHYSITIS (SEE ALSO 'OSTEOCHONDROSIS')

732.9 NOS
732.6 Juvenile
732.5 Juvenile calcaneal

641.2# APOPLEXIA UTEROPLACENTAL

5th digit: 641.2
0. Episode of care NOS or N/A
1. Delivered
3. Antepartum complication

436 APOPLEXY
V12.54 APOPLEXY HISTORY (HEALED) (OLD) WITHOUT RESIDUAL
0 APOPLEXY WITH RESIDUAL SEE 'LATE EFFECT', CEREBROVASCULAR DISEASE
0 APPARENT LIFE-THREATENING EVENT (ALTE) CODE INDIVIDUAL SYMPTOM(S)

APPENDICITIS

541 NOS
540.9 Acute
540.1 Acute with peritoneal abscess
540.0 Acute with peritonitis
540.0 Acute with rupture
540.9 Acute without peritonitis
006.8 Amebic
542 Chronic
540.9 Gangrenous
540.1 Gangrenous with peritoneal abscess
540.0 Gangrenous with peritonitis or rupture
542 Recurrent
542 Relapsing
541 Retrocecal
542 Subacute
541 Unqualified
540.1 With cecal abscess

V44.52 APPENDICO-VESICOSTOMY STATUS

APPENDIX, APPENDICEAL

751.2 Absence congenital
543.9 Atrophy
543.9 Disease other and NOS
543.9 Diverticulum
751.5 Duplication congenital
543.0 Hyperplasia lymphoid

APPENDIX, APPENDICEAL (continued)

863.85 Injury traumatic
863.95 Injury traumatic with open wound into cavity
908.1 Injury traumatic late effect
751.5 Megaloappendix congenital
752.89 Morgagni (male)
540.0 Rupture (with peritonitis)
751.5 Transposition congenital

APPETITE

307.59 Disorder psychogenic
783.0 Loss
300.11 Loss hysterical
307.59 Loss nonorganic origin
307.59 Loss psychogenic
307.52 Perverted nonorganic origin

521.10 APPROXIMAL WEAR

300.16 APPROXIMATE ANSWERS SYNDROME

784.69 APRAXIA (AUDITORY) (VISUAL) (ORGANIC)

438.81 APRAXIA (AUDITORY) (VISUAL) (ORGANIC) LATE EFFECT OF CEREBROVASCULAR DISEASE

742.3 AQUEDUCT OF SYLVIUS ATRESIA

0 AQUEDUCT OF SYLVIUS ATRESIA WITH SPINA BIFIDA SEE 'SPINA BIFIDA' WITH CEREBRAL DEGENERATION

331.4 AQUEDUCT OF SYLVIUS OBSTRUCTION (OCCLUSION)

331.4 AQUEDUCT OF SYLVIUS OBSTRUCTION (OCCLUSION) WITH DEMENTIA [**294.1#**]

5th digit: 294.1

0. Without behavioral disturbance or NOS
1. With behavioral disturbance

742.3 AQUEDUCT OF SYLVIUS OBSTRUCTION (OCCLUSION) CONGENITAL

741.0# AQUEDUCT OF SYLVIUS OBSTRUCTION (OCCLUSION) CONGENITAL WITH SPINA BIFIDA

5th digit: 741.0

0. Region NOS
1. Cervical region
2. Dorsal (thoracic) region
3. Lumbar region

AQUEOUS

364.04 Cells
364.04 Fibrin
364.04 Flare
365.83 Misdirection

0 ARACHNOIDITIS SEE ALSO 'MENINGITIS'

335.21 ARAN-DUCHENNE MUSCULAR ATROPHY

066.9 ARBOVIRUS INFECTION

> ***AIDS, ARC and symptomatic HIV infection are all reported with 042. This code should be sequenced as the principal diagnosis with an additional code for any manifestation. Exception: If the encounter is for an unrelated condition such as a trauma, sequence the trauma as the principal diagnosis, followed by the 042 code, and then the additional codes for any manifestations.***

042 ARC

042 ARC DUE TO HIV II [079.53]

503 ARC WELDER'S LUNG DISEASE

370.24 ARC WELDER'S SYNDROME (PHOTOKERATITIS)

734 ARCHES FALLEN

447.4 ARCUATE LIGAMENT (-CELIAC AXIS) SYNDROME

446.7 ARCUS AORTAE SYNDROME

743.43 ARCUS JUVENILIS

743.42 ARCUS JUVENILIS INTERFERING WITH VISION

371.41 ARCUS SENILIS

ARDS

518.5 NOS
507.0 Associated with aspiration pneumonia
514 Associated with hypostatic pneumonia
518.81 Associated with respiratory failure - acute in other conditions
518.84 Associated with respiratory failure - acute and chronic in other conditions
518.83 Associated with respiratory failure - chronic in other conditions
518.5 Associated with shock
518.82 Associated with other conditions
518.5 Following trauma and surgery
518.5 Traumatic or postsurgical
518.82 Other causes NEC

259.2 ARGENTAFFIN, ARGINTAFFINOMA SYNDROME

371.16 ARGENTOUS DEPOSITS CORNEA

270.6 ARGININE METABOLISM DISORDERS

270.6 ARGININOSUCCINATE SYNTHETASE OR LYASE DEFICIENCY

270.6 ARGININOSUCCINIC ACID METABOLISM DISORDERS

253.1 ARGONZ-DEL CASTILLO SYNDROME (NONPUERPERAL GALACTORRHEA AND AMENORRHEA

379.45 ARGYLL ROBERTSON PUPIL SYNDROME (ATYPICAL) (NONSYPHILITIC)

094.89 ARGYLL ROBERTSON PUPIL SYNDROME SYPHILITIC

371.16 ARGYRIA CORNEA

709.09 ARGYRIA SKIN FROM DRUG OR CORRECT SUBSTANCE PROPERLY ADMINISTERED

372.55 ARGYROSIS CONJUNCTIVAL

742.2 ARHINENCEPHALY CONGENITAL

621.30 ARIAS-STELLA PHENOMENON

315.1 ARITHMETICAL DISORDER SPECIFIC (DELAY IN DEVELOPMENT)

008.1 ARIZONA GROUP OF PARACOLON BACILLI GASTROENTERITIS

ARM

V49.60 Absence (acquired) - NOS
V49.66 Absence (acquired) - above elbow
V49.65 Absence (acquired) - below elbow
0 Absence congenital - lower see 'Forearm'
755.24 Absence congenital - upper with incomplete absence of distal elements
755.21 Absence congenital - upper with complete absence of distal elements
755.23 Absence congenital - upper with forearm (incomplete)
0 Amputation status see 'Amputation' status upper limb
728.2 Atrophy
903.9 Blood vessel injury NOS
903.8 Blood vessel injury multiple
903.8 Blood vessel injury specified NEC

ARM (continued)

736.89 Deformity (acquired) NEC
959.2 Injury (proximal)
V52.0 Prosthesis (fitting and adjustment) (removal)
755.22 Rudimentary
840.9 Separation (rupture) (tear) (laceration)
755.20 Shortening congenital
337.9 Shoulder syndrome see also 'Neuropathy Peripheral' autonomic
840.9 Strain (sprain) (avulsion) (hemarthrosis)

277.31 ARMENIAN DISEASE OR SYNDROME

ARNOLD CHIARI SYNDROME

348.4 Type I
741.0# Type II
5th digit: 741.0
0. Region NOS
1. Cervical region
2. Dorsal (thoracic) region
3. Lumbar region

742.0 Type III
742.2 Type IV

327.41 AROUSALS CONFUSIONAL

ARRHYTHMIA

427.9 NOS
427.9 Auricular
427.89 Bigeminy
426.9 Block NOS (see also 'Heart Block')
427.89 Bradycardia
779.81 Bradycardia neonatal
427.9 Cardiac
427.89 Coronary sinus
427.89 Ectopic
427.60 Extrasystolic
427.9 Juvenile
427.9 Nodal
997.1 Postoperative (during or resulting from a procedure)
306.2 Psychogenic
427.9 Reflex
0 See also 'Dysrhythmia'
427.9 Sinus
427.9 Supraventricular
427.9 Transitory
780.2 Vagal
427.9 Ventricular

416.0 ARRILLAGA-AYERZA SYNDROME (PULMONARY ARTERY SCLEROSIS WITH PULMONARY HYPERTENSION)

709.09 ARSENICAL PIGMENTATION DUE TO DRUG OR CORRECT SUBSTANCE PROPERLY ADMINISTERED

0 ARTERIAL SEE 'ARTERY, ARTERIAL'

447.9 ARTERIOLE DISORDER NOS

447.8 ARTERIOLE DISORDER OTHER NEC

537.89 ARTERIOMESENTERIC DUODENUM OCCLUSION SYNDROME

Do not use code 996.03, complication of a device, implant or graft mechanical cardiac, when the physician documents that arteriosclerosis has caused an occlusion of a bypass graft. In coding terms, this is considered to be a normal progression of arteriosclerosis rather than a complication of a graft. Assign code 414.0#, arteriosclerosis of bypass graft, coronary.

ARTERIOSCLEROSIS, ARTERIOSCLEROTIC

440.9 NOS
440.0 Aorta
424.1 Aortic valve
433.0# Basilar artery
5th digit: 433.0
0. Without cerebral infarction
1. With cerebral infarction

414.0# Bypass graft coronary
414.0# Bypass graft coronary with chronic complete or total occlusion [414.2]
5th digit: 414.0
2. Autologous vein bypass graft
3. Nonautologous biological bypass graft
4. Autologous artery bypass graft (gastroepiploic) (internal mammary)
5. Unspecified type of bypass graft
7. Bypass graft of transplanted heart

440.3# Bypass graft of the extremities
440.3# Bypass graft of the extremities with chronic complete or total occlusion [440.4]
5th digit: 440.3
0. Unspecified graft
1. Autologous vein bypass graft
2. Nonautologous biological bypass graft

429.2 Cardiovascular disease (nonhypertensive) [440.9]
433.1# Carotid artery
5th digit: 433.1
0. Without cerebral infarction
1. With cerebral infarction

437.0 Central nervous system
437.0 Cerebral
414.0# Coronary
414.0# Coronary with chronic complete or total occlusion [414.2]
5th digit: 414.0
0. Unspecified type of vessel, native or graft
1. Native coronary vessel
2. Autologous vein bypass graft
3. Nonautologous biological bypass graft
4. Autologous artery bypass graft (gastroepiploic) (internal mammary)
5. Unspecified type of bypass graft
6. Native vessel of transplanted heart
7. Bypass graft of transplanted heart

290.4# Dementia [437.0]
5th digit: 290.4
0. NOS
1. With delirium
2. With delusions
3. With depressed mood

ARTERIOSCLEROSIS, ARTERIOSCLEROTIC (continued)

440.2# Extremities arteries
440.2# Extremities arteries with chronic complete or total occlusion [440.4]
5th digit: 440.2
0. Unspecified
1. With intermittent claudication
2. With rest pain or rest pain and intermittent claudication
9. Other atherosclerosis extremities

> ***When coding arteriosclerosis of the extremities use an additional code, if applicable to identify chronic complete or total occlusion of the artery of the extremities (440.4.).***

440.24 Extremities arteries with ischemic gangrene or ischemic gangrene ulceration, or ulceration and intermittent claudication, rest pain [707.#(#)]
440.23 Extremities arteries with ulceration, or ulceration and intermittent claudication, rest pain [707.#(#)]
4th or 4th and 5th digit: 707
1#. Lower limb except decubitus
10. Unspecified
11. Thigh
12. Calf
13. Ankle
14. Heel and midfoot
15. Other parts of foot, toes
19. Other
8. Chronic of other specified site
9. Chronic site NOS

779.89 Fetus
440.9 Generalized
414.0# Heart disease (ASHD)
414.0# Heart disease (ASHD) with chronic complete or total occlusion [414.2]
5th digit: 414.0
0. Unspecified type of vessel, native or graft
1. Native coronary vessel
2. Autologous vein bypass graft
3. Nonautologous biological bypass graft
4. Autologous artery bypass graft (gastroepiploic) (internal mammary)
5. Unspecified type of bypass graft
6. Native vessel of transplanted heart
7. Bypass graft of transplanted heart

424.99 Heart valve unspecified

> ***648.5#: Use an additional code to identify the specific cardiovascular arteriosclerotic condition.***

648.5# Maternal - cardiovascular current (co-existent) in pregnancy
674.0# Maternal - cerebrovascular due to pregnancy
648.9# Maternal - other current (co-existent) in pregnancy
5th digit: 648.5, 9, 674.0
0. Episode of care NOS or N/A
1. Delivered
2. Delivered with postpartum complication
3. Antepartum complication
4. Postpartum complication

ARTERIOSCLEROSIS, ARTERIOSCLEROTIC (continued)

557.1 Mesenteric
424.0 Mitral valve
779.89 Newborn
440.8 Other specified arteries
433.9# Precerebral artery
433.8# Precerebral artery other specified
5th digit: 433.8-9
0. Without cerebral infarction
1. With cerebral infarction

416.0 Pulmonary idiopathic
416.0 Pulmonary chronic
424.3 Pulmonary valve
0 Renal arterioles see 'Hypertensive'
440.1 Renal artery
440.8 Retinal vascular changes [362.13]
440.8 Retinopathy vascular (changes) [362.13]
437.0 Spinal (cord)
424.2 Tricuspid valve
433.2# Vertebral artery
5th digit: 433.2
0. Without cerebral infarction
1. With cerebral infarction

0 ARTERIOSCLEROTIC SEE 'ARTERIOSCLEROSIS, ARTERIOSCLEROTIC'

747.60 ARTERIOVENOUS ARTERY NEC (ABERRANT) (ABSENCE) (AGENESIS) (ACCESSORY) (ANEURYSM) (DEFORMITY) (HYPOPLASIA) (MALPOSITION)

0 ARTERIOVENOUS COMPLICATION INTERNAL SHUNT OR FISTULA (SURGICALLY CREATED) SEE 'COMPLICATION' VASCULAR

ARTERIOVENOUS (A-V) MALFORMATION

437.3 Brain acquired
747.81 Brain congenital
430 Brain ruptured, subarachnoid
747.81 Cerebrovascular system congenital
746.85 Coronary artery congenital
747.6# Peripheral vascular system congenital (aberrant) (absence) (agenesis) (accessory) (aneurysm) (deformity) (hypoplasia) (malposition)
5th digit: 747.6
0. Peripheral vascular unspecified site
1. Gastrointestinal vessel
2. Renal vessel
3. Upper limb vessel
4. Lower limb vessel
9. Other specified site peripheral vascular

747.3 Pulmonary
743.58 Retina
747.82 Spinal vessel congenital
747.89 Other specified

996.73 ARTERIOVENOUS STEAL SYNDROME

747.60 ARTERIOVENOUS VEIN NEC (ABERRANT) (ABSENCE) (AGENESIS) (ACCESSORY) (ANEURYSM) (DEFORMITY) (HYPOPLASIA) (MALPOSITION)

A

ARTERITIS

447.6 NOS
446.20 Allergic
447.6 Aorta
446.7 Aortic arch
437.4 Brain
446.7 Branchial
446.7 Branchiocephalica
437.4 Cerebral
414.0# Coronary arteriosclerotic
414.0# Coronary arteriosclerotic with chronic complete or total occlusion [414.2]
5th digit: 414.0
0. Unspecified type of vessel, native or graft
1. Native coronary vessel
2. Autologous vein bypass graft
3. Nonautologous biological bypass graft
4. Autologous artery bypass graft (gastroepiploic) (internal mammary)
5. Unspecified type of bypass graft
6. Native vessel of transplanted heart
7. Bypass graft of transplanted heart

391.9 Coronary rheumatic
398.99 Coronary rheumatic chronic
446.5 Cranial (left) (right)
446.5 Giant cell
674.0# Maternal - cerebrovascular due to pregnancy
5th digit: 674.0
0. Episode of care NOS or N/A
1. Delivered
2. Delivered with postpartum complication
3. Antepartum complication
4. Postpartum complication

648.5#: Use an additional code to identify coronary arteritis.

648.5# Maternal - coronary current (co-existent) in pregnancy
5th Digit: 648.5
0. Episode of care NOS or N/A
1. Delivered
2. Delivered with postpartum complication
3. Antepartum complication
4. Postpartum complication

648.9#: Use an additional code to identify the specific arteritis.

648.9# Maternal - other current (co-existent) in pregnancy
5th digit: 648.9
0. Episode of care NOS or N/A
1. Delivered
2. Delivered with postpartum complication
3. Antepartum complication
4. Postpartum complication

ARTERITIS (continued)

446.0 Necrotizing
446.7 Obliterans
446.0 Poly
417.8 Pulmonary
362.18 Retinal
447.2 Suppurative
446.5 Temporal
446.7 Young female syndrome (obliterative brachiocephalic)

ARTERITIS SYPHILITIC

093.1 Aorta
093.1 Aortitis
094.89 Brain
093.89 Coronary artery
093.89 General

ARTERY, ARTERIAL

747.81 Anomaly - cerebral (aberrant) (absence) (agenesis) (accessory) (aneurysm) (atresia) (deformity) (hypoplasia)
746.85 Anomaly - coronary (absence) (agenesis) (accessory) (aneurysm) (atresia) (deformity) (hypoplasia) (malposition)
747.6# Anomaly - peripheral vascular NEC (aberrant) (absence) (agenesis) (accessory) (aneurysm) (deformity) (hypoplasia) (malposition)
5th digit: 747.6
0. Unspecified site
1. Gastrointestinal vessel
2. Renal vessel
3. Upper limb vessel
4. Lower limb vessel
9. Other specified site peripheral vascular

747.3 Anomaly - pulmonary (absence) (agenesis) (aneurysm) (hypoplasia) (malposition)
743.58 Anomaly - retinal (aneurysm) (atresia) (deformity) (hypoplasia)
747.82 Anomaly - spinal (aberrant) (aneurysm) (deformity) (hypoplasia)
747.5 Anomaly - umbilical (absence) (agenesis) (atresia) (hypoplasia)
440.2# Arteriosclerosis extremities (degeneration) (deformans) (arteritis)
440.2# Arteriosclerosis extremities (degeneration) (deformans) (arteritis) with chronic complete or total occlusion [440.4]
5th digit: 440.2
0. Unspecified
1. With intermittent claudication
2. With rest pain or rest pain and intermittent claudication
9. Other atherosclerosis extremities

ARTERY, ARTERIAL (continued)

When coding arteriosclerosis of the extremities use an additional code, if applicable to identify chronic complete or total occlusion of the artery of the extremities (440.4).

440.24 Arteriosclerosis extremities (degeneration) (deformans) (arteritis) with ischemic gangrene or ischemic gangrene and ulceration, or ulceration and intermittent claudication, rest pain [707.#(#)]

440.23 Arteriosclerosis extremities (degeneration) (deformans) (arteritis) with and ulceration, or ulceration and intermittent claudication, rest pain [707.#(#)]

440.24 Arteriosclerosis extremities with occlusion (degeneration) (deformans) (arteritis) with ischemic gangrene or ischemic gangrene and ulceration, or ulceration and intermittent claudication, rest pain [707.#(#)]

440.23 Arteriosclerosis extremities with occlusion (degeneration) (deformans) (arteritis) with ulceration, or ulceration and intermittent claudication, rest pain [707.#(#)]

4th or 4th and 5th digit: 707

1#. Lower limb except decubitus

10. Unspecified
11. Thigh
12. Calf
13. Ankle
14. Heel and midfoot
15. Other parts of foot, toes
19. Other

8. Chronic of other specified site
9. Chronic site NOS

440.3# Arteriosclerosis extremities bypass graft

440.3# Arteriosclerosis extremities bypass graft with chronic complete or total occlusion [440.4]

5th digit: 440.3

0. Unspecified graft
1. Autologous vein bypass graft
2. Nonautologous biological bypass graft

747.60 Atresia (anomaly NEC) congenital
747.3 Atresia pulmonary
790.91 Blood gas abnormal
277.39 Degeneration amyloid lardaceous
447.9 Disorders

648.9#: Use an additional code to identify the specific arterial disorder.

648.9# Disorders maternal current (co-existent) in pregnancy

5th digit: 648.9

0. Episode of care NOS or N/A
1. Delivered
2. Delivered with postpartum complication
3. Antepartum complication
4. Postpartum complication

447.8 Disorders other NEC
447.8 Fibromuscular hyperplasia
447.3 Fibromuscular hyperplasia renal

ARTERY, ARTERIAL (continued)

996.62 Graft complication - infection or inflammation
996.1 Graft complication - mechanical
996.74 Graft complication - other
447.8 Hyperplasia fibromuscular
447.3 Hyperplasia fibromuscular renal
0 Injury traumatic see specified artery, injury
443.9 Insufficiency (peripheral)
447.5 Necrosis
444.9 Obstruction or occlusion NEC (embolism) (infarction) (thrombosis)
447.1 Occlusion due to stricture or stenosis
444.22 Occlusion lower extremities
0 Occlusion lower extremities without thrombus or embolus see 'Artery, Arterial', arteriosclerosis extremities
444.21 Occlusion upper extremities
0 Occlusion upper extremities without thrombus or embolus see 'Artery, Arterial', arteriosclerosis extremities
447.2 Rupture due to erosion (ulceration)
0 Spasm see 'Spasm', artery, specified site
744.04 Stapedia (persistent)
447.1 Stricture
442.0 Upper extremity (aneurysm) (A-V fistula) (cirsoid) (false) (varicose)
447.2 Wall abscess

719.4# ARTHRALGIA

5th digit: 719.4

0. Site NOS
1. Shoulder region
2. Upper arm (elbow) (humerus)
3. Forearm (radius) (wrist) (ulna)
4. Hand (carpal) (metacarpal) (fingers)
5. Pelvic region and thigh (hip) (buttock) (femur)
6. Lower leg (fibula) (knee) (patella) (tibia)
7. Ankle and/or foot (metatarsals) (toes) (tarsals)
8. Other
9. Multiple

ARTHRITIS

716.9# NOS
716.2# Allergic
714.0 Atrophic
720.9 Atrophic spine
721.0 Cervical
716.3# Climacteric
098.50 Gonococcal
274.0 Gout
0 Hypertrophic see 'Osteoarthritis'

5th digit: 716.2-3, 9

0. Site NOS
1. Shoulder region
2. Upper arm (elbow) (humerus)
3. Forearm (radius) (wrist) (ulna)
4. Hand (carpal) (metacarpal) (fingers)
5. Pelvic region and thigh (hip) (buttock) (femur)
6. Lower leg (fibula) (knee) (patella) (tibia)
7. Ankle and/or foot (metatarsals) (toes) (tarsals)
8. Other (head) (neck) (rib) (skull) (trunk) (vertebrae)
9. Multiple

A

ARTHRITIS (continued)

711.9#	Infective
714.9	Inflammatory
721.3	Lumbar
721.3	Lumbosacral
716.3#	Menopausal
716.6#	Monoarticular
0	Nodosa see 'Arthritis Osteoarthritis'
721.3	Sacral
721.3	Sacrococcygeal
721.3	Sacroiliac
721.90	Spine NOS
721.2	Thoracic
716.4#	Transient
716.1#	Traumatic
716.8#	Other specified

5th digit: 711.9, 716.1-4, 6, 8
- **0. Site NOS**
- **1. Shoulder region**
- **2. Upper arm (elbow) (humerus)**
- **3. Forearm (radius) (wrist) (ulna)**
- **4. Hand (carpal) (metacarpal) (fingers)**
- **5. Pelvic region and thigh (hip) (buttock) (femur)**
- **6. Lower leg (fibula) (knee) (patella) (tibia)**
- **7. Ankle and/or foot (metatarsals) (toes) (tarsals)**
- **8. Other (head) (neck) (rib) (skull) (trunk) (vertebrae)**
- **9. Multiple**

Osteoarthritis, sometimes referred to as degenerative joint disease, is the most common type of arthritis. Classification is usually coded to localized (primary or secondary), or generalized.

ARTHRITIS OSTEOARTHRITIS (DEGENERATIVE)

715.9#	NOS
715.9#	Degenerative joint disease
715.3#	Localized
715.1#	Localized primary (by joint)
715.2#	Localized secondary (by joint)

5th digit: 715.1-3, 9
- **0. Site unspecified**
- **1. Shoulder region**
- **2. Upper arm (elbow) (humerus)**
- **3. Forearm (radius) (wrist) (ulna)**
- **4. Hand (carpal) (metacarpal) (fingers)**
- **5. Pelvic region and thigh (hip) (buttock) (femur)**
- **6. Lower leg (fibula) (knee) (patella) (tibia)**
- **7. Ankle and/or foot (metatarsals) (toes) (tarsals)**
- **8. Other specified except spine**

715.0# Generalized

5th digit: 715.0
- **0. Site unspecified**
- **4. Hand (carpal) (metacarpal) (fingers)**
- **9. Multiple**

715.8# Multiple sites (by joint) (not specified as generalized)

5th digit: 715.8
- **0. Site unspecified**
- **9. Multiple**

ARTHRITIS OSTEOARTHRITIS (DEGENERATIVE) OF SPINE: -WITH OSTEOPOROSIS [733.0#]

721.90	NOS
721.91	NOS with myelopathy (cord compression)
721.0	Cervical
721.1	Cervical with myelopathy (cord compression)
721.3	Lumbar
721.42	Lumbar with myelopathy (cord compression)
721.3	Lumbosacral
721.42	Lumbosacral with myelopathy (cord compression)
721.3	Sacral
721.42	Sacral with myelopathy (cord compression)
721.3	Sacrococcygeal
721.42	Sacrococcygeal with myelopathy (cord compression)
721.3	Sacroiliac
721.42	Sacroiliac with myelopathy (cord compression)
721.2	Thoracic
721.41	Thoracic with myelopathy (cord compression)
721.7	Traumatic

with osteoporosis [733.0#]

5th digit: 733.0
- **0. Unspecified**
- **1. Senile**
- **2. Idiopathic**
- **3. Disuse**
- **9. Drug induced**

ARTHRITIS RHEUMATOID

714.0	Adult
714.30	Juvenile chronic or unspecified
714.33	Juvenile monoarticular
714.32	Juvenile pauciarticular
714.31	Juvenile polyarticular acute
720.0	Spine
714.0	With myopathy [359.6]
714.0	With polyneuropathy [357.1]
714.2	With visceral or systemic involvement

ARTHRITIS OTHER SPECIFIED

253.0	Acromegalic [713.0]
039.8	Actinomycotic **[711.4#]**
117.6	Allescheriosis **[711.6#]**
277.39	Amyloid [713.7]
088.9	Arthropod borne disease **[711.8#]**
088.89	Arthropod borne disease other **[711.8#]**
117.3	Aspergilla **[711.6#]**
0	Bacterial see 'Arthritis' pyogenic
088.0	Bartonella **[711.8#]**
136.1	Behcet's syndrome **[711.2#]**

5th digit: 711.2, 4, 6, 8
- **0. Site NOS**
- **1. Shoulder region**
- **2. Upper arm (elbow) (humerus)**
- **3. Forearm (radius) (wrist) (ulna)**
- **4. Hand (carpal) (metacarpal) (fingers)**
- **5. Pelvic region and thigh (hip) (buttock) (femur)**
- **6. Lower leg (fibula) (knee) (patella) (tibia)**
- **7. Ankle and/or foot (metatarsals) (toes) (tarsals)**
- **8. Other (head) (neck) (rib) (skull) (trunk) (vertebrae)**
- **9. Multiple**

ARTHRITIS OTHER SPECIFIED (continued)

116.# Blastomycotic [711.6#]
4th digit: 116
0. Blastomycosis
1. Paracoccidioidomycosis
2. Lobomycosis

5th digit: 711.6
0. Site NOS
1. Shoulder region
2. Upper arm (elbow) (humerus)
3. Forearm (radius) (wrist) (ulna)
4. Hand (carpal) (metacarpal) (fingers)
5. Pelvic region and thigh (hip) (buttock) (femur)
6. Lower leg (fibula) (knee) (patella) (tibia)
7. Ankle and/or foot (metatarsals) (toes) (tarsals)
8. Other (head) (neck) (rib) (skull) (trunk) (vertebrae)
9. Multiple

081.1 Brill's disease [711.8#]
112.89 Candidal [711.6#]
133.8 Chiggers (due to) [711.8#]
134.1 Chigoe (sandflea) [711.8#]
117.2 Chromoblastomycotic [711.6#]
114.3 Coccidioidomycotic [711.6#]
5th digit: 711.6, 8
0. Site NOS
1. Shoulder region
2. Upper arm (elbow) (humerus)
3. Forearm (radius) (wrist) (ulna)
4. Hand (carpal) (metacarpal) (fingers)
5. Pelvic region and thigh (hip) (buttock) (femur)
6. Lower leg (fibula) (knee) (patella) (tibia)
7. Ankle and/or foot (metatarsals) (toes) (tarsals)
8. Other (head) (neck) (rib) (skull) (trunk) (vertebrae)
9. Multiple

The code in the left margin always sequences first. The additional code in brackets to the right of the description is sequenced second. Underlining shows the code number that corresponds to the underlined description. Underlining never implies correct sequencing.

094.0 Charcot's [713.5]
0 Chondrocalcinosis see 'Chondrocalcinosis'
556.# Colitis ulcerative (due to) [713.1]
4th digit: 556
0. Enterocolitis (chronic)
1. Ileocolitis (chronic)
2. Proctitis (chronic)
3. Proctosigmoiditis (chronic)
4. Pseudopolyposis of colon
5. Left-sided (chronic)
6. Universal (chronic)
8. Other ulcerative colitis
9. Ulcerative colitis (enteritis) unspecified

478.79 Cricoarytenoid cartilage

ARTHRITIS OTHER SPECIFIED (continued)

555.# Crohn's (due to Crohn's disease) [713.1]
5th digit: 555
0. Small intestine
1. Large intestine
2. Small intestine with large intestine
9. Unspecified site

117.5 Cryptococcal [711.6#]
275.49 Crystal induced - unspecified [712.9#]
0 Crystal induced - chondrocalcinosis see 'Chondrocalcinosis'
274.0 Crystal induced - gouty
275.49 Crystal induced - other specified [712.8#]
110.8 Dermatophytosis [711.6#]
079.83 Due to or associated with human parvovirus [711.5#]
079.83 Due to or associated with parvovirus B19 [711.5#]
5th digit: 711.5-6, 712.8-9
0. Site NOS
1. Shoulder region
2. Upper arm (elbow) (humerus)
3. Forearm (radius) (wrist) (ulna)
4. Hand (carpal) (metacarpal) (fingers)
5. Pelvic region and thigh (hip) (buttock) (femur)
6. Lower leg (fibula) (knee) (patella) (tibia)
7. Ankle and/or foot (metatarsals) (toes) (tarsals)
8. Other (head) (neck) (rib) (skull) (trunk) (vertebrae)
9. Multiple

279.0# Due to hypogammaglobulinemia [713.0]
5th digit: 279.0
0. Unspecified
1. Selective IGA
2. Selective IGM
3. Selective IGG
5. Increased IGM
6. Variable
9. Other

0 Dysenteric see 'Arthritis', postdysenteric
082.4# Ehrlichiosis [711.8#]
5th digit: 082.4
0. NOS
1. E. Chaffeensis
9. Other

5th digit: 711.8
0. Site NOS
1. Shoulder region
2. Upper arm (elbow) (humerus)
3. Forearm (radius) (wrist) (ulna)
4. Hand (carpal) (metacarpal) (fingers)
5. Pelvic region and thigh (hip) (buttock) (femur)
6. Lower leg (fibula) (knee) (patella) (tibia)
7. Ankle and/or foot (metatarsals) (toes) (tarsals)
8. Other (head) (neck) (rib) (skull) (trunk) (vertebrae)
9. Multiple

555.# Enteritis (due to Enteritis) [713.1]
4th digit: 555
0. Small intestine
1. Large intestine
2. Small intestine with large intestine
9. Unspecified site

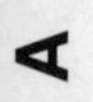

ARTHRITIS OTHER SPECIFIED (continued)

695.1 Erythema multiforme (due to) [713.3]
695.2 Erythema nodosum (due to) [713.3]
125.# Filarial **[711.7#]**
711.7# Helminthiasis
4th digit: 125
0. Bancroftian
1. Malayan
2. Loiasis
3. Onchocerciasis
4. Dipetalonemiasis
5. Mansonella ozzardi infection
6. Other specified
7. Dracontiasis
9. Unspecified

5th digit: 711.7
0. Site NOS
1. Shoulder region
2. Upper arm (elbow) (humerus)
3. Forearm (radius) (wrist) (ulna)
4. Hand (carpal) (metacarpal) (fingers)
5. Pelvic region and thigh (hip) (buttock) (femur)
6. Lower leg (fibula) (knee) (patella) (tibia)
7. Ankle and/or foot (metatarsals) (toes) (tarsals)
8. Other (head) (neck) (rib) (skull) (trunk) (vertebrae)
9. Multiple

282.49 Hemoglobinopathy (due to) [713.2]
275.0 Hemochromatosis (due to) [713.0]
286.0 Hemophilia VIII [713.2]
286.1 Hemophilia IX [713.2]
286.0 Hemophiliac [713.2]
287.0 Henoch Schonlein purpura (due to) [713.6]
134.2 Hirudiniasis **[711.8#]**
115.9# Histoplasmosis **[711.6#]**
5th digit: 115.9
0. Capsulatum
1. Duboisii
9. Unspecified

5th digit: 711.6, 8
0. Site NOS
1. Shoulder region
2. Upper arm (elbow) (humerus)
3. Forearm (radius) (wrist) (ulna)
4. Hand (carpal) (metacarpal) (fingers)
5. Pelvic region and thigh (hip) (buttock) (femur)
6. Lower leg (fibula) (knee) (patella) (tibia)
7. Ankle and/or foot (metatarsals) (toes) (tarsals)
8. Other (head) (neck) (rib) (skull) (trunk) (vertebrae)
9. Multiple

ARTHRITIS OTHER SPECIFIED (continued)

252.0# Hyperparathyroid [713.0]
5th digit: 252.0
0. NOS
1. Primary
2. Secondary non-renal
8. Other specified

244.# Hypothyroid acquired [713.0]
4th digit: 244
0. Postsurgical
1. Postablative (irradiation)
2. Iodine ingestion
3. PAS, phenylbut, resorcinol
8. Secondary NEC
9. NOS

243 Hypothyroid congenital (due to) [713.0]
085.9 Leishmaniasis **[711.8#]**
030.# Lepromatous **[711.4#]**
4th digit: 030
0. Type L
1. Type T
2. Group I
3. Group B
8. Other specified leprosy
9. NOS

5th digit: 711.4, 8
0. Site NOS
1. Shoulder region
2. Upper arm (elbow) (humerus)
3. Forearm (radius) (wrist) (ulna)
4. Hand (carpal) (metacarpal) (fingers)
5. Pelvic region and thigh (hip) (buttock) (femur)
6. Lower leg (fibula) (knee) (patella) (tibia)
7. Ankle and/or foot (metatarsals) (toes) (tarsals)
8. Other (head) (neck) (rib) (skull) (trunk) (vertebrae)
9. Multiple

100.# Leptospirosis **[711.8#]**
4th digit: 100
0. Icterohemorrhagica
9. Leptospirosis NOS

272.0 Lipoid disorder (due to) [713.0]
088.81 Lyme disease **[711.8#]**
117.4 Madura **[711.6#]**
084.9 Malarial **[711.8#]**
5th digit: 711.6, 8
0. Site NOS
1. Shoulder region
2. Upper arm (elbow) (humerus)
3. Forearm (radius) (wrist) (ulna)
4. Hand (carpal) (metacarpal) (fingers)
5. Pelvic region and thigh (hip) (buttock) (femur)
6. Lower leg (fibula) (knee) (patella) (tibia)
7. Ankle and/or foot (metatarsals) (toes) (tarsals)
8. Other (head) (neck) (rib) (skull) (trunk) (vertebrae)
9. Multiple

ARTHRITIS OTHER SPECIFIED (continued)

The code in the left margin always sequences first. The additional code in brackets to the right of the description is sequenced second. Underlining shows the code number that corresponds to the underlined description. Underlining never implies correct sequencing.

202.3# Malignant reticulosis (due to) [713.2]
5th digit: 202.3
0. NOS
1. Lymph nodes of head face neck
2. Lymph nodes intrathoracic
3. Lymph nodes abdominal
4. Lymph nodes axilla and upper limb
5. Lymph nodes inguinal region and lower limb
6. Lymph nodes intrapelvic
7. Spleen
8. Lymph nodes multiple sites

Code the specific maternal arthritis in addition to 648.7#. See 'Arthritis'.

648.7# Maternal current (co-existent) in pregnancy
5th digit: 648.7
0. Episode of care NOS or N/A
1. Delivered
2. Delivered with postpartum complication
3. Antepartum complication
4. Postpartum complication

277.31 Mediterranean Fever (due to) [713.7]
036.82 Meningococcal
133.9 Mites (due to) **[711.8#]**
117.7 Mucormycotic **[711.6#]**
203.0 Multiple myeloma (due to) [713.2]
110.8 Mycotic (epiderma) (actina) (nocardia) **[711.6#]**
118 Mycotic (opportunistic) **[711.6#]**
711.8# Myiasis [134.0]
094.0 Neuropathic joint disease [713.5]
711.4# Other bacterial
711.8# Parasitic or infectious
5th digit: 711.4, 6, 8
0. Site NOS
1. Shoulder region
2. Upper arm (elbow) (humerus)
3. Forearm (radius) (wrist) (ulna)
4. Hand (carpal) (metacarpal) (fingers)
5. Pelvic region and thigh (hip) (buttock) (femur)
6. Lower leg (fibula) (knee) (patella) (tibia)
7. Ankle and/or foot (metatarsals) (toes) (tarsals)
8. Other (head) (neck) (rib) (skull) (trunk) (vertebrae)
9. Multiple

ARTHRITIS OTHER SPECIFIED (continued)

132.9 Pediculosis **[711.8#]**
117.8 Phaehyphomycosis **[711.6#]**
103.9 Pinta **[711.8#]**
714.89 Poly (other specified)
009.0 Postdysenteric **[711.3#]**
714.4 Postrheumatic chronic
696.0 Psoriatic
5th digit: 711.3, 6, 8
0. Site NOS
1. Shoulder region
2. Upper arm (elbow) (humerus)
3. Forearm (radius) (wrist) (ulna)
4. Hand (carpal) (metacarpal) (fingers)
5. Pelvic region and thigh (hip) (buttock) (femur)
6. Lower leg (fibula) (knee) (patella) (tibia)
7. Ankle and/or foot (metatarsals) (toes) (tarsals)
8. Other (head) (neck) (rib) (skull) (trunk) (vertebrae)
9. Multiple

0 Pyogenic see 'Arthritis Other Specified,' septic pyogenic
083.0 Q fever **[711.8#]**
099.3 Reiter's disease **[711.1#]**
087.0 Relapsing fever **[711.8#]**
519.9 Respiratory disorder related [713.4]
390 Rheumatic acute
117.0 Rhinosporidiosis **[711.6#]**
082.8 Rickettsial lone star fever **[711.8#]**
083.8 Rickettsial other specified **[711.8#]**
083.2 Rickettsialpox **[711.8#]**
083.9 Rickettsiosis **[711.8#]**
082.0 Rocky mountain spotted fever **[711.8#]**
5th digit: 711.1, 6, 8
0. Site NOS
1. Shoulder region
2. Upper arm (elbow) (humerus)
3. Forearm (radius) (wrist) (ulna)
4. Hand (carpal) (metacarpal) (fingers)
5. Pelvic region and thigh (hip) (buttock) (femur)
6. Lower leg (fibula) (knee) (patella) (tibia)
7. Ankle and/or foot (metatarsals) (toes) (tarsals)
8. Other (head) (neck) (rib) (skull) (trunk) (vertebrae)
9. Multiple

056.71 Rubella
003.23 Salmonella

The code in the left margin always sequences first. The additional code in brackets to the right of the description is sequenced second. Underlining shows the code number that corresponds to the underlined description. Underlining never implies correct sequencing.

135 Sarcoid [713.7]

A

ARTHRITIS OTHER SPECIFIED (continued)

133.0 Scabies **[711.8#]**

711.0# Septic-pyogenic **[041.#(#)]**

4th or 4th and 5th digit code for organism: 041

- **.85 Aerobacter aerogenes**
- **.84 Anaerobes other**
- **.82 Bacteroides fragilis**
- **.83 Clostridium perfringens**
- **.4 E. coli (escherichia coli)**
- **.81 Eaton's agent**
- **.85 Enterobacter sakazakii**
- **.04 Enterococcus**
- **.3 Friedlander's bacillus**
- **.84 Gram-negative anaerobes**
- **.85 Gram-negative bacteria NOS**
- **.5 H. influenzae**
- **.86 H. pylori (helicobacter pylori)**
- **.3 Klebsiella**
- **.85 Mima polymorpha**
- **.81 Mycoplasma**
- **.81 Pleuropneumonia like organisms**
- **.2 Pneumococcus**
- **.6 Proteus (mirabilis) (morganii) (vulgaris)**
- **.7 Pseudomonas**
- **.85 Serratia (marcescens)**
- **.10 Staphylococcus unspecified**
- **.11 Staphylococcus aureus**
- **.19 Staphylococcus other**
- **.00 Streptococcus**
- **.01 Streptococcus group A**
- **.02 Streptococcus group B**
- **.03 Streptococcus group C**
- **.04 Streptococcus group D**
- **.05 Streptococcus group G**
- **.09 Streptococcus other**
- **.89 Other specified bacteria**

999.5 Serum sickness [713.6]
282.60 Sickle cell disease (anemia) [713.2]
282.5 Sickle cell trait arthritis [713.2]
134.9 Skin parasites **[711.8#]**
104.9 Spirochetal **[711.8#]**
104.0 Spirochetal (bejel) njoverna **[711.8#]**
104.8 Spirochetal other specified **[711.8#]**
117.1 Sporotrichosis **[711.6#]**

5th digit: 711.0, 6, 8

- **0. Site NOS**
- **1. Shoulder region**
- **2. Upper arm (elbow) (humerus)**
- **3. Forearm (radius) (wrist) (ulna)**
- **4. Hand (carpal) (metacarpal) (fingers)**
- **5. Pelvic region and thigh (hip) (buttock) (femur)**
- **6. Lower leg (fibula) (knee) (patella) (tibia)**
- **7. Ankle and/or foot (metatarsals) (toes) (tarsals)**
- **8. Other (head) (neck) (rib) (skull) (trunk) (vertebrae)**
- **9. Multiple**

094.0 Syphilitic (tabes dorsalis) [713.5]
336.0 Syringomyelic [713.5]
282.49 Thalassemia [713.2]

ARTHRITIS OTHER SPECIFIED (continued)

111.0 Tinea (dermatomycotic) **[711.6#]**
130.7 Toxoplasmosis **[711.8#]**
716.4# Transient
719.3# Transient palindromic
083.1 Trench mouth (quintan wolhynian) fever **[711.8#]**
131.8 Trichomonal **[711.8#]**
086.9 Trypanosoma **[711.8#]**

5th digit: 711.6, 8, 716.4, 719.3

- **0. Site NOS**
- **1. Shoulder region**
- **2. Upper arm (elbow) (humerus)**
- **3. Forearm (radius) (wrist) (ulna)**
- **4. Hand (carpal) (metacarpal) (fingers)**
- **5. Pelvic region and thigh (hip) (buttock) (femur)**
- **6. Lower leg (fibula) (knee) (patella) (tibia)**
- **7. Ankle and/or foot (metatarsals) (toes) (tarsals)**
- **8. Other**
- **9. Multiple**

015.0# Tuberculous **[711.4#]**

5th digit: 015.0

- **0. NOS**
- **1. Lab not done**
- **2. Lab pending**
- **3. Microscopy positive (in sputum)**
- **4. Culture positive - microscopy negative**
- **5. Culture negative - microscopy positive**
- **6. Culture and microscopy negative confirmed by other methods**

002.0 Typhoid **[711.3#]**
081.9 Typhus **[711.8#]**
082.1 Typhus boutonneuse (African) (Indian) (Mediterranean) **[711.8#]**
080 Typhus louse borne (epidemic) **[711.8#]**
081.0 Typhus murine **[711.8#]**
082.3 Typhus Queensland tick **[711.8#]**
081.2 Typhus scrub **[711.8#]**
082.2 Typhus Siberian **[711.8#]**
082.9 Typhus tick borne unspecified **[711.8#]**

5th digit: 711.3, 4, 8

- **0. Site NOS**
- **1. Shoulder region**
- **2. Upper arm (elbow) (humerus)**
- **3. Forearm (radius) (wrist) (ulna)**
- **4. Hand (carpal) (metacarpal) (fingers)**
- **5. Pelvic region and thigh (hip) (femur)**
- **6. Lower leg (fibula) (knee) (patella) (tibia)**
- **7. Ankle and/or foot (metatarsals) (toes) (tarsals)**
- **8. Other (head) (neck) (rib) (skull) (trunk) (vertebrae)**
- **9. Multiple**

A

ARTHRITIS OTHER SPECIFIED (continued)

556.# Ulcerative colitis (due to) [713.1]
4th digit: 556
0. Enterocolitis (chronic)
1. Ileocolitis (chronic)
2. Proctitis (chronic)
3. Proctosigmoiditis (chronic)
4. Pseudopolyposis of colon
5. Left-sided (chronic)
6. Universal (chronic)
8. Other ulcerative colitis
9. Ulcerative colitis (enteritis) unspecified

101 Vincent's angina **[711.8#]**
079.99 Viral NEC **[711.5#]**
056.71 Viral (rubella)
102.0 Yaws **[711.8#]**
716.8# Other specified
5th digit: 711.5, 8, 716.8
0. Site NOS
1. Shoulder region
2. Upper arm (elbow) (humerus)
3. Forearm (radius) (wrist) (ulna)
4. Hand (carpal) (metacarpal) (fingers)
5. Pelvic region and thigh (hip) (buttock) (femur)
6. Lower leg (fibula) (knee) (patella) (tibia)
7. Ankle and/or foot (metatarsals) (toes) (tarsals)
8. Other (head) (neck) (rib) (skull) (trunk) (vertebrae)
9. Multiple

V45.4 ARTHRODESIS STATUS
0 ARTHROFIBROSIS SEE 'ANKYLOSIS'
728.3 ARTHROGRYPOSIS
754.89 ARTHROGRYPOSIS MULTIPLEX CONGENITA
0 ARTHROPATHY SEE 'ARTHRITIS'
0 ARTHROPATHY SEPTIC SEE 'ARTHRITIS OTHER SPECIFIED' PYOGENIC
088.9 ARTHROPOD BORNE DISEASE
088.89 ARTHROPOD BORNE DISEASES OTHER SPECIFIED
134.1 ARTHROPOD INFESTATION
V64.43 ARTHROSCOPIC SURGICAL PROCEDURE CONVERTED TO OPEN PROCEDURE
995.21 ARTHUS PHENOMENON (REACTION) DUE TO DRUG, MEDICINAL OR BIOLOGICAL SUBSTANCE

ARTICULAR

718.0# Cartilage derangement
5th digit: 718.0
0. Site NOS
1. Shoulder region
2. Upper arm (elbow) (humerus)
3. Forearm (radius) (wrist) (ulna)
4. Hand (carpal) (metacarpal) (fingers)
5. Pelvic region and thigh (hip) (buttock) (femur)
7. Ankle and or foot (metatarsals) (toes) (tarsals)
8. Other specified sites
9. Multiple

717.9 Cartilage derangement knee
270.2 Cartilage disorder in ochronosis
524.63 Disc disorder (reducing or non reducing)

524.27 ARTICULATION DENTAL ARCH (ANTERIOR) (POSTERIOR) (REVERSE)
315.39 ARTICULATION DISORDER SPEECH DEVELOPMENTAL
V26.1 ARTIFICIAL INSEMINATION
V55.9 ARTIFICIAL OPENING UNSPECIFIED - CARE (CLOSURE) (TOILET) (ATTENTION)
V44.9 ARTIFICIAL OPENING UNSPECIFIED - STATUS
V55.8 ARTIFICIAL OPENING OTHER SPECIFIED - CARE (CLOSURE) (TOILET) (ATTENTION)
V44.8 ARTIFICIAL OPENING OTHER SPECIFIED - STATUS
V15.84 ASBESTOS EXPOSURE HISTORY
501 ASBESTOSIS
501 ASBESTOSIS LUNG (OCCUPATIONAL)
757.33 ASBOE-HANSEN'S DISEASE (INCONTINENTIA PIGMENTI)
127.0 ASCARIASIS
127.0 ASCARIDIASIS
127.0 ASCARIS LUMBRICOIDES INFECTION

ASCITES

789.59 NOS
789.59 Abdominal NOS
789.51 Cancerous (malignant) M8000/6
457.8 Chylous
125.9 Chylous - filarial
778.0 Congenital
653.7# Fetal causing fetopelvic disproportion
660.1# Fetal causing fetopelvic disproportion obstructing labor [653.7#]
5th digit: 653.7, 660.1
0. Episode of care unspecified or N/A
1. Delivered
3. Antepartum complication

719.0# Joint
719.3# Joint intermittent
5th digit: 719.0, 3
0. Site unspecified
1. Shoulder region
2. Upper arm (elbow) (humerus)
3. Forearm (radius) (wrist) (ulna)
4. Hand (carpal) (metacarpal) (fingers)
5. Pelvis thigh (hip) (buttock) (femur)
6. Lower leg (fibula) (knee) (patella) (tibia)
7. Ankle and/or foot (metatarsals) (toes) (tarsals)
8. Other
9. Multiple

789.51 Malignant
183.0 Malignant due to cancer of the ovary [789.51]
197.6 Malignant due to cancer of the retropertoneum and peritoneum [789.51]
789.59 Pseudochylous
095.2 Syphilitic
014.0# Tuberculous
5th digit: 014.0
0. NOS
1. Lab not pending
2. Lab pending
3. Microscopy positive (in sputum)
4. Culture positive - microscopy negative
5. Culture negative - microscopy positive
6. Culture and microscopy negative confirmed by other methods

A

117.4 ASCOMYCETES INFECTION
267 ASCORBIC ACID DEFICIENCY
795.02 ASC-H, CERVIX (ATYPICAL SQUAMOUS CELLS CANNOT EXCLUDE HIGH GRADE SQUAMOUS INTRAEPITHELIAL LESION)
795.01 ASC-US, CERVIX (ATYPICAL SQUAMOUS CELLS OF UNDETERMINED SIGNIFICANCE)
429.2 ASCVD (NONHYPERTENSIVE) WITH ARTERIOSCLEROSIS [440.9]
0 ASD (ATRIAL SEPTAL DEFECT) SEE 'ATRIAL', SEPTAL DEFECT
047.9 ASEPTIC MENINGITIS SYNDROME

ASEPTIC NECROSIS

733.40 Bone site unspecified
733.42 Femur (head and neck of)
733.49 Hand
733.42 Hip
733.41 Humerus (head)
733.45 Jaw
733.43 Medial femoral condyle
733.44 Talus
733.49 Other bone

414.0# ASHD (ARTERIOSCLEROTIC HEART DISEASE)
414.0# ASHD (ARTERIOSCLEROTIC HEART DISEASE) WITH CHRONIC COMPLETE OR TOTAL OCCLUSION [414.2]
5th digit: 414.0
0. Unspecified type of vessel, native or graft
1. Native coronary vessel
2. Autologous vein bypass graft
3. Nonautologous biological bypass graft
4. Autologous artery bypass graft (gastroepiploic) (internal mammary)
5. Unspecified type of bypass graft
6. Native vessel of transplanted heart
7. Bypass graft of transplanted heart

621.5 ASHERMAN'S SYNDROME
781.8 ASOMATOGNOSIA
299.8# ASPERGER'S DISORDER (SYNDROME)
5th digit: 299.8
0. Current or active state
1. Residual state
117.3 ASPERGILLOSIS
518.6 ASPERGILLOSIS ALLERGIC BRONCHOPULMONARY
117.3 ASPERGILLOSIS WITH EXTERNAL OTITIS [380.15]
300.00 ASPHYCTIC SYNDROME

The codes for fetal or newborn asphyxia cannot stand alone. Code the underlying cause of the asphyxia in addition to the 768.#. Sequence the asphyxia first, with the underlying cause second.

ASPHYXIA, ASPHYXIATION

799.01 NOS

BIRTH

768.9 Unspecified
768.6 Mild
768.6 Moderate
768.5 Severe
768.5 Severe with neurologic involvement

ASPHYXIA, ASPHYXIATION (continued)

768.9 Fetal affecting newborn

FOOD, MUCUS OR FOREIGN BODY INHALATION

933.1 NOS
934.8 Bronchioles
934.1 Bronchus main
933.1 Inhalation food choking, regurgitated, larynx
934.9 Inhalation liquid, lower respiratory tract
933.1 Inhalation phlegm choking, larynx
934.9 Inhalation vomitus, lower respiratory tract
933.1 Larynx
934.8 Lung
932 Nasal passages
933.0 Nasopharynx

For code 770.18, use an additional code to identify any secondary pulmonary hypertension (416.8), if applicable.

770.18 Newborn
933.0 Pharynx
934.9 Respiratory tract NOS
934.8 Respiratory tract other specified part
0 Suffocation see 'Suffocation'
933.0 Throat NOS
934.0 Trachea
770.18 Vaginal (fetus or newborn)

GASES, FUMES, OR VAPORS

987.9 Unspecified gas, fume, or vapor
987.5 Bromobenzyl cyanide
987.0 Butane
986 Carbon monoxide
987.6 Chlorine gas
987.5 Chloroacetophenone
987.4 Dichloromonofluoromethane
987.5 Ethyliodoacetate
987.4 Freon
987.7 Hydrocyanic acid gas
987.5 Lacrimogenic gas
987.2 Nitrogen dioxide
987.2 Nitrogen oxides
987.2 Nitrous fumes
987.8 Phosgene
987.8 Polyester fumes
987.0 Propane
0 Suffocation see 'Suffocation'
987.3 Sulfur dioxide
987.0 Other hydrocarbon gas
987.8 Other specified gas, fume or vapor

INTRAUTERINE

768.4 Live outcome - NOS onset
768.2 Live outcome - onset before labor
768.3 Live outcome - onset during labor and delivery
768.0 With fetal death - before onset of labor
768.1 With fetal death - during labor

MECHANICAL

994.7 NOS
0 During birth see 'Fetal Distress'
909.4 Late effect

ASPHYXIA, ASPHYXIATION (continued)

799.01 Pathological

ASPIRATION

997.3 Acid pulmonary (syndrome) (due to a procedure)
668.0# Acid pulmonary (syndrome) obstetrical
5th digit: 668.0
0. Episode of care NOS or N/A
1. Delivered
2. Delivered with postpartum complication
3. Antepartum complication
4. Postpartum complication

> ***For codes 770.12, 770.14, 770.16, 770.18, 770.86, use an additional code to identify any secondary pulmonary hypertension (416.8), if applicable.***

770.13 Amniotic fluid clear
770.14 Amniotic fluid clear with respiratory symptoms
770.17 Birth canal contents
770.18 Birth canal contents with respiratory symptoms
507.0 Bronchitis
770.10 Fetus or newborn
770.18 Fetus or newborn with respiratory symptoms
770.15 Fetus or newborn blood
770.16 Fetus or newborn blood with respiratory symptoms
0 Food, foreign body, or gasoline with asphyxiation see 'Asphyxiation Food, Mucus, or Foreign Body Inhalation'
770.11 Meconium (below vocal cords)
770.12 Meconium (below vocal cords) with respiratory symptoms

MUCUS

933.1 NOS
934.9 Into lower respiratory tract NOS
934.8 Into bronchioles
934.1 Into bronchus main
934.8 Into lung
934.0 Into trachea
934.8 Into other specified parts
770.17 Newborn
770.17 Vaginal (fetus or newborn)

PNEUMONIA / PNEUMONITIS

507.0 NOS
770.18 Fetal or newborn
770.16 Fetal or newborn with blood
770.14 Fetal or newborn with clear amniotic fluid
770.12 Fetal or newborn with meconium
770.12 Fetal or newborn with postnatal contents
507.0 Food regurgitated
506.0 Fumes or vapors (chemical) (acute)
507.0 Gastric secretions
516.8 Lipoid endogenous
507.1 Lipoid exogenous

> ***668.0#: When coding a maternal aspiration pneumonia/pneumonitis, use an additional code to show the type of aspiration.***

668.0# Obstetrical maternal
5th digit: 668.0
0. Episode of care NOS or N/A
1. Delivered
2. Delivered with postpartum complication
3. Antepartum complication
4. Postpartum complication

ASPIRATION (continued)

PNEUMONIA / PNEUMONITIS (continued)

507.1 Oils or essences
997.3 Postoperative
507.0 Vomitus
507.8 Other solids or liquids

ASPIRATION (continued)

770.85 Postnatal stomach contents
770.86 Postnatal stomach contents with respiratory symptoms
668.0# Pulmonary obstetrical (following anesthesia or other sedation in L&D)
5th digit: 668.0
0. Episode of care NOS or N/A
1. Delivered
2. Delivered with postpartum complication
3. Antepartum complication
4. Postpartum complication

997.3 Resulting from a procedure
770.18 Syndrome massive (of infant during birth)
770.12 Syndrome massive meconium (of infant during birth)
770.17 Vernix caseosa

V46.0 ASPIRATOR DEPENDENCE

V67.51 ASPIRIN DRUG FOLLOW UP EXAM - COMPLETED THERAPY

V58.66 ASPIRIN DRUG FOLLOW UP EXAM - CURRENT THERAPY

V58.83 ASPIRIN DRUG MONITORING ENCOUNTER

V58.83 ASPIRIN DRUG MONITORING ENCOUNTER WITH LONG TERM USE [V58.66]

307.9 ASTASIA

781.3 ASTASIA ATACTICA (CHOREIC) (PAROSXYSMAL TREPIDENT) (SPASTIC) (TREMBLING) (TREPIDAN)

300.11 ASTASIA HYSTERICAL

706.8 ASTEATOSIS (CUTIS)

780.99 ASTEREOGNOSIS

781.3 ASTERIXIS

379.22 ASTEROID HYALITIS

780.79 ASTHENIA

306.2 ASTHENIA NEUROCIRCULATORY

300.5 ASTHENIA PSYCHOGENIC

301.6 ASTHENIC PERSONALITY DISORDER

368.13 ASTHENOPIA

> ***Your choice of a fourth or fifth digit may significantly alter the meaning of your diagnosis. Note with asthma that the fourth digit clearly defines the type of asthma from unspecified to chronic obstructive with COPD. The fifth digit indicates with or without status, or with acute exacerbation.***

ASTHMA, ASTHMATIC

493.9# NOS
493.9# Allergic
493.0# Allergic rhinitis
493.0# Allergic with stated cause
493.0# Atopic
5th digit: 493.0, 9
0. NOS
1. With status asthmaticus
2. With (acute) exacerbation

ASTHMA, ASTHMATIC (continued)

493.90 Bronchitis
493.2# Bronchitis chronic
493.9# Bronchospasm
493.81 Bronchospasm exercise induced
493.0# Childhood
493.2# Chronic bronchitic
493.2# Chronic obstructive
493.2# Chronic obstructive with COPD
493.82 Cough variant
507.8 Detergent
518.3 Eosinophilia
493.81 Exercise induced bronchospasm
493.0# Extrinsic
V17.5 Family history
493.0# Hay
493.1# Infective
493.1# Intrinsic
493.1# Late-onset
500 Miners'
493.0# New Orleans (epidemic)
316 Psychogenic [493.9#]
5th digit: 493.0-2, 9
0. NOS
1. With status asthmaticus
2. With (acute) exacerbation

V71.89 Screening for suspected asthma
495.8 Wood
493.8# Other specified
5th digit: 493.8
1. Exercised induced bronchospasm
2. Cough variant

ASTIGMATISM

367.20 NOS
367.22 Irregular
367.21 Regular

755.67 ASTRAGALOSCAPHOID SYNOSTOSIS
191.9 ASTROBLASTOMA SITE NOS
0 ASTROBLASTOMA SITE SPECIFIED SEE 'CANCER', BY SITE M9430/3

Carcinomas and neoplasms should be coded by site if possible. Code by cell type, "site NOS", only if a site is not specified in the diagnosis. Otherwise, refer to the appropriate category of neoplasm for a more specific code. See 'Cancer' 'Cancer Metastatic', 'Carcinoma In Situ', 'Neoplasm Uncertain Behavior', 'Neoplasm Unspecified Nature', or 'Benign Neoplasm'.

ASTROCYTOMA

191.9 Site NOS
0 Site specified see 'Cancer', by site M9400/3
191.9 Anaplastic type site NOS
0 Anaplastic type site specified see 'Cancer', by site M9401/3
191.9 Fibrillary site NOS
0 Fibrillary site specified see 'Cancer', by site M9420/3
191.9 Gemistocytic site NOS
0 Gemistocytic site specified see 'Cancer', by site M9411/3
191.9 Pilocytic site NOS
0 Pilocytic site specified see 'Cancer', by site M9421/3

ASTROCYTOMA (continued)

191.9 Protoplasmic site NOS
0 Protoplasmic site specified see 'Cancer', by site M9410/3
237.5 Subependymal giant cell site NOS
0 Subependymal giant cell site specified see 'Neoplasm Uncertain Behavior', by site M9383/1

427.5 ASYSTOLE

ATAXIA, ATAXIC

781.3 NOS
303.## Alcoholic cerebellar [334.4]
4th digit: 303
0. Acute
9. Chronic

5th digit: 303
0. Unspecified
1. Continuous
2. Episodic
3. In remission

331.89 Brain
331.89 Brain with dementia [294.1#]
5th digit: 294.1
0. Without behavioral disturbance or NOS
1. With behavioral disturbance

334.3 Cerebellar
244.# Cerebellar hypothyroid [334.4]
334.2 Cerebellar Marie's (Sanger Brown) (myoclonica)
244.# Cerebellar myxedema [334.4]
4th digit: 244
0. Postsurgical
1. Postablative (irradiation)
2. Iodine ingestion
3. PAS, phenylbut, resorcinol
8. Secondary NEC
9. NOS

239.# Cerebellar neoplastic disease [334.4]
4th digit: 239
0. Digestive system, anal
1. Respiratory system
2. Bone, soft tissue, skin, (anal skin margin)
3. Breast
4. Bladder
5. Other genitourinary
6. Brain
7. Endocrine glands and other parts of nervous system
8. Other specified sites
9. Site unspecified

334.3 Cerebellar other
331.89 Cerebral
331.89 Cerebral with dementia [294.1#]
5th digit: 294.1
0. Without behavioral disturbance or NOS
1. With behavioral disturbance

A

ATAXIA, ATAXIC (continued)

250.6# Diabetic locomotor (progressive) [337.1]
5th digit: 250.6
0. Type II, adult-onset, non-insulin dependent (even if requiring insulin), or unspecified; controlled
1. Type I, juvenile-onset or insulin-dependent; controlled
2. Type II, adult-onset, non-insulin dependent (even if requiring insulin); uncontrolled
3. Type I, juvenile-onset or insulin-dependent; uncontrolled

334.0 Friedreich's
781.2 Gait
300.11 Hysterical
438.84 Late effect of cerebrovascular disease
094.0 Locomotor (progressive)
334.2 Marie's
094.0 Progressive locomotor
334.2 Sanger-Brown
334.0 Spinal hereditary
094.0 Spinal progressive locomotor
334.8 Telangiectasia syndrome (Louis Bar syndrome)

ATELECTASIS

518.0 NOS
770.5 Congenital partial
770.4 Congenital primary
770.5 Perinatal
997.3 Postoperative (symptomatic)
770.4 Primary perinatal
770.5 Secondary perinatal
011.8# Tuberculous
5th digit: 011.8
0. NOS
1. Lab not done
2. Lab pending
3. Microscopy positive (in sputum)
4. Culture positive - microscopy negative
5. Culture negative - microscopy positive
6. Culture and microscopy negative confirmed by other methods

742.59 ATELOMYELIA CONGENITAL

ATHEROEMBOLISM

445.02 Extremity lower (cholesterol) (microembolism)
445.01 Extremity upper (cholesterol) (microembolism)
445.81 Kidney (cholesterol) (microembolism)
445.81 Kidney (cholesterol) (microembolism) with renal failure acute [584.#]
4th digit: 584
5. With tubular necrosis
6. Renal cortical necrosis
7. Medullary (papillary) necrosis
8. Specified pathological lesion
9. Renal failure unspecified

445.81 Kidney (cholesterol) (microembolism) with kidney disease chronic [585.#]
4th digit: 585
1. Stage I
2. Stage II (mild)
3. Stage III (moderate)
4. Stage IV (severe)
5. Stage V
6. End stage
9. Unspecified stage

445.89 Other site (cholesterol) (microembolism)

437.0 ATHEROMA CEREBRAL ARTERIES
706.2 ATHEROMA SKIN

> ***Do not use code 996.03, complication of a device, implant or graft mechanical cardiac, when the physician documents that arteriosclerosis has caused an occlusion of a bypass graft. In coding terms, this is considered to be a normal progression of arteriosclerosis rather than a complication of a graft. Assign code 414.0#, arteriosclerosis of bypass graft, coronary.***

440.9 ATHEROSCLEROSIS NOS
440.3# ATHEROSCLEROSIS EXTREMITIES BYPASS GRAFT
440.3# ATHEROSCLEROSIS EXTREMITIES BYPASS GRAFT WITH CHRONIC COMPLETE OR TOTAL OCCLUSION [440.4]
5th digit: 440.3
0. Unspecified graft
1. Autologous vein bypass graft
2. Nonautologous biological bypass graft

440.2# ATHEROSCLEROSIS EXTREMITIES PERIPHERAL

440.2# ATHEROSCLEROSIS EXTREMITIES PERIPHERAL WITH CHRONIC COMPLETE OR TOTAL OCCLUSION [440.4]

5th digit: 440.2
- **0. Unspecified**
- **1. With intermittent claudication**
- **2. With rest pain or rest pain and intermittent claudication**
- **9. Other atherosclerosis extremities**

> *When coding atherosclerosis of the extremities use an additional code, if applicable to identify chronic complete or total occlusion of the artery of the extremities (440.4).*

440.24 ATHEROSCLEROSIS EXTREMITIES PERIPHERAL WITH ISCHEMIC GANGRENE OR ISCHEMIC GANGRENE AND ULCERATION, OR ULCERATION AND INTERMITTENT CLAUDICATION, REST PAIN [707.#(#)]

440.23 ATHEROSCLEROSIS EXTREMITIES PERIPHERAL WITH ULCERATION, OR ULCERATION AND INTERMITTENT CLAUDICATION, REST PAIN [707.#(#)]

4th or 4th and 5th digit: 707
- **1#. Lower limb except decubitus**
  - **10. Unspecified**
  - **11. Thigh**
  - **12. Calf**
  - **13. Ankle**
  - **14. Heel and midfoot**
  - **15. Other parts of foot, toes**
  - **19. Other**
- **8. Chronic of other specified site**
- **9. Chronic site NOS**

0 ATHEROSCLEROSIS RENAL ARTERIOLES SEE 'HYPERTENSIVE', RENAL DISEASE

0 ATHEROSCLEROSIS SEE 'ARTERIOSCLEROSIS, ARTERIOSCLEROTIC'

414.0# ATHEROSCLEROTIC HEART DISEASE

414.0# ATHEROSCLEROTIC HEART DISEASE WITH CHRONIC COMPLETE OR TOTAL OCCLUSION [414.2]

5th digit: 414.0
- **0. Unspecified type of vessel, native or graft**
- **1. Native coronary vessel**
- **2. Autologous vein bypass graft**
- **3. Nonautologous biological bypass graft**
- **4. Autologous artery bypass graft (gastroepiploic) (internal mammary)**
- **5. Unspecified type of bypass graft**
- **6. Native vessel of transplanted heart**
- **7. Bypass graft of transplanted heart**

781.0 ATHETOSIS (ACQUIRED)

333.79 ATHETOSIS (ACQUIRED) BILATERAL

333.6 ATHETOSIS (ACQUIRED) CONGENITAL (BILATERAL)

333.71 ATHETOSIS (ACQUIRED) DOUBLE

110.4 ATHLETE'S FOOT

0 ATHYROIDISM SEE 'HYPOTHYROIDISM'

779.89 ATONIA CONGENITAL

536.3 ATONIA DYSPEPSIA

661.2# ATONY UTERINE (INTRAPARTUM)

5th digit: 661.2
- **0. Episode of care NOS or N/A**
- **1. Delivered**
- **3. Antepartum**

666.1# ATONY UTERINE WITH HEMORRHAGE (POSTPARTUM)

5th digit: 666.1
- **0. Episode of care NOS or N/A**
- **1. Delivered**
- **3. Antepartum**

669.8# ATONY UTERINE WITHOUT HEMORRHAGE (POSTPARTUM)

5th digit: 669.8
- **0. Episode of care NOS or N/A**
- **1. Delivered**
- **2. Delivered with postpartum complication**
- **3. Antepartum**
- **4. Postpartum complication**

691.8 ATOPIC DERMATITIS

V15.09 ATOPY NEC

0 ATRESIA SEE ANATOMICAL SITE

759.89 ATRESIA NEC (CONGENITAL)

ATRIAL

429.89 Appendage clot

427.31 Fibrillation (paroxysmal)

427.32 Flutter

0 Infarction see 'Myocardial Infarction Acute'

427.61 Premature beats contractions or systoles

429.71 Septal defect acquired following myocardial infarction (>8 weeks) [414.8]

429.71 Septal defect acquired post MI acute (< 8 weeks) [410.##]

4th digit: 410
- **0. Anterolateral**
- **1. Anterior (wall) anteroapical anteroseptal other anterior**
- **2. Inferolateral**
- **3. Inferoposterior**
- **4. Inferior other**
- **5. Lateral apical, basolateral, posterolateral, lateral other**
- **6. Posterior (posterobasal)**
- **7. Subendocardial**
- **8. Atrium papillary or septum alone**
- **9. Unspecified**

5th digit: 410
- **0. Episode unspecified**
- **1. Initial episode**
- **2. Subsequent episode**

745.5 Septal defect ostium secundum type congenital

745.8 Septal defect ostium secundum type congenital sinus venosus

745.69 Septum absence congenital

745.7 Ventricular septal absence

757.4 ATRICHOSIS CONGENITAL

0 ATRIOVENTRICULAR BLOCK SEE 'HEART BLOCK'

745.69 ATRIOVENTRICULAR CANAL DEFECT CONGENITAL

745.69 ATRIUM COMMON CONGENITAL

745.5 ATRIUM SECUNDUM DEFECT CONGENITAL

709.09 ATROPHIA ALBA

701.8 ATROPHIA CUTIS SENILIS

ATROPHODERMA

701.9 Atrophoderma
701.3 Maculatum
701.8 Neuriticum

ATROPHY

0 See specified site
701.3 Blanche (of milian)
733.7 Bone (disuse)
728.2 Muscular (disuse)
797 Old age
359.1 Pseudohypertrophic

313.89 ATTACHMENT DISORDER REACTIVE OF INFANCY OR EARLY CHILDHOOD

ATTENTION DEFICIT DISORDER - (ADULT) (CHILD)

314.00 NOS
314.00 Inattentive
314.01 With hyperactivity/impulsiveness
314.8 With other specified manifestations

382.2 ATTICOANTRAL DISEASE CHRONIC (WITH POSTERIOR/SUPERIOR MARGINAL PERFORATION OF EAR DRUM)
0 ATTRITION GUM SEE 'GINGIVAL,' RECESSION
0 ATTRITION TEETH SEE 'TOOTH DISORDERS OF HARD TISSUES,' ATTRITION
786.59 ATYPICAL CHEST PAIN
413.1 ATYPICAL CHEST PAIN - CARDIAC ANGINA
795.02 ATYPICAL SQUAMOUS CELLS CANNOT EXCLUDE HIGH GRADE SQUAMOUS INTRAEPITHELIAL LESION, CERVIX (ASC-H)
795.01 ATYPICAL SQUAMOUS CELLS OF UNDETERMINED SIGNIFICANCE, CERVIX (ASC-US)
626.9 AUB (ABNORMAL UTERINE BLEEDING)

AUDITORY

433.8# Artery, internal occlusion
5th digit: 433.8
0. Without cerebral infarction
1. With cerebral infarction

744.01 Canal absence (congenital)
744.02 Canal atresia (congenital)
380.9 Canal disorder
959.09 Canal injury (external) (meatus)
315.32 Central processing disorder
388.43 Discrimination impairment
794.15 Function studies abnormal
388.5 Nerve atrophy
388.5 Nerve disorder
951.5 Nerve injury
388.40 Perception abnormal
388.45 Processing disorder NOS (acquired)
388.45 Processing disorder central development
388.44 Recruitment abnormality
V53.09 Substitution device fitting and adjustment

757.39 AUDRY'S SYNDROME (ACROPACHYDERMA)
078.89 AUJESZKY'S DISEASE

AURICLE EAR

744.01 Absence congenital
744.1 Accessory congenital
380.89 Calcification
380.30 Disorder
744.49 Fistula congenital
959.09 Injury
744.29 Prominence congenital
0 See also 'Ear', external

429.71 AURICULAR SEPTAL DEFECT
745.5 AURICULAR SEPTAL DEFECT CONGENITAL
350.8 AURICULOTEMPORAL NERVE DISORDER
350.8 AURICULOTEMPORAL SYNDROME
062.4 AUSTRALIAN ARBOENCEPHALITIS
062.4 AUSTRALIAN ENCEPHALITIS
062.4 AUSTRALIAN X DISEASE

299.0# AUTISTIC DISORDER
5th digit: 299.0
0. Current or active state
1. Residual state

799.89 AUTODIGESTION

AUTOIMMUNE DISEASE

279.4 NOS
283.0 Hemolytic (cold/warm type)
252.1 Parathyroid
245.2 Thyroid

799.89 AUTOINTOXICATION
337.3 AUTONOMIC DYSREFLEXIA
337.3 AUTONOMIC DYSREFLEXIA WITH DECUBITUS ULCER [707.0#]
5th digit: 707.0
0. NOS
1. Elbow
2. Upper back (shoulder blades)
3. Lower back (sacrum)
4. Hip
5. Buttock
6. Ankle
7. Heel
9. Other site (head)

337.3 AUTONOMIC DYSREFLEXIA WITH FECAL IMPACTION [560.39]

Urinary tract infection: Use additional code for the organism. See 'Bacterial Infection'.

337.3 AUTONOMIC DYSREFLEXIA WITH URINARY TRACT INFECTION [599.0]
337.9 AUTONOMIC NERVOUS SYSTEM DISORDER

AUTOSOME, AUTOSOMAL

758.5 Accessory congenital
758.0 Accessory - 21 or 22
758.1 Accessory - D1
758.2 Accessory - E3
758.0 Accessory - G
758.81 Accessory - sex
758.5 Anomalies other conditions

AUTOSOME, AUTOSOMAL (continued)

758.39 Deletion syndrome - NOS
758.31 Deletion syndrome - 5p
758.32 Deletion syndrome - 22q11.2
758.39 Deletion syndrome - other (Christchurch)
758.4 Translocation balanced in normal individual

780.99 AUTOTOPAGNOSIA

799.89 AUTOTOXEMIA

A-V (ARTERIOVENOUS) FISTULA

447.0 Acquired

648.9#: Use an additional code to identify the AV fistula.

648.9# Acquired maternal current (co-existent) in pregnancy
5th Digit: 648.9
0. Episode of care NOS or N/A
1. Delivered
2. Delivered with postpartum complication
3. Antepartum complication
4. Postpartum complication

900.01 Carotid artery common traumatic
900.00 Carotid artery traumatic
908.3 Carotid artery traumatic late effect
996.62 Complication (shunt) (surgically created) - infection or inflammation
996.1 Complication (shunt) (surgically created) - mechanical
996.74 Complication (shunt) (surgically created) - other
414.19 Heart acquired
417.0 Pulmonary vessels
747.3 Pulmonary vessels congenital
996.62 Shunt infection or inflammation

A-V (ARTERIOVENOUS) MALFORMATION

437.3 Brain acquired
747.81 Brain congenital
430 Brain ruptured, subarachnoid
094.87 Brain ruptured, syphilitic
747.81 Cerebrovascular system congenital
746.85 Coronary artery congenital
747.6# Peripheral vascular system congenital (aberrant) (absence) (agenesis) (accessory) (aneurysm) (deformity) (hypoplasia) (malposition)
5th digit: 747.6
0. Peripheral vascular unspecified site
1. Gastrointestinal vessel
2. Renal vessel
3. Upper limb vessel
4. Lower limb vessel
9. Other specified site peripheral vascular

747.3 Pulmonary
743.58 Retina
747.82 Spinal vessel congenital
747.89 Other specified

0 AV BLOCK SEE 'HEART BLOCK'
426.89 AV DISSOCIATION
427.89 AV NODAL RE-ENTRY (RE-ENTRANT) TACHYCARDIA
426.89 AV TACHYCARDIA NONPAROXYSMAL

AVASCULAR NECROSIS

733.40 Bone site unspecified
733.42 Femur (head and neck)
733.49 Hand
733.42 Hip
733.41 Humerus (head)
733.45 Jaw
733.43 Medial femoral condyle
733.44 Talus
733.49 Other bone

344.89 AVELLIS' SYNDROME
488 AVIAN INFLUENZA VIRUS
993.2 AVIATOR'S DISEASE
268.9 AVITAMINOSIS D
301.82 AVOIDANT PERSONALITY DISORDER

871.3 AVULSION EYE
871.3 AVULSION GLOBE
0 AVULSION INTERNAL ORGAN OR SITE SEE SPECIFIC ORGAN OR SITE, INJURY
0 AVULSION JOINT CAPSULE, LIGAMENT OR TENDON SEE 'SPRAIN', BY SITE
0 AVULSION OTHER SEE 'OPEN WOUND', BY SITE

780.02 AWARENESS TRANSIENT
502 AX GRINDER'S DISEASE
743.44 AXENFELD'S ANOMALY (SYNDROME)

AXILLA

729.9 Contracture
959.2 Injury
912.8 Injury other and unspecified superficial
912.9 Injury other and unspecified superficial infected

AXILLARY

444.21 Artery (embolism) (thrombosis) (occlusion) (infarction)
442.0 Artery aneurysm (ruptured) (cirsoid) (varix) (false)
440.2# Artery arteriosclerosis (degeneration) (deformans) (arteritis)
440.2# Artery arteriosclerosis (degeneration) (deformans) (arteritis) with chronic complete or total occlusion [440.4]
5th digit: 440.2
0. Unspecified
1. With intermittent claudication
2. With rest pain or rest pain and intermittent claudication
9. Other atherosclerosis extremities

AXILLARY (continued)

When coding arteriosclerosis of the extremities use an additional code, if applicable to identify chronic complete or total occlusion of the artery of the extremities (440.4).

440.24 Artery arteriosclerosis (degeneration) (deformans) (arteritis) with ischemic gangrene or ischemic gangrene and ulceration, or ulceration and intermittent claudication, rest pain [707.8]
440.23 Artery arteriosclerosis (degeneration) (deformans) (arteritis) with ulceration, or ulceration and intermittent claudication, rest pain [707.8]
440.3# Artery bypass graft arteriosclerosis (extremities)
440.3# Artery bypass graft arteriosclerosis (extremities) with chronic complete or total occlusion [440.4]
5th digit: 440.3
0. Unspecified graft
1. Autologous vein bypass graft
2. Nonautologous biological bypass graft

903.01 Artery injury
908.3 Artery injury late effect
903.01 Artery laceration traumatic (rupture) (hematoma) (avulsion) (aneurysm)
908.3 Artery laceration late effect
353.0 Nerve disorder
955.0 Nerve injury
353.0 Nerve neuritis

AXILLARY (continued)

903.02 Vein injury
908.3 Vein injury late effect
903.02 Vein laceration traumatic (rupture) (hematoma) (avulsion) (aneurysm)
908.3 Vein laceration late effect
451.89 Vein phlebitis
903.00 Vessel injury NOS
908.3 Vessel injury late effect
903.00 Vessel laceration (rupture) (hematoma) (avulsion) (aneurysm) unspecified
908.3 Vessel laceration late effect

756.89 AYALA'S DISEASE
416.0 AYERZA'S DISEASE OR SYNDROME (PULMONARY ARTERY SCLEROSIS WITH PULMONARY HYPERTENSION)
606.0 AZOOSPERMIA
334.8 AZOREAN DISEASE (OF THE NERVOUS SYSTEM)
790.6 AZOTEMIA
788.9 AZOTEMIA PRERENAL
588.0 AZOTEMIC OSTEODYSTROPHY

AZYGOS

748.69 Lobe fissure congenital (of lung)
901.89 Vein injury
908.4 Vein injury late effect
901.89 Vein laceration (rupture) (hematoma) (avulsion) (aneurysm) traumatic
908.4 Vein laceration late effect

V09.1 B-LACTAM ANTIBIOTICS RESISTANT INFECTION (SEE 'DRUG RESISTANCE' FOR COMPLETE LISTING)
695.1 BAADER'S SYNDROME (ERYTHEMA MULTIFORME EXUDATIVUM)
721.5 BAASTRUP'S SYNDROME
088.82 BABESIASIS
088.82 BABESIOSIS
448.0 BABINGTON'S DISEASE

BABINSKI

253.8 Frohlich syndrome (adiposogenital dystrophy)
344.89 Nageotte syndrome
093.89 Vaquez syndrome (cardiovascular syphilis)

0 BABY SEE 'INFANT'
791.9 BACILLURIA
005.89 BACILLUS CEREUS FOOD POISONING

BACK

> ***In order to code psychogenic pain or pain exclusively attributed to psychological factors, code first the site of the physical pain and use an additional code (307.80) to identify the psychogenic pain.***

307.80 Ache psychogenic
724.6 Ache sacroiliac
724.5 Ache vertebrogenic (postural)
724.9 Disorder other and unspecified
306.0 Disorder psychogenic (musculoskeletal)
959.19 Injury NOS
911.8 Injury superficial other and unspecified
911.9 Injury superficial other and unspecified infected
736.5 Knee (genu recurvatum)
724.2 Pain low back
724.5 Pain postural

> ***In order to code psychogenic pain or pain exclusively attributed to psychological factors, code first the site of the physical pain and use an additional code (307.80) to identify the psychogenic pain.***

307.80 Pain psychogenic
847.9 Separation (rupture) (tear) (laceration) unspecified
724.8 Stiff
847.9 Strain (sprain) (avulsion) (hemarthrosis) unspecified
846.9 Strain (sprain) low
724.8 Other symptoms referable to back

362.10 BACKGROUND RETINOPATHY
277.39 BACONY DEGENERATION (ANY SITE)

> ***Bacteremia: Use additional code for organism. See 'Bacterial Infection'.***

BACTEREMIA

790.7 NOS
031.2 Mycobacterium avium-intracellulare complex (MAC)
771.83 Newborn

BACTERIAL

040.89 Disease other specified
027.9 Disease zoonotic
027.8 Disease zoonotic other specified
008.5 Gastroenteritis

BACTERIAL (continued)

041.9 Infection
320.9 Meningitis
616.10 Vaginosis/vaginitis NOS

> ***Codes from this category are to be used as additional codes to identify bacterial agents in diseases that are classified elsewhere.***

BACTERIAL INFECTION

041.9 NOS
041.85 Aerobacter aerogenes
041.84 Anaerobes other
041.4 Bacillus coli
041.85 Bacillus coliform NEC
041.89 Bacillus NEC
041.82 Bacteroides fragilis
041.83 Clostridium perfringens
041.89 Coccus
041.4 E. coli
041.81 Eaton's agent
041.85 Enterobacter aerogenes
041.85 Enterobacter sakazakii
041.04 Enterococcus
041.84 Eubacterium
041.3 Friedlander's bacillus
041.84 Fusobacterium
041.89 Gardnerella
041.84 Gram-negative anaerobes
041.85 Gram-negative bacteria NOS
041.5 H. influenzae
041.86 H. pylori (helicobacter pylori)
041.86 Helicobacter pylori
041.5 Hemophilus
041.3 Klebsiella
041.85 Mima polymorpha
041.89 Mixed flora
041.81 Mycoplasma
041.84 Peptococcus
041.84 Peptostreptococcus
041.81 Pleuropneumonia like organisms
041.2 Pneumococcus
041.84 Propionibacterium
041.6 Proteus (mirabilis) (morganii) (vulgaris)
041.7 Pseudomonas
041.85 Serratia (marcescens)
041.10 Staphylococcus unspecified
041.11 Staphylococcus aureus
041.19 Staphylococcus other
041.00 Streptococcus
041.01 Streptococcus group A
041.02 Streptococcus group B
041.03 Streptococcus group C
041.04 Streptococcus group D (enterococcus)
041.05 Streptococcus group G
041.09 Streptococcus other
041.84 Treponema (denticola) (macrodenticum)
041.84 Veillonella
041.85 Vibrio vulnificus
041.89 Other specified bacteria

686.8 BACTERID, BACTERIDE (ANDREWS' PUSTULAR)

B

Bacteriuria: Use additional code for organism. See 'Bacterial Infection'.

BACTERIURIA

791.9 NOS
599.0 NOS with UTI
760.1 Affecting fetus or newborn
791.9 Asymptomatic
V81.5 Asymptomatic screening
646.5# Asymptomatic complicating pregnancy [791.9]
5th digit: 646.5
0. Episode of care NOS or N/A
1. Delivered
2. Delivered with postpartum complication
3. Antepartum complication
4. Postpartum complication

0 BACTEROIDES FRAGILIS SEE 'BACTERIAL INFECTION' OR SPECIFIED CONDITION
784.99 BAD BREATH
446.6 BAEHR-SCHIFFRIN DISEASE (THROMBOTIC THROMBOCYTOPENIC PURPURA)
528.5 BAELZ'S DISEASE
110.3 BAERENSPRUNG'S DISEASE (ECZEMA MARGINATUM)
495.1 BAGASSOSIS
085.1 BAGHDAD BOIL
446.5 BAGRATUNI'S SYNDROME (TEMPORAL ARTERITIS)
727.51 BAKER'S CYST (KNEE)
692.89 BAKER'S ITCH
756.89 BAKWIN KRIDA SYNDROME

BALANITIS

607.1 NOS
006.8 Amebic
112.2 Candidal
099.53 Chlamydial
099.0 Ducrey's bacillus
607.1 Gangrenous
098.0 Gonococcal acute
098.2 Gonococcal chronic
607.1 Nongonococcal
607.1 Phagedenic
099.8 Venereal NEC
607.81 Xerotica obliterans

607.1 BALANOPOSTHITIS
099.53 BALANOPOSTHITIS CHLAMYDIAL
007.0 BALANTIDIASIS
007.0 BALANTIDIASIS INTESTINAL
007.0 BALANTIDIUM COLI INTESTINAL INFECTION
307.0 BALBUTIES BALBUTIO
704.00 BALDNESS
205.3# BALFOURS DISEASE (CHLOROMA)
5th digit: 205.3
0. Without mention of remission
1. In remission

368.16 BALINT'S SYNDROME (PSYCHIC PARALYSIS OF VISUAL DISORIENTATION)
083.0 BALKAN GRIPPE

766.22 BALLANTYNE (-RUNGE) SYNDROME (POSTMATURITY)
V72.85 BALLISTOCARDIOGRAM
794.39 BALLISTOCARDIOGRAM ABNORMAL
V72.81 BALLISTOCARDIOGRAM PREOPERATIVE
993.2 BALLOON DISEASE
424.0 BALLOONING POSTERIOR LEAFLET SYNDROME
341.1 BALO'S CONCENTRIC SCLEROSIS
731.2 BAMBERGER MARIE DISEASE
288.66 BANDEMIA
0 BANDEMIA WITH LEUKEMIA SEE 'LEUKEMIA'
0 BANDEMIA WITH SPECIFED INFECTION SEE SPECIFIED INFECTION
661.4# BANDL'S RING COMPLICATING DELIVERY
5th digit: 661.4
0. Episode of care NOS or N/A
1. Delivered
3. Antepartum complication

023.1 BANGS DISEASE
995.1 BANNISTERS DISEASE
909.9 BANNISTERS LATE EFFECT
275.49 BANTAM ALBRIGHT MARTIN DISEASE (PSEUDOHYPOPARATHYROIDISM)
0 BANTI'S DISEASE OR SYNDROME SEE 'CIRRHOSIS'

BAR

755.67 Calcaneocuboid
755.67 Calcaneonavicular
755.67 Cubonavicular
600.90 Prostate

See 'LUTS' or 'Lower Urinary Tract Symptoms' for the additional code to identify the specific lower urinary tract symptoms.

600.91 Prostate with obstruction, retention or other lower urinary tract symptoms (LUTS)
755.67 Talocalcaneal

780.99 BARAGNOSIS
266.2 BARASHEH
305.4# BARBITURATE ABUSE (NONDEPENDENT)
304.1# BARBITURATE ADDICTION (DEPENDENT)
5th digit: 304.1, 305.4
0. NOS
1. Continuous
2. Episodic
3. In remission

707.9 BARCOO DISEASE (SEE ALSO 'ULCER, ULCERATION SKIN')
157.0 BARD - PIC CANCER
157.0 BARD-PIC SYNDROME (CARCINOMA HEAD OF PANCREAS)
759.89 BARDET-BIEDL (OBESITY, POLYDACTYLY AND MENTAL RETARDATION)
503 BARITOSIS
503 BARIUM LUNG DISEASE
267 BARLOW (-MOLLER) SYNDROME (INFANTILE SCURVY)
424.0 BARLOW'S SYNDROME (MITRAL VALVE PROLAPSE)
993.2 BARODONTALGIA
909.4 BARODONTALGIA LATE EFFECT

985.0 BAROMETER MAKER'S DISEASE

301.51 BARON MUNCHAUSEN SYNDROME

BAROTRAUMA

909.4 Late effect
993.2 Odontalgia
993.0 Otitic
993.1 Sinus

272.6 BARRAQUER SIMONS DISEASE (PROGRESSIVE LIPODYSTROPHY)

357.0 BARRE-GUILLAIN SYNDROME

723.2 BARRE LIEOU SYNDROME

738.3 BARREL CHEST

530.85 BARRETT'S SYNDROME (CHRONIC PEPTIC ULCER OF ESOPHAGUS)

530.5 BARSONY POLGAR SYNDROME (CORKSCREW ESOPHAGUS)

530.5 BARSONY TESCHENDORF SYNDROME (CORKSCREW ESOPHAGUS)

759.89 BARTH SYNDROME

BARTHOLIN

616.3 Abscess marsupialization (nonobstetrical)
616.89 Adenitis
616.3 Gland abscess (nonobstetrical)
616.2 Gland cyst (nonobstetrical)
616.89 Gland infection or inflammation

BARTHOLINITIS

098.0 Gonococcal acute
098.2 Gonococcal chronic
616.89 Suppurating

282.49 BART'S DISEASE

088.0 BARTONELLOSIS

255.13 BARTTER'S SYNDROME (SECONDARY HYPERALDOSTERONISM WITH JUXTAGLOMERULAR HYPERPLASIA)

173.# BASAL CELL CARCINOMA M8090/3

173.# BASAL CELL CARCINOMA FIBROEPITHELIAL TYPE M8093/3

4th digit: 173
0. Skin of lip
1. Eyelid including canthus
2. Skin of ear, auricular canal external, external meatus, pinna
3. Skin of unspecified parts of face, cheek external, chin, eyebrow, forehead, nose external
4. Scalp and skin of neck
5. Skin of trunk, axillary fold, perianal, abdominal wall, anus, back, breast (or mastectomy site), buttock
6. Skin upper limb, shoulder, arm, finger, forearm, hand
7. Skin lower limb, hip, ankle, foot, heel, knee, leg, thigh, toe, popliteal area
8. Other specified skin sites contiguous overlapping sites undetermined point of origin
9. Site NOS

The coding of cancers is complex. Coding by cell type is used only if the site is not specified.

173.# BASAL CELL CARCINOMA MORPHEA TYPE M8092/3

173.# BASAL CELL CARCINOMA MULTICENTRIC M8091/3

4th digit: 173
0. Skin of lip
1. Eyelid including canthus
2. Skin of ear, auricular canal external, external meatus, pinna
3. Skin of unspecified parts of face, cheek external, chin, eyebrow, forehead, nose external
4. Scalp and skin of neck
5. Skin of trunk, axillary fold, perianal, abdominal wall, anus, back, breast (or mastectomy site), buttock
6. Skin upper limb, shoulder, arm, finger, forearm, hand
7. Skin lower limb, hip, ankle, foot, heel, knee, leg, thigh, toe, popliteal area
8. Other specified skin sites contiguous overlapping sites undetermined point of origin
9. Site NOS

238.2 BASAL CELL TUMOR SITE NOS

0 BASAL CELL TUMOR SITE SPECIFIED SEE 'NEOPLASM UNCERTAIN BEHAVIOR', BY SITE M8090/1

333.90 BASAL GANGLION DISEASE

333.0 BASAL GANGLION DISEASE DEGENERATIVE

333.89 BASAL GANGLION DISEASE SPECIFIED NEC

794.7 BASAL METABOLIC RATE ABNORMAL

V72.6 BASAL METABOLIC RATE TESTING

199.1 BASALOID CARCINOMA SITE NOS

0 BASALOID CARCINOMA SITE SPECIFIED SEE 'CANCER', BY SITE M8123/3

757.31 BASAN'S DYSPLASIA

842.13 BASEBALL FINGER

242.00 BASEDOW'S DISEASE OR SYNDROME (EXOPHTHALMIC GOITER)

242.01 BASEDOW'S DISEASE WITH THYROTOXIC CRISIS OR STORM

583.89 BASEMENT MEMBRANE DISEASE NEC

446.21 BASEMENT MEMBRANE DISEASE NEC WITH PULMONARY HEMORRHAGE [583.81]

117.7 BASIDIOBOLUS INFECTION

BASILAR ARTERY

433.0# Arteriosclerosis (degeneration) (deformans) (arteritis)
433.0# Embolism thrombosis or obstruction
431 Hemorrhage (rupture)
433.0# Occlusion (thrombosis) (obstruction) (embolism) (narrowing) (stenosis)
433.3# Occlusion bilateral or with carotid and/or vertebral

5th digit: 433.0, 3
0. Without cerebral infarction
1. With cerebral infarction

435.0 Spasm
435.0 Syndrome (insufficiency)

903.1 BASILIC VEIN INJURY
451.82 BASILIC VEIN PHLEBITIS
377.04 BASOFRONTAL SYNDROME
288.59 BASOPENIA
194.3 BASOPHIL CARCINOMA SITE NOS
0 BASOPHIL CARCINOMA SITE SPECIFIED SEE 'CANCER', BY SITE M8300/3
288.65 BASOPHILIA
255.0 BASOPHILISM (CUSHING SYNDROME)
173.# BASOSQUAMOUS CARCINOMA (MULTICENTRIC) M8094/3
4th digit: 173
0. Skin of lip
1. Eyelid including canthus
2. Skin of ear, auricular canal external, external meatus, pinna
3. Skin of unspecified parts of face, cheek external, chin, eyebrow, forehead, nose external
4. Scalp and skin of neck
5. Skin of trunk, axillary fold, perianal, abdominal wall, anus, back, breast (or mastectomy site), buttock
6. Skin upper limb, shoulder, arm, finger, forearm, hand
7. Skin lower limb, hip, ankle, foot, heel, knee, leg, thigh, toe, popliteal area
8. Other specified skin sites contiguous overlapping sites undetermined point of origin
9. Site NOS

272.5 BASSEN KORNZWEIG RETINAL DYSTROPHY [362.72]
272.5 BASSEN KORNZWEIG SYNDROME (ABETALIPOPROTEINEMIA)
744.29 BAT EAR CONGENITAL
078.0 BATEMAN'S DISEASE
287.2 BATEMAN'S PURPURA
994.1 BATHING CRAMP
909.4 BATHING CRAMP LATE EFFECT
300.23 BATHOPHOBIA
330.1 BATTEN DISEASE (CEREBRAL LIPIDOSES WITH CEREBRORETINAL DYSTROPHY) [362.71]
359.21 BATTEN-STEINERT DISEASE OR SYNDROME

When the cause of an injury is stated to be abuse, multiple codes should be assigned if applicable, to identify any associated injuries. Sequence in the following order:

1. Type of abuse - child or adult (995.5, 995.8)

2. Type of injury

3. Nature of the abuse - see E-code directory 'Assault' (E904.0, E960-E966, E968)

4. Perpetrator of the abuse - see E-code directory 'Assault' (E967)

995.81 BATTERED ADULT (SPOUSE) SYNDROME
995.54 BATTERED CHILD (BABY) SYNDROME
V15.41 BATTERED HISTORY
995.81 BATTERED WIFE (SPOUSE) (WOMAN)

031.0 BATTEY DISEASE
571.5 BAUMGARTEN-CRUVEILHIER DISEASE OR SYNDROME (CIRRHOSIS OF LIVER)
571.5 BAUMGARTEN-CRUVEILHIER DISEASE (CIRRHOSIS OF LIVER) WITH ESOPHAGEAL VARICES [456.2#]
5th digit: 456.2
0. With bleeding
1. Without bleeding

503 BAUXITE-WORKERS DISEASE
094.1 BAYLE'S DISEASE (DEMENTIA PARALYTICA)
017.1# BAZIN'S DISEASE (PRIMARY) (SEE ALSO 'TUBERCULOSIS')
5th digit: 017.1
0. NOS
1. Lab not done
2. Lab unknown at present
3. Microscopy positive - (in sputum)
4. Culture positive - microscopy negative
5. Culture negative - microscopy positive
6. Culture and microscopy negative - confirmed by other methods

0 BBB (BUNDLE BRANCH BLOCK) SEE 'BUNDLE BRANCH BLOCK'
757.4 BEADED HAIR CONGENITAL
759.82 BEALS SYNDROME
300.5 BEARD'S DISEASE (NEURASTHENIA)
571.49 BEARN-KUNKEL (-SLATER) SYNDROME (LUPOID HEPATITIS)

BEAT
727.2 Elbow (occupational)
727.2 Hand (occupational)
727.2 Knee (occupational)

429.1 BEAU'S MYOCARDIAL DEGENERATION
429.1 BEAU'S SYNDROME
720.0 BECHTEREW-STRUMPELL-MARIE SYNDROME (ANKYLOSING SPONDYLITIS)
720.0 BECHTEREW'S ANKYLOSING SPONDYLITIS
433.8# BECK'S SYNDROME (ANTERIOR SPINAL ARTERY OCCLUSION)
5th digit: 433.8
0. Without cerebral infarction
1. With cerebral infarction

425.2 BECKER'S DISEASE IDIOPATHIC MURAL ENDOMYOCARDIAL
359.22 BECKER'S DISEASE MYOTONIA CONGENITA, RECESSIVE FORM
359.22 BECKER'S DYSTROPHY
759.89 BECKWITH (-WIEDEMANN) SYNDROME
079.98 BEDSONIA
079.88 BEDSONIA SPECIFIED NEC

V49.84 BED CONFINEMENT STATUS

707.0# BED SORE

707.0# BED SORE WITH GANGRENE [785.4]

5th digit: 707.0

0. NOS
1. Elbow
2. Upper back (shoulder blades)
3. Lower back (sacrum)
4. Hip
5. Buttock
6. Ankle
7. Heel
9. Other site (head)

788.36 BEDWETTING

989.5 BEE STING

995.0 BEE STING WITH ANAPHYLAXIS [989.5]

242.0# BEGBIE'S EXOPHTHALMIC GOITER

5th digit: 242.0

0. Without mention of thyrotoxic crisis or storm
1. With mention of thyrotoxic crisis or storm

0 BEHAVIORAL DISORDER SEE 'CONDUCT DISORDER'

V40.9 BEHAVIORAL PROBLEM

V40.3 BEHAVIORAL PROBLEM OTHER SPECIFIED

136.1 BEHCET'S DISEASE WITH VULVA ULCER [616.51]

136.1 BEHCET'S SYNDROME

0 BEHCET'S SYNDROME ARTHRITIS SEE 'ARTHRITIS OTHER SPECIFIED', BEHCET'S SYNDROME

362.50 BEHR'S DISEASE

111.2 BEIGEL'S WHITE PIEDRA

104.0 BEJEL

720.0 BEKHTEREV'S ANKYLOSING SPONDYLITIS

720.0 BEKHTEREV-STRUMPELL-MARIE SYNDROME (ANKYLOSING SPONDYLITIS)

0 BELCHING SEE 'ERUCTATION'

296.0# BELL'S AFFECTIVE PSYCHOSIS

5th digit: 296.0

0. NOS
1. Mild
2. Moderate
3. Severe without mention of psychotic behavior
4. Severe specified as with psychotic behavior
5. In partial or NOS remission
6. In full remission

351.0 BELL'S PALSY

791.0 BENCE JONES PROTEINURIA ABNORMAL

993.3 BENDS

909.4 BENDS LATE EFFECT

344.89 BENEDIKT'S SYNDROME (PARALYSIS)

348.2 BENIGN INTRACRANIAL HYPERTENSION

0 BENIGN LESION SEE 'BENIGN NEOPLASM'

BENIGN NEOPLASM

215.5 Abdomen connective tissue

210.7 Adenoid tissue

227.0 Adrenal gland

211.9 Alimentary tract

211.5 Ampulla of vater

211.4 Anal canal or sphincter

211.4 Anus (canal)

216.5 Anus skin (margin) (perianal)

211.3 Appendix

212.1 Arytenoid cartilage

210.8 Arytenoid fold

215.7 Back connective tissue

221.2 Bartholin's gland

223.3 Bladder

215.# Blood vessel

4th digit: 215

0. Head, face, neck
2. Upper limb including shoulder
3. Lower limb including hip
4. Thorax
5. Abdomen (wall), gastric, gastrointestinal, intestine, stomach
6. Pelvis, buttock, groin, inguinal region, perineum
7. Trunk NOS, back NOS, flank NOS
8. Other specified sites
9. Site NOS

213.# Bone and articular cartilage

4th digit: 213

0. Skull, face, upper jaw
1. Lower jaw NOS
2. Spine
3. Rib, sternum, clavicle
4. Upper limb long bones, scapula
5. Upper limb short bones
6. Pelvis, sacrum, coccyx
7. Lower limb long bone
8. Lower limb short bone
9. Site NOS

225.0 Brain

210.6 Branchial cleft (vestiges)

610.0 Breast cyst

610.2 Breast fibroadenosis

610.1 Breast fibrocystic disease

217 Breast glandular

610.8 Breast sebaceous cyst

217 Breast soft and connective tissues

212.3 Bronchus

210.4 Buccal mucosa

215.# Bursa

4th digit: 215

0. Head, face, neck
2. Upper limb including shoulder
3. Lower limb including hip
4. Thorax
5. Abdomen (wall), gastric, gastrointestinal, intestine, stomach
6. Pelvis buttock groin inguinal region perineum
7. Trunk NOS, back NOS, flank NOS
8. Other specified sites
9. Site NOS

215.6 Buttock connective tissue

211.1 Cardia of stomach

211.1 Cardiac orifice

B

BENIGN NEOPLASM (continued)

212.3 Carina
227.5 Carotid body
213.# Cartilage articular
4th digit: 213
0. Skull, face, upper jaw
1. Lower jaw NOS
2. Spine
3. Rib, sternum, clavicle
4. Upper limb long bones, scapula
5. Upper limb short bones
6. Pelvis, sacrum, coccyx
7. Lower limb long bone
8. Lower limb short bone
9. Site NOS

225.3 Cauda equina
211.3 Cecum
225.0 Cerebellopontine angle
225.2 Cerebral meninges
219.0 Cervix stump
224.6 Choroid
224.0 Ciliary body
221.2 Clitoris
227.6 Coccygeal body
211.3 Colon
211.4 Colon rectosigmoid
211.5 Common bile duct
224.3 Conjunctiva
215.# Connective tissue (soft tissue)
4th digit: 215
0. Head, face, neck
2. Upper limb including shoulder
3. Lower limb including hip
4. Thorax
5. Abdomen (wall), gastric, gastrointestinal, intestine, stomach
6. Pelvis, buttock, groin, inguinal region, perineum
7. Trunk NOS, back NOS, flank NOS
8. Other specified sites
9. Site NOS

224.4 Cornea
222.1 Corpus cavernosum
225.1 Cranial nerves
227.3 Craniobuccal pouch
212.1 Cricoid cartilage
212.1 Cuneiform cartilage
211.5 Cystic duct
211.9 Digestive other and unspecified parts
211.2 Duodenum
212.0 Ear (middle)
216.2 Ear external
212.0 Ear internal
227.9 Endocrine
227.6 Endocrine aortic body and paraganglia
227.5 Endocrine carotid body
220 Endocrine ovary
211.6 Endocrine pancreas
222.0 Endocrine testes
227.8 Endocrine other
219.1 Endometrium
222.3 Epididymis
212.1 Epiglottis (suprahyoid) (unspecified)
210.6 Epiglottis anterior aspect
211.0 Esophagus
212.0 Ethmoid sinus
212.0 Eustachian tube

BENIGN NEOPLASM (continued)

224.9 Eye
224.6 Eye choroid
224.0 Eye ciliary body
224.3 Eye conjunctiva
224.4 Eye cornea
224.0 Eye eyeball
215.0 Eye eyelid (cartilage)
216.1 Eye eyelid (skin)
224.2 Eye iris
224.7 Eye lacrimal duct
224.2 Eye lacrimal gland
224.6 Eye nevus choroidal
225.1 Eye optic nerve
224.1 Eye orbit
213.0 Eye orbital bone
224.5 Eye retina
228.03 Eye retinal hemangioma
224.0 Eye sclera
224.0 Eye uveal tract
224.8 Eye other specified
215.0 Eyelid cartilage
216.1 Eyelid skin
215.0 Face connective tissue
213.0 Facial bones
221.0 Fallopian tube
210.6 Fauces
215.7 Flank connective tissue
210.0 Frenulum labii
212.0 Frontal sinus
211.1 Fundus of stomach
219.1 Fundus uterine
211.5 Gallbladder
211.9 Gastrointestinal tract NOS
215.5 Gastrointestinal tract connective tissue
221.9 Genital female
221.2 Genital female external
221.8 Genital female other
222.9 Genital male
222.8 Genital male other
221.9 Genitourinary tract female NOS
222.9 Genitourinary tract male NOS
211.9 GI tract
210.4 Gingiva
222.1 Glans penis
227.6 Glomus jugulare
212.1 Glottis
215.4 Great vessels (thorax)
215.6 Groin connective tissue
210.4 Gum
215.0 Head connective tissue
212.7 Heart
211.4 Hemorrhoidal zone
211.5 Hepatic duct
212.3 Hilus lung
215.3 Hip connective tissue
216.7 Hip skin
215.5 Hypochondrium
210.8 Hypopharynx
227.3 Hypophysis
211.3 Ileocecal valve
211.2 Ileum
215.6 Inguinal region

BENIGN NEOPLASM (continued)

211.9 Intestine
215.5 Intestine connective tissue
211.3 Intestine large
211.2 Intestine small
229.8 Intrathoracic
224.0 Iris
211.7 Islets of langerhans (islet cell tumor)
213.1 Jaw lower bone
211.2 Jejunum

> *If a lesion is removed and the pathologist is unsure of malignancy or if it is undergoing malignant changes at the time (requiring more extensive study or procedures), code a neoplasm of uncertain behavior.*

213.# Joint cartilage

4th digit: 213
- **0. Skull, face, upper jaw**
- **1. Lower jaw NOS**
- **2. Spine**
- **3. Rib, sternum, clavicle**
- **4. Upper limb long bones, scapula**
- **5. Upper limb short bones**
- **6. Pelvis, sacrum, coccyx**
- **7. Lower limb long bone**
- **8. Lower limb short bone**
- **9. Site NOS**

223.0 Kidney
223.1 Kidney renal pelvis
221.2 Labia
210.4 Labial commissure
224.7 Lacrimal duct
224.2 Lacrimal gland
210.8 Laryngopharynx
212.1 Larynx
215.# Ligament

4th digit: 215
- **0. Head, face, neck**
- **2. Upper limb including shoulder**
- **3. Lower limb including hip**
- **4. Thorax**
- **5. Abdomen (wall), gastric, gastrointestinal, intestine, stomach**
- **6. Pelvis, buttock, groin, inguinal region, perineum**
- **7. Trunk NOS, back NOS, flank NOS**
- **8. Other specified sites**
- **9. Site NOS**

210.0 Lip
210.4 Lip labial commissure
216.0 Lip skin
211.5 Liver biliary passages
213.1 Lower jaw bone
215.3 Lower limb and hip connective tissue
212.3 Lung
229.0 Lymph nodes
210.7 Lymphadenoid tissue
210.2 Major salivary glands
212.0 Maxillary sinus
212.5 Mediastinum
225.2 Meninges cerebral
225.4 Meninges spinal
211.8 Mesentery
211.8 Mesocolon
210.6 Mesopharynx

BENIGN NEOPLASM (continued)

210.3 Mouth floor
210.4 Mouth other and unspecified parts
215.# Muscle

4th digit: 215
- **0. Head, face, neck**
- **2. Upper limb including shoulder**
- **3. Lower limb including hip**
- **4. Thorax**
- **5. Abdomen (wall), gastric, gastrointestinal, intestine, stomach**
- **6. Pelvis, buttock, groin, inguinal region, perineum**
- **7. Trunk NOS, back NOS, flank NOS**
- **8. Other specified sites**
- **9. Site NOS**

219.1 Myometrium
212.0 Nares
229.8 Nasal
212.0 Nasal cartilage
212.0 Nasal cavities
471.8 Nasal polyp accessory sinus
212.0 Nasal septum
210.7 Nasal septum posterior
212.0 Nasal sinuses
216.3 Nasal skin
224.7 Nasolacrimal duct
210.7 Nasopharynx
215.0 Neck connective tissue
225.0 Nervous system brain
225.2 Nervous system meninges unspecified
225.9 Nervous system part unspecified
225.3 Nervous system spinal cord
225.4 Nervous system spinal meninges
225.8 Nervous system other specified sites
229.8 Nose
216.3 Nose skin
225.1 Olfactory nerve or bulb
211.8 Omentum
225.1 Optic nerve
210.4 Oral cavity NOS
210.4 Oral mucosa
224.1 Orbit
213.0 Orbital (bone)
210.6 Oropharynx other parts
229.8 Other
220 Ovary
620.0 Ovary cyst follicular
221.0 Oviduct
210.4 Palate (hard) (soft)
211.6 Pancreas
211.7 Pancreas islets of langerhans
227.6 Para-aortic body
221.0 Parametrium
227.1 Parathyroid gland
223.89 Paraurethral glands
210.2 Parotid gland
215.6 Pelvis connective tissue
222.1 Penis
212.7 Pericardium
215.6 Perineum connective tissue

B

BENIGN NEOPLASM (continued)

213.# Periosteum
4th digit: 213
0. Skull, face, upper jaw
1. Lower jaw NOS
2. Spine
3. Rib, sternum, clavicle
4. Upper limb long bones, scapula
5. Upper limb short bones
6. Pelvis, sacrum, coccyx
7. Lower limb long bone
8. Lower limb short bone
9. Site NOS

215.# Peripheral nerves and ganglia
4th digit: 215
0. Head, face, neck
2. Upper limb including shoulder
3. Lower limb including hip
4. Thorax
5. Abdomen (wall), gastric, gastrointestinal, intestine, stomach
6. Pelvis, buttock, groin, inguinal region, perineum
7. Trunk NOS, back NOS, flank NOS
8. Other specified sites
9. Site NOS

210.7 Pharyngeal tonsil
210.9 Pharynx
227.4 Pineal gland
227.3 Pituitary gland
212.4 Pleura
210.8 Postcricoid region
222.1 Prepuce
222.2 Prostate
600.20 Prostate adenoma

See 'LUTS' or 'Lower Urinary Tract Symptoms' for the additional code to identify the specific lower urinary tract symptoms.

600.21 Prostate adenoma with urinary obstruction, retention or other lower urinary tract symptoms
222.2 Prostate with urinary incontinence [788.3#]
5th digit: 788.3
0. Unspecified
1. Urge incontinence
2. Stress, male
3. Mixed urge and stress
4. Without sensory awareness
5. Post-void dribbling
6. Nocturnal enuresis
7. Continuous leakage
8. Overflow incontinence
9. Other

221.2 Pudendum
211.1 Pylorus
210.8 Pyriform fossa
227.3 Rathke's pouch
211.4 Rectosigmoid junction
211.4 Rectum and anal canal
223.1 Renal pelvis
223.1 Renal pelvis (calyces)
212.8 Respiratory other specified site
212.9 Respiratory site unspecified
224.5 Retina
228.03 Retinal hemangioma

BENIGN NEOPLASM (continued)

211.8 Retroperitoneum and peritoneum
210.4 Salivary gland (minor) (unspecified)
210.2 Salivary gland major
224.0 Sclera
222.4 Scrotum skin
227.3 Sella turcica
222.8 Seminal vesicle
215.2 Shoulder connective tissue
216.6 Shoulder skin
212.0 Sinus - ethmoidal, frontal, maxillary, sphenoidal
216.# Skin
4th digit: 216
0. Lip skin
1. Eyelid including canthus
2. Ear external (auricle) (pinna)
3. Face (cheek) (nose) (eyebrow)
4. Scalp, neck
5. Trunk (back) (chest) (breast)
6. Upper limb including shoulder
7. Lower limb including hip
8. Other specified sites
9. Skin NOS

222.# Skin other male genital
4th digit: 222
0. Testis
1. Penis
2. Prostate
3. Epididymis
4. Scrotum
8. Other specified sites
9. Site unspecified

213.0 Skull, face and upper jaw bones
222.8 Spermatic cord
212.0 Sphenoidal sinus
211.5 Sphincter of oddi
225.3 Spinal cord
225.4 Spinal meninges
211.9 Spleen NEC
211.1 Stomach
215.5 Stomach connective tissue
210.2 Sublingual gland
210.2 Submandibular salivary gland
227.0 Suprarenal gland
215.# Synovia
215.# Tendon (sheath)
4th digit: 215
0. Head, face, neck
2. Upper limb including shoulder
3. Lower limb including hip
4. Thorax
5. Abdomen (wall), gastric, gastrointestinal, intestine, stomach
6. Pelvis, buttock, groin, inguinal region, perineum
7. Trunk NOS, back NOS, flank NOS
8. Other specified sites
9. Site NOS

222.0 Testis
229.8 Thoracic
215.4 Thoracic connective tissue
215.4 Thoracic great vessels
210.9 Throat
212.6 Thymus
226 Thyroid
212.1 Thyroid cartilage
210.1 Tongue

BENIGN NEOPLASM (continued)

210.1 Tonsil lingual
210.5 Tonsil palatine
210.7 Tonsil pharyngeal
210.6 Tonsil fossa
210.6 Tonsillar pillars
212.2 Trachea (tracheobronchial)
215.7 Trunk connective tissue
216.5 Trunk skin
215.2 Upper limb connective tissue
212.9 Upper respiratory
223.2 Ureter
223.3 Ureter orifice of bladder
223.81 Urethra
223.3 Urethra orifice of bladder
223.89 Urinary organs other specified
223.9 Urinary organs
219.9 Uterus
219.1 Uterus body
219.0 Uterus cervix uteri
219.1 Uterus endometrium
219.1 Uterus fundus
221.0 Uterus ligaments
219.1 Uterus myometrium
221.0 Uterus tube
219.8 Uterus other specified part
224.0 Uveal tract
210.4 Uvula
221.1 Vagina
210.6 Vallecula
213.2 Vertebral column
221.9 VesicovaginaL
221.2 Vestibular (Bartholin's) gland
212.1 Vocal cords (true) (false)
221.2 Vulva
210.2 Wharton's duct
227.6 Zuckerkandl's organ

694.5 BENIGN PEMPHIGUS

See 'LUTS' or 'Lower Urinary Tract Symptoms' for the additional code to identify the specific lower urinary tract symptoms.

600.90 BENIGN PROSTATE HYPERPLASIA NOS
600.91 BENIGN PROSTATE HYPERPLASIA NOS WITH URINARY OBSTRUCTION, RETENTION OR OTHER LOWER URINARY TRACT SYMPTOMS
600.20 BENIGN PROSTATE HYPERPLASIA LOCALIZED
600.21 BENIGN PROSTATE HYPERPLASIA LOCALIZED WITH URINARY OBSTRUCTION, RETENTION OR OTHER LOWER URINARY TRACT SYMPTOMS
600.00 BENIGN PROSTATE HYPERTROPHY
600.01 BENIGN PROSTATE HYPERTROPHY WITH URINARY OBSTRUCTION, RETENTION OR OTHER LOWER URINARY TRACT SYMPTOMS

333.93 BENIGN SHUDDERING ATTACKS
208.9# BENNET'S LEUKEMIA M9800/3
5th digit: 208.9
0. Without mention of remission
1. In remission

379.22 BENSON'S DISEASE
305.4# BENZODIAZEPINE ABUSE (NONDEPENDENT)
304.1# BENZODIAZEPINE ADDICTION (DEPENDENT)
5th digit: 304.1, 305.4
0. NOS
1. Continuous
2. Episodic
3. In remission

288.2 BEQUEZ CESAR (STEINBRINCK-CHEDIAK-HIGASHI) (CONGENITAL GIGANTISM OF PEROXIDASE GRANULES)
V62.82 BEREAVEMENT UNCOMPLICATED (REASON FOR ENCOUNTER)
300.11 BERGERON'S HYSTEROEPILEPSY
265.0 BERIBERI
265.0 BERIBERI CARDIOMYOPATHY [425.7]
265.0 BERIBERI CEREBRAL DEGENERATION DISEASE [331.7]
265.0 BERIBERI POLYNEUROPATHY [357.4]
921.3 BERLIN'S DISEASE
921.3 BERLIN'S EDEMA (RETINA)
337.9 BERNARD-HORNER SYNDROME SEE ALSO 'NEUROPATHY PERIPHERAL' AUTONOMIC
255.41 BERNARD-SERGENT SYNDROME (ACUTE ADRENOCORTICAL INSUFFICIENCY)
287.1 BERNARD-SOULIER THROMBOPATHY DUE TO QUALITATIVE PLATELET DEFECTS
355.1 BERNHARDT - ROTH SYNDROME
428.0 BERNHEIM'S SYNDROME
430 BERRY ANEURYSM RUPTURED
123.8 BERTIELLIASIS
756.15 BERTOLOTTI'S SYNDROME (SACRALIZATION OF FIFTH LUMBAR VERTEBRA)
503 BERYLLIOSIS
503 BERYLLIOSIS (OCCUPATIONAL)
135 BESNIER-BOECK-SCHAUMANN DISEASE OR SYNDROME (SARCOIDOSIS)
362.76 BEST'S DISEASE
302.1 BESTIALITY
255.2 BETA 3 HYDROXYSTEROID DEHYDROGENASE DEFICIENCY
255.2 BETA 11 HYDROXYLASE DEFICIENCY
277.2 BETA-AMINO-ISOBUTYRICACIDURIA AMINO ACID DISTURBANCE (METABOLIC)
V69.3 BETTING AND GAMBLING PROBLEM
117.1 BEURMANN'S DISEASE (SPOROTRICHOSIS)
935.2 BEZOAR GASTRIC
936 BEZOAR INTESTINE
784.69 BIANCHI'S SYNDROME (APHASIA-APRAXIA-ALEXIA SYNDROME)
276.9 BICARBONATE ABNORMAL FINDINGS

B

BICEPS, BICIPITAL

891.2 Femori tendon laceration
880.23 Tendon laceration
727.62 Tendon rupture (long head) nontraumatic
726.12 Tendonitis

759.89 BIEDL-BARDET SYNDROME (OBESITY, POLYDACTYLY AND MENTAL RETARDATION)
330.1 BIELSCHOWSKY'S DISEASE
759.89 BIEMOND'S SYNDROME (OBESITY, POLYDACTYLY AND MENTAL RETARDATION)
281.0 BIERMER'S ANEMIA
695.4 BIETT'S DISEASE
755.66 BIFID DIGIT
289.4 BIG SPLEEN SYNDROME
427.89 BIGEMINY
256.4 BILATERAL POLYCYSTIC OVARIAN SYNDROME

BILE DUCT

751.61 Absence (common) (congenital)
576.8 Adhesions
751.60 Anomaly NOS
751.69 Anomaly other specified
576.2 Atresia
751.61 Atresia congenital
576.8 Atrophy
576.8 Contraction
576.8 Cyst
576.9 Disorders
576.8 Disorders other specified
751.69 Duplication congenital
576.4 Fistula
576.8 Hypertrophy (stasis) (cyst)
751.61 Hypoplasia congenital
868.02 Injury traumatic
868.12 Injury traumatic with open wound into cavity
908.1 Injury late effect
751.61 Obstruction (occlusion) congenital
751.61 Obstruction (occlusion) congenital with jaundice [774.5]
0 Obstruction (occlusion) due to gallstone see 'Choledocholithiasis'
576.2 Obstruction (occlusion) without mention of calculus
576.3 Perforation
996.69 Prosthesis complication - infection or inflammation
996.59 Prosthesis complication - mechanical
996.79 Prosthesis complication - other
576.3 Rupture (non traumatic)
0 Stenosis (stricture) (occlusion) with calculus see 'Choledocholithiasis'
576.2 Stenosis (stricture) (occlusion) without calculus
576.8 Ulcer

791.4 BILE IN URINE
0 BILHARZIASIS SEE 'SCHISTOSOMA, SCHISTOSOMIASIS'

BILIARY

751.61 Atresia congenital
571.6 Cirrhosis
574.20 Colic
574.21 Colic with obstruction
V58.82 Drainage tube fitting
751.69 Duct duplication of congenital
575.8 Dyskinesia

BILIARY (continued)

576.2 Obstruction
751.61 Obstruction congenital

> ***646.8#: Specify the maternal complication with an additional code.***

646.8# Problem complicating pregnany
5th digit: 646.8
0. Episode of care unspecified or N/A
1. Delivered
2. Delivered with postpartum complication
3. Antepartum complication
4. Postpartum complication

576.9 Tract disorder
793.3 Tract filling defect

277.4 BILIRUBIN ABNORMAL FINDING
277.4 BILIRUBIN EXCRETION DISORDER
791.4 BILIURIA
741.9# BILLROTH'S MENINGOCELE
5th digit: 741.9
0. Region NOS
1. Cervical
2. Dorsal
3. Lumbar

346.2# BING HORTON SYNDROME
5th digit: 346.2
0. Without mention intractable migraine
1. With intractable migraine

BINOCULAR VISION

368.34 Abnormal retinal correspondence
368.30 Disorder
368.33 Fusion with defective stereopsis
368.31 Suppression
368.32 Without fusion

290.12 BINSWANGERS DEMENTIA
259.2 BIORCK (-THORSON) SYNDROME (MALIGNANT CARCINOID)
277.6 BIOTINDTDASE DEFICIENCY

BIPOLAR DISORDER

296.80 NOS
296.7 Atypical NOS
296.7 Circular type I
296.7 Circular type, current or most recent episode NOS
296.5# Circular type, current or most recent episode depressed
296.4# Circular type, current or most recent episode manic
296.6# Circular type, current or most recent episode mixed
5th digit: 296.4-6
0. NOS
1. Mild
2. Moderate
3. Severe without mention of psychotic behavior
4. Severe specified as with psychotic behavior
5. In partial or NOS remission
6. In full remission

BIPOLAR DISORDER (continued)

296.7 Type I, current or most recent episode NOS
296.5# Type I, current or most recent episode depressed
296.4# Type I, current or most recent episode hypomanic
296.4# Type I, current or most recent episode manic
296.6# Type I, current or most recent episode mixed

5th digit: 296.4-6
0. NOS
1. Mild
2. Moderate
3. Severe without mention of psychotic behavior
4. Severe specified as with psychotic behavior
5. In partial or NOS remission
6. In full remission

296.89 Type II
296.8# Other manic depressive

5th digit: 296.8
0. Unspecified
1. Atypical manic
2. Atypical depressive
9. Other (mixed)

754.82 BIRD CHEST CONGENITAL
495.2 BIRD FANCIERS' LUNG
271.8 BIRD'S DISEASE (OXALURIA)
767.9 BIRTH INJURY NOS (SEE ALSO SPECIFIED INJURY)
767.9 BIRTH TRAUMA NOS (SEE ALSO SPECIFIED TRAUMA)
757.32 BIRTHMARKS CONGENITAL
0 BIRTHWEIGHT HIGH SEE 'LARGE BABY'
0 BIRTHWEIGHT LOW, NORMAL GESTATION SEE 'LIGHT FOR DATES'
0 BIRTHWEIGHT LOW, PREMATURE INFANT SEE 'PREMATURE INFANT'
273.8 BISALBUMINEMIA

> ***All bites and stings are coded as venomous or nonvenomous. Nonvenomous bites are classified by type of injury. If with laceration or puncture code to 'Open Wound'. If skin is intact, code to 'Contusion'. Nonvenomous insects, however, are considered superficial injuries and are found under 'Insect Bite' in Easy Coder. Venomous insect bites can be found under the category, 'Sting Venomous', or 'Bites Venomous'.***

BITE NONVENOMOUS

0 Animal skin intact see 'Contusion', by site
0 Animal with laceration or puncture see 'Open Wound', by site
133.8 Chigger (red bug)
0 Flea see 'Insect Bite Nonvenomous', by site
0 Human skin surface intact see 'Contusion', by site
0 Human laceration or puncture see 'Open Wound', by site, complicated
0 Insect see 'Insect Bite Nonvenomous', by site or 'Insect Bite Venomous'
0 Tick see 'Insect Bite Nonvenomous', by site

BITE VENOMOUS

989.5 Ant (fire ant)
995.0 Ant (fire ant) with anaphylaxis [989.5]
989.5 Black Widow spider
995.0 Black Widow spider with anaphylaxis [989.5]
989.5 Brown spider
995.0 Brown spider with anaphylaxis [989.5]
989.5 Centipede
995.0 Centipede with anaphylaxis [989.5]
989.5 Copperhead snake
995.0 Copperhead snake with anaphylaxis [989.5]
989.5 Coral snake
995.0 Coral snake with anaphylaxis [989.5]
989.5 Fer de Lance
995.0 Fer de Lance with anaphylaxis [989.5]
989.5 Gila monster
995.0 Gila monster with anaphylaxis [989.5]
909.1 Late effect
909.9 Late effect with anaphylaxis
989.5 Lizard
995.0 Lizard with anaphylaxis [989.5]
989.5 Rattlesnake
995.0 Rattlesnake with anaphylaxis [989.5]
989.5 Sea snake
995.0 Sea snake with anaphylaxis [989.5]
989.5 Snake venomous
995.0 Snake venomous with anaphylaxis [989.5]
989.5 Tarantula
995.0 Tarantula with anaphylaxis [989.5]
989.5 Venomous
989.5 Viper
995.0 Viper with anaphylaxis [989.5]
989.5 Water Moccasin
995.0 Water Moccasin with anaphylaxis [989.5]

264.1 BITOT'S SPOT IN YOUNG CHILD
020.9 BLACK DEATH
921.0 BLACK EYE
924.20 BLACK HEEL
500 BLACK LUNG DISEASE OR SYNDROME
923.20 BLACK PALM
111.3 BLACK PIEDRA
284.01 BLACKFAN DIAMOND ANEMIA OR SYNDROME (CONGENITAL HYPOPLASTIC ANEMIA)
706.1 BLACKHEAD
780.2 BLACKOUT
084.8 BLACKWATER FEVER
989.5 BLACK WIDOW SPIDER BITE (SYNDROME)
995.0 BLACK WIDOW SPIDER BITE WITH ANAPHYLAXIS [989.5]

B

Bladder disorders with incontinence (retention): When coding the disorders below, code the disorder first, then add the appropriate additional code for the incontinence (retention) - 788.2#, 788.3#, or 625.6. The disorder sequences before the incontinence (retention). For example, the codes for bladder wall hemorrhage with stress incontinence, female would be; 596.7 (bladder hemorrhage) and 625.6, (stress incontinence).

BLADDER :
-WITH INCONTINENCE [788.3#]
-WITH STRESS INCONTINENCE, FEMALE [625.6]
-WITH URINARY RETENTION [788.2#]

V45.74 Absence postsurgical
344.61 Acontractile
596.8 Adhesion (sphincter)
596.4 Atony or inertia
344.61 Atony or inertia neurogenic
596.8 Atrophy
344.61 Autonomic hyperreflexia
596.8 Calcification
594.1 Calculus
594.0 Calculus in diverticulum
596.4 Compliance high
596.52 Compliance low
596.8 Contracted
596.0 Contracture acquired disorder
344.61 Cord
596.8 Deformity
596.59 Detrusor instability
596.55 Detrusor sphincter dyssynergia

WITH INCONTINENCE [788.3#]
5th digit: 788.3
0. Unspecified
1. Urge incontinence
2. Stress, male
3. Mixed urge and stress
4. Without sensory awareness
5. Post-void dribbling
6. Nocturnal enuresis
7. Continuous leakage
8. Overflow incontinence
9. Other

WITH RETENTION [788.2#]
5th digit: 788.2
0. Unspecified
1. Incomplete bladder emptying
9. Other specified retention

Bladder disorders with incontinence (retention): When coding the disorders below, code the disorder first, then add the appropriate additional code for the incontinence (retention) - 788.2#, 788.3#, or 625.6. The disorder sequences before the incontinence (retention). For example, the codes for bladder wall hemorrhage with stress incontinence, female would be; 596.7 (bladder hemorrhage) and 625.6, (stress incontinence).

BLADDER :
-WITH INCONTINENCE [788.3#]
-WITH STRESS INCONTINENCE, FEMALE [625.6]
-WITH URINARY RETENTION [788.2#] (continued)

596.8 Dilatation
654.4# Dilatation maternal complicating pregnancy
660.2# Dilatation maternal complicating pregnancy obstructing labor [654.4#]

5th digit: 654.4
0. Episode of care NOS or N/A
1. Delivered
2. Delivered with postpartum complication
3. Antepartum complication
4. Postpartum complication

5th digit: 660.2
0. Episode of care NOS or N/A
1. Delivered
3. Antepartum complication

596.9 Disorder
596.59 Disorder detrusor instability
596.59 Disorder functional
0 Disorder neurogenic see under specific neurogenic disorder
596.8 Disorder specified NEC
596.3 Diverticulitis
596.3 Diverticulum
594.0 Diverticulum with calculus
596.8 Eversion
596.8 Fibrosis
595.1 Fibrosis interstitial
595.1 Fibrosis panmural

WITH INCONTINENCE [788.3#]
5th digit: 788.3
0. Unspecified
1. Urge incontinence
2. Stress, male
3. Mixed urge and stress
4. Without sensory awareness
5. Post-void dribbling
6. Nocturnal enuresis
7. Continuous leakage
8. Overflow incontinence
9. Other

WITH RETENTION [788.2#]
5th digit: 788.2
0. Unspecified
1. Incomplete bladder emptying
9. Other specified retention

> ***Bladder disorders with incontinence (retention): When coding the disorders below, code the disorder first, then add the appropriate additional code for the incontinence (retention) - 788.2#, 788.3#, or 625.6. The disorder sequences before the incontinence (retention). For example, the codes for bladder wall hemorrhage with stress incontinence, female would be; 596.7 (bladder hemorrhage) and 625.6, (stress incontinence).***

BLADDER :
-WITH INCONTINENCE [788.3#]
-WITH STRESS INCONTINENCE, FEMALE [625.6]
-WITH URINARY RETENTION [788.2#]
(continued)

793.5	Filling defect
596.2	Fistula NOS
619.0	Fistula female, bladder and genital tract
596.1	Fistula intestinovesical
596.2	Fistula vesical NEC
794.9	Function abnormal finding
596.59	Functional disorder other
596.8	Hemorrhage
596.7	Hemorrhage bladder wall
595.0	Hemorrhage due to acute cystitis
0	Hernia female see 'Cystocele', female
596.8	Hernia male
596.51	Hyperactive
596.7	Hyperemia
344.61	Hyperflexia detrusor
596.54	Hyperreflexia (autonomic)
344.61	Hyperreflexia (autonomic) with cauda equina
596.51	Hypertonicity (of sphincter)
596.8	Hypertrophy
596.4	Hypotonicity
639.2	Injury following abortion, ectopic or molar pregnancy
665.5#	Injury - obstetrical

5th digit: 665.5
- **0. Episode of care NOS or N/A**
- **1. Delivered**
- **4. Postpartum complication**

867.0	Injury traumatic
867.1	Injury traumatic with open wound into cavity
908.2	Injury traumatic late effect
596.59	Instability detrusor
596.9	Lesion
596.8	Leukoplakia vesical
596.52	Low compliance

WITH INCONTINENCE [788.3#]
5th digit: 788.3
- **0. Unspecified**
- **1. Urge incontinence**
- **2. Stress, male**
- **3. Mixed urge and stress**
- **4. Without sensory awareness**
- **5. Post-void dribbling**
- **6. Nocturnal enuresis**
- **7. Continuous leakage**
- **8. Overflow incontinence**
- **9. Other**

WITH RETENTION [788.2#]
5th digit: 788.2
- **0. Unspecified**
- **1. Incomplete bladder emptying**
- **9. Other specified retention**

> ***Bladder disorders with incontinence (retention): When coding the disorders below, code the disorder first, then add the appropriate additional code for the incontinence (retention) - 788.2#, 788.3#, or 625.6. The disorder sequences before the incontinence (retention). For example, the codes for bladder wall hemorrhage with stress incontinence, female would be; 596.7 (bladder hemorrhage) and 625.6, (stress incontinence).***

BLADDER :
-WITH INCONTINENCE [788.3#]
-WITH STRESS INCONTINENCE, FEMALE [625.6]
-WITH URINARY RETENTION [788.2#]
(continued)

596.8	Malacoplakia
596.0	Neck contracture
788.30	Neck syndrome
596.8	Necrosis
596.54	Neurogenic NOS
344.61	Neurogenic with cauda equina
596.0	Obstruction neck
997.5	Obstruction neck postoperative [596.0]
596.0	Obstruction vesicourethral orifice
596.51	Overactive
788.9	Pain
596.53	Paralysis
596.54	Paralysis neurogenic (sensory)
344.61	Paralysis neurogenic (sensory) with cauda equina
596.54	Paralysis spastic (sensory)
344.61	Paralysis spastic (sensory) with cauda equina
596.53	Paralysis sphincter
596.53	Paralysis vesical
0	Prolapse female see 'Cystocele', female
596.8	Prolapse male
794.9	Radioisotope study abnormal
596.59	Relaxation
596.59	Relaxation vesical
V43.5	Replacement (artificial) (prosthesis)
788.20	Retention NEC
596.6	Rupture nontraumatic
867.0	Rupture traumatic
794.9	Scan abnormal
V76.3	Screening cancer (mass)
596.8	Spasm
596.0	Sphincter contracture
596.0	Stenosis
596.0	Stenosis bladder neck (acquired)
596.0	Stricture bladder neck
788.9	Tenesmus

WITH INCONTINENCE [788.3#]
5th digit: 788.3
- **0. Unspecified**
- **1. Urge incontinence**
- **2. Stress, male**
- **3. Mixed urge and stress**
- **4. Without sensory awareness**
- **5. Post-void dribbling**
- **6. Nocturnal enuresis**
- **7. Continuous leakage**
- **8. Overflow incontinence**
- **9. Other**

WITH RETENTION [788.2#]
5th digit: 788.2
- **0. Unspecified**
- **1. Incomplete bladder emptying**
- **9. Other specified retention**

B

BLADDER CONGENITAL

753.8 Absence
753.8 Accessory
753.9 Anomaly NOS
753.8 Anomaly other specified
753.6 Atresia (neck)
753.9 Deformity NOS
753.8 Dilatation
763.1 Dilatation with obstructed labor affecting fetus or newborn
753.8 Diverticulum
753.5 Ectopic
753.5 Exstrophy
753.5 Extroversion
756.71 Hernia congenital (female) (male)
753.6 Obstruction neck
753.6 Obstruction vesicourethral orifice
756.71 Prolapse (female) (male)
753.6 Stenosis (neck)

701.3 BLANCHE (OF MILIAN) ATROPHY

BLAST

921.3 Blindness
0 Concussion see 'Blast', injury
869.0 Injury NOS
869.1 Injury NOS with open wound
0 Injury abdomen or thorax see anatomical site, injury
850.9 Injury brain (see also 'Concussion')
0 Injury brain with skull fracture see 'Fracture', skull
951.5 Injury ear (acoustic nerve trauma)
872.61 Injury ear (acoustic nerve trauma) with tympanic membrane perforation traumatic
872.71 Injury ear (acoustic nerve trauma) with tympanic membrane perforation traumatic complicated
0 Injury internal organs see specific organ, injury
861.20 Injury lung
388.11 Injury otitic (explosive)
0 Syndrome see 'Blast', injury

116.0 BLASTOMYCES (AJELLOMYCES) DERMATITIDIS INFECTION
116.2 BLASTOMYCES LOBOI INFECTIONS

BLASTOMYCOSIS

116.1 Brazilian
116.0 Cutaneous
116.0 Dermatitis
116.0 Disseminated
116.2 Keloidal
116.2 Lobo's
116.0 North American
116.1 Paracoccidioid block
116.0 Pulmonary primary
116.1 South American

709.8 BLEB
379.63 BLEB ASSOCIATED ENDOPHTHALMITIS
V45.69 BLEB FILTERING, EYE (POSTGLAUCOMA) (STATUS)
997.99 BLEB FILTERING, EYE (POSTGLAUCOMA) (STATUS) WITH COMPLICATION
997.99 BLEB FILTERING, EYE (POSTGLAUCOMA) (STATUS) POST CATARACT EXTRACTION
492.0 BLEB LUNG
770.5 BLEB LUNG CONGENITAL

379.60 BLEBITIS POSTPROCEDURAL INFLAMMATION (INFECTION) NOS
379.61 BLEBITIS POSTPROCEDURAL INFLAMMATION (INFECTION) STAGE 1
379.62 BLEBITIS POSTPROCEDURAL INFLAMMATION (INFECTION) STAGE 2
379.63 BLEBITIS POSTPROCEDURAL INFLAMMATION (INFECTION) STAGE 3

BLEEDING

569.3 Anal
628.0 Anovulatory cycle
448.9 Capillary
0 Coagulation defect see 'Coagulation Defect'
286.9 Disorder
621.1 Due to subinvolution uterus
666.2# Due to subinvolution uterus puerperal

5th digit: 666.2

0. Episode of care NOS or N/A
2. Delivered
4. Postpartum complication

388.69 Ear
627.0 Excessive menopausal onset - menorrhagia
626.3 Excessive menstrual onset - menorrhagia pubertal
286.9 Familial (see also 'Coagulation Defect')
626.7 Following intercourse
578.9 GI cause unspecified
523.8 Gums
455.8 Hemorrhoids NOS (see also 'Hemorrhoids')
626.6 Intermenstrual irregular
626.5 Intermenstrual regular
998.11 Intraoperative complicating a procedure
626.4 Irregular menstrual NEC
627.0 Menopausal
627.4 Menopausal artificial (induced)
627.1 Menopausal post
626.0 Menstrual - absence
626.9 Menstrual - disorder
306.52 Menstrual - disorder psychogenic
626.8 Menstrual - disorder other
626.2 Menstrual - excessive heavy periods
627.0 Menstrual - excessive menopausal
626.3 Menstrual - excessive onset of puberty
627.0 Menstrual - excessive premenopausal
V25.3 Menstrual - extraction
626.1 Menstrual - infrequent
626.4 Menstrual - irregular
627.1 Menstrual - postmenopausal bleeding
626.5 Menstrual - regular
V25.3 Menstrual - regulation
626.1 Menstrual - scanty
626.8 Menstrual - suppression
626.8 Menstrual - other specified
528.9 Mouth
611.79 Nipple
784.7 Nosebleed
528.9 Oral soft tissue
626.5 Ovulation
626.7 Postcoital
627.1 Postmenopausal
998.11 Postoperative complicating a procedure

BLEEDING (continued)

666.1# Postpartum (atonic)
666.2# Postpartum delayed or secondary
666.0# Postpartum third stage
5th digit: 666.0-2
0. Episode of care NOS or N/A
2. Delivered
4. Postpartum complication

626.3 Pubertal excessive (menstrual onset)
569.3 Rectal
784.8 Throat
790.92 Time abnormal finding
286.9 Time prolonged coagulation defect - (see also 'Coagulation Defect')
789.9 Umbilical
772.3 Umbilical cord stump after birth
626.9 Uterine NOS
627.0 Uterine climacteric
626.8 Uterine dysfunctional (DUB)
621.1 Uterine subinvolution
666.2# Uterine subinvolution puerperal
5th digit: 666.2
0. Episode of care NOS or N/A
2. Delivered
4. Postpartum complication

626.6 Uterine unrelated to menstrual cycle
623.8 Vaginal NOS
641.9# Vaginal NOS in pregnancy
641.2# Vaginal abruptio placentae in pregnancy
641.1# Vaginal placenta previa in pregnancy
5th digit: 641.1-2, 9
0. Episode of care NOS or N/A
1. Delivered
3. Antepartum complication

626.7 Vaginal postcoital irregular
625.8 Vicarious menstruation

BLENNORRHEA

098.0 NOS (acute)
098.40 Adultorum
523.40 Alveolaris
098.2 Chronic or duration of 2 months or over
098.40 Gonnococcal (neonatorum)
771.6 Inclusion (neonatal) (newborn)
098.40 Neonatorum

BLEPHARITIS

373.00 NOS
373.02 Squamous
373.01 Ulcerative

374.34 BLEPHAROCHALASIS

BLEPHAROCONJUNCTIVITIS

372.20 NOS
372.21 Angular
372.22 Contact

374.46 BLEPHAROPHIMOSIS
374.89 BLEPHAROPLEGIA
0 BLEPHAROPTOSIS SEE 'PTOSIS OF THE EYE'
333.81 BLEPHAROSPASM
333.85 BLEPHAROSPASM DUE TO DRUGS
362.62 BLESSIG'S CYST

631 BLIGHTED OVUM
631 BLIGHTED OVUM WITH COMPLICATION DURING TREATMENT [639.#]
639.# BLIGHTED OVUM WITH COMPLICATION FOLLOWING TREATMENT
4th digit: 639
0. Genital tract and pelvic infection
1. Delayed or excessive hemorrhage
2. Damage to pelvic organs and tissue
3. Renal failure
4. Metabolic disorders
5. Shock
6. Embolism
8. Other specified complication
9. Unspecified complication

BLIND/BLINDNESS

0 Color see 'Blind/Blindness - Color'
377.75 Cortical
368.10 Day
V19.0 Family history (blindness)
360.42 Hypertensive eye
360.41 Hypotensive eye
300.11 Hysterical
369.4 Legal - USA definition
369.00 Legal - WHO definition
579.2 Loop syndrome (postoperative)
0 Night see 'Night Blindness'
369.60 One eye
784.69 Psychic
306.7 Psychogenic
363.31 Sun (solar)
368.12 Temporary (transient)
369.01 Total both eyes
950.9 Traumatic

Code first hearing and/or visual impairment.

V49.85 With deafness (combined visual hearing impairment) (dual sensory impairment)

BLIND/BLINDNESS - COLOR

368.54 Achromatopsia (total)
368.55 Acquired
368.52 Deutan defect (green)
V19.0 Family history
368.54 Monochromatic (cone) (rod)
368.51 Protan defect (red)
368.54 Total
368.53 Tritan defect (blue)
368.59 Other

374.45 BLINK REFLEX DEFICIENT

BLISTER

919.2 Site NOS
919.3 Site NOS infected
911.2 Abdominal wall
911.3 Abdominal wall Infected
916.2 Ankle
916.3 Ankle infected
911.2 Anus
911.3 Anus infected
912.2 Arm upper
912.3 Arm upper infected
912.2 Axilla
912.3 Axilla infected

B

B

BLISTER (continued)

911.2 Back
911.3 Back infected
911.2 Breast
911.3 Breast infected
911.2 Buttock
911.3 Buttock infected
916.2 Calf
916.3 Calf infected
910.2 Cheek
910.3 Cheek infected
911.2 Chest wall
911.3 Chest wall infected
910.2 Ear
910.3 Ear infected
913.2 Elbow
913.3 Elbow infected
910.2 Face
910.3 Face infected
915.2 Finger
915.3 Finger infected
911.2 Flank
911.3 Flank infected
917.2 Foot
917.3 Foot infected
913.2 Forearm
913.3 Forearm infected
911.2 Groin
911.3 Groin infected
910.2 Gum
910.3 Gum infected
914.2 Hand
914.3 Hand infected
917.2 Heel
917.3 Heel infected
916.2 Hip
916.3 Hip infected
911.2 Interscapular region
911.3 Interscapular region infected
916.2 Knee
916.3 Knee infected
911.2 Labia
911.3 Labia infected
906.2 Late effect
916.2 Leg
916.3 Leg infected
910.2 Lip
910.3 Lip infected
919.2 Multiple
919.3 Multiple infected
910.2 Neck
910.3 Neck infected
910.2 Nose
910.3 Nose infected
911.2 Penis
911.3 Penis infected
911.2 Perineum
911.3 Perineum infected
910.2 Scalp
910.3 Scalp infected
912.2 Scapular region
912.3 Scapular region infected
911.2 Scrotum
911.3 Scrotum infected
912.2 Shoulder
912.3 Shoulder infected

BLISTER (continued)

911.2 Testis
911.3 Testis infected
916.2 Thigh
916.3 Thigh infected
910.2 Throat
910.3 Throat infected
915.2 Thumb
915.3 Thumb infected
917.2 Toe
917.3 Toe infected
911.2 Trunk
911.3 Trunk infected
911.2 Vagina
911.3 Vagina infected
911.2 Vulva
911.3 Vulva infected
913.2 Wrist
913.3 Wrist infected
919.2 Other sites
919.3 Other sites infected

787.3 BLOATING ABDOMINAL
757.33 BLOCH SIEMENS SYNDROME
757.33 BLOCH SULZBERGER INCONTINENTIA PIGMENTI
307.9 BLOCQ'S SYNDROME (ASTASIA-ABASIA)

BLOOD

V70.4 Alcohol test
790.7 Culture positive (abnormal findings)
289.9 Disorder NOS
V18.3 Disorder family history
V12.3 Disorder personal history
306.8 Disorder psychogenic
V78.9 Disorder screening
V78.8 Disorder screening other specified
289.89 Disorder specified NEC
V59.0# Donor non-autogenous
5th digit: V59.0
1. Whole
2. Stem cells
9. Other

0 Donor self donation - code underlying disease
289.9 Dyscrasia
776.9 Dyscrasia fetus or newborn NEC
289.9 Forming organ disorder NOS
V12.3 Forming organ disorder history
289.89 Forming organ disorder NEC
790.91 Gas level abnormal
790.29 Glucose abnormal findings
790.29 Glucose high
251.2 Glucose low
578.1 In feces
792.1 In feces occult
608.82 In semen
578.1 In stool
792.1 In stool occult
599.7 In urine
772.0 Loss fetal
762.1 Loss maternal affecting fetus or newborn
790.6 Nitrogen derivatives abnormal
796.2 Pressure elevated
0 Pressure elevated with hypertension see 'Hypertension'
796.4 Pressure fluctuating

BLOOD (continued)

796.2 Pressure labile
0 Pressure labile with hypertension see 'Hypertension'
796.3 Pressure low reading
V72.86 Rh typing encounter
371.12 Staining cornea
790.29 Sugar abnormal findings
790.29 Sugar high
251.2 Sugar low
V70.4 Test medicolegal
V58.83 Test therapeutic drug monitoring encounter
V58.83 Test therapeutic drug monitoring encounter with long term drug use [V58.6#]

5th digit: V58.6

1. Anticoagulants
2. Antibiotics
3. Antiplatelets/antithrombotics
4. Anti-inflammatories non-steroidal (NSAID)
5. Steroids
6. Aspirin
7. Insulin
9. Other

V58.2 Transfusion without reported diagnosis
V72.86 Type encounter (Rh typing)
656.2# Type incompatibility maternal complicating pregnancy - ABO
656.1# Type incompatibility maternal complicating pregnancy - anti-D antibodies (RH)
656.1# Type incompatibility maternal complicating pregnancy - rhesus (RH)
656.2# Type incompatibility maternal complicating pregnancy - other specified

5th digit: 656.1-2

0. Episode of care unspecified or N/A
1. Delivered
3. Antepartum complication

773.1 Type reaction ABO hemolytic perinatal
773.2 Type reaction hemolytic perinatal
773.0 Type reaction RH hemolytic perinatal
747.60 Vessel atresia NEC (congenital)
459.9 Vessel disorder
0 Vessel injury see 'Blood Vessel Injury'
0 Vessel graft complication see 'Complication' vascular
459.9 Vessel occlusion NEC
V43.4 Vessel replacement (artificial) (prosthesis) (vessel)
459.0 Vessel rupture spontaneous
V42.89 Vessel transplant status

> ***Injury of a blood vessel can be a laceration, A-V fistula, aneurysm, or hematoma. Use the injury code found by anatomical site (the name of the blood vessel).***

> ***The blood vessels below are those vaguely defined, poorly specified vessels in general body areas. Specific artery and vein injuries can be found under their anatomical name. For example carotid artery or aorta.***

BLOOD VESSEL INJURY

0 See specified blood vessel or anatomical site
902.9 Abdomen and pelvis
902.87 Abdomen and pelvis multiple
902.89 Abdomen and pelvis other
902.87 Abdomen multiple

BLOOD VESSEL INJURY (continued)

903.5 Digital
900.9 Head NOS
900.9 Head and neck NOS
900.82 Head and neck multiple
900.89 Head and neck multiple other
908.4 Late effect - abdomen and pelvis vessels
908.3 Late effect - head and neck vessels
908.3 Late effect - lower extremity and unspecified vessels
908.4 Late effect - thorax vessels
908.3 Late effect - upper extremity vessels
904.8 Lower extremity unspecified
904.7 Lower extremity multiple
904.7 Lower extremity other specified
900.9 Neck NOS
902.9 Pelvis NOS
902.87 Pelvis and abdomen multiple
902.87 Pelvis multiple
901.9 Thorax
901.83 Thorax multiple
903.9 Upper extremity unspecified
903.8 Upper extremity multiple
903.8 Upper extremity other specified
904.9 Site unspecified

610.1 BLOODGOOD'S DISEASE
757.39 BLOOM (-MACHACEK) (-TORRE) SYNDROME
732.4 BLOUNT-BARBER SYNDROME (TIBIA VARA)
732.4 BLOUNT'S DISEASE (TIBIA VARA)
802.6 BLOW OUT FRACTURE ORBIT CLOSED
802.7 BLOW OUT FRACTURE ORBIT OPEN
491.2# BLUE BLOATER (SYNDROME)

5th digit: 491.2

0. NOS
1. With (acute) exacerbation
2. With acute bronchitis

270.0 BLUE DIAPER SYNDROME
746.9 BLUE DISEASE (CONGENITAL HEART ANOMALY)
381.02 BLUE DRUM SYNDROME
216.# BLUE NEVUS M8780/0
173.# BLUE NEVUS MALIGNANT M8780/3

4th digit: 173, 216

0. Lip skin
1. Eyelid including canthus
2. Ear external (auricle) (pinna)
3. Face (cheek) (nose)
4. Scalp, neck
5. Trunk, back, chest
6. Upper limb including shoulder
7. Lower limb including hip
8. Other specified sites
9. Skin NOS

756.51 BLUE SCLERA AND FRAGILITY OF BONE WITH DEAFNESS
756.51 BLUE SCLERA SYNDROME
445.02 BLUE TOE SYNDROME

862.8 BLUNT CHEST TRAUMA
862.9 BLUNT CHEST TRAUMA WITH OPEN WOUND (INTRATHORACIC)
908.0 BLUNT CHEST TRAUMA LATE EFFECT
0 BLUNT TRAUMA INTERNAL ORGANS SEE SPECIFIC ORGAN, INJURY

368.8 BLURRED VISION
782.62 BLUSHING EXCESSIVE
273.1 BMH (BENIGN MONOCLONAL HYPERGAMMAGLOBULINEMIA)
0 BMI (BODY MASS INDEX) SEE BODY MASS INDEX
794.7 BMR ABNORMAL
V65.0 BOARDER (SEEKING CONSULTATION) ACCOMPANYING SICK PERSON
704.8 BOCKHART'S IMPETIGO (SUPERFICIAL FOLLICULITIS)
046.2 BODECHTEL GUTTMANN DISEASE
334.8 BODER-SEDGWICK SYNDROME (ATAXIA-TELANGIECTASIA)
V15.85 BODY FLUID EXPOSURE HISTORY
V49.89 BODY IMPAIRMENT (ENTIRE)
132.1 BODY LICE

V85.#(#): These codes are for use in persons over 20 years old.

V85.#(#) BODY MASS INDEX (BMI) ADULT

4th or 4th and 5th digit: V85

- **0. Less than 19**
- **1. 19-24**
- **2#. 25-29**
  - **1. 25.0-25.9**
  - **2. 26.0-26.9**
  - **3. 27.0-27.9**
  - **4. 28.0-28.9**
  - **5. 29.0-29.9**
- **3#. 30-39**
  - **0. 30.0-30.9**
  - **1. 31.0-31.9**
  - **2. 32.0-32.9**
  - **3. 33.0-33.9**
  - **4. 34.0-34.9**
  - **5. 35.0-35.9**
  - **6. 36.0-36.9**
  - **7. 37.0-37.9**
  - **8. 38.0-38.9**
  - **9. 39.0-39.9**
- **4. 40 and over**

V85.5#: These codes are for use in persons age 2-20 years old. These percentiles are based on the growth charts published by the Centers for Disease Control and Prevention (CDC).

V85.5# BODY MASS INDEX (BMI) PEDIATRIC

5th digit: V85.5

- **1. Less than 5th percentile for age**
- **2. 5th percentile to less than 85th percentile for age**
- **3. 85th percentile to less than 95th percentile for age**
- **4. Greater than or equal to 95th percentile for age**

307.3 BODY ROCKING

135 BOECK'S DISEASE (SARCOIDOSIS)
530.4 BOERHAAVE'S SYNDROME (SPONTANEOUS ESOPHAGEAL RUPTURE)
0 BOIL SEE 'CARBUNCLE'
238.72 BOMFORD RHOADS ANEMIA

BONE

756.9 Absence congenital
756.9 Agenesis
733.99 Atrophy - NOS
733.7 Atrophy - due to disuse
733.99 Atrophy - due to infection
733.99 Atrophy - posttraumatic
738.9 Deformity (acquired)
738.8 Deformity (acquired) other specified
733.91 Development arrested
733.90 Disorder (and cartilage)
733.29 Disorder (and cartilage) fibrocystic
733.99 Disorder (and cartilage) other specified NEC
648.7# Disorder back, pelvis and lower limbs maternal current (co-existent) in pregnancy

5th digit: 648.7

- **0. Episode of care NOS or N/A**
- **1. Delivered**
- **2. Delivered with postpartum complication**
- **3. Antepartum complication**
- **4. Postpartum complication**

V59.2 Donor non - autogenous
0 Donor self - donation, code underlying disease
756.59 Fibrosis (diffuse) congenital
733.29 Fibrous dysplasia (monostotic)
756.54 Fibrous dysplasia polyostotic congenital
794.9 Function study abnormal
996.67 Graft complication - infection or inflammation
996.49 Graft complication – mechanical **[V43.6#]**

5th digit: V43.6

- **0. Site unspecified**
- **1. Shoulder**
- **2. Elbow**
- **3. Wrist**
- **4. Hip**
- **5. Knee**
- **6. Ankle**
- **9. Other**

996.78 Graft complication - other
996.67 Growth stimulator complication - infection or inflammation
996.49 Growth stimulator complication – mechanical **[V43.6#]**

5th digit: V43.6

- **0. Site unspecified**
- **1. Shoulder**
- **2. Elbow**
- **3. Wrist**
- **4. Hip**
- **5. Knee**
- **6. Ankle**
- **9. Other**

996.78 Growth stimulator complication - other
733.99 Hyperplasia
733.99 Hypertrophy
756.9 Hypoplasia NOS

BONE (continued)

730.9# Infection
5th digit: 730.9
0. Site NOS
1. Shoulder region
2. Upper arm (elbow) (humerus)
3. Forearm (radius) (wrist) (ulna)
4. Hand (carpal) (metacarpal) (fingers)
5. Pelvic region (hip) (buttock) (femur)
6. Lower leg (fibula) (knee) (patella) (tibia)
7. Ankle and foot (metatarsals) (toes) (tarsals)
8. Other (head) (neck) (rib) (skull) (trunk) (vertebrae)
9. Multiple

284.9 Marrow absence - NOS (idiopathic)
284.89 Marrow aplasia - acquired (secondary)
284.09 Marrow absence – congenital (hereditary)
284.01 Marrow aplasia - congenital
289.9 Marrow disorder
V59.3 Marrow donor non - autogenous
0 Marrow donor self - donation code underlying disease
284.9 Marrow failure
284.89 Marrow failure - acquired
284.09 Marrow failure - congenital
996.85 Marrow graft-versus-host disease (acute) (chronic)
289.9 Marrow hyperplasia
284.9 Marrow hypoplasia
284.09 Marrow hypoplasia - congenital
287.30 Marrow megakaryocytic
289.89 Marrow necrosis
996.85 Marrow transplant failure
V42.81 Marrow transplant status
794.9 Scan abnormal
V59.2 Tissue donor non - autogenous
0 Tissue donor self - donation code underlying disease
V42.4 Tissue transplant status

BONE SPUR

726.91 NOS
726.73 Calcaneus
726.39 Elbow
726.73 Foot
726.4 Hand
726.73 Heel
726.5 Hip
726.5 Iliac crest
726.60 Knee
726.91 Nose
726.33 Olecranon
726.69 Prepatellar or subpatellar
726.4 Wrist
726.8 Other specified site

0 BONIFIL'S DISEASE SEE 'HODGKIN'S' DISEASE
758.6 BONNEVIE ULLRICH SYNDROME
386.19 BONNIER'S SYNDROME
780.79 BONVALE DAM FEVER
0 BORDERLINE GLAUCOMA SEE 'GLAUCOMA', BORDERLINE
301.83 BORDERLINE PERSONALITY DISORDER
759.89 BORJESON-FORRSMAN-LEHMANN SYNDROME

062.9 BORNA DISEASE
074.1 BORNHOLM DISEASE (EPIDEMIC PLEURODYNIA)
477.9 BOSTOCK'S DISEASE (SEE ALSO 'HAY FEVER')
048 BOSTON EXANTHEM

BOTULISM

005.1 NOS (food poisoning)
040.42 NOS non foodborne
005.1 Food poisoning
040.41 Infant
040.42 Non-foodborne
005.1 With myasthenia [358.1]
040.42 Wound

536.1 BOUCHARD'S DISEASE (MYOPATHIC GASTRIC DILATATION)
298.3 BOUFFEE DELIRANTE
391.9 BOUILLAUD'S SYNDROME (RHEUMATIC HEART DISEASE)
759.5 BOURNEVILLE (-PRINGLE) SYNDROME (TUBEROUS SCLEROSIS)
082.1 BOUTONNEUSE FEVER
736.21 BOUTONNIERE DEFORMITY FINGER (ACQUIRED)
427.2 BOUVERET-HOFFMANN SYNDROME (PAROXYSMAL TACHYCARDIA)

BOWEL

787.99 Habits change
564.9 Hyperactive syndrome
0 Inflammatory see 'Enteritis'
639.2 Injury post abortive
564.1 Irritable syndrome
557.# Ischemic syndrome
4th digit: 557
0. Acute
1. Chronic
9. Unspecified transient

0 Locked see 'Bowel', obstruction
564.81 Neurogenic
560.9 Obstruction (stenosis) (stricture) (occlusion)
751.1 Obstruction congenital and infantile
560.81 Obstruction due to adhesions
560.89 Obstruction due to mural thickening
560.31 Obstruction gallstone
997.4 Obstruction post op
560.81 Obstruction post op due to adhesions
579.3 Short syndrome
787.5 Sounds abnormal
787.5 Sounds absent
787.5 Sounds hyperactive
560.2 Volvulus (torsion) (strangulation)

232.9 BOWEN'S DISEASE SITE UNSPECIFIED
0 BOWEN'S DISEASE SITE SPECIFIED SEE 'CARCINOMA IN SITU' SKIN BY SITE M8081/2

BOWLEG

736.42 Acquired
754.44 Congenital
268.1 Rachitic

371.31 BOWMAN'S MEMBRANE RUPTURE
371.31 BOWMAN'S MEMBRANE FOLDS AND RUPTURE
0 BOXER'S FRACTURE SEE 'FRACTURE', METACARPAL
004.2 BOYD'S DYSENTERY - GROUP C SHIGELLA (SHIGELLA BOYDII)

B

203.0#	BOZZOLO'S MULTIPLE MYELOMA M9730/3 **5th digit: 203.0** **0. Without mention of remission** **1. In remission**

BPH (BENIGN PROSTATE HYPERTROPHY)

600.00	NOS
600.00	With bladder neck obstruction [596.0]

> ***See 'LUTS' or 'Lower Urinary Tract Symptoms' for the additional code to identify the specific lower urinary tract symptoms.***

600.01	With urinary obstruction, retention or other lower urinary tract symptoms
V53.7	BRACE DEVICE (ORTHOPEDIC) FITTING AND ADJUSTMENT

B

BRACHIAL

442.0	Artery aneurysm (ruptured) (cirsoid) (varix) (false)
440.2#	Artery arteriosclerosis (degeneration)
440.2#	Artery arteriosclerosis (degeneration) with chronic complete or total occlusion [440.4] **5th digit: 440.2** **0. Unspecified** **1. With intermittent claudication** **2. With rest pain or rest pain and intermittent claudication** **9. Other atherosclerosis extremities**

> ***When coding arteriosclerosis of the extremities use an additional code, if applicable to identify chronic complete or total occlusion of the artery of the extremities (440.4).***

440.24	Artery arteriosclerosis (degeneration) with ischemic gangrene or ischemic gangrene ulceration, or ulceration and intermittent claudication, rest pain [707.8]
440.23	Artery arteriosclerosis (degeneration) with ulceration, or ulceration and intermittent claudication, rest pain [707.8]
440.3#	Artery bypass graft arteriosclerosis - extremities
440.3#	Artery bypass graft arteriosclerosis - extremities with chronic complete or total occlusion [440.4] **5th digit: 440.3** **0. Unspecified graft** **1. Autologous vein bypass graft** **2. Nonautologous biological bypass graft**
444.21	Artery embolism (thrombosis) (occlusion) (infarction)
903.1	Artery injury
908.3	Artery injury late effect
903.1	Blood vessels injury
903.1	Blood vessels laceration traumatic (rupture) (hematoma) (avulsion) (aneurysm)
908.3	Blood vessels laceration late effect
723.4	Neuritis
353.0	Plexus disorders (nondiscogenic)
742.8	Plexus displacement congenital
953.4	Plexus injury
767.6	Plexus injury birth trauma
353.0	Plexus syndrome
0	Radiculitis discogenic see 'Cervical Disc Disorder'
723.4	Radiculitis nondiscogenic
451.83	Vein phlebitis

> ***Injury to nerve includes laceration, traumatic neuroma, or lesion in continuity. Search for these codes by anatomical site or name.***

759.89	BRACHMAN-DE LANGE SYNDROME (AMSTERDAM DWARF, MENTAL RETARDATION AND BRACHYCEPHALY)
756.0	BRACHYCEPHALY HEMIFACIAL
759.89	BRACHYMORPHISM ECTOPIA LENTIS
078.82	BRADLEY'S DISEASE (EPIDEMIC VOMITING)

BRADYCARDIA

427.89	Unspecified
427.81	Chronic
779.81	Newborn
779.81	Neonatal
768.9	Neonatal NOS due to birth asphyxia
768.6	Neonatal mild or moderate due to birth asphyxia
768.5	Neonatal severe due to birth asphyxia
427.89	Nodal
997.1	Postoperative (during or resulting from a procedure)
337.0	Reflex
427.89	Sinoatrial
427.81	Sinoatrial chronic
427.89	Sinus
427.81	Sinus persistent (severe)
427.81	Tachycardia syndrome
427.89	Vagal
427.81	With PAT
277.6	BRADYKINASE 1 DEFICIENCY
277.5	BRAILSFORD MORQUIO SYNDROME (MUCOPOLYSACCHARIDOSIS IV)
732.3	BRAILSFORD'S DISEASE RADIAL HEAD
732.5	BRAILSFORD'S DISEASE TARSAL SCAPHOID

BRAIN

794.01	Abnormal echoencephalogram
794.02	Abnormal electroencephalogram (EEG)
794.00	Abnormal function study
794.09	Abnormal scan
740.0	Absence - congenital
742.2	Absence - specified part congenital
742.2	Agenesis - specified part congenital
742.9	Anomaly NOS congenital
742.4	Anomaly multiple NOS congenital
742.2	Aplasia - specified part congenital
331.9	Atrophy
331.9	Atrophy with dementia **[294.1#]**
290.10	Atrophy - NOS with dementia presenile
331.0	Atrophy - Alzheimer's
331.0	Atrophy - Alzheimer's with dementia **[294.1#]**
331.11	Atrophy - circumscribed Pick's
331.11	Atrophy - circumscribed Pick's with dementia **[294.1#]**
331.19	Atrophy - circumscribed other
331.19	Atrophy - circumscribed other with dementia **[294.1#]**
742.4	Atrophy - congenital
331.2	Atrophy - senile
331.2	Atrophy – senile with dementia **[294.1#]** **5th digit: 294.1** **0. Without behavioral disturbance or NOS** **1. With behavioral disturbance**

BRAIN (continued)

348.4 Compression
767.0 Compression due to hemorrhagic injury at birth
0 Concussion see 'Cerebral', concussion
348.9 Condition
348.8 Condition other specified
851.8# Contusion NOS (with hemorrhage)
851.9# Contusion NOS with open intracranial wound (with hemorrhage)
851.4# Contusion brain stem (with hemorrhage)
851.5# Contusion brain stem with open intracranial wound (with hemorrhage)
851.4# Contusion cerebellum (with hemorrhage)
851.5# Contusion cerebellum with open intracranial wound (with hemorrhage)
851.0# Contusion cerebral cortex (with hemorrhage)
851.1# Contusion cerebral cortex with open intracranial wound (with hemorrhage)
851.0# Contusion cortex (cerebral) (with hemorrhage)
851.1# Contusion cortex (cerebral) with open intracranial wound (with hemorrhage)
851.4# Contusion occipital lobe (with hemorrhage)
851.5# Contusion occipital lobe with open intracranial wound (with hemorrhage)

5th digit: 851.0-9
0. Level of consciousness (LOC) NOS
1. No LOC
2. LOC < 1 hr
3. LOC 1 - 24 hrs
4. LOC > 24 hrs with return to prior level
5. LOC > 24 hrs without return to prior level: or death before regaining consciousness, regardless of duration of LOC
6. LOC duration NOS
9. With concussion NOS

348.9 Damage
348.1 Damage - anoxic
768.7 Damage – anoxic, hypoxic ischemic in newborn
0 Damage - child NEC see 'Cerebral', palsy
767.0 Damage - due to birth injury
997.01 Damage - resulting from a procedure
348.8 Death
742.9 Deformity congenital
742.2 Deformity reduction congenital
0 Degeneration see 'Cerebral', degeneration
0 Disease inflammatory see 'Encephalitis'
348.9 Disease organic
437.0 Disease organic arteriosclerotic
331.2 Disease senile
331.2 Disease senile with dementia [294.1#]

5th digit: 294.1
0. Without behavioral disturbance or NOS
1. With behavioral disturbance

996.63 Electrode complication - infection or inflammation
996.2 Electrode complication - mechanical
996.75 Electrode complication - other
794.00 Function study abnormal (see also 'Brain', abnormal)
0 Hemorrhage see 'Hemorrhage', brain
742.2 Hypoplasia

BRAIN (continued)

854.## Injury NOS

4th digit: 854
0. Without mention of open intracranial wound
1. With mention of open intracranial wound

5th digit: 854
0. Level of consciousness NOS
1. No LOC
2. LOC < 1 hr
3. LOC 1 - 24 hrs
4. LOC > 24 hrs with return to prior level
5. LOC > 24 hrs without return to prior level: or death before regaining consciousness, regardless of duration of LOC
6. LOC duration NOS
9. With concussion NOS

348.8 Lesion
742.9 Lesion congenital
437.9 Lesion vascular NOS
437.1 Lesion vascular degenerative
437.2 Lesion vascular hypertensive
V12.54 Lesion vascular old without residual
0 Lesion vascular with residual see 'Late Effect', cerebrovascular disease
348.8 Mass
V53.02 Neuropacemaker fitting and adjustment
0 Occlusion see 'Infarction', by site
0 Palsy see 'Cerebral', palsy
794.09 Scan abnormal
341.9 Sclerosis (general) (lobular)
331.0 Sclerosis lobar atrophic
331.0 Sclerosis lobar atrophic with dementia [294.1#]

5th digit: 294.1
0. Without behavioral disturbance or NOS
1. With behavioral disturbance

SOFTENING (NECROTIC) (PROGRESSIVE)

434.9# NOS

5th digit: 434.9
0. Without cerebral infarction
1. With cerebral infarction

437.0 Arteriosclerotic
742.4 Congenital
434.1# Embolic
431 Hemorrhagic
434.0# Thrombotic

5th digit: 434.0, 1
0. Without cerebral infarction
1. With cerebral infarction

SYNDROME

310.9 NOS
291.2 Chronic alcoholic
319 Congenital
310.9 Organic
310.2 Postcontusional
310.2 Posttraumatic
293.9 Posttraumatic psychotic
293.0 Posttraumatic psychotic - acute
294.8 Posttraumatic psychotic - chronic
293.1 Posttraumatic psychotic - subacute

B

BRAIN (continued)

SYNDROME (continued)

310.9 Psycho-organic
294.9 Psychotic
290.0 Senile
290.10 With presenile brain disease
294.9 With psychosis, psychotic reaction

BRAIN STEM

348.4 Compression
851.4# Contusion (with hemorrhage)
851.5# Contusion with open intracranial wound (with hemorrhage)
5th digit: 851.4-5
0. Level of consciousness NOS
1. No LOC
2. LOC< 1 hr
3. LOC 1 - 24 hrs
4. LOC > 24 hrs with return to prior level
5. LOC >24 hrs without return to prior level: or death before regaining consciousness, regardless of duration of LOC
6. LOC duration NOS
9. With concussion NOS

348.4 Herniation
434.91 Infarction
434.11 Infarction embolic
997.02 Infarction iatrogenic
0 Infarction old with residual see 'Late Effect', cerebrovascular disease
V12.54 Infarction old without residual
997.02 Infarction postoperative
434.01 Infarction thrombotic
851.6# Laceration (with hemorrhage)
851.7# Laceration with open intracranial wound (with hemorrhage)
5th digit: 851.6-7
0. Level of consciousness NOS
1. No LOC
2. LOC < 1 hr
3. LOC 1 - 24 hrs
4. LOC > 24 hrs with return to prior level
5. LOC > 24 hrs without return to prior level: or death before regaining consciousness, regardless of duration of LOC
6. LOC duration NOS
9. With concussion NOS

744.41 BRANCHIAL ARCH SYNDROME

BRANCHIAL CLEFT

744.42 Cyst congenital
744.41 Fistula
744.41 Sinus or fistula congenital
744.41 Vestige

686.8 BRANDT'S SYNDROME (ACRODERMATITIS ENTEROPATHICA)

644.1# BRAXTON HICKS CONTRACTIONS
5th digit: 644.1
0. Episode of care NOS or N/A
3. Antepartum complication

985.8 BRAZIERS DISEASE
116.1 BRAZILIAN BLASTOMYCOSIS

569.3 BRBPR (BRIGHT RED BLOOD PER RECTUM)

061 BREAKBONE FEVER

BREAST

793.8# Abnormal x-ray, ultrasound, thermography
5th digit: 793.8
0. Unspecified
1. Mammographic microcalcification
9. Other abnormal findings (calcification) (calculus)

757.6 Absence congenital (or nipple)
V45.71 Absence postsurgical
757.6 Accessory congenital (or nipple)
675.9# And nipple infection maternal due to pregnancy
675.8# And nipple infection other specified maternal due to pregnancy
757.9 Anomaly NOS
611.4 Atrophy
676.3# Atrophy puerperal
5th digit: 675.8-9, 676.3
0. Episode of care NOS or N/A
1. Delivered
2. Delivered with postpartum complication
3. Antepartum complication
4. Postpartum complication

V50.1 Augmentation (elective) (for unacceptable cosmetic appearance)
259.1 Buds (premature)
793.89 Calcification - mammographic
793.89 Calculus - mammographic
0 Cancer see 'Cancer', breast
V76.10 Cancer screening unspecified
V76.11 Cancer screening mammogram for high risk patient
V76.12 Cancer screening mammogram NEC
V76.19 Cancer screening specified type NEC
611.79 Discharge (male) (female)
610.1 Disease cystic chronic
610.1 Disease fibrocystic
611.0 Disease inflammatory
676.9# Disorder lactating NOS maternal due to pregnancy
676.8# Disorder lactating other maternal due to pregnancy
676.3# Disorder other and unspecified maternal due to pregnancy
5th digit: 676.3, 8-9
0. Episode of care NOS or N/A
1. Delivered
2. Delivered with postpartum complication
3. Antepartum complication
4. Postpartum complication

611.9 Disorder nonpuerperal NOS
611.8 Disorder nonpuerperal other specified
611.8 Droop (cooper's)
611.8 Duct occlusion nonpuerperal
610.4 Ductal ectasia
778.7 Engorgement newborn
676.2# Engorgement maternal due to pregnancy
676.8# Feeding difficulty maternal due to pregnancy
5th digit: 676.2, 8
0. Episode of care NOS or N/A
1. Delivered
2. Delivered with postpartum complication
3. Antepartum complication
4. Postpartum complication

BREAST (continued)

610.2 Fibroadenosis
610.1 Fibrocystic disease
610.3 Fibrosclerosis
611.8 Hematoma nontraumatic nonpuerperal
611.1 Hyperplasia nonpuerperal
611.1 Hypertrophy nonpuerperal
757.6 Hypoplasia congenital
996.69 Implant complication - infection or inflammation
996.54 Implant complication - mechanical
996.79 Implant complication - other
V52.4 Implant - fitting and adjustment
V50.1 Implant - insertion admission
V52.4 Implant - removal admission
V45.83 Implant - removal status
V43.82 Implant - status
611.79 Induration nonpuerperal
611.8 Infarction nonpuerperal
675.9# Infection nipple maternal due to pregnancy
675.8# Infection nipple maternal other due to pregnancy

5th digit: 675.8-9
0. Episode of care NOS or N/A
1. Delivered
2. Delivered with postpartum complication
3. Antepartum complication
4. Postpartum complication

959.19 Injury
911.8 Injury other and unspecified superficial
911.9 Injury other and unspecified superficial infected
611.72 Mass or lump nonpuerperal
793.81 Microcalcification mammographic
611.71 Pain
611.71 Pain psychogenic [307.80]
611.8 Pendulous
V50.1 Reduction (elective) (for unacceptable cosmetic appearance)
V50.41 Removal prophylactic
611.8 Subinvolution (postlactational) (postpartum) nonpuerperal
757.6 Supernumerary congenital (or nipple)
611.79 Symptoms other
757.6 Tissue ectopic
611.0 Ulcer

784.99 BREATH FOUL (FETID)
312.81 BREATH HOLDING CHILD
786.9 BREATH HOLDING SPELL

BREATHING

V57.0 Exercises
786.09 Labored
784.99 Mouth
524.59 Mouth causing malocclusion
786.09 Periodic
327.22 Periodic high altitude

102.9 BREDA'S DISEASE

BREECH

652.2# Delivery
763.0 Delivery and extraction affecting fetus or newborn
660.0# Delivery obstructing labor [**652.2#**]

5th digit: 652.2, 660.0
0. Episode of care NOS or N/A
1. Delivered
3. Antepartum complication

BREECH (continued)

669.6# Delivery with breech extraction
669.6# Extraction

5th digit: 669.6
0. Episode of care NOS or N/A
1. Delivered

761.7 Presentation affecting fetus or newborn before L&D
652.2# Presentation buttocks, complete or frank
660.0# Presentation buttocks, complete or frank obstructing labor [**652.2#**]
652.8# Presentation footling or incomplete
660.0# Presentation footling or incomplete obstructing labor [**652.8#**]
652.6# Presentation with multiple gestation
660.0# Presentation with multiple gestation obstructing labor [**652.6#**]
652.1# Presentation converted to cephalic presentation (or other malpresentation)
660.0# Presentation converted to cephalic presentation (or other malpresentation) obstructing labor [**652.1#**]

5th digit: 652.1-2, 6, 8, 660.0
0. Episode of care NOS or N/A
1. Delivered
3. Antepartum complication

624.09 BREISKY'S DISEASE (KRAUROSIS VULVAE)

289.2 BRENNEMANN'S SYNDROME

BRENNER TUMOR

220 Site NOS
0 Site specified see 'Benign Neoplasm', by site M9000/0
236.2 Borderline malignancy site NOS
0 Borderline malignancy site specified see 'Neoplasm Uncertain Behavior', by site M9000/1
183.0 Malignant site NOS
0 Malignant site specified see 'Cancer', by site M9000/3

032.0 BRETONNEAU'S DISEASE (DIPHTHERITIC MALIGNANT ANGINA)
631 BREUS MOLE
631 BREUS MOLE WITH COMPLICATION DURING TREATMENT [**639.#**]
639.# BREUS MOLE WITH COMPLICATION FOLLOWING TREATMENT

4th digit: 639
0. Genital tract and pelvic infection
1. Delayed or excessive hemorrhage
2. Damage to pelvic organs and tissue
3. Renal failure
4. Metabolic disorders
5. Shock
6. Embolism
8. Other specified complication
9. Unspecified complication

756.16 BREVIOCOLLIS
569.3 BRIGHT RED BLOOD PER RECTUM (BRBPR)
583.9 BRIGHT'S DISEASE (SEE ALSO 'NEPHRITIS')
0 BRIGHT'S DISEASE ARTERIOSCLEROTIC SEE 'HYPERTENSIVE', RENAL DISEASE

B

202.0# BRILL SYMMERS DISEASE
5th digit: 202.0
0. NOS
1. Lymph nodes of head, face, neck
2. Lymph nodes intrathoracic
3. Lymph nodes abdominal
4. Lymph nodes axilla and upper limb
5. Lymph nodes inguinal region and lower limb
6. Lymph nodes intrapelvic
7. Spleen
8. Lymph nodes multiple sites

B

081.1 BRILL ZINSSER DISEASE
081.0 BRILL'S RECRUDESCENT TYPHUS - FLEA BORNE
081.1 BRILL'S RECRUDESCENT TYPHUS - LOUSE BORNE
151.9 BRINTON'S DISEASE (LEATHER BOTTLE STOMACH)
002.9 BRION-KAYSER DISEASE
300.81 BRIQUET'S DISORDER OR SYNDROME

BRISSAUD'S

244.# Infantilism
4th digit: 244
0. Postsurgical
1. Postablative (irradiation)
2. Iodine ingestion
3. PAS, phenylbut, resorcinol
8. Secondary NEC
9. NOS

243 Infantilism congenital
244.9 Meige syndrome (infantile myxedema)
307.23 Tic (motor verbal)

272.2 BROAD-BETALIPOPROTEINEMIA

BROAD LIGAMENT

752.19 Absence congenital
752.19 Accessory congenital
752.10 Anomaly congenital
752.19 Atresia congenital
620.8 Cyst or polyp
620.9 Disorder noninflammatory
620.8 Disorder specified NEC
620.7 Hematoma (hematocele)
620.8 Infarction
867.6 Injury (traumatic)
867.7 Injury (traumatic) with open wound
639.2 Injury post abortive
620.6 Laceration syndrome
620.8 Polyp
620.8 Rupture

518.0 BROCK'S SYNDROME (ATELECTASIS DUE TO ENLARGED LYMPH NODES)

BROCQ'S DISEASE

694.0 Herpetic dermatitis
698.3 Lichen simplex chronicus
691.8 Neurodermatitis (atopic) (diffuse)
696.2 Parapsoriasis
698.2 Prurigo

730.1# BRODIE'S JOINT DISEASE
5th digit: 730.1
0. Site NOS
1. Shoulder region
2. Upper arm (elbow) (humerus)
3. Forearm (radius) (wrist) (ulna)
4. Hand (carpal) (metacarpal) (fingers)
5. Pelvic region and thigh (hip) (buttock) (femur)
6. Lower leg (fibula) (knee) (patella) (tibia)
7. Ankle and/or foot (metatarsals) (toes)
8. Other (head) (neck) (rib) (skull) (vertebrae)
9. Multiple

429.83 BROKEN HEART SYNDROME
705.89 BROMHIDROSIS
349.82 BROMIDISM (BROMISM) ACUTE DUE TO CORRECT SUBSTANCE PROPERLY ADMINISTERED
0 BROMIDISM (BROMISM) ACUTE DUE TO OVERDOSE OR POISONING SEE 'TABLE OF DRUGS AND CHEMICALS'
304.1# BROMIDISM (BROMISM) CHRONIC
5th digit: 304.1
0. NOS
1. Continuous
2. Episodic
3. In remission

0 BRONCHIAL SEE 'BRONCHUS, BRONCHIAL'

BRONCHIECTASIS

494.# NOS
748.61 Congenital
494.# Fusiform
494.# Postinfectious
494.# Recurrent
4th digit: 494
0. Without acute exacerbation
1. With acute exacerbation

011.5# Tuberculous
5th digit: 011.5
0. NOS
1. Lab not done
2. Lab pending
3. Microscopy positive (in sputum)
4. Culture positive - microscopy negative
5. Culture negative - microscopy positive
6. Culture and microscopy negative confirmed by other methods

494.# With COPD
4th digit: 494
0. Without acute exacerbation
1. With acute exacerbation

When coding an infection, use an additional code, [041.#(#)], to identify the organism. See 'Bacterial Infection'.

BRONCHIOLITIS

ACUTE (SUBACUTE) (INFECTIOUS)

466.19 NOS
466.19 Catarrhal
466.11 Due to RSV (respiratory syncytial virus)
466.11 Due to RSV (respiratory syncytial virus) with bronchospasm or obstruction
487.1 Influenzal
466.19 With bronchospasm or obstruction
466.19 Due to other specified organism

BRONCHIOLITIS (continued)

491.8 Chronic
491.8 Obliterans
996.84 Obliterans status post lung transplant
516.8 Obliterans with organizing pneumonia (BOOP)
506.4 Obliterative due to fumes and vapors chronic

BRONCHITIS QUICK REFERENCE

490 NOS
466.0 Acute
493.9# Allergic NOS
493.0# Allergic with stated cause

5th digit: 493.0, 9
0. NOS
1. With status asthmaticus
2. With (acute) exacerbation

493.## Asthmatic (acute)

4th or 4th and 5th digit: 493
0. Extrinsic (or allergic with stated cause)
1. Intrinsic
2. Chronic obstructive with COPD
8#. Other specified
1. Exercised induced bronchospasm
2. Cough variant
9. NOS (or allergic cause not stated)

5th digit: 493.0-2, 9
0. NOS
1. With status asthmaticus
2. With (acute) exacerbation

491.9 Chronic
491.2# Chronic obstructive
491.2# Emphysematous

5th digit: 491.2
0. NOS
1. With (acute) exacerbation
2. With acute bronchitis

490 With tracheitis (tracheobronchitis)
466.0 With tracheitis (tracheobronchitis) acute
491.8 With tracheitis (tracheobronchitis) chronic

BRONCHITIS

934.1 Arachidic
507.0 Aspiration food or vomitus
493.2# Asthmatic (chronic)

5th digit: 493.2
0. NOS
1. With status asthmaticus
2. With (acute) exacerbation

466.19 Capillary acute (with bronchospasm or obstruction)
491.8 Capillary chronic
011.3# Caseous (tuberculous)

5th digit: 011.3
0. NOS
1. Lab not done
2. Lab pending
3. Microscopy positive (in sputum)
4. Culture positive - microscopy negative
5. Culture negative - microscopy positive
6. Culture and microscopy negative confirmed by other methods

104.8 Castellani's
490 Catarrhal
466.0 Catarrhal acute
491.0 Catarrhal chronic
506.0 Chemical (or fumes)(vapor) acute
506.4 Chemical (or fumes)(vapor) chronic
466.0 Croupous
466.0 Exudative (fibrinous) (membranous) (pseudomembranous) acute or subacute
502 Moulder's
466.0 Mucopurulent (purulent) acute
491.1 Mucopurulent (purulent) chronic
491.8 Obliterans
491.2# Obstructive (chronic)

5th digit: 491.2
0. NOS
1. With (acute) exacerbation
2. With acute bronchitis

493.2# Obstructive asthmatic chronic

5th digit: 493.2
0. NOS
1. With status asthmaticus
2. With (acute) exacerbation

491.1 Pituitious
466.0 Pneumococcal acute or subacute (with bonchospasm or obstruction)
466.0 Pseudomembranous
508.8 Radiation
490 Simple
491.8 Ulcerative
487.1 With influenza, flu, grippe

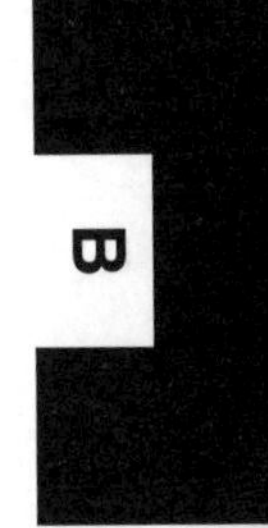

If the diagnosis is not specified as acute on the record, select the chronic or NOS code. If the medical record indicates that the patient sought care due to an exacerbation of a chronic condition, consult the physician for further documentation.

BRONCHITIS ACUTE

466.0 NOS
507.0 Aspiration food or vomitus
493.## Asthmatic
4th or 4th and 5th digit: 493
0. Extrinsic (or allergic with stated cause)
1. Intrinsic
2. Chronic obstructive with COPD
8#. Other specified
1. Exercised induced bronchospasm
2. Cough variant
9. NOS (or allergic cause not stated)
5th digit: 493.0-2, 9
0. NOS
1. With status asthmaticus
2. With (acute) exacerbation

466.19 Capillary (with bronchospasm or obstruction)
466.0 Catarrhal
506.0 Chemical (or fumes)
466.0 Croupous
466.0 Exudative (fibrinous) (membranous) (pseudomembranous)(septic)
466.0 Mucopurulent (purulent)
466.0 Pneumococcal (viral)(purulent)
508.8 Radiation
466.0 Simple
466.0 Subacute
466.0 With bronchospasm
466.0 With tracheitis (tracheobronchitis)

If the diagnosis is not specified as acute on the record, select the chronic or NOS code. If the medical record indicates that the patient sought care due to an exacerbation of a chronic condition, consult the physician for further documentation.

BRONCHITIS CHRONIC

491.9 NOS
493.2# Asthmatic obstructive
5th digit: 493.2
0. NOS
1. With status asthmaticus
2. With (acute) exacerbation

491.8 Capillary
491.0 Catarrhal
506.4 Chemical (or fumes)
506.4 Due to fumes and vapors

BRONCHITIS CHRONIC (continued)

491.2# Emphysematous
5th digit: 491.2
0. NOS
1. With (acute) exacerbation
2. With acute bronchitis

491.1 Fetid
502 Moulder's
491.1 Mucopurulent (purulent)
491.8 Obliterans
491.2# Obstructive (chronic)
5th digit: 491.2
0. NOS
1. With (acute) exacerbation
2. With acute bronchitis

493.2# Obstructive asthmatic chronic
5th digit: 493.2
0. NOS
1. With status asthmaticus
2. With (acute) exacerbation

491.1 Pituitous
508.8 Radiation
V81.3 Screening
491.0 Simple
491.0 Smokers'
487.1 With influenza, flu, grippe
491.8 With tracheobronchitis or tracheitis
491.8 Other specified

485 BRONCHOALVEOLITIS
519.19 BRONCHOCELE MEANING DILATATION OF BRONCHUS
240.9 BRONCHOCELE MEANING GOITER
530.89 BRONCHOESOPHAGEAL FISTULA
117.9 BRONCHOHEMISPOROSIS
518.89 BRONCHOLITHIASIS
748.3 BRONCHOMALACIA
112.89 BRONCHOMONILIASIS

BRONCHOPNEUMONIA (SEE ALSO 'PNEUMONIA')

485 NOS
466.19 With acute bronchiolitis
466.11 With acute bronchiolitis due to RSV (respiratory syncytial virus)

When coding an infection, use an additional code, [041.#(#)], to identify the organism. See 'Bacterial Infection'.

466.19 With acute bronchiolitis due to other infectious organism
491.8 With chronic bronchiolitis

518.6 BRONCHOPULMONARY ASPERGILLOSIS ALLERGIC
519.19 BRONCHOPULMONARY DISEASE
770.7 BRONCHOPULMONARY DYSPLASIA ARISING IN PERINATAL PERIOD

> ***Bronchospasm is an integral part of asthma and should be coded only if the underlying disease is not identified.***

BRONCHOSPASM

519.11 NOS
519.11 Acute
493.81 Exercise induced
0 With asthma see 'Asthma'
0 With bronchitis see 'Bronchitis'
466.11 With bronchiolitis (acute) due to RSV (respiratory syncytial virus)

> ***When coding an infection, use an additional code, [041.#(#)], to identify the organism. See 'Bacterial Infection'.***

466.19 With bronchiolitis (acute) due to other infectious organism
496 WIth chronic obstructive pulmonary disease (COPD)
0 With emphysema see 'Emphysema'

519.19 BRONCHOSTENOSIS

BRONCHUS, BRONCHIAL

748.3 Absence, agenesis or atresia (congenital)
901.89 Blood vessel injury
519.19 Calcification
519.19 Compression
519.19 Congestion
519.19 Constriction
519.19 Contraction
519.19 Contracture
519.19 Deformity acquired
494.# Dilatation
519.19 Disease
494.# Diverticulum acquired
4th digit: 494
0. Without acute exacerbation
1. With acute exacerbation

748.3 Diverticulum congenital
519.19 Erosion
862.21 Injury
862.31 Injury with open wound
908.0 Injury late effect
519.19 Obstruction
519.19 Ossification
519.19 Paralysis
748.3 Rudimentary tracheal congenital
519.11 Spasm
519.19 Stenosis
748.3 Stenosis congenital
519.19 Ulcer

255.41 BRONZE DISEASE (ADDISON'S) (SKIN)

275.0 BRONZED DIABETES (IRON)
959.09 BROW INJURY
652.4# BROW PRESENTATION
652.6# BROW PRESENTATION WITH MULTIPLE GESTATION
660.0# BROW PRESENTATION WITH MULTIPLE GESTATION OBSTRUCTING LABOR [652.6#]
5th digit: 652.4, 6, 660.0
0. Episode of care NOS or N/A
1. Delivered
3. Antepartum complication

344.89 BROWN SEQUARD'S SYNDROME

989.5 BROWN SPIDER BITE
995.0 BROWN SPIDER BITE WITH ANAPHYLAXIS [989.5]
756.59 BROWN SPOT SYNDROME
378.61 BROWN'S (TENDON SHEATH) SYNDROME

BRUCELLA

023.1 Abortus infection
023.3 Canis infection
023.9 Infection
023.8 Infection other
023.0 Melitensis infection
023.2 Suis infection
V74.8 Screening exam

759.89 BRUCK DE LANGE SYNDROME
733.99 BRUCK'S DISEASE
746.89 BRUGADA SYNDROME
125.1 BRUG'S FILARIASIS
757.39 BRUGSCH'S SYNDROME (ACROPACHYDERMA)
285.8 BRUHL'S DISEASE
285.8 BRUHL'S SPLENIC ANEMIA WITH FEVER
0 BRUISE SEE 'CONTUSION'
772.6 BRUISING FETUS OR NEWBORN
785.9 BRUIT ARTERIAL
279.04 BRUTON'S X-LINKED AGAMMAGLOBULINEMIA
306.8 BRUXISM
327.53 BRUXISM SLEEP RELATED
770.7 BUBBLY LUNG SYNDROME

BUBO

289.3 NOS
099.0 Chancroidal
099.1 Climatic
098.89 Gonococcal
099.0 Hemophilus ducreyi
099.8 Indolent
099.8 Inguinal
099.8 Phagedenic
099.1 Tropical
099.8 Venereal

0 BUBONOCELE SEE 'HERNIA', INGUINAL
020.0 BUBONIC PLAGUE
528.9 BUCCAL CAVITY DISEASE
732.1 BUCHANAN'S JUVENILE OSTEOCHONDROSIS
733.3 BUCHEM'S SYNDROME (HYPEROSTOSIS CORTICALIS)

BUCKET HANDLE TEAR

717.0 Cartilage (old)
717.0 Knee (old)
836.0 Medial meniscus acute

453.0 BUDD - CHIARI SYNDROME (HEPATIC VEIN THROMBOSIS)
648.9# BUDD - CHIARI SYNDROME (HEPATIC VEIN THROMBOSIS) MATERNAL CURRENT (CO-EXISTENT) IN PREGNANCY [453.0]
5th digit: 648.9
0. Episode of care NOS or N/A
1. Delivered
2. Delivered with postpartum complication
3. Antepartum complication
4. Postpartum complication

B

B

495.2 BUDGERIGAR-FANCIERS' DISEASE
717.89 BUDINGER-LUDLOFF-LAWEN DISEASE OR SYNDROME
443.1 BUERGER'S DISEASE
431 BULBAR ARTERY HEMORRHAGE (RUPTURE)
335.22 BULBAR PALSY PROGRESSIVE
344.89 BULBAR PALSY SUPRANUCLEAR NEC
745.0 BULBAR SEPTUM DEFECT
335.22 BULBAR SYNDROME
436 BULBAR SYNDROME LATERAL
756.0 BULGING FONTANELS
783.6 BULIMIA
307.51 BULIMIA NERVOSA
307.51 BULIMIA NONORGANIC
787.7 BULKY STOOLS
709.8 BULLA(AE)
082.8 BULLIS FEVER SYNDROME

BULLOUS

694.9 Dermatoses
646.8# Dermatoses herpes gestationis
5th digit: 646.8
0. Episode of care NOS or N/A
1. Delivered
2. Delivered with postpartum complication
3. Antepartum complication
4. Postpartum complication

694.8 Dermatoses other specified
684 Impetigo
371.23 Keratopathy corneal
384.01 Myringitis acute without otitis media
694.5 Pemphigoid

790.6 BUN AND CREATINE ELEVATED

BUNDLE BRANCH BLOCK

426.50 NOS
426.53 Bifascicular NOS
426.53 Bilateral NOS
426.3 Left NOS
426.2 Left anterior fascicular
426.3 Left anterior with left posterior
426.3 Left complete
426.2 Left hemiblock
426.2 Left posterior fascicular
0 Left with right see 'Bundle Branch Block', right
426.4 Right NOS
426.53 Right with left NOS (incomplete) (main stem)
426.52 Right with left anterior fascicular
426.54 Right with left anterior with left posterior
426.53 Right with left fascicular NOS
426.51 Right with left posterior fascicular
426.54 Trifascicular
426.4 Wilson's type

426.7 BUNDLE OF KENT SYNDROME (ANOMALOUS ATRIOVENTRICULAR EXCITATION)
040.81 BUNGPAGGA
727.1 BUNION
066.3 BUNYAMWERA FEVER (VIRAL)

BUPHTHALMOS

743.20 Congenital
743.22 Keratoglobus congenital
743.22 Megalocornea congenital
743.21 Simple congenital
743.22 With other ocular anomalies congenital

272.3 BURGER-GRUTZ SYNDROME (ESSENTIAL FAMILIAL HYPERLIPEMIA)
577.8 BURKE'S SYNDROME (PANCREATIC INSUFFICIENCY AND CHRONIC NEUTROPENIA)

BURKITT'S

200.2# Lymphoma
200.2# Tumor site M9750/3
5th digit: 200.2
0. NOS, extranodal and solid organ sites
1. Lymph nodes of head, face, neck
2. Lymph nodes intrathoracic
3. Lymph nodes abdominal
4. Lymph nodes axilla and upper limb
5. Lymph nodes inguinal region and lower limb
6. Lymph nodes intrapelvic
7. Spleen
8. Lymph nodes multiple sites

"Rule of Nines": A general guideline to estimate percentage of body surface.

each arm =9%, each leg = 18%, anterior trunk = 18%, posterior trunk = 18%, genitalia = 9%.

BURN

949.# NOS site or NOS percentage of body surface
4th digit: 949
0. Unspecified degree
1. Erythema (first degree)
2. Blisters (second degree)
3. Full thickness skin (third degree NOS)
4. Necrosis of underlying tissues (deep third degree) without loss of a body part
5. Necrosis of underlying tissues (deep third degree) with loss of a body part

BURN (continued)

Code 948.## is recommended as an additional code to specify the percentage of body surface involved.

948.## Classified according to % of body surface

4th digit: 948

0. **Burn (any degree) involving less than 10%**
1. **Burn (any degree) 10-19 %**
2. **Burn (any degree) 20-29 %**
3. **Burn (any degree) 30-39 %**
4. **Burn (any degree) 40-49 %**
5. **Burn (any degree) 50-59 %**
6. **Burn (any degree) 60-69 %**
7. **Burn (any degree) 70-79 %**
8. **Burn (any degree) 80-89 %**
9. **Burn (any degree) 90 % or more**

5th digit: 948

0. **With third degree less than 10% or unspecified**
1. **With third degree 10-19%**
2. **With third degree 20-29%**
3. **With third degree 30-39%**
4. **With third degree 40-49%**
5. **With third degree 50-59%**
6. **With third degree 60-69%**
7. **With third degree 70-79%**
8. **With third degree 80-89%**
9. **With third degree 90% or more of body surface**

940.# Eye and adnexa

4th digit: 940

0. **Chemical burn of eyelids and periocular area**
1. **Other burns of eyelids and periocular area**
2. **Alkaline chemical burn cornea and conjunctiva**
3. **Acid chemical burn of cornea and conjunctival**
4. **Other burn of cornea and conjunctival**
5. **Burn with resulting rupture and destruction of eyeball**
9. **Unspecified burn of eye and adnexa**

BURN (continued)

941.## Head, neck, face

4th digit: 941

0. **Unspecified degree**
1. **Erythema (first degree)**
2. **Blisters (second degree)**
3. **Full thickness skin (third degree NOS)**
4. **Necrosis of underlying tissues (deep third degree) without loss of a body part**
5. **Necrosis of underlying tissues (deep, third degree) with loss of a body part**

5th digit: 941

0. **Face and head unspecified site**
1. **Ear (any part)**
2. **Eye (with other parts of face, head, and neck)**
3. **Lip (s)**
4. **Chin**
5. **Nose (septum)**
6. **Scalp (any part)**
7. **Forehead and cheek**
8. **Neck**
9. **Multiple sites (except with eye) of face, head, neck**

958.3 Infected

947.# Internal organs (chemical)

4th digit: 947

0. **Mouth and pharynx; gum, tongue**
1. **Larynx, trachea, lung**
2. **Esophagus**
3. **Gastrointestinal tract; colon, rectum, small intestine, stomach**
4. **Vagina, uterus**
8. **Other specified sites**
9. **Unspecified sites**

906.9 Late effect - unspecified site
906.5 Late effect - eye, face, head, neck
906.6 Late effect - wrist, hand
906.7 Late effect - other extremities
906.8 Late effect - other specified sites

945.## Lower limb, thigh, knee, ankle, foot, toe

4th digit: 945

0. **Unspecified degree**
1. **Erythema (first degree)**
2. **Blisters (second degree)**
3. **Full thickness skin (third degree NOS)**
4. **Necrosis of underlying tissues (deep third degree) without loss of a body part**
5. **Necrosis of underlying tissues (deep third degree) with loss of a body part**

5th digit: 945

0. **Lower limb (leg) unspecified site**
1. **Toe (s) (nail)**
2. **Foot**
3. **Ankle**
4. **Lower leg**
5. **Knee**
6. **Thigh (any part)**
9. **Multiple sites of lower limb (s)**

BURN (continued)

946.# Multiple specified site
4th digit: 946
0. Unspecified degree
1. Erythema (first degree)
2. Blisters (second degree)
3. Full thickness skin (third degree NOS)
4. Necrosis of underlying tissues (deep third degree) without loss of a body part
5. Necrosis of underlying tissues (deep third degree) with loss of a body part

692.7# Sunburn
5th digit: 692.7
1. NOS (first degree)
6. Second degree
7. Third degree

692.82 Sunburn tanning bed

942.## Trunk, chest, wall, abdominal wall, back, genitalia
4th digit: 942
0. Unspecified degree
1. Erythema (first degree)
2. Blisters (second degree)
3. Full thickness skin (third degree NOS)
4. Necrosis of underlying tissues (deep third degree) without loss of a body part
5. Necrosis of underlying tissues (deep third degree) with loss of a body part

5th digit: 942
0. Trunk unspecified site
1. Breast
2. Chest wall excluding breast and nipple
3. Abdominal wall
4. Back (any part)
5. Genitalia
9. Other and multiple sites of trunk

943.## Upper limb except wrist and hand
4th digit: 943
0. Unspecified degree
1. Erythema (first degree)
2. Blisters (second degree)
3. Full thickness skin (third degree NOS)
4. Necrosis of underlying tissues (deep third degree) without loss of a body part
5. Necrosis of underlying tissues (deep, third degree) with loss of a body part

5th digit: 943
0. Upper limb unspecified site
1. Forearm
2. Elbow
3. Upper arm
4. Axilla
5. Shoulder
6. Scapular region
9. Multiple except wrist and hand

BURN (continued)

944.## Wrist and hand, fingers, thumbs
4th digit: 944
0. Unspecified degree
1. Erythema (first degree)
2. Blisters (second degree)
3. Full thickness skin (third degree NOS)
4. Necrosis of underlying tissues (deep third degree) without loss of a body part
5. Necrosis of underlying tissues (deep third degree) with loss of a body part
5th digit: 944
0. Hand unspecified site
1. Single digit [finger (nail)] other than thumb
2. Thumb (nail)
3. Two or more digits not including thumb
4. Two or more digits including thumb
5. Palm
6. Back of hand
7. Wrist
8. Multiple sites of wrist (s) and hand(s)

BURN LATE EFFECT

906.9 Unspecified site
906.5 Eye, face, head, neck
906.6 Wrist, hand
906.7 Other extremities
906.8 Other specified sites

732.3 BURN'S DISEASE (LOWER ULNA)
275.42 BURNETT'S SYNDROME (MILK-ALKALI)
253.3 BURNIER'S SYNDROME HYPOPHYSEAL DWARFISM
266.2 BURNING FEET SYNDROME
782.0 BURNING SENSATION SKIN

BURSA

727.82 Calcification
756.9 Deformity congenital
727.9 Disorder
727.89 Disorder other

BURSITIS

727.3 NOS
726.71 Achilles
726.90 Adhesive site unspecified
726.79 Ankle
726.5 Buttock
726.79 Calcaneal
727.82 Calcification
727.2 Carpenter's occupational
726.63 Collateral ligament - fibula
726.62 Collateral ligament - tibia
275.4 Crystal induced
726.19 Deltoid
726.2 Duplay's
726.33 Elbow
727.2 Elbow occupational
726.63 Fibular
726.63 Fibular collateral ligament
726.8 Finger
726.79 Foot
098.52 Gonococcal

BURSITIS (continued)

274.0	Gouty
726.4	Hand
727.2	Hand occupational
726.4	Hand or wrist
726.5	Hip
726.69	Infrapatellar
726.5	Ischiogluteal
726.60	Knee
727.2	Knee occupational
727.2	Occupational origin
726.33	Olecranon
726.61	Pes anserinus
478.29	Pharyngeal
727.51	Popliteal
726.65	Prepatellar
727.3	Radiohumeral
726.19	Scapulohumeral
726.0	Scapulohumeral adhesive
726.10	Shoulder
726.0	Shoulder adhesive
726.19	Subacromial
726.0	Subacromial adhesive
726.19	Subcoracoid
726.19	Subdeltoid
726.0	Subdeltoid adhesive
726.69	Subpatellar
095.7	Syphilitic
726.62	Tibial
726.62	Tibial collateral ligament
726.79	Toe
726.5	Trochanteric
726.4	Wrist
0	See also 'Tendinitis'

031.1 BURULI ULCER

695.89 BURY'S DISEASE (ERYTHEMA ELEVATUM DIUTINUM)

710.1 BUSCHKE'S DISEASE (SCLERODERMA)

710.1 BUSCHKE'S DISEASE (SCLERODERMA) WITH LUNG INVOLVEMENT [517.2]

710.1 BUSCHKE'S DISEASE (SCLERODERMA) WITH MYOPATHY [359.6]

730.1# BUSQUET'S DISEASE

5th digit: 730.1
- **0. Site NOS**
- **1. Shoulder region**
- **2. Upper arm (elbow) (humerus)**
- **3. Forearm (radius) (wrist) (ulna)**
- **4. Hand (carpal) (metacarpal) (fingers)**
- **5. Pelvic region and thigh (hip) (buttock) (femur)**
- **6. Lower leg (fibula) (knee) (patella) (tibia)**
- **7. Ankle and/or foot (metatarsals) (toes)**
- **8. Other (head) (neck) (rib) (skull) (vertebrae)**
- **9. Multiple**

117.5 BUSSE BUSCHKE'S DISEASE (CRYPTOCOCCOSIS)

959.19 BUTTOCK INJURY

911.8 BUTTOCK INJURY SUPERFICIAL

911.9 BUTTOCK INJURY SUPERFICIAL INFECTED

085.1 BUTTON BISKRA DELHI ORIENTAL

736.21 BUTTONHOLE HAND

616.10 BV (BACTERIAL VAGINOSIS/VAGINITIS NOS)

066.3 BWAMBA FEVER (VIRAL)

Do not use code 996.03, complication of a device, implant or graft mechanical cardiac, when the physician documents that arteriosclerosis has caused an occlusion of a bypass graft. In coding terms, this is considered to be a normal progression of arteriosclerosis rather than a complication of a graft. Assign code 414.0#, arteriosclerosis of a bypass graft, coronary.

B

BYPASS GRAFT

998.2 Accidental puncture or laceration during procedure
414.0# Arteriosclerosis coronary
414.0# Arteriosclerosis coronary with chronic complete or total occlusion [414.2]
5th digit: 414.0
2. Autologous vein bypass graft
3. Nonautologous biological bypass graft
4. Autologous artery bypass graft (gastroepiploic) (internal mammary)
5. Unspecified type of bypass graft
7. Bypass graft of transplanted heart

440.3# Arteriosclerosis extremities
440.3# Arteriosclerosis extremities with chronic complete or total occlusion [440.4]
5th digit: 440.3
0. Unspecified graft
1. Autologous vein bypass graft
2. Nonautologous biological bypass graft

BYPASS GRAFT (continued)

414.0# Coronary arteriosclerosis
414.0# Coronary arteriosclerosis with chronic complete or total occlusion [414.2]
5th digit: 414.0
2. Autologous vein bypass graft
3. Nonautologous biological bypass graft
4. Autologous artery bypass graft (gastroepiploic) (internal mammary)
5. Unspecified type of bypass graft
7. Bypass graft of transplanted heart

996.61 Coronary artery - infection or inflammation
996.03 Coronary artery - mechanical complication
996.72 Coronary artery - other complication
V45.81 Coronary - status
997.02 CVA (infarction) post op iatrogenic
V45.3 Intestinal - status
410.## MI acute during procedure
4th digit: 410
0. Anterior lateral
1. Anterior
2. Inferior lateral
3. Inferior posterior
4. Inferior other
5. Lateral
6. Posterior
7. Subendocardial
8. Other site
9. Site NOS
5th digit: 410
0. Episode of care
1. Initial episode of care
2. Subsequent episode of care

415.11 Pulmonary embolism infarction postop iatrogenic
998.31 Wound dehiscence internal
998.32 Wound dehiscence external
998.59 Wound infection

504 BYSSINOSIS
958.5 BYWATERS SYNDROME
908.6 BYWATERS SYNDROME LATE EFFECT

005.2 C. WELCHII FOOD POISONING

795.82 CA 125 ELEVATED (CANCER ANTIGEN 125)

0 CA IN SITU SEE 'CARCINOMA IN SITU', BY SITE

0 CA METASTATIC SEE 'CANCER', BY SITE, METASTATIC OR 'CANCER METASTATIC'

0 CA SEE 'CANCER', BY SITE

CABG (CORONARY ARTERY BYPASS GRAFT)

998.2 Accidental puncture or laceration during procedure
414.0# Arteriosclerosis
414.0# Arteriosclerosis with chronic complete or total occlusion [414.2]

5th digit: 414.0
2. Autologous vein bypass graft
3. Nonautologous biological bypass graft
4. Autologous artery bypass graft (gastroepiploic) (internal mammary)
5. Unspecified type of bypass graft
7. Bypass graft of transplanted heart

996.61 Complication - infection or inflammation
996.03 Complication - mechanical
996.72 Complication - other specified
997.02 CVA (Infarction) post op iatrogenic
410.## MI acute during procedure

4th digit: 410
0. Anterior lateral
1. Anterior
2. Inferior lateral
3. Inferior posterior
4. Inferior other
5. Lateral
6. Posterior
7. Subendocardial
8. Other site
9. Site NOS

5th digit: 410
0. Episode of care
1. Initial episode of care
2. Subsequent episode of care

415.11 Pulmonary embolism infarction postop iatrogenic
V45.81 Status
998.32 Wound dehiscence external
998.31 Wound dehiscence internal
998.59 Wound infection

799.4 Cachexia – Code first underlying condition, if known

799.4 CACHEXIA

0 CACHEXIA CANCEROUS OR MALIGNANT SEE 'CANCER', BY SITE, MALIGNANT

276.51 CACHEXIA DEHYDRATION

799.4 CACHEXIA DUE TO MALNUTRITION

414.0# CAD (CORONARY ARTERY DISEASE)
414.0# CAD (CORONARY ARTERY DISEASE) WITH CHRONIC COMPLETE OR TOTAL OCCLUSION [414.2]

5th digit: 414.0
0. Unspecified type of vessel, native or graft
1. Native coronary vessel
2. Autologous vein bypass graft
3. Nonautologous biological bypass graft
4. Autologous artery bypass graft (gastroepiploic) (internal mammary)
5. Unspecified type of bypass graft
6. Native vessel of transplanted heart
7. Bypass graft of transplanted heart

709.09 CAFE' AU LAIT SPOTS
305.9# CAFFEINE ABUSE NONDEPENDENT

5th digit: 305.9
0. Unspecified
1. Continuous
2. Episodic
3. In remission

756.59 CAFFEY'S SYNDROME (INFANTILE CORTICAL HYPEROSTOSIS)

993.3 CAISSON DISEASE

909.4 CAISSON DISEASE LATE EFFECT

0 CALCANEAL SEE 'CALCANEUS, CALCANEAL'

845.02 CALCANEOFIBULAR SEPARATION (RUPTURE) (TEAR) (LACERATION)

845.02 CALCANEOFIBULAR STRAIN (SPRAIN) (AVULSION) (HEMARTHROSIS)

755.67 CALCANEONAVICULAR BAR

CALCANEUS, CALCANEAL

732.5 Apophysitis (juvenile)
755.67 Coalition
736.76 Deformity other (acquired)
726.73 Spur

275.49 CALCAREOUS DEGENERATION NEC

502 CALCICOSIS LUNG (OCCUPATIONAL)

727.82 CALCIFIC TENDINITIS

726.11 CALCIFIC TENDINITIS SHOULDER

275.40 CALCIFICATION GENERAL

275.40 CALCIFICATION METASTATIC

0 CALCIFICATION SEE ANATOMICAL SITE

275.49 CALCINOSIS

709.3 CALCINOSIS CIRCUMSCRIPTA

709.3 CALCINOSIS CUTIS

275.49 CALCINOSIS INTERVERTEBRALIS **[722.9#]**

5th digit: 722.9
0. Unspecified
1. Cervical
2. Thoracic
3. Lumbar

275.49 CALCIPHYLAXIS

246.0 CALCITONIN HYPERSECRETION

CALCIUM

275.41 Deficiency
269.3 Deficiency (dietary)
275.49 Degeneration NEC
275.42 Excess
275.49 Infiltrate (muscle)

CALCIUM (continued)

275.40 Metabolic disorder NOS
252.0# Metabolic disorder hyperparathyroid
5th digit: 252.0
0. NOS
1. Primary
2. Secondary non-renal
8. Other specified
252.1 Metabolic disorder hypoparathyroid
252.9 Metabolic disorder parathyroid gland disorder
252.8 Metabolic disorder parathyroid gland disorder other specified
268.2 Metabolic disorders with osteomalacia
268.0 Metabolic disorders with rickets active
268.1 Metabolic disorders with rickets late effect
268.9 Metabolic disorders with vitamin D deficiency
275.40 Thesaurismosis

CALCULUS, CALCULOUS

543.9 Appendix
0 Bile duct (any) see 'Choledocholithiasis'
594.1 Bladder
594.0 Bladder diverticulum
793.89 Breast - mammographic
518.89 Bronchus
0 Cholesterol (pure) (solitary) see 'Cholelithiasis'
372.54 Conjunctiva
523.6 Dental (subgingival) (supragingival)
592.9 Disease
608.89 Epididymis
0 Gallbladder see 'Cholelithiasis'
751.69 Gallbladder congenital
0 Hepatic (duct) see 'Choledocholithiasis'
560.39 Intestine (obstructed)
592.0 Kidney
753.3 Kidney congenital
592.0 Kidney staghorn
274.11 Kidney uric acid
375.57 Lacrimal passages
0 Liver (impacted) see 'Choledocholithiasis'
518.89 Lung
478.19 Nose
577.8 Pancreatic (duct)
527.5 Parotid gland
602.0 Prostate
592.0 Renal
753.3 Renal congenital
274.11 Renal uric acid
527.5 Salivary system
608.89 Seminal vesicle
592.0 Staghorn kidney
527.5 Stensen's duct
527.5 Sublingual (duct) (gland)
750.26 Sublingual (duct) (gland) congenital
527.5 Submaxillary (duct) (gland)
594.8 Suburethral
474.8 Tonsil
523.6 Tooth, teeth
608.89 Tunica vaginalis
592.1 Ureter
594.2 Urethral
274.11 Uric acid kidney
592.9 Urinary
594.9 Urinary tract lower unspecified
594.8 Urinary tract lower other

CALCULUS, CALCULOUS (continued)

623.8 Vagina
594.1 Vesical (impacted)
527.5 Wharton's duct

916.8 CALF INJURY OTHER AND UNSPECIFIED SUPERFICIAL
916.9 CALF INJURY OTHER AND UNSPECIFIED SUPERFICIAL INFECTED
0 CALIFORNIA DISEASE SEE 'COCCIDIOIDOMYCOSIS'
062.5 CALIFORNIA VIRUS ENCEPHALITIS
371.03 CALIGO CORNEA
700 CALLUS
732.1 CALVE-LEGG-PERTHES SYNDROME (OSTEOCHONDROSIS FEMORAL CAPITAL)
732.1 CALVE (-PERTHES) OSTEOCHONDROSIS FEMORAL CAPITAL
755.59 CAMPTODACTYLY (CONGENITAL)
008.43 CAMPYLOBACTER INFECTION INTESTINE
756.59 CAMURATI-ENGELMANN DIAPHYSEAL SCLEROSIS
752.89 CANAL OF NUCK ANOMALY SPECIFIED (DEFORMITY)
375.31 CANALICULITIS LACRIMAL ACUTE
375.41 CANALICULITIS LACRIMAL CHRONIC
743.65 CANALICULUS LACRIMALIS ABSENCE CONGENITAL
330.0 CANAVAN'S DISEASE

CANCER

Symptoms of a malignancy such as pain or nausea should not replace the cancer code(s). Sequence the cancer first and the cancer associated pain 338.3 or nausea second.

199.1 NOS or by morphology
199.1 NOS metastatic
195.2 Abdomen cavity, organ viscera, ill- defined (non GI)
198.89 Abdomen cavity, organ viscera, ill- defined (non GI) metastatic
173.5 Abdomen skin
198.2 Abdomen skin metastatic
173.5 Abdomen wall ill-defined
198.2 Abdomen wall ill-defined metastatic
171.5 Abdomen wall soft tissue
198.89 Abdomen wall soft tissue metastatic
195.8 Abdominopelvic
198.89 Abdominopelvic metastatic
160.9 Accessory sinus
197.3 Accessory sinus metastatic
170.4 Acromion
198.5 Acromion metastatic
147.1 Adenoid
198.89 Adenoid metastatic
183.9 Adnexa (uterine) NEC
198.82 Adnexa (uterine) NEC metastatic
183.8 Adnexa (uterine) other specified sites
183.8 Adnexa (uterine) overlapping sites
194.0 Adrenal cortex
194.0 Adrenal gland
194.0 Adrenal medulla
198.7 Adrenal metastatic

CANCER (continued)

159.9 Alimentry canal ill-defined
197.8 Alimentry tract ill-defined metastatic

143.9 Alveolar (alveolus) NOS
198.89 Alveolar (alveolus) NOS metastatic
143.9 Alveolar (alveolus) mucosa NOS
143.1 Alveolar (alveolus) mucosa lower
198.89 Alveolar (alveolus) mucosa metastatic
143.0 Alveolar (alveolus) mucosa upper
170.1 Alveolar ridge or process (upper or lower) (odontogenic)
198.5 Alveolar ridge or process (upper or lower) (odontogenic) metastatic

If an encounter is for chemotherapy or radiotherapy, sequence the therapy first, with the cancer as an additional code.

156.2 Ampulla of vater
197.8 Ampulla of vater metastatic

159.1 Angiosarcoma of spleen
170.8 Ankle bone
198.5 Ankle bone metastatic
173.7 Ankle skin
198.2 Ankle skin metastatic

154.8 Anorectum
197.5 Anorectum metastatic

164.2 Anterior mediastinum
197.1 Anterior mediastinum metastatic

160.2 Antrum maxillary (highmore)
197.3 Antrum maxillary (highmore) metastatic
151.2 Antrum pyloric
197.8 Antrum pyloric metastatic
160.1 Antrum tympanicum
197.3 Antrum tympanicum metastatic

154.3 Anus NOS
197.5 Anus NOS metastatic
154.2 Anus canal
197.5 Anus canal metastatic
173.5 Anus canal skin
172.5 Anus canal skin melanoma
198.2 Anus canal skin metastaic
172.5 Anus margin melanoma
V10.06 Anus personal history
173.5 Anus skin
198.2 Anus skin metastatic
154.2 Anus sphincter
197.5 Anus sphincter metastatic
173.5 Anus sphincter skin
172.5 Anus sphincter skin melanoma
198.2 Anus sphincter skin metastatic
154.8 Anus undetermined origin overlapping

194.6 Aortic body
198.89 Aortic body metastatic

153.5 Appendix
197.5 Appendix metastatic

Use an additional code to identify estrogen receptor status. V86.0 Estrogen receptor positive status (ER+) or V86.1 Estrogen receptor negative status (ER-).

174.0 Areola female soft tissue
175.0 Areola male soft tissue
198.81 Areola metastatic

CANCER (continued)

173.6 Arm skin
198.2 Arm skin metastatic
171.2 Arm soft tissue
198.89 Arm soft tissue metastatic

170.9 Articular cartilage
198.5 Articular cartilage metastatic

148.2 Aryepiglottic fold NOS (hypopharyngeal) (marginal zone)
198.89 Aryepiglottic fold NOS (hypopharyngeal) (marginal zone) metastatic
161.1 Aryepiglottic fold laryngeal aspect
197.3 Aryepiglottic fold laryngeal aspect metastatic

161.3 Arytenoid cartilage
197.3 Arytenoid cartilage metastatic

170.8 Astragalus
198.5 Astragalus metastatic

173.2 Auditory canal external
198.2 Auditory canal external metastatic
160.1 Auditory tube internal
197.3 Auditory tube internal metastatic
147.2 Auditory tube opening
198.89 Auditory tube opening metastatic

195.1 Axilla ill-defined
198.89 Axilla ill-defined metastatic
196.3 Axilla nodes metastatic
171.4 Axilla soft tissue
198.89 Axilla soft tissue metastatic

195.8 Back ill-defined
198.89 Back ill-defined metastatic
173.5 Back skin
198.2 Back skin metastatic

When an encounter is for placement of radioactive implants, use the code for the cancer, rather than the encounter codes.

171.7 Back soft tissue
198.89 Back soft tissue metastatic

184.1 Bartholin gland
198.82 Bartholin gland metastatic

191.0 Basal ganglia
198.3 Basal ganglia metastatic

156.1 Bile duct common
156.1 Bile duct cystic
156.1 Bile duct extrahepatic
156.1 Bile duct hepatic
155.1 Bile duct intrahepatic
156.9 Bile duct intrahepatic and extrahepatic
197.8 Bile duct metastatic

155.1 Biliary canaliculi intrahepatic
155.1 Biliary canals interlobular
155.1 Biliary gall duct intrahepatic
197.8 Biliary metastatic
156.1 Biliary passages NOS
155.1 Biliary passages intrahepatic
156.9 Bilary tract

188.9 Bladder
188.3 Bladder anterior wall
188.1 Bladder dome
188.2 Bladder lateral wall
198.1 Bladder metastatic

C

CANCER (continued)

188.5	Bladder neck
V10.51	Bladder personal history
188.4	Bladder posterior wall
188.0	Bladder trigone
188.7	Bladder urachus
188.5	Bladder urethral orifice
188.9	Bladder wall NOS
188.8	Bladder other specified sites
171.#	Blood vessel **4th digit: 171** **0. Head, face, neck** **2. Upper limb including shoulder** **3. Lower limb including hip** **4. Thorax** **5. Abdomen (wall), gastric, gastrointestinal, intestine, stomach** **6. Pelvis, buttock, groin, inguinal region, perineum** **7. Trunk NOS, back NOS, flank NOS** **8. Other specified sites** **9. Site NOS**
198.89	Blood vessel metastatic

731.3: Use an additional code to identify major osseous defect, if applicable.

170.#	Bone and articular cartilage **4th digit: 170** **0. Skull and face** **1. Mandible** **2. Vertebral column** **3. Ribs, sternum, clavicle** **4. Scapula, long bones of upper limb** **5. Short bones of upper limb** **6. Pelvic bones, sacrum, coccyx** **7. Long bones of lower limb** **8. Short bones of lower limb** **9. Site NOS**
198.5	Bone and articular cartilage metastatic
170.9	Bone NOS
198.5	Bone NOS metastatic
170.8	Bone cuboid
198.5	Bone cuboid metastatic
170.5	Bone hands
198.5	Bone hands metastatic
170.9	Bone limb NOS
198.5	Bone limb NOS metastatic
170.7	Bone lower limb long bones

Symptoms of a malignancy such as pain or nausea should not replace the cancer code(s). Sequence the cancer first and the cancer associated pain 338.3 or nausea second.

170.8	Bone lower limb short bones
198.5	Bone lower limb short or long metastatic
170.1	Bone mandible (odontogenic)
198.5	Bone mandible metastatic
202.90	Bone marrow
198.5	Bone marrow metastatic
170.0	Bone maxilla (odontogenic)
198.5	Bone maxilla (odontogenic) metastatic
198.5	Bone or marrow metastatic
170.8	Bone patella
198.5	Bone patella metastatic
V10.81	Bone personal history

CANCER (continued)

170.3	Bone ribs sternum
198.5	Bone ribs sternum metastatic
170.0	Bone skull
198.5	Bone skull metastatic
170.2	Bone spine
198.5	Bone spine metastatic
170.4	Bone upper limb long bones
170.5	Bone upper limb short bones
198.5	Bone upper limb short or long bones metastatic
170.2	Bone vertebra
198.5	Bone vertebra metastatic
196.3	Brachial nodes metastatic
191.9	Brain NOS
198.3	Brain NOS metastatic
191.6	Brain cerebellum
198.3	Brain cerebellum metastatic
191.0	Brain cerebrum (except lobes or ventricles)
198.3	Brain cerebrum (except lobes or ventricles) metastatic
191.1	Brain cerebrum frontal lobe
198.3	Brain cerebrum frontal lobe metastatic
191.4	Brain cerebrum occipital lobe
198.3	Brain cerebrum occipital lobe metastatic
191.3	Brain cerebrum parietal lobe
198.3	Brain cerebrum parietal lobe metastatic
191.2	Brain cerebrum temporal lobe
198.3	Brain cerebrum temporal lobe metastatic
191.8	Brain overlapping sites
V10.85	Brain personal history
191.7	Brain stem
198.3	Brain stem metastatic
191.5	Brain ventricles
198.3	Brain ventricles metastatic
191.8	Brain other parts
198.3	Brain other parts metastatic
146.8	Branchial cleft
198.89	Branchial cleft metastatic

Use an additional code to identify estrogen receptor status. V86.0 Estrogen receptor positive status (ER+) or V86.1 Estrogen receptor negative status (ER-).

174.#	Breast female connective soft tissue **4th digit: 174** **0. Nipple and areola** **1. Central portion** **2. Upper inner quadrant** **3. Lower inner quadrant** **4. Upper outer quadrant** **5. Lower outer quadrant** **6. Axillary tail** **8. Mastectomy site, inner lower midline outer upper ectopic sites contiguous overlapping sites undetermined** **9. Breast (female) site NOS**
198.81	Breast female connective soft tissue metastatic
175.9	Breast male NOS or ectopic tissue
198.81	Breast male NOS or ectopic tissue metastatic
175.0	Breast male areola
198.81	Breast male areola metastatic
175.0	Breast male nipple
198.81	Breast male nipple metastatic
175.0	Breast male soft tissue
198.81	Breast male soft tissue metastatic
V10.3	Breast personal history

CANCER (continued)

173.5	Breast skin
173.5	Breast skin mastectomy site
198.2	Breast skin metastatic
174.8	Breast tissue mastectomy site
198.81	Breast tissue mastectomy site, metastatic
183.3	Broad ligament
198.82	Broad ligament mestastatic
196.1	Bronchopulmonary nodes metastatic
162.9	Bronchus
162.5	Bronchus lower lobe
162.2	Bronchus main bronchus
197.0	Bronchus metastatic
162.4	Bronchus middle lobe
V10.11	Bronchus personal history
162.8	Bronchus undetermined origin
162.3	Bronchus upper lobe
145.9	Buccal cavity NOS
198.89	Buccal metastatic
145.0	Buccal mucosa
145.1	Buccal sulcus (upper) (lower)
171.#	Bursa

4th digit: 171

0. Head, face, neck
2. Upper limb including shoulder
3. Lower limb including hip
4. Thorax
5. Abdomen (wall), gastric, gastrointestinal, intestine, stomach
6. Pelvis, buttock, groin, inguinal region, perineum
7. Trunk NOS, back NOS, flank NOS
8. Other specified sites
9. Site NOS

198.89	Bursa metastatic
173.5	Buttocks skin
198.2	Buttocks skin metastatic
171.6	Buttocks soft tissue
198.89	Buttocks soft tissue metastatic
170.8	Calcaneous
198.5	Calcaneous metastatic
155.1	Canaliculi biliferi
197.8	Canaliculi biliferi metastatic
173.1	Canthus skin
198.2	Canthus skin metastatic

If treatment is directed towards the metastatic site, then that site is coded first, even if the primary site is known.

199.1	Carcinoma
199.0	Carcinomatosis
151.0	Cardia (gastric)
197.8	Cardia (gastric) metastatic
164.1	Cardiac
198.89	Cardiac metastatic
151.0	Cardiac orifice (stomach)
197.8	Cardiac orifice (stomach) metastatic
151.0	Cardio-esophageal junction
197.8	Cardio-esophageal junction metastatic

CANCER (continued)

162.2	Carina
197.0	Carina - bronchus metastatic
197.3	Carina - trachea metastatic
194.5	Carotid body
198.89	Carotid body metastatic
170.5	Carpal bone
198.5	Carpal bone metastatic
192.2	Cauda equina
198.3	Cauda equina metastatic
192.9	Central nervous system
198.4	Central nervous system metastatic
191.6	Cerebellopontine angle
198.3	Cerebellopontine angle metastatic
191.6	Cerebellum
198.3	Cerebellum metastatic
191.0	Cerebral cortex
198.3	Cerebral cortex metastatic
192.1	Cerebral meninges
198.4	Cerebral meninges metastatic
191.7	Cerebral peduncle
198.3	Cerebral peduncle metastatic
191.1	Cerebrum frontal lobe
198.3	Cerebrum frontal lobe metastatic
191.4	Cerebrum occipital lobe
198.3	Cerebrum occipital lobe metastatic
191.3	Cerebrum parietal lobe
198.3	Cerebrum parietal lobe metastatic
191.2	Cerebrum temporal lobe
198.3	Cerebrum temporal lobe metastatic
196.0	Cervical nodes metastatic
196.0	Cervicofacial nodes metastatic
180.9	Cervix
180.0	Cervix canal
180.0	Cervix endocervix
180.1	Cervix exocervix
198.82	Cervix metastatic
V10.41	Cervix personal history
180.8	Cervix squamocolumnar junction
180.8	Cervix stump
180.8	Cervix other specified sites
195.0	Cheek ill-defined
145.0	Cheek inner aspect
198.89	Cheek inner aspect or ill-defined metastatic
173.3	Cheek skin (external)
198.2	Cheek skin (external) metastatic
195.1	Chest wall ill-defined
198.89	Chest wall ill-defined metastatic
173.5	Chest wall skin
198.2	Chest wall skin metastatic
173.3	Chin skin
198.2	Chin skin metastatic
147.3	Choanae posterior margin
198.89	Choanae posterior margin metastatic
181	Choriocarcinoma
186.9	Choriocarcinoma male
181	Chorioepithelioma

C

CANCER (continued)

190.6	Choroid
198.4	Choroid metastatic
191.5	Choroid plexus
198.3	Choroid plexus metastatic
190.0	Ciliary body
198.4	Ciliary body metastatic
170.3	Clavicle
198.5	Clavicle metastatic
184.3	Clitoris
198.82	Clitoris metastatic
154.8	Cloacogenic zone
197.5	Cloacogenic zone metastatic
192.9	CNS
198.4	CNS metastatic
194.6	Coccygeal body
198.89	Coccygeal body metastatic
170.6	Coccyx
198.5	Coccyx metastatic
153.9	Colon
153.5	Colon appendix
153.6	Colon ascending
153.4	Colon cecum
153.2	Colon descending
153.0	Colon hepatic flexure
153.4	Colon ileocecal valve
153.2	Colon left
197.5	Colon metastatic
V10.00	Colon personal history
154.0	Colon rectosigmoid
153.6	Colon right
153.3	Colon sigmoid
153.7	Colon splenic flexure
153.1	Colon transverse
153.8	Colon undetermined site
154.0	Colon with rectum
153.8	Colon other specified site
156.1	Common duct
197.8	Common duct metastatic
190.3	Conjunctiva
198.4	Conjunctiva metastatic
171.#	Connective tissue
	4th digit: 171
	0. Head, face, neck
	2. Upper limb including shoulder
	3. Lower limb including hip
	4. Thorax
	5. Abdomen (wall), gastric, gastrointestinal, intestine, stomach
	6. Pelvis, buttock, groin, inguinal region, perineum
	7. Trunk NOS, back NOS, flank NOS
	8. Other specified sites
	9. Site NOS
198.89	Connective tissue metastatic
190.4	Cornea
198.4	Cornea metastatic
182.0	Cornu
198.82	Cornu metastatic

CANCER (continued)

191.8	Corpus callosum
198.3	Corpus callosum metastatic
187.3	Corpus cavernosum
198.82	Corpus cavernosum metastatic
191.0	Corpus striatum
198.3	Corpus striatum metastatic

If encounter is for chemotherapy or radiotherapy and a complication of the therapy develops, sequence the therapy first, the complication second, then the cancer.

170.3	Costal cartilage
198.5	Costal cartilage metastatic
170.3	Costovertebral joint
198.5	Costovertebral joint metastatic
191.9	Cranial fossa
198.3	Cranial fossa metastatic
192.0	Cranial nerves
198.4	Cranial nerves metastatic
194.3	Craniobuccal pouch
198.89	Craniobuccal pouch metastatic
194.3	Craniopharyngeal tract
198.89	Craniopharyngeal tract metastatic
161.3	Cricoid cartilage
197.3	Cricoid cartilage metastatic
190.0	Crystalline lens
198.4	Crystalline lens metastatic
170.8	Cuboid
198.5	Cuboid metastatic
158.8	Cul de sac (Douglas)
197.6	Cul de sac (Douglas) metastatic
170.8	Cuneiform ankle
198.5	Cuneiform ankle metastatic
161.3	Cuneiform cartilage
197.3	Cuneiform cartilage metastatic
170.5	Cuneiform wrist
198.5	Cuneiform wrist metastatic
156.1	Cystic duct
197.8	Cystic duct metastatic
171.4	Diaphragm
198.89	Diaphragm metastatic
159.8	Digestive organ sites NEC
197.8	Digestive organ sites NEC metastatic
199.0	Disseminated
199.0	Disseminated metasatic
157.3	Duct of Santorini
197.8	Duct of Santorini metastatic
157.3	Duct of Wirsung
197.8	Duct of Wirsung metastatic
152.8	Duodenojejunal junction
197.4	Duodenojejunal junction metastatic
152.0	Duodenum
197.4	Duodenum metastatic
192.1	Dura (mater)
198.4	Dura (mater) metastatic

CANCER (continued)

171.0 Ear cartilage
198.89 Ear cartilage metastatic
160.1 Ear inner
160.1 Ear middle
V10.22 Ear middle (inner) personal history
173.2 Ear skin
198.2 Ear skin metastatic
164.1 Endocardium
198.89 Endocardium metastatic

180.0 Endocervical canal
180.0 Endocervical gland
198.82 Endocervical metastatic

194.9 Endocrine gland
198.89 Endocrine gland metastatic
157.4 Endocrine islets langerhans
197.8 Endocrine islets langerhans metastatic
183.0 Endocrine ovary
198.6 Endocrine ovary metastatic

If treatment is directed toward the metastatic site, then that site is coded first, even if the primary site is known.

186.9 Endocrine testis descended
198.82 Endocrine testis metastatic
186.0 Endocrine testis undescended
164.0 Endocrine thymus
198.89 Endocrine thymus metastatic
194.8 Endocrine other and multiple glands
198.89 Endocrine other and multiple glands metastatic

182.0 Endometrium
198.82 Endometrium metastatic

164.1 Epicardium
198.89 Epicardium metastatic

187.5 Epididymis
198.82 Epididymis metastatic
V10.48 Epididymis personal history

161.1 Epiglottis NOS
197.3 Epiglottis NOS metastatic
146.4 Epiglottis anterior only oropharynx
198.89 Epiglottis anterior only oropharynx metastatic
146.4 Epiglottis free border (margin)
198.89 Epiglottis free border (margin) metastatic
161.1 Epiglottis posterior
197.3 Epiglottis posterior metastatic
161.1 Epiglottis suprahyoid portion or NOS
197.3 Epiglottis suprahyoid portion or NOS metastatic

196.3 Epitrochlear nodes metastatic

150.9 Esophagus
150.2 Esophagus abdominal segment
151.0 Esophagus abdominal segment adenocarcinoma
151.0 Esophagus cardioesophageal
150.0 Esophagus cervical segment
150.5 Esophagus distal third
150.5 Esophagus lower third
151.0 Esophagus lower third adenocarcinoma
197.8 Esophagus metastatic
150.4 Esophagus middle third
150.8 Esophagus overlapping sites
V10.03 Esophagus personal history
150.3 Esophagus proximal third

CANCER (continued)

150.1 Esophagus thoracic segment
150.3 Esophagus upper third
150.8 Esophagus other specified

170.0 Ethmoid bone (cartilage) (joint) (periosteum)
198.5 Ethmoid bone (cartilage) (joint) (periosteum) metastatic
160.3 Ethmoid sinus
197.3 Ethmoid sinus metastatic

160.1 Eustachian tube
197.3 Eustachian tube metastatic

V71.1 Evaluation none found

173.2 External auditory canal skin
198.2 External auditory canal skin metastatic

156.1 Extrahepatic bile duct
156.2 Extrahepatic bile duct ampulla of vater
197.8 Extrahepatic bile duct metastatic

190.1 Extraocular muscle
198.4 Extraocular muscle metastatic

Symptoms of a malignancy such as pain or nausea should not replace the cancer code(s). Sequence the cancer first and the cancer associated pain 338.3 or nausea second.

190.# Eye

4th digit: 190

0. Eyeball
1. Orbit soft tissue
2 Lacrimal gland
3. Conjunctiva
4. Cornea
5. Retina
6. Choroid
7. Lacrimal duct
8. Other specified or overlapping
9. NOS

V10.84 Eye history of malignant neoplasm
190.0 Eye lens
198.4 Eye metastatic
170.0 Eye orbit bone
198.5 Eye orbit bone metastatic
190.1 Eye orbit connective tissue
V10.84 Eye personal history
190.8 Eye undetermined site
190.8 Eye other specified sites

190.0 Eyeball (internal structures)
190.0 Eyeball ciliary body
198.4 Eyeball metastatic

173.3 Eyebrow skin
198.2 Eyebrow skin metastatic

171.0 Eyelid cartilage
198.89 Eyelid cartilage metastatic
173.1 Eyelid skin
198.2 Eyelid skin metastatic

195.0 Face ill-defined
198.89 Face ill-defined metastatic
173.3 Face skin other unspecified parts
198.2 Face skin other unspecified parts metastatic

170.0 Facial bones
198.5 Facial bones metastatic

183.2 Fallopian tube
198.82 Fallopian tube metastatic

C

CANCER (continued)

161.1 False cords
197.3 False cords metastatic

192.1 Falx (cerebelli) (cerebri)
198.4 Falx (cerebelli) (cerebri) metastatic

0 Family history see 'Family History', CA, by site

When a primary site has been resected, and the current encounter is for recurrence in the original site, sequence the primary site first.

171.# Fascia
198.89 Fascia metastatic

171.# Fat
4th digit: 171
0. Head, face, neck
2. Upper limb including shoulder
3. Lower limb including hip
4. Thorax
5. Abdomen (wall), gastric, gastrointestinal, intestine, stomach
6. Pelvis, buttock, groin, inguinal region, perineum
7. Trunk NOS, back NOS, flank NOS
8. Other specified sites
9. Site NOS

198.89 Fat metastatic

196.5 Femoral lymph nodes metastatic

170.7 Femur
198.5 Femur metastatic

170.7 Fibula
198.5 Fibula metastatic

173.6 Finger skin
198.2 Finger skin metastatic
171.2 Finger soft tissue
198.89 Finger soft tissue metastatic

195.8 Flank ill-defined
198.89 Flank metastatic
171.7 Flank soft tissue

170.8 Foot bone
198.5 Foot bone metastatic
173.7 Foot skin
198.2 Foot skin metastatic
171.3 Foot soft tissue
198.89 Foot soft tissue metastatic

173.6 Forearm skin
198.2 Forearm skin metastatic
171.2 Forearm soft tissue
198.89 Forearm soft tissue metastatic

173.3 Forehead skin
198.2 Forehead skin metastatic

187.1 Foreskin
198.82 Foreskin metastatic

147.2 Fossa of Rosenmuller
198.89 Fossa of Rosenmuller metastatic

170.0 Frontal bone (cartilage) (joint) (periosteum)
198.5 Frontal bone (cartilage) (joint) (periosteum) metastatic
191.1 Frontal lobe
198.3 Frontal lobe metastatic

CANCER (continued)

160.4 Frontal sinus
197.3 Frontal sinus metastatic

182.0 Fundus uterine
198.82 Fundus uterine metastatic

156.0 Gallbladder
156.8 Gallbladder extra hepatic ducts (overlapping)
197.8 Gallbladder metastatic

156.1 Gall duct extrahepatic
155.1 Gall duct intrahepatic
197.8 Gall duct metastatic

171.# Ganglia
4th digit: 171
0. Head, face, neck
2. Upper limb including shoulder
3. Lower limb including hip
4. Thorax
5. Abdomen (wall), gastric, gastrointestinal, intestine, stomach
6. Pelvis, buttock, groin, inguinal region, perineum
7. Trunk NOS, back NOS, flank NOS
8. Other specified sites
9. Site NOS

198.89 Ganglia metastatic
192.0 Ganglia cranial
198.4 Ganglia cranial metastatic

184.0 Gartner's duct
198.82 Gartner's duct metastatic

If treatment is directed toward the metastatic site, then that site is coded first, even if the primary site is known.

151.9 Gastric
151.4 Gastric body
151.0 Gastric cardiac orifice
150.2 Gastric cardiac orifice squamous cell
151.0 Gastric cardioesophageal junction
150.5 Gastric cardioesophageal junction squamous cell
151.3 Gastric fundus
151.6 Gastric greater curvature
151.5 Gastric lesser curvature
197.8 Gastric metastatic
151.8 Gastric overlapping undetermined
151.2 Gastric pyloric antrum
151.1 Gastric pylorus
171.5 Gastric soft tissue

171.5 Gastrointestinal soft tissue
159.9 Gastrointestinal tract
197.8 Gastrointestinal tract metastatic
V10.00 Gastrointestinal tract personal history

199.0 Generalized cancer unspecified site

184.8 Genital organs female other specified site
V10.40 Genital organs female personal history
184.9 Genital organs female site NOS
187.9 Genital organs male
198.82 Genital organs metastatic

184.4 Genitalia female external
198.82 Genitalia female external metastatic

184.9 Genitourinary tract female NOS
198.82 Genitourinary tract female NOS metastatic

CANCER (continued)

V10.00 GI tract personal history

143.1 Gingiva lower
198.89 Gingiva metastatic
143.8 Gingiva sites overlapping
143.0 Gingiva upper

187.2 Glans penis
198.82 Glans penis metastatic

191.0 Globus pallidus
198.3 Globus pallidus metastatic

194.6 Glomus jugulare
198.89 Glomus jugulare metastatic

146.4 Glossoepiglottic fold
198.89 Glossoepiglottic fold metastatic

146.2 Glossopalatine fold
198.89 Glossopalatine fold metastatic

161.0 Glottis
161.0 Glottis larynx
197.3 Glottis metastatic

171.4 Great vessels
198.89 Great vessels metastatic

184.1 Greater vestibular gland
198.82 Greater vestibular gland metastatic

195.3 Groin ill-defined
198.89 Groin ill-defined metastatic
196.5 Groin lymph nodes metastatic
173.5 Groin skin
198.2 Groin skin metastatic
171.6 Groin soft tissue
198.89 Groin soft tissue metastatic

143.9 Gum
198.89 Gum metastatic
143.1 Gum lower
170.1 Gum lower jaw odontogenic
198.5 Gum lower jaw odontogenic metastatic
198.89 Gum lower metastatic
143.0 Gum upper
198.89 Gum upper metastatic
170.0 Gum upper jaw odontogenic
198.5 Gum upper jaw odontogenesis metastatic
143.8 Gum other site
198.89 Gum other site metastatic

170.5 Hand bones
198.5 Hand bones metastatic
173.6 Hand skin
198.2 Hand skin metastatic
171.2 Hand soft tissue
198.89 Hand soft tissue metastatic

145.2 Hard palate
198.89 Hard palate metastatic

195.0 Head ill-defined
198.89 Head ill-defined metastatic

164.1 Heart
198.89 Heart metastatic
164.8 Heart overlapping sites

154.2 Hemorrhoidal zone
197.5 Hemorrhoidal zone metastatic

CANCER (continued)

156.1 Hepatic duct
197.8 Hepatic duct metastatic
153.0 Hepatic flexure
197.5 Hepatic flexure metastatic
155.0 Hepatoblastoma primary
155.0 Hepatocellular primary

162.2 Hilus of lung
197.0 Hilus of lung metastatic

173.7 Hip skin
198.2 Hip skin metastatic

191.2 Hippocampus
198.3 Hippocampus metastatic

0 History see 'History'

170.4 Humerus
198.5 Humerus metastatic

171.5 Hypochondrium soft tissue
198.89 Hypochondrium soft tissue metastatic

196.6 Hypogastric nodes metastatic

148.9 Hypopharynx
148.2 Hypopharynx aryepiglottic fold
198.89 Hypopharynx metastatic
148.0 Hypopharynx postcricoid region
148.3 Hypopharynx posterior wall
148.1 Hypopharynx pyriform sinus
148.9 Hypopharynx wall NOS
148.8 Hypopharynx other sites

194.3 Hypophysis
198.89 Hypophysis metastatic

191.0 Hypothalamus
198.3 Hypothalamus metastatic

152.2 Ileum
153.4 Ileum ileocecal valve
197.4 Ileum metastatic

196.6 Iliac nodes metastatic

170.6 Ilium
198.5 Ilium metastatic

203.8# Immunoproliferative
5th digit: 203.8
0. Without mention of remission
1. In remission

196.3 Infraclavicular nodes metastatic

195.3 Inguinal region ill-defined
198.89 Inguinal region metastatic
171.6 Inguinal region soft tissue
198.89 Inguinal region soft tissue metastatic

196.1 Intercostal nodes metastatic
0 Interdental papillae see 'Cancer', gum

196.2 Intestinal nodes metastatic

159.0 Intestinal tract
197.8 Intestinal tract metastatic
171.5 Intestinal tract soft tissue

195.2 Intra abdominal ill-defined (non GI)
198.89 Intra abdominal ill-defined (non GI) metastatic
196.2 Intra abdominal nodes metastatic

196.6 Intrapelvic nodes metastatic

C

CANCER (continued)

195.1	Intrathoracic ill-defined
198.89	Intrathoracic ill-defined metastatic
196.1	Intrathoracic metastatic
163.9	Intrathoracic pleura
197.2	Intrathoracic pleura metastatic
163.0	Intrathoracic pleura parietal
163.1	Intrathoracic pleura visceral
163.8	Intrathoracic pleura undetermined
164.8	Intrathoracic thymus heart mediastinum undetermined
190.0	Iris
198.4	Iris metastatic
170.6	Ischium
198.5	Ischium metastatic

If treatment is directed towards the primary site, sequence that site first.

170.1	Jaw bone
170.1	Jaw bone lower
198.5	Jaw bone metastatic
170.0	Jaw bone upper
195.0	Jaw ill-defined
198.89	Jaw ill-defined metastatic
152.1	Jejunum
197.4	Jejunum metastatic
189.0	Kidney
198.0	Kidney metastatic
189.0	Kidney parenchyma
V10.52	Kidney personal history
189.9	Kidney ureter
173.7	Knee (popliteal) skin
198.2	Knee (popliteal) skin metastatic
184.1	Labia majora
198.82	Labia metastatic
184.2	Labia minora
140.6	Labial commissure
198.89	Labial commissure or sulcus metastatic
145.1	Labial sulcus mouth (upper) (lower)
190.7	Lacrimal duct
198.4	Lacrimal duct metastatic
190.2	Lacrimal gland
198.4	Lacrimal gland metastatic
153.9	Large intestine
197.5	Large intestine metastatic
V10.05	Large intestine personal history
161.#	Larynx

4th digit: 161
- **0. Glottic, commissure**
- **1. Supraglottic, areyepiglottic fold, false cords**
- **2. Subglottic**
- **3. Cartilage**
- **8. Other specified sites**
- **9. Site unspecified**

197.3	Larynx metastatic
V10.21	Larynx personal history
173.7	Leg skin
198.2	Leg skin metastatic
171.3	Leg soft tissue
198.89	Leg soft tissue metastatic

CANCER (continued)

182.0	Leiomyosarcoma
190.0	Lens eye
198.4	Lens eye metastatic
171.#	Ligament except uterine

4th digit: 171
- **0. Head, face, neck**
- **2. Upper limb including shoulder**
- **3. Lower limb including hip**
- **4. Thorax**
- **5. Abdomen (wall), gastric, gastrointestinal, intestine, stomach**
- **6. Pelvis, buttock, groin, inguinal region, perineum**
- **7. Trunk NOS, back NOS, flank NOS**
- **8. Other specified sites**
- **9. Site NOS**

198.89	Ligament except uterine metastatic
141.3	Linguae frenulum
198.89	Linguae frenulum metastatic
141.6	Lingual tonsil
198.89	Lingual tonsil metastatic
140.6	Lip commissure
198.89	Lip commissure metastatic
140.5	Lip frenulum
140.4	Lip frenulum lower
198.89	Lip frenulum metastatic
140.3	Lip frenulum upper
149.9	Lip ill defined
140.5	Lip inner
140.5	Lip inner buccal mucosa
140.5	Lip inner oral aspect
140.1	Lip lower
140.4	Lip lower buccal mucosa
140.1	Lip lower external
140.4	Lip lower frenulum
140.4	Lip lower inner aspect
140.1	Lip lower lipstick area
140.4	Lip lower mucosa
140.4	Lip lower oral aspect
140.1	Lip lower vermilion border
198.89	Lip metastatic
173.0	Lip skin
198.2	Lip skin metastatic
140.0	Lip upper
140.3	Lip upper buccal mucosa
140.0	Lip upper external
140.3	Lip upper frenulum
140.3	Lip upper inner aspect
140.0	Lip upper lipstick area
140.3	Lip upper mucosa
140.3	Lip upper oral aspect
140.0	Lip upper vermilion border
140.9	Lip vermilion border external
140.9	Lip vermilion border lipstick area
140.8	Lip other overlapping sites
149.8	Lip other overlapping sites with oral cavity
155.1	Liver intraheptic bile ducts
197.7	Liver metastatic
V10.07	Liver personal history
155.0	Liver primary
155.2	Liver undetermined primary or secondary

CANCER (continued)

171.3 Lower limb and hip soft tissue
198.89 Lower limb and hip soft tissue metastatic
195.5 Lower limb ill-defined
198.89 Lower limb ill-defined metastatic
173.7 Lower limb skin
198.2 Lower limb skin metastatic

162.5 Lower lobe bronchus
197.0 Lower lobe bronchus metastatic

170.5 Lunate
198.5 Lunate metastatic

162.9 Lung
162.9 Lung bronchus
162.8 Lung bronchus undetermined origin
162.5 Lung lower lobe
197.0 Lung metastatic
162.4 Lung middle lobe
V10.11 Lung personal history
162.3 Lung upper lobe

202.9# Lymph node (any site) primary
5th digit: 202.9
0. NOS, extranodal and solid organ sites
1. Lymph nodes of head, face, neck
2. Lymph nodes intrathoracic
3. Lymph nodes abdominal
4. Lymph nodes axilla and upper limb
5. Lymph nodes inguinal region and lower limb
6. Lymph nodes intrapelvic
7. Spleen
8. Lymph nodes multiple sites

196.# Lymph node metastatic
4th digit: 196
0. Head, face, neck, cervical, supraclavicular
1. Intrathoracic, bronchopulmonary, mediastinal, tracheobronchial
2. Intra abdominal, mesenteric, retroperitoneal
3. Axilla, upper limb, brachial, intraclavicular, pectoral
5. Lower limb, inguinal, femoral, groin, tibial
6. Intrapelvic, hypogastric, iliac, parametrial
8. Multiple sites
9. Lymph nodes NOS

202.9# Lymphoid histiocytic tissue
200.1# Lymphosarcoma
5th digit: 200.1, 202.9
0. NOS, extranodal and solid organ sites
1. Lymph nodes of head, face, neck
2. Lymph nodes intrathoracic
3. Lymph nodes abdominal
4. Lymph nodes axilla and upper limb
5. Lymph nodes inguinal region and lower limb
6. Lymph nodes intrapelvic
7. Spleen
8. Lymph nodes multiple sites

170.0 Malar bone (cartilage) (joint) (periosteum)
198.5 Malar bone (cartilage) (joint) (periosteum) metastatic

187.8 Male genital other
198.82 Male genital other metastatic

CANCER (continued)

199.1 Malignancy NOS

170.1 Mandible
198.5 Mandible metastatic

202.90 Marrow bone
198.5 Marrow bone metastatic

173.5 Mastectomy site breast skin
198.2 Mastectomy site breast skin, metastatic
174.8 Mastectomy site breast tissue
198.81 Mastectomy site breast tissue, metastatic

160.1 Mastoid air cells
197.3 Mastoid air cells metastatic

170.1 Maxilla inferior
198.5 Maxilla metastatic
170.0 Maxilla superior
160.2 Maxillary antrum
197.3 Maxillary antrum metastatic
160.2 Maxillary sinus
197.3 Maxillary sinus metastatic

152.3 Meckel's diverticulum
197.4 Meckel's diverticulum metastatic

196.1 Mediastinal nodes metastatic

164.9 Mediastinum
164.2 Mediastinum anterior
197.1 Mediastinum metastatic
164.3 Mediastinum posterior

194.0 Medulla adrenal
198.7 Medulla adrenal metastatic
191.7 Medulla oblongata
198.3 Medulla oblongata metastatic

172.# Melanoma skin
4th digit: 172
0. Lip
1. Eyelid including canthus
2. Ear (auricle) auricular canal external (acoustic) meatus pinna
3. Unspecified parts of face external, cheek, chin, eyebrow, forehead, nose, temple
4. Scalp and neck
5. Trunk, axilla, breast, groin, perianal skin, perineum, umbilicus
6. Upper limb including shoulder
7. Lower limb including hip
8. Other specified skin sites, contiguous or overlapping, undetermined point of origin
9. Site unspecified

Symptoms of a malignancy such as pain or nausea should not replace the cancer code(s). Sequence the cancer first and the cancer associated pain 338.3 or nausea second.

192.1 Meninges cerebral
198.4 Meninges cerebral metastatic
192.3 Meninges spinal cord
198.4 Meninges spinal cord metastatic

196.2 Mesenteric nodes metastatic

158.8 Mesentery
197.6 Mesentery metastatic

C

CANCER (continued)

158.8 Mesocolon
197.6 Mesocolon metastatic

183.3 Mesovarium
198.82 Mesovarium metastatic

170.5 Metacarpals
198.5 Metacarpals metastatic

170.8 Metatarsal
198.5 Metatarsal metastatic

199.1 Metastatic site NOS

191.7 Midbrain
198.3 Midbrain metastatic

162.4 Middle lobe bronchus
197.0 Middle lobe bronchus metastatic

145.9 Mouth
144.0 Mouth anterior to premolar-canine junction
145.0 Mouth cheek
144.9 Mouth floor
144.0 Mouth floor anterior
144.1 Mouth floor lateral
144.8 Mouth floor other sites
145.2 Mouth hard palate
198.89 Mouth metastatic
145.6 Mouth retromolar
145.5 Mouth roof
145.3 Mouth soft palate
147.3 Mouth soft palate posterior portion
145.4 Mouth uvula
145.1 Mouth vestibule
145.8 Mouth other specified area

199.0 Multiple cancers
203.0# Multiple myeloma
5th digit: 203.0
0. Without mention of remission
1. In remission

171.# Muscle
4th digit: 171
0. Head, face, neck
2. Upper limb including shoulder
3. Lower limb including hip
4. Thorax
5. Abdomen (wall), gastric, gastrointestinal, intestine, stomach
6. Pelvis, buttock, groin, inguinal region, perineum
7. Trunk NOS, back NOS, flank NOS
8. Other specified sites
9. Site NOS

198.89 Muscle metastatic

164.1 Myocardium
198.89 Myocardium metastatic

182.0 Myometrium
198.82 Myometrium metastatic

170.0 Nasal bone (cartilage) (joint) (periosteum)
198.5 Nasal bone metastatic
160.0 Nasal cartilage
197.3 Nasal cartilage metastatic
160.0 Nasal cavity
160.9 Nasal cavity accessory sinuses
160.3 Nasal cavity ethmoidal sinus

CANCER (continued)

160.4 Nasal cavity frontal sinus
160.2 Nasal cavity maxillary sinus
197.3 Nasal cavity metastatic
160.8 Nasal cavity origin undetermined
160.5 Nasal cavity sphenoidal sinus
147.3 Nasal choanae (posterior margin)
198.89 Nasal choanae (posterior margin) metastatic
160.0 Nasal conchae nasal turbinates
197.3 Nasal conchae nasal turbinates metastatic
192.0 Nasal olfactory bulb
198.4 Nasal olfactory bulb metastatic
160.0 Nasal septum
197.3 Nasal septum metastatic
147.3 Nasal septum posterior margin
198.89 Nasal septum posterior margin metastatic
170.0 Nasal turbinate bone
198.5 Nasal turbinate bone metastatic
160.0 Nasal turbinate mucosa
197.3 Nasal turbinate mucosa metastatic
160.0 Nasal vestibule
197.3 Nasal vestibule metastatic

190.7 Nasolacrimal duct
198.4 Nasolacrimal duct metastatic

147.9 Nasopharynx
147.3 Nasopharynx anterior wall
147.3 Nasopharynx floor
147.2 Nasopharynx fossa of Rosenmuller
147.2 Nasopharynx lateral wall
198.89 Nasopharynx metastatic
147.1 Nasopharynx posterior wall
147.0 Nasopharynx superior wall (roof)
147.9 Nasopharynx wall NOS
147.8 Nasopharynx other specified sites

170.8 Navicular ankle
198.5 Navicular ankle or hand metastatic
170.5 Navicular hand

195.0 Neck ill-defined
198.89 Neck ill-defined metastatic
173.4 Neck skin
198.2 Neck skin metastatic

171.# Nerve (peripheral) (sympathetic) (parasympathetic)
4th digit: 171
0. Head, face, neck
2. Upper limb including shoulder
3. Lower limb including hip
4. Thorax
5. Abdomen (wall), gastric, gastrointestinal, intestine, stomach
6. Pelvis, buttock, groin, inguinal region, perineum
7. Trunk NOS, back NOS, flank NOS
8. Other specified sites
9. Site NOS

198.89 Nerve (peripheral) (sympathetic) (parasympathetic) metastatic

192.0 Nerve cranial
198.4 Nerve cranial metastatic

192.9 Nervous system
198.4 Nervous system metastatic
192.8 Nervous system other specified sites

CANCER (continued)

> *Use an additional code to identify estrogen receptor status. V86.0 Estrogen receptor positive status (ER+) or V86.1 Estrogen receptor negative status (ER-).*

174.0	Nipple female soft tissue
175.0	Nipple male soft tissue
198.81	Nipple soft tissue metastatic
195.0	Nose ill defined
198.89	Nose ill defined metastatic
160.0	Nose internal
197.3	Nose internal metastatic
173.3	Nose skin external
172.3	Nose skin melanoma
198.2	Nose skin melanoma metastatic
198.2	Nose skin metastatic
V71.1	Observation none found
196.6	Obturator nodes metastatic
170.0	Occipital bone (cartilage) (joint) (periosteum)
198.5	Occipital bone (cartilage) (joint) (periosteum) metastatic
191.4	Occipital lobe
198.3	Occipital lobe metastatic
192.0	Olfactory bulb
198.4	Olfactory bulb metastatic
158.8	Omentum
197.6	Omentum metastatic
192.0	Optic nerve
198.4	Optic nerve metastatic
145.9	Oral cavity NOS
149.9	Oral cavity ill-defined
198.89	Oral cavity metastatic
V10.02	Oral cavity personal history
149.8	Oral cavity other specified
170.0	Orbit bone (cartilage) (joint) (periosteum)
198.5	Orbit bone (cartilage) (joint) (periosteum) metastatic
190.1	Orbit connective tissue
198.4	Orbit connective tissue metastatic
190.1	Orbit retrobulbar
198.4	Orbit retrobulbar metastatic
146.9	Oropharynx
146.5	Oropharynx junctional region
146.6	Oropharynx lateral wall
146.7	Oropharynx posterior wall
198.89	Oropharynx metastatic
146.2	Oropharynx tonsillar pillars anterior
146.8	Oropharynx other specified sites
183.0	Ovary
198.6	Ovary metastatic
V10.43	Ovary personal history
183.2	Oviduct
198.82	Oviduct metastatic
145.5	Palate
145.2	Palate hard
145.5	Palate junction of hard and soft
198.89	Palate metastatic
145.3	Palate soft
147.3	Palate soft posterior portion

CANCER (continued)

146.2	Palatoglossal arch
198.89	Palatoglossal arch metastatic
146.2	Palatopharyngeal arch
198.89	Palatopharyngeal arch metastatic
157.9	Pancreas
157.1	Pancreas body
157.3	Pancreas ducts
157.8	Pancreas ectopic tissue
157.0	Pancreas head
157.4	Pancreas islets of langerhans
197.8	Pancreas metastatic
157.3	Pancreas santorini duct
157.2	Pancreas tail
157.8	Pancreas undetermined site
157.3	Pancreas Wirsung duct
194.6	Para aortic body
198.89	Para aortic body metastatic
194.6	Paraganglia related
198.89	Paraganglia related metastatic
196.6	Parametrial nodes metastatic
183.4	Parametrium
198.82	Parametrium metastatic
194.1	Parathyroid gland
198.89	Parathyroid gland metastatic
189.4	Paraurethral glands
198.1	Paraurethral glands metastatic
170.0	Parietal bone (cartilage) (joint) (periosteum)
198.5	Parietal bone (cartilage) (joint) (periosteum) metastatic
191.3	Parietal lobe
198.3	Parietal lobe metastatic
158.8	Parietal peritoneum
197.6	Parietal peritoneum metastatic
163.0	Parietal pleura
197.2	Parietal pleura metastatic
142.0	Parotid gland
198.89	Parotid gland metastatic

> ***When two primary sites are found, sequence the site receiving the most treatment first.***

183.3	Parovarian region
198.82	Parovarian region metastatic
170.8	Patella
198.5	Patella metastatic
196.3	Pectoral nodes metastatic
158.8	Pelvic peritoneum
197.6	Pelvic peritoneum metastatic
195.3	Pelvis ill-defined
198.89	Pelvis ill-defined metastatic
171.6	Pelvis soft tissue
198.89	Pelvis soft tissue metastatic
187.4	Penis
187.3	Penis body
187.2	Penis glans
198.82	Penis metastatic
187.4	Penis skin

C

CANCER (continued)

158.0	Periadrenal tissue
197.6	Periadrenal tissue metastatic
164.1	Pericardium
198.89	Pericardium metastatic
158.0	Perinephric tissue
197.6	Perinephric tissue metastatic
173.5	Perineum skin
198.2	Perineum skin metastatic
171.6	Perineum soft tissue
198.89	Perineum soft tissue metastatic
158.0	Perirenal tissue
197.6	Perirenal tissue metastatic
158.9	Peritoneum
158.8	Peritoneum cul-de-sac
158.8	Peritoneum mesentery
197.6	Peritoneum metastatic
158.8	Peritoneum omentum
158.8	Peritoneum specified parts
170.8	Phalanges foot
198.5	Phalanges foot metastatic
170.5	Phalanges hand
198.5	Phalanges hand metastatic
146.3	Pharyngoepiglottic fold anterior and medial surface
198.89	Pharyngoepiglottic fold anterior and medial surface metastatic
149.0	Pharynx
149.9	Pharynx ill defined
198.89	Pharynx metastatic
V10.02	Pharynx personal history
147.2	Pharynx recess
149.1	Pharynx Waldeyer's ring
149.8	Pharynx other specified
194.4	Pineal gland
198.89	Pineal gland metastatic
170.5	Pisiform
198.5	Pisiform metastatic
194.3	Pituitary and craniopharyngeal duct
198.89	Pituitary metastatic
181	Placenta
198.82	Placenta metastatic
163.9	Pleura
197.2	Pleura metastatic
163.8	Pleura other specified sites
194.8	Pluriglandular involvement
198.89	Pluriglandular involvement metastatic
191.7	Pons
198.3	Pons metastatic
196.5	Popliteal lymph nodes metastatic
171.3	Popliteal soft tissue
198.89	Popliteal soft tissue metastatic
164.3	Posterior mediastinum
197.1	Posterior mediastinum metastatic
187.1	Prepuce
198.82	Prepuce metastatic
151.1	Prepylorus
197.8	Prepylorus metastatic

C

CANCER (continued)

195.3	Presacral region ill defined
198.89	Presacral region ill defined metastatic

When encounter is for a complication of a surgical procedure to resect a cancer, sequence the complication first and the cancer as an additional code.

185	Prostate
198.82	Prostate metastatic
V10.46	Prostate personal history
170.6	Pubis
198.5	Pubis metastatic
184.4	Pudendum
198.82	Pudendum metastatic
151.1	Pylorus (canal)
197.8	Pylorus (canal) metastatic
148.1	Pyriform sinus
198.89	Pyriform sinus metastatic
170.4	Radius
198.5	Radius metastatic
194.3	Rathke's pouch
198.89	Rathke's pouch metastatic
154.0	Rectosigmoid (junction)
197.5	Rectosigmoid (junction) metastatic
154.8	Rectosigmoid (junction) overlapping sites
158.8	Rectouterine pouch
197.6	Rectouterine pouch metastatic
195.3	Rectovaginal (septum) ill-defined
198.89	Rectovaginal metastatic
195.3	Rectovaginal rectovesical overlapping sites
195.3	Rectovesical (septum) ill-defined
198.89	Rectovesical (septum) ill-defined metastatic
154.1	Rectum
154.1	Rectum ampulla
197.5	Rectum metastatic
V10.06	Rectum (rectosigmoid junction) (anus) personal history
154.8	Rectum undetermined
189.1	Renal pelvis
198.0	Renal pelvis metastatic
V10.53	Renal pelvis personal history
165.8	Respiratory and intrathoracic other specified sites
197.3	Respiratory and intrathoracic other specified sites metastatic
V10.29	Respiratory and intrathoracic organs personal history other
165.9	Respiratory organ or system ill defined
197.3	Respiratory organ or system ill defined metastatic
V10.20	Respiratory organ or system personal history
165.9	Respiratory tract
165.9	Respiratory tract ill-defined sites
197.3	Respiratory tract metastatic
165.8	Respiratory tract other specified sites
190.5	Retina
198.4	Retina metastatic
190.5	Retinoblastoma
190.1	Retrobulbar
198.4	Retrobulbar metastatic

CANCER (continued)

158.0 Retrocecal tissue
197.6 Retrocecal tissue metastatic
196.2 Retroperitoneal nodes metastatic

158.0 Retroperitoneum
197.6 Retroperitoneum metastatic

170.3 Ribs
198.5 Ribs metastatic

183.5 Round ligament
198.82 Round ligament metastatic

195.3 Sacrococcygeal region ill-defined
198.89 Sacrococcygeal region ill-defined metastatic

170.6 Sacrum
198.5 Sacrum metastatic

> ***When treatment is directed toward a secondary site, even if the primary site is known, sequence the secondary site first.***

142.9 Salivary gland
145.9 Salivary gland (minor gland)
198.89 Salivary gland metastatic
142.8 Salivary gland other
142.2 Salivary gland sublingual
142.1 Salivary gland submandibular or submaxillary

196.0 Scalene nodes metastatic

173.4 Scalp skin
198.2 Scalp skin metastatic

170.5 Scaphoid of hand
198.5 Scaphoid of hand metastatic

170.4 Scapula
198.5 Scapula metastatic

190.0 Sclera
198.4 Sclera metastatic

0 Screening see 'Cancer Screening'

187.7 Scrotum (skin)
198.82 Scrotum (skin) metastatic

173.# Sebaceous glands
4th digit: 173
0. Skin of lip
1. Eyelid including canthus
2. Skin of ear auricular canal external meatus pinna
3. Skin of unspecified parts of face, cheek, chin, eyebrow, forehead, nose external
4. Scalp and skin of neck
5. Skin trunk, axilla, perianal, abdominal wall, anus, back, breast (or mastectomy site), buttock
6. Skin upper limb, shoulder, arm, finger, hand
7. Skin lower limb, hip, ankle, foot, knee, leg, thigh, toe, popliteal area
8. Other specified skin sites, contiguous sites, undetermined point of origin
9. Site NOS

198.2 Sebaceous gland metastatic

CANCER (continued)

194.3 Sella turcica pituitary
198.89 Sella turcica pituitary metastatic

170.5 Semilunar
198.5 Semilunar metastatic

187.8 Seminal vesicle
198.82 Seminal vesicle metastatic

173.6 Shoulder skin
198.2 Shoulder skin metastatic

154.0 Sigmoid (rectosigmoid)
153.3 Sigmoid flexure
197.5 Sigmoid metastatic

199.1 Simplex site NOS

160.9 Sinus accessory
197.3 Sinus accessory metastatic
160.3 Sinus ethmoidal
197.3 Sinus ethmoidal metastatic
V10.22 Sinus ethmoidal personal history
160.4 Sinus frontal
197.3 Sinus frontal metastatic
V10.22 Sinus frontal personal history
160.2 Sinus maxillary
197.3 Sinus maxillary metastatic
V10.22 Sinus maxillary personal history

> ***When the reason for an encounter is to evaluate the extent of a cancer already diagnosed, you may code the cancer again as the reason for encounter, rather than just the symptoms.***

V10.22 Sinus personal history
160.5 Sinus sphenoidal
197.3 Sinus sphenoidal metastatic
V10.22 Sinus sphenoidal personal history

258.02 Sipple's syndrome (medullary thyroid carcinoma-pheochromocytoma)

173.# Skin
4th digit: 173
0. Skin of lip
1. Eyelid including canthus
2. Ear (auricle) auricular canal external (acoustic)
3. Unspecified parts of face, cheek external, chin, eyebrow, forehead, nose external, temple
4. Scalp and neck
5. Trunk, axilla, breast (or mastectomy site), buttock, groin, perianal skin, perineum, umbilicus
6. Upper limb including shoulder
7. Lower limb including hip
8. Other specified skin sites, contiguous or overlapping, undetermined point of origin
9. Site NOS

198.2 Skin metastatic
V10.83 Skin (other) personal history

170.0 Skull calvarium
198.5 Skull calvarium metastatic

152.3 Small bowel meckel's diverticulum
197.4 Small bowel metastatic
152.9 Small bowel other or undetermined
152.8 Small bowel other undetermined sites overlapping

C

CANCER (continued)

145.3	Soft palate
198.89	Soft palate metastatic
147.3	Soft palate posterior portion
187.6	Spermatic cord
198.82	Spermatic cord metastatic
170.0	Sphenoid bone (cartilage) (joint) (periosteum)
198.5	Sphenoid bone (cartilage) (joint) (periosteum) metastatic
160.5	Sphenoid sinus
197.3	Sphenoid sinus metastatic
156.1	Sphincter of oddi
197.8	Sphincter of oddi metastatic
192.2	Spinal cord
198.3	Spinal cord metastatic
192.3	Spinal meninges
198.4	Spinal meninges metastatic
198.5	Spine - metastatic
170.6	Spine - sacrum, coccyx
170.2	Spine - spinal column, vertebra
159.1	Spleen
159.1	Spleen angiosarcoma
159.1	Spleen fibrosarcoma
200.17	Spleen lymphosarcoma
197.8	Spleen metastatic
200.07	Spleen reticulosarcoma (lymphoma)
170.3	Sternum
198.5	Sternum metastatic

If encounter is for chemotherapy or radiotherapy and a complication of the therapy develops, sequence the therapy first, the complication second, then the cancer.

151.9	Stomach
151.4	Stomach body
151.0	Stomach cardiac orifice
150.2	Stomach cardiac orifice squamous cell
151.0	Stomach cardioesophageal junction
150.5	Stomach cardioesophageal squamous cell
151.3	Stomach fundus
151.6	Stomach greater curvature
151.5	Stomach lesser curvature
197.8	Stomach metastatic
151.8	Stomach other undetermined overlapping
V10.04	Stomach personal history
151.2	Stomach pyloric antrum
151.1	Stomach pylorus
171.5	Stomach soft tissue
161.2	Subglottis larynx
197.3	Subglottis larynx metastatic
142.2	Sublingual gland
198.89	Sublingual gland metastatic
142.1	Submandibular gland
198.89	Submandibular gland metastatic
142.1	Submaxillary gland
198.89	Submaxillary gland metastatic

CANCER (continued)

173.# Sudoriferous sudoriparous glands

4th digit: 173

0. Skin of lip
1. Eyelid including canthus
2. Ear (auricle) auricular canal external (acoustic)
3. Unspecified parts of face, cheek external, chin, eyebrow, forehead, nose external, temple
4. Scalp and neck
5. Trunk, axilla, breast (or mastectomy site), buttock, groin, perianal skin, perineum, umbilicus
6. Upper limb including shoulder
7. Lower limb including hip
8. Other specified skin sites, contiguous or overlapping, undetermined point of origin
9. Site NOS

198.2	Sudoriferous sudoriparous glands metastatic
145.1	Sulcus buccal upper lower
145.1	Sulcus labial upper lower
198.89	Sulcus metastatic
196.0	Supraclavicular gland metastatic
195.0	Supraclavicular region ill-defined
198.89	Supraclavicular region ill-defined metastatic
161.1	Supraglottis
197.3	Supraglottis metastatic
194.0	Suprarenal gland
198.7	Suprarenal gland metastatic

173.# Sweat gland

4th digit: 173

0. Lip skin
1. Eyelid including canthus
2. Ear (auricle) auricular canal external (acoustic)
3. Unspecified parts of face, cheek external, chin, eyebrow, forehead, nose external, temple
4. Scalp and neck
5. Trunk, axilla, breast (or mastectomy site), buttock, groin, perianal skin, perineum, umbilicus
6. Upper limb including shoulder
7. Lower limb including hip
8. Other specified skin sites, contiguous or overlapping, undetermined point of origin
9. Site NOS

198.2 Sweat gland metastatic

171.# Synovia

4th digit: 171

0. Head, face, neck
2. Upper limb including shoulder
3. Lower limb including hip
4. Thorax
5. Abdomen (wall), gastric, gastrointestinal, intestine, stomach
6. Pelvis, buttock, groin, inguinal region, perineum
7. Trunk NOS, back NOS, flank NOS
8. Other specified sites
9. Site NOS

198.89 Synovia metastatic

CANCER (continued)

170.8 Talus
198.5 Talus metastatic

191.8 Tapetum
198.3 Tapetum metastatic

170.8 Tarsal bone
198.5 Tarsal bone metastatic

173.3 Temple skin
198.2 Temple skin metastatic

170.0 Temporal bone (cartilage) (joint) (periosteum)
198.5 Temporal bone (cartilage) (joint) (periosteum) metastatic
191.2 Temporal lobe
198.3 Temporal lobe metastatic
191.2 Temporal lobe uncus
198.3 Temporal lobe uncus metastatic

171.# Tendon (sheath)

4th digit: 171

0. Head, face, neck
2. Upper limb including shoulder
3. Lower limb including hip
4. Thorax
5. Abdomen (wall), gastric, gastrointestinal, intestine, stomach
6. Pelvis, buttock, groin, inguinal region, perineum
7. Trunk NOS, back NOS, flank NOS
8. Other specified sites
9. Site NOS

198.89 Tendon (sheath) metastatic

192.1 Tentorium
198.4 Tentorium metastatic

186.9 Testis NOS
186.9 Testis choriocarcinoma
186.0 Testis choriocarcinoma undescended
186.9 Testis descended
186.0 Testis ectopic undescended
198.82 Testis metastatic
V10.47 Testis personal history
186.0 Testis retained
186.9 Testis scrotal
186.0 Testis undescended
186.9 Testis other and unspecified

191.0 Thalamus
198.3 Thalamus metastatic

195.5 Thigh ill defined
198.89 Thigh ill defined metastatic
173.7 Thigh skin
198.2 Thigh skin metastatic
171.3 Thigh soft tissue
198.89 Thigh soft tissue metastatic

195.1 Thorax ill defined
198.89 Thorax metastatic
171.4 Thorax soft tissue

149.0 Throat
198.89 Throat metastatic

164.0 Thymus
198.89 Thymus metastatic
V10.29 Thymus personal history

CANCER (continued)

193 Thyroglossal duct
198.89 Thyroglossal duct metastatic

161.3 Thyroid cartilage
197.3 Thyroid cartilage metastatic
193 Thyroid gland
198.89 Thyroid gland metastatic
V10.87 Thyroid personal history

170.7 Tibia
198.5 Tibia metastatic

196.5 Tibial lymph nodes metastatic

195.5 Toe ill defined
198.89 Toe ill defined metastatic
173.7 Toe skin
198.2 Toe skin metastatic
171.3 Toe soft tissue
198.89 Toe soft tissue metastatic

141.9 Tongue
141.4 Tongue anterior two-thirds
141.1 Tongue anterior two thirds, dorsal surface
141.3 Tongue anterior two thirds, ventral surface
141.0 Tongue base
141.0 Tongue base dorsal
141.1 Tongue dorsal
141.1 Tongue dorsal midline
141.0 Tongue dorsal surface of base
141.0 Tongue fixed part
141.5 Tongue junctional zone
141.2 Tongue lateral border
141.6 Tongue lingual tonsil
198.89 Tongue metastatic
141.4 Tongue mobile part NOS
V10.01 Tongue personal history
141.2 Tongue tip
141.3 Tongue ventral
141.8 Tongue other overlapping
141.8 Tongue overlapping origin not determined

Symptoms of a malignancy such as pain or nausea should not replace the cancer code(s). Sequence the cancer first and the cancer associated pain 338.3 or nausea second.

146.0 Tonsil
146.0 Tonsil faucial
141.6 Tonsil lingual
198.89 Tonsil or tonsillar metastatic
146.0 Tonsil oropharynx faucial
146.0 Tonsil oropharynx palatine
146.0 Tonsil palatine
147.1 Tonsil pharyngeal
146.1 Tonsillar fossa
146.1 Tonsillar fossa oropharynx
146.2 Tonsillar pillars

195.8 Torso other specified sites ill defined
198.89 Torso other specified sites ill defined metastatic

162.0 Trachea
162.0 Trachea cartilage
197.3 Trachea metastatic
162.0 Trachea mucosa
V10.12 Trachea personal history

C

CANCER (continued)

162.8	Tracheobronchial NOS
197.3	Tracheobronchial NOS metastatic
196.1	Tracheobronchial nodes metastatic
170.5	Trapezium, trapezoid
198.5	Trapezium, trapezoid metastatic
195.8	Trunk ill defined
198.89	Trunk ill defined metastatic
173.5	Trunk skin
198.2	Trunk skin metastatic
171.7	Trunk soft tissue
198.89	Trunk soft tissue metastatic
183.8	Tubo ovarian
198.82	Tubo ovarian metastatic
187.8	Tunica vaginalis
198.82	Tunica vaginalis metastatic
170.0	Turbinate bone (cartilage) (joint) (periosteum)
198.5	Turbinate bone (cartilage) (joint) (periosteum) metastatic
160.1	Tympanic cavity
197.3	Tympanic cavity metastatic
170.4	Ulna
198.5	Ulna metastatic
173.5	Umbilicus skin
198.2	Umbilicus skin metastatic
170.5	Unciform
198.5	Unciform metastatic
191.2	Uncus
198.3	Uncus metastatic
199.1	Undifferentiated type site unspecified
165.0	Upper airway
197.3	Upper airway metastatic
195.4	Upper limb ill defined
198.89	Upper limb ill defined metastatic
171.2	Upper limb shoulder soft tissue
198.89	Upper limb shoulder soft tissue metastatic
173.6	Upper limb skin
198.2	Upper limb skin metastatic
165.0	Upper respiratory tract
197.3	Upper respiratory tract metastatic
189.2	Ureter
198.1	Ureter metastatic
188.6	Ureteric orifice bladder
198.1	Ureteric orifice bladder metastatic
189.1	Ureteropelvic junction
198.0	Ureteropelvic junction metastatic
189.3	Urethra
198.1	Urethra metastatic
188.5	Urethra orifice of bladder
189.9	Urinary organs
V10.50	Urinary organs unspecified personal history
198.1	Urinary organs metastatic
V10.59	Urinary organs other specified personal history
189.8	Urinary organs overlapping sites
189.9	Urinary system NOS
198.1	Urinary system NOS metastatic

CANCER (continued)

183.8	Utero ovarian
198.82	Utero ovarian metastatic
183.4	Uterosacral ligament
198.82	Uterosacral ligament metastatic

When both a primary and secondary site are present and treated equally, sequence the primary site first.

179	Uterus
182.0	Uterus body corpus
180.9	Uterus cervix
182.0	Uterus cornu
182.0	Uterus fundus
182.1	Uterus isthmus
183.4	Uterus ligament
182.1	Uterus lower segment
198.82	Uterus metastatic
V10.42	Uterus personal history (excluding cervix)
183.2	Uterus tube
182.8	Uterus other specified site
190.0	Uveal tract
198.4	Uveal tract metastatic
145.4	Uvula
198.89	Uvula metastatic
184.0	Vagina
198.82	Vagina metastatic
184.9	Vagina septum
184.0	Vagina vault
146.3	Vallecula
198.89	Vallecula metastatic
187.6	Vas deferens (spermatic cord)
198.82	Vas deferens (spermatic cord) metastatic
191.5	Ventricles choroid plexus
198.3	Ventricles choroid plexus metastatic
191.5	Ventricles floor of ventricle
198.3	Ventricles floor of ventricle metastatic
161.1	Ventricular bands, supraglottis
197.3	Ventricular bands, supraglottis metastatic
140.9	Vermilion border
140.1	Vermilion border lip lower
140.0	Vermilion border lip upper
198.89	Vermilion border metastatic
170.2	Vertebra
198.5	Vertebra metastatic
170.6	Vertebra - sacrum, coccyx
198.5	Vertebra - sacrum, coccyx metastatic
184.9	Vesicovaginal
198.82	Vesicovaginal metastatic
184.9	Vesicovaginal septum
198.82	Vesicovaginal septum metastatic
163.1	Visceral pleural
197.2	Visceral pleural metastatic
161.0	Vocal cords true
161.1	Vocal cords false
197.3	Vocal cords metastatic (true) (false)
170.0	Vomer (cartilage) (joint) (periosteum)
198.5	Vomer metastatic (cartilage) (joint) (periosteum)

C

CANCER (continued)

184.4 Vulva
198.82 Vulva metastatic
149.1 Waldeyer's ring
198.89 Waldeyer's ring metastatic
142.1 Wharton's duct
198.89 Wharton's duct metastatic
170.3 Xiphoid
198.5 Xiphoid metastatic
194.6 Zuckerkandl's organ
198.89 Zuckerkandl's organ metastatic
170.0 Zygomatic bone
198.5 Zygomatic bone metastatic

795.82 CANCER ANTIGEN 125 ELEVATED (CA 125)

> ***If treatment is directed toward the metastatic site, then that site is coded first, even if the primary site is known.***
>
> ***When both a primary and secondary site are present and treated equally, sequence the primary site first.***

CANCER METASTATIC

199.1 Site NOS

197.# Digestive

4th digit: 197
- **4. Small intestine, duodenum**
- **5. Large intestine, rectum**
- **6. Retroperitoneum and peritoneum**
- **7. Liver, specified as secondary**
- **8. Other digestive organs and spleen**

196.# Lymph node metastatic

4th digit: 196
- **0. Head, face, neck, cervical, supraclavicular**
- **1. Intrathoracic, bronchopulmonary, mediastinal, tracheobronchial**
- **2. Intraabdominal, mesenteric, retroperitoneal**
- **3. Axilla, upper limb, brachial, intraclavicular, pectoral**
- **5. Lower limb, inguinal, femoral, groin, tibial**
- **6. Intrapelvic hypogastric iliac parametrial**
- **8. Multiple sites**
- **9. Lymph nodes NOS**

197.# Respiratory

4th digit: 197
- **0. Lung, bronchus**
- **1. Mediastinum**
- **2. Pleura**
- **3. Other respiratory organs, trachea**

198.#(#) Other specified sites

4th or 4th and 5th digit: 198
- **0. Kidney**
- **1. Other urinary organs**
- **2. Skin and skin of breast (or mastectomy site skin)**
- **3. Brain and spinal cord**
- **4. Other parts of nervous system, meninges (cerebral) (spinal)**
- **5. Bone and bone marrow**
- **6. Ovary**
- **7. Adrenal gland**
- **8#. Other specified sites**
  - **81. Breast soft tissue**
  - **82. Genital organs**
  - **89. Other**

CANCER SCREENING

V76.9 NOS
V76.3 Bladder
V76.89 Blood
V76.10 Breast unspecified
V76.11 Breast mammogram for high risk patient
V76.12 Breast mammogram NEC
V76.19 Breast specified type NEC
V76.2 Cervix
V76.51 Colon
V76.51 Colorectal
V76.50 Intestinal - unspecified
V76.51 Intestinal - colon
V76.52 Intestinal - small
V76.89 Lymph (gland) (node)
V76.81 Nervous system
V76.42 Oral cavity
V76.46 Ovary
V76.44 Prostate
V76.41 Rectal cancer
V76.0 Respiratory organs
V76.43 Skin
V76.45 Testis
V76.47 Vagina
V76.49 Other sites
V76.89 Other neoplasms (benign) (tumors)

528.1 CANCRUM ORIS

112.5 CANDIDEMIA

CANDIDIASIS

112.9 Unspecified site
112.2 Balanitis
112.5 Disseminated
112.81 Endocarditis
112.85 Enteritis
112.84 Esophagitis
771.7 Infection neonatal
112.3 Intertrigo
112.85 Intestine
112.4 Lung
112.83 Meningitis
112.0 Mouth
112.3 Nails
112.3 Onychia
112.0 Oral
112.82 Otitis externa
112.3 Perionyxis (paronychia)
112.4 Pneumonia
112.2 Pyelonephritis
112.3 Skin
112.5 Systemic
112.2 Urinary tract
112.2 Urogenital other
112.2 UTI
112.1 Vulvovaginitis
112.89 Other specified site NEC

136.8 CANDIRU INFESTATION

528.2 CANKER SORE

504 CANNABINOSIS

C

305.2# CANNABIS ABUSE NONDEPENDENT
304.3# CANNABIS ADDICTION DEPENDENT

5th digit: 304.3, 305.2
0. NOS
1. Continuous
2. Episodic
3. In remission

128.8 CAPILLARIA HEPATICA INFECTION
127.5 CAPILLARIA PHILIPPINENSIS INFECTION
127.5 CAPILLARIASIS
128.8 CAPILLARIASIS HEPATICA

CAPILLARY

277.39 Degeneration amyloid lardaceous
448.9 Disease

648.9#: Use an additional code to identify the capillary disease.

648.9# Disease maternal current (co-existent) in pregnancy

5th digit: 648.9
0. Episode of care NOS or N/A
1. Delivered
2. Delivered with postpartum complication
3. Antepartum complication
4. Postpartum complication

287.8 Fragility (hereditary)
448.9 Hemorrhage (thrombosis) hyperpermeability

714.81 CAPLAN (-COLINET) SYNDROME
434.0# CAPSULAR THROMBOSIS SYNDROME

5th digit: 434.0
0. Without cerebral infarction
1. With cerebral infarction

CAPSULITIS

726.90 Site unspecified
726.5 Hip
726.60 Knee
387.8 Labyrinthine
726.0 Shoulder (adhesive)
726.4 Wrist
0 Site specified see 'Bursitis'

767.19 CAPUT SUCCEDANEUM
087.1 CARAPATA DISEASE
271.8 CARBOHYDRATE-DEFICIENT GLYCOPROTEIN SYNDROME (CDGS)
271.9 CARBOHYDRATE TRANSPORT AND METABOLISM DISORDER
271.8 CARBOHYDRATE TRANSPORT AND METABOLISM DISORDER - OTHER SPECIFIED
786.09 CARBON DIOXIDE NARCOSIS
276.2 CARBON DIOXIDE RETENTION
276.9 CARBONATE ABNORMAL FINDINGS

CARBUNCLE

680.9 Site unspecified
680.2 Abdominal wall
680.6 Ankle
680.5 Anus
680.3 Arm (any part except hand)
680.3 Axilla
680.2 Back (any part except buttocks)
680.2 Breast
680.5 Buttocks

CARBUNCLE (continued)

680.2 Chest wall
607.2 Corpus cavernosum
680.0 Ear (any part)
680.0 External auditory canal
373.13 Eyelid
680.0 Face
680.4 Finger (any)
680.2 Flank
680.7 Foot
680.3 Forearm
616.4 Genitalia female nonobstetrical
608.4 Genitalia male
680.5 Gluteal region
680.2 Groin
680.4 Hand
680.8 Head (any part except face)
680.7 Heel
680.6 Hip
680.6 Knee
375.31 Lacrimal system
680.6 Leg (except foot)
680.9 Multiple site
680.1 Neck
680.0 Nose
680.0 Nose septum
376.01 Orbit
680.2 Pectoral region
607.2 Penis
680.2 Perineum
680.0 Pinna
680.8 Scalp
608.4 Scrotum
680.3 Shoulder
680.0 Temple region
608.4 Testis
680.6 Thigh
680.4 Thumb
680.7 Toe
680.2 Trunk
680.2 Umbilicus
608.4 Vas deferens
616.4 Vulva nonobstetrical
680.4 Wrist

795.81 CARCINOEMBRYONIC ANTIGEN ELEVATED (CEA)
453.1 CARCINOGENIC THROMBOPHLEBITIS SYNDROME

CARCINOID

238.9 Site NOS
0 Site specified see 'Neoplasm Uncertain Behavior', by site
199.1 Composite site NOS
0 Composite site specified see 'Cancer', by site M8244/3
236.2 Strumal site NOS
0 Strumal site specified see 'Neoplasm Uncertain Behavior', by site M9091/1
259.2 Syndrome
238.9 Tumor site NOS
0 Tumor site specified see 'Neoplasm Uncertain Behavior', by site M8240/1

C

CARCINOID (continued)

199.1 Tumor (malignant) site NOS
0 Tumor (malignant) site specified see 'Cancer', by site M8240/3

199.1 Tumor argentaffin malignant site NOS
0 Tumor argentaffin malignant site specified see 'Cancer', by site M8241/1

238.9 Tumor argentaffin site NOS
0 Tumor argentaffin site specified see 'Neoplasm Uncertain Behavior', by site M8241/1

199.1 Tumor nonargentaffin malignant site NOS
0 Tumor nonargentaffin malignant site specified see 'Cancer', by site M8242/1

238.9 Tumor nonargentaffin site NOS
0 Tumor nonargentaffin site specified see 'Neoplasm Uncertain Behavior', by site M8242/1

0 CARCINOMA SITE SPECIFIED SEE 'CANCER', BY SITE M8010/3

CARCINOMA IN SITU QUICK REFERENCE

230.# Digestive organs
4th digit: 230
- **0. Lip, oral cavity, pharynx, marginal zone**
- **1. Esophagus**
- **2. Stomach**
- **3. Colon**
- **4. Rectum**
- **5. Anal canal**
- **6. Anus, unspecified**
- **7. Other and unspecified parts of intestine**
- **8. Liver and biliary system**
- **9. Other and unspecified digestive organs**

233.#(#) Genitourinary and breast
4th or 4th and 5th digit: 233
- **0. Breast**
- **1. Cervix uteri**
- **2. Other and unspecified parts of uterus**
- **3#. Other and unspecified female genital organs**
  - **0. Unspecified**
  - **1. Vagina**
  - **2. Vulva**
  - **9. Other**
- **4. Prostate**
- **5. Penis**
- **6. Other and unspecified male genital organs**
- **7. Bladder**
- **9. Other and unspecified urinary organs**

231.# Respiratory
4th digit: 231
- **0. Larynx, arytenoid/cricoid/cuneiform/ thyroid cartilage, epiglottis (suprahyoid), vocal cords**
- **1. Trachea**
- **2. Bronchus and lung, carina, hilus of lung**
- **8. Other specified parts of respiratory system: nasal cavities, middle ear, pleura, accessory sinus**
- **9. Respiratory system (organ) NOS**

CARCINOMA IN SITU QUICK REFERENCE (continued)

232.# Skin
4th digit: 232
- **0. Lip**
- **1. Eyelid including canthus**
- **2. Ear external, auditory canal**
- **3. Skin of other and unspecified parts of face**
- **4. Scalp, skin of neck**
- **5. Skin of trunk except scrotum: abdominal wall, anus, anal margin, axillary fold, back, breast, buttock, chest wall, groin, perineum**
- **6. Skin of upper limb, shoulder**
- **7. Skin of lower limb, hip**
- **8. Other specified skin site: nose NOS**
- **9. Skin site NOS**

234.# Other and unspecified parts
4th digit: 234
- **0. Eye**
- **8. Other specified sites: endocrine gland (any), eyelid cartilage, optic nerve, orbit bone**
- **9. Site NOS: CA in situ NOS**

CARCINOMA IN SITU

234.9 NOS
230.8 Ampulla of vater
230.5 Anal canal
230.6 Anus
232.5 Anus skin (margin) (perinal)
230.3 Appendix
230.0 Aryepiglottic fold
231.0 Aryepiglottic fold, laryngeal aspect
230.0 Aryepiglottic hypopharyngeal
230.0 Aryepiglottic marginal
231.0 Arytenoid cartilage
232.5 Axillary fold skin
230.8 Biliary system
233.7 Bladder
230.2 Body of stomach
233.0 Breast
232.5 Breast skin
231.2 Bronchus
232.5 Buttock skin
230.2 Cardia of stomach
230.2 Cardiac orifice
231.2 Carina
230.3 Cecum
233.1 Cervix (stump)
232.5 Chest wall skin
230.3 Colon
230.4 Colon rectosigmoid
230.8 Common bile duct
234.0 Conjunctiva
234.0 Cornea
231.0 Cricoid cartilage
231.0 Cuneiform cartilage
230.8 Cystic duct
230.7 Digestive intestine other
230.9 Digestive organs other and unspecified
230.7 Duodenum
232.2 Ear external
231.8 Ear internal
234.8 Endocrine

C

CARCINOMA IN SITU (continued)

231.0	Epiglottis
231.0	Epiglottis posterior
231.0	Epiglottis suprahyoid
230.1	Esophagus
234.0	Eye
234.8	Eyelid cartilage
232.1	Eyelid skin
232.1	Eyelid skin canthus
232.3	Face skin other and unspecified parts
230.2	Fundus of stomach
230.8	Gallbladder
230.9	Gastrointestinal
233.30	Genitourinary organ female NOS
233.39	Genitourinary organ female NEC
233.6	Genitourinary organ male NEC
230.0	Gingiva
232.5	Groin skin
230.8	Hepatic duct
231.2	Hilus of lung
232.7	Hip lower limb skin
230.0	Hypopharyngeal
230.0	Hypopharynx
230.3	Ileocecal valve
230.7	Ileum
230.7	Intestine small NOS
230.7	Jejunum
230.3	Large intestine
231.0	Larynx
230.0	Lip
232.0	Lip skin
230.8	Liver
231.2	Lung
230.0	Marginal
231.8	Middle ear
230.0	Mouth
230.0	Mouth floor
231.8	Nasal cavities
230.0	Nasopharynx
232.4	Neck skin
234.8	Optic nerve
234.8	Orbit (bone)
230.0	Oropharynx
230.9	Pancreas
230.0	Parotid gland in situ
233.5	Penis
232.5	Perineum skin
231.8	Pleura
233.4	Prostate
230.2	Pylorus
230.4	Rectosigmoid junction
230.4	Rectum
231.9	Respiratory
231.8	Respiratory other
230.0	Salivary gland or duct
232.4	Scalp
232.6	Shoulder upper limb skin
231.8	Sinus (accessory)
232.9	Skin
232.8	Skin other specified sites
230.7	Small intestine
230.8	Sphincter of oddi
230.9	Spleen
230.2	Stomach
231.0	Thyroid
231.0	Thyroid cartilage

CARCINOMA IN SITU (continued)

230.0	Tongue
231.1	Trachea
231.1	Tracheobronchial
232.5	Trunk skin
232.5	Umbilicus skin
233.9	Urinary organ NEC
233.2	Uterus
233.31	Vagina
233.39	Vaginal vesicovaginal septum
234.8	Vesicorectal
231.0	Vocal cords
233.32	Vulva
230.0	Wharton's duct
234.8	Other specified sites

0	CARCINOMA METASTATIC SITE SPECIFIED SEE 'CANCER', BY SITE, METASTATIC M8010/6
0	CARCINOMA SIMPLEX SITE SPECIFIED SEE 'CANCER', BY SITE M8231/3
0	CARCINOMA SKIN APPENDAGE SITE SPECIFIED SEE 'CANCER' SKIN BY SITE M8231/3
0	CARCINOMA UNDIFFERENTIATED TYPE SITE SPECIFIED SEE 'CANCER', BY SITE M8020/3
0	CARCINOMA VENTRICULI SEE 'CANCER', STOMACH
199.0	CARCINOMATOSIS SITE NOS M8010/6
0	CARCINOMATOSIS SITE SPECIFIED SEE 'CANCER', BY SITE M8010/3
199.1	CARCINOSARCOMA EMBRYONAL TYPE SITE NOS
0	CARCINOSARCOMA EMBRYONAL TYPE SITE SPECIFIED SEE 'CANCER', BY SITE M8981/3
199.1	CARCINOSARCOMA SITE NOS
0	CARCINOSARCOMA SITE SPECIFIED SEE 'CANCER' BY SITE M8980/3

CARDIAC

996.83	Allograft vasculopathy
746.87	Apex malposition congenital
428.1	Asthma (syndrome)
429.1	Atrophy (see also 'Myocardial', degeneration)
996.09	Catheter complication mechanical
V58.82	Catheter nonvascular adjustment
V58.81	Catheter vascular adjustment
426.9	Conduction delay (ventricular)
861.01	Contusion
861.11	Contusion with open wound
908.0	Contusion late effect
0	Defibrillator see 'Cardiac Defibrillator'
V53.39	Device other specified - fitting and adjustment
V45.00	Device unspecified - in situ status
V45.09	Device other specified - in situ status
785.3	Dullness (increased) (decreased)
0	Dysrhythmia see 'Dysrhythmias' or by specified dysrhythmia
428.9	Failure
779.89	Failure fetus or newborn
794.30	Function study abnormal
429.3	Hypertrophy
746.89	Hypertrophy congenital
861.00	Injury NOS
861.10	Injury NOS with open wound into thorax
908.0	Injury NOS late effect
429.4	Insufficiency following cardiac surgery

CARDIAC (continued)

861.02 Laceration
861.12 Laceration with open wound into chest
908.0 Laceration late effect
306.2 Neurosis psychogenic
0 Pacemaker see 'Cardiac Pacemaker'

> ***When code V57.89 is assigned as the principal diagnosis, a secondary code (s) should be assigned to identify and explain the condition(s) requiring the rehabilitation services.***
>
> ***V57.89 Cardiac rehabilitation due to myocaridial infaction less than 8 weeks [410.#2] or greater than 8weeks [414.##].***

V57.89 Rehabilitation
V57.89 Rehabilitation secondary to MI (< 8 weeks) **[410.#2]**
4th digit: 410.#2
0. Anterior lateral
1. Anterior
2. Inferior lateral
3. Inferior posterior
4. Inferior other
5. Lateral
6. Posterior
7. Subendocardial
8. Other site
9. Site NOS
V57.89 Rehabilitation secondary to MI (> 8 weeks) with CAD with chronic complete or total occlussion **[414.0#]** [414.2]
5th digit: 414.0
0. Unspecified type of vessel, native or graft
1. Native coronary vessel
2. Autologous vein bypass graft
3. Nonautologous biological bypass graft
4. Autologous artery bypass graft (gastroepiploic) (internal mammary)
5. Unspecified type of bypass graft
6. Native vessel of transplanted heart
7. Bypass graft of transplanted heart
794.39 Stress test abnormal NOS
423.3 Tamponade
746.89 Valve atresia
746.89 Valve hypertrophy NEC congenital
746.89 Vein atresia
746.89 Vein hypoplasia

> ***Cardiac arrest is not an acceptable principal diagnosis by most carriers. As a general rule, code first the disease or condition which led immediately to the arrest. Exception: If the reason the patient presented was the arrest.***

CARDIAC ARREST

427.5 NOS
997.1 During or resulting from a procedure [427.5]
779.85 Fetus
639.8 Following abortion
668.1# Following anesthesia (or failure) L&D
669.4# Following obstetrical surgery or procedure or delivery
5th digit: 668.1, 669.4
0. Episode of care NOS or N/A
1. Delivered
2. Delivered with postpartum complication
3. Antepartum complication
4. Postpartum complication

CARDIAC ARREST (continued)

V12.53 History sudden (successfully resuscitated)
779.85 Newborn
V12.53 Sudden history (successfully resuscitated)

CARDIAC DEFIBRILLATOR

996.61 Complication - infection or inflammation
996.04 Complication - mechanical
996.72 Complication - other
V53.32 Fitting and adjustment
V45.02 In situ (automatic implantable)

CARDIAC PACEMAKER

V53.31 Battery replacement
996.61 Complication - infection or inflammation
996.01 Complication - mechanical (breakdown) (perforation) (displaced)
996.72 Complication - other
V53.31 Fitting and adjustment
V45.01 In situ status
996.01 Malfunction (breakdown) (perforation) (displaced)
V53.31 Reprogramming
429.4 Syndrome

416.0 CARDIACOS NEGROS SYNDROME
747.49 CARDINAL VEIN LEFT POSTERIOR PERSISTENT CONGENITAL
530.89 CARDIO-ESOPHAGEAL RELAXATION
530.81 CARDIOCHALASIA
793.2 CARDIOGRAM ABNORMAL

CARDIOMEGALY

429.3 NOS
746.89 Congenital
271.0 Glycogen
402.#0 Hypertensive
4th digit: 402.#0
0. Malignant
1. Benign
9. NOS

402.#1 Hypertensive with heart failure **[428.#(#)]**
4th digit: 402.#1
0. Malignant
1. Benign
9. NOS

4th digit: 428
0. Congestive
1. Left
2#. Systolic
3#. Diastolic
4#. Combined systolic and diastolic
9. NOS

5th digit: 428.2-4
0. NOS
1. Acute
2. Chronic
3. Acute on chronic

429.3 Idiopathic

CARDIOMYOPATHY

425.4 NOS
425.5 Alcoholic
429.1 Arteriosclerotic [440.9]
425.5 Cobalt-beer
425.3 Congenital
425.4 Congestive
425.4 Constrictive

CARDIOMYOPATHY (continued)

425.4 Familial
274.82 Gouty
402.#0 Hypertensive
4th digit: 402.#0
0. Malignant
1. Benign
9. NOS

402.#1 Hypertensive with heart failure [**428.#(#)**]
4th digit: 402.#1
0. Malignant
1. Benign
9. NOS

4th digit: 428
0. Congestive
1. Left
2#. Systolic
3#. Diastolic
4#. Combined systolic and diastolic
9. NOS
5th digit: 428.2-4
0. NOS
1. Acute
2. Chronic
3. Acute on chronic

425.4 Hypertrophic
425.1 Hypertrophic obstructive
746.84 Hypertrophic obstructive congenital
425.4 Idiopathic
425.2 Idiopathic mural
414.8 Ischemic
425.4 Newborn
425.3 Newborn congenital
425.4 Nonobstructive
425.2 Obscure of africa
425.4 Obstructive
425.4 Primary
425.4 Restrictive
425.9 Secondary
429.83 Stress induced
429.83 Takotsubo
425.9 Toxic NEC

CARDIOMYOPATHY OTHER

277.39 Amyloid [425.7]
265.0 Beri Beri [425.7]
086.0 Chagas' disease
425.3 Elastomyofibrosis
425.0 Endomyocardial fibrosis
334.0 Friedreich's (ataxia) [425.8]
271.0 Glycogenic (cardiac) [425.7]
487.8 Influenza [425.8]

When coding a maternal cardiomyopathy complicating pregnancy, 648.6#, use an additional code to identify the cardiomyopathy.

648.6# Maternal current (co-existent) in pregnancy [425.9]
5th digit: 648.6
0. Episode of care NOS or N/A
1. Delivered
2. Delivered with postpartum complication
3. Antepartum complication
4. Postpartum complication

CARDIOMYOPATHY OTHER (continued)

674.5# Maternal peripartum or postpartum
5th digit: 674.5
0. Episode of care NOS or N/A
1. Delivered
2. Delivered with postpartum complication
3. Antepartum complication
4. Postpartum complication

277.39 Metabolic amyloid [425.7]
277.9 Metabolic NEC [425.7]
277.5 Mucopolysaccharidosis [425.7]
359.1 Muscular dystrophy [425.8]
359.21 Myotonia atrophica [425.8]
265.0 Nutritional (beriberi) [425.7]
269.9 Nutritional malnutrition [425.7]
135 Sarcoid [425.8]
242.## Thyrotoxic [425.7]
4th digit: 242
0. Diffuse
1. Uninodular
2. Multinodular
3. Nodular unspecified
4. Ectopic thyroid nodular
8. Other specified
9. NOS
5th digit: 242
0. Without mention of thyrotoxic crisis or storm
1. With mention of thyrotoxic crisis or storm

017.9# Tuberculous [425.8]
5th digit: 017.9
0. Unspecified
1. Lab not done
2. Lab pending
3. Microscopy positive (in sputum)
4. Culture positive - microscopy negative
5. Culture negative - microscopy positive
6. Culture and microscopy negative confirmed by other methods

306.2 CARDIONEUROSIS
746.87 CARDIOPTOSIS
427.5 CARDIOPULMONARY ARREST
416.9 CARDIOPULMONARY DISEASE, CHRONIC
278.8 CARDIOPULMONARY OBESITY SYNDROME
428.9 CARDIORENAL FAILURE (CHRONIC)
404.90 CARDIORENAL SYNDROME
779.85 CARDIORESPIRATORY COLLAPSE NEWBORN
769 CARDIORESPIRATORY DISTRESS SYNDROME (IDIOPATHIC) NEWBORN
799.1 CARDIORESPIRATORY FAILURE
V47.2 CARDIORESPIRATORY PROBLEMS OTHER
530.0 CARDIOSPASM
750.7 CARDIOSPASM CONGENITAL
423.1 CARDIOSYMPHYSIS

CARDIOVASCULAR

794.30 Abnormal function study
794.31 Abnormal electrocardiogram (ECG) (EKG)
794.39 Abnormal other study
425.4 Collagenosis

CARDIOVASCULAR (continued)

785.51 Collapse
779.85 Collapse newborn
V81.2 Conditons unspecified screening
429.2 Disease
429.2 Disease arteriosclerotic [440.9]
746.9 Disease congenital
V17.49 Disease family history
402.#0 Disease hypertensive (arteriosclerotic)
402.#1 Disease hypertensive (arteriosclerotic) with heart failure [428.#(#)]

4th digit: 402.#1
0. Malignant
1. Benign
9. NOS

4th digit: 428
0. Congestive
1. Left
2#. Systolic
3#. Diastolic
4#. Combined systolic and diastolic
9. NOS

5th digit: 428.2-4
0. NOS
1. Acute
2. Chronic
3. Acute on chronic

V12.50 Disease history unspecified
V12.59 Disease history other specified

> ***When coding a maternal cardiovascular disease complicating pregnancy, 648.6#, use an additional code to identify the condition.***

648.6# Disease maternal current (co-existent) in pregnancy

5th digit: 648.6
0. Episode of care NOS or N/A
1. Delivered
2. Delivered with postpartum complication
3. Antepartum complication
4. Postpartum complication

306.2 Disorder (system) psychogenic
306.2 Neurosis psychogenic
404.90 Renal syndrome
785.9 Symptom other

272.7 CARDIOVASORENAL SYNDROME

CARDITIS

429.89 NOS
074.20 Coxsackie
0 Hypertensive see 'Cardiomyopathy'
036.40 Meningococcal
429.89 Other (nonhypertensive)
391.9 Rheumatic acute
398.90 Rheumatic chronic

V60.5 CARE HOLIDAY RELIEF
V62.2 CAREER CHOICE PROBLEM
0 CARIES DENTAL SEE 'DENTAL', CARIES
757.1 CARINI'S SYNDROME (ICHTHYOSIS CONGENITA)

631 CARNEOUS MOLE
631 CARNEOUS MOLE WITH COMPLICATION DURING TREATMENT [639.#]
639.# CARNEOUS MOLE WITH COMPLICATION FOLLOWING TREATMENT

4th digit: 639
0. Genital tract and pelvic infection
1. Delayed or excessive hemorrhage
2. Damage to pelvic organs and tissue
3. Renal failure
4. Metabolic disorders
5. Shock
6. Embolism
8. Other specified complication
9. Unspecified complication

CARNITINE DEFICIENCY

277.81 NOS
277.83 Due to hemodialysis
277.82 Due to inborn errors of metabolism
277.83 Due to valproic acid therapy
277.83 Iatrogenic (due to procedure)
277.85 Palmitoyltransferase (CPT1, CPT2)
277.85 Palmityl transferase (CPT1, CPT2)
277.81 Primary
277.84 Secondary other specified

270.5 CARNOSINEMIA

CAROTID ARTERY

437.3 Aneurysm - internal NOS (intracranial portion)
442.81 Aneurysm - internal extracranial portion
433.1# Arteriosclerosis

5th digit: 433.1
0. Without cerebral infarction
1. With cerebral infarction

237.3 Body tumor site NOS
0 Body tumor site specified see 'Neoplasm Uncertain Behavior', by site M8980/3
996.62 Bypass graft complication - infection or inflammation
996.1 Bypass graft complication - mechanical
996.74 Bypass graft complication - other
433.1# Disease (ulcerative)
443.21 Dissection
433.1# Embolism thrombosis

5th digit: 433.1
0. Without cerebral infarction
1. With cerebral infarction

447.8 Hyperplasia

> ***Injury of a blood vessel can be a laceration, A-V fistula, aneurym or hematoma. Use the injury code found by anatomical site (the name of the blood vessel).***

900.00 Injury - NOS
900.01 Injury - common
900.02 Injury - external
900.03 Injury - internal
908.3 Injury - late effect
433.1# Occlusion (obstruction) (thrombosis) (embolism) (stenosis)
433.3# Occlusion bilateral or with basilar and/or vertebral artery

5th digit: 433.1, 3
0. Without cerebral infarction
1. With cerebral infarction

CAROTID ARTERY (continued)

337.0 Pain
337.0 Sinus syncope
435.8 Spasm
435.8 Syndrome (internal)

337.0 CAROTID BODY OR SINUS SYNDROME
259.8 CAROTID GLAND DISEASE
V53.39 CAROTID SINUS PACEMAKER FITTING AND ADJUSTMENT
V45.09 CAROTID SINUS PACEMAKER IN SITU
337.0 CAROTIDYNIA
278.3 CAROTINEMIA

CARPAL

755.21 Absence with complete absence of distal elements
755.28 Absence with incomplete absence of distal elements
755.56 Accessory bone
755.28 Agenesis
755.28 Or metacarpals agenesis
842.01 Separation (rupture) (tear) (laceration)
842.01 Strain (sprain) (avulsion) (hemarthrosis)
354.0 Tunnel syndrome

759.89 CARPENTER'S SYNDROME

CARPOMETACARPAL JOINT DISLOCATION

833.04 Carpometacarpal closed
833.14 Carpometacarpal open

833.05 Metacarpal bone proximal closed
833.15 Metacarpal bone proximal open

833.03 Midcarpal closed
833.13 Midcarpal open

842.11 CARPOMETACARPAL STRAIN (SPRAIN)
781.7 CARPOPEDAL SPASM

CARRIER (SUSPECTED)

V02.2 Amebiasis
V02.0 Cholera
V83.81 Cystic fibrosis gene
V02.4 Diphtheria
V02.2 Endamoeba histolytica
V02.3 Gastrointestinal other pathogens
V83.89 Genetic defect
V02.7 Gonorrhea
V02.61 HAA (hepatitis Australian-antigen)
V83.01 Hemophilia A
V83.02 Hemophilia A - symptomatic
V02.60 Hepatitis viral NOS
V02.61 Hepatitis viral B (HAA) (serum)
V02.62 Hepatitis viral C
V02.69 Hepatitis viral other
V02.59 Meningococcal
V02.3 Salmonella
V02.61 Serum hepatitis
V02.3 Shigella
V02.59 Staphylococcal
V02.51 Streptococcus group B
V02.52 Streptococcus other
V02.1 Typhoid
V02.60 Viral hepatitis NOS
V02.61 Viral hepatitis B (HAA) (serum)
V02.62 Viral hepatitis C
V02.69 Viral hepatitis other

CARRIER (SUSPECTED) (continued)

V83.89 Other defective gene
V02.59 Other specified bacterial disease
V02.9 Other specified infectious organism
V02.8 Other venereal disease

088.0 CARRION'S DISEASE (BARTONELLOSIS)

CARTILAGE

756.9 Agenesis
733.99 Atrophy (infectional) (joint)
733.99 Calcification (postinfectional)
748.3 Cleft congenital
718.0# Derangement (articular) old
718.3# Derangement (articular) - recurrent

5th digit: 718.0, 3
0. Site unspecified
1. Shoulder region
2. Upper arm (elbow) (humerus)
3. Forearm (radius) (wrist) (ulna)
4. Hand (carpal) (metacarpal) (fingers)
5. Pelvic region (hip) (buttock) (femur)
6. Lower leg (fibula) (knee) (patella) (tibia)
7. Ankle and/or foot (metatarsals) (toes) (tarsals)
8. Other
9. Multiple

717.9 Derangement knee - NOS old
0 Derangement knee - meniscus see 'Meniscus', knee tear
717.5 Derangement knee - semilunar old
733.90 Disease or disorder
733.99 Disease or disorder - specified NEC

CARUNCLE

372.00 Conjunctiva
373.00 Eyelid
616.89 Labium
375.30 Lacrimal
599.3 Urethra
616.89 Vagina

537.6 CASCADE STOMACH
259.2 CASSIDY (-SCHOLTE) SYNDROME (MALIGNANT CARCINOID)

CAST

V54.89 Aftercare
0 Application see specific injury
V54.89 Change
V54.89 Checking
V53.7 Fitting and adjustment
V54.89 Removal
557.1 Syndrome (body cast) (mesenteric artery ischemia)

104.8 CASTELLANI'S DISEASE
281.0 CASTLE'S DEFICIENCY
281.0 CASTLE'S DEFICIENCY WITH <u>SPINAL CORD DEGENERATION</u> [336.2]
266.2 CASTLE'S DEFICIENCY WITHOUT ANEMIA
266.2 CASTLE'S DEFICIENCY WITHOUT ANEMIA OR SPINAL CORD DEGENERATION

0 CAT BITE SEE 'OPEN WOUND', BY SITE
758.31 CAT CRY SYNDROME
V72.5 CAT SCAN
794.09 CAT SCAN BRAIN ABNORMAL

078.3	CAT SCRATCH FEVER
0	CATAPLEXY SEE 'NARCOLEPSY'

CATARACT

366.9	NOS
V45.61	Extraction status with artificial lens status [V43.1]
998.82	Fragments in eye following surgery
V80.2	Screening

CATARACT NONSENILE (INFANTILE) (JUVENILE) (PRESENILE)

366.00	NOS
366.09	Combined forms
366.03	Cortical
998.82	Fragments in eye following surgery
366.03	Lamellar
366.04	Nuclear
366.01	Subcapsular polar anterior
366.02	Subcapsular polar posterior
366.03	Zonular
366.09	Other forms

CATARACT SENILE

366.10	NOS
366.19	Combined forms
366.12	Coronary
366.15	Cortical
V45.61	Extraction status with artificial lens status [V43.1]
998.82	Fragments in eye following surgery
366.18	Hypermature
366.12	Immature
366.12	Incipient
366.17	Mature
366.18	Morgagni
366.16	Nuclear
366.11	Pseudoexfoliation of lens capsule
366.12	Punctate
V80.2	Screening
366.13	Subcapsular polar anterior
366.14	Subcapsular polar posterior
366.17	Total
366.12	Water clefts
366.19	Other forms

CATARACT TRAUMATIC

366.20	NOS
V45.61	Extraction status with artificial lens status [V43.1]
998.82	Fragments in eye following surgery
366.21	Localized opacities
366.23	Partially resolved
V80.2	Screening
366.22	Total

CATARACT OTHER ETIOLOGIES

366.46	Associated with radiation and other physical influences
275.40	Calcinosis (due to) [366.42]
743.31	Capsular and subcapsular congenital
360.24	Chalcosis [366.34]
363.20	Choroiditis (chronic) [366.32]
366.30	Complicata
743.30	Congenital
743.32	Cortical and zonular congenital
756.0	Craniofascial dysostosis [366.44]
366.34	Degenerative (in degenerative disorder)

CATARACT OTHER ETIOLOGIES (continued)

250.5#	Diabetic [366.41] **5th digit: 250.5** **0. Type II, adult-onset, non-insulin dependent (even if requiring insulin), or unspecified; controlled** **1. Type I, Juvenile-onset or insulin-dependent; controlled** **2. Type II, adult-onset, non-insulin dependent (even if requiring insulin); uncontrolled** **3. Type I, juvenile-onset or insulin-dependent; uncontrolled**
366.45	Drug induced
998.82	Fragments in eye following surgery
271.1	Galactosemic [366.44]
365.9	Glaucoma [366.31]
366.31	Glaucomatous flecks (subcapsular)
252.1	Hypoparathyroidism (due to) [366.42]
363.0#	Inflammatory (choroiditis) (retinitis) [366.32] **5th digit: 363.0** **0. Focal NOS** **1. Focal juxtapapillary** **3. Focal posterior pole** **4. Focal peripheral** **5. Focal juxtapapillary with retinochoroiditis** **6. Focal macular** **7. Focal posterior pole with retinochorioditis** **8. Focal peripheral retinochorioditis**
366.32	Inflammatory (disorder)
364.10	Iridocyclitis (due to) [366.33]
366.8	Lens calcification
360.21	Myopic (degenerative) [366.34]
359.21	Myotonic [366.43]
743.33	Nuclear congenital
743.39	Other congenital
362.74	Pigmentary retinal dystrophy [366.34]
366.46	Radiation and other physical influences (associated)
366.50	Secondary
366.30	Secondary to ocular disorders
250.5#	Snowflake [366.41] **5th digit: 250.5** **0. Type II, adult-onset, non-insulin dependent (even if requiring insulin), or unspecified; controlled** **1. Type I, juvenile-onset or insulin-dependent; controlled** **2. Type II, adult-onset, non-insulin dependent (even if requiring insulin); uncontrolled** **3. Type I, juvenile-onset or insulin-dependent; uncontrolled**
360.24	Sunflower [366.34]
275.49	Tetanic due to calcinosis [366.42]
252.1	Tetanic due to hypothyroidism [366.42]
743.34	Total and subtotal congenital
366.45	Toxic
366.33	With neovascularization
743.32	Zonular congenital
366.03	Zonular juvenile

366.16	CATARACTA BRUNESCENS
366.30	CATARACTA COMPLICATA

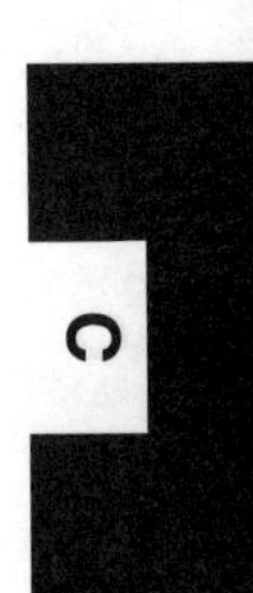

462 CATARRHAL ANGINA

781.99 CATATONIA (ACUTE)

293.89 CATATONIA DISORDER IN CONDITIONS CLASSIFIED ELSEWHERE

293.89 CATATONIA DUE TO OR ASSOCIATED WITH PHYSICAL CONDITION

0 CATATONIA WITH AFFECTIVE PSYCHOSIS SEE 'MANIC DEPRESSIVE PSYCHOSIS'

0 CATATONIA WITH SCHIZOPHRENIA SEE 'SCHIZOPHRENIA'

791.9 CATECHOLAMINES ABNORMAL

255.6 CATECHOLAMINE SECRETION BY PHEOCHROMOCYTOMA

791.9 CATECHOLAMINES URINARY ELEVATION

CATHETER

998.2 Accidental laceration or puncture (during a procedure)

V58.82 Aftercare - nonvascular NEC

V58.81 Cardiac - aftercare

V58.81 Cardiac - care (fitting) (adjustment) (removal) (replacement) (toilet) (cleansing)

996.61 Cardiac complication - infection or inflammation

996.09 Cardiac complication - mechanical

996.72 Cardiac complication - other specified

0 Dialysis see 'Catheter', hemodialysis

V56.1 Hemodialysis (extracorporeal) - aftercare

V56.1 Hemodialysis (extracorporeal) - care (fitting) (adjustment) (removal) (replacement) (toilet) (cleansing)

996.62 Hemodialysis (extracorporeal) complication - infection or inflammation

996.1 Hemodialysis (extracorporeal) complication - mechanical

996.73 Hemodialysis (extracorporeal) complication - other specified

0 Ostomy complication see specified ostomy

V56.2 Peritoneal dialysis - aftercare

V56.2 Peritoneal dialysis - care (fitting) (adjustment) (removal) (replacement) (toilet) (cleansing)

996.68 Peritoneal dialysis complication - infection or inflammation

996.56 Peritoneal dialysis complication - mechanical

996.79 Peritoneal dialysis complication - other specified

999.31 Other infection - Use an additional code to identify the specified infection such as septicemia, (038.#(#)).

999.31 Related bloodstream infection (CRBSI)

996.63 Spinal complication - infection or inflammation

996.2 Spinal complication - mechanical

996.75 Spinal complication - other specified

V53.6 Urinary - aftercare

V53.6 Urinary - care (fitting) (adjustment) (removal) (replacement) (toilet) (cleansing)

996.64 Urinary indwelling complication - infection or inflammation

996.31 Urinary indwelling complication - mechanical

996.76 Urinary indwelling complication - other specified

CATHETER (continued)

V58.81 Vascular NEC - aftercare

V58.81 Vascular NEC - care (fitting) (adjustment) (removal) (replacement) (toilet) (cleansing)

996.62 Vascular NEC (arterial) (arteriovenous dialysis) (venous) complication - infection or inflammation

996.1 Vascular NEC (arterial) (arteriovenous dialysis) (venous) complication - mechanical

996.74 Vascular NEC (arterial) (arteriovenous dialysis) (venous) complication - other specified

996.63 Ventricular shunt complication - infection or inflammation

996.2 Ventricular shunt complication - mechanical

996.75 Ventricular shunt complication - other specified

996.69 Other specified catheter complication - infection or inflammation

996.59 Other specified catheter complication - mechanical

996.79 Other specified catheter complication - other specified

CAUDA EQUINA

742.59 Development defective

806.6# Spinal cord injury with fracture closed

806.7# Spinal cord injury with fracture open

5th digit: 806.6-7

0. Cord injury unspecified

1. Complete cauda equina injury

2. Other cauda equina injury

9. With other spinal cord injury

952.4 Spinal cord injury without fracture

344.60 Syndrome (old) (cause other or unspecified)

344.61 Syndrome (old) (cause other or unspecified) with neurogenic bladder

738.7 CAULIFLOWER EAR

CAUSALGIA (SYNDROME)

355.9 NOS

355.71 Lower limb

354.4 Upper limb

359.3 CAVARE'S FAMILIAL PERIODIC PARALYSIS

228.0# CAVERNOUS NEVUS

5th digit: 228.0

0. Site NOS

1. Skin and subcutaneous tissue

2. Intracranial structures

3. Retina

4. Intra abdominal structures

9. Other sites

437.6 CAVERNOUS SINUS SYNDROME

325 CAVERNOUS SINUS THROMBOSIS

326 CAVERNOUS SINUS THROMBOSIS LATE EFFECT

736.75 CAVOVARUS FOOT DEFORMITY (ACQUIRED)

754.59 CAVOVARUS FOOT DEFORMITY CONGENITAL

736.73 CAVUS FOOT

754.71 CAVUS FOOT CONGENITAL

736.74 CAVUS FOOT WITH CLAW FOOT

694.4 CAZENAVE'S PEMPHIGUS

271.8 CDG (CONGENITAL DISORDER OF GLYCOSYLATION)

271.8 CDGS (CARBOHYDRATE-DEFICIENT GLYCOPROTEIN SYNDROME)

795.81 CEA (CARCINOEMBRYONIC ANTIGEN) ELEVATED

0 CECITIS SEE 'APPENDICITIS'

CECOSTOMY

V53.5 Care - device
V55.4 Care - stoma
V55.4 Catheter care
V55.4 Closure
569.60 Complication - NOS
569.62 Complication - mechanical
569.69 Complication - other
569.69 Fistula
569.69 Hernia

> ***When coding an infection of an ostomy, use an additional code to specify the organism. See 'Bacterial Infection'***

569.61 Infection
569.61 Infection with cellulitis of abdomen [682.2]
569.61 Infection with septicemia [**038.#(#)**]

4th or 4th and 5th Digit Code for Organism: 038

.9 NOS
.3 Anaerobic
.3 Bacteroides
.3 Clostridium
.42 E. coli
.49 Enterobacter aerogenes
.40 Gram negative
.49 Gram negative other
.41 Hemophilus influenzae
.2 Pneumococcal
.49 Proteus
.43 Pseudomonas
.44 Serratia
.10 Staphylococcal NOS
.11 Staphylococcal aureus
.19 Staphylococcal other
.0 Streptococcal (anaerobic)
.49 Yersinia enterocolitica
.8 Other specified

569.62 Malfunction
569.69 Prolapse
V55.4 Removal or replacement
V44.4 Status

CECUM

751.2 Absence congenital
V45.72 Absence postsurgical
564.89 Atony
751.2 Atresia (congenital)
564.89 Dilatation
569.9 Disease
562.10 Diverticulum
751.5 Diverticulum congenital
751.5 Duplication congenital
564.9 Hypermobility
863.89 Injury (traumatic)
863.99 Injury (traumatic) with open wound
560.9 Obstruction (see also 'Intestine, Intestinal', obstruction)
211.3 Polyp
751.4 Rotation (failure) (incomplete) (insufficient) congenital
564.89 Stasis

CELIAC

442.84 Artery (aneurysm) (A-V fistula) (cirsoid) (false) (varicose) (ruptured)
447.4 Artery compression syndrome
648.9# Artery compression syndrome maternal current (co-existent) in pregnancy [447.4]

5th digit: 648.9
0. Episode of care NOS or N/A
1. Delivered
2. Delivered with postpartum complication
3. Antepartum complication
4. Postpartum complication

902.20 Artery injury NOS
902.24 Artery injury other NEC
908.4 Artery injury late effect
902.24 Axis injury other specified branches
908.4 Axis injury late effect
902.24 Axis laceration (rupture) (hematoma) (avulsion) (aneurysm) traumatic
908.4 Axis laceration late effect
447.4 Axis syndrome
579.0 Crisis
579.0 Disease (infantilism) (rickets)
579.0 Disease sprue
579.1 Disease sprue - tropical
954.1 Ganglion or plexus injury
579.0 Syndrome

709.09 CELLULAR TISSUE DISEASE NEC

> ***Cellulitis, 681-682, associated with or secondary to a superficial injury, open wound, burn, or bites requires two codes. Report one for the injury complicated and one for the cellulitis. Sequencing of the two codes depends on the circumstances of admission to a doctor's office or hospital.***

CELLULITIS:

-WITH ORGANISM KNOWN [041.#(#)]

682.9 NOS
682.2 Abdominal wall
040.0 Anaerobic
566 Anal
682.6 Ankle
611.0 Areola
682.3 Arm
682.3 Axilla
682.2 Back
682.5 Back buttock
611.0 Breast
675.1# Breast complicating pregnancy and the puerperium

5th digit: 675.1
0. Episode of care NOS or N/A
1. Delivered
2. Delivered with postpartum complication
3. Antepartum complication
4. Postpartum complication

611.0 Breast nipple
614.4 Broad ligament
614.3 Broad ligament acute
614.4 Broad ligament chronic
682.5 Buttock
569.61 Cecostomy with cellulitis of abdomen [682.2]
569.5 Cecum
540.1 Cecum with appendicitis

C

CELLULITIS: (continued)
-WITH ORGANISM KNOWN [041.#(#)]

616.0 Cervix
682.0 Cheek external
528.3 Cheek internal
682.2 Chest wall
682.0 Chin
569.61 Colostomy with cellulitis of abdomen [682.2]
607.2 Corpus cavernosum

In order to correctly code diabetic cellulitis, you must use an additional code to identify the specified site of the cellulitis. For example: Staphylococcal diabetic cellulitis foot 250.80, 682.7 and 041.10.

250.8# Diabetic
5th digit: 250.8
0. Type II, adult-onset, non-insulin dependent (even if requiring insulin), or unspecified; controlled
1. Type I, juvenile-onset or insulin-dependent; controlled
2. Type II, adult-onset, non-insulin dependent (even if requiring insulin); uncontrolled
3. Type I, juvenile-onset or insulin-dependent; uncontrolled

When coding an infection, use an additional code, [041.#(#)], to identify the organism.

681.9 Digit
614.4 Douglas' cul-de-sac NOS
614.3 Douglas' cul-de-sac acute
614.4 Douglas' cul-de-sac chronic
998.59 Drainage site postoperative
380.10 Ear external auditory canal
380.11 Ear pinna
569.61 Enterostomy with cellulitis of abdomen [682.2]
035 Erysipelas (see also 'Erysipelas')
530.86 Esophagostomy
373.13 Eyelid
682.0 Face
681.01 Felon
681.00 Finger
681.02 Finger onychia and paronychia
682.2 Flank

999.39 Other infection - Use an additional code to identify the specified infection such as septicemia, (038.#(#)).

999.39 Following vaccination
682.7 Foot
681.10 Foot - toe
681.11 Foot - toe onychia and paronychia
682.3 Forearm
682.0 Forehead
785.4 Gangrenous (see also 'Gangrene')
536.41 Gastrostomy with cellulitis of abdomen [682.2]
616.9 Genital organ female (see also 'Abscess', by site)
608.4 Genital organ male
478.71 Glottis
682.5 Gluteal region
098.0 Gonococcal NEC
682.2 Groin

CELLULITIS: (continued)
-WITH ORGANISM KNOWN [041.#(#)]

682.4 Hand
681.00 Hand - finger
681.02 Hand - finger onychia
681.00 Hand - thumb
682.8 Head (except face)
682.7 Heel
682.6 Hip
569.61 Ileostomy with cellulitis of abdomen [682.2]
566 Ischiorectal
682.0 Jaw
569.61 Jejunostomy with cellulitis of abdomen [682.2]
682.6 Knee
616.10 Labium majus minus (see also 'Vaginitis')
478.71 Larynx
682.6 Leg
528.5 Lip
611.0 Mammary gland
528.3 Mouth (floor)
681.9 Nail NOS (finger) (toe)
478.19 Nasal cavity
478.21 Nasopharynx
682.2 Navel
771.4 Navel cord newborn
682.1 Neck
611.0 Nipple
682.0 Nose external
681.02 Onychia finger
681.11 Onychia toe
376.01 Orbital
998.59 Ostomy external
682.8 Other specified site
528.3 Palate (soft)
681.02 Paronychia finger
681.11 Paronychia toe
682.2 Pectoral region
614.4 Pelvis
614.4 Pelvis chronic
614.4 Pelvis female
614.3 Pelvis female - acute
614.4 Pelvis female - chronic
016.7# Pelvis female - tuberculous
5th digit: 016.7
0. Unspecified
1. Lab not done
2. Lab pending
3. Microscopy positive (in sputum)
4. Culture positive - microscopy negative
5. Culture negative - microscopy positive
6. Culture and microscopy negative confirmed by other methods

639.0 Pelvis following abortion ectopic or molar pregnancy
567.21 Pelvis male
670.0# Pelvis maternal due to pregnancy
5th digit: 670.0
0. Episode of care NOS or N/A
2. Delivered with postpartum complication
4. Postpartum complication

0 Pelvis with abortion see 'Abortion', by type, with infection
0 Pelvis with ectopic pregnancy see 'Ectopic Pregnancy'
0 Pelvis with molar pregnancy see 'Molar Pregnancy'

CELLULITIS: (continued)

-WITH ORGANISM KNOWN [041.#(#)]

607.2 Penis
566 Perianal
682.2 Perineum
566 Perirectal
475 Peritonsillar
597.0 Periurethral
0 Periuterine see 'Cellulitis', pelvic
478.21 Pharynx or nasopharynx
682.9 Phlegmonous NEC
380.11 Pinna
614.4 Pouch of Douglas (chronic)
614.3 Pouch of Douglas acute
566 Rectal
611.0 Retromammary
0 Retroperitoneal see 'Peritonitis'
614.4 Round ligament
614.3 Round ligament - acute
614.4 Round ligament - chronic
682.8 Scalp
704.8 Scalp dissecting
608.4 Scrotum
608.0 Seminal vesicle
682.3 Shoulder
682.9 Skin NEC
017.0# Skin and subcutaneous cellular tissue - tuberculous (primary)

5th digit: 017.0
0. Unspecified
1. Lab not done
2. Lab pending
3. Microscopy positive (in sputum)
4. Culture positive - microscopy negative
5. Culture negative - microscopy positive
6. Culture and microscopy negative confirmed by other methods

608.4 Spermatic cord
682.0 Submandibular region
527.3 Submandibular gland
528.3 Submaxillary
527.3 Submaxillary gland
682.0 Submental
527.3 Submental gland
682.0 Temple (region)
608.4 Testis
682.6 Thigh
681.00 Thumb
681.10 Toe
681.11 Toe onychia and paronychia
475 Tonsil
519.01 Tracheostomy with cellulitis of neck [682.1]
682.2 Trunk
608.4 Tunica vaginalis
771.4 Umbilical cord - newborn
682.2 Umbilicus
0 Vagina see 'Vaginitis'
608.4 Vas deferens
478.5 Vocal cord
616.10 Vulva (see also 'Vulvitis')
682.4 Wrist
682.8 Other specified site

CELLULITIS: (continued)

-WITH ORGANISM KNOWN [041.#(#)]

4th or 4th and 5th digit code for organism: 041
.85 Aerobacter aerogenes
.84 Anaerobes other
.82 Bacteroides fragilis
.83 Clostridium perfringens
.4 E. coli (escherichia coli)
.81 Eaton's agent
.85 Enterobacter sakazakii
.04 Enterococcus
.3 Friedlander's bacillus
.84 Gram-negative anaerobes
.85 Gram-negative bacteria NOS
.5 H. influenzae
.86 H. pylori (helicobacter pylori)
.3 Klebsiella
.85 Mima polymorpha
.81 Mycoplasma
.81 Pleuropneumonia like organisms
.2 Pneumococcus
.6 Proteus (mirabilis) (morganii) (vulgaris)
.7 Pseudomonas
.85 Serratia (marcescens)
.10 Staphylococcus unspecified
.11 Staphylococcus aureus
.19 Staphylococcus other
.00 Streptococcus
.01 Streptococcus group A
.02 Streptococcus group B
.03 Streptococcus group C
.04 Streptococcus group D
.05 Streptococcus group G
.09 Streptococcus other
.89 Other specified bacteria

213.# CEMENTOBLASTOMA BENIGN M9273/0
213.# CEMENTOMA NOS M9272/0
213.# CEMENTOMA GIGANTIFORM M9276/0

4th digit: 213
0. Skull, face, upper jaw
1. Lower jaw (or site unspecified)

523.40 CEMENTOPERIOSTITIS
520.4 CEMENTUM APLASIA AND HYPOPLASIA
521.5 CEMENTUM HYPERPLASIA
989.5 CENTIPEDE BITE
995.0 CENTIPEDE BITE WITH ANAPHYLAXIS [989.5]
315.32 CENTRAL AUDITORY PROCESSING DISORDER
359.0 CENTRAL CORE DISEASE
341.8 CENTRAL DEMYELINATION OF CORPUS CALLOSUM
063.2 CENTRAL EUROPEAN ENCEPHALITIS
999.31 CENTRAL LINE COMPLICATION - INFECTION OR INFLAMMATION
996.1 CENTRAL LINE COMPLICATION - MECHANICAL
996.74 CENTRAL LINE COMPLICATION - OTHER
794.00 CENTRAL NERVOUS SYSTEM ABNORMAL FUNCTION STUDY
779.2 CENTRAL NERVOUS SYSTEM DYSFUNCTION NEWBORN NOS
338.0 CENTRAL PAIN SYNDROME
341.8 CENTRAL PONTINE MYELINOSIS

C

362.31 CENTRAL RETINAL ARTERY OCCLUSION
362.35 CENTRAL RETINAL VEIN OCCLUSION
365.63 CENTRAL RETINAL VEIN OCCLUSION CAUSING GLAUCOMA [362.35]
362.41 CENTRAL SEROUS RETINOPATHY
524.55 CENTRIC OCCLUSION MAXIMUM INTERCUSPATION OF TEETH
359.0 CENTRONUCLEAR MYOPATHY
0 CEPHALGIA SEE 'HEADACHE'
920 CEPHALHEMATOMA (TRAUMATIC)
767.19 CEPHALHEMATOMA BIRTH TRAUMA (CEPHALEMATOCELE) (CALCIFIED)

903.1 CEPHALIC VEIN (ARM) INJURY
451.82 CEPHALIC VEIN PHLEBITIS
652.1# CEPHALIC VERSION
660.0# CEPHALIC VERSION OBSTRUCTING LABOR **[652.1#]**

5th digit: 652.1, 660.0
0 Episode of care NOS or N/A
1. Delivered
3. Antepartum complication

653.4# CEPHALOPELVIC DISPROPORTION NOS
660.1# CEPHALOPELVIC DISPROPORTION OBSTRUCTING LABOR NOS **[653.4#]**

5th digit: 653.4, 660.1
0. Episode of care NOS or N/A
1. Delivered
3. Antepartum complication

V09.1 CEPHALOSPORINS RESISTANT INFECTION (SEE 'DRUG RESISTANCE' FOR COMPLETE LISTING)
120.3 CERCARIAE OF SCHISTOSOMA INFECTION

CEREBELLAR

742.2 Absence (congenital)
433.8# Artery occlusion
433.8# Artery thrombosis (embolism) (deformans)

5th digit: 433.8
0. Without cerebral infarction
1. With cerebral infarction

334.3 Ataxia
334.0 Ataxia Friedrich's
334.2 Ataxia Marie's
334.3 Ataxia other
331.9 Atrophy
331.9 Atrophy with dementia **[294.1#]**

5th digit: 294.1
0. Without behavioral disturbance or NOS
1. With behavioral disturbance

851.4# Contusion (with hemorrhage)
851.5# Contusion with open intracranial wound (with hemorrhage)

5th digit: 851.4-5
0. Level of consciousness (LOC) NOS
1. No LOC
2. LOC < 1 hr
3. LOC 1 - 24 hrs
4. LOC > 24 hrs with return to prior level
5. LOC > 24 hrs without return to prior level: or death before regaining consciousness, regardless of duration of LOC
6. LOC duration NOS
9. With concussion NOS

CEREBELLAR (continued)

334.2 Degeneration primary (hereditary) (sporadic)
431 Hemorrhage (rupture)
674.0# Hemorrhage maternal complicating pregnancy

5th digit: 674.0
0. Episode of care NOS or N/A
1. Delivered
2. Delivered with postpartum complication
3. Antepartum complication
4. Postpartum complication

434.91 Infarction
434.11 Infarction embolic
434.01 Infarction thrombotic
851.6# Laceration (with hemorrhage)
851.7# Laceration with open intracranial wound (with hemorrhage)

5th digit: 851.6-7
0. Level of consciousness NOS
1. No LOC
2. LOC < 1 hr
3. LOC 1 - 24 hrs
4. LOC > 24 hrs with return to prior level
5. LOC > 24 hrs without return to prior level: or death before regaining consciousness, regardless of duration of LOC
6. LOC duration NOS
9. With concussion NOS

433.8# Occlusion

5th digit: 433.8
0. Without cerebral infarction
1. With cerebral infarction

741.0# CEREBELLOMEDULLARY MALFORMATION SYNDROME

5th digit: 741.0
0. Region NOS
1. Cervical region
2. Dorsal (thoracic) region
3. Lumbar region

CEREBRAL

437.3 Aneurysm NOS
747.81 Aneurysm (A-V) congenital
430 Aneurysm (A-V) ruptured
094.87 Aneurysm (A-V) ruptured syphilitic
437.3 Aneurysm-internal carotid artery NOS or intracranial portion
348.1 Anoxia
668.2# Anoxia maternal following anesthesia or other sedation in L&D
669.4# Anoxia maternal following obstetrical surgery

5th digit: 668.2, 669.4
0. Episode of care NOS or N/A
1. Delivered
2. Delivered with postpartum complication
3. Antepartum complication
4. Postpartum complication

437.0 Arteriosclerosis (degeneration) (deformans) (arteritis)
437.4 Arteritis

CEREBRAL (continued)

747.81 Artery atresia (congenital)
435.8 Artery insufficiency (spasm) with TIA
434.9# Artery occlusion
435.9 Artery spasm - unspecified artery
435.8 Artery spasm - other specified artery
434.0# Artery thrombosis

5th digit: 434.0, 9
0. Without cerebral infarction
1. With cerebral infarction

331.89 Ataxia
331.89 Ataxia with dementia [294.1#]
437.0 Atherosclerosis
331.9 Atrophy with dementia [294.1#]
290.10 Atrophy with dementia presenile
331.0 Atrophy - Alzheimer's
331.0 Atrophy - Alzheimer's with dementia [294.1#]
331.11 Atrophy - circumscribed Pick's
331.11 Atrophy - circumscribed Pick's with dementia [294.1#]
331.19 Atrophy - circumscribed other
331.19 Atrophy - circumscribed other with dementia [294.1#]
742.4 Atrophy - congenital
331.2 Atrophy - senile
331.2 Atrophy – senile with dementia [294.1#]

5th digit: 294.1
0. Without behavioral disturbance or NOS
1. With behavioral disturbance

436 Attack
780.39 Attack - toxic
348.8 Calcification (cortex)
437.0 Calcification artery
853.0# Compression traumatic
853.1# Compression traumatic with open intracranial wound

5th digit: 853.0-1
0. Level of consciousness (LOC) NOS
1. No LOC
2. LOC < 1 hr
3. LOC 1 - 24 hrs
4. LOC > 24 hrs with return to prior level of consciousness
5. LOC > 24 hrs without return to prior level: or death before regaining consciousness, regardless of duration of LOC
6. LOC duration NOS
9. With concussion NOS

Cerebral concussion results from a blow to the head, and may be coded as a trauma. Code it as a trauma until the physician states that the active phase of the concussion has subsided and the symptoms are no longer organic in nature. As long as the documentation states that the patient's symptoms are directly resultant from a concussion, use a trauma code.

CONCUSSION

850.9 NOS
850.0 No loss of consciousness (LOC)
850.5 LOC unspecified duration
850.11 LOC 30 minutes or less
850.12 LOC 31 to 59 minutes
850.2 LOC 1-24 hours
850.3 LOC >24 hours with complete recovery
850.4 LOC >24 hours without return to pre-existing level of consciousness

CEREBRAL (continued)

Post-concussion syndrome is a neurological condition resulting from the concussion trauma. ICD-9 assigns it to a non-psychotic mental disorder. Post-concussion syndrome cannot be assigned a trauma code (850.#).

CONTUSION

851.8# NOS (with hemorrhage)
851.9# NOS with open intracranial wound (with hemorrhage)
851.4# Brain stem (with hemorrhage)
851.5# Brain stem with open intracranial wound (with hemorrhage)
851.4# Cerebellar (with hemorrhage)
851.5# Cerebellar with open intracranial wound (with hemorrhage)
851.0# Cortex (with hemorrhage)
851.1# Cortex with open intracranial wound (with hemorrhage)
851.4# Occipital lobe (with hemorrhage)
851.5# Occipital lobe with open intracranial wound (with hemorrhage)
851.8# Parietal lobe (with hemorrhage)
851.9# Parietal lobe with open intracranial wound (with hemorrhage)
851.8# Other (with hemorrhage)
851.9# Other with open intracranial wound (with hemorrhage)

5th digit: 851.0-1, 4-5, 8-9
0. Level of consciousness (LOC) NOS
1. No LOC
2. LOC < 1 hr
3. LOC 1 - 24 hrs
4. LOC > 24 hrs with return to prior level of consciousness
5. LOC > 24 hrs without return to prior level: or death before regaining consciousness, regardless of duration of LOC
6. LOC duration NOS
9. With concussion NOS

CEREBRAL (continued)

0 Crisis see 'Cerebrovascular Disease'
348.0 Cyst
742.4 Cyst congenital

DEGENERATION

331.9 NOS
331.9 NOS with dementia [294.1#]

5th digit: 294.1
0. Without behavioral disturbance or NOS
1. With behavioral disturbance

437.0 Arteriosclerotic
330.9 Childhood
330.8 Childhood other specified
742.4 Congenital
348.0 Cystic
046.1 Jakob Creutzfeldt
330.2 Lipidoses generalized
046.3 Progressive (multifocal) (encephalopathy)

C

CEREBRAL (continued)

DEGENERATION (continued)

331.2 Senile
331.2 Senile with dementia [**294.1#**]
5th digit: 294.1
0. Without behavioral disturbance or NOS
1. With behavioral disturbance

046.1 Spongiform (subacute)
331.89 Other
331.89 Other with dementia [**294.1#**]
5th digit: 294.1
0. Without behavioral disturbance or NOS
1. With behavioral disturbance

CEREBRAL (continued)

779.2 Depression neonatal
348.9 Disease
437.9 Disease arterial
348.30 Dysfunction
348.30 Dysrhythmia
348.5 Edema
348.5 Edema anoxic
434.1# Embolism
5th digit: 434.1
0. Without cerebral infarction
1. With cerebral infarction

348.8 Fungus
253.0 Gigantism syndrome
0 Hematoma, see 'Cerebral', hemorrhage
431 Hemorrhage
767.0 Hemorrhage fetus or newborn birth trauma (intrapartum hypoxia/anoxia)
853.0# Hemorrhage traumatic
853.1# Hemorrhage traumatic with open intracranial wound
5th digit: 853.0-1
0. Level of consciousness (LOC) NOS
1. No LOC
2. LOC < 1 hr
3. LOC 1 - 24 hrs
4. LOC >24 hrs with return to prior level
5. LOC > 24 hrs without return to prior level: or death before regaining consciousness, regardless of duration of LOC
6. LOC duration NOS
9. With concussion NOS

348.1 Hypoxia
997.01 Hypoxia during or resulting from a procedure
0 Hypoxia fetal or newborn see 'Anoxia/Anoxic'
668.2# Hypoxia maternal following anesthesia or other sedation in L&D
669.4# Hypoxia maternal following obstetrical surgery
5th digit: 668.2, 669.4
0. Episode of care NOS or N/A
1. Delivered
2. Delivered with postpartum complication
3. Antepartum complication
4. Postpartum complication

434.91 Infarction
434.11 Infarction embolic
434.01 Infarction thrombotic
779.1 Irritability other and unspecified of newborn

CEREBRAL (continued)

779.2 Ischemia NOS of newborn
437.1 Ischemia (chronic)
437.0 Ischemia arteriosclerotic
767.0 Ischemia due to birth trauma
435.9 Ischemia intermittent (transient)
0 Ischemia intrauterine see 'Fetal – Infant's Record', distress
435.8 Ischemias transient other specified
851.2# Laceration (cortex) (with hemorrhage)
851.3# Laceration (cortex) with open intracranial wound (with hemorrhage)
851.8# Laceration other (with hemorrhage)
851.9# Laceration other with open intracranial wound (with hemorrhage)
5th digit: 851.2-3, 8-9
0. Level of consciousness (LOC) NOS
1. No LOC
2. LOC < 1 hr
3. LOC 1 - 24 hrs
4. LOC > 24 hrs with return to prior level
5. LOC > 24 hrs without return to prior level: or death before regaining consciousness, regardless of duration of LOC
6. LOC duration NOS
9. With concussion NOS

348.8 Lesion
330.1 Lipidoses
330.1 Lipidoses with dementia [**294.1#**]
5th digit: 294.1
0. Without behavioral disturbance or NOS
1. With behavioral disturbance

0 Nerve see 'Cranial', nerve
434.9# Occlusion artery
5th digit: 434.9
0. Without cerebral infarction
1. With cerebral infarction

PALSY

333.71 Athetoid (Vogt's disease)
343.9 Congenital
343.0 Diplegic
343.1 Hemiplegic
343.# Infantile
4th digit: 343
0. Paraplegic (diplegic)
1. Hemiplegic
2. Quadriplegic
3. Monoplegic
4. Hemiplegic (postnatal) NOS
8. Other specified
9. NOS

343.3 Monoplegic
437.8 Noninfantile, noncongenital
343.0 Paraplegic
343.2 Quadriplegic
343.9 Spastic
344.89 Spastic noninfantile, noncongenital
094.89 Syphilitic
090.49 Syphilitic congenital
343.2 Tetraplegic

CEREBRAL (continued)

341.9 Sclerosis (general) (lobular)
331.0 Sclerosis lobar atrophic
331.0 Sclerosis lobar atrophic with dementia [294.1#]
5th digit: 294.1
0. Without behavioral disturbance or NOS
1. With behavioral disturbance

436 Seizure
434.0# Thrombosis artery
5th digit: 434.0
0. Without cerebral infarction
1. With cerebral infarction

671.5# Thrombosis (venous sinus) maternal due to pregnancy
5th digit: 671.5
0. Episode of care NOS or N/A
1. Delivered
2. Delivered with postpartum complication
3. Antepartum complication
4. Postpartum complication

434.91 Vascular accident acute
V53.01 Ventricle (communicating) shunt fitting and adjustment
V45.2 Ventricle (communicating) shunt in situ
747.81 Vessels anomalies (congenital)

759.89 CEREBROHEPATORENAL SYNDROME

CEREBROSPINAL FLUID

792.0 Abnormal
V45.2 Drainage device (presence of) status
997.09 Leakage at lumbar puncture site
388.61 Otorrhea
349.81 Rhinorrhea
V53.01 Shunt fitting
V45.2 Shunt status

Remember, CVA, stroke and cerebral infarction with occlusion NOS are all indexed to code 434.91. Do not use code 436.

CEREBROVASCULAR

434.91 Accident
434.91 Accident - aborted
434.11 Accident - embolic
0 Accident - hemorrhagic see 'Hemorrhage', brain
V12.54 Accident - history without residual
435.9 Accident - impending (transient ischemic attack)
434.91 Accident - ischemic
434.91 Accident - lacunar infarct
0 Accident - late effect see 'Late Effect', cerebrovascular disease
0 Accident - old with residual see 'Late Effect', cerebrovascular disease
V12.54 Accident - old without residual
997.02 Accident - postop iatrogenic
434.01 Accident - thrombotic
435.9 Accident - transient ischemic attack (TIA)
437.7 Amnesia transient global
747.81 Anomalies
0 Crisis see 'Cerebrovascular', disease
437.9 Disease
437.0 Disease arteriosclerotic
437.1 Disease ischemic generalized NEC
0 Disease late effect see 'Late Effect', cerebrovascular disease

CEREBROVASCULAR (continued)

437.1 Disease occlusive
437.8 Disease other
674.0# Disorder (puerperium) maternal due pregnancy
5th digit: 674.0
0. Episode of care NOS or N/A
1. Delivered
2. Delivered with postpartum complication
3. Antepartum complication
4. Postpartum complication

437.1 Insufficiency acute
435.9 Insufficiency acute with transient neurological signs
434.9# Occlusion
5th digit: 434.9
0. Without cerebral infarction
1. With cerebral infarction

437.0 Occlusion diffuse
747.81 System anomalies - congenital

272.7 CEROID STORAGE DISEASE

CERTIFICATE ISSUE

V68.09 Death
V68.01 Disability
V68.09 Fitness
V68.09 Incapacity
V68.09 Medical

380.4 CERUMEN IMPACTED

CERVICAL

744.43 Auricle congenital
723.4 Brachial radicular syndrome
952.0# Cord injury
806.0# Cord injury with closed fracture
806.1# Cord injury with open fracture
5th digit: 806.0-1, 952.0
0. C1-C4 with cord injury NOS
1. C1-C4 with complete cord lesion
2. C1-C4 with anterior cord syndrome
3. C1-C4 with central cord lesion
4. C1-C4 with incomplete cord lesion NOS or posterior cord syndrome
5. C5-C7 with cord injury NOS
6. C5-C7 complete lesion of cord
7. C5-C7 with anterior cord syndrome
8. C5-C7 with central cord syndrome
9. C5-C7 with incomplete cord lesion NOS or posterior

0 Disc disorder see 'Cervical Disc Disorder'
722.0 Disc herniation (HNP)
722.71 Disc herniation (HNP) with myelopathy
744.43 Ear congenital
722.0 Nerve compression - discogenic
722.71 Nerve compression - discogenic with myelopathy
723.4 Nerve compression - root (by scar tissue) NEC
722.81 Nerve compression - root postoperative
723.2 Posterior, sympathetic syndrome
0 Radiculitis (discogenic) see 'Cervical Disc' disorder
723.4 Radiculitis (nondiscogenic)
723.9 Region disorder NEC
739.1 Region segmental or somatic dysfunction
756.2 Rib
353.0 Rib syndrome (nondiscogenic)
953.0 Root injury (nerve)
353.2 Root lesions NEC (nondiscogenic)

C

CERVICAL (continued)

723.0 Spinal stenosis
723.9 Spine disorder (nondiscogenic)
337.0 Sympathetic dystrophy or paralysis syndrome
954.0 Sympathetic nerve injury
723.8 Syndrome NEC
847.0 Traumatic syndrome (acute) NEC
0 Uterus see 'Cervix'

When coding back disorders due to degeneration, displacement or HNP of the intervertebral disc, it is important to distinguish whether these conditions are with or without myelopathy. Myelopathy refers to functional disturbances and/or pathological changes in the spinal cord that result from compression.

CERVICAL DISC DISORDER

722.91 Unspecified
722.91 Calcification or discitis
722.4 Disease/degeneration
722.71 Disease/degeneration - with myelopathy
722.0 Displacement (herniation) (HNP) (protrusion) (rupture)
722.71 Displacement (herniation) (HNP) (protrusion) (rupture) with myelopathy
722.71 Syndrome
722.91 Other specified

723.1 CERVICALGIA (NECK PAIN) (NONDISCOGENIC)

CERVICITIS

616.0 NOS
760.8 Affecting newborn or fetus
616.0 Atrophic or senile (nonobstetrical)
616.0 Ectropion cervical
616.0 Eversion cervix
098.15 Gonorrhea (acute)
0 Gravid see 'Pregnancy Complications', maternal conditions
616.89 Inflammatory disease (other)
616.0 Nonobstetrical
095.8 Syphilitic
131.09 Trichomonal
016.7# Tuberculous

5th digit: 016.7
0. NOS
1. Lab not done
2. Lab pending
3. Microscopy positive (in sputum)
4. Culture positive - microscopy negative
5. Culture negative - microscopy positive
6. Culture and micro negative confirmed by other methods

744.49 CERVICOAURAL FISTULA CONGENITAL
723.3 CERVICOBRACHIAL SYNDROME (DIFFUSE)
723.2 CERVICOCRANIAL SYNDROME
353.2 CERVICODORSAL OUTLET SYNDROME
739.1 CERVICOTHORACIC REGION SEGMENTAL OR SOMATIC DYSFUNCTION

CERVIX (UTERI)

V45.77 Absence acquired
752.49 Absence congenital
622.3 Adhesion (band)
752.49 Agenesis congenital
622.10 Anaplasia

CERVIX (UTERI) (continued)

752.40 Anomaly congenital
752.49 Anomaly congenital other specified
795.02 ASC-H (atypical squamous cells cannot exclude high grade squamous intraepithelial lesion)
795.01 ASC-US (atypical squamous cells of undetermined significance)
622.4 Atresia
752.49 Atresia congenital
622.8 Atrophy (senile)
795.02 Atypical squamous cells cannot exclude high grade squamous intraepithelial lesion (ASC-H)
795.01 Atypical squamous cells of undetermined significance (ASC-US)
622.10 Atypism
622.8 Calcification (uteri)
622.3 Cicatrix (postpartum)
622.4 Contracture
752.49 Contracture congenital
622.8 Cyst
795.06 Cytologic evidence of malignancy
616.0 Disorder inflammatory
622.9 Disorder noninflammatory
622.8 Disorder noninflammatory specified NEC
0 Displacement see 'Uterus, uterine', displacement
622.10 Dyskeratosis
622.10 Dysplasia
622.11 Dysplasia - CIN I
622.12 Dysplasia - CIN II
233.1 Dysplasia - CIN III
V13.22 Dysplasia - history
622.11 Dysplasia - mild
622.12 Dysplasia - moderate
233.1 Dysplasia - severe
622.0 Ectropion
622.10 Epidermidization
622.0 Erosion
622.0 Erosion and ectropion
622.0 Eversion
622.8 Fibrosis
621.6 Flexion
622.8 Hemorrhage
795.04 HGSIL cervix (high grade squamous intraepithelial lesion)
795.04 High grade squamous intraepithelial lesion (HGSIL)
795.05 High risk <u>human</u> <u>papillomavirus</u> (<u>HPV</u>) DNA test positive <u>[079.4]</u>
622.10 Hyperkeratosis
0 Hyperplasia see 'Cervix', dysplasia
752.49 Hyperplasia congenital
622.6 Hypertrophic elongation
622.5 Incompetence (nonpregnant)
761.0 Incompetent affecting fetus or newborn
639.2 Injury postabortive
867.4 Injury (traumatic)
867.5 Injury (traumatic) with open wound
233.1 Intraepithelial glandular neoplasia
622.11 Intraepithelial neoplasia I
622.12 Intraepithelial neoplasia II
233.1 Intraepithelial neoplasia III
622.2 Leukoplakia
795.03 LGSIL cervix (low grade squamous intraepithelial lesion)
795.03 Low grade squamous intraepithelial lesion (LGSIL)
795.09 Low risk <u>human</u> <u>papillomavirus</u> (<u>HPV</u>) DNA test positive <u>[079.4]</u>
616.81 Mucositis (ulcerative)

CERVIX (UTERI) (continued)

622.4 Occlusion
084.0 Occlusion by falciparum malaria
752.49 Occlusion congenital
622.3 Old laceration
0 Pap smear abnormal see 'Pap Smear'
622.7 Polyp
219.0 Polyp adenomatous
622.7 Polyp mucous or unspecified
622.4 Stricture and stenosis
752.49 Stricture or stenosis congenital
622.8 Stump healed
618.84 Stump prolapse
622.0 Ulcer

CERVIX COMPLICATING PREGNANCY CHILDBIRTH OR PUERPERIUM

654.6# Abnormality or atresia
660.2# Abnormality or atresia obstructing labor **[654.6#]**
654.6# Cicatrix
660.2# Cicatrix obstructing labor **[654.6#]**
661.0# Dilation failure
654.5# Incompetence
660.2# Incompetence obstructing labor **[654.5#]**
654.6# Rigid
660.2# Rigid obstructing labor **[654.6#]**
654.6# Stenosis
660.2# Stenosis obstructing labor **[654.6#]**
654.6# Surgery previous
660.2# Surgery previous obstructing labor **[654.6#]**
654.6# Tumor
660.2# Tumor obstructing labor **[654.6#]**
654.6# Polyp
660.2# Polyp obstructing labor **[654.6#]**

5th digit: 654.5-6
0. Episode of care NOS or N/A
1. Delivered
2. Delivered with postpartum complication
3. Antepartum complication
4. Postpartum complication

5th digit: 660.2, 661.0
0. Episode of care NOS or N/A
1. Delivered
3. Antepartum complication

> ***When coding a cesarean section, code the reason that the cesarean was done. Use the codes below only if the cesarean itself is a complicating factor.***

CESAREAN

763.4 Delivery affecting fetus or newborn
674.3# Postoperative infection

5th digit: 674.3
0. Episode of care unspecified or N/A
2. Delivered with postpartum complication
4. Postpartum complication

654.2# Section previous complicating childbirth
660.2# Section previous obstructing labor **[654.2#]**

5th digit: 654.2, 660.2
0. Episode of care NOS or N/A
1. Delivered
3. Antepartum complication

CESAREAN (continued)

654.8# Section previous surgery to rectum complicating childbirth
660.2# Section previous surgery to rectum obstructing labor **[654.8#]**

5th digit: 654.8
0. Episode of care NOS or N/A
1. Delivered
2. Delivered with postpartum complication
3. Antepartum complication
4. Postpartum complication

5th digit: 660.2
0. Episode of care NOS or N/A
1. Delivered
3. Antepartum complication

763.4 Section affecting fetus or newborn
762.1 Section damage to placenta affecting fetus or newborn
763.89 Section scar previous affecting fetus or newborn
669.7# Section without mention of indication

5th digit: 669.7
0. Episode of care NOS or N/A
1. Delivered

674.1# Section wound dehiscence

5th digit: 674.1
0. NOS
2. Delivered with postpartum complication
4. Postpartum complication

344.89 CESTAN - CHENAIS SYNDROME
433.8# CESTAN - RAYMOND SYNDROME

5th digit: 433.8
0. Without cerebral infarction
1. With cerebral infarction

022.9 CHABERT'S DISEASE
759.89 CGF (CONGENITAL GENERALIZED FIBROMATOSIS)

CHAGAS' DISEASE

086.2 Unspecified
V75.3 Screening exam
086.0 With heart involvement
086.1 With other organ involvement
086.2 Without mention of organ involvement

530.81 CHALASIA (CARDIAC SPHINCTER)
373.2 CHALAZION

CHALCOSIS

360.24 NOS (globe)
371.15 Cornea
360.24 Crystalline lens [366.34]
360.24 Retina

502 CHALICOSIS LUNG (OCCUPATIONAL)
360.34 CHAMBER ANGLE FLAT
364.77 CHAMBER ANGLE RECESSION (IRIS AND CILIARY BODY)
091.2 CHANCRE CONJUNCTIVA (PRIMARY SYPHILITIC)
099.0 CHANCRE DUCREY'S
091.2 CHANCRE EYELID (PRIMARY SYPHILITIC)
091.0 CHANCRE GENITAL
099.0 CHANCRE SIMPLE
099.0 CHANCRE SOFT
114.1 CHANCRIFORM SYNDROME COCCIDIOIDOMYCOSIS

C

099.0 CHANCROID

647.2# CHANCROID MATERNAL CURRENT (CO-EXISTENT) IN PREGNANCY [099.0]

5th digit: 647.2

0. Episode of care NOS or N/A
1. Delivered
2. Delivered with postpartum complication
3. Antepartum complication
4. Postpartum complication

655.4# CHANCROID MATERNAL (WITH KNOWN/SUSPECTED DAMAGE TO FETUS)

5th digit: 655.4

0. Episode of care NOS or N/A
1. Delivered
3. Antepartum complication

066.8 CHANDIPURA FEVER
732.7 CHANDLER'S OSTEOCHONDRITIS DISSECANS, HIP
787.99 CHANGE BOWEL HABITS
066.0 CHANGUINOLA FEVER
301.9 CHARACTER DISORDER NOS

C

CHARCOT('S)

094.0 Arthritis tabes or syphilitic [713.5]
094.0 Joint disease [713.5]
250.6# Joint diabetic [713.5]

5th digit: 250.6

0. Type II, adult-onset, non-insulin dependent (even if requiring insulin), or unspecified; controlled
1. Type I, juvenile-onset or insulin-dependent; controlled
2. Type II, adult-onset, non-insulin dependent (even if requiring insulin); uncontrolled
3. Type I, juvenile-onset or insulin-dependent; uncontrolled

356.1 Marie tooth (scoliosis) [737.43]
443.9 Syndrome - angina cruris
443.9 Syndrome - intermittent claudication

When coding atherosclerosis of the extremities use an additional code, if applicable to identify chronic complete or total occlusion of the artery of the extremities (440.4).

440.21 Syndrome - intermittent claudication due to atherosclerosis
440.3# Syndrome - intermittent claudication due to bypass graft atherosclerosis
440.3# Syndrome - intermittent claudication due to bypass graft atherosclerosis with chronic complete or total occlusion [440.4]

5th digit: 440.3

0. Unspecified graft
1. Autologous vein bypass graft
2. Nonautologous biological bypass graft

CHARCOT('S) (continued)

648.9#: Use an additional code to identify the specific type of Charcot's syndrome.

648.9# Syndrome - maternal current (co-existent) in pregnancy

5th digit: 648.9

0. Episode of NOS or N/A
1. Delivered
2. Delivered with postpartum complication
3. Antepartum complication
4. Postpartum complication

337.0 Weiss-Baker syndrome

759.89 CHARGE ASSOCIATION (SYNDROME)
102.9 CHARLOUIS' DISEASE
267 CHEADLE (-MOLLER) (-BARLOW) SYNDROME (INFANTILE SCURVY)
288.2 CHEDIAK STEINBRINCK (HIGASHI) SYNDROME

CHEEK

528.9 Biting
738.19 Deformity
744.9 Deformity congenital
528.9 Disease (inner)
959.09 Injury
925.1 Injury crush
910.8 Injury other and unspecified superficial
910.9 Injury other and unspecified superficial infected

495.8 CHEESE WASHERS' LUNG

CHEILITIS

528.5 NOS
692.72 Actinic acute due to sun
692.74 Actinic chronic due to sun
692.82 Actinic due to radiation (except sun)
702.0 Actinic solar keratosis
528.5 Acute or chronic
528.5 Angular
528.5 Catarrhal
528.5 Exfoliative
528.5 Gangrenous
528.5 Glandularis apostematosa
351.8 Granulomatosa
528.5 Infectional
528.5 Membranous
351.8 Miescher's
692.7# Sunburn

5th digit: 692.7

1. NOS (first degree)
6. Second degree
7. Third degree

692.82 Sunburn tanning bed
528.5 Suppurative
528.5 Ulcerative
528.5 Vesicular

749.2# CHEILOPALATOSCHISIS

5th digit: 749.2

0. Cleft palate with cleft lip unspecified
1. Cleft palate unilateral complete
2. Cleft palate unilateral incomplete
3. Cleft palate bilateral complete
4. Cleft palate bilateral incomplete
5. Cleft palate other combinations

Code	Term
749.1#	CHEILOSCHISIS

5th digit: 749.1
0. Cleft NOS
1. Cleft unilateral complete
2. Cleft unilateral incomplete
3. Cleft bilateral complete
4. Cleft bilateral incomplete

Code	Term
528.5	CHEILOSIS
705.81	CHEIROPOMPHOLYX
701.4	CHELOID
0	CHEMICAL BURN SEE 'BURN', BY SITE
0	CHEMICAL BURN INGESTED AGENT SEE 'BURN', INTERNAL ORGANS, BY SITE
V82.5	CHEMICAL POISONING AND OTHER CONTAMINATION SCREENING

If a patient is administered chemotherapy at the time of port-o-cath or hickman catheter insertion, assign code V58.11 as the principal diagnosis and the malignancy as the secondary code.

If chemotherapy is not administered at the same time as the catheter insertion code the malignancy as the principal diagnosis.

CHEMOTHERAPY

Code	Term
V58.11	Admission
V58.11	Chemoembolization therapy
995.29	Complication
V66.2	Convalescence
V58.11	Encounter
V67.2	Follow up exam
V58.11	Intra-arterial
V58.11	Maintenance
V58.69	Status current
V07.39	CHEMOTHERAPEUTIC AGENT ADMINISTRATION PROPHYLACTIC NEC
V58.11	CHEMOTHERAPEUTIC AGENT MAINTENANCE FOLLOWING DISEASE

CHEST

Code	Term
786.7	Abnormal percussion
786.9	Congestion
862.8	Crushed
908.0	Crushed late effect
738.3	Deformity acquired
786.59	Discomfort
519.9	Disease (respiratory)
754.89	Flat congenital NEC
754.81	Funnel congenital
786.6	Mass or swelling
786.9	Symptoms NEC
862.8	Trauma (with injury to intrathoracic organs)
862.9	Trauma with open wound (with injury to intrathoracic organs)
908.0	Trauma late effect
V58.82	Tube fitting (adjustment) (replacement) (cleansing)
754.89	Wall deformity congenital
959.11	Wall injury
911.8	Wall injury other and unspecified superficial
911.9	Wall injury other and unspecified superficial infected
786.52	Wall pain anterior
786.52	Wall syndrome (anterior)
793.1	X-ray abnormal (lung) (shadow)
V71.2	X-ray for suspected tuberculosis
V72.5	X-ray routine

CHEST PAIN

Code	Term
786.50	NOS
786.59	Atypical
413.1	Atypical - angina
786.51	Midsternal
786.59	Musculoskeletal
786.59	Noncardiac
786.52	Pleuritic
786.51	Precordial
786.59	Pressure
786.51	Substernal
786.59	Tightness
786.04	CHEYNE STOKES RESPIRATION

For coding purposes, CHF and right ventricular failure are considered to be synonymous and both are assigned a 4th digit of "0". Left ventricular failure is not the same as CHF. Left ventricular failure is assigned a 4th digit of "1".

CHF (CONGESTIVE HEART FAILURE)

Code	Term
428.0	NOS
428.0	Acute
0	Acute left ventricular see 'Heart Failure', left
0	Acute left ventricular with pulmonary edema see 'Heart Failure', left
428.0	Acute with pulmonary edema
428.0	Combined left-right sided
428.0	Compensated
428.0	Decompensated (right congestive)
997.1	During a procedure
779.89	Fetus or newborn
402.91	Hypertensive NOS [428.0]
402.11	Hypertensive benign [428.0]
402.01	Hypertensive malignant [428.0]
0	Hypertensive heart and chronic kidney disease with and without heart failure see 'Hypertensive', heart and chronic kidney disease
0	Left ventricular see 'Heart Failure'

Cardiac complications post-op are divided into two types: Immediate post-op (surgery to discharge), 997.1, and late or following discharge, 429.4.

Code	Term
997.1	Post op (resulting from a procedure) [428.0]
997.1	Post op heart surgery - immediate
429.4	Post op heart surgery - late
398.91	Rheumatic
391.8	Rheumatic acute or active
398.91	Rheumatic chronic or inactive (with chorea)
428.0	Right secondary to left
392.0	Sydenham's chorea with heart involvement
402.91	With hypertensive cardiomyopathy [428.0]
402.11	With hypertensive cardiomyopathy benign [428.0]
402.01	With hypertensive cardiomyopathy malignant [428.0]

CHF (CONGESTIVE HEART FAILURE) OBSTETRICAL

635.7# Complicating abortion
5th digit: 635.7
0. Unspecified
1. Incomplete
2. Complete

669.4# Complicating labor and delivery

648.6#, Use an additional code to specify the congestive heart failure. See 'CHF'.

648.6# Current (co-existent) in pregnancy
668.1# Due to anesthesia, other sedation in L&D
5th digit: 648.6, 668.1, 669.4
0. Episode of care NOS
1. Delivered w/ or w/o mention antepartum condition
2. Delivered with mention of postpartum complication
3. Antepartum complication
4. Postpartum complication

639.8 Following abortion

CHIARI

453.0 Disease (hepatic vein thrombosis)
676.6# Frommel syndrome maternal due to pregnancy
5th digit: 676.6
0. Episode of care NOS
1. Delivered w/ or w/o mention antepartum condition
2. Delivered with mention of postpartum complication
3. Antepartum complication
4. Postpartum complication

348.4 Malformation type I
741.0# Malformation type II
5th digit: 741.0
0. Region NOS
1. Cervical region
2. Dorsal (thoracic) region
3. Lumbar region

742.0 Malformation type III
742.2 Malformation type IV
453.0 Syndrome (hepatic vein thrombosis)

368.41 CHIASMATIC SYNDROME
116.0 CHICAGO DISEASE (NORTH AMERICAN BLASTOMYCOSIS)
0 CHICKENPOX SEE 'VARICELLA'
085.4 CHICLERO ULCER
133.8 CHIGGERS
767.19 CHIGNON (DUE TO VACUUM EXTRACTION)
111.2 CHIGNON (WHITE PIEDRA)
134.1 CHIGOE INFESTATION
066.3 CHIKUNGUNYA FEVER (VIRAL)
751.4 CHILAIDITI'S SYNDROME (SUBPHRENIC DISPLACEMENT, COLON)
991.5 CHILBLAINS
909.4 CHILBLAINS LATE EFFECT

When the cause of an injury is stated to be abuse, multiple codes should be assigned if applicable, to identify any associated injuries. Sequence in the following order:

1. Type of abuse - child or adult (995.5, 995.8)

2. Type of injury

3. Nature of the abuse - see E-code directory 'Assault' (E904.0, E960-E966, E968)

4. Perpetrator of the abuse - see E-code directory 'Assault' (E967)

CHILD

995.5# Abuse (victim)
5th digit: 995.5
0. Unspecified
1. Emotional/psychological (deprivation)
2. Neglect (nutritional), desertion
3. Sexual
4. Physical
5. Shaken infant syndrome
9. Other abuse and neglect, multiple forms

V62.83 Abuse - counseling of perpetrator non-parental of physical/sexual abuse
V61.22 Abuse - counseling of perpetrator parental
V61.21 Abuse - counseling of victim
V71.81 Abuse - evaluation (alleged)
V71.6 Abuse - evaluation for battery (alleged)
V71.81 Abuse - evaluation for neglect (alleged)
V71.5 Abuse - evaluation for sexual (alleged)
V15.4# Abuse history
5th digit: V15.4
1. Physical abuse, rape, sexual
2. Emotional abuse, neglect
9. Other psychological trauma

995.52 Desertion
995.5# Maltreatment syndrome
5th digit: 995.5
0. Unspecified
1. Emotional/psychological (deprivation)
2. Neglect (nutritional), desertion
3. Sexual
4. Physical
5. Shaken infant syndrome
9. Other abuse and neglect, multiple forms

780.99 CHILLS
780.6 CHILLS WITH FEVER

CHIN

744.89 Absence congenital
524.05 Hyperplasia
524.06 Hypoplasia
959.09 Injury
996.69 Prosthesis complication - infection or inflammation
996.59 Prosthesis complication - mechanical
996.79 Prosthesis complication - other

121.1 CHINESE LIVER FLUKE DISEASE

277.39 CHITNOUS DEGENERATION

CHLAMYDIA

079.98 Infection (organism)
079.88 Infection other specified chlamydial
483.1 Pneumonia
V73.98 Screening chlamydial unspecified
V73.88 Screening chlamydial other specified
099.50 Trachomatis infection unspecified
099.52 Trachomatis anus
099.53 Trachomatis bladder [595.4]
099.53 Trachomatis cervix [616.0]
099.54 Trachomatis epididymis [604.91]
099.54 Trachomatis genitourinary specified NEC
099.53 Trachomatis genitourinary lower
099.54 Trachomatis pelvic inflammatory disease [614.9]
099.56 Trachomatis perihepatic
099.56 Trachomatis peritoneum
099.51 Trachomatis pharynx
099.52 Trachomatis rectum
099.54 Trachomatis testis [604.91]
099.53 Trachomatis vagina [616.11]
099.53 Trachomatis vulvitis [616.11]
099.53 Trachomatis vulvovaginitis [616.11]
099.59 Venereal specified site NEC

CHLOASMA

709.09 NOS
709.09 Cachecticorum
709.09 Ephelides
374.52 Eyelid
709.09 Idiopathic
709.09 Symptomatic
709.09 Vaginal

276.9 CHLORIDE ABNORMAL FINDINGS

748.0 CHOANAL ATRESIA CONGENITAL
748.0 CHOANAL OCCLUSION

617.1 CHOCOLATE CYST OVARY

933.1 CHOKING (FOOD REGURGITATED) (PHLEGM)
784.99 CHOKING SENSATION

155.1 CHOLANGIOCARCINOMA SITE NOS

0 CHOLANGIOCARCINOMA SITE SPECIFIED SEE 'CANCER', BY SITE M8160/3

CHOLANGITIS

576.1 NOS
576.1 Acute
576.1 Ascending (sclerosing) (secondary) (recurrent)
576.1 Chronic
571.6 Chronic nonsuppurative
571.6 Chronic nonsuppurative with esophageal varices [456.2#]

5th digit: 456.2
0. With bleeding
1. Without bleeding

576.1 Suppurative

575.9 CHOLECYSTIC DISEASE

> ***A combination code is used to classify two diagnoses or a diagnosis with its manifestation or complication. For example, 574.00, cholecystitis acute with cholelithiasis.***

CHOLECYSTITIS

575.10 NOS
574.4# NOS - with choledocholithiasis
574.1# NOS - with cholelithiasis
574.7# NOS - with cholelithiasis and choledocholithiasis
575.0 Acute
574.3# Acute - with choledocholithiasis
574.0# Acute - with cholelithiasis
574.6# Acute - with cholelithiasis and choledocholithiasis
575.12 Acute and chronic
574.8# Acute and chronic - with cholelithiasis and choledocholithiasis
575.11 Chronic
574.4# Chronic - with choledocholithiasis
574.1# Chronic - with cholelithiasis
574.7# Chronic - with cholelithiasis and choledocholithiasis
575.12 Chronic and acute
574.8# Chronic and acute with cholelithiasis and choledocholithiasis

5th digit: 574.0, 1, 3, 4, 6-8
0. Without obstruction
1. With obstruction

0 Emphysematous see 'Cholecystitis', acute
0 Gangrenous see 'Cholecystitis', acute
0 Suppurative see 'Cholecystitis', acute

CHOLEDOCHAL CYST

576.8 NOS
751.69 NOS congenital

CHOLEDOCHOLITHIASIS

574.5# NOS
574.9# NOS with cholelithiasis
574.4# With cholecystitis NOS
574.3# With cholecystitis acute
574.6# With cholecystitis acute - with cholelithiasis
574.8# With cholecystitis acute and chronic- with cholelithiasis
574.4# With cholecystitis chronic
574.7# With cholecystitis chronic - with cholelithiasis

5th digit: 574.3-9
0. Without obstruction
1. With obstruction

CHOLELITHIASIS

574.2# NOS
646.8# NOS complicating pregnancy **[574.2#]**
574.9# NOS with choledocholithiasis

5th digit: 646.8
0. Episode of care unspecified or N/A
1. Delivered
2. Delivered with postpartum complication
3. Antepartum complication
4. Postpartum complication

5th digit: 574.2, 9
0. Without obstruction
1. With obstruction

CHOLELITHIASIS (continued)

574.1# With cholecystitis NOS
574.0# With cholecystitis acute
574.6# With cholecystitis acute - with choledocholithiasis
574.8# With cholecystitis acute and chronic- with choledocholithiasis
574.1# With cholecystitis chronic
574.7# With cholecystitis chronic - with choledocholithiasis

5th digit: 574.0, 1, 6-9
0. Without obstruction
1. With obstruction

782.4 CHOLEMIA

567.81 CHOLEPERITONITIS

CHOLERA

001.9 NOS
985.4 Antimonial
V02.0 Carrier
V01.0 Exposure
V74.0 Scrooning exam
V06.0 Typhoid paratyphoid vaccination
V03.0 Vaccination
001.0 Vibrio
001.1 Vibrio el tor

576.8 CHOLESTASIS

573.8 CHOLESTASIS DUE TO TOTAL PARENTERAL NUTRITION (TPN)

CHOLESTEATOMA

385.30 NOS
385.31 Attic
385.35 Diffuse (cholesteatosis)
380.21 Externa
385.32 Middle ear
385.33 Middle ear and mastoid
383.32 Postmastoidectomy

385.35 CHOLESTEATOSIS DIFFUSE

385.82 CHOLESTERIN GRANULOMA MIDDLE EAR AND MASTOID

CHOLESTEROL

272.9 Abnormal (serum level)
272.0 Elevated (high)
272.2 Elevated with high triglycerides
0 Embolism see 'Atheroembolism'
593.81 Embolization syndrome (embolus renal arteriole due to aortic arteriosclerosis) [440.0]
272.9 Metabolism disorder
V77.91 Screening

575.6 CHOLESTEROLOSIS GALLBLADDER

0 CHOLESTEROLOSIS MIDDLE EAR SEE 'CHOLESTEATOMA'

733.99 CHONDRITIS

380.03 CHONDRITIS AURICLE OR PINNA

733.6 CHONDRITIS COSTAL

CHONDROBLASTOMA

213.# NOS M9230/0
170.# Malignant M9230/3

4th digit: 170, 213
0. Skull, face, upper jaw
1. Lower jaw NOS
2. Spine
3. Rib, sternum, clavicle
4. Upper limb of long bones, scapula
5. Upper limb of short bones
6. Pelvis, sacrum, coccyx
7. Lower limb of long bone
8. Lower limb of short bone
9. Site NOS

CHONDROCALCINOSIS

275.49 Crystal deposition - NOS **[712.3#]**
275.49 Crystal deposition - dicalcium phosphate **[712.1#]**
275.49 Crystal deposition - pyrophosphate crystals **[712.2#]**

5th digit: 712.1-3
0. Site NOS
1. Shoulder region
2. Upper arm (elbow) (humerus)
3. Forearm (radius) (wrist) (ulna)
4. Hand (carpal) (metacarpal) (fingers)
5. Pelvic region and thigh (hip) (buttock) (femur)
6. Lower leg (fibula) (knee) (patella) (tibia)
7. Ankle and/or foot (metatarsals) (toes) (tarsals)
8. Other (head) (neck) (rib) (skull) (trunk) (vertebrae)
9. Multiple

380.00 CHONDRODERMATITIS NODULARIS HELICIS (SEE ALSO 'PERICHONDRITIS EAR')

CHONDRODYSPLASIA

756.4 NOS
756.4 Angiomatose
756.59 Calcificans congenita
756.59 Epiphysialis punctata
756.4 Hereditary deforming
277.86 Rhizomelic punctata

756.4 CHONDRODYSTROPHIA (FETALIS) CONGENITAL

756.4 CHONDRODYSTROPHY CONGENITAL

359.23 CHONDRODYSTROPHY MYOTONIC CONGENITAL

756.55 CHONDROECTODERMAL DYSPLASIA SYNDROME

CHONDROMA

213.# NOS M9220/0
213.# Juxtacortical M9221/0

4th digit: 213
0. Skull, face, upper jaw
1. Lower jaw NOS
2. Spine
3. Rib, sternum, clavicle
4. Upper limb long bones, scapula
5. Upper limb short bones
6. Pelvis, sacrum, coccyx
7. Lower limb long bone
8. Lower limb short bone
9. Site NOS

CHONDROMALACIA

733.92 NOS
733.92 Localized
717.7 Localized patella
733.92 Systemic
733.92 Tibial plateau

238.0 CHONDROMATOSIS SITE NOS

0 CHONDROMATOSIS SITE SPECIFIED SEE 'NEOPLASM UNCERTAIN BEHAVIOR', BY SITE M9220/1

CHONDROSARCOMA

170.# Chrondrosarcoma M9220/3
170.# Juxtacortical M9221/3
170.# Mesenchymal M9240/3

4th digit: 170
0. Skull and face
1. Mandible
2. Vertebral column
3. Ribs, sternum, clavicle
4. Scapula, long bones of upper limb
5. Short bones of upper limb
6. Pelvic bones, sacrum, coccyx
7. Long bones lower limb
8. Short bones lower limb
9. Site NOS

848.42 CHONDROSTERNAL SEPARATION (RUPTURE) (TEAR) (LACERATION)

848.42 CHONDROSTERNAL STRAIN (SPRAIN) (AVULSION) (HEMARTHROSIS)

429.5 CHORDAE TENDINEAE RUPTURE

429.5 CHORDAE TENDINEAE RUPTURE (POST INFARCTION) [410.90]

607.89 CHORDEE (NONVENEREAL)

752.63 CHORDEE CONGENITAL

478.5 CHORDITIS

CHORDOMA

199.1 Site NOS
0 Site specified see 'Cancer', by site M9370/3

CHOREA

275.1 Athetosis-agitans syndrome
333.5 Hemiballism (US)
333.4 Huntington's
333.5 Other
333.5 Paroxysmal choreo-athetosis
344.89 Posthemiplegic
392.9 Rheumatic acute
392.0 Rheumatic with heart involvement acute

333.5 CHOREOATHETOSIS PAROXYSMAL

236.1 CHORIOADENOMA (DESTRUENS) M9100/1

762.7 CHORIOAMNIONITIS AFFECTING FETUS OR NEWBORN

0 CHORIOAMNIONITIS SEE 'AMNIONITIS'

Carcinomas and neoplasms should be coded by site if possible. Code by cell type, "site NOS", only if a site is not specified in the diagnosis. Otherwise, refer to the appropriate category of neoplasm for a more specific code. See 'Cancer' 'Cancer Metastatic', 'Neoplasm Uncertain Behavior', 'Neoplasm Unspecified Nature', or 'Benign Neoplasm'.

CHORIOCARCINOMA

181 NOS M9100/3
199.1 Combined with teratoma site NOS
0 Combined with teratoma site specified see 'Cancer', by site M9101/3
181 Female site NOS
0 Female site specified see 'Cancer', by site M9101/3
186.9 Male site NOS
0 Male site specified see 'Cancer', by site M9101/3

181 CHORIOEPITHELIOMA NOS M9100/3

762.9 CHORION AND AMNION ABNORMALITY AFFECTING FETUS OR NEWBORN

762.8 CHORION AND AMNION ABNORMALITIES OTHER SPECIFIED AFFECTING FETUS OR NEWBORN

CHORIORETINAL SCAR

363.30 NOS
363.35 Disseminated
743.53 Degeneration congenital
363.32 Macular
363.34 Peripheral
363.33 Posterior pole

CHORIORETINITIS

363.20 NOS
363.10 Disseminated
363.00 Focal
363.01 Focal juxtapapillary (and choroiditis)
363.03 Focal other posterior pole (and choroiditis)
363.04 Focal peripheral (and choroiditis)
0 Histoplasma see 'Histoplasma'
363.21 Pars planitis
362.18 Perivasculitis
0 See also 'Retinitis'
090.0 Syphilitic congenital early [363.13]
095.8 Syphilitic congenital late [363.13]
091.51 Syphilitic secondary
130.2 Toxoplasmosis
017.3# Tuberculous [363.13]

5th digit: 017.3
0. NOS
1. Lab not done
2. Lab unknown at present
3. Microscopy positive - (in sputum)
4. Culture positive - microscopy negative
5. Culture negative - microscopy positive
6. Culture and microscopy negative - confirmed by other methods

C

CHOROID, CHOROIDAL

363.43 Angioid streaks
433.8# Artery obstruction or occlusion
433.8# Artery thrombosis (embolism) (deformans)
5th digit: 433.8
0. Without cerebral infarction
1. With cerebral infarction

363.40 Atrophy
363.42 Atrophy diffuse secondary
0 Atrophy hereditary see 'Choroid, Choroidal', dystrophy hereditary
363.41 Atrophy senile
743.59 Defect congenital
363.40 Degeneration
363.70 Detachment
363.72 Detachment hemorrhagic
363.71 Detachment serous
363.9 Disorder
363.8 Disorder other specified

DYSTROPHY HEREDITARY

363.50 NOS
363.57 Atrophic (generalized gyrate)
363.54 Central gyrate
363.53 Central partial
363.54 Central total
363.55 Choroideremia
363.53 Circinate
363.51 Circumpapillary partial
363.52 Circumpapillary total
363.56 Diffuse sclerosis
363.57 Generalized gyrate atrophy
363.52 Helicoid
363.56 Sclerosis
363.54 Serpiginous
363.56 Other diffuse or generalized partial
363.57 Other diffuse or generalized total

CHOROID, CHOROIDAL (continued)

363.61 Hemorrhage
363.62 Hemorrhage expulsive
362.16 Neovascularization
224.6 Nevus
363.63 Rupture
363.30 Scar
363.35 Scar disseminated
363.33 Scar of posterior pole
363.34 Scar peripheral
363.31 Scar solar
363.40 Sclerosis
363.56 Sclerosis diffuse hereditary

349.2 CHOROID PLEXUS CALCIFICATION

CHOROIDITIS

363.20 NOS
363.00 Focal
363.10 Disseminated
363.11 Disseminated posterior pole (and chorioretinitis)
363.12 Disseminated peripheral (and chorioretinitis)
363.13 Disseminated generalized (and chorioretinitis)
091.51 Syphilitic secondary
017.3# Tuberculous [363.13]
5th digit: 017.3
0. NOS
1. Lab not done
2. Lab unknown at present
3. Microscopy positive - (in sputum)
4. Culture positive - microscopy negative
5. Culture negative - microscopy positive
6. Culture and microscopy negative - confirmed by other methods

0 See also 'Retinitis' or 'Chorioretinitis'

758.39 CHRISTCHURCH CHROMOSOME ANOMALY
720.30 CHRISTIAN-WEBER NODULAR NONSUPPURATIVE PANNICULITIS
277.89 CHRISTIAN'S DISEASE (SYNDROME) (CHRONIC HISTIOCYTOSIS X)
286.1 CHRISTMAS DISEASE
705.89 CHROMHIDROSIS
117.2 CHROMOBLASTOMYCOSIS
117.2 CHROMOMYCOSIS
194.3 CHROMOPHOBE CARCINOMA SITE NOS
0 CHROMOPHOBE CARCINOMA SITE SPECIFIED SEE 'CANCER', BY SITE M8270/3
758.39 CHROMOSOME 4 SHORT ARM DELETION SYNDROME
758.81 CHROMOSOME ACCESSORY - SEX CHROMOSOME
758.5 CHROMOSOME ACCESSORY - NEC
795.2 CHROMOSOME ANALYSIS ABNORMAL
758.9 CHROMOSOME ANOMALY - UNSPECIFIED CHROMOSOME
758.9 CHROMOSOME ANOMALY - MOSAICS
758.81 CHROMOSOME ANOMALY - MOSAICS SEX CHROMOSOME
758.81 CHROMOSOME ANOMALY - SEX CHROMOSOME
758.89 CHROMOSOME ANOMALY - OTHER
V82.4 CHROMOSOME ANOMALY SCREENING (MATERNAL POSTNATAL)
0 CHRONIC BRONCHITIS SEE 'BRONCHITIS CHRONIC'
416.9 CHRONIC COR PULMONALE
357.81 CHRONIC INFLAMMATORY DEMYELINATING POLYNEUROPATHY (CIDP)

When a patient is admitted in acute respiratory failure due to acute exacerbation of a chronic respiratory condition, sequence the failure before the chronic disease.

When a patient is admitted in respiratory failure due to a non respiratory condition, sequence that condition before the respiratory failure.

CHRONIC OBSTRUCTIVE PULMONARY DISEASE (COPD)

496 NOS
491.22 Acute bronchitis
491.21 Acute exacerbation
518.5 Acute exacerbation - ARDS [496]
415.0 Acute exacerbation - cor pulmonale [496]
486 Acute exacerbation - pneumonia [496]
512.8 Acute exacerbation - pneumothorax [496]
415.19 Acute exacerbation - pulmonary embolus [496]
415.11 Acute exacerbation - pulmonary embolus post op or iatrogenic [496]
518.81 Acute exacerbation - respiratory failure [496]
491.21 Decompensated
495.6 Fungal (thermophilic) (actinomycete) (other)
495.4 With allergic alveolitis (aspergillus clavatus)
495.9 With allergic alveolitis and pneumonitis
493.2# With asthma
5th digit: 493.2
0. NOS
1. With status asthmaticus
2. With (acute) exacerbation

494.# With bronchiectasis
4th digit: 494
0. NOS
1. With (acute) exacerbation

491.2# With bronchitis (chronic)
5th digit: 491.2
0. NOS
1. With (acute) exacerbation
2. With acute bronchitis
496 With bronchospasm
492.8 With emphysema
492.0 With emphysema bullous
491.21 With (acute) exacerbation

338.4 CHRONIC PAIN SYNDROME
446.4 CHURG-STRAUSS SYNDROME
457.8 CHYLOCELE
0 CHYLOCELE FILARIAL SEE 'FILARIASIS
608.84 CHYLOCELE TUNICA VAGINALIS
791.1 CHYLURIA
125.1 CHYLURIA DUE TO BRUGIA (WUCHERERIA) MALAYI
125.0 CHYLURIA DUE TO WUCHERERIA BANCROFTI
791.1 CHYLURIA NONFILARIAL ABNORMAL

CICATRIX

709.2 NOS
474.8 Adenoid
525.8 Alveolar process
569.49 Anus
380.89 Auricle
576.8 Bile duct

CICATRIX (continued)

596.8 Bladder
733.99 Bone
348.8 Brain
622.3 Cervix postpartum
654.6# Cervix pregnancy or childbirth
660.2# Cervix pregnancy or childbirth obstructing labor [**654.6#**]
5th digit: 654.6
0. Episode of care unspecified or N/A
1. Delivered
2. Delivered with postpartum complication
3. Antepartum complication
4. Postpartum complicatION

5th digit: 660.2
0. Episode of care unspecified or N/A
1. Delivered
3. Antepartum complication
363.30 Chorioretinal - NOS
363.35 Chorioretinal - disseminated
743.53 Chorioretinal - degeneration congenital
363.32 Chorioretinal - macular
363.34 Chorioretinal - peripheral
363.33 Chorioretinal - posterior pole NEC
576.8 Common duct
757.39 Congenital
372.64 Conjunctiva
709.2 Contracture
371.00 Cornea
537.3 Duodenum (bulb)
530.3 Esophagus
374.46 Eyelid
478.29 Hypopharynx
717.5 Knee, semilunar cartilage
375.53 Lacrimal canaliculi
375.56 Lacrimal duct acquired
375.55 Lacrimal duct neonatal
375.52 Lacrimal punctum
375.54 Lacrimal sac
478.79 Larynx
518.89 Lung
363.32 Macular
363.35 Macular - disseminated
363.34 Macular - peripheral
385.89 Middle ear
528.9 Mouth
728.89 Muscle
375.56 Nasolacrimal duct acquired
375.55 Nasolacrimal duct neonatal
478.29 Nasopharynx
528.9 Palate (soft)
607.89 Penis
602.8 Prostate
569.49 Rectum
363.30 Retina - NOS
363.35 Retina - disseminated
743.53 Retina - degeneration congenital
363.32 Retina - macular
363.34 Retina - peripheral
363.33 Retina - posterior pole NEC
608.89 Seminal vesicle
709.2 Skin
686.8 Skin infected
478.29 Throat
529.8 Tongue

CICATRIX (continued)

474.8 Tonsil
478.9 Trachea
593.89 Ureter
599.84 Urethra
621.8 Uterus
623.4 Vagina
478.5 Vocal cord
709.2 Wrist constricting (annular)

357.81 CIDP (CHRONIC INFLAMMATORY DEMYELINATING POLYNEUROPATHY)

374.89 CILIA ABSENCE CONGENITAL
743.63 CILIA AGENESIS ABSENCE CONGENITAL

364.57 CILIARY BODY DEGENERATIVE CHANGES (ATROPHY)
364.9 CILIARY BODY DISEASE
364.89 CILIARY BODY DISEASE OR DISORDER SPECIFIED NEC
364.41 CILIARY BODY HEMORRHAGE
362.16 CILIARY BODY NEOVASCULARIZATION

622.11 CIN I (CERVICAL INTRAEPITHELIAL NEOPLASIA I)
622.12 CIN II (CERVICAL INTRAEPITHELIAL NEOPLASIA II)
233.1 CIN III (CERVICAL INTRAEPITHELIAL NEOPLASIA III)

CIRCADIAN RHYTHM SLEEP DISORDER

327.32 Advanced sleep phase
291.82 Alcohol induced
327.31 Delayed sleep phase
292.85 Drug induced
780.55 Disruption of 24 hr sleep wake cycle
327.34 Free-running type
327.33 Irregular sleep-wake type
327.35 Jet lag type
307.45 Nonorganic
327.30 Organic NOS

> *327.37: Code first the underlying medical or mental disorder.*

327.37 Organic disorder in conditions classified elsewhere
327.39 Organic other
327.35 Rapid time zone change syndrome
327.36 Shift work type

799.89 CIRCULATION FAILURE
747.83 CIRCULATION FETAL PERSISTENT
794.39 CIRCULATION TIME ABNORMAL

CIRCULATORY

747.9 Anomaly NOS (congenital)
747.89 Anomaly NEC specified site (congenital)
785.59 Collapse
779.85 Collapse newborn
639.5 Collapse post pregnancy (abortive) (ectopic) (molar)
V12.50 Disease history unspecified
V12.59 Disease history other specified
760.3 Disease maternal, chronic affecting fetus or newborn
093.9 Disease syphilitic
090.5 Disease syphilitic congenital
459.9 Disorder

CIRCULATORY (continued)

> *648.9#: Use an additional code to identify circulatory disorders.*

648.9# Disorder maternal current (co-existent) in pregnancy

5th digit: 648.9

0. Episode of care NOS or N/A
1. Delivered
2. Delivered with postpartum complication
3. Antepartum complication
4. Postpartum complication

459.89 Disorder other specified
459.9 Insufficiency
779.85 Insufficiency newborn
459.9 Obstruction
747.89 System absence congenital
747.9 System anomaly NOS (congenital)
747.89 System anomaly NEC specified site (congenital)

629.2# CIRCUMCISION FEMALE GENITAL MUTILATION (CUTTING) STATUS

5th digit: 629.2

0. Unspecified
1. Type I (clitorectomy)
2. Type II (clitorectomy with excision of labia minora)
3. Type III (infibulation)
9. Type IV or other

V50.2 CIRCUMCISION ROUTINE OR RITUAL (ELECTIVE)

CIRRHOSIS:

-WITH ESOPHAGEAL VARICES [456.2#]

571.2 Alcoholic (liver)
571.5 Baumgarten-Cruveilhier
571.6 Biliary
121.1 Biliary due to clonorchiasis
121.3 Biliary due to flukes
331.9 Brain
331.9 Brain with dementia [294.1#]

5th digit: 294.1

0. Without behavioral disturbance or NOS
1. With behavioral disturbance

571.5 Cardiac
571.2 Cardiac alcoholic
571.6 Charcot's
571.6 Cholangitic (cholestatic)
624.2 Clitoris (hypertrophic)
777.8 Congenital (due to failure of obliteration of umbilical vein)
571.5 Congestive (liver)
571.2 Congestive alcoholic (liver)
571.5 Cryptogenic (liver)
571.2 Cryptogenic alcoholic (liver)
571.8 Fatty (liver)
571.0 Fatty alcoholic (liver)
571.2 Florid
571.5 Glisson's (liver)
571.2 Glisson's alcoholic (liver)

-WITH ESOPHAGEAL VARICES [456.2#]

5th digit: 456.2

0. With bleeding
1. Without bleeding

CIRRHOSIS: (continued)

-WITH ESOPHAGEAL VARICES [456.2#]

571.6 Hanot's
571.5 Hobnail (liver)
571.2 Hobnail alcoholic (liver)
571.6 Intrahepatic
571.5 Juvenile (liver)
571.2 Juvenile alcoholic (liver)
587 Kidney
571.5 Laennec's (liver)
571.2 Laennec's alcoholic (liver)
571.5 Liver NOS
515 Lung
571.5 Macronodular (liver)
571.2 Macronodular alcoholic (liver)
084.9 Malarial
571.5 Micronodular (liver)
571.2 Micronodular alcoholic (liver)
587 Nephrotic
571.6 Obstructive (biliary) (extrahepatic) (intrahepatic)
620.8 Ovarian
084.9 Paludal
577.8 Pancreas (duct)
275.0 Pigmentary (iron)
571.5 Portal (liver)
571.2 Portal alcoholic (liver)
571.5 Posthepatitic
571.5 Postnecrotic (liver)
571.2 Postnecrotic alcoholic (liver)
571.6 Primary (intrahepatic)
515 Pulmonary
587 Renal
571.5 Septal
289.51 Spleen
571.5 Splenomegalic (liver)
571.2 Splenomegalic alcoholic (liver)
535.4 Stomach
571.6 Todd's
571.5 Without mention of alcohol
571.6 Xanthomatous (biliary)
272.2 Xanthomatous (biliary) due to xanthomatosis

-WITH ESOPHAGEAL VARICES [456.2#]
5th digit: 456.2
0. With bleeding
1. Without bleeding

270.6 CITRULLINE METABOLISM DISORDERS
270.6 CITRULLINEMIA
709.09 CIVATTE'S POIKILODERMA

> ***Use additional code to identify kidney transplant status, if applicable.***

585.# CKD (CHRONIC KIDNEY DISEASE)
4th digit: 585
1. Stage I
2. Stage II (mild)
3. Stage III (moderate)
4. Stage IV (severe)
5. Stage V
6. End stage
9. Unspecified stage

117.2 CLADOSPORIDIUM CARRIONII INFECTION

111.1 CLADOSPORIUM SPECIES INFECTION
117.8 CLADOSPORIUM TRICHOIDES INFECTION
577.8 CLARKE-HADFIELD SYNDROME (PANCREATIC INFANTILISM)
704.2 CLASTOTHRIX
337.9 CLAUDE BERNARD-HORNER SYNDROME SEE ALSO 'NEUROPATHY PERIPHERAL' AUTONOMIC
352.6 CLAUDE'S SYNDROME

CLAUDICATION

> ***When coding atherosclerosis of the extremities use an additional code, if applicable to identify chronic complete or total occlusion of the artery of the extremities (440.4).***

440.21 Due to atherosclerosis
440.3# Due to atherosclerosis of a bypass graft extremities
440.3# Due to atherosclerosis of a bypass graft extremities with chronic complete or total occlusion [440.4]
5th digit: 440.3
0. Unspecified graft
1. Autologous vein bypass graft
2. Nonautologous biological bypass graft

443.9 Intermittent NOS
453.8 Intermittent venous
443.9 Peripheral vascular disease

300.29 CLAUSTROPHOBIA
738.8 CLAVICLE DEFORMITY ACQUIRED
755.51 CLAVICLE DEFORMITY CONGENITAL
700 CLAVUS
736.74 CLAW FOOT ACQUIRED
736.06 CLAW HAND ACQUIRED
735.5 CLAW TOE ACQUIRED
229.9 CLEAR CELL ADENOFIBROMA SITE NOS
0 CLEAR CELL ADENOFIBROMA SITE SPECIFIED SEE 'BENIGN NEOPLASM', BY SITE M8313/0

CLEFT

755.58 Hand congenital
749.1# Lip
749.0# Palate
5th digit: 749.0-1
0. NOS
1. Unilateral complete
2. Unilateral incomplete
3. Bilateral complete
4. Bilateral incomplete

749.2# Palate with cleft lip
5th digit: 749.2
0. Palate with cleft lip unspecified
1. Palate unilateral complete
2. Palate unilateral incomplete
3. Palate bilateral complete
4. Palate bilateral incomplete
5. Palate other combinations

752.89 Scrotum
749.02 Uvula

755.59 CLEIDOCRANIAL DYSOSTOSIS
763.89 CLEIDOTOMY, FETAL

C

348.8 CLERAMBAULT'S AUTOMATISM SYNDROME
297.8 CLERAMBAULT'S EROTOMANIA SYNDROME
766.22 CLIFFORD'S SYNDROME (POSTMATURITY)
608.89 CLIMACTERIC MALE
627.2 CLIMACTERIC SYNDROME (FEMALE)
099.1 CLIMATIC BUBO
796.4 CLINICAL FINDINGS OTHER ABNORMAL

CLITORIS, CLITORAL

752.49 Absence (agenesis) (stricture) congenital
752.49 Anomaly NEC
752.49 Hooded congenital
752.49 Hyperplasia congenital
255.2 Hypertrophy - adrenogenital
624.2 Hypertrophy - nonendocrine
256.1 Hypertrophy - ovarian androgen secretion
959.14 Injury NOS

751.5 CLOACAL ANOMALY
154.8 CLOACOGENIC CARCINOMA SITE NOS
0 CLOACOGENIC CARCINOMA SITE SPECIFIED SEE 'CANCER', BY SITE M8124/3
121.1 CLONORCHIOSIS
121.1 CLONORCHIOSIS BILIARY CIRRHOSIS DUE TO
524.20 CLOSED BITE

CLOSTRIDIUM

008.45 Difficile
005.2 Food poisoning perfringens
005.2 Food poisoning welchii
005.3 Food poisoning other specified type
040.0 Histolyticum
771.89 Intra-amniotic infection of fetus [041.84]
040.0 Oedematiens
041.83 Perfringens
771.89 Perinatal infection of fetus [041.84]
038.3 Septicemia
040.0 Septicum
004.0 Sordellii
040.0 Welchii infection (perfringens)

286.3 CLOTTING FACTOR DEFICIENCY OTHER
473.0 CLOUDY ANTRUM, ANTRA
792.5 CLOUDY (HEMODIALYSIS) (PERITONEAL) DIALYSIS EFFLUENT
757.31 CLOUSTON'S SYNDROME (HIDROTIC ECTODERMAL DYSPLASIA)
756.0 CLOVERLEAF SKULL

CLUB

736.29 Finger acquired
754.89 Finger congenital
736.71 Foot acquired
754.70 Foot congenital
754.51 Foot equinovarus
736.07 Hand acquired
754.89 Hand congenital
703.8 Nail acquired
757.5 Nail congenital

781.5 CLUBBING FINGER
315.4 CLUMSINESS SYNDROME

CMV (CYTOMEGALOVIRUS INFECTIONS)

078.5 CMV
771.1 Congenital or perinatal
V01.79 Exposure
078.5 Hepatitis [573.1]
078.5 Inclusion disease (generalized)
078.5 Pneumonia [484.1]

794.00 CNS ABNORMAL FUNCTION STUDY
779.2 CNS DYSFUNCTION NEWBORN NOS
786.09 CO 2 (CARBON DIOXIDE) NARCOSIS

COAGULATION

790.92 Delay NEC
286.9 Disorder
286.7 Factor deficiency acquired
776.0 Factor deficiency acquired newborn
286.9 Factor deficiency congenital
776.2 Newborn intravascular disseminated
790.92 Study abnormal
790.92 Time prolonged

COAGULATION DFFECT

286.9 NOS
0 Abortion (in) see 'Abortion', by type with hemorrhage
286.7 Acquired (any)
641.3# Antepartum or intrapartum causing hemorrhage
5th digit: 641.3
0. Episode of care NOS or N/A
1. Delivered
3. Antepartum

762.1 Antepartum or intrapartum affecting fetus or newborn
286.3 Congenital NEC

649.3#: Use an additional code to identify the specific coagulation defect.

649.3# Deficiency complicating pregnancy not associated with antepartum hemorrhage
5th digit: 649.3
0. Episode of care NOS or N/A
1. Delivered
2. Delivered with postpartum complication
3. Antepartum
4. Postpartum complication

286.7 Due to liver disease
286.7 Due to vitamin K deficiency
286.7 Hypoprothrombinemia acquired
776.3 Neonatal other transient
666.3# Postpartum
5th digit: 666.3
0. Episode of care unspecified or N/A
2. Delivered with postpartum complication
4. Postpartum complication

286.3 Other specified type NEC

286.6 COAGULOPATHY CONSUMPTION
727.2 COAL MINER'S ELBOW
500 COAL WORKERS' PNEUMOCONIOSIS
747.10 COARCTATION AORTA CONGENITAL
747.3 COARCTATION PULMONARY ARTERY CONGENITAL
362.12 COATS' SYNDROME
790.6 COBALT ABNORMAL BLOOD LEVEL

305.6# COCAINE ABUSE (NONDEPENDENT)
304.2# COCAINE ADDICTION (DEPENDENT)
5th digit: 304.2, 305.6
0. NOS
1. Continuous
2. Episodic
3. In remission

760.75 COCAINE AFFECTING FETUS OR NEWBORN - ASYMPTOMATIC
779.5 COCAINE AFFECTING FETUS OR NEWBORN - WITH WITHDRAWAL SYMPTOMS
0 COCCIDIOIDAL DISEASE SEE 'COCCIDIOIDOMYCOSIS'

COCCIDIOIDOMYCOSIS

114.9 NOS
114.1 Cutaneous primary
114.3 Disseminated
114.1 Extrapulmonary primary
114.3 Granuloma
114.4 Granuloma lung
114.2 Meninges
114.2 Meningitis
114.0 Pneumonial
114.3 Prostate
114.3 Other forms progressive
114.5 Pulmonary
114.0 Pulmonary acute primary
114.4 Pulmonary chronic secondary
114.4 Pulmonary residual
114.3 Specified site NEC

0 COCCIDIOIDOSIS SEE 'COCCIDIOIDOMYCOSIS'
007.2 COCCIDIOSIS INTESTINAL
791.9 COCCIURIA
791.9 COCCUS IN URINE
0 COCCUS SEE 'BACTERIAL INFECTION' OR SPECIFIED CONDITION
724.79 COCCYGODYNIA

COCCYX, COCCYGEAL

724.70 Disorder
724.79 Disorder NEC
724.71 Hypermobility
959.19 Injury NOS
665.6# Injury obstetrical
5th digit: 665.6
0. Episode of care NOS or N/A
1. Delivered
4. Postpartum complication

724.79 Pain
847.4 Separation (rupture) (tear) (laceration)
847.4 Strain (sprain) (avulsion) (hemarthrosis)

085.1 COCHIN-CHINA ULCER
759.89 COCKAYNE'S SYNDROME (MICROENCEPHALY AND DWARFISM)
757.39 COCKAYNE-WEBER SYNDROME (EPIDERMOLYSIS BULLOSA)
V14.5 CODEINE ALLERGY HISTORY
495.8 COFFEE WORKERS' LUNG
759.89 COFFIN-LOWRY SYNDROME
370.52 COGAN'S SYNDROME (NONSYPHILITIC INTERSTITIAL KERATITIS)

294.9 COGNITIVE DISORDER
438.0 COGNITIVE DISORDER LATE EFFECT OF CEREBROVASCULAR DISEASE
0 COGNITIVE IMPAIRMENT DUE TO CONCUSSION, SEE 'CONCUSSION'
0 COGNITIVE IMPAIRMENT WITH INTRACRANIAL INJURY, SEE SPECIFIED INTRACRANIAL INJURY
907.0 COGNITIVE IMPAIRMENT LATE EFFECT OF INTRACRANIAL INJURY
331.83 COGNITIVE IMPAIRMENT MILD, SO STATED
331.83 COGNITIVE IMPAIRMENT MILD, SO STATED WITH DEMENTIA **[294.1#]**
5th digit: 294.1
0. Without behavioral disturbance or NOS
1. With behavioral disturbance

793.1 COIN LESION (LUNG)

COLD

460 NOS
283.0 Agglutinin disease or hemoglobinuria
283.2 Agglutinin hemoglobinuria paroxysmal
477.9 Allergic (see also 'Rhinitis', allergic)
460 Common
460 Common due to RSV (respiratory syncytial virus) [079.6]
487.1 Grippy
460 Head common
283.0 Hemagglutinin disease chronic
487.1 Influenzal
991.9 Injury effect of reduced temperature
909.4 Injury effect of reduced temperature - late effect
991.8 Injury effect of reduced temperature - other specified
778.2 Injury syndrome of newborn
780.99 Intolerance
782.0 Sense absence
283.0 Type hemolytic anemia (secondary) (symptomatic)
V04.7 Vaccination

791.9 COLIBACILLURIA

COLIC

789.0# NOS
789.0# Abdominal
543.9 Appendicular
789.0# Infantile
5th digit: 789.0
0. Unspecified site
1. Upper right quadrant
2. Upper left quadrant
3. Lower right quadrant
4. Lower left quadrant
5. Periumbilic
6. Epigastric
7. Generalized
9. Other specified site (multiple)

788.0 Kidney unknown etiology
564.9 Mucous
316 Mucous psychogenic [564.9]

C

C

COLIC (continued)

789.0# Recurrent
5th digit: 789.0
0. Unspecified site
1. Upper right quadrant
2. Upper left quadrant
3. Lower right quadrant
4. Lower left quadrant
5. Periumbilic
6. Epigastric
7. Generalized
9. Other specified site (multiple)

788.0 Renal
788.0 Ureter
599.84 Urethral

902.26 COLICA DEXTRA INJURY

COLITIS

558.9 Unspecified
558.9 Acute
564.9 Adaptive
558.3 Allergic
558.3 Allergic due to ingested foods [V15.0#]
5th digit: V15.0
1. Peanuts
2. Milk products
3. Eggs
4. Seafood
5. Other foods

006.2 Amebic nondysenteric
022.2 Anthrax
007.0 Balantidial
558.9 Chronic
007.2 Coccidial
007.4 Cryptosporidial
007.5 Cyclosporiasis
558.9 Dietary
V65.3 Dietary counseling and surveillance
558.1 Due to radiation
557.0 Fulminant
558.9 Functional
007.1 Giardial
009.0 Gangrenous
555.1 Granulomatous
0 Infectious see 'Enteritis' by specified organism
009.0 Infectious (septic)
009.1 Infectious origin presumed
564.9 Irritable
306.4 Irritable bowel psychogenic
564.1 Irritable bowel syndrome
557.9 Ischemic - NOS
557.0 Ischemic - acute
557.1 Ischemic - chronic
557.1 Ischemic - due to mesenteric artery insufficiency
564.9 Membranous (mucous) (adaptive) (spastic)
316 Membranous (mucous) (adaptive) (spastic) psychogenic [564.9]
564.9 Mucous
316 Mucous psychogenic [564.9]
009.0 Necrotic
006.2 Nondysenteric amebic
558.9 Noninfectious
007.8 Protozoal other specified
007.9 Protozoal unspecified
008.45 Pseudomembranous
564.9 Pseudomucinous

COLITIS (continued)

306.4 Psychogenic
555.1 Regional
555.1 Segmental
009.0 Septic (see also 'Enteritis' by specific organism)
564.9 Spastic colon
316 Spastic colon psychogenic [564.9]
008.41 Staphylococcus
005.0 Staphylococcus due to food
557.0 Thromboulcerative
558.2 Toxic
555.1 Transmural
014.8# Tuberculosis (ulcerative)
5th digit: 014.8
0. NOS
1. Lab not done
2. Lab pending
3. Microscopy positive (in sputum)
4. Culture positive - microscopy negative
5. Culture negative - microscopy positive
6. Culture and microscopy negative confirmed by other methods

556.# Ulcerative
4th digit: 556
0. Enterocolitis (chronic)
1. Ileocolitis (chronic)
2. Proctitis (chronic)
3. Proctosigmoiditis (chronic)
4. Pseudopolyposis of colon
5. Left-sided (chronic)
6. Universal (chronic)
8. Other ulcerative colitis
9. Ulcerative colitis (enteritis) unspecified

COLLAGEN

710.9 Disease NEC
446.20 Disease vascular
446.21 Disease vascular - Goodpasture's

> ***648.9#: Use an additional code to identify the specific collagen disease.***

648.9# Disease vascular - maternal current (co-existent) in pregnancy
5th digit: 648.9
0. Episode of care NOS or N/A
1. Delivered
2. Delivered with postpartum complication
3. Antepartum complication
4. Postpartum complication

446.29 Disease vascular - specified NEC
V50.1 Injection, cosmetic

425.4 COLLAGENOSIS CARDIOVASCULAR

780.2 COLLAPSE

459.89 COLLATERAL CIRCULATION (VENOUS) ANY SITE
0 COLLATERAL LIGAMENT RUPTURE SEE 'SPRAIN'

352.6 COLLET SICARD SYNDROME

701.3 COLLOID ATROPHY DEGENERATIVE

709.3 COLLOID MILIUM

COLOBOMA

743.59 Choroid congenital
743.52 Fundus congenital
743.46 Iris congenital
743.36 Lens congenital
743.62 Lids congenital
377.23 Optic (disc)
743.57 Optic disc congenital
743.56 Retina congenital
743.47 Sclera congenital
743.49 Other specified

> *Injury to internal organs, lung, spleen, liver or kidney, can be a contusion, laceration, tear, or rupture. Use the injury code found under the anatomical site.*

COLON

751.2 Absence congenital
V45.72 Absence postsurgical
751.3 Aganglionosis congenital
564.89 Atony functional
751.2 Atresia congenital
V76.51 Cancer screening
564.7 Dilatation
751.3 Dilatation congenital
560.89 Dilatation mechanical obstruction
306.4 Dilatation psychogenic
569.9 Disorder
751.3 Disorder congenital
564.9 Disorder functional
751.3 Disorder functional congenital
564.81 Disorder functional neurogenic
564.89 Disorder functional other specified
306.4 Disorder psychogenic
562.10 Diverticulum
751.5 Diverticulum congenital
211.3 Dysplasia
564.9 Hyperactive
564.9 Hypermobility
564.9 Hypermotility
564.9 Hypersensitive
863.4# Injury
863.5# Injury with open wound

5th digit: 863.4-5
- **0. Colon unspecified site**
- **1. Ascending (right) colon**
- **2. Transverse colon**
- **3. Descending (left)S colon**
- **4. Sigmoid colon**
- **5. Rectum**
- **6. Multiple sites in colon and rectum**
- **9. Other**

908.1 Injury late effect
560.0 Invagination
564.1 Irritable
557.# Ischemia

4th digit: 557
- **0. Acute**
- **1. Chronic**
- **9. Unspecified transient**

569.89 Lesion
751.4 Malrotation congenital
560.9 Obstruction (occlusion) due to stenosis or stricture
560.89 Obstruction sympathicotonic

COLON (continued)

211.3 Polyp adenomatous
569.89 Polyp nonadenomatous
V12.72 Polyp history
211.4 Polyp rectosigmoid junction, adenomatous
556.4 Pseudopolyposis
564.9 Spastic
564.89 Stasis
751.5 Transposition congenital
560.2 Volvulus (torsion) (strangulation)

COLOR BLINDNESS

368.54 Achromatopsia (total)
368.55 Acquired
368.52 Deutan defect (green)
368.54 Monochromatic (cone) (rod)
368.51 Protan defect (red)
368.53 Tritan defect (blue)
368.59 Other

COLOSTOMY

V53.5 Belt fitting and adjustment
V55.3 Care
V55.3 Catheter adjustment or repositioning
V55.3 Catheter removal or replacement
V55.3 Closure
569.60 Complication - NOS
569.62 Complication - mechanical
569.69 Complication - other
569.69 Fistula
569.69 Hernia

> *When coding an infection of an ostomy, use an additional code to specify the organism. See 'Bacterial Infection'*

569.61 Infection
569.61 Infection with cellulitis of abdomen [682.2]
569.61 Infection with septicemia [**038.#(#)**]

4th or 4th and 5th Digit Code for Organism: 038
- **.9 NOS**
- **.3 Anaerobic**
- **.3 Bacteroides**
- **.3 Clostridium**
- **.42 E. coli**
- **.49 Enterobacter aerogenes**
- **.40 Gram negative**
- **.49 Gram negative other**
- **.41 Hemophilus influenzae**
- **.2 Pneumococcal**
- **.49 Proteus**
- **.43 Pseudomonas**
- **.44 Serratia**
- **.10 Staphylococcal NOS**
- **.11 Staphylococcal aureus**
- **.19 Staphylococcal other**
- **.0 Streptococcal (anaerobic)**
- **.49 Yersinia enterocolitica**
- **.8 Other specified**

569.62 Malfunction
569.69 Prolapse
V44.3 Status
V55.3 Toilet stoma
569.62 Valve malfunction

625.1 COLPOSPASM

C

COMA

780.01 Coma
250.2# Diabetic hyperosmolar non ketotic
250.3# Diabetic hypoglycemic
250.3# Diabetic insulin
250.3# Diabetic ketoacidotic
5th digit: 250.2-3
0. Type II, adult-onset, non-insulin dependent (even if requiring insulin), or unspecified; controlled
1. Type I, juvenile-onset or insulin-dependent; controlled
2. Type II, adult-onset, non-insulin dependent (even if requiring insulin); uncontrolled
3. Type I, Juvenile-onset or insulin-dependent; uncontrolled

0 Due to hepatitis see 'Hepatitis'
780.39 Eclamptic
572.2 Hepatic (chronic liver disease)
251.0 Hyperinsulinism organic
251.0 Hypoglycemic non-diabetic
251.0 Hypoglycemic non-diabetic, iatrogenic
251.0 Insulin non-diabetic
779.2 Neonatal
780.09 Other alteration of consciousness
780.02 Transient alteration of awareness
0 Uremic see 'Uremia'
780.03 Vegetative state persistent
0 See also 'Alteration Of Consciousness'

0 COMATOSE SEE 'COMA'
0 COMBAT FATIGUE SEE 'STRESS REACTION'
255.41 COMBINED GLUCOCORTICOID WITH MINERALOCORTICOID DEFIECIENCY
279.2 COMBINED IMMUNITY DEFICIENCY SYNDROME
266.2 COMBINED SYSTEM DISEASE (OF SPINAL CORD) [336.2]
281.0 COMBINED SYSTEM DISEASE (OF SPINAL CORD) WITH ANEMIA [266.2]
706.1 COMEDO

Use an additional code to identify estrogen receptor status. V86.0 Estrogen receptor positive status (ER+) or V86.1 Estrogen receptor negative status (ER-).

COMEDOCARCINOMA

174.9 Site NOS
0 Site specified see 'Cancer', by site M8501/3
174.# Breast soft tissue
4th digit: 174
0. Nipple and areola
1. Central portion
2. Upper inner quadrant
3. Lower inner quadrant
4. Upper outer quadrant
5. Lower outer quadrant
6. Axillary tail
8. Mastectomy site, inner, lower, midline, outer, upper, ectopic sites, contiguous, overlappiing sites, undetermined
9. Breast (female) site NOS

0 Noninfiltrating site specified see 'Ca In Situ', by site M8501/2
233.2 Noninfiltrating site NOS

610.4 COMEDOMASTITIS
745.69 COMMON ATRIUM CONGENITAL
868.02 COMMON DUCT INJURY (TRAUMATIC)
868.12 COMMON DUCT INJURY (TRAUMATIC) WITH OPEN WOUND
0 COMMON DUCT OBSTRUCTION SEE 'BILE DUCT', OBSTRUCTION
0 COMMON DUCT STONE SEE 'CHOLEDOCHOLITHIASIS'
921.3 COMMOTIO RETINAE
V01.9 COMMUNICABLE DISEASES EXPOSURE UNSPECIFIED
V01.89 COMMUNICABLE DISEASE EXPOSURE OTHER
433.8# COMMUNICATING POSTERIOR ARTERY OCCLUSION
5th digit: 433.8
0. Without cerebral infarction
1. With cerebral infarction

307.9 COMMUNICATION DISORDER NOS
V40.1 COMMUNICATION PROBLEM
0 COMMOTIO CEREBRI SEE 'CONCUSSION'

COMPARTMENT SYNDROME

729.7# Nontraumatic
5th digit: 729.7
1. Upper extremity
2. Lower extremity
3. Abdomen
9. Other sites

908.6 Late effect (anterior) (deep) (posterior) (tibial)
958.9# Traumatic
5th digit: 958.9
0. Unspecified
1. Upper extremity
2. Lower extremity including buttocks
3. Abdomen
9. Other sites

V65.5 COMPLAINT UNFOUNDED (FEARED CONDITION)
279.8 COMPLEMENT C1-C9 DEFICIENCY

COMPLICATION OF A DEVICE, IMPLANT OR GRAFT - MECHANICAL

A mechanical complication may be a break down (mechanical) displacement, leakage, obstruction, perforation, or protusion of an implanted device.

996.0# Cardiac
5th digit: 996.0
0. Unspecified device, implant or graft
1. Cardiac pacemaker (electrode)
2. Heart valve prosthesis
3. Coronary bypass graft
Aortocoronary graft
Arterial occlusion
4. Cardiac defibrillator (automatic implantable)
9. Other
Artificial heart
Cardiac catheter
Cardiac stent

996.2 Central nervous system
Brain electrode
Dorsal column stimulator
Intrathecal infusion pump
Pacemaker brain
Pacemaker phrenic nerve
Peripheral nerve graft
Spinal column electrode
Ventricular shunt

COMPLICATION OF A DEVICE, IMPLANT OR GRAFT – MECHANICAL (continued)

996.3# Genitourinary

5th digit: 996.3

0. Unspecified device, implant or graft

1. Due to urethral (indwelling catheter)

2. Due to intrauterine contraceptive device

IUD (imbedded, displacement, perforation)

9. Other

Catheter cystostomy
Graft NEC
Penile prosthesis
Ureteral repair (graft)
Vas deferens prosthesis/reconstruction

996.4# Orthopedic internal **[V43.6#]**

5th digit: 996.4

0. Unspecified device, implant or graft

Internal fixation nail, rod or plate

1. Loosening prosthetic joint

Aseptic loosening

2. Dislocation prosthetic joint

Instability, subluxation

3. Implant failure prosthetic joint

Breakage, fracture

4. Periprosthetic fracture around prosthetic joint

5. Periprosthetic osteolysis

> ***731.3: Use an additional code to identify major osseous defect, if applicable.***

6. Articular bearing surface wear prosthetic joint

Breakage, fracture

7. Other mechanical complication of prosthetic joint

9. Other mechanical complication of other device implant or graft

Bone graft
Cartilage graft
External fixation with internal components
Muscle graft
Tendon graft

5th digit: V43.6

0. Site unspecified
1. Shoulder
2. Elbow
3. Wrist
4. Hip
5. Knee
6. Ankle
9. Other

0 Ostomy see specific ostomy

996.1 Vascular

Access device
A-V fistula or shunt
Aortic (bifurcation) graft (replacement)
Arterial graft
Blood vessel graft
Carotid artery bypass
Central line
Arteriovenous dialysis catheter
Femoral popliteal bypass graft
Infusion pump
Intraaortic balloon
Umbrella vena cava

COMPLICATION OF A DEVICE, IMPLANT OR GRAFT - MECHANICAL (continued)

996.5# Other specified

5th digit: 996.5

1. Due to corneal graft (rejection/ reaction)

2. Due to graft of other tissue not elsewhere classified

Graft NEC
Skin graft failure or rejection
Tissue NEC

3. Due to ocular lens prosthesis

4. Due to breast prosthesis

Breast capsule
Mammary implant

5. Due to artificial skin graft and decellularized allodermis

6. Due to peritoneal dialysis catheter

7. Due to insulin pump

9. Due to other implant (internal device) not elsewhere classified

Bile duct prosthesis
Catheter NEC
Chin prosthesis
Contraceptive device subdermal
Electrode implant NEC
Eye (globe) prosthesis
Gastrointestinal device
Implant NEC
Mechanical device NEC
Non-absorbable surgical material
Orbital globe implant
Pacemaker NEC
PE tube
Prosthetic device NEC
Reimplantation NEC
Respiratory
Shunt NEC
Stent NEC
Tooth implant
Tympanostomy tube

> ***Do not assume that a condition is a post-op complication. It must be perfectly clear that the condition developed directly as a result of surgery or medical care. The doctor must document in the record that the condition was due to a procedure.***

COMPLICATION OF AN INTERNAL PROSTHESIS IMPLANT OR GRAFT - INFECTION OR INFLAMMATION

996.60 Unspecified internal prosthesis implant or graft

996.61 Cardiac

Arterial
Artificial heart
Coronary artery bypass graft
Coronary stent
Defibrillator
Electrode
Heart assist device
Heart valve prosthesis
Pacemaker
Pulse generator
Subcutaneous pocket

> ***999.31 Other infection - Use an additional code to identify the specified infection such as septicemia, (038.#(#)).***

999.31 Central venous catheter

Central line
Hickman catheter
Peripherally inserted central catheter (PICC)
Triple lumen catheter

C

COMPLICATION OF AN INTERNAL PROSTHESIS IMPLANT OR GRAFT - INFECTION OR INFLAMMATION (continued)

996.65 Genitourinary other
IUD
Penile prosthesis
Vas deferens prosthesis

996.66 Joint prosthesis internal

996.63 Nervous system
Spinal catheter
Catheter ventricular shunt
Brain electrode
Peripheral nerve graft
Ventricular shunt

996.67 Orthopedic other internal
Bone growth stimulator
External fixation with internal components
Orthopedic NEC
Nail, pins, rods, plate or screws

0 Ostomy see specific ostomy

996.68 Peritonoal dialysis catheter-exit site

996.64 Urinary catheter (indwelling)
Urethral catheter

996.62 Vascular
A-V fistula or shunt
Arterial NEC
Arterial renal dialysis
Carotid artery graft
Catheter vascular (peripheral venous)
Arteriovenous dialysis catheter
Infusion pump
Intraaortic balloon
Vascular access device

996.69 Other internal prosthesis
Bile duct implant
Breast implant
Catheter NEC
Chin implant
Contraceptive device subdermal
Corneal implant NEC
Eye (orbit) implant
Gastrointestinal NEC
Insulin pump
Ocular lens implant
PE tube
Respiratory
Skin graft
Tooth implant
Tympanostomy tube

Non-mechancial complications are abnormal body reactions due to the presence of a properly functioning device, implant or graft these conditions include: embolism, fibrosis, infection, inflammation, hemorrhage, pain, stenosis, rejection and thrombosis.

COMPLICATION OF AN INTERNAL PROSTHETIC DEVICE, IMPLANT OR GRAFT - OTHER SPECIFIED (EMBOLUS) (FIBROSIS) (HEMORRHAGE) (PAIN) (STENOSIS) (THROMBUS)

Use an additional code to identify the complication such as pain. See 'Pain'.

996.70 Unspecified internal prosthesis implant or graft, other specified complication

COMPLICATION OF AN INTERNAL PROSTHETIC DEVICE, IMPLANT OR GRAFT - OTHER SPECIFIED (EMBOLUS) (FIBROSIS) (HEMORRHAGE) (PAIN) (STENOSIS) (THROMBUS) (continued)

996.72 Cardiac
Artificial heart
Cardiac stent
Coronary artery bypass graft
Coronary stent
Defibrillator
Electrodes
Heart assist device
Pacemaker
Pacemaker subcutaneous pocket

996.76 Genitourinary
IUD
Penile prosthesis
Urethral catheter
Urinary indwelling catheter
Vas deferens prosthesis

996.71 Heart valve prosthesis

996.75 Nervous system
Brain electrodes
Spinal catheter
Ventricular shunt

Use an additional code to identify the complication such as pain. See 'Pain'.

V43.6# Prosthetic joint- Use an additional code to identify the specified joint. See ' Prosthesis' joint .

996.77 Orthopedic joint prosthesis internal

996.78 Orthopedic other
Bone growth stimulator
External fixation with internal components
Nail, rod or plate (internal)

0 Ostomy see specific ostomy

996.73 Renal dialysis
Dialysis catheter
Vascular catheter NEC

996.74 Vascular
Arterial
A-V fistula or shunt
Blood vessel graft
Carotid artery graft
Catheter NEC
Central line
Infusion pump
Intraaortic balloon
Vascular access device

996.79 Other
Bile duct implant
Breast implant
Catheter NEC
Catheter peritoneal dialysis
Chin implant
Contraceptive device subdermal
Corneal graft
Eye prosthesis implant
Gastrointestinal NEC
Insulin pump
Ocular lens
Orbital
PE tube
Respiratory
Skin graft NEC
Tooth implant
Tympanostomy tube

When coding a complication of an organ transplant, use an additional code to identify the nature of the complication, such as CMV infection [078.5].

COMPLICATION ORGAN TRANSPLANT

996.80 Organ unspecified
996.85 Bone marrow
996.83 Heart
996.87 Intestines
996.81 Kidney
996.82 Liver
996.84 Lung
996.86 Pancreas
996.89 Organ other specified

COMPLICATION REATTACHED EXTREMITY OR BODY PART - INFECTION OR REJECTION

996.90 Unspecified reattached extremity or body part extremity
996.93 Finger (s)
996.95 Foot and toe(s)
996.91 Forearm
996.92 Hand
996.96 Lower extremity other and unspecified
996.94 Upper extremity other and unspecified
996.99 Other specified body part

Do not assume that a condition is a post-op complication. It must be perfectly clear that the condition developed directly as a result of surgery or medical care. The doctor must document in the record that the condition was due to a procedure.

COMPLICATIONS AFFECTING SPECIFIED BODY SYSTEMS NOT ELSEWHERE CLASSIFIED

997.6# Amputation stump (late)
5th digit: 997.6
0. Unspecified complication
1. Neuroma
2. Infection (chronic)
9. Other

997.1 Cardiac
Cardiac arrest/insufficiency
Cardiorespiratory failure
Heart failure

997.4 Digestive system
Anastomosis intestinal
Bariatric surgery
Hepatic failure
Intestinal obstruction
Postoperative NEC
Stomach banding
Stomach stapling

997.0# Nervous system
5th digit: 997.0
0. NOS
1. Central nervous system
Anoxic brain damage
Cerebral hypoxia
2. Cerebrovascular infarction or hemorrhage
Iatrogenic stroke
Postoperative stroke
9. Other

0 Ostomy malfunction see specific ostomy

COMPLICATIONS AFFECTING SPECIFIED BODY SYSTEMS NOT ELSEWHERE CLASSIFIED (continued)

997.2 Peripheral vascular
Phlebitits
Postoperative NEC
Thrombophlebitis

997.3 Respiratory
Mendelson's syndrome
Pneumonia (aspiration)
Postoperative NEC

997.5 Urinary
Anastomosis urinary tract
Anuria
Cystostomy malfunction
Nephrostomy malfunction
Oliguria
Postcystoscopic
Postoperative NEC
Pyelogram
Renal failure/insufficiency
Tubular necrosis (acute)
Ureterostomy malfunction
Urethrostomy malfunction

997.7# Vascular
5th digit: 997.7
1. Mesenteric artery
2. Renal artery
9. Other vessels

997.2 Vascular peripheral
Phlebitits
Postoperative NEC
Thrombophlebitis

997.9# Other
5th digit: 997.9
1. Hypertension
9. Other
Elephantiasis or lymphedema
Vitreous touch syndrome
Other body system NEC

When coding an infection, use an additional code, [041.#(#)], to identify the organism. See 'Bacterial Infection'.

COMPLICATIONS OTHER OF PROCEDURES NOT ELSEWHERE CLASSIFIED

998.9 Unspecified complication not elsewhere classified
Surgical procedure
Therapeutic misadventure of surgical treatment

998.7 Acute reaction to foreign substance accidentally left during a procedure
Talc granuloma

998.31 Disruption of internal operative wound
Burst stitches/sutures
Disruption of internal suture
Wound dehiscence

998.32 Disruption of external operative wound
Burst stitches/sutures
Wound dehiscence

998.6 Fistula persistent postoperative
998.4 Foreign body accidentally left during a procedure
998.12 Hematoma
998.11 Hemorrhage

998.5# Infection postoperative
5th digit: 998.5
1. Seroma
9. Other
Abscess postoperative
Septicemia postoperative

998.2 Laceration or puncture accidental during a procedure
By Catheter or other instrument during a procedure (blood vessel) (nerve) (organ)

C

COMPLICATIONS OTHER OF PROCEDURES NOT ELSEWHERE CLASSIFIED (continued)

998.83 Non-healing surgical wound
0 Ostomy see specific ostomy
998.13 Seroma complicating procedure
998.51 Seroma infected postoperative
998.0 Shock postoperative
Collapse NOS
Shock (hypovolemic)
998.83 Surgical wound non-healing
998.8# Other specified complications of procedures not elsewhere classified
5th digit: 998.8
1. Emphysema (subcutaneous)
2. Cataract fragments
3. Non-healing surgical wound
9. Other complications of procedure NEC

> ***Do not assume that a condition is a post-op complication. It must be perfectly clear that the condition developed directly as a result of surgery or medical care. The doctor must document in the record that the condition was due to a procedure.***

C

COMPLICATIONS OF MEDICAL CARE NOT ELSEWHERE CLASSIFIED

999.9 Other and unspecified complications of medical care not elsewhere classified
Unspecified misadventure
Dialysis NEC
During dialysis
Electroshock therapy
Extracorporeal circulation
Hyperalimentation therapy
Infusion / perfusion procedure NEC
Inhalation therapy
Injection procedure
Therapeutic misadventure
Therapy NEC
Ultrasound therapy
Vaccination NEC
Ventilation therapy
999.6 ABO incompatibility in infusion perfusion or transfusion
999.1 Air embolism
To any site following infusion perfusion or transfusion
999.4 Anaphylactic shock due to serum
Allergic anaphylactic shock
Vaccination anaphylaxis
999.0 General vaccinia
999.7 RH incompatibility reaction in infusion perfusion or transfusion

> ***999.39 Other infection - Use an additional code to identify the specified infection such as septicemia, (038.#(#)).***

999.39 Other infection following infusion, injection, transfusion, or vaccination
General localized infection
Infection NEC
Infusion infection/sepsis
Sepsis NEC
Septicemia
Vaccination cellulitis
Vaccinia localized
999.5 Other serum reaction
Allergic reaction
Protein sickness
Serum sickness / rash / intoxication
Urticaria due to serum

COMPLICATIONS OF MEDICAL CARE NOT ELSEWHERE CLASSIFIED (continued)

999.8 Other transfusion reaction
Blood (lymphocytes) (plasma)
Shock or reaction
Transfusion reaction NOS
999.2 Other vascular complications following infusion, perfusion, or transfusion
Embolism / thrombus
Phlebitis thrombophlebitis

0 COMPLICATION OF LABOR AND DELIVERY SEE SPECIFIED COMPLICATION, OR 'LABOR AND DELIVERY COMPLICATIONS'

909.3 COMPLICATION OF SURGICAL AND MEDICAL CARE LATE EFFECT

COMPOUND PRESENTATION

652.8# NOS
660.0# NOS obstructing labor [652.8#]
652.6# With multiple gestation
660.0# With multiple gestation obstructing labor [652.6#]
5th digit: 652.6, 8, 660.0
0. Episode of care unspecified or N/A
1. Delivered
3. Antepartum complication

993.3 COMPRESSED AIR DISEASE
344.60 COMPRESSION CAUDA EQUINA SYNDROME
344.61 COMPRESSION CAUDA EQUINA SYNDROME WITH NEUROGENIC BLADDER
0 COMPRESSION NERVE SEE SPECIFIC NERVE, DISORDER
724.9 COMPRESSION OF SPINAL NERVE ROOT NEC (NONVERTEBRAL) (NONDISCOGENIC)
958.5 COMPRESSION SYNDROME
301.4 COMPULSIVE PERSONALITY DISORDER
423.2 CONCATO'S PERICARDIAL POLYSEROSITIS
568.82 CONCATO'S DISEASE PERITONEAL
309.81 CONCENTRATION CAMP SYNDROME
368.12 CONCENTRIC FADING
560.39 CONCRETION INTESTINE

> ***Cerebral concussion results from a blow to the head, and should be coded as a trauma. Code it as a trauma until the physician states that the active phase of the concussion has subsided and the symptoms are no longer organic in nature. As long as the documentation states that the patient's symptoms are directly resultant from a concussion, use a trauma code.***

CONCUSSION

850.9 NOS
0 Injury internal organs (except cerebral) see specific organ, injury
850.11 LOC 30 minutes or less
850.12 LOC 31 to 59 minutes
850.2 LOC 1-24 hours
850.3 LOC >24 hours with complete recovery
850.4 LOC >24 hours without return to pre-existing conscious level
850.5 LOC unspecified duration
850.0 No loss of consciousness
V71.89 Observation for suspected
310.2 Syndrome

117.7 CONDIOBOLUS INFECTION
V49.89 CONDITIONS INFLUENCING HEALTH STATUS OTHER SPECIFIED
799.89 CONDITIONS OTHER ILL-DEFINED

CONDUCT DISORDER

312.9 NOS
312.89 NOS unspecified onset
312.82 NOS adolescent onset
312.81 NOS childhood onset
309.3 Adjustment reaction
312.0# Aggressive
5th digit: 312.0
0. NOS
1. Mild
2. Moderate
3. Severe

301.3 Aggressive intermittent
312.23 Aggressive socialized
312.4 Delinquency neurotic
312.9 Disruptive behavior NOS
312.3# Explosive disorder
5th digit: 312.3
4. Intermittent impulse control
5. Isolated impulse control

312.31 Gambling pathological
312.30 Impulse control disorder
312.39 Impulse control disorder other specified
312.9 Juvenile delinquency
312.32 Kleptomania
312.4 Mixed with emotion disturbance
312.33 Pyromania
312.2# Socialized
312.1# Unaggressive
5th digit: 312.1-2
0. NOS
1. Mild
2. Moderate
3. Severe

312.21 Unaggressive socialized
312.8# Other specified NEC
5th digit: 312.8
1. Childhood onset
2. Adolescent onset
9. Unspecified onset

426.9 CONDUCTION DELAY (CARDIAC) (VENTRICULAR)

CONDYLOMA

078.10 NOS
078.11 Acuminatum
098.0 Gonorrheal
091.3 Latum
091.3 Syphilitic (venereal) (latum)
090.0 Syphilitic congenital

701.8 CONFLUENT AND RETICULATE PAPILLOMATOSIS

CONFUSION

298.9 NOS
293.0 Acute due to conditions classified elsewhere
290.3 Acute with senile dementia
291.0 Alcoholic
292.81 Drug-induced
298.2 Psychogenic
298.2 Reactive

372.41 CONFUSIONAL AROUSALS

CONGENITAL

0 See specified condition or anatomical site
286.3 Afibrinogenemia
776.5 Anemia due to blood loss
V19.5 Anomalies family history
759.9 Anomaly
759.7 Anomaly multiple NOS
759.89 Anomaly other specified
327.25 Central alveolar hypoventilation
779.9 Debility
759.7 Deformity multiple NOS
717.5 Discoid meniscus (knee)
799.89 Disease NEC
757.31 Ectodermal dysplasia
352.6 Facial diplegia syndrome
759.89 Generalized fibromatosis (CGF)
271.8 Glycosylation disorder
282.0 Hemolytic anemia spherocytic
243 Hypothyroidism
757.0 Lymphedema
759.89 Muscular hypertrophy-cerebral syndrome
751.62 Polycystic disease liver
759.7 Syndrome affecting more than one system
759.89 Syndrome affecting more than one system, specified type NEC

CONGENITAL CONDITIONS COMPLICATING PREGNANCY

When coding a maternal cardiovascular disease complicating pregnancy, 648.5#, use an additional code to identify the condition.

648.5# Cardiovascular disorder maternal
648.5# Heart disease maternal
654.0# Uterine abnormality complicating pregnancy
660.2# Uterine abnormality complicating pregnancy obstructing labor [654.0#]
5th digit: 648.5, 654.0
0. Episode of care NOS or N/A
1. Delivered
2. Delivered With postpartum complication
3. Antepartum complication
4. Postpartum complication

5th digit: 660.2
0. Episode of care NOS or N/A
1. Delivered
3. Antepartum

0 CONGESTION SEE SPECIFIED SITE OR CONDITION

For coding purposes, CHF and right ventricular failure are considered to be synonymous. Both are assigned a 4th digit of "0". Left ventricular failure is not the same as CHF. Left ventricular failure is assigned a 4th digit of "1".

CONGESTIVE HEART FAILURE (CHF)

428.0 NOS
428.0 Acute
0 Acute left ventricular see 'Heart Failure' left
0 Acute left ventricular with pulmonary edema see 'Heart Failure' left
428.0 Acute with pulmonary edema
428.0 Combined left-right sided
428.0 Compensated

C

CONGESTIVE HEART FAILURE (CHF) (continued)

428.0 Decompensated (right congestive)
997.1 During a procedure
779.89 Fetus or newborn
402.91 Hypertensive NOS [428.0]
402.11 Hypertensive benign [428.0]
402.01 Hypertensive malignant [428.0]
0 Hypertensive heart and chronic kidney disease with and without heart failure see 'Hypertensive', heart and chronic kidney disease
0 Left ventricular see 'Heart Failure'
997.1 Post op resulting from a procedure [428.0]
997.1 Post op heart surgery - immediate
429.4 Post op heart surgery - late
398.91 Rheumatic
391.8 Rheumatic acute or active
398.91 Rheumatic chronic or inactive (with chorea)
428.0 Right secondary to left
392.0 Sydenham's chorea with heart involvement
402.91 With hypertensive cardiomyopathy [428.0]
402.11 With hypertensive cardiomyopathy benign [428.0]
402.01 With hypertensive cardiomyopathy malignant [428.0]

CONGESTIVE HEART FAILURE (CHF) OBSTETRICAL

635.7# Complicating abortion
5th digit: 635.7
0. Unspecified
1. Incomplete
2. Complete

669.4# Complicating labor and delivery
668.1# Due to anesthesia, other sedation in L&D
639.8 Following abortion
648.6# Maternal current (co-existent)
5th digit: 648.6, 668.1, 669.4
0. Episode of care NOS or N/A
1. Delivered
2. Delivered with postpartum complication
3. Antepartum complication
4. Postpartum complication

759.4 CONJOINED TWINS

CONJUGATE GAZE

378.85 Anomalies of divergence
378.83 Convergence insufficiency or palsy
378.84 Excess or spasm
378.81 Palsy
378.87 Skew deviation
378.82 Spasm

CONJUNCTIVA, CONJUNCTIVAL

918.2 Abrasion
372.63 Adhesions (extensive)
372.62 Adhesions and strands (localized)
372.74 Aneurysm
372.55 Argyrosis
372.89 Atrophy
372.54 Calcification
372.73 Chemosis
372.54 Concretions
372.71 Congestion
372.75 Cyst
372.50 Degeneration
277.39 Degeneration amyloid [372.50]
372.56 Deposits

CONJUNCTIVA, CONJUNCTIVAL (continued)

372.89 Discharge
372.9 Disease (see also 'Conjunctivitis')
372.9 Disorder
372.89 Disorder other
372.73 Edema
372.89 Emphysema
372.02 Folliculosis acute
372.61 Granuloma
372.72 Hemorrhage
372.71 Hyperemia
372.73 Hypertrophy lymphoid
918.2 Injury superficial
372.55 Pigmentations
379.93 Redness
372.64 Scarring (post enucleation)
372.62 Strands
372.74 Vascular abnormalities
372.53 Xerosis
264.0 Xerosis vitamin A
264.1 Xerosis vitamin A deficiency with Bitot's spot

CONJUNCTIVITIS

372.30 NOS
372.00 Acute
372.05 Acute atopic
372.03 Acute catarrhal
372.02 Acute follicular
077.3 Acute follicular adenoviral
077.4 Acute follicular epidemic hemorrhagic
077.8 Acute follicular newcastle
077.2 Acute follicular pharynconjunctival
372.03 Acute mucopurulent
372.04 Acute pseudomembranous
372.01 Acute serous
372.14 Allergic
372.05 Anaphylactic
372.03 Angular
077.4 Apollo
372.30 Bacterial
372.01 Chemical
372.05 Chemical allergic
0 Chemical meaning corrosion see 'Burn', eye and adnexa
077.98 Chlamydial
0 Chlamydial trachomatis see 'Trachoma'
372.10 Chronic
372.14 Chronic allergic other
372.12 Chronic follicular
372.11 Chronic simple
372.13 Chronic vernal
032.81 Diphtheritic
372.05 Dust (due to)
370.31 Eczematous
077.4 Enterovirus type 70
077.4 Epidemic hemorrhagic
077.1 Epidemic keratoconjunctivitis
695.1 Erythema multiforme [372.33]
125.9 Filarial [372.15]
077.3 Follicular adenoviral
076.1 Follicular trachomatous
370.34 Glare
098.49 Gonococcal
098.40 Gonococcal neonatal
076.1 Granular trachomatous
077.4 Hemorrhagic (acute) (epidemic)

CONJUNCTIVITIS (continued)

054.43 Herpetic simplex
053.21 Herpetic zoster
077.0 Inclusion
771.6 Inclusion neonatal
372.03 Influenzal
372.03 Koch weeks
085.5 Leishmaniasis [372.15]
372.05 Light
372.05 Medicamentosa
372.04 Membranous acute
036.89 Meningococcal
372.02 Morax Axenfeld
771.6 Neonatal
077.8 Newcastle
360.14 Nodosa
077.3 Of beal
085.5 Parasitic mucocutaneous leishmaniasis [372.15]
077.0 Paratrachoma
372.02 Parinaud's
694.61 Pemphigoid
372.39 Petrificans
077.2 Pharyngoconjunctival fever
370.31 Phlyctenular
372.30 Pneumococcal
099.3 Reiter's [372.33]
695.3 Rosacea [372.31]
V74.4 Screening exam (bacterial)
077.99 Serous viral
372.30 Staphylococcal
372.30 Streptoccal, streptococcus
372.04 Sun lamp
077.0 Swimming pool
095.8 Syphilis [372.10]
130.1 Toxoplasmosis
372.39 Traumatic NEC
017.3# Tuberculous [370.31]

5th digit: 017.3
0. NOS
1. Lab not done
2. Lab pending
3. Microscopy positive (in sputum)
4. Culture positive - microscopy negative
5. Culture negative - microscopy positive
6. Culture and micro negative confirmed by other methods

021.3 Tularemic
372.13 Vernal
370.32 Vernal limbar and corneal involvement [372.13]
077.99 Viral
077.4 Viral acute hemorrhagic
077.8 Viral other
372.39 Other

372.81 CONJUNCTIVOCHALASIS

099.3 CONJUNCTIVOURETHROSYNOVIAL SYNDROME
099.3 CONJUNCTIVOURETHROSYNOVIAL SYNDROME WITH ARTHROPATHY [711.1#]

5th digit: 711.1
0. Site NOS
1. Shoulder region
2. Upper arm (elbow) (humerus)
3. Forearm (radius) (wrist) (ulna)
4. Hand (carpal) (metacarpal) (fingers)
5. Pelvic region and thigh (hip) (buttock) (femur)
6. Lower leg (fibula) (knee) (patella) (tibia)
7. Ankle and/or foot (metatarsals) (toes) (tarsals)
8. Other (head) (neck) (rib) (skull) (trunk) (vertebrae)
9. Multiple

099.3 CONJUNCTIVOURETHROSYNOVIAL SYNDROME WITH CONJUNCTIVITIS [372.33]
710.9 CONNECTIVE TISSUE DISEASE NEC (SEE ALSO 'COLLAGEN')
255.12 CONN-LOUIS SYNDROME (PRIMARY ALDOSTERONISM)
255.12 CONN'S SYNDROME (PRIMARY ALDOSTERONISM)
082.1 CONOR AND BRUCH'S BOUTONNEUSE FEVER
756.59 CONRADI (-HUNERMANN) DISEASE OR SYNDROME (CHONDRODYSPLASIA CALCIFICANS CONGENITA)
V19.7 CONSANGUINITY FAMILY HISTORY

CONSTIPATION

564.00 NOS
564.09 Atonic
564.09 Drug induced
564.09 Neurogenic
306.4 Psychogenic [**564.0#**]

5th digit: 564.0
0. Unspecified
1. Slow transit
2. Outlet dysfunction
9. Other

564.02 Outlet dysfunction
564.00 Simple
564.01 Slow transit
564.09 Spastic
564.09 Other specified

CONSTITUTIONAL STATE

V21.2 Adolescence
V21.0 Development rapid growth
V21.9 In development
V21.8 In development other specified
V21.1 Puberty

286.4 CONSTITUTIONAL THROMBOPATHY
0 CONSULTATION SEE 'COUNSELING'
0 CONTACT DERMATITIS SEE 'DERMATITIS CONTACT'
371.82 CONTACT LENS CAUSING CORNEAL DISORDER
V53.1 CONTACT LENSES FITTING AND ADJUSTMENT
0 CONTACT WITH COMMUNICABLE DISEASE SEE 'EXPOSURE'
051.2 CONTAGIOUS PUSTULAR DERMATITIS

CONTRACEPTION, CONTRACEPTIVE

ADVICE / COUNSELING

V25.09 Family planning
V25.04 Family planning natural to avoid pregnancy
V25.03 Postcoital emergency (with prescription)
V25.03 Prescription or use - emergency postcoital
V25.02 Prescription or use - foams, creams or other agents
V25.01 Prescription or use - oral contraceptive
V25.09 Tuboplasty (proposed)
V25.09 Vasectomy (proposed)
V25.09 Other specified NEC

MANAGEMENT

V25.9 Unspecified
V25.02 Diaphragm fitting
V15.7 History
V25.43 Implantable subdermal - checking, reinsertion or removal
V45.52 Implantable subdermal - in situ
V25.5 Implantable subdermal - insertion
V25.02 Injection
V25.49 Injection repeat
V25.42 IUD checking, reinsertion or removal
V45.51 IUD in situ
V25.1 IUD insertion
V25.3 Menstrual regulation
V25.01 Oral prescription
V25.03 Oral prescription emergency postcoital
V25.41 Oral repeat prescription
V25.02 Prescription foams, creams
V25.03 Prescription emergency postcoital
V25.02 Prescription other specified agent NEC
V25.49 Prescription other specified agent NEC - repeat
V25.8 Sperm count post-vasectomy
V25.2 Sterilization
V25.40 Surveillance
V25.2 Tuboplasty encounter
V25.2 Vasectomy encounter
V25.49 Other specified contraceptive method NEC
V45.59 Other specified device in situ
V25.8 Other specified NEC

0 CONTRACTURE/CONTRACTION SEE ANATOMICAL SITE OR SPECIFIED CONDITION

V64.1 CONTRAINDICATION CAUSING CANCELLATION OF PROCEDURE

> ***A contusion is a collection of blood under the surface of the skin with the skin surface intact resulting from an injury. Do not code contusions when they accompany a fracture, dislocation, laceration, or a crush injury. Rather, use a code from these categories since contusions are considered to be incidental to the greater injury. For contusions of nerves or internal organs, use the"injury code found under the specific anatomical sites.***

CONTUSION

924.9 NOS
922.2 Abdomen wall or muscle
868.00 Abdominal organ unspecified
868.10 Abdominal organ unspecified with open wound
868.09 Abdominal organ other or multiple
868.19 Abdominal organ other or multiple with open wound
921.9 Adnexa eye
868.01 Adrenal gland
868.11 Adrenal gland with open wound

CONTUSION (continued)

924.21 Ankle
924.20 Ankle and foot
923.9 Arm
923.10 Arm lower
923.09 Arm and shoulder
923.8 Arm multiple sites
923.03 Arm upper
920 Auditory canal (external) (meatus)
920 Auricle ear
923.02 Axillary region
923.09 Axillary region and shoulder
923.09 Axillary region and upper arm
922.31 Back
868.02 Bile duct
868.12 Bile duct with open wound
924.9 Bone unspecified
851.8# Brain NOS (with hemorrhage)
851.9# Brain NOS with open intracranial wound (with hemorrhage)
851.0# Brain cortex (with hemorrhage)
851.1# Brain cortex with open intracranial wound (with hemorrhage)
851.4# Brain stem (cerebellum) (occipital lobe) (with hemorrhage)
851.5# Brain stem (cerebellum) (occipital lobe) with open intracranial wound (with hemorrhage)
851.8# Brain other (with hemorrhage)
851.9# Brain other with open intracranial wound (with hemorrhage)
922.0 Breast
920 Brow
922.32 Buttock
921.1 Canthus
861.01 Cardiac
861.11 Cardiac with open wound into thorax
952.4 Cauda equina (spine)
851.4# Cerebellum (with hemorrhage)
851.5# Cerebellum with open intracranial wound (with hemorrhage)
851.8# Cerebral (with hemorrhage)
851.9# Cerebral with open intracranial wound (with hemorrhage)
851.0# Cerebral cortex (with hemorrhage)
851.1# Cerebral cortex with open intracranial wound (with hemorrhage)

5th digit: 851.0-1, 4-5, 8-9
- **0. Level of consciousness (LOC) NOS**
- **1. No LOC**
- **2. LOC < 1 hr**
- **3. LOC 1 - 24 hrs**
- **4. LOC > 24 hrs with return to prior level of consciousness**
- **5. LOC > 24 hrs without return to prior level: or death before regaining consciousness, regardless of duration of LOC**
- **6. LOC duration NOS**
- **9. With concussion NOS**

920 Cheek
922.1 Chest (wall)
920 Chin
922.4 Clitoris
921.1 Conjunctiva
952.4 Conus medullaris (spine)
921.3 Cornea
922.4 Corpus cavernosum

CONTUSION (continued)

851.0# Cortex – brain (cerebral) (with hemorrhage)

851.1# Cortex – brain (cerebral) with open intracranial wound (with hemorrhage)

5th digit: 851.0-1

- **0. Level of consciousness (LOC) NOS**
- **1. No LOC**
- **2. LOC < 1 hr**
- **3. LOC 1 - 24 hrs**
- **4. LOC > 24 hrs with return to prior level of consciousness**
- **5. LOC > 24 hrs without return to prior level: or death before regaining consciousness, regardless of duration of LOC**
- **6. LOC duration NOS**
- **9. With concussion NOS**

922.1	Costal region
920	Ear (auricle)
923.11	Elbow
923.10	Elbow with forearm
922.4	Epididymis
922.2	Epigastric region
924.5	Extremity lower
924.4	Extremity lower multiple sites
923.9	Extremity upper
923.8	Extremity upper multiple sites
921.9	Eye
921.0	Eye and adnexa (black eye)
921.3	Eyeball
921.1	Eyelid
920	Face
922.2	Femoral triangle
772.6	Fetus or newborn
923.3	Finger
923.3	Fingernail
922.2	Flank
924.20	Foot or foot and ankle
923.10	Forearm
923.10	Forearm and elbow
920	Forehead
868.02	Gallbladder
868.12	Gallbladder with open wound
922.4	Genital organs external
921.3	Globe (eye)
922.2	Groin
920	Gum
923.20	Hand
920	Head
861.01	Heart
861.11	Heart with open wound of thorax
924.20	Heel
924.01	Hip
924.00	Hip with thigh
922.2	Iliac region
922.2	Inguinal region
922.33	Interscapular region
862.8	Intrathoracic organs multiple
862.9	Intrathoracic organs multiple, with open wound into cavity
921.3	Iris (eye)
866.01	Kidney
866.11	Kidney with open wound into cavity
924.11	Knee
924.10	Knee with lower leg

CONTUSION (continued)

922.4	Labia
921.1	Lacrimal apparatus, gland or sac
920	Larynx
906.3	Late effect
924.5	Leg
924.10	Leg lower
924.4	Leg multiple sites
921.3	Lens
920	Lingual
920	Lip
864.01	Liver
864.11	Liver with open wound
922.31	Lumbar region
861.21	Lung
861.31	Lung with open wound
920	Malar region
920	Mandibular joint area
920	Mastoid region
851.8#	Membrane - brain (with hemorrhage)
851.9#	Membrane - brain with open intracranial wound (with hemorrhage)

5th digit: 851.8-9

- **0. Level of consciousness (LOC) NOS**
- **1. No LOC**
- **2. LOC < 1 hr**
- **3. LOC 1 - 24 hrs**
- **4. LOC > 24 hrs with return to prior level of consciousness**
- **5. LOC > 24 hrs without return to prior level: or death before regaining consciousness, regardless of duration of LOC**
- **6. LOC duration NOS**
- **9. With concussion NOS**

922.1	Midthoracic region
920	Mouth
862.8	Multiple intrathoracic organs
862.9	Multiple intrathoracic organs with open wound into cavity
924.8	Multiple sites
924.4	Multiple sites lower limb
922.8	Multiple sites trunk
923.8	Multiple sites upper limb
924.9	Muscle site unspecified
861.01	Myocardial
861.11	Myocardial with open wound of thorax
920	Nasal (septum)
920	Neck
920	Nose
851.4#	Occipital lobe (with hemorrhage)
851.5#	Occipital lobe with open intracranial wound (with hemorrhage)

5th digit: 851.4-5

- **0. Level of consciousness (LOC) NOS**
- **1. No LOC**
- **2. LOC < 1 hr**
- **3. LOC 1 - 24 hrs**
- **4. LOC > 24 hrs with return to prior level of consciousness**
- **5. LOC > 24 hrs without return to prior level: or death before regaining consciousness, regardless of duration of LOC**
- **6. LOC duration NOS**
- **9. With concussion NOS**

920	Occipital region

CONTUSION (continued)

921.2	Orbital area
920	Palate
851.8#	Parietal lobe (with hemorrhage)
851.9#	Parietal lobe with open intracranial wound (with hemorrhage)

5th digit: 851.8-9

0. Level of consciousness (LOC) NOS
1. No LOC
2. LOC < 1 hr
3. LOC 1 - 24 hrs
4. LOC > 24 hrs with return to prior level of consciousness
5. LOC > 24 hrs without return to prior level: or death before regaining consciousness, regardless of duration of LOC
6. LOC duration NOS
9. With concussion NOS

920	Parietal region
922.9	Pelvis
922.4	Penis
861.01	Pericardium
861.11	Pericardium with open wound of thorax
922.4	Perineum
921.1	Periocular
921.2	Periorbital
868.03	Peritoneum
868.13	Peritoneum with open wound
920	Pharynx
924.11	Popliteal space
922.4	Prepuce
922.4	Pubic region
922.4	Pudenda
861.21	Pulmonary
861.31	Pulmonary with open wound
924.00	Quadriceps femoralis
866.01	Renal
866.11	Renal with open wound into cavity
921.2	Retrobulbar
868.04	Retroperitoneum
868.14	Retroperitoneum with open wound
922.1	Rib
922.32	Sacral region
920	Salivary ducts or gland
920	Scalp
923.01	Scapula
923.09	Scapula and shoulder
923.01	Scapular region
921.3	Sclera (eye)
922.4	Scrotum
923.00	Shoulder
923.09	Shoulder and arm multiple sites
923.00	Shoulder region
924.9	Skin unspecified site
920	Skull
922.4	Spermatic cord
952.4	Spinal cord cauda equina
952.4	Spinal cord conus medullaris
865.01	Spleen
865.11	Spleen with open wound into cavity
922.1	Sternal region
921.1	Subconjunctival
924.9	Subcutaneous unspecified site
920	Submaxillary region
920	Submental region

CONTUSION (continued)

924.9	Subperiosteal
923.3	Subungual fingernail
923.3	Subungual thumbnail
924.3	Subungual toenail
920	Supraclavicular fossa
920	Supraorbital
920	Temple
922.4	Testis
924.00	Thigh
924.00	Thigh and hip
922.1	Thorax
920	Throat
923.3	Thumb
923.3	Thumbnail
924.3	Toe
924.3	Toenail
920	Tongue
922.9	Trunk
922.8	Trunk multiple sites
922.4	Tunica vaginalis
920	Tympanum
920	Uvula
922.4	Vagina
920	Vocal cord
922.4	Vulva
923.21	Wrist
923.20	Wrist and hand

743.57 CONUS (CONGENITAL)

371.60 CONUS ACQUIRED

336.8 CONUS MEDULLARIS SYNDROME

CONVALESCENCE

V66.9	Unspecified
V66.2	Following chemotherapy
V66.6	Following combined treatment
V66.4	Following fracture
V66.3	Following mental disorder
V66.3	Following psychotherapy
V66.1	Following radiotherapy
V66.0	Following surgery
V66.5	Following other treatment

When using code V66.7, code the terminal illness first.

V66.7	For end-of-life, hospice or terminal care
V66.7	For palliative care

378.84 CONVERGENCE EXCESS OR SPASM

378.83 CONVERGENCE INSUFFICIENCY OR PALSY

300.11 CONVERSION DISORDER

300.11 CONVERSION HYSTERIA OR REACTION

CONVULSIONS

780.39	NOS
780.39	Brain, cerebral, cerebrospinal
780.39	Disorder or state
780.39	Due to ether anesthetic correct substance correctly administered
780.39	Eclamptic
0	Epileptic see 'Epilepsy, Epileptic'
780.39	Epileptiform, epileptoid
780.31	Febrile NOS (simple)
780.32	Febrile complex
780.39	Generalized

CONVULSIONS (continued)

780.39 Infantile
779.0 Newborn
780.39 Nonepileptic unknown etiology or unspecified
780.39 Recurrent
780.39 Repetitive
780.39 Spasmodic
780.39 Uncinate

255.2 COOKE-APERT-GALLAIS SYNDROME (ADRENOGENITAL)
282.49 COOLEY'S (ERYTHROBLASTIC) ANEMIA
610.1 COOPER'S DISEASE
611.8 COOPER'S DROOP BREAST

COORDINATION

315.4 Developmental disorder
781.3 Lack of

When a patient is admitted in acute respiratory failure due to acute exacerbation of a chronic respiratory condition, sequence the failure before the chronic disease.

When a patient is admitted in respiratory failure due to a non respiratory condition, sequence that condition before the respiratory failure.

COPD (CHRONIC OBSTRUCTIVE PULMONARY DISEASE)

496 NOS
491.22 Acute bronchitis
491.21 Acute exacerbation
518.5 Acute exacerbation - ARDS [496]
415.0 Acute exacerbation - cor pulmonale [496]
486 Acute exacerbation - pneumonia [496]
512.8 Acute exacerbation - pneumothorax [496]
415.19 Acute exacerbation - pulmonary embolus [496]
415.11 Acute exacerbation - pulmonary embolus post op or iatrogenic [496]
518.81 Acute exacerbation - respiratory failure [496]
491.21 Decompensated
495.6 Fungal (thermophilic) (actinomycete) (other)
495.4 With allergic alveolitis (aspergillus clavatus)
495.9 With allergic alveolitis and pneumonitis
493.2# With asthma
5th digit: 493.2
0. NOS
1. With status asthmaticus
2. With (acute) exacerbation

494.# With bronchiectasis
4th digit: 494
0. NOS
1. With (acute) exacerbation

491.2# With bronchitis (chronic)
5th digit: 491.2
0. NOS
1. With (acute) exacerbation
2. With acute bronchitis

496 With bronchospasm
492.8 With emphysema
492.0 With emphysema bullous
491.21 With (acute) exacerbation

790.6 COPPER ABNORMAL BLOOD LEVEL
275.1 COPPER METABOLISM DISORDER
989.5 COPPERHEAD SNAKE BITE
995.0 COPPERHEAD SNAKE BITE WITH ANAPHYLAXIS [989.5]

560.39 COPROLITH
302.89 COPROPHILIA
277.1 COPROPORPHYRIA HEREDITARY

745.7 COR BILOCULARE ATRIAL AND VENTRICULAR SEPTUM ABSENCE
415.0 COR PULMONALE ACUTE
416.9 COR PULMONALE CHRONIC
416.9 COR PULMONALE SYNDROME
746.82 COR TRIATRIATUM CONGENITAL
745.3 COR TRILOCULARE BIATRIATUM
745.69 COR TRILOCULARE BIVENTRICULARE

Injury of a tendon, joint capsule, or ligament can be a separation, tear, laceration, avulsion, strain, sprain, or hemarthrosis. You can find this under 'Sprain' also.

840.1 CORACOCLAVICULAR SEPARATION (RUPTURE) (TEAR) (LACERATION)
840.1 CORACOCLAVICULAR STRAIN (SPRAIN) (AVULSION) (HEMARTHROSIS)
840.2 CORACOHUMERAL SEPARATION (RUPTURE) (TEAR) (LACERATION)
840.2 CORACOHUMERAL STRAIN (SPRAIN) (AVULSION) (HEMARTHROSIS)
989.5 CORAL SNAKE BITE
995.0 CORAL SNAKE BITE WITH ANAPHYLAXIS [989.5]
607.1 CORBUS' DISEASE
762.5 CORD COMPRESSION (AROUND NECK) (ENTANGLEMENT) (KNOT) (TORSION) AFFECTING FETUS OR NEWBORN
762.4 CORD PROLAPSED (PRESENTATION) AFFECTING FETUS OR NEWBORN
762.6 CORD CONDITION OTHER AFFECTING FETUS OR NEWBORN
743.46 CORECTOPIA CONGENITAL
495.3 CORKHANDLER'S LUNG
530.5 CORKSCREW ESOPHAGUS
700 CORN

CORNEA, CORNEAL

918.1 Abrasion
371.81 Anesthesia and hypoesthesia
743.9 Anomalies NOS
743.41 Anomalies of size and shape congenital
743.49 Anomalies specified NEC
371.16 Argentous deposits
371.03 Caligo
371.30 Changes membrane
371.41 Changes senile

DEFORMITY

371.70 NOS
743.9 NOS congenital
371.71 Ectasia
371.72 Descemetocele
371.73 Staphyloma

C

CORNEA, CORNEAL (continued)

DEGENERATION

371.40 NOS
371.44 Calcerous
371.41 Dellen
371.41 Hyaline
371.46 Nodular
371.48 Peripheral
371.41 Senile

CORNEA, CORNEAL (continued)

371.41 Dellen

DEPOSIT

371.10 NOS
371.15 Associated with metabolic disorders
371.16 Argentous
<u>270.0</u> In <u>cystinosis</u> [371.15]
277.5 In <u>mucopolysaccharidosis</u> [371.15]

CORNEA, CORNEAL (continuod)

371.72 Descemetocele

DISORDER

371.9 NOS
371.82 Due to contact lens
371.89 Other specified

CORNEA, CORNEAL (continued)

743.41 Distortion congenital
V59.5 Donor non-autogenous

DYSTROPHY

371.50 NOS
371.52 Anterior other
371.57 Combined
371.56 Crystalline
371.57 Endothelial (Fuch's)
371.53 Granular
371.51 Juvenile epithelial
371.54 Lattice
371.55 Macular
371.52 Microscopic cystic
371.58 Polymorphous
371.58 Posterior
371.52 Ring like
371.56 Stromal

CORNEA, CORNEAL (continued)

371.71 Ectasia

EDEMA

371.20 NOS
371.21 Idiopathic
371.22 Secondary
371.23 Bullous keratopathy
371.24 Due to wearing contact lenses

CORNEA, CORNEAL (continued)

371.42 Erosion recurrent
371.44 Facet
996.69 Graft complication - infection or inflammation
996.51 Graft complication - mechanical
996.79 Graft complication - other
371.57 Guttata

CORNEA, CORNEAL (continued)

054.43 Herpes disciform (simplex)
054.43 Herpes simplex
053.21 Herpes zoster
371.89 Hypertrophy
371.81 Hyperesthesia
371.81 Hypoesthesia
371.20 Infiltrate
370.9 Inflammation
370.00 Inflammation with ulcer
371.82 Injury (superficial) due to contact lens
918.1 Laceration superficial
371.04 Leucoma central
371.02 Macula
371.03 Macula interfering with central vision
371.30 Membrane change
371.01 Nebula

NEOVASCULARIZATION

370.60 NOS
370.61 Localized
370.62 Pannus
370.63 Deep vascularization
370.64 Ghost vessels

OPACITY

371.00 NOS
371.03 Central
743.43 Congenital
743.42 Congenital interfering with vision
371.01 Minor
371.02 Peripheral

CORNEA, CORNEAL (continued)

<u>**017.3#**</u> Phthisical <u>tuberculous</u> [371.05]

5th digit: 017.3
0. NOS
1. Lab not done
2. Lab pending
3. Microscopy positive (in sputum)
4. Culture positive - microscopy negative
5. Culture negative - microscopy positive
6. Culture and microscopy negative confirmed by other methods

PIGMENTATIONS

371.10 NOS
371.11 Anterior
371.13 Posterior
371.12 Stromal

CORNEA, CORNEAL (continued)

743.41 Plana
371.00 Scar
264.6 Scar due to vitamin A deficiency
370.54 Sclerosis
371.73 Staphyloma
V45.69 Status postsurgical
V42.5 Transplant (status)

ULCER

370.00 NOS
370.03 Central
264.3 Due to vitamin A deficiency

CORNEA, CORNEAL (continued)

ULCER (continued)

370.04 Hypopyon ulcer
370.01 Marginal
370.07 Mooren's ulcer
370.05 Mycotic
370.06 Perforated
370.02 Ring
370.04 Serpiginous

CORNEA, CORNEAL (continued)

371.40 Xerosis

759.89 CORNELIA DE LANGE'S SYNDROME (AMSTERDAM DWARF, MENTAL RETARDATION, AND BRACHYCEPHALY)

700 CORNS

700 CORNS AND CLAVUS

079.89 CORONA-VIRUS INFECTION

079.82 CORONA-VIRUS SARS ASSOCIATED INFECTION

V01.82 CORONA-VIRUS SARS ASSOCIATED INFECTION EXPOSURE

480.3 CORONA-VIRUS SARS ASSOCIATED INFECTION PNEUMONIA

CORONARY

V45.82 Angioplasty status (PTCA)
746.85 Artery absence congenital
746.85 Artery anomalous origin or communication
414.11 Artery aneurysm
414.0# Artery disease (arteriosclerosis) (deformans) (arteritis)
414.0# Artery disease (arteriosclerosis) (deformans) (arteritis) with chronic complete or total occlusion [414.2]

5th digit: 414.0
0. Unspecified type of vessel, native or graft
1. Native coronary vessel
2. Autologous vein bypass graft
3. Nonautologous biological bypass graft
4. Autologous artery bypass graft (gastroepiploic) (internal mammary)
5. Unspecified type of bypass graft
6. Native vessel of transplanted heart
7. Bypass graft of transplanted heart

414.12 Artery dissection
411.81 Artery embolism (thrombosis) acute
0 Artery embolism (thrombosis) with infarction see 'MI (myocardial infarction) Acute'
414.0# Atherosclerosis
414.0# Atherosclerosis with chronic complete or total occlusion [414.2]

5th digit: 414.0
0. Unspecified type of vessel, native or graft
1. Native coronary vessel
2. Autologous vein bypass graft
3. Nonautologous biological bypass graft
4. Autologous artery bypass graft (gastroepiploic) (internal mammary)
5. Unspecified type of bypass graft
6. Native vessel of transplanted heart
7. Bypass graft of transplanted heart

CORONARY (continued)

414.0# Bypass graft arteriosclerosis
414.0# Bypass graft arteriosclerosis with chronic complete or total occlusion [414.2]

5th digit: 414.0
2. Autologous vein bypass graft
3. Nonautologous biological bypass graft
4. Autologous artery bypass graft (gastroepiploic) (internal mammary)
5. Unspecified type of bypass graft
7. Bypass graft of transplanted heart

996.61 Bypass graft complication - infection or inflammation
996.03 Bypass graft complication - mechanical (leakage) (obstruction) (perforation)
996.72 Bypass graft complication - other
V45.81 Bypass status
414.9 Disease ischemic
746.85 Disease ischemic congenital
093.20 Disease ostial syphilitic
411.89 Failure
411.89 Insufficiency acute
414.8 Insufficiency chronic
411.1 Insufficiency or intermediate syndrome
411.81 Obstruction (occlusion) acute without infarction
0 Obstruction (occlusion) acute with infarction see 'MI (Myocardial Infarction) Acute'
0 Obstruction (occlusion) chronic without infarction due to atherosclerosis see 'Coronary', artery disease
996.61 Stent complication - infection inflammation
996.09 Stent complication - mechanical
996.72 Stent complication - other
411.89 Syndrome acute
0 Syndrome acute with MI - see 'MI (Myocardial Infarction) Acute'
746.89 Vein anomaly

620.2 CORPUS ALBICANS CYST

742.2 CORPUS CALLOSUM ABSENCE CONGENITAL

341.8 CORPUS CALLOSUM CENTRAL DYMYELINATION

CORPUS CAVERNOSUM

607.89 Atrophy (fibrosis) (ulcer) (hypertrophy)
607.89 Calcification
607.2 Cellulitis (abscess) (boil) (carbuncle)
607.89 Fibrosis
607.82 Hematoma (hemorrhage) nontraumatic
959.13 Injury
607.82 Thrombosis

620.1 CORPUS LUTEUM CYST OR HEMATOMA

620.1 CORPUS LUTEUM CYST RUPTURE

0 CORRIGAN'S DISEASE SEE 'AORTA, AORTIC (VALVE) INSUFFICIENCY'

V53.7 CORSET FITTING AND ADJUSTMENT ORTHOPEDIC

0 CORTICAL ATROPHY SEE 'BRAIN', ATROPHY

377.75 CORTICAL BLINDNESS

255.41 CORTICOADRENAL INSUFFICIENCY (DEFICIENCY) (HYPOFUNCTION)

255.2 CORTICOSEXUAL SYNDROME

255.2 CORTICOSTEROID METABOLISM DISORDER NEC

334.8 CORTICOSTRIATAL SPINAL DEGENERATION

255.8 CORTISOL BINDING GLOBULIN ABNORMALITY

255.0 CORTISOL OVERPRODUCTION

0 CORYNEBACTERIUM DIPHTHERIAE INFECTION SEE 'DIPHTHERIA'
460 CORYZA ACUTE
V50.9 COSMETIC SURGERY UNSPECIFIED (ELECTIVE)
V50.8 COSMETIC SURGERY OTHER (ELECTIVE)
959.11 COSTAL REGION INJURY NEC
524.60 COSTEN'S SYNDROME (COMPLEX)
0 COSTIVENESS SEE 'CONSTIPATION'

COSTOCHONDRAL

959.11 Injury
733.6 Junction syndrome
786.52 Pain
739.8 Segmental or somatic dysfunction

733.6 COSTOCHONDRITIS
353.0 COSTOCLAVICULAR SYNDROME (NONDISCOGENIC)
739.8 COSTOVERTEBRAL REGION SEGMENTAL OR SOMATIC DYSFUNCTION
798.0 COT DEATH
297.1 COTARD'S SYNDROME (DELUSIONAL DISORDER)
362.83 COTTON WOOL SPOTS RETINAL
724.3 COTUGNO'S SCIATICA

COUGH

786.2 NOS
306.1 Psychogenic
491.0 Smokers'
493.82 Variant asthma
786.3 With hemorrhage

Coumadin, Digoxin, chemotherapy drugs, and any other drug with a risk of adverse reaction is considered to be high-risk medication. Code V67.51 is used to identify patients that have completed high risk medication therapy.

V58.83 COUMADIN DRUG MONITORING ENCOUNTER
V58.83 COUMADIN DRUG MONITORING ENCOUNTER WITH LONG TERM USE [V58.61]
V67.51 COUMADIN FOLLOW UP EXAM - COMPLETED THERAPY
V58.61 COUMADIN FOLLOW UP EXAM - CURRENT THERAPY

COUNSELING

V62.83 Abuse - counseling of perpetrator non-parental/non-spousal of physical/sexual abuse
V62.89 Abuse - counseling of victim of other specified abuse NEC
V62.83 Abuse child - counseling of perpetrator non-parental of physical/sexual abuse
V61.22 Abuse child - counseling of perpetrator parental
V61.21 Abuse child - counseling of victim
V61.12 Abuse spousal (partner) - counseling of perpetrator
V61.11 Abuse spousal (partner) - counseling of victim
V61.29 Adopted child problem
V65.42 Alcohol abuse
V65.8 Breast implant removal (elective)

CONTRACEPTION

V25.03 Emergency postcoital (with prescription)
V25.09 Family planning
V25.04 Family planning natural to avoid pregnancy
V25.03 Postcoital emergency (with prescription)

COUNSELING (continued)

CONTRACEPTION (continued)

V25.03 Prescription or use - emergency postcoital
V25.01 Prescription or use - oral contraceptive
V25.02 Prescription or use - foams, creams or other agents
V25.09 Tuboplasty (proposed)
V25.09 Vasectomy (proposed)
V25.09 Other specified NEC

COUNSELING (continued)

V65.3 Use an additional code to identify body mass index (BMI), if known. See 'Body Mass Index'.

V65.3 Diet
V65.42 Drug abuse
V65.49 Education
V65.41 Exercise
V65.49 Explanation of investigative findings
V25.09 Family planning
V26.41 Family planning natural procreative
V25.04 Family planning natural to avoid pregnancy
V65.8 For other reasons
V61.29 Foster child problem
V26.33 Genetic
V65.45 Gonorrhea
V65.49 Health
V65.44 HIV
V65.43 Injury prevention
V60.6 Institutional resident
V65.49 Instruction
V65.46 Insulin pump training
V65.49 Lab or results of studies
V65.2 Malingerer
V61.10 Marital problems NOS
V61.10 Marital relationship problem
V65.9 Medical NOS
V65.8 Medical other
V65.49 Medication
V61.20 Parent - child problem, unspecified
V61.20 Parent - child relationship problem
V61.10 Partner relationship problem
V65.5 Patient with feared complaint in whom no diagnosis made
V65.8 Patient/person for other reasons
V65.11 Pediatric pre-birth visit for expectant mother
V65.0 Person accompanying sick person
V65.19 Person consulting on behalf of another person
V65.19 Person other than patient
V26.41 Procreative using natural family planning
V26.49 Procreative other
V65.49 Sex NEC
V65.45 Sexually transmitted disease
V61.8 Sibling relationship problem
V65.49 Smoking cessation
V65.42 Substance abuse
V65.45 Syphilis
V65.49 Treatment plan
V65.49 Without complaint or sickness
V65.40 Other NEC
V65.49 Other specified

427.89 COUPLED RHYTHM
759.6 COWDEN SYNDROME
597.89 COWPERITIS
131.02 COWPERITIS TRICHOMONAL

051.0 COWPOX
999.0 COWPOX FROM VACCINATION

COXA

732.1 Plana hip and pelvis juvenile
736.31 Valga
755.61 Valga congenital
736.32 Vara
755.62 Vara congenital

COXSACKIE

074.20 Carditis
074.22 Endocarditis
047.0 Meningitis
074.23 Myocarditis
074.21 Pericarditis
079.2 Virus infection (infecting agent)
074.8 Virus other specified diseases

CPD

653.4# NOS
660.1# NOS obstructing labor [**653.4#**]
655.0# Due to anencephaly, hydrocephaly, spina bifida (suspected/known affecting management of mother)
5th digit: 653.4, 655.0, 660.1
0. Episode of care NOS or N/A
1. Delivered
3. Antepartum complication

790.5 CPK ELEVATED
277.85 CPT1, CPT2 DEFICIENCY (CARNITINE PALMITOYLTRANSFERASE)

> *'Crack baby': Code on baby's record only. Do not code mother's abuse/dependence with these codes.*

760.75 CRACK AFFECTING FETUS OR NEWBORN VIA PLACENTA OR BREAST MILK (CRACK BABY) - ASYMPTOMATIC
779.5 CRACK AFFECTING FETUS OR NEWBORN VIA PLACENTA OR BREAST MILK (CRACK BABY) - WITH WITHDRAWAL SYMPTOMS
521.81 CRACKED TOOTH
873.63 CRACKED TOOTH DUE TO TRAUMA
873.73 CRACKED TOOTH DUE TO TRAUMA COMPLICATED
690.11 CRADLE CAP (SEBORRHEA CAPITIS)

CRAMP

729.82 NOS
789.0# Abdominal
5th digit: 789.0
0. Unspecified site
1. Upper right quadrant
2. Upper left quadrant
3. Lower right quadrant
4. Lower left quadrant
5. Periumbilic
6. Epigastric
7. Generalized
9. Other specified site (multiple)

994.1 Bathing
729.82 Extremity (lower) (upper) NEC
992.2 Heat
300.11 Hysterical
0 Intestinal see 'Cramp', abdominal
327.52 Leg – sleep related
625.3 Menstrual

CRAMP (continued)

729.82 Muscle
994.1 Muscle due to immersion
307.89 Psychogenic
276.1 Salt depletion
327.52 Sleep related leg
789.06 Stomach
300.89 Telegraphers' (typist)
333.84 Telegraphers' (typist) organic
625.8 Uterine
625.3 Uterine menstrual
333.84 Writers'
300.89 Writers' psychogenic

CRANIAL

352.9 Nerve atrophy
352.9 Nerve disorder
951.9 Nerve injury
767.7 Nerve injury due to birth trauma
907.1 Nerve injury late effect
352.6 Nerve palsies multiple
756.0 Suture delayed closure
756.0 Suture premature closure
755.55 Suture premature fusion (Apert's syndrome)

763.89 CRANIOCLASIS, FETAL
376.44 CRANIOFACIAL DEFORMITIES WITH ASSOCIATED ORBIT DEFORMITY
756.0 CRANIOFACIAL DYSOSTOSIS
759.4 CRANIOPAGUS
237.0 CRANIOPHARYNGIOMA SITE NOS
0 CRANIOPHARYNGIOMA SITE SPECIFIED SEE 'NEOPLASM UNCERTAIN BEHAVIOR', BY SITE M9350/1
740.1 CRANIORACHISCHISIS CONGENITAL
756.0 CRANIOSYNOSTOSIS
763.89 CRANIOTOMY, FETAL
723.2 CRANIOVERTEBRAL SYNDROME
738.19 CRANIUM DEFORMITY
0 CRANIUM DEFORMITY CONGENITAL SEE SPECIFIC DEFORMITY

> ***999.31 Other infection - Use an additional code to identify the specified infection such as septicemia, (038.#(#)).***

999.31 CRBSI (CATHETER-RELATED BLOODSTREAM INFECTION)
790.6 CREATINE AND BUN ELEVATED
790.5 CREATINE PHOSPHOKINASE (CPK) ABNORMAL
126.9 CREEPING ERUPTION NOS

CREPITUS

719.6# Joint
5th digit: 719.6
0. Site NOS
1. Shoulder region
2. Upper arm (elbow) (humerus)
3. Forearm (radius) (wrist) (ulna)
4. Hand (carpal) (metacarpal) (fingers)
5. Pelvic region and thigh (hip) (buttock) (femur)
6. Lower leg (fibula) (knee) (patella) (tibia)
7. Ankle and/or foot (metatarsals) (toes) (tarsals)
8. Other
9. Multiple

C

CREPITUS (continued)

518.1 Subcutaneous - nontraumatic
998.81 Subcutaneous - surgical
958.7 Subcutaneous - traumatic

243 CRETINISM (ATHYROTIC) (ENDEMIC)
246.1 CRETINISM GOITROUS (SPORADIC)
046.1 CREUTZFELDT-JAKOB CEREBRAL DEGENERATION
046.1 CREUTZFELDT-JAKOB CEREBRAL DEGENERATION WITH DEMENTIA [294.1#]
5th digit: 294.1
0. Without behavioral disturbance or NOS
1. With behavioral disturbance

046.1 CREUTZFELDT-JAKOB DISEASE (SYNDROME) (NEW VARIANT)
758.31 CRI DU CHAT SYNDROME
798.0 CRIB DEATH SYNDROME
199.1 CRIBRIFORM CARCINOMA SITE NOS
0 CRIBRIFORM CARCINOMA SITE SPECIFIED SEE 'CANCER', BY SITE M8201/3

CRICOID

748.3 Cartilage anomaly (absence) congenital
748.3 Cartilage posterior cleft congenital
748.3 Cleft (posterior) congenital

787.20 CRICOPHARYNGEAL SYNDROME
277.4 CRIGLER NAJJAR SYNDROME (CONGENITAL HYPERBILIRUBINEMIA)
0 CRISIS ASTHMATIC SEE 'ASTHMA'
0 CRISIS HYPERTENSIVE SEE 'HYPERTENSION, HYPERTENSIVE'
351.8 CROCODILE TEARS SYNDROME
443.89 CROCQ'S ACROCYANOSIS

CROHN'S DISEASE

555.9 NOS
555.1 Large intestine
555.0 Small intestine
555.2 Small intestine and large intestine

211.3 CRONKHITE-CANADA SYNDROME
524.27 CROSSBITE (ANTERIOR) (POSTERIOR)
464.4 CROUP (SYNDROME)
464.4 CROUPOUS ANGINA
756.0 CROUZON'S CRANIOFACIAL DYSOSTOSIS
790.95 CRP ELEVATED (C-REACTIVE PROTEIN)
710.1 CRST SYNDROME (CUTANEOUS SYSTEMIC SCLEROSIS)
710.1 CRST SYNDROME (CUTANEOUS SYSTEMIC SCLEROSIS) WITH LUNG INVOLVEMENT [517.2]
710.1 CRST SYNDROME (CUTANEOUS SYSTEMIC SCLEROSIS) WITH MYOPATHY [359.6]
049.8 CRUCHET'S ENCEPHALITIS LETHARGICA

CRUCIATE LIGAMENT (KNEE)

717.83 Anterior - disruption (old)
717.9 Anterior - relaxation
844.2 Anterior - sprain (rupture) (strain) (tear) acute
717.84 Posterior - disruption (old)
717.9 Posterior - relaxation
844.2 Posterior - sprain (rupture) (strain) (tear) acute

443.9 CRURAL ANGINA

When coding crush injuries it is necessary to report any additional injuries such as fractures, lacerations, open wounds and concussions.

CRUSH INJURY

929.9 Site unspecified
928.21 Ankle
927.9 Arm
927.03 Arm upper
927.8 Arm multiple sites
927.02 Axillary region
926.11 Back
926.19 Breast
926.12 Buttock
925.1 Cheek
862.8 Chest
925.1 Ear
927.11 Elbow
926.0 External genitalia
925.1 Face
927.3 Finger
928.20 Foot
927.10 Forearm
927.20 Hand
928.20 Heel
928.01 Hip
0 Internal organs see specific organ, injury
928.11 Knee
926.0 Labia
925.2 Larynx
906.4 Late effect
928.9 Leg
928.10 Leg lower
928.8 Leg multiple sites
929.0 Multiple sites NEC
925.2 Neck
926.0 Penis
925.2 Pharynx
925.1 Scalp
927.01 Scapular region
926.0 Scrotum
927.00 Shoulder
927.09 Shoulder and arm multiple sites
958.5 Syndrome
908.6 Syndrome late effect
926.0 Testis
928.00 Thigh
925.2 Throat
928.3 Toe (s)
925.2 Tonsil
926.9 Trunk
926.8 Trunk multiple sites
926.19 Trunk other sites
926.0 Vulva
927.21 Wrist

861.20 CRUSHED LUNG SYNDROME
690.11 CRUSTA LACTEA
571.5 CRUVEILHIER-BAUMGARTEN SYNDROME (CIRRHOSIS OF LIVER)
335.21 CRUVEILHIER'S DISEASE
086.2 CRUZ-CHAGAS DISEASE (SEE ALSO 'CHAGAS' DISEASE')

780.95 CRYING CONTINUOUS EXCESSIVE CHILD, ADOLESCENT OR ADULT
780.92 CRYING CONTINUOUS EXCESSIVE NEWBORN, INFANT OR BABY
273.2 CRYOGLOBULINEMIA MIXED
569.49 CRYPTITIS (ANAL) (RECTAL)

CRYPTOCOCCOSIS

117.5 NOS
117.5 European
117.5 Neoformans infection
117.5 Pulmonary
117.5 Systemic

743.06 CRYPTOPHTHALMOS CONGENITAL
752.51 CRYPTORCHISM CONGENITAL
007.4 CRYPTOSPORIDIA INFECTION
495.6 CRYPTOSTROMA CORTICALE ALVEOLITIS

CRYSTALLOPATHY

275.49 NOS [712.9#]
275.49 Chondrocalcinosis - calcium pyrophosphate crystals [712.2#]
275.49 Chondrocalcinosis - dicalcium phosphate [712.1#]
275.49 Chondrocalcinosis - unspecified [712.3#]
274.0 Gouty
274.0 Uric acid
275.49 Other specified [712.8#]

5th digit: 712.1-3, 8-9
0. Site NOS
1. Shoulder region
2. Upper arm (elbow) (humerus)
3. Forearm (radius) (wrist) (ulna)
4. Hand (carpal) (metacarpal) (fingers)
5. Pelvic region and thigh (hip) (buttock) (femur)
6. Lower leg (fibula) (knee) (patella) (tibia)
7. Ankle and/or foot (metatarsals) (toes) (tarsals)
8. Other (head) (neck) (rib) (skull) (trunk) (vertebrae)
9. Multiple

791.9 CRYSTALLURIA
791.9 CRYSTALLURIA ELEVATED URINE LEVELS
791.9 CRYSTALS URINE ABNORMAL
388.61 CSF OTORRHEA
349.81 CSF RHINORRHEA
701.0 CSILLAG'S LICHEN SCLEROSUS ET ATROPHICUS
794.09 CT BRAIN ABNORMAL
354.0 CTS (CARPAL TUNNEL SYNDROME)
354.2 CUBITAL TUNNEL SYNDROME
736.01 CUBITUS VALGUS
755.59 CUBITUS VALGUS CONGENITAL
736.02 CUBITUS VARUS
755.59 CUBITUS VARUS CONGENITAL
162.3 CUIFFINI-PANCOAST SYNDROME (CARCINOMA, PULMONARY APEX) M8010/3

CULTURE ABNORMAL FINDINGS

790.7 Blood
795.39 Microbiologic NEC
795.39 Nasal
795.39 Skin lesion NEC

CULTURE ABNORMAL FINDINGS (continued)

792.0 Spinal fluid
795.39 Sputum
792.1 Stool
795.39 Throat
791.9 Urine
795.39 Wound
795.39 NEC

V62.4 CULTURE DEPRIVATION
309.29 CULTURE SHOCK
117.7 CUNNINGHAMELLA INFECTION
530.5 CURLING ESOPHAGUS
359.21 CURSCHMANN'S (-BATTEN) (-STEINERT) DISEASE OR SYNDROME

CUSHING'S SYNDROME

255.0 NOS
255.2 Due to adrenal hyperplasia
255.0 Iatrogenic
255.0 Idiopathic
962.0 Overdose or wrong substance given or taken
255.0 Pituitary dependent
255.0 With myopathy [359.5]

0 CUT SEE 'LACERATION', BY SITE
702.8 CUTANEOUS HORN
126.9 CUTANEOUS LARVA MIGRANS
782.2 CUTANEOUS NODULE
956.4 CUTANEOUS SENSORY NERVE INJURY LOWER LIMB
955.5 CUTANEOUS SENSORY NERVE INJURY UPPER LIMB
V44.51 CUTANEOUS-VESICOSTOMY STATUS
277.39 CUTIS AMYLOID DEGENERATION
701.8 CUTIS LAXA SENILIS

Remember, CVA, stroke and cerebral infarction with occlusion NOS are all indexed to code 434.91. Do not use code 436.

CVA (CEREBROVASCULAR ACCIDENT)

434.91 NOS
434.91 Acute
434.11 Embolic
V17.1 Family history
0 Hemorrhagic see 'Hemorrhage', brain
V12.54 History without residual
997.02 Iatrogenic
435.9 Impending (transient ischemic attack)
434.91 Ischemic
434.91 Lacunar infarct

LATE EFFECT

438.9 Unspecified
438.81 Apraxia
438.84 Ataxia
438.0 Cognitive defect
438.82 Dysphagia [787.2#]

5th digit: 787.2
0. Unspecified
1. Oral phase
2. Oropharyngeal phase
3. Pharyngeal phase
4. Pharyngoesophageal phase
9. Other

C

CVA (CEREBROVASCULAR ACCIDENT) (continued)

LATE EFFECT (continued)

438.83 Facial droop
438.83 Facial weakness
438.2# Paralytic - hemiplegia or hemiparesis
438.4# Paralytic - monoplegia lower limb
438.3# Paralytic - monoplegia upper limb
5th digit: 438.2-4
0. Unspecified side
1. Dominant side
2. Nondominant side

438.5# Paralytic - other syndrome
5th digit: 438.5
0. Unspecified side
1. Dominant side
2. Nondominant side
3. Bilateral

Use additional code to identify the altered sensation.

438.6 Sensation alteration
438.1# Speech and language deficit
5th digit: 438.1
0. Unspecified
1. Aphasia
2. Dysphasia
9. Other

438.85 Vertigo

Use additional code to identify the visual disturbance.

438.7 Vision disturbance
438.89 Other specified

CVA (CEREBROVASCULAR ACCIDENT) (continued)

0 Old with residual see 'CVA', late effect
V12.54 Old without residual
997.02 Postoperative
434.01 Thrombotic
435.9 Transient ischemic attack (TIA)

279.06 CVID (COMMON VARIABLE IMMUNODEFICIENCY)
266.2 CYANOCOBALAMIN DEFICIENCY (NUTRITIONAL)
770.83 CYANOPATHY NEWBORN

CYANOSIS, CYANOTIC

782.5 NOS
770.83 Attacks perinatal period
770.83 Congenital
372.71 Conjunctiva
289.7 Enterogenous
770.83 Newborn
362.10 Retinal

CYCLITIS

364.00 Acute subacute
098.41 Gonococcal
054.44 Herpes simplex
053.22 Herpes zoster
363.21 Posterior
364.01 Primary
364.02 Recurrent

CYCLITIS (continued)

364.03 Secondary infectious
364.04 Secondary noninfectious
0 See also 'Iridocyclitis'

378.44 CYCLOPHORIA
367.51 CYCLOPLEGIA
007.5 CYCLOSPORIASIS
301.13 CYCLOTHYMIC DISORDER
378.33 CYCLOTROPIA
733.99 CYRIAX'S (SLIPPING RIB) SYNDROME

When you assign a code for cyst; refer first to the type, and then to the site. Most cysts are not neoplastic and are classified to disease of the specified anatomical site. This does not apply to cysts which are neoplastic in nature.

CYST

474.8 Adenoid (infected)
255.8 Adrenal gland
518.89 Air lung
526.2 Alveolar process
762.8 Amnion affecting fetus or newborn
658.8# Amniotic complicating childbirth
5th digit: 658.8
0. Episode of care NOS or N/A
1. Delivered
3. Antepartum complication

364.62 Anterior chamber - exudative
364.60 Anterior chamber - idiopathic
364.61 Anterior chamber - implantation
478.19 Antrum
569.49 Anus
522.8 Apical (periodontal)
543.9 Appendix
348.0 Arachnoid
478.79 Arytenoid
706.2 Auricle
727.51 Baker's knee
<u>015.2#</u> Baker's knee <u>tuberculous</u> [727.51]
5th digit: 015.2
0. NOS
1. Lab not done
2. Lab pending
3. Microscopy positive (in sputum)
4. Culture positive - microscopy
5. Culture negative - microscopy positive
6. Culture and microscopy negative confirmed by other methods

616.2 Bartholin's gland (duct)
576.8 Bile duct
596.8 Bladder
362.62 Blessig's
733.2# Bone
5th digit: 733.2
0. Unspecified (localized)
1. Solitary or unicameral
2. Aneurysmal
9. Other

0 Bone jaw see 'Cyst', jaw, by type
348.0 Brain (see also 'Cyst Congenital' and 'Cyst of the Nervous System')
0 Brain hydatid see 'Echinococcus'

	CYST (continued)
610.0	Breast - benign
610.0	Breast - blue dome
610.4	Breast - involution
611.5	Breast - milk
610.0	Breast - nipple
610.0	Breast - pedunculated
610.8	Breast - sebaceous
610.0	Breast - solitary
610.0	Breast - traumatic
620.8	Broad ligament (nonpregnant)
518.89	Bronchogenic (mediastinal) (sequestration)
528.4	Buccal
599.89	Bulbourethral
727.49	Bursa
629.1	Canal of nuck acquired
372.75	Canthus
0	Cartilage (joint) see 'Joint Derangement'
336.8	Cauda equina
348.0	Cavum septi pellucidi NEC
348.0	Cerebral
348.0	Cerebral meninges
622.8	Cervix
617.1	Chocolate (ovary)
576.8	Choledochal
658.8#	Chorion complicating pregnancy **5th digit: 658.8** **0. Episode of care NOS or N/A** **1. Delivered** **3. Antepartum complication**
348.0	Choroid plexus
457.8	Chyle mesentery
364.62	Ciliary body - exudative
364.60	Ciliary body - idiopathic
364.61	Ciliary body - implantation
364.60	Ciliary body - iris
624.8	Clitoris
733.20	Coccyx (see 'Cyst', bone)
0	Colloid thyroid gland see 'Goiter'
0	Colloid third ventricle brain see 'cyst congenital', cerebral
569.89	Colon
576.8	Common bile duct
0	Congenital see 'Cyst Congenital'
372.75	Conjunctival
371.23	Cornea
348.0	Corpora quadrigemina
620.2	Corpus albicans (ovary)
620.1	Corpus luteum ovary (ruptured)
599.89	Cowper's gland
253.8	Craniobuccal pouch
253.8	Craniopharyngeal pouch
575.8	Cystic duct
123.1	Cysticercus (any site)
526.0	Dental primordial (keratocyst)
522.8	Dental root
526.0	Dentigerous
526.0	Dentigerous mandible
526.0	Dentigerous maxilla
522.8	Dentoalveolar
709.8	Dermoid implantation skin NEC
623.8	Dermoid implantation vagina
624.8	Dermoid implantation vulva

	CYST (continued)
528.4	Dermoid mouth
528.4	Dermoid oral soft tissue
685.1	Dermoid sacrococcygeal
685.0	Dermoid sacrococcygeal with abscess
0	Dermoid see 'Benign Neoplasm', by site
0	Dermoid with malignant transformation see 'Cancer', by site
348.0	Dura cerebral
349.2	Dura spinal
706.2	Ear (external)
122.9	Echinococcal (see 'Echinococcus Infection')
621.8	Endometrial
617.9	Endometrial ectopic
706.2	Epidermal (inclusion) (see also 'Cyst' skin)
706.2	Epidermoid (inclusion) (see also 'Cyst' skin)
528.4	Epidermoid (inclusion) mouth
528.4	Epidermoid mouth
0	Epidermoid other than skin see 'Cyst', by site
608.89	Epididymis
478.79	Epiglottis
259.8	Epiphysis cerebri
706.2	Epithelial inclusion (skin)
530.89	Esophagus
478.19	Ethmoid sinus
364.62	Eye - anterior chamber exudative
364.60	Eye - anterior chamber idiopathic
364.61	Eye - anterior chamber implantation
372.75	Eye - canthus
371.23	Eye - cornea
364.62	Eye - iris exudative
364.60	Eye - iris idiopathic
364.61	Eye - iris implantation
364.55	Eye - iris miotic pupillary margin
360.13	Eye - iris parasitic
379.39	Eye - lens
373.2	Eye - meibomian gland
377.54	Eye - optic chiasm (see also 'Optic Chiasm')
361.19	Eye - ora serrata
379.8	Eye - retention
361.19	Eye - retinal pseudocyst
361.19	Eye - retinal other
379.19	Eye - sclera
379.29	Eye - vitreous humor
706.2	Eyebrow
374.84	Eyelid
373.13	Eyelid infected
374.84	Eyelid sweat gland or duct
573.8	Falciform ligament liver (inflammatory)
620.8	Fallopian tube
526.1	Fissural of jaw
526.0	Follicular dentigerous
620.0	Follicular ovarian
478.19	Frontal sinus
575.8	Gallbladder
0	Ganglion see 'Ganglion'
568.89	Gas mesentery
629.89	Genital organ female NEC
523.8	Gingiva
374.84	Gland of moll
526.1	Globulomaxillary
620.0	Graafian follicle ovary
620.2	Granulosal lutein
0	Hemangiomatous see 'Hemangioma'
0	Hydatid fallopian tube see 'Cyst Congenital', hydatid
0	Hydatid see 'Echinococcus'
623.8	Hymen

C

CYST (continued)

478.26	Hypopharynx
253.8	Hypophysis, hypophyseal (duct)
253.8	Hypophysis cerebri
526.1	Incisor
526.1	Incisor canal
0	Inclusion - see 'Benign Neoplasm', by site
706.2	Inclusion - skin
728.89	Intraligamentous knee
348.0	Intramedullary
364.62	Iris - exudative
364.60	Iris - idiopathic
364.61	Iris - implantation
364.55	Iris - miotic pupillary margin
360.13	Iris - parasitic
362.62	Iwanoff's
526.#	Jaw (bone)

4th digit: 526
0. Odontogenic
1. Fissural
2. Aneurysmal, hemorrhagic, NOS, other, and traumatic

526.89	Jaw (bone) latent
706.2	Keratin
593.2	Kidney acquired
727.51	Knee (baker's)
717.5	Knee meniscus
624.8	Labium (majus) (minus)
624.8	Labium sebaceous
375.43	Lacrimal apparatus
375.12	Lacrimal gland and cystic degeneration
478.79	Larynx
379.39	Lens (eye)
717.89	Ligamentous knee
528.5	Lip (gland)
573.8	Liver
122.8	Liver echinococcal
122.0	Liver echinococcal - granulosis
122.5	Liver echinococcal - multilocularis
518.89	Lung
492.0	Lung giant bullous
620.1	Lutein
228.1	Lymphangiomatous
528.4	Lymphoepithelial mouth
362.54	Macular (degeneration) (hole or pseudohole)
0	Malignant see 'Cancer', by site
610.0	Mammary gland
611.5	Mammary gland (milk)
526.2	Mandible
526.2	Maxilla
478.19	Maxillary sinus
526.1	Median anterior maxillary
526.1	Median palatal
373.2	Meibomian (gland)
717.5	Meniscus knee
457.8	Mesentery chyle
568.89	Mesentery (mesenteric gas)
568.89	Mesothelial peritoneum
568.89	Mesothelial pleura (peritoneal)
528.4	Mouth
528.4	Mouth - Epstein's pearl
523.8	Mouth - gingival
529.8	Mouth - tongue
383.31	Mucosal mastoidectomy complication
383.31	Mucosal postmastoidectomy cavity
239.5	Multilocular ovary

CYST (continued)

621.8	Myometrium
616.0	Nabothian (gland) (nonobstetrical)
478.19	Nasal antrum
478.19	Nasal cavity
478.19	Nasal septum
478.19	Nasal sinus
733.20	Nasal turbinate
528.4	Nasoalveolar mouth
528.4	Nasolabial
526.1	Nasopalatine
478.26	Nasopharynx
0	Nervous system see 'Cyst of the Nervous System'
706.2	Nose (skin of)
213.1	Odontogenic calcifying
213.0	Odontogenic calcifying upper jaw (bone)
526.0	Odontogenic developmental
568.89	Omentum (lesser)
377.54	Optic chiasm (see also 'Optic Chiasm')
528.4	Oral soft tissue (implantation)
361.19	Ora serrata
376.81	Orbital
0	Oropharyngeal see 'Cyst Oropharyngeal'
763.89	Ovarian affecting fetus or newborn
654.4#	Ovarian complicating pregnancy or childbirth
660.2#	Ovarian complicating pregnancy and causing obstructed labor **[654.4#]**

5th digit: 654.4
0. Episode of care NOS or N/A
1. Delivered
2. Delivered with postpartum complication
3. Antepartum complication
4. Postpartum complication

5th digit: 660.2
0. Episode of care NOS or N/A
1. Delivered
3. Antepartum complication

763.1	Ovarian with obstructed labor affecting fetus or newborn
620.2	Ovary
617.1	Ovary - chocolate
752.0	Ovary - congenital
620.2	Ovary - corpus albicans
620.1	Ovary - corpus luteum (hemorrhage) (ruptured)
220	Ovary - cystadenoma
620.2	Ovary - cystoma simple
220	Ovary - dermoid
620.2	Ovary - due to involution failure
617.1	Ovary - endometrial cystoma
620.0	Ovary - graafian follicle
620.0	Ovary - follicular
620.2	Ovary - hemorrhagic
620.1	Ovary - lutein
239.5	Ovary - multilocular
220	Ovary - neoplastic
620.8	Ovary - oviduct
220	Ovary - pseudomucinous
256.4	Ovary - polycystic (Stein-leventhal syndrome)
620.2	Ovary - retention
617.1	Ovary - sampson's
620.2	Ovary - serous
256.4	Ovary - stein leventhal
620.2	Ovary - theca-lutein
620.2	Ovary - twisted
620.2	Ovary - other
620.8	Oviduct

CYST (continued)

526.1 Palatine of jaw
526.1 Palatine of papilla
577.2 Pancreas
593.2 Paranephric
136.9 Parasitic NEC
252.8 Parathyroid gland
620.8 Paratubal (fallopian)
599.89 Paraurethral duct
527.6 Parotid gland
364.64 Pars plana exudative
364.63 Pars plana primary
763.89 Pelvic affecting fetus or newborn
654.4# Pelvic complicating pregnancy or childbirth
660.2# Pelvic complicating pregnancy and causing obstructed labor **[654.4#]**

5th digit: 654.4
- **0. Episode of care NOS or N/A**
- **1. Delivered**
- **2. Delivered with postpartum complication**
- **3. Antepartum complication**
- **4. Postpartum complication**

5th digit: 660.2
- **0. Episode of care NOS or N/A**
- **1. Delivered**
- **3. Antepartum complication**

763.1 Pelvic with obstructed labor affecting fetus or newborn
607.89 Penis (sebaceous)
522.8 Periapical
746.89 Pericardial (congenital)
423.8 Pericardial acquired (secondary)
624.8 Perineum - female
355.9 Perineural (Tarlov's)
522.8 Periodontal
577.2 Peripancreatic
593.2 Peripelvic (lymphatic)
593.2 Perirenal
568.89 Peritoneal
457.8 Peritoneal chylous
478.26 Pharyngeal bursa
478.26 Pharynx
478.26 Pharynx wall
685.1 Pilonidal
173.5 Pilonidal malignant
685.0 Pilonidal with abscess
253.8 Pituitary (duct) (gland)
519.8 Pleura
727.51 Popliteal
727.51 Popliteal synovial
348.0 Porencephalic
685.1 Postanal infected
685.0 Postanal with abscess
383.31 Postmastoidectomy cavity (mucosal cyst)
607.89 Prepuce
526.0 Primordial (jaw)

CYST (continued)

600.3 Prostate
600.3 Prostate with urinary incontinence **[788.3#]**

5th digit: 788.3
- **0. Unspecified**
- **1. Urge incontinence**
- **2. Stress, male**
- **3. Mixed urge and stress**
- **4. Without sensory awareness**
- **5. Post-void dribbling**
- **6. Nocturnal enuresis**
- **7. Continuous leakage**
- **8. Overflow incontinence**
- **9. Other**

600.3 Prostate with urinary retention **[788.2#]**

5th digit: 788.2
- **0. Unspecified**
- **1. Incomplete bladder emptying**
- **9. Other specified retention**

624.8 Pudenda (sweat glands)
364.55 Pupillary miotic
624.8 Pupillary sebaceous
522.8 Radicular
522.8 Radiculodental
527.6 Ranula (mouth floor)
253.8 Rathke's pouch
569.49 Rectum (epithelium) (mucous)
593.2 Renal acquired
591 Renal calyceal or pyelogenic
522.8 Residual (radicular)
620.2 Retention ovary
706.2 Retention skin
360.13 Retinal
362.54 Retinal macular
360.13 Retinal parasitic
361.13 Retinal primary
361.19 Retinal pseudocyst
361.14 Retinal secondary
361.19 Retinal other
568.89 Retroperitoneal
685.1 Sacrococcygeal (dermoid)
685.0 Sacrococcygeal (dermoid) with abscess
527.6 Salivary gland or duct
617.1 Sampson's
379.19 Sclera
706.2 Sebaceous
610.8 Sebaceous - breast
374.84 Sebaceous - eyelid
629.89 Sebaceous - genital organ female
608.89 Sebaceous - genital organ male
706.2 Sebaceous - gland (duct)
706.2 Sebaceous - scrotum
717.5 Semilunar cartilage (knee) old
608.89 Seminal vesicle
620.2 Serous (ovary)
478.19 Sinus (antral) (ethmoidal) (frontal) (maxillary) (nasal)
599.89 Skene's gland
706.2 Skin
610.8 Skin - breast
706.2 Skin - ear (external)
374.84 Skin - eyelid
216.3 Skin - face neoplastic
629.89 Skin - genital organ female
608.89 Skin - genital organ male

C

C

CYST (continued)

216.3	Skin - nose neoplastic
706.2	Skin - scrotum
705.89	Skin - sweat gland or duct
608.89	Spermatic cord
478.19	Sphenoid sinus
349.2	Spinal meninges
733.20	Spine (bone)
289.59	Spleen
348.0	Subarachnoid
348.0	Subdural cerebral
349.2	Subdural spinal cord
527.6	Sublingual gland
527.6	Submaxillary gland
599.89	Suburethral
255.8	Suprarenal gland
348.0	Suprasellar
705.89	Sweat gland or duct
337.9	Sympathetic nervous system
727.40	Synovial
727.51	Synovial popliteal space
355.9	Tarlov's
727.42	Tendon (sheath)
608.89	Testis
620.2	Theca lutein of ovary
478.26	Thornwaldt's
254.8	Thymus
246.2	Thyroid
0	Thyroid adenomatous see 'Goiter' nodular
0	Thyroid colloid see 'Goiter'
226	Thyroid with cystadenoma
529.8	Tongue
474.8	Tonsil
522.8	Tooth (dental root)
478.26	Tornwaldt's
620.8	Tubo ovarian
614.1	Tubo ovarian inflammatory
608.89	Tunica vaginalis
733.20	Turbinate (nose)
607.89	Tyson's gland
593.89	Ureter
593.89	Ureterovesical orifice
599.84	Urethra
599.89	Urethral gland
620.8	Uterine ligament
621.8	Uterus
386.8	Utricle ear
599.89	Utricle prostate
599.89	Utriculus masculinus
623.8	Vagina
478.79	Vallecula
348.0	Ventricle (neuroepithelial)
599.89	Verumontanum
596.8	Vesical orifice
379.29	Vitreous humor
624.8	Vulva
624.8	Vulva sebaceous gland
624.8	Vulvovaginal gland
706.2	Wen

CYST CONGENITAL

752.11	Accessory fallopian tube
759.1	Adrenal glands
753.7	Allantoic
751.69	Bile duct (choledochal)
742.4	Brain colloid third ventricle

CYST CONGENITAL (continued)

744.42	Branchial cleft
752.11	Broad ligament (embryonic)
748.4	Bronchogenic (mediastinal) (sequestration)
752.41	Canal of nuck
746.89	Celomic (pericardium)
742.4	Cerebral
751.69	Choledochal
742.4	Colloid brain third ventricle
742.3	Dandy-Walker
0	Dandy-Walker with spina bifida see 'Spina Bifida'
752.11	Embryonic - broad ligament
752.41	Embryonic - cervix
752.11	Embryonic - fallopian tubes
752.41	Embryonic - hymen
752.11	Embryonic - uterine ligament
752.3	Embryonic - uterus
752.41	Embryonic - vagina
751.5	Enteric
751.5	Enterogenous
748.3	Epiglottis
752.11	Epoophoron
750.4	Esophagus
743.39	Eye lens
743.54	Eye posterior segment
743.03	Eye retention
752.11	Fallopian tube accessory
752.11	Fimbrial
752.41	Gartner's duct
752.41	Genitalia female embryonic
752.89	Hydatid cyst of Morgagni
752.11	Hydatid cyst of morgagni - fallopian tubes
752.41	Hymen embryonal
751.5	Intestine (small)
753.11	Kidney
0	Kidney cystic (disease of) see 'Kidney Congenital', cystic disease
0	Kidney polycystic (disease of) see 'Kidney Congenital', polycystic
748.3	Larynx
743.39	Lens
751.62	Liver
748.4	Lung (cystic) (polycystic)
748.8	Mediastinum
752.89	Mesonephric duct
752.89	Morgagni (hydatid)
750.26	Mouth (sublingual) (submaxillary gland)
752.89	Mullerian duct
742.59	Neuroenteric
751.8	Omentum
752.0	Ovary
752.11	Oviduct
751.7	Pancreas
752.11	Paroophoron
752.11	Parovarian
752.69	Penis (sebaceous)
746.89	Pericardium
753.8	Periurethral (tissue)
742.4	Porencephalic
744.47	Preauricular
752.69	Prepuce
753.11	Renal single
759.0	Spleen
750.26	Sublingual
750.26	Submaxillary gland
759.2	Thymus gland

CYST CONGENITAL (continued)

759.2 Thyroglossal duct
759.2 Thyrolingual duct
750.19 Tongue
759.89 Umbilicus
753.7 Urachus
753.4 Ureterovesical orifice
752.3 Uterus embryonal
752.41 Vagina embryonal
752.41 Vulva
752.89 Wolffian

CYST OF THE EYE AND PERIORBITAL STRUCTURES

364.62 Anterior chamber exudative
364.60 Anterior chamber idiopathic
364.61 Anterior chamber implantation
372.75 Canthus
364.62 Ciliary body exudative
364.60 Ciliary body idiopathic
364.61 Ciliary body implantation
372.75 Conjunctival
371.23 Cornea
379.8 Eye retention
374.84 Eyelid
364.62 Iris exudative
364.60 Iris idiopathic
364.61 Iris implantation
364.55 Iris miotic pupillary margin
360.13 Iris parasitic
375.12 Lacrimal gland and cystic degeneration
379.39 Lens
362.54 Macular (degeneration) (hole or pseudohole)
373.2 Meibomian gland
377.54 Optic chiasm (see also 'Optic Chiasm')
361.19 Ora serrata
376.81 Orbital
364.64 Pars plana exudative
364.63 Pars plana primary
379.8 Retention
360.13 Retinal
360.13 Retinal parasitic
361.13 Retinal primary
361.19 Retinal pseudocyst
361.14 Retinal secondary
361.19 Retinal other
379.19 Sclera
379.29 Vitreous humor

CYST OF THE NERVOUS SYSTEM

348.0 Arachnoid
336.8 Cauda equina
348.0 Cavum septi pellucidi NEC
348.0 Cerebral meninges
348.0 Choroid plexus
348.0 Corpora quadrigemina
348.0 Dura cerebral
349.2 Dura spinal
348.0 Porencephalic
349.2 Spinal meninges
348.0 Subarachnoid
793.0 Subarachnoid intrasellar abnormal radiological study
348.0 Subdural cerebral
349.2 Subdural spinal cord
348.0 Ventricle (neuroepithelial)

CYST OROPHARYNGEAL

526.2 Alveolar process (jaw bone)
526.0 Dentigerous (mandible) (maxilla)
526.1 Fissural of jaw
526.1 Globulomaxillary
478.26 Hypopharynx
526.1 Incisor
526.1 Incisor canal
526.2 Jaw
526.2 Jaw aneurysmal
526.1 Jaw fissural
526.2 Jaw hemorrhagic
526.2 Jaw traumatic
526.1 Median anterior maxillary
526.1 Median palatal
523.8 Mouth gingival
478.19 Nasal (antrum) (cavity) (sinus) (septum)
526.1 Nasopalatine
526.0 Odontogenic developmental
526.1 Palatine of jaw
526.1 Palatine of papilla
527.6 Parotid gland
478.26 Pharyngeal bursa
478.26 Pharynx
526.0 Primordial (jaw)
522.8 Radicular
522.8 Radiculodental
522.8 Residual (radicular)
478.19 Sinus (antral) (ethmoidal) (frontal) (maxillary) (nasal)
478.19 Sphenoid sinus
478.26 Thornwaldt's
474.8 Tonsil

Carcinomas and neoplasms should be coded by site if possible. Code by cell type, "site NOS", only if a site is not specified in the diagnosis. Otherwise, refer to the appropriate category of neoplasm for a more specific code. See 'Cancer' 'Cancer Metastatic', 'Carcinoma In Situ', 'Neoplasm Uncertain Behavior', 'Neoplasm Unspecified Nature', or 'Benign Neoplasm'.

CYSTADENOCARCINOMA

199.1 Site NOS
0 Site specified see 'Cancer', by site M8440/3
155.1 Bile duct site NOS
0 Bile duct site specified see 'Cancer', by site M8161/3
183.0 Mucinous site NOS
0 Mucinous site specified see 'Cancer', by site M8470/3
183.0 Papillary mucinous site NOS
0 Papillary mucinous site specified see 'Cancer', by site M8471/3
0 Papillary site specified see 'Cancer', by site M8450/3
183.0 Papillary serous site NOS
0 Papillary serous site specified see 'Cancer', by site M8460/3
174.9 Serous site NOS
0 Serous site specified see 'Cancer', by site M8441/3

C

> ***Carcinomas and neoplasms should be coded by site if possible. Code by cell type, "site NOS", only if a site is not specified in the diagnosis. Otherwise, refer to the appropriate category of neoplasm for a more specific code. See 'Cancer' 'Cancer Metastatic', 'Carcinoma In Situ', 'Neoplasm Uncertain Behavior', 'Neoplasm Unspecified Nature', or 'Benign Neoplasm'.***

CYSTADENOMA

229.9 Site NOS
0 Site specified see 'Benign Neoplasm', by site M8440/0
211.5 Bile duct site NOS
0 Bile duct site specified see 'Benign Neoplasm', by site M8161/0
220 Mucinous site NOS
0 Mucinous (borderline malignancy) site specified see 'Neoplasm Uncertain Behavior' M8470/1
236.2 Mucinous (borderline malignancy) site NOS
0 Mucinous site specified see 'Benign Neoplasm', by site M8470/0
220 Papillary site NOS
0 Papillary site specified see 'Benign Neoplasm', by site M8450/0
236.2 Papillary (borderline malignancy) site NOS M8450/1
0 Papillary (borderline malignancy) site specified see 'Neoplasm Uncertain Behavior', by site
236.2 Papillary mucinous (borderline malignancy) site NOS
0 Papillary mucinous (borderline malignancy) site specified see 'Neoplasm Uncertain Behavior', by site M8471/1
220 Papillary mucinous site NOS
0 Papillary mucinous site specified see 'Benign Neoplasm', by site M8471/0
236.2 Papillary serous (borderline malignancy) site NOS
0 Papillary serous (borderline malignancy) site specified see 'Neoplasm Uncertain Behavior', by site M8460/1
220 Papillary serous site NOS
0 Papillary serous site specified site specified see 'Benign Neoplasm', by site M8460/0
236.2 Serous (borderline malignancy) site NOS
0 Serous (borderline malignancy) site specified see 'Neoplasm Uncertain Behavior' by site M8441/1
229.9 Serous site NOS
0 Serous site specified see 'Benign Neoplasm', by site M8441/0

270.4 CYSTATHIONINE METABOLISM DISTURBANCES
270.4 CYSTATHIONINEMIA, CYSTATHIONINURIA
123.1 CYSTICERCIASIS
123.1 CYSTICERCUS CELLULOSAE INFECTION

CYSTIC

902.24 Artery injury
908.4 Artery injury late effect
742.4 Brain degeneration congenital
610.1 Breast disease
620.1 Corpora lutea
575.8 Duct adhesion (atrophy) (cyst) (ulcer) (dyskinesia)
575.8 Duct atresia
751.61 Duct atresia congenital
576.8 Duct atrophy

CYSTIC (continued)

0 Duct calculus see 'Cholelithiasis'
751.69 Duct duplication congenital
575.2 Duct obstruction (occlusion) (stenosis) (stricture)
751.61 Duct obstruction (occlusion) congenital
0 Duct obstruction (occlusion) (stenosis) (stricture) with calculus see 'Cholecystitis'
575.8 Duct disorders other specified
575.4 Duct perforation
576.0 Duct stump syndrome
743.03 Eyeball congenital

> ***When coding an infection, use an additional code, [041.#(#)], to identify the organism. See 'Bacterial Infection'.***

277.0# Fibrosis

5th digit: 277.0

- **0. NOS**
- **1. With meconium ileus**
- **2. With pulmonary manifestations**
- **3. With gastrointestinal manifestations**
- **9. With other manifestations**

V83.81 Fibrosis gene carrier
V77.6 Fibrosis screening
228.1 Hygroma
0 Kidney disease congenital see 'Kidney Congenital'
751.62 Liver disease congenital
518.89 Lung acquired
748.4 Lung congenital
0 Mass see 'Cyst'
610.1 Mastitis, chronic
620.2 Ovary NOS
751.7 Pancreas disease congenital
717.5 Semilunar cartilage disease
902.39 Vein injury
908.4 Vein injury late effect
902.39 Vein laceration (rupture) (hematoma) (avulsion) (aneurysm) traumatic
908.4 Vein laceration late effect

123.1 CYSTICERCOSIS
270.0 CYSTINE STORAGE METABOLISM DISORDER
270.0 CYSTINOSIS
270.0 CYSTINURIA

CYSTITIS

595.9 NOS
039.8 Actinomycotic [595.4]
595.0 Acute
595.0 Acute hemorrhagic
595.89 Allergic
006.8 Amebic [595.4]
120.9 Bilharziasis (due to) [595.4]
595.89 Bullous emphysematous glandularis
595.2 Chronic
595.1 Chronic interstitial
099.53 Chlamydial lower genitourinary sites
595.81 Cystica
032.84 Diphtheritic
122.3 Echinococcus granulosus [595.4]
122.6 Echinococcus multicularis [595.4]
595.89 Emphysematous
595.3 Follicular
595.89 Gangrenous
098.11 Gonococcal (acute)
098.31 Gonococcal chronic

CYSTITIS (continued)

595.1 Interstitial chronic
595.82 Irradiation

646.6#: Specify the maternal cystitis with an additional code.

646.6# Maternal complicating pregnancy
5th digit: 646.6
0. Episode of care NOS or N/A
1. Delivered
2. Delivered with postpartum complication
3. Antepartum complication
4. Postpartum complication

112.2 Monilial
595.2 Subacute
595.1 Submucous
131.09 Trichomonal
595.3 Trigonitis
016.1# Tuberculous [595.4]
5th digit: 016.1
0. NOS
1. Lab not done
2. Lab pending
3. Microscopy positive (in sputum)
4. Culture positive - microscopy negative
5. Culture negative - microscopy positive
6. Culture and microscopy negative confirmed by other methods

595.1 Ulcerative
595.89 Other specified

CYSTOCELE

618.#(#) Female
618.#(#) Female with stress incontinence [625.6]
618.#(#) Female with other urinary incontinence **[788.3#]**
4th digit: 618
0#. Without uterine prolapse
2. With incomplete uterine prolapse
3. With complete uterine prolapse
4. Uterine prolapse unspecified
5th digit: 618.0
1. Midline (NOS)
2. Lateral (paravaginal)
5th digit: 788.3
1. Urge incontinence
3. Mixed urge and stress
4. Without sensory awareness
5. Post-void dribbling
6. Nocturnal enuresis
7. Continuous leakage
8. Overflow incontinence
9. Other

596.8 Male

CYSTOCELE OBSTETRICAL

763.89 Affecting fetus or newborn
654.4# Complicating pregnancy
660.2# Obstructing labor **[654.4#]**
5th digit: 654.4
0. Episode of care NOS or N/A
1. Delivered
2. Delivered with postpartum complication
3. Antepartum complication
4. Po stpartum complication
5th digit: 660.2
0. Episode of care NOS or N/A
1. Delivered
3. Antepartum complication

763.1 Obstructing labor affecting fetus or newborn

594.1 CYSTOLITHIASIS

596.53 CYSTOPLEGIA

CYSTOSARCOMA PHYLLODES

174.9 Malignant site NOS
0 Malignant site specified see 'Cancer', by site M9020/3
239.3 Site NOS
0 Site specified see 'Neoplasm Uncertain Behavior', by site M9020/1

When coding an infection of an ostomy, use an additional code to specify the organism. See 'Bacterial Infection'

CYSTOSTOMY

V55.5 Care
V55.5 Catheter adjustment or repositioning
996.39 Catheter complication mechanical
V55.5 Catheter removal or replacement
V55.5 Closure
996.39 Complication catheter mechanical
997.5 Complication stoma
V53.6 Device fitting and adjustment
997.5 Malfunction
V55.5 Removal or change
V44.50 Status - NOS
V44.52 Status - appendico-vesicostomy
V44.51 Status - cutaneous-vesicostomy
V44.59 Status - other
V55.5 Toilet stoma

C

618.09 CYSTOURETHROCELE (FEMALE) (WITHOUT UTERINE PROLAPSE)

618.09 CYSTOURETHROCELE (FEMALE) (WITHOUT UTERINE PROLAPSE) WITH STRESS INCONTINENCE [625.6]

618.09 CYSTOURETHROCELE (FEMALE) (WITHOUT UTERINE PROLAPSE) WITH OTHER URINARY INCONTINENCE [788.3#]

5th digit: 788.3

1. Urge incontinence
3. Mixed urge and stress
4. Without sensory awareness
5. Post-void dribbling
6. Nocturnal enuresis
7. Continuous leakage
8. Overflow incontinence
9. Other

C

CYTOMEGALOVIRUS INFECTIONS

078.5 NOS
771.1 Congenital or perinatal
V01.79 Exposure
078.5 Hepatitis [573.1]
078.5 Inclusion disease (generalized)
078.5 Pneumonia [484.1]

289.9 CYTOPENIA

238.72 CYTOPENIA REFRACTORY WITH MULTILINEAGE DYSPLASIA (RCMD)

238.72 CYTOPENIA REFRACTORY WITH MULTILINEAGE DYSPLASIA AND RINGED SIDEROBLASTS (RCMD-RS)

719.06 CZERNY'S PERIODIC HYDRARTHROSIS OF THE KNEE

306.2 DA COSTA'S SYNDROME (NEUROCIRCULATORY ASTHENIA)

074.1 DAAE (-FINSEN) EPIDEMIC PLEURODYNIA

DACRYOADENITIS

375.00 NOS
375.01 Acute
375.02 Chronic

DACRYOCYSTITIS

375.30 NOS
375.32 Acute
375.42 Chronic
771.6 Neonatal
771.6 Ophthalmia neonatorum
375.33 Phlegmonous

375.57 DACRYOLITH

375.11 DACRYOPS

375.56 DACRYOSTENOSIS

DACTYLITIS

282.62 Sickle cell
282.64 Sickle cell Hb-C
282.62 Sickle cell Hb-SS
282.69 Sickle cell specified NEC

136.0 DACTYLOLYSIS SPONTANEA

282.49 DAMESHEK'S SYNDROME (ERYTHROBLASTIC ANEMIA)

281.0 DANA-PUTNAM SYNDROME (SCLEROSIS SUBACUTE WITH PERNICIOUS ANEMIA) [336.2]

686.8 DANBOLT (-CLOSS) SYNDROME (ACRODERMATITIS ENTEROPATHICA)

297.8 DANCING DISEASE

690.18 DANDRUFF

742.3 DANDY WALKER SYNDROME (ATRESIA, FORAMEN OF MAGENDIE)

741.0# DANDY WALKER SYNDROME (ATRESIA, FORAMEN OF MAGENDIE) WITH SPINA BIFIDA

5th digit: 741.0
0. Region NOS
1. Cervical region
2. Dorsal (thoracic region)
3. Lumbar region

030.1 DANIELSSEN'S ANESTHETIC LEPROSY

756.83 DANLOS' SYNDROME

695.0 DARIER'S ERYTHEMA ANNULARE CENTRIFUGUM

757.39 DARIER'S KERATOSIS FOLLICULARIS CONGENITAL

135 DARIER-ROUSSY SARCOID

264.8 DARIER'S VITAMIN A DEFICIENCY

368.63 DARK ADAPTATION CURVE ABNORMAL

0 DARLING'S DISEASE SEE 'HISTOPLASMOSIS'

744.29 DARWIN'S TUBERCLE CONGENITAL

425.0 DAVIES' DISEASE

425.0 DAVIES' ENDOMYOCARDIAL FIBROSIS

733.99 DAVIES-COLLEY SYNDROME (SLIPPING RIB)

046.2 DAWSON'S INCLUSION BODY ENCEPHALITIS

368.10 DAY BLINDNESS

117.1 DE BEURMANN-GOUGEROT SPOROTRICHOSIS

789.2 DEBOVE'S SPLENOMEGALY

727.04 DE QUERVAIN'S TENDINITIS

245.1 DE QUERVAIN'S THYROIDITIS

641.3# DEAD FETUS SYNDROME

5th digit: 641.3
0. Episode of care NOS or N/A
1. Delivered
3. Antepartum complication

389.7 DEAF NONSPEAKING NEC

DEAFNESS

389.9 NOS
744.03 Congenital
V19.2 Family history hearing loss
300.11 Hysterical
388.02 Ischemic (transient)
389.12 Neural bilateral
306.7 Psychogenic
951.5 Traumatic
0 See also 'Hearing Loss'

Code first hearing and/or visual impairment.

V49.85 With blindness (combined visual hearing impairment) (dual sensory impairment)
756.51 With blue sclera and fragility of bone

DEATH

348.8 Brain
V68.09 Certificate issue
768.0 Fetal due to asphyxia or anoxia before onset of labor and/or unspecified time
768.1 Fetal due to asphyxia or anoxia during labor
779.6 Fetal due to induced abortion
779.6 Fetal due to termination of pregnancy
V17.41 History family sudden cardiac
V12.53 History resuscitated
798.2 In 24 hours from onset of symptoms unexplained
798.1 Instantaneous cause unknown
761.6 Maternal affecting fetus or newborn
674.9# Maternal sudden (unknown cause) due to pregnancy

5th digit: 674.9
0. NOS
2. Delivered with postpartum complication
4. Postpartum complication

V17.41 Sudden cardiac family history
V12.53 Sudden cardiac history successfully resuscitated
798.0 Sudden infant syndrome (SIDS)
0 Sudden infant syndrome (SIDS) near miss - code individual symptom(s)
798.9 Unattended
798.2 Unexplained < 24 hours from onset of symptoms

DEBILITY

799.3 NOS
780.79 Asthenic
779.9 Congenital
300.5 Nervous
797 Senile

874.9 DECAPITATION

993.3 DECOMPRESSION SICKNESS

909.4 DECOMPRESSION SICKNESS LATE EFFECT

D

DECUBITUS (ULCER)

707.0# NOS
707.0# With cellulitis [682.#]
5th digit: 707.0
0. NOS
1. Elbow
2. Upper back (shoulder blades)
3. Lower back (sacrum)
4. Hip
5. Buttock
6. Ankle
7. Heel
9. Other site (head)
4th digit: 682
0. Face
1. Neck
2. Trunk
3. Upper arm and forearm
4. Hand, except fingers and thumb
5. Buttock
6. Leg, except foot
7. Foot, except toes
8. Other specified sites
9. Unspecified site
707.0# With gangrene [785.4]
5th digit: 707.0
0. NOS
1. Elbow
2. Upper back (shoulder blades)
3. Lower back (sacrum)
4. Hip
5. Buttock
6. Ankle
7. Heel
9. Other site (head)

0 DEER FLY BITE, SEE 'INSECT BITE NONVENOMOUS', BY SITE
021.9 DEER FLY TULAREMIA (SEE ALSO 'TULAREMIA')
255.2 DEFEMINIZATION SYNDROME
286.6 DEFIBRINATION SYNDROME
639.1 DEFIBRINATION SYNDROME POST ABORTION OR ECTOPIC/MOLAR PREGNANCY

DEFICIENCY

V48.0 Head
V47.0 Internal organs
V48.1 Neck
V48.1 Trunk

DEFORMITY

738.9 NOS (acquired)
759.9 NOS congenital
759.7 Multiple congenital
738.8 Other specified site (acquired)
0 See also anatomical site

0 DEGENERATIVE ARTHRITIS SEE 'OSTEOARTHRITIS'
701.3 DEGENERATIVE COLLOID ATROPHY

DEGENERATIVE DISC DISEASE

722.6 Site NOS
722.70 Site NOS with myelopathy
722.4 Cervical
722.71 Cervical with myelopathy
722.52 Lumbar (lumbosacral)
722.73 Lumbar (lumbosacral) with myelopathy
722.51 Thoracic (thoracolumbar)
722.72 Thoracic (thoracolumbar) with myelopathy

DEGENERATIVE JOINT DISEASE (DJD)

715.90 Site unspecified
715.97 Ankle and/or foot (metatarsals) (toes) (tarsals)
715.93 Forearm (radius) (wrist) (ulna)
715.94 Hand (carpal) (metacarpal) (fingers)
715.96 Leg lower (fibula) (knee) (patella) (tibia)
715.95 Leg upper (pelvic region) (thigh) (hip) (buttock) (femur)
715.95 Pelvic region and thigh (hip) (buttock) (femur)
715.91 Shoulder region
721.90 Spine - NOS
721.0 Spine - cervical
721.3 Spine - lumbar or lumbosacral
721.2 Spine - thoracic
715.92 Upper arm (elbow) (humerus)
715.98 Other specified

709.3 DEGENERATIVE SKIN DISORDER
0 DEGLOVING INJURY SEE 'OPEN WOUND', BY SITE
447.8 DEGOS' DISEASE OR SYNDROME
784.99 DEGLUTITION PARALYSIS

DEHISCENCE OF WOUND POST OP

998.32 NOS
674.2# Episiotomy
998.32 External
998.31 Internal
674.2# Perineal obstetrical
674.1# Uterine obstetrical
5th digit: 674.1-2
0. Episode of care NOS or N/A
2. Delivered with mention of postpartum complication
4. Postpartum condition or complication

> ***When a patient is admitted and treated for dehydration, and the treatment is directed only at that condition, the dehydration would be the principal diagnosis, regardless of the underlying condition.***

276.51 DEHYDRATION
778.4 DEHYDRATION FEVER NEWBORN
775.5 DEHYDRATION NEWBORN
276.50 DEHYDRATION VOLUME DEPLETION
276.0 DEHYDRATION WITH HYPERNATREMIA
276.1 DEHYDRATION WITH HYPONATREMIA
386.19 DEITERS' NUCLEUS SYNDROME
338.0 DEJERINE-ROUSSY SYNDROME
356.0 DEJERINE SOTTAS DISEASE
333.0 DEJERINE THOMAS SYNDROME
759.89 DE LANGE'S SYNDROME (AMSTERDAM DWARF, MENTAL RETARDATION AND BRACHYCEPHALY) (CORNELIA)
756.0 DELAYED CLOSURE CRANIAL SUTURES
783.42 DELAYED MILESTONES CHILD (LATE TALKER) (LATE WALKER)
606.0 DEL CASTILLO SYNDROME (GERMINAL APLASIA)
359.89 DELEAGE'S DISEASE
758.39 DELETION SYNDROME – NOS
758.31 DELETION SYNDROME – 5p
758.32 DELETION SYNDROME – 22q11.2
758.39 DELETION SYNDROME – CONSTITUTIONAL 5q DELETION
758.39 DELETION SYNDROME – OTHER
085.1 DELHI BOIL

DELINQUENCY CONDUCT DISORDER

312.2 Group
312.9 Juvenile
312.4 Neurotic

DELIRIUM

780.09 NOS
291.0 Alcoholic
292.81 Drug induced [**304.##**]
4th digit: 304
0. Opioid
1. Sedative, hypnotic or anxiolytic
2. Cocaine
3. Cannabis
4. Amphetamine type
5. Hallucinogenic
6. Other specified
7. Mixed with opioid
8. Mixed
9. NOS

5th digit: 304
0. NOS
1. Continuous
2. Episodic
3. In remission

293.0 Due to conditions classified elsewhere
780.39 Eclamptic
293.1 Subacute (transient) (organic) (psychosis)
293.81 Transient organic with delusions
293.82 Transient organic with hallucinations
291.0 Tremens (DT'S) (alcohol withdrawal delirium)
0 See also 'Psychosis'

> ***650, Normal delivery refers to the delivery episode of care only. If a complication of pregnancy is no longer present at the time of delivery, the delivery itself is still assigned 650 as the principal diagnosis.***

DELIVERY

V39.1 NOS - born before admission to hospital (code on infant's record)
V39.0# NOS - born in hospital (code on infant's record)
5th digit: V39.0
0. Delivered
1. Delivered by cesarean section

V39.2 NOS - born outside hospital, not hospitalized (code on infant's record)
763.0 Affecting fetus or newborn - breech delivery and extraction
763.6 Affecting fetus or newborn - rapid second stage
669.7# Cesarean without indication
V23.49 Difficult previous affecting current pregnancy
669.5# Forceps or vacuum extraction
5th digit: 669.5, 7
0. Episode of care NOS or N/A
1. Delivered

650 Normal in complicated or uncomplicated pregnancy - single liveborn (code on mother's record) [V27.0]
644.2# Premature
5th digit: 644.2
0. Episode of care NOS or N/A
1. Delivered

V23.41 Premature previous affecting current pregnancy

DELIVERY (continued)

V30.1 Single liveborn - born before admission to hospital (code on infant's record)
V30.0# Single liveborn - born in hospital (code on infant's record)
5th digit: V30.0
0. Delivered
1. Delivered by cesarean section

V30.2 Single liveborn - born outside hospital, not hospitalized (code on infant's record)
V27.0 Single liveborn (code on mother's record)
V27.1 Single stillborn (code on mother's record)
V31.# Twin mate, liveborn - not born in hospital (code on infant's record)
4th digit: V31
1. Born before admission to hospital
2. Born outside hospital and not hospitalized

V31.0# Twin mate, liveborn - born in hospital (code on infant's record)
5th digit: V31.0
0. Delivered
1. Delivered by cesarean section

V32.# Twin mate, stillborn - not born in hospital (code on infant's record)
4th digit: V32
1. Born before admission to hospital
2. Born outside hospital and not hospitalized

V32.0# Twin mate, stillborn - born in hospital (code on infant's record)
5th digit: V32.0
0. Delivered
1. Delivered by cesarean section

V33.# Twin unspecified - not born in hospital (code on infant's record)
4th digit: V33
1. Born before admission to hospital
2. Born outside hospital and not hospitalized

V33.0# Twin unspecified - born in hospital (code on infant's record)
5th digit: V33.0
0. Delivered
1. Delivered by cesarean section

V27.2 Twins both liveborn (code on mother's record)
V27.3 Twins one liveborn and one stillborn (code on mother's record)
V27.4 Twins both stillborn (outcome code on mother's record)
V34.# Other multiple, mates all liveborn - not born in hospital (code on infant's record)
4th digit: V34
1. Born before admission to hospital
2. Born outside hospital and not hospitalized

V34.0# Other multiple, mates all liveborn - born in hospital (code on infant's record)
5th digit: V34 .0
0. Delivered
1. Delivered by cesarean section

V35.# Other multiple, mates all stillborn - not born in hospital (code on infant's record)
4th digit: V35
1. Born before admission to hospital
2. Born outside hospital and not hospitalized

D

DELIVERY (continued)

V35.0# Other multiple, mates all stillborn - born in hospital (code on infant's record)
5th digit: V35.0
0. Delivered
1. Delivered by cesarean section

V36.# Other multiple, mates live and stillborn - not born in hospital (code on infant's record)
4th digit: V36
1. Born before admission to hospital
2. Born outside hospital and not hospitalized

V36.0# Other multiple, mates live and stillborn - born in hospital (code on infant's record)
5th digit: V36.0
0. Delivered
1. Delivered by cesarean section

V37.# Other multiple, unspecified - not born in hospital (code on infant's record)
4th digit: V37
1. Born before admission to hospital
2. Born outside hospital and not hospitalized

V37.0# Other multiple, unspecified - born in hospital (code on infant's record)
5th digit: V37.0
0. Delivered
1. Delivered by cesarean section

V27.5 Other multiple birth all liveborn (outcome code on mother's record)
V27.6 Other multiple birth some liveborn (code on mother's record)
V27.7 Other multiple birth all stillborn (code on mother's record)
V27.9 Outcome of delivery unspecified (code on mother's record)

644.2# Premature
5th digit: 644.2
0. Episode of care NOS or N/A
1. Delivered

763.6 Rapid second stage affecting fetus or newborn
0 See also 'Pregnancy Complications, Delivery Problems'
0 See also 'Labor And Delivery Complications'

DELIVERY DELAYED

658.3# After artificial rupture of membranes
658.2# After Spontaneous rupture of membranes
662.1# Birth NEC
5th digit: 658.2-3, 662.1
0. Episode of care NOS or N/A
1. Delivered
3. Antepartum complication

763.89 Birth NEC affecting fetus or newborn
662.3# Birth of second twin, triplet, etc.
5th digit: 662.3
0. Episode of care NOS or N/A
1. Delivered
3. Antepartum complication

763.89 Birth of second twin, triplet, etc. affecting fetus or newborn

D

DELUSIONAL DISORDER

297.1 NOS
297.2 Paraphrenia
300.29 Parasitosis
297.3 Shared paranoid disorder
297.3 Shared psychotic disorder
297.0 Simple paranoid state
297.1 Systematized (grandiose)
293.81 Transient in conditions classified elsewhere
297.8 Other specified

DELUSIONAL SYNDROME

291.5 Alcohol induced (see also 'Psychosis Alcoholic')
290.42 Arteriosclerotic [437.0]
292.11 Drug induced (see also 'Psychosis Drug Induced')
293.81 Organic (transient)

117.8 DEMATIACIOUS FUNGI INFECTION

DEMENTIA

> ***294.1# Dementia in conditions classified elsewhere, is used only as a secondary code. Code first any underlying physical condition. Some of the physical conditions often accompaning dementia are provided for you. For those not listed here, look up the code for the condition and report it first followed by code 294.1#.***

294.8 NOS
042 AIDS **[294.1#]**
5th digit: 294.1
0. Without behavioral disturbance or NOS
1. With behavioral disturbance

291.2 Alcohol-induced persisting
331.0 Alzheimer's (senile) (presenile) **[294.1#]**
5th digit: 294.1
0. Without behavioral disturbance or NOS
1. With behavioral disturbance

299.1# Aphonia syndrome of childhood
5th digit: 299.1
0. Active state
1. Residual state

> ***290.#(#), Dementia: Code first any associated neurological condition.***

290.4# Arteriosclerosis [437.0]
5th digit: 290.4
0. NOS
1. With delirium
2. With delusions
3. With depressed mood

330.1 Cerebral lipidoses [294.1#]
5th digit: 294.1
0. Without behavioral disturbance or NOS
1. With behavioral disturbance

294.8 Dialysis [E879.1]
985.8 Dialysis due to aluminum overload [294.8] [E879.1]
293.9 Dialysis transient [E879.1]
292.82 Drug-induced persisting

DEMENTIA (continued)

345.## Epileptic **[294.1#]**
4th digit: 345
0. Generalized nonconvulsive
1. Generalized convulsive
4. Partial, with impairment of consciousness
5. Partial, without impairment of consciousness
6. Infantile spasms
7. Epilepsia partialis continua
8. Other forms
9. Unspecified, NOS

5th digit: 345
0. Without mention of intractable epilepsy
1. With intractable epilepsy

5th digit: 294.1
0. Without behavioral disturbance or NOS
1. With behavioral disturbance

345.3 Epileptic grand mal status **[294.1#]**
345.2 Epileptic petit mal status **[294.1#]**
331.19 Frontal other **[294.1#]**
331.19 Frontotemporal other **[294.1#]**
275.1 Hepatolenticular degeneration **[294.1#]**
042 HIV **[294.1#]**
333.4 Huntington's chorea **[294.1#]**
046.1 Jakob Creutzfeldt (new variant) (presenile) **[294.1#]**
5th digit: 294.1
0. Without behavioral disturbance or NOS
1. With behavioral disturbance

331.82 Lewy bodies **[294.1#]**
-0 Multi-infarct see 'Dementia', arteriosclerotic
340 Multiple sclerosis **[294.1#]**
0 Neurosyphilis see 'Neurosyphilis'
090.40 Paralytica juvenilis
331.82 Parkinsonism **[294.1#]**
333.0 Pelizaeus-Merzbacher disease **[294.1#]**
331.11 Pick's disease **[294.1#]**
446.0 Polyarteritis nodosa **[294.1#]**
5th digit: 294.1
0. Without behavioral disturbance or NOS
1. With behavioral disturbance

290 .#(#), Dementia: Code first any associated neurological condition.

PRESENILE

290.10 NOS
290.11 With delirium
290.12 With delusions
290.13 With depression

DEMENTIA (continued)

SENILE

290.0 NOS
290.20 Delusional
290.21 Depressive
090.40 Paralytica juvenilis
290.20 Paranoid type
094.1 Syphilitic **[294.1#]**
5th digit: 294.1
0. Without behavioral disturbance or NOS
1. With behavioral disturbance

290.3 With acute confusional state
290.3 With delirium

DEMENTIA (continued)

294.1# Dementia in conditions classified elsewhere, is used only as a secondary code. Code first any underlying physical condition. Some of the physical conditions often accompaning dementia are provided for you. For those not listed here, look up the code for the condition and report it first followed by code 294.1#.

094.1 Syphilitic **[294.1#]**
5th digit: 294.1
0. Without behavioral disturbance or NOS
1. With behavioral disturbance

290.4# Vascular [437.0]
5th digit: 290.4
0. NOS
1. With delirium
2. With delusions
3. With depressed mood

275.1 Wilson's disease **[294.1#]**
5th digit: 294.1
0. Without behavioral disturbance or NOS
1. With behavioral disturbance

133.8 DEMODEX FOLLICULORUM INFESTATION
341.9 DEMYELINATING DISEASE OR SYNDROME (CENTRAL NERVOUS SYSTEM)
341.8 DEMYELINATING DISEASE OR SYNDROME (CENTRAL NERVOUS SYSTEM) OTHER SPECIFIED NEC
357.81 DEMYELINATING POLYNEURITIS CHRONIC INFLAMMATORY

DENGUE
061 NOS
V73.5 Fever screening exam
065.4 Hemorrhagic fever

307.9 DENIAL VISUAL HALLUCINATION SYNDROME
520.2 DENS EVAGINATUS (INVAGINATUS)
520.2 DENS IN DENTE

D

DENTAL

524.7# Alveolar anomaly
5th digit: 524.7
0. Unspecified (mandible) (maxilla)
1. Maxillary hyperplasia
2. Mandibular hyperplasia
3. Maxillary hypoplasia
4. Mandibular hypoplasia
5. Vertical displacement
6. Occlusal plane deviation
9. Other specified

524.2# Arch relationship anomaly (malocclusion)
5th digit: 524.2
0. Unspecified
1. Angle's class I
2. Angle's class II
3. Angle's class III
4. Open anterior occlusal
5. Open posterior occlusal
6. Excessive horizontal overlap
7. Reverse articulation, crossbite
8. Interarch distance
9. Other

525.60 Bridge defect
523.6 Calculus subgingival
523.6 Calculus supragingival
521.0# Caries
5th digit: 521.0
0. Unspecified
1. Limited to enamel
2. Extending into dentine
3. Extending into pulp
4. Arrested
5. Odontoclasia
6. Pit and fissure origin (primary)
7. Smooth surface origin (primary)
8. Root surface (primary)
9. Other

525.60 Crown defect
525.60 Filling defect
525.7# Implant failure
5th digit: 525.7
1. Oseointegration (hemorrhagic) (iatrogenic) (due to systemic disease or poor bone quality) (pre-integration NOS) (pre-osseointegration)
2. Post-oseointegration biological (due to lack of attached gingival) (due to post occlusal trauma) (parafunctional habits) (periodontal infection) (poor oral hygiene) (iatrogenic) (systemic disease)
3. Post-oseointegration mechanical (dental prosthesis failure) (fracture)
9. Other endosseous (NOS)

V52.3 Prosthetic device (fitting and adjustment) (removal)
522.2 Pulp calcification

DENTAL (continued)

V45.84 Restoration status
525.6# Restoration unsatisfactory
5th digit: 525.6
0. Unspecified
1. Open margins
2. Unrepairable overhanging materials
3. Fractured material without loss of material
4. Fractured material with loss of material
5. Contour incompatible with oral health
6. Allergy
7. Poor aesthetics
9. Other

525.3 Root retained
V49.82 Sealant status

520.6 DENTIA PRAECOX

DENTIN

522.3 Irregular (pulp)
520.5 Opalescent
522.3 Secondary (pulp)
521.89 Sensitive

520.5 DENTINAL DYSPLASIA
521.5 DENTINAL HYPERPLASIA
520.4 DENTINAL PAPILLA CALCIFICATION
520.5 DENTINOGENESIS IMPERFECTA
213.# DENTINOMA M9271/0
4th digit: 213
0. Skull, face, upper jaw
1. Lower jaw

520.6 DENTITION DISORDER (OBSTRUCTED) (DELAYED) (NEONATAL) (PREMATURE)
524.7# DENTOALVEOLAR ANOMALIES
5th digit: 524.7
0. Unspecified (mandible) (maxilla)
1. Maxillary hyperplasia
2. Mandibular hyperplasia
3. Maxillary hypoplasia
4. Mandibular hypoplasia
5. Vertical displacement
6. Occlusal plane deviation
9. Other specified

524.5# DENTOFACIAL ABNOMALITIES FUNCTIONAL
5th digit: 524.5
0. Unspecified
1. Abnormal jaw closure
2. Limited mandibular range of motion
3. Deviation in opening and closing of mandible
4. Insufficient anterior guidance
5. Centric occlusion maximum intercuspation discrepancy
6. Nonworking side interference
7. Lack of posterior occlusal support
9. Other

524.9 DENTOFACIAL ANOMALIES
524.8# DENTOFACIAL ANOMALIES OTHER SPECIFIED
5th digit: 524.8
1. Anterior soft tissue impingement
2. Posterior soft tissue impingement
9. Other

528.9 DENTURE SORE

V52.3 DENTURES FITTING AND ADJUSTMENT

DEPENDENCE

V46.0 Aspirator (mechanical)
V45.1 Hemodialysis
V46.8 Hyperbaric chamber
V46.9 Machine
V46.2 Oxygen therapy
V45.1 Peritoneal dialysis
V46.8 Possum
V45.1 Renal dialysis machine
V46.1# Respirator (ventilator)

5th digit: V46.1
1. Status
2. Encounter during power failure
3. Encounter for weaning from
4. Mechanical complication

0 Substance see 'Substance Abuse' or specified substance

301.59 DEPENDENT PERSONALITY

300.6 DEPERSONALIZATION DISORDER OR SYNDROME

V25.02 DEPO-PROVERA INJECTION

V25.49 DEPO-PROVERA INJECTION REPEAT

DEPRESSION

311 NOS
296.82 Disorder atypical (psychosis)
296.3# Disorder recurrent episode (psychosis)
296.2# Disorder single episode (psychosis)
292.84 Drug induced
296.3# Endogenous (psychotic) recurrent episode (psychosis)
296.2# Endogenous (psychotic) single episode
296.3# Involutional recurrent (psychosis)
296.2# Involutional single episode or unspecified

5th digit: 296.2-3
0. Unspecified
1. Mild
2. Moderate
3. Severe without mention of psychotic behavior
4. Severe specified as with psychotic behavior
5. In partial or unspecified remission
6. In full remission

648.4# Maternal current (co-existent) in pregnancy

5th digit: 648.4
0. Episode of care NOS
1. Delivered with or without mention of antepartum condition
2. Delivered with mention of postpartum complication
3. Antepartum condition
4. Postpartum complication

296.2# Monopolar (single episode or unspecified)
296.3# Monopolar recurrent

5th digit: 296.2-3
0. Unspecified
1. Mild
2. Moderate
3. Severe without mention of psychotic behavior
4. Severe specified as with psychotic behavior
5. In partial or unspecified remission
6. In full remission

DEPRESSION (continued)

648.4# Postpartum - (blues)
648.4# Postpartum - depression NOS [311]
648.4# Postpartum psychotic - recurrent [**296.3#**]
648.4# Postpartum psychotic - single episode [**296.2#**]

5th digit: 648.4
0. Episode of care NOS
1. Delivered with or without mention of antepartum condition
2. Delivered with mention of postpartum complication
3. Antepartum condition
4. Postpartum complication

5th digit: 296.2-3
0. Unspecified
1. Mild
2. Moderate
3. Severe without mention of psychotic behavior
4. Severe specified as with psychotic behavior
5. In partial or unspecified remission

300.4 Reactive
298.0 Reactive psychotic
V79.0 Screening
293.83 Transient (organic) (psychosis) (alcoholic) (drugs)
300.4 With anxiety

DEPRESSIVE

311 Disorder unspecified
296.82 Disorder atypical (psychosis)
311 Disorder NEC
300.4 Neurotic state
301.12 Personality disorder chronic
298.0 Psychosis reactive
296.3# Psychosis recurrent major episode
296.2# Psychosis single episode or unspecified

5th digit: 296.2-3
0. Unspecified
1. Mild
2. Moderate
3. Severe without mention of psychotic behavior
4. Severe specified as with psychotic behavior
5. In partial or unspecified remission
6. In full remission

300.4 Reaction
309.1 Reaction prolonged (adjustment reaction)
290.43 Syndrome arteriosclerotic [437.0]

727.04 DEQUERVAIN TENDONITIS

245.1 DEQUERVAIN THYROIDITIS

0 DERANGEMENT JOINT SEE 'JOINT', DERANGEMENT

272.8 DERCUM'S SYNDROME (ADIPOSIS DOLOROSA)

300.6 DEREALIZATION (NEUROTIC)

757.39 DERMAL HYPOPLASIA

D

DERMATITIS

692.9	Unspecified
692.82	Ab Igne
692.70	Actinic solar
692.72	Actinic solar - acute
692.74	Actinic solar - chronic
692.75	Actinic solar - porokeratosis, disseminated superficial (DSAP)
692.89	Actinic other
698.4	Artefacta
316	Artefacta psychogenic [698.4]
691.8	Atopic
701.8	Atrophicans (diffusa)
701.3	Atrophicans maculosa
694.9	Bullous
694.9	Bullosa
692.6	Bullosa striata pratensis
120.3	Cercarial cutaneous
991.5	Congelationis
0	Contact see 'Dermatitis Contact'
695.2	Contusiformis
032.85	Diphtheritica
692.82	Due to other radiation
692.3	Due to drugs and medicines applied to skin
693.0	Due to drugs and medicines ingested
692.5	Due to food in contact with skin
693.1	Due to food ingested
693.9	Due to substances - unspecified ingested
693.0	Due to substances - specified ingested
693.8	Due to substances - other ingested
625.8	Dysmenorrheica
690.8	Eczematous infectious
692.9	Eczematous NEC
695.89	Epidemica
695.81	Erysipelatosa
695.89	Exfoliativa
695.81	Exfoliativa (infantum) neonatorum
0	Eyelid see 'Dermatitis Eyelid'
698.4	Factitia (artefacta)
704.8	Follicularis
646.8#	Gestationis

5th digit: 646.8
- **0. Episode of care NOS or N/A**
- **1. Delivered**
- **2. Delivered with postpartum complication**
- **3. Antepartum complication**
- **4. Postpartum complication**

694.0	Herpetiformis
694.2	Herpetiformis juvenile
694.5	Herpetiformis senile
692.89	Hiemalis
690.12	Infantile
690.8	Infectiosa eczematoides
686.9	Infectious (staphylococcal) (streptococcal)
690.8	Infectious (staphylococcal) (streptococcal) eczematoid
695.89	Intertriginous superficial due to heat/moisture/friction
709.1	Lichenoides purpurica pigmentosa
692.3	Medicamentosa applied to skin
693.0	Medicamentosa ingested
694.0	Multiformis
694.2	Multiformis juvenile
694.5	Multiformis senile

DERMATITIS (continued)

691.8	Neurogenic
694.0	Neurotica
706.1	Papillaris capillitii
695.3	Perioral
694.0	Polymorpha dolorosa
694.0	Pruriginosa
694.2	Psoriasiform nodularis
316	Psychogenic [692.9]
686.00	Purulent
686.00	Pyococcal, pyococcide
686.09	Pyocyaneus
686.00	Pyogenica
690.10	Seborrheic
690.10	Seborrheic external ear [380.13]
690.11	Seborrheic capitis
690.11	Seborrheic capitis external ear [380.13]
690.12	Seborrheic infantile
690.12	Seborrheic infantile external ear [380.13]
690.18	Seborrheic other
690.18	Seborrheic other external ear [380.13]
686.00	Septic
0	Solar see 'Dermatitis Solar'
459.81	Stasis
459.81	Stasis ulcerated [**707.#(#)**]

4th or 4th and 5th digit: 707
- **1#. Lower limb except decubitus**
  - **0. Unspecified**
  - **1. Thigh**
  - **2. Calf**
  - **3. Ankle**
  - **4. Heel and midfoot**
  - **5. Other parts of foot, toes**
  - **9. Other**
- **8. Chronic of other specified site**
- **9. Chronic site NOS**

454.1	Stasis varicose
459.12	Stasis varicose due to postphlebitic syndrome
459.13	Stasis varicose due to postphlebitic syndrome with ulcer
459.12	Stasis varicose secondary to deep vein thrombosis
454.2	Stasis varicose ulcerated
454.8	Stasis varicose with edema
454.8	Stasis varicose with pain
454.8	Stasis varicose with swelling
454.8	Stasis varicose with other complications
709.8	Traumatic NEC
694.0	Trophoneurotica
686.8	Vegetans
117.2	Verrucosa

DERMATITIS CONTACT QUICK REFERENCE

692.9	NOS
692.4	Chemical products
692.0	Detergents
692.3	Drugs and medicines (in contact with skin)
692.5	Food (in contact with skin)
692.1	Oils and greases
692.6	Plants (except food)

D

DERMATITIS CONTACT QUICK REFERENCE (continued)

692.7# Solar radiation
5th digit: 692.7
0. NOS
1. Sunburn NOS (first degree)
2. Acute due to solar radiation
3. Actinic reticuloid and actinic granuloma
4. Chronic due to solar radiation
5. Disseminated superficial actinic porokeratosis (DSAP))
6. Sunburn second degree
7. Sunburn third degree
9. Other due to solar radiation

692.2 Solvents
686.00 Suppurative
692.8# Other specified
5th digit: 692.8
1. Due to cosmetics
2. Due to other radiation (tanning bed)
3. Due to metals, jewelry
4. Due to animal (cat) (dog) dander and hair
9. Other substances or transient temperature

DERMATITIS CONTACT

692.9 NOS
692.2 Acetone
692.4 Acids
692.4 Adhesive plaster (tape)
692.4 Alcohol (in contact with skin)
692.4 Alkalis
692.9 Allergy
692.4 Ammonia (household) (liquid)
692.84 Animal (cat) (dog) dander or hair
692.3 Arnica (in contact with skin)
692.4 Arsenic
692.89 Blister beetle
692.89 Caterpillar
692.4 Caustics
692.5 Cereal (in contact with skin)
692.2 Chlorocompound
692.5 Coffee (in contact with skin)
692.89 Cold weather
692.81 Cosmetics
692.2 Cyclohexane
692.81 Deodorant
692.0 Detergents
692.4 Dichromates
692.3 Drugs and medicines (in contact with skin)
692.89 Dyes
692.2 Ester
373.32 Eyelids
692.5 Fish (in contact with skin)
692.5 Flour (in contact with skin)
692.5 Fruit (in contact with skin)
692.3 Fungicides (in contact with skin)
692.84 Fur
692.2 Glycol
692.1 Grease
692.89 Hot weather or places
692.2 Hydrocarbons
692.82 Infrared rays
692.4 Insecticides

DERMATITIS CONTACT (continued)

692.3 Iodine (in contact with skin)
692.3 Iodoform (in contact with skin)
692.83 Jewelry
692.3 Keratolytics (in contact with skin)
692.2 Ketone group
692.6 Lacquer tree [Rhus Verniciflua]
692.82 Light, except sun
692.5 Meat (in contact with skin)
692.3 Mercurials (in contact with skin)
692.83 Metals
692.5 Milk (in contact with skin)
692.3 Neomycin (in contact with skin)
692.4 Nylon
692.1 Oil
692.2 Paint
692.3 Pediculocides (in contact with skin)
692.4 Petroleum
692.3 Phenols (in contact with skin)
692.6 Plants
692.3 Plasters medicated (in contact with skin)
692.4 Plastic
692.6 Poison ivy [RHUS toxicodendron]
692.6 Poison oak [RHUS diversiloba]
692.6 Poison sumac [RHUS venenata]
692.6 Poison vine [RHUS radicans]
692.89 Preservatives
692.6 Primrose [Primula]
692.82 Radioactive substances
692.6 Ragweed [Senecio Jacobae]
692.4 Rubber
692.3 Scabicides (in contact with skin)
0 Solar see 'Dermatitis Solar'
692.3 Topical medications (in contact with skin)
692.2 Turpentine
692.82 Ultraviolet rays, except sun
692.82 X-ray
692.4 Other chemical products
692.82 Other radiation
692.89 Other substances

DERMATITIS EYELID

039.3 Actinomycotic [373.5]
373.32 Contact and allergic
373.31 Eczematous
110.8 Dermatophytic [373.5]
054.41 Herpes simplex
053.20 Herpes zoster
684 Impetigo [373.5]
030.0 Lepromatous [373.4]
017.0# Lupus vulgaris (tuberculous) [373.4]
5th digit: 017.0
0. Unspecified
1. Lab not done
2. Lab pending
3. Microscopy positive (in sputum)
4. Culture positive - microscopy negative
5. Culture negative - microscopy positive
6. Culture and microscopy negative confirmed by other methods

111.9 Mycotic [373.5]
373.5 Other infective
999.0 Post vaccination [373.5]

D

DERMATITIS EYELID (continued)

017.0# Tuberculous [373.4]

5th digit: 017.0

0. Unspecified
1. Lab not done
2. Lab pending
3. Microscopy positive (in sputum)
4. Culture positive - microscopy negative
5. Culture negative - microscopy positive
6. Culture and microscopy negative confirmed by other methods

051.0 Vaccinia [373.5]
102.9 Yaws [373.4]

DERMATITIS SOLAR

692.70 NOS
692.73 Actinic reticuloid and actinic granuloma
692.72 Acute due to solar radiation
692.72 Acute solar skin damage NOS
692.72 Berloque
692.74 Chronic due to solar radiation
692.74 Chronic solar skin damage NOS
692.75 Disseminated superficial actinic porokeratosis (DSAP)
692.74 Elastosis
692.72 Photoallergic response
692.72 Phototoxic response
692.72 Polymorphus light eruption
692.79 Skin damage NOS
692.7# Sunburn

5th digit: 692.7

1. NOS (first degree)
6. Second degree
7. Third degree

692.79 Other

134.0 DERMATOBIA (HOMINIS) INFESTATION
374.87 DERMATOCHALASIS
216.# DERMATOFIBROMA NOS M8832/0

4th digit: 216

0. Lip skin
1. Eyelid including canthus
2. Ear external (auricle) (pinna)
3. Face (cheek) (nose)
4. Scalp, neck
5. Trunk, back, chest
6. Upper limb including shoulder
7. Lower limb including hip
8. Other specified sites
9. Skin unspecified

238.2 DERMATOFIBROMA PROTUBERANS SITE NOS
0 DERMATOFIBROMA PROTUBERANS SEE 'NEOPLASM UNCERTAIN BEHAVIOR', SKIN, BY SITE M8832/1
171.9 DERMATOFIBROSARCOMA SITE NOS
0 DERMATOFIBROSARCOMA SITE SPECIFIED SEE 'CANCER', SKIN, BY SITE M8832/3
757.2 DERMATOGLYPHIC ANOMALIES CONGENITAL
708.3 DERMATOGRAPHIA
111.9 DERMATOMYCOSIS
111.8 DERMATOMYCOSIS OTHER SPECIFIED
710.3 DERMATOMYOSITIS
110.1 DERMATOPHYTIC ONYCHIA

110.# DERMATOPHYTOSIS

4th digit: 110

0. Scalp and beard
1. Nail (unguium)
2. Hand (manuum)
3. Groin and perianal (cruris)
4. Foot (pedis)
5. Body (corporus)
6. Deep seated (granuloma trichophyticum)
8. Other specified site
9. Unspecified site

698.8 DERMATOPIELINOSIS
701.0 DERMATOSCLEROSIS LOCALIZED

DERMATOSIS

709.9 NOS
691.8 Atopic
694.9 Bullous
694.8 Bullous other
690.8 Erythematosquamous
695.89 Exfoliativa
698.4 Factitial
098.89 Gonococcal
694.0 Herpetiformis
694.2 Herpetiformis juvenile
694.5 Herpetiformis senile
694.8 Linear IGA
709.8 Menstrual
695.89 Neutrophilic, acute febrile
709.8 Papulosa nigra
709.00 Pigmentary NEC
0 Pregnancy see 'PUPP'
709.09 Progressive pigmentary
316 Psychogenic [709.9]
709.3 Senile NEC
690.10 Unna's (seborrheic dermatitis)

DERMOID CYST

229.9 Site NOS
0 Site specified see 'Benign Neoplasm', by site M9084/0
183.0 With malignant transformation site NOS
0 With malignant transformation site specified see 'Cancer', by site M9084/3

655.5# DES (KNOWN) (SUSPECTED) DAMAGE TO FETUS COMPLICATING PREGNANCY MANAGEMENT

5th digit: 655.5

0. Episode of care unspecified or N/A
1. Delivered
3. Antepartum complication

760.76 DES TRANSMITTED VIA PLACENTA OR BREAST MILK AFFECTING FETUS OR NEWBORN
371.32 DESCEMET'S MEMBRANE FOLDS
371.33 DESCEMET'S MEMBRANE RUPTURE
371.72 DESCEMETOCELE
V07.1 DESENSITIZATION ALLERGY
0 DESERT RHEUMATISM SEE 'COCCIDIOIDOMYCOSIS'
995.84 DESERTION ADULT
995.52 DESERTION CHILD (NEWBORN)

238.1 DESMOID TUMOR SITE UNSPECIFIED
0 DESMOID TUMOR (ABDOMINAL) SITE SPECIFIED SEE 'NEOPLASM UNCERTAIN BEHAVIOR' OTHER AND UNSPECIFIED SITES CONNECTIVE AND OTHER TISSUE M8822/1
0 DESMOID TUMOR (EXTRA-ABDOMINAL) SITE SPECIFIED SEE 'NEOPLASM UNCERTAIN BEHAVIOR' OTHER AND UNSPECIFIED SITES CONNECTIVE AND OTHER TISSUE M8821/1
362.43 DETACHMENT RETINAL PIGMENT EPITHELIUM HEMORRHAGIC
977.3 DETERRENT ALCOHOL
270.0 DE TONI-FANCONI (-DEBRE) SYNDROME (CYSTINOSIS)
596.59 DETRUSOR INSTABILITY
596.55 DETRUSOR SPHINCTER DYSSYNERGIA
368.52 DEUTAN DEFECT
368.52 DEUTERANOMALY
368.52 DEUTERANOPIA
117.4 DEUTEROMYCETES INFECTION
0 DEUTSCHLANDER'S SEE 'FRACTURE' FOOT

DEVELOPMENTAL DISORDER

315.9 NOS
314.1 Associated with hyperkinesia
315.4 Clumsiness syndrome
315.4 Coordination
783.42 Delay milestones in childhood (late walker) (late talker)
783.40 Delay physiological in childhood
V79.9 Handicaps screening
V79.3 Handicaps in early childhood screening
V79.8 Handicaps other specified screening
783.40 Inadequate in childhood

Use an additional code to indentify the type of hearing loss. See 'HEARING LOSS'.

315.34 Language due to hearing loss
315.31 Language expressive
315.32 Language receptive (receptive-expressive) (mixed)
315.9 Learning NOS
315.2 Learning other specified
315.1 Mathematics
315.5 Mixed
315.39 Phonological (speech) (reading)
783.9 Physiological developmental problem
315.00 Reading
315.39 Reading phonological
783.43 Short stature

Use an additional code to indentify the type of hearing loss. See 'HEARING LOSS'.

315.34 Speech due to hearing loss
315.39 Speech phonological
315.09 Spelling
V20.2 Testing (child) (infant)
315.31 Word deafness (delay in development)
315.2 Written expression
315.2 Other specified learning disorder
315.09 Other specified reading or spelling disorder
315.39 Other specified speech or language disorder
315.8 Other specified delay in development

696.4 DEVERGIE'S PITYRIASIS RUBRA PILARIS

470 DEVIATED NASAL SEPTUM (ACQUIRED)
V53.90 DEVICE UNSPECIFIED FITTING AND ADJUSTMENT
V53.99 DEVICE OTHER FITTING AND ADJUSTMENT
341.0 DEVIC'S NEUROMYELITIS OPTICA
074.1 DEVIL'S GRIP
746.87 DEXTROCARDIA
759.3 DEXTROCARDIA WITH VISCERA
110.3 DHOBIE ITCH

Type I (insulin - dependent) diabetics cannot produce enough insulin to sustain life. Type II (non-insulin dependent) diabetics produce insulin, but have problems utilizing it. Though they may be taking insulin on a day - to - day basis, they are still considered to be non-insulin dependent and therefore, type II diabetics. The physician must document the type for the record to be coded. Use the additional code, V58.67 long-term (current) insulin use for Type II diabetics that take insulin on a day – to – day basis.

DIABETES, DIABETIC

250.0# NOS
250.0# Uncomplicated
250.9# Unspecified complication
0 Acidosis see 'Diabetes, Diabetic', ketoacidosis

5th digit: 250
0. Type II, adult-onset, non-insulin dependent (even if requiring insulin), or unspecified; controlled
1. Type I, juvenile-onset or insulin-dependent; controlled
2. Type II, adult-onset, non-insulin dependent (even if requiring insulin); uncontrolled
3. Type I, juvenile-onset or insulin-dependent; uncontrolled

250.4# Acute renal failure [584.#]

4th digit: 584
5. With tubular necrosis
6. Renal cortical necrosis
7. Medullary (papillary) necrosis
8. Specified pathological lesion
9. Renal failure unspecified

250.6# Amyotrophy syndrome [353.1]
250.7# Angiopathy (peripheral) [443.81]
250.6# Arthropathy (neurogenic) [713.5]
790.29 Asymptomatic

Diabetic blindness requires a second code for the amount of impairment. See "Vision Impairment" for second code.

250.5# Blindness
250.0# Brittle
250.5# Cataract [366.41]

5th digit: 250
0. Type II, adult-onset, non-insulin dependent (even if requiring insulin), or unspecified; controlled
1. Type I, juvenile-onset or insulin-dependent; controlled
2. Type II, adult-onset, non-insulin dependent (even if requiring insulin); uncontrolled
3. Type I, juvenile-onset or insulin-dependent; uncontrolled

D

Type I (insulin - dependent) diabetics cannot produce enough insulin to sustain life. Type II (non-insulin dependent) diabetics produce insulin, but have problems utilizing it. Though they may be taking insulin on a day - to - day basis, they are still considered to be non-insulin dependent and therefore, type II diabetics. The physician must document the type for the record to be coded. Use the additional code, V58.67 long-term (current) insulin use for Type II diabetics that take insulin on a day – to – day basis.

DIABETES, DIABETIC (continued)

790.29 Chemical
250.4# Chronic renal failure (kidney disease) **[585.#]**
4th digit: 585
1. Stage I
2. Stage II (mild)
3. Stage III (moderate)
4. Stage IV (severe)
5. Stage V
6. End stage
9. Unspecified stage

250.7# Circulatory disorder peripheral
250.2# Coma hyperosmolar (non ketotic)
250.3# Coma hypoglycemic
250.3# Coma insulin
250.3# Coma ketoacidotic
250.6# Dorsal sclerosis [340]
5th digit: 250
0. Type II, adult-onset, non-insulin dependent (even if requiring insulin), or unspecified; controlled
1. Type I, juvenile-onset or insulin-dependent; controlled
2. Type II, adult-onset, non-insulin dependent (even if requiring insulin); uncontrolled
3. Type I, juvenile-onset or insulin-dependent; uncontrolled

258.1 Dwarfism obesity syndrome
V18.0 Family history

Diabetic gangrene [785.4] requires code 250.7# before code 785.4. Remember, the code to the left of the description always sequences first.

250.7# Gangrene [785.4]
250.6# Gastroparalysis [536.3]
250.6# Gastroparesis [536.3]
5th digit: 250
0. Type II, adult-onset, non-insulin dependent (even if requiring insulin), or unspecified; controlled
1. Type I, juvenile-onset or insulin-dependent; controlled
2. Type II, adult-onset, non-insulin dependent (even if requiring insulin); uncontrolled
3. Type I, juvenile-onset or insulin-dependent; uncontrolled

648.8# Gestational
5th digit: 648.8
0. Episode of care unspecified or N/A
1. Delivered
2. Delivered with postpartum complication
3. Antepartum complication
4. Postpartum complication

DIABETES, DIABETIC (continued)

250.5# Glaucoma [365.44]
250.4# Glomerulosclerosis (intercapillary) [581.81]
250.8# Glycogenosis, secondary [259.8]
250.2# Hyperosmolar (non ketotic) coma
250.3# Hyperosmolar (ketoacidotic) coma
250.2# Hyperosmolarity
250.4# Hypertension-nephrosis syndrome [581.81]
250.8# Hypoglycemia
250.3# Hypoglycemic coma
250.8# Hypoglycemic shock
253.5 Insipidus
588.1 Insipidus nephrogenic
250.3# Insulin coma
250.5# Iritis [364.42]
250.1# Ketoacidosis
250.3# Ketoacidosis coma
250.4# Kimmelstiel Wilson disease [581.81]
250.8# Lancereaux's [261]
790.29 Latent (chemical)
250.8# Lipoidosis [272.7]
0 Macular edema see 'Diabetes, Diabetic', retinopathy
250.5# Macular edema cystoid [362.53]
5th digit: 250
0. Type II, adult-onset, non-insulin dependent (even if requiring insulin), or unspecified; controlled
1. Type I, juvenile-onset or insulin-dependent; controlled
2. Type II, adult-onset, non-insulin dependent (even if requiring insulin); uncontrolled
3. Type I, juvenile-onset or insulin-dependent; uncontrolled

775.0 Maternal affecting infant (with hypoglycemia)

648.0#: Specify the maternal diabetes with an additional code for the specific diabetes. See 'Diabetes, Diabetic'.

648.0# Maternal current (co-existent) in pregnancy
648.8# Maternal gestational
5th digit: 648.0, 648.8
0. Episode of care unspecified or N/A
1. Delivered
2. Delivered with postpartum complication
3. Antepartum complication
4. Postpartum complication

250.6# Mononeuritis NOS [355.9]
250.6# Mononeuritis lower limb [355.8]
250.6# Mononeuritis upper limb [354.9]
250.8# Necrobiosis lipoidica diabeticorum [709.3]
775.1 Neonatal
588.1 Nephrogenic
5th digit: 250
0. Type II, adult-onset, non-insulin dependent (even if requiring insulin), or unspecified; controlled
1. Type I, juvenile-onset or insulin-dependent; controlled
2. Type II, adult-onset, non-insulin dependent (even if requiring insulin); uncontrolled
3. Type I, juvenile-onset or insulin-dependent; uncontrolled

D

Type I (insulin - dependent) diabetics cannot produce enough insulin to sustain life. Type II (non-insulin dependent) diabetics produce insulin, but have problems utilizing it. Though they may be taking insulin on a day - to - day basis, they are still considered to be non-insulin dependent and therefore, type II diabetics. The physician must document the type for the record to be coded. Use the additional code, V58.67 long-term (current) insulin use for Type II diabetics that take insulin on a day – to – day basis.

DIABETES, DIABETIC (continued)

250.4# Nephritis [583.81]
250.4# Nephritis with nephrotic syndrome [581.81]
250.4# Nephropathy [583.81]
250.4# Nephrosis [581.81]
250.4# Nephrotic syndrome [581.81]
250.6# Neuralgia [357.2]
250.6# Neurological manifestations
250.6# Neuropathy NOS [357.2]
250.6# Neuropathy mononeuritis site NOS [355.9]
250.6# Neuropathy mononeuritis lower limb [355.8]
250.6# Neuropathy mononeuritis upper limb [354.9]
250.6# Neuropathy peripheral autonomic [337.1]
250.6# Neuropathy polyneuropathy [357.2]
775.1 Newborn infant syndrome
790.29 Nonclinical
250.8# Osteopathy [731.8]
250.8# Osteomyelitis [731.8] **[730.0#]**

5th digit: 250
0. Type II, adult-onset, non-insulin dependent (even if requiring insulin), or unspecified; controlled
1. Type I, juvenile-onset or insulin-dependent; controlled
2. Type II, adult-onset, non-insulin dependent (even if requiring insulin); uncontrolled
3. Type I, juvenile-onset or insulin-dependent; uncontrolled

5th digit: 730.0
0. Site NOS
1. Shoulder region
2. Upper arm (elbow) (humerus)
3. Forearm (radius) (wrist) (ulna)
4. Hand (carpal) (metacarpal) (fingers)
5. Pelvic region (hip) (buttock) (femur) and thigh
6. Lower leg (fibula) (knee) (patella) (tibia)
7. Ankle and or foot (metatarsals) (toes) (tarsals)
8. Other (head) (neck) (rib) (skull) (trunk) (vertebrae)
9. Multiple

DIABETES, DIABETIC (continued)

250.7# Peripheral vascular disease [443.81]
253.5 Pituitary
250.6# Polyneuropathy [357.2]
250.0# Poorly controlled

5th digit: 250
0. Type II, adult-onset, non-insulin dependent (even if requiring insulin), or unspecified; controlled
1. Type I, juvenile-onset or insulin-dependent; controlled
2. Type II, adult-onset, non-insulin dependent (even if requiring insulin); uncontrolled
3. Type I, juvenile-onset or insulin-dependent; uncontrolled

271.4 Renal glycosuria
0 Retinal edema see 'Diabetes, Diabetic', retinopathy
250.5# Retinal hemorrhage (microaneurysms) [362.01]
250.5# Retinitis [362.01]
250.5# Retinopathy **[362.0#]**
250.5# Retinopathy with macular or retinal edema **[362.0#]** [362.07]

4th digit: 362.0
1. Background or NOS
2. Proliferative
3. Nonproliferative NOS
4. Nonproliferative mild
5. Nonproliferative moderate
6. Nonproliferative severe

V77.1 Screening
251.8 Steroid induced
790.29 Stress
250.4# Renal disease [583.81]
790.29 Subclinical
790.29 Subliminal
250.8# Ulcer **[707.#(#)]**
250.6# Ulcer - neuropathic **[707.#(#)]**
250.7# Ulcer - peripheral vascular **[707.#(#)]**

5th digit: 250
0. Type II, adult-onset, non-insulin dependent (even if requiring insulin), or unspecified; controlled
1. Type I, juvenile-onset or insulin-dependent; controlled
2. Type II, adult-onset, non-insulin dependent (even if requiring insulin); uncontrolled
3. Type I, juvenile-onset or insulin-dependent; uncontrolled

4th or 4th and 5th digit: 707
1#. Lower limb except decubitus
0. Unspecified
1. Thigh
2. Calf
3. Ankle
4. Heel and midfoot
5. Other parts of foot, toes
9. Other
8. Chronic of other specified site
9. Chronic site NOS

D

DIABETES, DIABETIC (continued)

588.1 Vaso-pressin resistant
250.9# With complications (unspecified)
250.7# With circulatory (peripheral) manifestations
250.2# With coma hyperosmolar
250.3# With coma other (hypoglycemic) (insulin)
250.1# With ketoacidosis
250.6# With neurological manifestations
250.5# With ophthalmic manifestations
250.4# With renal manifestations
250.8# With other specified manifestations
250.8# Xanthoma [272.2]

5th digit: 250
0. Type II, adult-onset, non-insulin dependent (even if requiring insulin), or unspecified; controlled
1. Type I, juvenile-onset or insulin-dependent; controlled
2. Type II, adult-onset, non-insulin dependent (even if requiring insulin); uncontrolled
3. Type I, juvenile-onset or insulin-dependent; uncontrolled

> *V56.#, Admission for dialysis, should be assigned as the principal diagnosis when the encounter is for the sole purpose of dialysis. Use an additional code for the condition for which dialysis is performed.*

DIALYSIS

V56.31 Adequacy testing hemodialysis
V56.32 Adequacy testing peritoneal
V56.0 Admission/encounter for - extracorporeal treatment
V56.8 Admission/encounter for - peritoneal treatment
996.62 A-V fistula or shunt complication - infection or inflammation
996.1 A-V fistula or shunt complication - mechanical
996.74 A-V fistula or shunt complication - other
999.9 Complication NOS medical (hemodialysis) (renal)
294.8 Dementia [E879.1]
985.8 Dementia due to aluminum overload [294.8] [E879.1]
293.9 Dementia transient [E879.1]
276.9 Disequilibrium [E879.1]
792.5 Effluent cloudy (hemodialysis) (peritoneal)
V56.31 Extracorporeal adequacy testing
V56.1 Extracorporeal catheter care (removal) (replacement) (toilet) (cleansing)
996.62 Extracorporeal catheter complication - infection or inflammation
996.1 Extracorporeal catheter complication - mechanical
996.73 Extracorporeal catheter complication - other
V45.1 Extracorporeal status
V56.0 Extracorporeal treatment encounter (intermittent)
V45.1 Hemodialysis status
V56.32 Peritoneal adequacy testing
V56.2 Peritoneal catheter care (removal) (replacement) (toilet) (cleansing)
996.68 Peritoneal catheter complication - infection or inflammation, exit site
996.56 Peritoneal catheter complication - mechanical
996.79 Peritoneal catheter complication - other
V45.1 Peritoneal status
V56.8 Peritoneal treatment encounter (intermittent)
0 Preparation - code underlying condition

DIALYSIS (continued)

V56.1 Renal catheter care (removal) (replacement) (toilet) (cleansing)
996.62 Renal catheter complication - infection or inflammation
996.1 Renal catheter complication - mechanical
996.73 Renal catheter complication - other
V45.1 Renal status
V56.0 Renal treatment encounter (intermittent)

284.01 DIAMOND BLACKFAN ANEMIA (SYNDROME) (CONGENITAL HYPOPLASTIC ANEMIA)

287.2 DIAMOND-GARDENER SYNDROME (AUTOERYTHROCYTE SENSITIZATION)

691.0 DIAPER DERMATITIS
691.0 DIAPER RASH
289.7 DIAPHORASE DEFICIENCY
780.8 DIAPHORESIS

DIAPHRAGM

756.6 Absence (congenital)
756.6 Defect congenital
551.3 Defect hernia with gangrene
519.4 Disorder
756.6 Eventration congenital
V25.02 Fitting for contraception
756.6 Hernia congenital
862.0 Injury
862.1 Injury with open wound into cavity
908.0 Injury late effect
519.4 Paralysis
519.4 Relaxation

519.4 DIAPHRAGMITIS
733.99 DIAPHYSITIS

DIARRHEA

787.91 NOS
787.91 Acute
558.3 Allergic
558.3 Allergic due to ingested foods [**V15.0#**]

5th digit: V15.0
1. Peanuts
2. Milk products
3. Eggs
4. Seafood
5. Other foods

007.0 Balantidial
787.91 Cachectic NEC
787.91 Chronic
007.2 Coccidial
007.4 Cryptosporidial
007.5 Cyclosporiasis
787.91 Dietetic
008.2 Due to enterobacter aerogenes
787.91 Due to irritating foods
009.2 Dysenteric
787.91 Dyspeptic
009.3 Endemic
009.2 Epidemic
787.91 Fermentative
007.9 Flagellate
564.5 Functional
007.1 Giardial
009.2 Infectious
009.3 Infectious origin presumed
787.91 Inflammatory

DIARRHEA (continued)

787.91 Noninfectious
558.9 Noninfectious due to gastroenteritis or colitis
564.4 Post gastrectomy or post vagotomy
564.4 Post op GI surgery
007.# Protozoal
4th digit: 007
0. Balantidiasis
1. Giardiasis
2. Coccidiosis
3. Trichomoniasis
4. Cryptosporidiosis
5. Cyclosporiasis
8. Other specified
9. Unspecified

306.4 Psychogenic (cyclical)
009.2 Travelers
007.3 Trichomonal
008.8 Viral

DIASTASIS

733.99 Cranial bones
756.0 Cranial bones congenital
728.84 Muscle
728.84 Rectus abdominis
665.8# Rectus abdominis complicating pregnancy
5th digit: 665.8
0. Episode of care NOS or N/A
1. Delivered
2. Delivered with postpartum complication
3. Antepartum complication
4. Postpartum complication

756.79 Rectus abdominis congenital

742.51 DIASTEMATOMYELIA SPINAL CORD CONGENITAL
428.4# DIASTOLIC AND SYSTOLIC HEART FAILURE
429.9 DIASTOLIC DYSFUNCTION
428.3# DIASTOLIC HEART FAILURE
5th digit: 428.3-4
0. NOS
1. Acute
2. Chronic
3. Acute on chronic

502 DIATOMACEOUS EARTH DISEASE (OCCUPATIONAL)
732.5 DIAZ'S OSTEOCHONDROSIS ASTRAGALUS
963.1 DIBROMOMANNITOL
286.6 DIC (SYNDROME)
776.2 DIC NEWBORN
759.4 DICEPHALUS
V74.8 DICK SCREENING EXAM
121.8 DICROCOELIUM DENDRITICUM INFECTION
253.8 DIENCEPHALOHYPOPHYSEAL SYNDROME
V69.1 DIET AND EATING HABITS PROBLEM

V65.3 Use an additional code to identify body mass index (BMI), if known. See 'Body Mass Index'.

V65.3 DIET COUNSELING
760.76 DIETHYLSTILBESTROL (DES) TRANSMITTED VIA PLACENTA OR BREAST MILK AFFECTING FETUS OR NEWBORN

537.84 DIEULAFOY LESION (HEMORRHAGIC) DUODENUM
530.82 DIEULAFOY LESION (HEMORRHAGIC) ESOPHAGUS
569.86 DIEULAFOY LESION (HEMORRHAGIC) INTESTINE
537.84 DIEULAFOY LESION (HEMORRHAGIC) STOMACH
0 DIEULAFOY'S ULCER SEE 'ULCER', PYLORIC
151.9 DIFFUSE CARCINOMA SITE NOS
0 DIFFUSE CARCINOMA SITE SPECIFIED SEE 'CANCER', BY SITE M8145/3
723.3 DIFFUSE CERVICOBRACHIAL SYNDROME
496 DIFFUSE OBSTRUCTIVE PULMONARY SYNDROME
286.6 DIFFUSE OR DISSEMINATED DIC SYNDROME
279.11 DIGEORGE'S SYNDROME (THYMIC HYPOPLASIA)

DIGESTIVE

V45.79 Absence organ or tract acquired
751.8 Absence organ or tract congenital
751.2 Absence organ or tract congenital - lower
750.8 Absence organ or tract congenital - upper
536.9 Disorder
564.9 Disorder functional NOS
306.4 Disorder psychogenic
V12.70 History of disease
V12.79 History of disease other specified
751.8 Organs NOS duplication (malposition) congenital
V47.3 Problem other
751.9 System anomaly NOS - congenital
751.8 System anomalies other specified- congenital
751.8 System atresia
777.9 System disorder perinatal
777.8 System disorder perinatal other specified
787.99 System symptoms
V55.4 Tract artificial opening care (other)

756.51 DIGHTON'S SYNDROME
0 DIGIT SEE 'FINGER' OR 'THUMB' OR 'TOE'

DIGITAL

903.5 Artery injury
908.3 Artery or blood vessel injury or laceration late effect
903.5 Blood vessels injury
903.5 Blood vessels laceration (rupture) (hematoma) (avulsion) (aneurysm) traumatic
955.6 Nerve injury
907.4 Nerve injury late effect

207.0# DI GUGLIELMO'S DISEASE OR SYNDROME (ERYTHREMIC MYELOSIS) M9841/3
5th digit: 207.0
0. Without mention of remission
1. With mention of remission

796.0 DILANTIN TOXICITY - ASYMPTOMATIC
0 DILANTIN TOXICITY - SYMPTOMATIC SEE DRUGS AND CHEMICALS (APPENDIX B) OR 'POISONING MEDICINAL'
305.3# DIMETHYLTRYPTAMINE (DMT) ABUSE (NONDEPENDENT)
304.5# DIMETHYLTRYPTAMINE (DMT) ADDICTION (DEPENDENT)
5th digit: 304.5, 305.3
0. Unspecified
1. Continuous
2. Episodic
3. In remission

D

759.6 DIMITRI-STURGE-WEBER ENCEPHALOCUTANEOUS ANGIOMATOSIS
125.4 DIPETALONEMA PERSTANS INFECTION
125.6 DIPETALONEMA STREPTOCERCA INFECTION
125.4 DIPETALONEMIASIS
752.69 DIPHALLUS

DIPHTHERIA, DIPHTHERITIC

032.9 NOS
032.0 Angina gangrenous
032.0 Angina malignant
032.0 Angina membranous
032.0 Angina phlegmonous
032.2 Anterior nasal
V02.4 Carrier
032.81 Conjunctival
032.85 Cutaneous
032.84 Cystitis
032.0 Faucial
032.9 Infection
032.3 Laryngeal
032.82 Myocarditis
032.1 Nasopharyngeal
032.83 Peritonitis
0 Polyneuropathy see 'Polyneuropathy', diphtheritic
V74.3 Screening exam
032.3 Tracheitis
032.89 Other
V03.5 Vaccination single
V06.5 Vaccination tetanus - diptheria

0 DIPHTHERITIC SEE 'DIPHTHERIA, DIPHTHERITIC'

123.4 DIPHYLLOBOTHRIASIS INTESTINAL
123.4 DIPHYLLOBOTHRIUM INFECTION (ADULT)
123.5 DIPHYLLOBOTHRIUM LARVAE INFECTION
388.41 DIPLACUSIS

DIPLEGIA

344.1 Acquired lower limb (old)
438.53 Acquired lower limb (old) - late effect of cerebrovascular disease [344.1]
344.2 Acquired upper limb (old)
438.53 Acquired upper limb (old) - late effect of cerebrovascular disease [344.2]
343.0 Congenital

123.8 DIPLOGONOPORUS INFECTION (GRANDIS)
368.2 DIPLOPIA
368.15 DIPLOPIA REFRACTIVE
303.9# DIPSOMANIA
5th digit: 303.9
0. NOS
1. Continuous
2. Episodic
3. In remission

123.8 DIPYLIDIUM INFECTION (CANINUM)
125.6 DIROFILARIA INFECTION
307.52 DIRT EATING CHILD

Use additional code(s) to identify: specific examination(s), screening and testing performed.

V68.01 DISABILITY CERTIFICATE ISSUE

0 DISARTICULATION SEE 'AMPUTATION'

When coding back disorders due to degeneration, displacement or HNP of the intervertebral disc, it is important to distinguish whether these conditions are with or without myelopathy. Myelopathy refers to functional disturbances and/or pathological changes in the spinal cord that result from compression.

722.10 Lumbar disc herniation (HNP)

722.73 Lumbar disc herniation (HNP) with myelopathy

DISC (INTERVERTEBRAL)

0 Bulge see 'Disc (Intervertebral)', displacement, by site

CALCIFICATION OR DISCITIS

722.90 NOS
722.91 Cervical
722.93 Lumbar (lumbosacral)
722.92 Thoracic (thoracolumbar)

DEGENERATIVE DISEASE (DEGENERATION)

722.6 Site NOS
722.70 Site NOS with myelopathy
722.4 Cervical
722.71 Cervical with myelopathy
722.52 Lumbar (lumbosacral)
722.73 Lumbar (lumbosacral) with myelopathy
722.51 Thoracic (thoracolumbar)
722.72 Thoracic (thoracolumbar) with myelopathy

DISORDER

722.90 Unspecified
722.70 Unspecified with myelopathy

DISPLACEMENT (RUPTURE)

722.2 Site NOS
722.70 Site NOS with myelopathy
722.0 Cervical
722.71 Cervical with myelopathy
722.10 Lumbar
722.73 Lumbar with myelopathy
722.11 Thoracic
722.72 Thoracic with myelopathy

HERNIATION

722.2 Site NOS
722.70 Site NOS with myelopathy
722.0 Cervical
722.71 Cervical with myelopathy
722.10 Lumbar
722.73 Lumbar with myelopathy
722.11 Thoracic
722.72 Thoracic with myelopathy

DISC (INTERVERTEBRAL) (continued)

0 Slipped see 'Disc (Intervertebral)', displacement, by site

0 DISCHARGE SEE BY ANATOMICAL SITE
722.9# DISCITIS (INTERVERTEBRAL)
5th digit: 722.9
0. Unspecified
1. Cervical
2. Thoracic
3. Lumbar

373.34 DISCOID LUPUS ERYTHEMATOSUS EYELID
717.5 DISCOID MENISCUS - OLD

V62.4 DISCRIMINATION (POLITICAL) (RELIGIOUS) (SEX)

0 DISEASE SEE BY ANATOMICAL SITE OR SPECIFIED DISORDER

799.9 DISEASE UNDIAGNOSED CAUSE OF MORBIDITY AND MORTALITY

276.9 DISEQUILIBRIUM (ELECTROLYTES) SYNDROME

276.9 DISEQUILIBRIUM DUE TO DIALYSIS [E879.1]

V48.6 DISFIGUREMENT HEAD

V48.7 DISFIGUREMENT NECK

V48.7 DISFIGUREMENT TRUNK

299.1# DISINTEGRATIVE DISORDER OF CHILDHOOD

5th digit: 299.1

0. Current or active state

1. Residual state

799.89 DISINTERGRATION COMPLETE OF BODY

In coding multiple injuries, sequence the most severe injury first. Open dislocations sequence before closed dislocations.

For pathological dislocations, look under "Dislocation Pathological".

DISLOCATION

839.8 NOS closed
839.9 NOS open

831.04 Acromioclavicular closed
831.14 Acromioclavicular open

837.0 Ankle closed
837.1 Ankle open

839.8 Arm closed
839.9 Arm open
839.8 Arm multiple and ill-defined closed
839.9 Arm multiple and ill-defined open

837.0 Astragalus closed
837.1 Astragalus open

839.01 Atlanto axial closed
839.11 Atlanto axial open
839.01 Atlas closed
839.11 Atlas open
839.02 Axis closed
839.12 Axis open

839.8 Back closed
839.9 Back open
839.8 Back multiple and ill-defined closed
839.9 Back multiple and ill-defined open

723.8 Bell-Daly

839.61 Breast bone closed
839.71 Breast bone open

833.00 Carpal (bone) closed
833.10 Carpal (bone) open

833.04 Carpometacarpal closed
833.14 Carpometacarpal open

DISLOCATION (continued)

839.0# Cervical spine (vertebra) closed
839.1# Cervical spine (vertebra) open

5th digit: 839.0-1

0. Cervical vertebra unspecified
1. First cervical vertebra
2. Second cervical vertebra
3. Third cervical vertebra
4. Fourth cervical vertebra
5. Fifth cervical vertebra
6. Sixth cervical vertebra
7. Seventh cervical vertebra
8. Multiple cervical vertebra

756.19 Cervical spine (vertebra) congenital
723.8 Cervical spine (vertebra) pathologic or recurrent

0 Chiropractic see 'Lesion', nonallopathic

831.04 Clavicle closed
831.14 Clavicle open

839.41 Coccyx closed
839.51 Coccyx open
724.79 Coccyx pathologic or recurrent

831.04 Collar bone closed
831.14 Collar bone open

831.09 Coracoid closed
831.19 Coracoid open

839.69 Costal cartilage closed
839.79 Costal cartilage open

839.69 Costochondral closed
839.79 Costochondral open

839.69 Cricoarytenoid articulation closed
839.79 Cricoarytenoid articulation open

839.69 Cricothyroid (cartilage) articulation closed
839.79 Cricothyroid (cartilage) articulation open

718.7# Developmental

5th digit: 718.7

0. Site unspecified
1. Shoulder region
2. Upper arm (elbow) (humerus)
3. Forearm (radius) (wrist) (ulna)
4. Hand (carpal) (metacarpal) (fingers)
5. Pelvic region (hip) (buttock) (femur)
6. Lower leg (fibula) (knee) (patella) (tibia)
7. Ankle and or foot (metatarsals) (toes) (tarsals)
8. Other
9. Multiple

385.23 Ear ossicles

832.0# Elbow closed
832.1# Elbow open

5th digit: 832.0-1

0. Unspecified
1. Anterior
2. Posterior
3. Medial
4. Lateral
9. Other

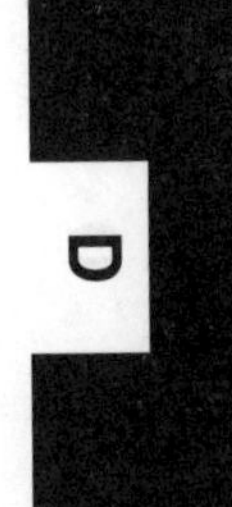

DISLOCATION (continued)

754.89 Elbow congenital
718.72 Elbow developmental
832.01 Elbow nursemaid's
718.22 Elbow pathological
718.32 Elbow recurrent old

360.81 Eye or eyeball
376.36 Eye or eyeball lateral

0 Femur distal end see 'Dislocation', knee
0 Femur proximal end see 'Dislocation', hip

837.0 Fibula distal end closed
837.1 Fibula distal end open
0 Fibula proximal end see 'Dislocation', knee

834.00 Finger closed
834.02 Finger closed interphalangeal
834.01 Finger closed metacarpophalangeal
718.74 Finger developmental
834.10 Finger open
834.12 Finger open interphalangeal
834.11 Finger open metacarpophalangeal
718.24 Finger pathological
718.34 Finger recurrent old

838.## Foot
4th digit: 838
0. Closed
1. Open

5th digit: 838
0. Foot unspecified
1. Tarsal (bone) joint unspecified
2. Midtarsal (joint)
3. Tarsometatarsal (bone)
4. Metatarsal (bone) joint unspecified
5. Metatarsophalangeal (joint)
6. Interphalangeal (joint) foot
9. Other

718.77 Foot developmental
718.27 Foot pathological
718.37 Foot recurrent

831.09 Glenoid closed
831.19 Glenoid open

839.8 Hand closed
839.9 Hand open
839.8 Hand multiple and ill-defined closed
839.9 Hand multiple and ill-defined open

835.## Hip
4th digit: 835
0. Closed
1. Open

5th digit: 835
0. Unspecified
1. Posterior
2. Obturator
3. Anterior

754.30 Hip congenital
754.31 Hip congenital bilateral
754.35 Hip congenital with subluxation of other hip
718.75 Hip developmental
996.42 Hip joint prosthesis [V43.64]

DISLOCATION (continued)

665.6# Hip, maternal, birthing trauma
5th digit: 665.6
0. Episode of care unspecified or N/A
1. Delivered
4. Postpartum complication

718.25 Hip pathological
718.35 Hip recurrent old
V82.3 Hip (congenital) screening

0 Humerus distal see 'Dislocation', elbow
831.0# Humerus proximal closed
831.1# Humerus proximal open
5th digit: 831.0-1
0. Unspecified
1. Anterior
2. Posterior
3. Inferior

385.23 Incus

831.01 Infracoracoid closed
831.11 Infracoracoid open

839.69 Innominate (pubic junction) (sacral junction) closed
839.79 Innominate (pubic junction) (sacral junction) open

0 Intercarpal see 'Dislocation', wrist

834.02 Interphalangeal finger or hand closed
834.12 Interphalangeal finger or hand open

838.06 Interphalangeal foot or toe closed
838.16 Interphalangeal foot or toe open

830.0 Jaw closed (cartilage) (meniscus) (TMJ)
830.1 Jaw open (cartilage) (meniscus) (TMJ)
524.69 Jaw recurrent

836.5# Knee closed
836.6# Knee open
5th digit: 836.5-6
0. Unspecified
1. Anterior
2. Posterior
3. Medial
4. Lateral end
9. Other or rotatory

754.41 Knee congenital with genu recurvatum
718.76 Knee developmental
718.26 Knee pathological
836.59 Knee rotatory closed
836.69 Knee rotatory open
718.36 Knee recurrent old

375.16 Lacrimal gland
905.6 Late effect

839.8 Leg closed
839.9 Leg open

379.32 Lens (crystalline) (complete) (partial)
379.33 Lens anterior
743.37 Lens congenital
379.34 Lens posterior
921.3 Lens traumatic

839.20 Lumbar vertebra closed
839.30 Lumbar vertebra open
839.20 Lumbosacral closed

DISLOCATION (continued)

839.30 Lumbosacral open
756.19 Lumbosacral congenital
724.6 Lumbosacral pathologic or recurrent

0 Lunate see 'Dislocation', wrist

830.0 Mandible closed (TMJ)
830.1 Mandible open (TMJ)

830.0 Maxilla (inferior) closed
830.1 Maxilla (inferior) open

834.01 Metacarpal (bone) distal end closed
834.11 Metacarpal (bone) distal end open
833.05 Metacarpal (bone) proximal end closed
833.15 Metacarpal (bone) proximal end open

834.01 Metacarpophalangeal closed
834.11 Metacarpophalangeal open

838.04 Metatarsal (bone) closed
838.14 Metatarsal (bone) open

838.05 Metatarsophalangeal closed
838.15 Metatarsophalangeal open

833.03 Midcarpal closed
833.13 Midcarpal open

838.02 Midtarsal closed
838.12 Midtarsal open

0 Monteggia's see 'Dislocation', hip

839.8 Multiple and ill-defined closed
839.9 Multiple and ill-defined open

837.0 Navicular foot closed
837.1 Navicular foot open

0 Neck see 'Dislocation', cervical spine

0 Nelaton's see 'Dislocation', ankle

832.01 Nursemaid's elbow
831.0# Nursemaid's shoulder

5th digit: 831.0
0. Unspecified
1. Anterior
2. Posterior
3. Inferior
4. Acromioclavicular
9. Scapula

839.69 Nose closed
839.79 Nose open

839.01 Occiput from atlas closed
839.11 Occiput from atlas open

996.53 Ocular implant

836.3 Patella closed
836.4 Patella open
755.64 Patella congenital
718.76 Patella developmental
718.26 Patella pathologic
718.36 Patella recurrent old

DISLOCATION (continued)

718.2# Pathological

5th digit: 718.2
0. Site unspecified
1. Shoulder region
2. Upper arm (elbow) (humerus)
3. Forearm (radius) (wrist) (ulna)
4. Hand (carpal) (metacarpal) (fingers)
5. Pelvic region (hip) (buttock) (femur)
6. Lower leg (fibula) (knee) (patella) (tibia)
7. Ankle and or foot (metatarsals) (toes) (tarsals)
8. Other
9. Multiple

724.8 Pathological spine - NOS
724.6 Pathological spine - lumbosacral joint
724.6 Pathological spine - sacroiliac joint

839.69 Pelvis closed
839.79 Pelvis open

0 Phalanx of foot or toe see 'Dislocation', toe
0 Phalanx of hand see 'Dislocation', finger

832.01 Radial head closed
832.11 Radial head open

833.02 Radiocarpal closed
833.12 Radiocarpal open

833.01 Radioulnar distal end closed
833.11 Radioulnar distal end open
0 Radioulnar proximal end see 'Dislocation', elbow

833.00 Radius distal end closed
833.10 Radius distal end open
0 Radius proximal end see 'Dislocation', elbow

718.3# Recurrent

5th digit: 718.3
0. Site unspecified
1. Shoulder region
2. Upper arm (elbow) (humerus)
3. Forearm (radius) (wrist) (ulna)
4. Hand (carpal) (metacarpal) (fingers)
5. Pelvic region (hip) (buttock) (femur)
6. Lower leg (fibula) (knee) (patella) (tibia)
7. Ankle and or foot (metatarsals) (toes) (tarsals)
8. Other
9. Multiple

724.9 Recurrent spine - NOS
724.6 Recurrent spine - lumbosacral joint
724.6 Recurrent spine - sacroiliac joint

839.69 Rib closed
839.79 Rib open
756.3 Rib congenital
718.28 Rib pathological
718.38 Rib recurrent old

836.59 Rotatory (knee) closed
836.69 Rotatory (knee) open

839.42 Sacroiliac closed
839.52 Sacroiliac open
755.69 Sacroiliac congenital
724.6 Sacroiliac pathologic or recurrent

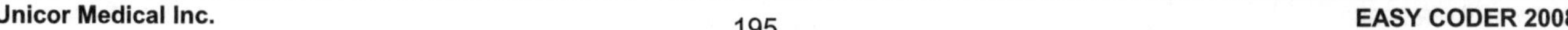

DISLOCATION (continued)

839.42 Sacrum closed
839.52 Sacrum open

837.0 Scaphoid foot closed
837.1 Scaphoid foot open
833.00 Scaphoid wrist closed
833.10 Scaphoid wrist open

831.09 Scapula closed
831.19 Scapula open

839.69 Septal cartilage (nose) closed
839.79 Septal cartilage (nose) open
470 Septum nasal (old)

831.0# Shoulder closed
831.1# Shoulder open
831.0# Shoulder nursemaid's

5th digit: 831.0-1
0. Unspecified
1. Anterior
2. Posterior
3. Inferior
4. Acromioclavicular
9. Scapula

718.71 Shoulder developmental
718.21 Shoulder pathologic
718.31 Shoulder recurrent

838.00 Smith's epiphyseal closed
838.10 Smith's epiphyseal open

839.40 Spine NOS closed
839.50 Spine NOS open
756.19 Spine NOS congenital
724.8 Spine NOS pathologic
724.9 Spine NOS recurrent
767.4 Spine or spinal cord birth trauma

0 Spontaneous see 'Dislocation', pathological

839.61 Sternoclavicular closed
839.71 Sternoclavicular open

839.61 Sternum closed
839.71 Sternum open

831.01 Subglenoid closed
831.11 Subglenoid open

838.## Subtalar
838.## Tarsal

4th digit: 838
0. Closed
1. Open

5th digit: 838
0. Foot unspecified
1. Tarsal (bone) joint unspecified
2. Midtarsal (joint)
3. Tarsometatarsal (bone) joint unspecified
4. Metatarsal (bone) joint unspecified
5. Metatarsophalangeal (joint)
6. Interphalangeal (joint) foot
9. Other

718.77 Tarsal developmental
718.27 Tarsal pathologic
718.37 Tarsal recurrent

837.0 Tarsonavicular closed
837.1 Tarsonavicular open

DISLOCATION (continued)

830.0 Temporomandibular closed
830.1 Temporomandibular open
524.69 Temporomandibular recurrent

839.21 Thoracic vertebra closed
839.31 Thoracic vertebra open
724.8 Thoracic pathologic
724.9 Thoracic recurrent

839.69 Thyroid cartilage closed
839.79 Thyroid cartilage open

837.0 Tibia distal end closed
837.1 Tibia distal end open
0 Tibia proximal end see 'Dislocation', knee

838.06 Toe interphalangeal closed
838.16 Toe interphalangeal open
718.77 Toe(s) developmental
838.09 Toe(s) other closed
838.19 Toe(s) other open
718.27 Toe(s) pathological
718.37 Toe(s) recurrent old

839.69 Trachea closed
839.79 Trachea open

833.09 Ulna distal end closed
833.19 Ulna distal end open
0 Ulna proximal end see 'Dislocation', elbow

0 Vertebra – non-traumatic see 'Intervertebral Disc', displacement

839.40 Vertebra NOS closed
839.50 Vertebra NOS open
756.19 Vertebra NOS or other congenital
724.8 Vertebra NOS or other pathological
724.9 Vertebra NOS or other recurrent old
839.49 Vertebra other closed
839.59 Vertebra other open

833.## Wrist

4th digit: 833
0. Closed
1. Open

5th digit: 833
0. Unspecified part
1. Radioulnar
2. Radiocarpal
3. Midcarpal
4. Carpometacarpal
5. Metacarpal
9. Other

718.73 Wrist developmental
718.23 Wrist pathological
718.33 Wrist recurrent old

839.61 Xiphoid cartilage closed
839.71 Xiphoid cartilage open

839.69 Other specified bone closed
839.79 Other specified bone open

0 DISORDER SEE BY ANATOMICAL SITE OR SPECIFIED DISORDER

0 DISPROPORTIONS INDICATING CARE IN PREGNANCY SEE 'PREGNANCY COMPLICATIONS', DISPROPORTIONS

D

DISSECTION

441.0# Aortic (ruptured)
5th digit: 441.0
0. Unspecified site
1. Thoracic
2. Abdominal
3. Thoracoabdominal

443.21 Carotid artery
414.12 Coronary artery
443.22 Iliac artery
443.23 Renal artery
459.9 Vascular
443.24 Vertebral artery
443.29 Other artery

286.6 DISSEMINATED INTRAVASCULAR COAGULATION
776.2 DISSEMINATED INTRAVASCULAR COAGULATION IN NEWBORN
031.2 DISSEMINATED MYCOBACTERIUM AVIUM-INTRACELLULARE COMPLEX (DMAC)
446.6 DISSEMINATED PLATELET THROMBOSIS SYNDROME
692.75 DISSEMINATED SUPERFICIAL ACTINIC POROKERATOSIS (DSAP)

378.87 DISSOCIATED DEVIATION OF EYE MOVEMENT
300.15 DISSOCIATIVE DISORDER OR REACTION
300.14 DISSOCIATIVE IDENTITY DISORDER
743.63 DISTICHIASIS CONGENITAL
524.22 DISTO OCCLUSION (DIVISION I OR II)

DISTOMIASIS

121.9 NOS
120.9 Hemic
121.1 Hepatic due to clonorchis sinensis
121.4 Intestinal
121.2 Pulmonary

> *Use additional code to identify the altered sensation.*

438.6 DISTURBANCE OF SENSATION LATE EFFECT OF CVA
782.0 DISTURBANCE OF SKIN SENSATION

733.7 DISUSE ATROPHY BONE
728.2 DISUSE ATROPHY MUSCLE
307.81 DITTHOMSKA SYNDROME
788.42 DIURESIS
993.3 DIVERS' PALSY OR PARALYSIS
909.4 DIVERS' PALSY OR PARALYSIS LATE EFFECT
378.85 DIVERGENCE ANOMALIES (EYE MOVEMENT)

0 DIVERTICULA SEE ANATOMICAL SITE

DIVERTICULITIS

596.3 Bladder
562.1# Colon (large bowel) (intestine)
562.1# Colon with abscess [569.5]
562.1# Colon with peritonitis [567.9]
562.1# Colon with peritonitis pneumococcal [567.1]
562.1# Colon with peritonitis suppurative [567.29]
562.1# Colon with peritonitis other type [567.89]
5th digit: 562.0, 1
1. Without hemorrhage
3. With hemorrhage

DIVERTICULITIS (continued)

562.0# Duodenum
562.0# Ileum
562.0# Jejunum
562.0# Small intestine
562.0# Small intestine with abscess [569.5]
562.0# Small intestine with peritonitis [567.9]
562.0# Small intestine with peritonitis pneumococcal [567.1]
562.0# Small intestine with peritonitis suppurative [567.29]
562.0# Small intestine with peritonitis other type [567.89]
5th digit: 562.0, 1
1. Without hemorrhage
3. With hemorrhage

DIVERTICULOSIS

562.1# Colon
562.1# Colon (large bowel) (intestine)
562.1# Colon with abscess [569.5]
562.1# Colon with peritonitis [567.9]
562.1# Colon with peritonitis pneumococcal [567.1]
562.1# Colon with peritonitis suppurative [567.29]
562.1# Colon with peritonitis other type [567.89]
562.0# Duodenum
562.0# Ileum
562.0# Jejunum
562.0# Small intestine
562.0# Small intestine with abscess [569.5]
562.0# Small intestine with peritonitis [567.9]
562.0# Small intestine with peritonitis pneumococcal [567.1]
562.0# Small intestine with peritonitis suppurative [567.29]
562.0# Small intestine with peritonitis other type [567.89]
5th digit: 562.0
0. Without hemorrhage
2. With hemorrhage

0 DIVERTICULUM SEE ANATOMICAL SITE
V61.0 DIVORCE (REASON FOR ENCOUNTER)
386.12 DIX-HALLPIKE NEUROLABYRINTHITIS

DIZZINESS

780.4 NOS
300.11 Hysterical
306.9 Psychogenic [780.4]

DJD (DEGENERATIVE JOINT DISEASE)

715.90 Site unspecified
715.97 Ankle and/or foot (metatarsals) (toes) (tarsals)
715.93 Forearm (radius) (wrist) (ulna)
715.94 Hand (carpal) (metacarpal) (fingers)
715.96 Lower leg (fibula) (knee) (patella) (tibia)
715.95 Pelvic region and thigh (hip) (buttock) (femur)
715.91 Shoulder region
721.90 Spine - NOS
721.0 Spine - cervical
721.3 Spine - lumbar or lumbosacral
721.2 Spine - thoracic
715.92 Upper arm (elbow) (humerus)
715.98 Other specified

D

250.1# DKA (DIABETIC KETOACIDOSIS)
250.3# DKA (DIABETIC KETOACIDOSIS) COMA
5th digit: 250.1, 3
0. Type II, adult-onset, non-insulin dependent (even if requiring insulin), or unspecified; controlled
1. Type I, juvenile-onset or insulin-dependent; controlled
2. Type II, adult-onset, non-insulin dependent (even if requiring insulin); uncontrolled
3. Type I, juvenile-onset or insulin-dependent; uncontrolled

031.2 DMAC (DISSEMINATED MYCOBACTERIUM AVIUM INTRACELLULARE COMPLEX)
289.53 DOAN-WISEMAN SYNDROME (PRIMARY SPLENIC NEUTROPENIA)
0 DOG BITE SEE 'OPEN WOUND', BY SITE
123.8 DOG TAPEWORM (INFECTION)
093.1 DOHLE-HELLER AORTITIS
288.2 DOHLE BODY-PANMYELOPATHIC SYNDROME
754.0 DOLICHOCEPHALY
751.5 DOLICHOCOLON DIVERTICULUM CONGENITAL
759.82 DOLICHOSTENOMELIA
259.8 DONOHUE'S SYNDROME (LEPRECHAUNISM)

Tissue or organ donor: Do not use V59 for self-donation (autogenous donation). Rather, code the underlying condition.

DONOR NON-AUTOGENOUS

V59.0# Blood
5th digit: V59.0
1. Whole
2. Stem cells
9. Other

V59.2 Bone
V59.3 Bone marrow
V59.5 Cornea
V59.7# Egg (oocyte) (ovum)
4th digit: V59.7
0. Unspecified
1. Under age 35, NOS or anonymous recipient
2. Under age 35, designated recipient
3. Age 35 and over, NOS or anonymous recipient
4. Age 35 and over, designated recipient
V70.8 Exam - potential donor organ or tissue
V59.4 Kidney
V59.6 Liver
V59.8 Lung
V59.8 Lymphocyte
V59.9 Organ NOS
V59.8 Organ other specified
V59.1 Skin
59.8 Sperm
V59.9 Tissue NOS
V59.8 Tissue other specified

099.2 DONOVANOSIS
496 DOPS - DIFFUSE OBSTRUCTIVE PULMONARY SYNDROME

DORSAL COLUMN STIMULATOR

996.63 Complication - infection or inflammation
996.2 Complication - mechanical (displaced) (failed)
996.75 Complication - other
V53.02 Fitting or adjustment

722.11 DORSAL DISC DISPLACEMENT
722.72 DORSAL DISC DISPLACEMENT WITH MYELOPATHY
953.1 DORSAL ROOT INJURY (NERVE)
0 DORSAL SEE THORACIC
436 DORSOLATERAL MEDULLARY SYNDROME
333.71 DOUBLE ATHETOSIS SYNDROME
759.4 DOUBLE MONSTER
368.2 DOUBLE VISION
360.81 DOUBLE WHAMMY SYNDROME
758.0 DOWN'S SYNDROME (MONGOLISM)
V19.5 DOWN'S SYNDROME (MONGOLISM) FAMILY HISTORY
V28.0 DOWN'S SYNDROME SCREENING – AMNIOCENTESIS (ANTENATAL)
V06.1 DPT (DTaP) VACCINATION
V06.3 DPT WITH POLIO VACCINATION
V06.2 DPT WITH TAB VACCINATION
125.7 DRACONTIASIS
125.7 DRACUNCULUS MEDINENSIS INFECTION
282.1 DRESBACH'S SYNDROME (ELLIPTOCYTOSIS)
117.8 DRESCHLERA HAWAIIENSIS INFECTION
118 DRESCHLERA INFECTION TO COMPROMISED HOST ONLY
V58.30 DRESSING CHANGE NONSURGICAL AFTERCARE
V58.31 DRESSING CHANGE SURGICAL AFTERCARE
283.2 DRESSLER'S HEMOGLOBINURIA SYNDROME
429.4 DRESSLER'S POSTCARDIOTOMY SYNDROME
411.0 DRESSLER'S SYNDROME (POSTMYOCARDIAL INFARCTION)
527.7 DROOLING, EXCESSIVE

DROP

736.29 Finger
736.79 Foot
735.8 Toe
736.05 Wrist

782.3 DROPSY
789.59 DROPSY ABDOMEN
428.0 DROPSY HEART SEE ALSO 'CHF'
994.1 DROWNING AND NONFATAL SUBMERSION
909.4 DROWNING AND NONFATAL SUBMERSION LATE EFFECT
780.09 DROWSINESS

Abuse versus dependence is the major distinction to make when coding for a patient with an alcohol or drug problem. Addiction is dependence.

DRUG

796.0 Abnormal levels (blood) (urine) (other tissue)
0 Abuse see 'Drug Abuse'
995.20 Adverse effect NEC to correct substance properly administered
995.27 Allergy NOS
995.29 Complication NOS

DRUG (continued)

995.20 Damage
692.3 Eruption fixed applied to skin
693.0 Eruption fixed ingested
995.27 Hypersensitivity NOS (properly administered)
995.27 Intolerance to correct substance properly administered
995.27 Intoxication to correct substance properly administered
292.9 Intoxication unspecified mental disorder
292.89 Intoxication other specified mental disorder
292.2 Intoxication pathological with brief psychosis
977.9 Overdose unspecified
995.20 Reaction NOS (properly administered)
995.27 Reaction allergic (properly administered)
V70.3 Screen administrative
V70.4 Screen medicolegal
796.0 Test abnormal (blood) (urine) (other tissue)
V70.3 Test administrative
V70.4 Test medicolegal
V58.83 Test monitoring encounter
V58.83 Test monitoring encounter with long term drug use [V58.6#]
V58.6# Therapy long-term - current
V58.83 Therapy monitoring encounter
V58.83 Therapy monitoring encounter with long term drug use [V58.6#]

5th digit: V58.6
1. Anticoagulants
2. Antibiotics
3. Antiplatelets/antithrombotics
4. Anti-inflammatories non-steroidal (NSAID)
5. Steroids
6. Aspirin
7. Insulin
9. Other

V58.11 Therapy status chemotherapy antineoplastic
V58.12 Therapy status immunotherapy antineoplastic

> ***Substance abuse describes the practice of using drugs or alcohol to excess without reaching the state of physical dependence.***

> ***Substance dependence is addiction. Dependence involves the loss of control and judgment and/or the inability to use in moderation. Dependence is marked by compulsive physical demands which are triggered by further ingestion.***

DRUG ABUSE

304.## Dependent (addiction)

4th digit: 304
0. Opioid
1. Sedative, hypnotic or anxiolytic
2. Cocaine
3. Cannabis
4. Amphetamine type
5. Hallucinogenic
6. Other specified
7. Mixed with opioid
8. Mixed
9. NOS

5th digit: 304
0. NOS
1. Continuous
2. Episodic
3. In remission

DRUG ABUSE (continued)

304.8# Dependent polysubstance (addiction)

5th digit: 304.8
0. NOS
1. Continuous
2. Episodic
3. In remission

V11.8 History
305.## Nondependent (abuse)

4th digit: 305
0. Alcohol
2. Cannabis
3. Hallucinogen
4. Sedative, hypnotic or anxiolytic
5. Opioid
6. Cocaine
7. Amphetamine type
8. Antidepressant type
9. Mixed or other specified

5th digit: 305
0. NOS
1. Continuous
2. Episodic
3. In remission

305.9# Nondependent polysubstance (abuse)

5th digit: 305.9
0. NOS
1. Continuous
2. Episodic
3. In remission

> ***648.3# : Code the specific maternal drug abuse or dependence with an additional code. See 'Abuse' drug.***

DRUG ABUSE COMPLICATING PREGNANCY

648.3# Maternal current (co-existent)

5th digit: 648.3
0. Episode of care unspecified or N/A
1. Delivered
2. Delivered with postpartum complication
3. Antepartum complication
4. Postpartum complication

655.5# Maternal with suspected damage to fetus

5th digit: 655.5
0. Episode of care unspecified or N/A
1. Delivered
3. Antepartum complication

D

DRUG INDUCED MENTAL DISORDERS (WITH ASSOCIATED DRUG DEPENDENCE)

292.9 NOS [304.##]
292.84 Affective syndrome organic [304.##]
292.83 Amnesia persisting [304.##]
292.89 Anxiety [304.##]
305.3 Bad trip (LSD) (hallucinogenic)
292.81 Delirium [304.##]
292.11 Delusional psychosis [304.##]
292.82 Dementia persisting [304.##]
292.84 Depression [304.##]
292.12 Hallucinatory psychosis [304.##]
292.89 Intoxication [304.##]
292.2 Intoxication pathological (resulting in brief psychotic state) [304.##]
292.84 Mood disorder [304.##]
292.11 Paranoid state [304.##]
292.89 Personality [304.##]
292.9 Psychosis NOS [304.##]
292.89 Sexual dysfunction [304.##]
292.85 Sleep disorder [304.##]
292.0 Withdrawal syndrome [304.##]
292.89 Other specified mental disorder [304.##]

4th digit: 304
0. Opioid
1. Sedative, hypnotic or anxiolytic
2. Cocaine
3. Cannabis
4. Amphetamine type
5. Hallucinogenic
6. Other specified
7. Mixed with opioid
8. Mixed
9. NOS

5th digit: 304
0. Unspecified
1. Continuous
2. Episodic
3. In remission

DRUG REACTION

292.2 Unspecified with brief psychosis (unexpected)
292.2 Idiosyncratic resulting in brief psychotic state
763.5 Maternal affecting fetus or newborn
779.4 Newborn specific to newborn
292.2 Pathologic resulting in brief psychotic state

Never use a code for drug resistance as a principal diagnosis. These should be used as additional codes only.

Do not assign these codes solely on the basis of lab reports. Only the physician can diagnose an infection with a drug resistant organism.

Sequencing of drug resistant organisms: the disease or complication code is first, followed by the organism code (if known), followed by the V09. Code.

DRUG RESISTANCE

V09.90 Drugs NOS
V09.91 Drugs multiple NOS
V09.4 Amikacin
V09.4 Aminoglycosides NEC
V09.5# Amodiaquine
V09.8# Amodiquin
V09.0 Amoxicillin
V09.0 Ampicillin
V09.7# Antimycobacterial agents NEC
V09.2 Azithromycin
V09.0 Azlocillin
V09.1 Aztreonam
V09.1 B-lactam antibiotics NEC
V09.0 Bacampicillin
V09.8# Bacitracin
V09.8# Benznidazole
V09.7# Capreomycin
V09.0 Carbenicillin
V09.1 Cefaclor
V09.1 Cefadroxil
V09.1 Cefamandole
V09.1 Cefatetan
V09.1 Cefazolin
V09.1 Cefonicid
V09.1 Cefoperazone
V09.1 Ceforanide
V09.1 Cefotaxime
V09.1 Cefoxitin
V09.1 Ceftazidine
V09.1 Ceftizoxime
V09.1 Ceftriaxone
V09.1 Cefuroxime
V09.1 Cephaloglycin
V09.1 Cephaloridine
V09.1 Cephalosporins NEC
V09.1 Cephalothin
V09.1 Cephapirin
V09.1 Cephradine

5th digit: V09.5, 7, 8
0. Without resistance to multiple drugs of this class
1. With resistance to multiple drugs of this class

DRUG RESISTANCE (continued)

V09.8# Chloramphenicol
V09.5# Chloraquine
V09.8# Chlorguanide
V09.8# Chloroquine
V09.8# Chlorproguanil
V09.3 Chlortetracycline
V09.5# Cinoxacin
V09.5# Ciprofloxacin
V09.2 Clarithromycin
V09.8# Clindamycin
V09.5# Clioquinol
V09.7# Clofazimine
V09.0 Cloxacillin
V09.0 Cyclacillin
V09.7# Cycloserine
V09.7# Dapsone (DZ)
V09.3 Demeclocycline
V09.0 Dicloxacillin
V09.3 Doxycycline
V09.1 Ecphalexin
V09.5# Enoxacin
V09.2 Erythromycin
V09.7# Ethambutol (EMB)
V09.7# Ethionamide (ETA)
V09.5# Fluoroquinolones
V09.4 Gentamicin
V09.8# Halofantrine
V09.1 Imipenem
V09.5# Iodoquinol
V09.7# Isoniazid (INH)
V09.4 Kanamycin
V09.2 Macrolides NEC
V09.6 Mafenide
V09.8# Mefloquine
V09.8# Melassoprol
V09.3 Methacycline
V09.0 Methicillin-resistant staphyloccus aureus (MRSA)
V09.8# Methenamine
V09.8# Metronidazole
V09.0 Mexlocillin
V09.3 Minocycline
V09.91 Multiple drug resistant organisms NOS
V09.0 Nafcillin
V09.5# Nalidixic acid
V09.2 Natamycin
V09.4 Neomycin
V09.4 Netilmicin
V09.8# Nimorazole
V09.8# Nitrofurantoin
V09.8# Nitrofurtimox
V09.5# Norfloxacin
V09.2 Nystatin
V09.5# Ofloxacin
V09.2 Oleandomycin
V09.0 Oxacillin
V09.3 Oxytetracycline
V09.7# Para-amino salicylic acid (PAS)
V09.4 Paromomycin
V09.0 Penicillin (G) (V) (VK)
V09.8# Pentamidine

5th digit: V09.5, 7-8
0. Without resistance to multiple drugs of this class
1. With resistance to multiple drugs of this class

DRUG RESISTANCE (continued)

V09.0 Piperacillin
V09.5# Primaquine
V09.8# Proguanil
V09.7# Pyrazinamide (PZA)
V09.8# Pyrimethamine/sulfalene
V09.8# Pyrimethamine/sulfodoxine
V09.5# Quinacrine
V09.8# Quinidine
V09.8# Quinine
V09.5# Quinolones NEC
V09.7# Rifabutin
V09.7# Rifampin (RIF)
V09.7# Rifamycin
V09.3 Rolitetracycline
V09.8# Spectinomycin
V09.2 Spiramycin
V09.4 Streptomycin (SM)
V09.6 Sulfacetamide
V09.6 Sulfacytine
V09.6 Sulfadiazine
V09.6 Sulfadoxine
V09.6 Sulfamethoxazole
V09.6 Sulfapyridine
V09.6 Sulfasalizine
V09.6 Sulfisoxazole
V09.6 Sulfonamides
V09.7# Sulfoxone
V09.3 Tetracycline
V09.3 Tetracyclines NEC
V09.8# Thiamphenicol
V09.0 Ticarcillin
V09.8# Tinidazole
V09.4 Tobramycin
V09.8# Triamphenicol
V09.8# Trimethoprim
V09.8# Vancomycin (glycopeptide) (intermediate or resistant staphylococcus aureus) (resistant enterococcus)
V09.8# Other specified drugs NEC

5th digit: V09.5, 7-8
0. Without resistance to multiple drugs of this class
1. With resistance to multiple drugs of this class

DRUG WITHDRAWAL

292.0 Symptoms or syndrome
779.5 Symptoms or syndrome newborn or infant of dependent mother

303.0# DRUNKENNESS ACUTE IN ALCOHOLISM
305.0# DRUNKENNESS NONDEPENDENT

5th digit: 303.0, 305.0
0. Unspecified
1. Continuous
2. Episodic
3. In remission

291.4 DRUNKENNESS PATHOLOGIC

DRUSEN

362.57 Degenerative
362.77 Hereditary
377.21 Optic disc

375.15 DRY EYE SYNDROME
701.1 DRY SKIN SYNDROME
526.5 DRY SOCKET
692.75 DSAP (DISSEMINATED SUPERFICIAL ACTINIC POROKERATOSIS)
291.0 DT'S
300.14 DUAL PERSONALITY DISORDER
378.71 DUANE'S SYNDROME (DUANE-STILLING-TURK SYNDROME) (OCULAR RETRACTION)
626.8 DUB
277.4 DUBIN-JOHNSON SYNDROME (CONSTITUTIONAL HYPERBILIRUBINEMIA)
277.4 DUBIN-SPRINZ SYNDROME (CONSTITUTIONAL HYPERBILIRUBINEMIA)
049.8 DUBINI'S ELECTRIC CHOREA
090.5 DUBOIS' THYMUS GLAND (ABSCESS)

DUCHENNE'S

335.21 Aran muscular atrophy
094.0 Disease
094.0 Locomotor ataxia
359.1 Muscular dystrophy
335.22 Paralysis
359.1 Pseudohypertrophy muscles
335.22 Syndrome

747.89 DUCTUS ARTERIOSUS ABSENCE CONGENITAL
747.0 DUCTUS ARTERIOSUS DEFORMITY
795.79 DUFFY ANTIGEN POSITIVE
694.0 DUHRING'S DISEASE (DERMATITIS HERPETIFORMIS)
057.8 DUKES FILATOW DISEASE
085.0 DUMDUM FEVER
564.2 DUMPING SYNDROME
536.8 DUMPING SYNDROME NONSURGICAL
0 DUODENAL SEE 'DUODENUM, DUODENAL'

DUODENUM, DUODENAL

V45.72 Absence (acquired) (postoperative)
751.1 Atresia (absence) congenital
568.0 Band due to adhesion
564.89 Dilatation
537.9 Disorder
537.89 Disorder other specified NEC
562.00 Diverticula
751.5 Diverticula congenital
535.6# Duodenitis
5th Digit : 535.6
0. Without hemorrhage
1. With hemorrhage

793.4 Filling defect
537.4 Fistula
537.2 Ileus chronic
863.21 Injury traumatic
863.31 Injury traumatic with open wound
908.1 Injury traumatic late effect
564.89 Irritability
537.3 Obstruction
751.1 Obstruction congenital
0 Obstruction due to ulcer see 'Ulcer', duodenal
537.89 Prolapse

DUODENUM, DUODENAL (continued)

537.89 Reflux
537.89 Rupture
564.89 Spasm
537.3 Stenosis (stricture) (volvulus) (cicatrix)
751.1 Stenosis (stricture) (cicatrix) congenital
532.## Ulcer
532.## Ulcer due to helicobacter pylori [041.86]
316 Ulcer psychogenic [**532.##**]
4th digit: 532
0. Acute with hemorrhage
1. Acute with perforation
2. Acute with hemorrhage and perforation
3. Acute
4. Chronic or unspecified with hemorrhage
5. Chronic or unspecified with perforation
6. Chronic or unspecified with hemorrhage and perforation
7. Chronic
9. Unspecified as acute or chronic

5th digit: 532
0. Without obstruction
1. Obstructed

537.3 Volvulus
751.5 Web (congenital)

726.2 DUPLAY'S DISEASE OR SYNDROME
781.6 DUPRE'S SYNDROME (MENINGISM)
728.6 DUPUYTREN'S CONTRACTURE OF PALMAR FASCIA
998.2 DURAL TEAR
099.1 DURAND-NICOLAS-FAVRE CLIMATIC BUBO
746.5 DUROZIEZ'S CONGENITAL MITRAL STENOSIS
086.9 DUTTON'S TRYPANOSOMIASIS
453.4# DVT (DEEP VEIN THROMBOSIS)
5th digit: 453.4
0. NOS
1. Proximal (femoral) (iliac) (popliteal) (thigh) (upper leg NOS)
2. Distal (calf) (peroneal) (tibial) (lower leg NOS)

DWARFISM

259.4 Unspecified
756.4 Achondroplasia
759.7 Intrauterine
253.3 Lorain levi
263.2 Nutritional
253.3 Pituitary
259.8 Progeria
316 Psychosocial factors [259.4]
588.0 Renal

283.9 DYKE YOUNG SYNDROME (ACQUIRED MACROCYTIC HEMOLYTIC ANEMIA)
255.9 DYSADRENOCORTISM
255.3 DYSADRENOCORTISM HYPERFUNCTION
255.41 DYSADRENOCORTISM HYPOFUNCTION
784.5 DYSARTHRIA
337.9 DYSAUTONOMIA

440.21 DYSBASIA ANGIOSCLEROTICA DUE TO ATHEROSCLEROSIS

440.21 DYSBASIA ANGIOSCLEROTICA DUE TO ATHEROSCLEROSIS WITH CHRONIC COMPLETE OR TOTAL OCCLUSION [440.4]

315.1 DYSCALCULIA (DELAY IN DEVELOPMENT)

0 DYSCHEZIA SEE 'CONSTIPATION'

756.4 DYSCHONDROPLASIA CONGENITAL

756.4 DYSCHONDROPLASIA WITH HEMANGIOMATA

783.43 DYSCHONDROSTEOSIS WITH SHORT STATURE HOMEBOX GENE (SHOX)

709.0# DYSCHROMIA

5th digit: 709.0

0. Unspecified
1. Vitiligo
9. Other dyschromia

289.9 DYSCRASIA BLOOD

004.0 DYSENTERIAE SHIGELLA

009.2 DYSENTERIC DIARRHEA

DYSENTERY

009.2 Unspecified
006.0 Amebic acute
006.1 Amebic chronic
0 Bacillary see 'Dysentery', shigella
007.0 Balantidiasis
009.0 Catarrhal
007.2 Coccidiosis
007.4 Cryptosporidial
007.5 Cyclosporiasis
007.1 Giardiasis
009.0 Hemorrhagic
009.0 Infectious
009.0 Infectious (hemorrhagic)
007.3 Intestinal trichomoniasis
007.2 Isospora (belli) (hominis)
007.# Protozoal

4th digit: 007

0. Balantidiasis
1. Giardiasis
2. Coccidiosis
3. Trichomoniasis
4. Cryptosporidiosis
5. Cyclosporiasis
8. Other specified
9. Unspecified

004.9 Shigella
004.2 Shigella boydii (group C)
004.0 Shigella dysenteriae (group A) (Schmitz) (shiga)
004.1 Shigella flexneri (group B)
004.3 Shigella sonnei (group D)
004.8 Shigella other specified
007.3 Trichomoniasis intestinal

780.4 DYSEQUILIBRIUM

286.3 DYSFIBRINOGENEMIA

626.8 DYSFUNCTIONAL UTERINE BLEEDING (HEMORRHAGE)

279.06 DYSGAMMAGLOBULINEMIA (ACQUIRED) (CONGENITAL) (PRIMARY)

DYSGERMINOMA

183.0 Female site NOS
0 Female site specified see 'Cancer', by site M9060/3
186.9 Male site NOS
0 Male site specified see 'Cancer', by site M9060/3

705.81 DYSHIDROSIS

795.09 DYSKARYOTIC CERVICAL SMEAR (PAP)

Dyskinesia due to drugs need an additional E-Code assigned to specify the specific drug causing the adverse effect in therapeutic use. Also assign an additional 3rd code to show the condition the patient is taking the drug for.

DYSKINESIA

781.3 NOS
530.5 Esophagus
300.11 Hysterical
564.89 Intestinal
333.85 Neuroleptic induced tardive
333.82 Orofacial
333.85 Orofacial due to drugs
307.9 Psychogenic
333.85 Subacute, due to drugs
333.85 Tardive
333.85 Tardive neuroleptic induced

784.5 DYSLALIA

315.39 DYSLALIA DEVELOPMENT

784.61 DYSLEXIA

315.02 DYSLEXIA DEVELOPMENTAL (DELAY IN DEVELOPMENT)

272.4 DYSLIPIDEMIA

625.3 DYSMENORRHEA

306.52 DYSMENORRHEA PSYCHOGENIC

277.7 DYSMETABOLIC SYNDROME X

277.7 DYSMETABOLIC SYNDROME X WITH CARDIOVASCULAR DISEASE **[414.0#]**

277.7 DYSMETABOLIC SYNDROME X WITH CARDIOVASCULAR DISEASE WITH CHRONIC COMPLETE OR TOTAL OCCLUSION **[414.0#] [414.2]**

5th digit: 414.0
- **0. Unspecified type of vessel, native or graft**
- **1. Native coronary vessel**
- **2. Autologous vein bypass graft**
- **3. Nonautologous biological bypass graft**
- **4. Autologous artery bypass graft (gastroepiploic) (internal mammary)**
- **5. Unspecified type of bypass graft**
- **6. Native vessel of transplanted heart**
- **7. Bypass graft of transplanted heart**

277.7 DYSMETABOLIC SYNDROME X WITH OBESITY AND BODY MASS INDEX 25 AND ABOVE **[278.0#] [V85.#(#)]**

5th digit: 278.0
- **0. NOS**
- **1. Morbid (severe)**

These codes are for use in persons over 20 years old.

4th or 4th and 5th digit: V85
- **2#. 25-29**
  - **1. 25.0-25.9**
  - **2. 26.0-26.9**
  - **3. 27.0-27.9**
  - **4. 28.0-28.9**
  - **5. 29.0-29.9**
- **3#. 30-39**
  - **0. 30.0-30.9**
  - **1. 31.0-31.9**
  - **2. 32.0-32.9**
  - **3. 33.0-33.9**
  - **4. 34.0-34.9**
  - **5. 35.0-35.9**
  - **6. 36.0-36.9**
  - **7. 37.0-37.9**
  - **8. 38.0-38.9**
  - **9. 39.0-39.9**
- **4. 40 and over**

300.7 DYSMORPHIC BODY DISORDER

784.3 DYSNOMIA

625.0 DYSPAREUNIA

608.89 DYSPAREUNIA MALE

302.76 DYSPAREUNIA PSYCHOGENIC

536.3 DYSPEPSIA ATONIC

536.8 DYSPEPSIA DISORDERS OTHER SPECIFIED FUNCTION OF STOMACH

564.89 DYSPEPSIA INTESTINAL

306.4 DYSPEPSIA PSYCHOGENIC (CYCLICAL)

787.2# DYSPHAGIA

438.82 DYSPHAGIA LATE EFFECT OF CEREBROVASCULAR DISEASE **[787.2#]**

5th digit: 787.2
- **0. Unspecified**
- **1. Oral phase**
- **2. Oropharyngeal phase**
- **3. Pharyngeal phase**
- **4. Pharyngoesophageal phase**
- **9. Other (cervical) (neurogenic)**

288.1 DYSPHAGOCYTOSIS CONGENITAL

784.5 DYSPHASIA

438.12 DYSPHASIA LATE EFFECT CEREBROVASCULAR DISEASE

784.49 DYSPHONIA

625.4 DYSPHORIA PREMENSTRUAL

374.52 DYSPIGMENTATION EYELID

253.9 DYSPITUITARISM

DYSPLASIA

770.7 Bronchopulmonary perinatal

CERVIX (UTERI)

795.02 ASC-H (atypical squamous cannot exclude high grade squamous intraepithelial lesion)

795.01 ASC-US (atypical squamous cells of undetermined significance)

622.11 CIN I

622.12 CIN II

233.1 CIN III

795.04 HGSIL (high grade squamous intraepithelial lesion)

V13.22 History

795.03 LGSIL (low grade squamous intraepithelial lesion)

622.11 Mild

622.12 Moderate

233.1 Severe

DYSPLASIA (continued)

211.3 Colon

756.56 Epiphyseal multiple

289.89 Erythroid NEC

0 High grade focal see 'Benign Neoplasm', by site

289.89 Myeloid NEC

602.3 Prostate - PIN I

602.3 Prostate - PIN II

233.4 Prostate - PIN III

623.0 Vagina - VAIN I

623.0 Vagina - VAIN II

233.31 Vagina - VAIN III

233.31 Vagina severe

624.01 Vulva - VIN I

624.02 Vulva - VIN II

233.32 Vulva - VIN III

624.01 Vulva mild

624.02 Vulva moderate

233.32 Vulva severe

D

786.09 DYSPNEA (PAROXYSMAL) (NOCTURNAL)
0 DYSPNEA ASTHMATIC SEE 'ASTHMA'
428.1 DYSPNEA CARDIAC

> *770.89: Use additional code to specify condition.*

770.89 DYSPNEA NEWBORN
306.1 DYSPNEIC DISORDER PSYCHOGENIC
781.3 DYSPRAXIA
315.4 DYSPRAXIA SYNDROME
286.3 DYSPROTHROMBINEMIA
337.3 DYSREFLEXIA AUTONOMIC
337.3 DYSREFLEXIA AUTONOMIC WITH DECUBITUS ULCER [**707.0#**]

5th digit: 707.0
- **0. NOS**
- **1. Elbow**
- **2. Upper back (shoulder blades)**
- **3. Lower back (sacrum)**
- **4. Hip**
- **5. Buttock**
- **6. Ankle**
- **7. Heel**
- **6. Other site (head)**

337.3 DYSREFLEXIA AUTONOMIC WITH FECAL IMPACTION [560.39]

> *Urinary tract infection: Use additional code for organism. See 'Bacterial Infection'.*

337.3 DYSREFLEXIA AUTONOMIC WITH URINARY TRACT INFECTION [599.0]

> *Cardiac dysrhythmia , 427.9, is a non-specific diagnosis. Always code the specific type of dysrhythmia when possible.*

DYSRHYTHMIAS

427.31 Atrial fibrillation (paroxysmal)
427.32 Atrial flutter
427.61 Atrial premature beats contractions or systoles
427.89 Atrial tachycardia
427.0 Atrial tachycardia paroxysmal
316 Atrial tachycardia paroxysmal psychogenic [427.0]
427.89 Bigeminy
427.2 Bouveret-Hoffmann syndrome
427.81 Bradycardia chronic
779.81 Bradycardia neonatal
337.0 Bradycardia reflex
427.89 Bradycardia sinus
427.81 Bradycardia sinus persistent (severe)
427.89 Bradycardia vagal
427.81 Bradycardia with PAT
427.9 Cardiac NOS
427.5 Cardiac arrest NOS
427.89 Cardiac other specified
337.0 Carotid sinus syncope
348.30 Cerebral
427.89 Coronary sinus arrhythmia
348.30 Cortical
427.89 Ectopic arrhythmia
427.61 Ectopic auricular beats
427.60 Ectopic beats
427.69 Ectopic ventricular beats
427.60 Extrasystoles

DYSRHYTHMIAS (continued)

427.31 Fibrillation atrial
427.41 Fibrillation ventricular
427.32 Flutter atrial
427.42 Flutter ventricular
0 Following abortion see 'Abortion'
0 Following ectopic or molar pregnancy see 'Ectopic Pregnancy' or 'Molar Pregnancy'
427.60 Junctional premature contraction
429.4 Late effect of cardiac surgery
427.60 Nodal premature contraction
427.61 PAC's (premature atrial contractions)
429.4 Pacemaker syndrome
427.2 Paroxysmal tachycardia
427.0 Paroxysmal tachycardia atrial
427.0 Paroxysmal tachycardia supraventricular
427.1 Paroxysmal tachycardia ventricular
427.0 PAT (paroxysmal atrial tachycardia)
316 PAT (paroxysmal atrial tachycardia) psychogenic [427.0]
429.4 Postcardiotomy syndrome
997.1 Postoperative (during or resulting from a procedure)
429.4 Postvalvulotomy syndrome
427.61 Premature atrial contractions
427.69 Premature beats other
427.60 Premature junctional contractions
427.60 Premature nodal contraction
427.69 Premature ventricular contractions
427.69 PVC's (premature ventricular contraction)
427.81 Sick sinus syndrome (SSS)
427.81 Sinoatrial node dysfunction
427.89 Sinus bradycardia
427.81 Sinus bradycardia persistent
427.81 Sinus bradycardia severe
427.61 Supraventricular premature beats
427.89 Supraventricular tachycardia
427.0 Supraventricular tachycardia paroxysmal
427.81 Tachybrady syndrome
785.0 Tachycardia
427.89 Tachycardia atrial
427.0 Tachycardia atrial paroxysmal
427.0 Tachycardia AV paroxysmal
427.81 Tachycardia bradycardia syndrome
427.0 Tachycardia junctional paroxysmal
779.82 Tachycardia neonatal
427.2 Tachycardia paroxysmal
427.89 Tachycardia supraventricular
427.0 Tachycardia supraventricular paroxysmal
427.1 Tachycardia ventricular
427.41 Tachycardia ventricular fibrillation
427.42 Tachycardia ventricular flutter
427.1 Tachycardia ventricular paroxysmal
427.1 V tach
427.1 V tach paroxysmal
427.69 Ventricular escape beats
427.41 Ventricular fibrillation
427.42 Ventricular flutter
427.69 Ventricular premature beats (contractions)
427.69 Ventricular premature contractions
427.5 Ventricular standstill
427.1 Ventricular tachycardia
427.1 Ventricular tachycardia paroxysmal
427.89 Wandering (atrial) pacemaker

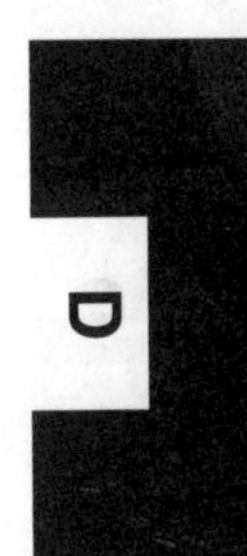

307.47 DYSSOMNIA NONORGANIC ORIGIN
780.56 DYSSOMNIA ORGANIC ORIGIN
289.4 DYSSPLENISM
334.2 DYSSYNERGIA CEREBELLARIS MYOCLONICA
300.4 DYSTHYMIC DISORDER
661.2# DYSTOCIA CERVICAL COMPLICATING LABOR AND DELIVERY
660.9# DYSTOCIA WITH OBSTRUCTED LABOR
660.4# DYSTOCIA SHOULDER OBSTRUCTING LABOR

5th digit: 660.4, 9, 661.2
0. Episode of care unspecified or N/A
1. Delivered
3. Antepartum complication

654.9# DYSTOCIA SYNDROME (DYSTROPHIA)

5th digit: 654.9
0. Episode of care unspecified or N/A
1. Delivered
2. Delivered with postpartum complication
3. Antepartum complication
4. Postpartum complication

333.72 DYSTONIA ACUTE DUE TO DRUGS
333.72 DYSTONIA ACUTE NEUROLEPTIC INDUCED
333.6 DYSTONIA DEFORMANS PROGRESSIVA
333.6 DYSTONIA MUSCULORUM DEFORMANS
333.79 DYSTONIA TORSION ACQUIRED
333.6 DYSTONIA TORSION GENETIC
333.79 DYSTONIA TORSION SYMPTOMATIC
359.21 DYSTROPHIA MYOTONICA
703.8 DYSTROPHIA UNGUIUM
337.0 DYSTROPHY CERVICAL SYMPATHETIC (CAUSALGIA)
270.8 DYSTROPHY OCULOCEREBRORENAL
337.2# DYSTROPHY REFLEX/POSTTRAUMATIC SYMPATHETIC

5th digit: 337.2
0. Unspecified
1. Upper limb
2. Lower limb
9. Other specified site

788.1 DYSURIA
306.53 DYSURIA PSYCHOGENIC

D

0 E COLI SEE 'BACTERIAL INFECTION' OR SPECIFIED CONDITION
756.71 EAGLE-BARRETT SYNDROME
362.18 EALES' DISEASE OR SYNDROME

EAR

V45.79 Absence acquired
0 Absence congenital see 'Ear Anomaly'
388.70 Ache
0 Anomaly see 'Ear Anomaly'
388.9 Atrophy
380.50 Canal obstruction
388.60 Discharge
388.69 Discharge blood
388.61 Discharge cerebrospinal fluid
V80.3 Diseases screening
384.20 Drum perforation (see also 'Tympanic Membrane Perforation')
V72.19 Exam
0 External ear see also 'Pinna'
380.31 Hematoma auricle
388.69 Hemorrhage
380.10 Infection external NOS (see also 'Otitis Externa')
386.30 Infection inner NOS (see also 'Labyrinthitis')
382.9 Infection middle (see also 'Otitis Media')
380.11 Infection pinna acute
698.9 Itching
388.8 Mass
388.10 Noise effects (to inner ear)
388.70 Pain
388.71 Pain otogenic
388.72 Pain referred
V50.3 Piercing (elective)
381.81 Pressure (eustachian)
V41.3 Problem other specified
380.12 Swimmer's
380.4 Wax

EAR ANOMALY

744.3 NOS
744.00 NOS with impairment of hearing
744.09 Absence
744.01 Absence external ear
744.21 Absence lobe
744.04 Absence ossicles
744.02 Canal atresia
744.3 Deformity NOS
744.02 External ear other with impairment of hearing
744.05 Inner ear
744.03 Middle ear except ossicles
744.1 Supernumerary (ear) (lobule)
744.09 Other specified causing impairment of hearing

EAR DISORDER

388.9 Unspecified
388.00 Degenerative
380.9 External
380.89 External other
388.9 Inner chronic NEC
385.9 Middle (and mastoid)
385.10 Middle (and mastoid) adhesive
385.89 Middle (and mastoid) other
388.00 Vascular
388.8 Other specified NEC

EAR INFECTION

380.10 External NOS (see also 'Otitis Externa')
035 External (acute) erysipelas [380.13]
684 External (acute) impetiginous [380.13]
690.10 External seborrheic dermatitis NOS [380.13]
690.11 External seborrheic dermatitis capitis [380.13]
690.12 External seborrheic dermatitis infantile [380.13]
690.18 External seborrheic dermatitis other [380.13]
386.30 Inner NOS (see also 'Labyrinthitis')
382.9 Middle see 'Otitis Media'

EAR INJURY

959.09 Unspecified
388.11 Blast trauma (inner ear)
925.1 Crushing
910.8 Other and unspecified superficial
910.9 Other and unspecified superficial infected

EAR OSSICLES

744.04 Anomalies congenital
385.23 Discontinuity
385.23 Dislocation
385.22 Impaired mobility
385.21 Impaired mobility - malleus
385.22 Impaired mobility - other
385.24 Partial loss or necrosis

388.70 EARACHE
780.94 EARLY SATIETY
062.2 EASTERN EQUINE ENCEPHALITIS

EATING DISORDER

307.50 NOS
307.1 Anorexia nervosa
307.59 Appetite loss psychogenic
307.51 Bulimia nervosa
783.3 Difficulties mismanagement
783.6 Excessive
307.59 Infancy or early childhood nonorganic
307.59 Infantile nonorganic
307.59 Loss of appetite nonorganic
307.52 Pica
V69.1 Problem
307.50 Psychogenic NEC
307.53 Rumination disorder
307.54 Vomiting psychogenic
307.59 Other

EATON LAMBERT SYNDROME

005.1 Botulism [358.1]
244.# Hypothyroid [358.1]

4th digit: 244
0. Postsurgical
1. Postablative (irradiation)
2. Iodine ingestion
3. PAS, phenylbut, resorcinol
8. Secondary NEC
9. NOS

281.0 Pernicious anemia [358.1]

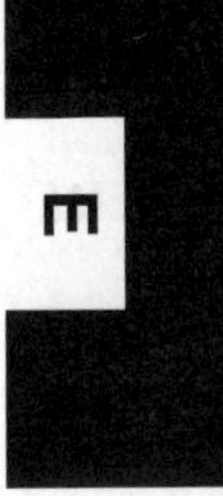

EATON LAMBERT SYNDROME (continued)

<u>**242.##**</u> <u>Thyrotoxic</u> [358.1]
4th digit: 242
0. Toxic diffuse goiter
1. Toxic uninodular goiter
2. Toxic multinodular goiter
3. Toxic nodular goiter unspecified
4. From ectopic thyroid nodule
8. Of other specified origin
9. Without goiter or other cause
5th digit: 242
0. Without storm
1. With storm

0 EATON'S AGENT SEE 'BACTERIAL INFECTION' OR SPECIFIED CONDITION
002.2 EBERTH'S TYPHOID FEVER
065.8 EBOLA HEMORRHAGIC FEVER
078.89 EBOLA INFECTION (VIRUS)
746.2 EBSTEIN'S ANOMALY (HEART)
<u>**250.4#**</u> EBSTEIN'S NEPHROTIC SYNDROME (<u>DIABETIC</u>) [581.81]
5th digit: 250.4
0. Type II, adult-onset, non-insulin dependent (even if requiring insulin), or unspecified; controlled
1. Type I, juvenile-onset or insulin-dependent; controlled
2. Type II, adult-onset, non-insulin dependent (even if requiring insulin); uncontrolled
3. Type I, juvenile-onset or insulin-dependent; uncontrolled

746.2 EBSTEIN'S SYNDROME (DOWNWARD DISPLACEMENT, TRICUSPID VALVE INTO RIGHT VENTRICLE)

ECCHYMOSES

459.89 NOS
372.72 Conjunctiva
921.0 Eye (traumatic)
921.1 Eyelid (traumatic)
772.6 Fetus or newborn
459.89 Multiple
772.6 Newborn
782.7 Spontaneous
0 Traumatic see 'Contusion', by site

216.# ECCRINE ACROSPIROMA M8402/0
216.# ECCRINE DERMAL CYLINDROMA M8200/0
216.# ECCRINE SPIRADENOMA M8403/0
4th digit: 216
0. Lip (skin of)
1. Eyelid including canthus
2. Ear (external) (auricle) (pinna)
3. Face (cheek) (nose)
4. Scalp, neck
5. Trunk, back, chest
6. Upper limb including shoulder
7. Lower limb including hip
8. Other specified sites
9. Skin unspecified

794.31 ECG ABNORMAL
0 ECHINOCOCCIASIS SEE 'ECHINOCOCCUS'

ECHINOCOCCUS GRANULOSUS INFECTION

122.4 Unspecified
122.0 Liver
122.1 Lung
122.2 Thyroid
122.3 Other

ECHINOCOCCUS INFECTION

122.9 Unspecified
122.8 Liver
122.9 Lung
122.9 Thyroid
122.9 Other

ECHINOCOCCUS INFECTION OF ORBIT (EYE)

<u>122.9</u> <u>Unspecified</u> [376.13]
<u>122.3</u> <u>Granulosus</u> [376.13]
<u>122.6</u> <u>Multilocularis</u> [376.13]

ECHINOCOCCUS MULTILOCULARIS INFECTION

122.7 Unspecified
122.5 Liver
122.6 Lung
122.6 Thyroid
122.6 Other

121.8 ECHINOSTOMA ILOCANUM INFECTION
078.89 ECHO VIRUS DISEASE NEC
079.1 ECHO VIRUS IN DISEASES CLASSIFIED ELSEWHERE
047.1 ECHO VIRUS MENINGITIS

ECHOCARDIOGRAM

793.2 Abnormal
V72.81 Preoperative
V72.85 Screening

794.01 ECHOENCEPHALOGRAM ABNORMAL
793.#(#) ECHOGRAM ABNORMAL FINDINGS (NONSPECIFIC) NEC
4th or 4th <u>and</u> 5th digit: 793
0. Skull and head
1. Lung field
2. Other intrathoracic
3. Biliary tract
4. Gastrointestinal tract
5. Genitourinary organs
6. Abdominal area including retroperitoneum
7. Musculoskeletal system
8#. Breast
80. Unspecified
81. Mammographic microcalcification
89. Other abnormal findings (calcification) (calculus)
9#. Other
91. Inconclusive due to excess body fat
99. Other abnormal findings (placenta) (skin) (subcutaneous)

When using code 793.91, Image test inconclusive due to excess body fat, use additional code to identify body mass index (BMI) which can be found at 'Body Mass Index'.

E

780.39 ECLAMPSIA (COMA) (CONVULSIONS) (DELIRIUM) (NOT ASSOCIATED WITH CHILDBIRTH)
780.39 ECLAMPSIA MALE
642.6# ECLAMPSIA MATERNAL
642.7# ECLAMPSIA MATERNAL WITH PRE-EXISTING HYPERTENSION

5th digit: 642.6-7
0. Episode of care NOS or N/A
1. Delivered
2. Delivered with postpartum complications
3. Antepartum complication
4. Postpartum complication

V15.87 ECMO (EXTRACORPOREAL MEMBRANE OXYGENATION) HISTORY
V60.9 ECONOMIC CIRCUMSTANCE (REASON FOR ENCOUNTER)
V60.8 ECONOMIC CIRCUMSTANCE OTHER SPECIFIED
049.8 ECONOMO'S ENCEPHALITIS LETHARGICA

ECTASIA

448.9 Capillary
538.82 Gastric antral vascular (GAVE) without hemorrhage
538.83 Gastric antral vascular (GAVE) with hemorrhage
593.89 Kidney
448.9 Papillary
527.8 Salivary gland (duct)

ECTHYMA

686.8 Unspecified
051.2 Contagiosum
686.09 Gangrenosum
051.2 Infectiosum

757.31 ECTODERMAL DYSPLASIA CONGENITAL
746.87 ECTOPIA CORDIS

ECTOPIC

255.0 ACTH syndrome
427.61 Auricular beats
427.60 Beats
259.3 Hormone secretion NEC

KIDNEY

753.3 Unspecified
654.4# Pregnancy (childbirth)
660.2# Pregnancy (childbirth) obstructing labor **[654.4#]**

5th digit: 654.4
0. Episode of care unspecified or N/A
1. Delivered
2. Delivered with postpartum complication
3. Antepartum complication
4. Postpartum complication

5th digit: 660.2
0. Episode of care unspecified or N/A
1. Delivered
3. Antepartum complication

ORGANS CONGENITAL

751.8 Abdominal viscera
756.79 Abdominal viscera due to defect in anterior abdominal wall
759.1 Adrenal gland
753.5 Bladder
748.69 Bone and cartilage in lung
742.4 Brain
757.6 Breast tissue

ECTOPIC (continued)

ORGANS CONGENITAL (continued)

746.87 Cardium
742.4 Cerebrum
746.87 Cordis
617.9 Endometrium
751.69 Gallbladder
750.7 Gastric mucosa
743.37 Lentis
752.0 Ovary congenital
751.7 Pancreas
750.26 Sebaceous glands mouth
752.51 Testis
759.2 Thyroid
753.5 Vesicae

PREGNANCY (RUPTURED) (UNRUPTURED)

633.90 NOS
761.4 NOS affecting fetus or newborn
633.90 NOS with complication during treatment **[639.#]**
639.# NOS with complication following treatment
633.91 NOS with intrauterine pregnancy
633.91 NOS with intrauterine pregnancy with complication during treatment **[639.#]**
633.00 Abdominal
761.4 Abdominal affecting fetus or newborn
633.00 Abdominal with complication during treatment **[639.#]**
639.# Abdominal with complication following treatment
633.01 Abdominal with intrauterine pregnancy
633.01 Abdominal with intrauterine pregnancy with complication during treatment **[639.#]**
761.4 Affecting fetus or newborn
639.# Complication following treatment
633.80 Cornual
761.4 Cornual affecting fetus or newborn
633.80 Cornual with complication during treatment **[639.#]**
639.# Cornual with complication following treatment
633.81 Cornual with intrauterine pregnancy
633.81 Cornual with intrauterine pregnancy with complication during treatment **[639.#]**
633.20 Ovarian
761.4 Ovarian affecting fetus or newborn
633.20 Ovarian with complication during treatment **[639.#]**
639.# Ovarian with complication following treatment
633.21 Ovarian with intrauterine pregnancy
633.21 Ovarian with intrauterine pregnancy with complication during treatment **[639.#]**
633.10 Tubal
761.4 Tubal affecting fetus or newborn
633.10 Tubal with complication during treatment **[639.#]**
639.# Tubal with complication following treatment
633.11 Tubal with intrauterine pregnancy
633.11 Tubal with intrauterine pregnancy with complication during treatment **[639.#]**

4th digit: 639
0. Genital tract and pelvic infection
1. Delayed or excessive hemorrhage
2. Damage to pelvic organs and tissue
3. Renal failure
4. Metabolic disorders
5. Shock
6. Embolism
8. Other specified complication
9. Unspecified complication

E

ECTOPIC (continued)

PREGNANCY (RUPTURED) (UNRUPTURED) (continued)

633.80	Other
761.4	Other affecting fetus or newborn
633.80	Other with complication during treatment [**639.#**]
639.#	Other with complication following treatment
633.81	Other with intrauterine pregnancy
633.81	Other with intrauterine pregnancy with complication during treatment [**639.#**]

4th digit: 639

0. Genital tract and pelvic infection
1. Delayed or excessive hemorrhage
2. Damage to pelvic organs and tissue
3. Renal failure
4. Metabolic disorders
5. Shock
6. Embolism
8. Other specified complication
9. Unspecified complication

SECRETION

259.3	ADH
259.3	Adrenalin
255.0	Adrencorticotropin
259.3	Epinephrine
259.3	Hormone NEC
259.3	Norepinephrine
259.3	Pituitary (posterior)

ECTOPIC (continued)

427.69	Ventricular beats

ECTROMELIA

755.4	Unspecified
755.30	Lower limb
755.20	Upper limb

ECTROPION

569.49	Anal
622.0	Cervical
616.0	Cervical with cervicitis
374.10	Eyelid
374.14	Eyelid - cicatricial
743.62	Eyelid - congenital
374.12	Eyelid - mechanical
374.11	Eyelid - senile
374.13	Eyelid - spastic
364.54	Eyelid - uvea
528.5	Lip
750.26	Lip congenital
569.49	Rectal
599.84	Urethral

ECZEMA

692.9	NOS
692.9	Allergic
706.8	Asteatotic
691.8	Atopic
692.9	Contact NEC
692.9	Dermatitis NEC
705.81	Dyshydrotic

ECZEMA (continued)

380.22	Ear (external)
691.8	Flexural
274.89	Gouty
054.0	Herpeticum herpes simplex
701.8	Hypertrophicum
684	Impetiginous
690.12	Infantile (seborrheic) (intertriginous)
692.9	Intertriginous NEC
690.12	Intertriginous infantile (seborrheic)
691.8	Intrinsic
692.9	Lichenified NEC
110.3	Marginatum
692.9	Nummular
316	Psychogenic [692.9]
316	Psychogenic atopic [691.8]
686.8	Pustular
690.18	Seborrheic
690.12	Seborrheic infantile
692.79	Solar
454.1	Stasis (lower extremity)
454.2	Stasis (lower extremity) with ulcer
454.8	Stasis varicose with edema
454.8	Stasis varicose with pain
454.8	Stasis varicose with swelling
454.8	Stasis varicose with other complications
279.12	Thrombocytopenia syndrome
999.0	Vaccinatum
698.3	Verrucosum callosum

756.51	EDDOWES' SYNDROME (BRITTLE BONES AND BLUE SCLERA)

EDEMA

782.3	NOS
995.1	Allergic
909.9	Allergic late effect
348.5	Cerebral
372.73	Conjunctiva
0	Corneal see 'Cornea, Corneal', edema
374.82	Eyelid
782.3	Extremities lower
454.8	Extremities lower due to varicose vein
459.2	Extremities lower due to venous obstruction
629.89	Genitalia - female NOS
608.86	Genitalia - male NOS
478.6	Glottic
478.6	Laryngeal
782.3	Leg
454.8	Leg due to varicose vein
459.2	Leg due to venous obstruction
757.0	Leg hereditary
782.3	Localized NOS
782.3	Lower extremities
454.8	Lower extremities due to varicose vein
459.2	Lower extremities due to venous obstruction

E

EDEMA (continued)

362.83 Macular
362.53 Macular cystoid
250.5# Macular diabetic cystoid [362.53]
250.5# Macular diabetic with retinopathy [**362.0#**] [362.07]

5th digit: 250.5
- **0. Type II, adult-onset, non-insulin dependent (even if requiring insulin), or unspecified; controlled**
- **1. Type I, juvenile-onset or insulin-dependent; controlled**
- **2. Type II, adult-onset, non-insulin dependent (even if requiring insulin); uncontrolled**
- **3. Type I, juvenile-onset or insulin-dependent; uncontrolled**

4th digit: 362.0
- **1. Background or NOS**
- **2. Proliferative**
- **3. Nonproliferative NOS**
- **4. Nonproliferative mild**
- **5. Nonproliferative moderate**
- **6. Nonproliferative severe**

040.0 Malignant
778.5 Neonatorum
778.5 Newborn other and unspecified
262 Nutritional without mention of dyspigmentation of skin and hair
376.33 Orbital
577.8 Pancreatic
782.3 Pedal
607.83 Penile
478.25 Pharynx or nasopharynx
782.3 Pitting

PULMONARY

514 NOS
518.4 Acute
507.0 Acute aspiration
428.1 Acute cardiogenic
506.1 Acute chemical or fumes
518.4 Acute due to pneumonia
518.4 Acute postoperative
428.0 Acute with CHF (right heart failure)
402.91 Acute with hypertensive heart failure - NOS
402.11 Acute with hypertensive heart failure - benign
402.01 Acute with hypertensive heart failure - malignant
428.1 Acute with left heart failure
518.5 Adult respiratory distress syndrome associated with shock
507.0 Associated with aspiration pneumonia [518.82]
514 Associated with hypostatic pneumonia
518.81 Associated with respiratory failure - acute in other conditions
518.84 Associated with respiratory failure - acute and chronic in other conditions
518.83 Associated with respiratory failure - chronic in other conditions
518.82 Associated with other conditions
514 Chronic
518.4 Due to ARDS [518.82]
518.4 Due to ARDS drug overdose
518.5 Due to ARDS post op with shock
518.5 Due to ARDS traumatic [518.4]
508.9 Due to external agents - unspecified
508.8 Due to external agents - other

EDEMA (continued)

PULMONARY (continued)

508.1 Due to radiation chronic
508.0 Due to radiation pneumonitis
518.4 Due to renal disease chronic [**585.#**]

4th digit: 585
- **1. Stage I**
- **2. Stage II (mild)**
- **3. Stage III (moderate)**
- **4. Stage IV (severe)**
- **5. Stage V**
- **6. End stage**
- **9. Unspecified stage**

518.5 Due to shock lung
518.5 Due to shock traumatic
518.5 Following trauma and surgery
518.4 Postoperative acute
518.4 Postoperative acute due to fluid overload [276.6]
391.8 Rheumatic acute
398.91 Rheumatic chronic
392.0 Rheumatic with chorea
428.## With heart disease or failure

4th digit: 428
- **0. Congestive**
- **1. Left**
- **2#. Systolic**
- **3#. Diastolic**
- **4#. Combined systolic and diastolic**
- **9. NOS**

5th digit: 428.2-4
- **0. NOS**
- **1. Acute**
- **2. Chronic**
- **3. Acute on chronic**

EDEMA (continued)

581.9 Renal
362.83 Retinal (localized) (macular) (peripheral)
362.53 Retinal (localized) (macular) (peripheral) cystoid
250.5# Retinal diabetic with retinopathy [**362.0#**] [362.07]

5th digit: 250.5
- **0. Type II, adult-onset, non-insulin dependent (even if requiring insulin), or unspecified; controlled**
- **1. Type I, juvenile-onset or insulin-dependent; controlled**
- **2. Type II, adult-onset, non-insulin dependent (even if requiring insulin); uncontrolled**
- **3. Type I, juvenile-onset or insulin-dependent; uncontrolled**

4th digit: 362.0
- **1. Background or NOS**
- **2. Proliferative**
- **3. Nonproliferative NOS**
- **4. Nonproliferative mild**
- **5. Nonproliferative moderate**
- **6. Nonproliferative severe**

608.86 Scrotal
336.1 Spinal cord arterial

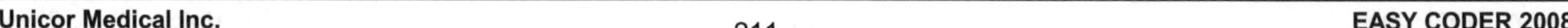

EDEMA (continued)

459.3# Stasis
459.1# Stasis due to deep vein thrombosis
5th digit: 459.1, 3
0. NOS
1. With ulcer
2. With inflammation
3. With ulcer and inflammation
9. With other complication

478.6 Subglottic
478.6 Supraglottic
782.3 Toxic
782.3 Unknown etiology
478.6 Vocal cords
624.8 Vulva (acute)

520.0 EDENTIA

525.1# EDENTIA ACQUIRED **[525.##]**
5th digit: 525.1
0. Unspecified
1. Due to trauma
2. Due to periodontal disease
3. Due to caries
9. Other
4th digit: 525
4. Complete or NOS
5. Partial
5th digit: 525
0. Unspecified
1. Class I
2. Class II
3. Class III
4. Class IV

524.30 EDENTIA CAUSING MALOCCLUSION

525.1# EDENTULISM DUE TO TRAUMA, EXTRACTION OR DISEASE **[525.##]**
5th digit: 525.1
0. Unspecified
1. Due to trauma
2. Due to periodontal disease
3. Due to caries
9. Other
4th digit: 525
4. Complete or NOS
5. Partial
5th digit: 525
0. Unspecified
1. Class I
2. Class II
3. Class III
4. Class IV

992.2 EDSALL'S DISEASE
V62.3 EDUCATIONAL CIRCUMSTANCE (HANDICAP) CAUSING ENCOUNTER
758.2 EDWARD'S SYNDROME

EEG

794.02 Abnormal
V72.83 Preoperative
V72.85 Screening

537.89 EFFERENT LOOP SYNDROME
704.02 EFFLUVIUM TELOGEN
306.2 EFFORT SYNDROME (AVIATORS') (PSYCHOGENIC)

EFFUSION

490 Bronchial (see also 'Bronchitis')
348.5 Cerebral
719.0# Joint
719.3# Joint intermittent
5th digit: 719.0, 3
0. Site unspecified
1. Shoulder region
2. Upper arm (elbow) (humerus)
3. Forearm (radius) (wrist) (ulna)
4. Hand (carpal) (metacarpal) (fingers)
5. Pelvis thigh (hip) (buttock) (femur)
6. Lower leg (fibula) (knee) (patella) (tibia)
7. Ankle and/or foot (metatarsals) (toes) (tarsals)
8. Other
9. Multiple

423.9 Pericardial
420.90 Pericardial acute
568.82 Peritoneal chronic
789.59 Peritoneal chronic ascites
511.9 Pleural - unspecified
511.9 Pleural - fetus or newborn
197.2 Pleural - malignant
511.9 Pleural - pleurisy NOS
997.3 Pleural - post op
511.1 Pleural - pneumococcal [041.2]
511.1 Pleural - staphylococcal **[041.1#]**
5th digit: 041.1
0. Unspecified
1. Aureus
9. Other

511.1 Pleural - streptococcal **[041.0#]**
5th digit: 041.0
0. NOS
1. Group A
2. Group B
3. Group C
4. Group D (enterococcus)
5. Group G
9. Other strep

862.29 Pleural - traumatic without open wound
862.39 Pleural - traumatic with open wound
012.0# Pleural - tuberculous
010.1# Pleural - tuberculous primary progressive
5th digit: 010.1, 012.0
0. Unspecified
1. Lab not done
2. Lab pending
3. Microscopy positive (in sputum)
4. Culture positive - microscopy negative
5. Culture negative - microscopy positive
6. Culture and microscopy negative confirmed by other methods

0 Pulmonary see 'Effusion', pleural
322.9 Spinal (see also 'Meningitis')

530.81 EGERD (ESOPHAGEAL GASTROINTESTINAL DISEASE)

V59.7# EGG DONOR (OOCYTE) (OVUM)
4th digit: V59.7
0. Unspecified
1. Under age 35, NOS or anonymous recipient
2. Under age 35, designated recipient
3. Age 35 and over, NOS or anonymous recipient
4. Age 35 and over, designated recipient

756.83 EHLERS DANLOS SYNDROME

082.4# EHRLICHIOSIS INFECTION
5th digit: 082.4
0. NOS
1. E. Chaffeensis
9. Other

111.0 EICHSTEDT'S PITYRIASIS VERSICOLOR

EIGHTH

388.5 Cranial nerve disorder (atrophy) (degeneration)
951.5 Cranial nerve injury
094.86 Nerve neuritis (syphilitic)

745.4 EISENMENGER'S DEFECT, SYNDROME OR COMPLEX (VENTRICULAR SEPTAL DEFECT)

EJACULATE/EJACULATORY

792.2 Abnormal
608.82 Bloody
752.9 Duct anomaly nos
752.89 Duct anomaly nec
752.89 Duct atresia (absence) (agenesis) (congenital)
608.89 Duct obstruction
608.89 Painful
306.59 Painful psychogenic
302.75 Premature
608.87 Retrograde

333.94 EKBOM'S SYNDROME (RESTLESS LEG)

EKG

794.31 Abnormal
412 M.I. diagnosed, but presenting no symptoms
V71.7 Normal (evaluation for suspected heart disease)
V72.81 Preoperative exam

756.51 EKMAN'S SYNDROME (BRITTLE BONES AND BLUE SCLERA)

215.# ELASTOFIBROMA M8820/0
4th digit: 215
0. Head, face, neck
2. Upper limb including shoulder
3. Lower limb including hip
4. Thorax
5. Abdomen (wall), gastric, gastrointestinal, intestine, stomach
6. Pelvis, buttock, groin, inguinal region, perineum
7. Trunk NOS, back NOS, flank NOS
8. Other specified sites
9. Site unspecified

701.8 ELASTOIDOSIS CUTANEA NODULARIS
757.39 ELASTOMA JUVENILE

ELASTOSIS

701.8 NOS
701.1 Perforans serpiginosa
701.8 Senilis
692.74 Solar

ELBOW

736.00 Deformity acquired
726.30 Inflammation (enthesopathy)
959.3 Injury
913.8 Injury other and unspecified superficial
913.9 Injury other and unspecified superficial infected
719.82 Joint calcification
718.92 Joint ligament relaxation
0 Joint ligament tear see 'Sprain'
0 Joint see also 'Joint'
718.12 Loose body
726.39 Other specified inflammation
V54.81 Replacement aftercare [V43.62]
V43.62 Replacement status
841.9 Separation (rupture) (tear) (laceration)
841.8 Separation (rupture) (tear) (laceration) other specified sites
841.9 Strain (sprain) (avulsion) (hemarthrosis)
841.8 Strain (sprain) (avulsion) (hemarthrosis) other specified sites

Injury of a tendon joint capsule, or ligament can be a separation, tear, laceration, avulsion, strain, sprain, or hemarthrosis. You can find this under 'Sprain' also.

ELECTIVE SURGERY

V50.9 Procedure unspecified
V50.8 Other specified surgery

266.2 ELECTRIC FEET SYNDROME
0 ELECTRICAL BURN SEE 'BURN', BY SITE
994.8 ELECTRICAL SHOCK NONFATAL
909.4 ELECTRICAL SHOCK LATE EFFECT
794.31 ELECTROCARDIOGRAM ABNORMAL
994.8 ELECTROCUTION
909.4 ELECTROCUTION LATE EFFECT
794.02 ELECTROENCEPHALOGRAM (EEG) ABNORMAL

ELECTROLYTE

791.9 Abnormal level - urinary
276.9 Disorder (imbalance) NEC
276.9 Disorder (imbalance) uremic
276.2 Imbalance acidosis
276.3 Imbalance alkalosis
643.1# Imbalance associated with hyperemesis in pregnancy
5th digit: 643.1
0. Episode of care unspecified or N/A
1. Delivered
3. Antepartum complication

669.0# Imbalance complicating L&D
5th digit: 669.0
0. Episode of care unspecified or N/A
1. Delivered
2. Delivered with postpartum complication
3. Antepartum complication
4. Postpartum complication

639.4 Imbalance following abortion/ectopic/molar pregnancy
775.5 Imbalance newborn (transitory)
791.9 Level abnormal - urinary
775.5 Neonatal transitory disturbance NEC

794.17 ELECTROMYOGRAM ABNORMAL EXCLUDES EYE
794.12 ELECTRO-OCULOGRAM ABNORMAL (EOG)
794.11 ELECTRORETINOGRAM (ERG) ABNORMAL

237.71 ELEPHANT MAN SYNDROME

ELEPHANTIASIS

457.1 NOS
125.1 Due to brugia (wuchereria) malayi
125.0 Due to wuchereria bancrofti
125.9 Filarial
457.1 Nonfilarial
757.0 Nonfilarial congenital
374.83 Nonfilarial eyelid
624.8 Nonfilarial vulva
457.0 Post mastectomy
997.99 Surgical

352.4 ELEVENTH CRANIAL NERVE DISORDERS (ATROPHY)

951.6 ELEVENTH CRANIAL NERVE INJURY

ELLIPTOCYTOSIS

282.1 NOS (congenital) (hereditary)
282.7 HB-C (disease)
282.7 Hemoglobin disease
282.60 Sickle-cell disease (anemia)
0 Sickle-cell disease (anemia) with crisis see 'Sickle Cell'
282.5 Sickle-cell trait

756.55 ELLIS-VAN CREVELD SYNDROME (CHONDROECTODERMAL DYSPLASIA)

251.5 ELLISON-ZOLLINGER (GASTRIC HYPERSECRETION WITH PANCREATIC ISLET CELL TUMOR)

309.22 EMANCIPATION ADJUSTMENT REACTION (ADOLESCENT) (EARLY ADULT)

EMBOLISM

958.0 Air (any site)
999.1 Air following infusion, perfusion or transfusion
908.6 Air following trauma late effect
444.1 Aorta
444.0 Aorta abdominal
444.0 Aorta bifurcation
444.0 Aorta saddle
444.1 Aorta thoracic
444.0 Aortoiliac
444.9 Artery NOS
444.22 Artery lower extremity

When assigning code 449, use an additional code to identify the site of the embolism (433.0-433.9) (444.0-444.9).

449 Artery pyemic (septic)
415.12 Artery pyemic pulmonary
449 Artery septic (pyemic)
444.89 Artery specified site NEC
444.21 Artery upper extremity
433.8# Auditory artery internal
433.0# Basilar artery
433.3# Basilar artery bilateral or multiple
444.89 Bladder artery
444.21 Brachial artery
434.1# Brain
448.9 Capillary
0 Cardiac acute with infarction see 'Myocardial Infarction Acute'
5th digit: 433.0, 3, 8, 434.1
0. Without cerebral infarction
1. With cerebral infarction

EMBOLISM (continued)

433.1# Carotid artery
433.3# Carotid artery bilateral or multiple
433.8# Cerebellar artery
434.1# Cerebral artery or vein
997.02 Cerebral artery postoperative NEC
0 Cholesterol see 'Atheroembolsim'
433.8# Choroidal artery
433.8# Communicating posterior artery
0 Complicating abortion see 'Abortion', by type, with embolism
0 Complicating ectopic pregnancy see 'Ectopic Pregnancy', by site with complication
0 Complicating molar pregnancy see 'Molar Pregnancy', by type with complication
0 Coronary artery or vein acute with infarction see 'Myocardial Infarction Acute'
411.81 Coronary artery or vein acute without MI
0 Due to a device see 'Complication Of A Device, Implant Or Graft - Other Specified'
434.1# Encephalomalacia
5th digit: 433.1, 3, 8, 434.1
0. Without cerebral infarction
1. With cerebral infarction

444.22 Extremity artery NOS
444.22 Extremity artery lower
444.21 Extremity artery upper
453.4# Extremity vein lower deep
5th digit: 453.4
0. NOS
1. Proximal (femoral) (iliac) (popliteal) (thigh) (upper leg NOS)
2. Distal (calf) (peroneal) (tibial) (lower leg NOS)

0 Eye see 'Retinal Artery Occlusion'
958.1 Fat (cerebral) (pulmonary) (systemic)
958.1 Fat following trauma
908.6 Fat following trauma late effect
444.22 Femoral artery
453.8 Femoral vein
453.41 Femoral vein deep
639.6 Following abortion
639.6 Following ectopic or molar pregnancy
0 Heart acute with infarction see 'Myocardial Infarction Acute'
453.0 Hepatic (vein)
433.8# Hypophyseal artery
444.81 Iliac (artery)
453.41 Iliac vein deep
444.81 Iliofemoral
557.0 Intestine (artery) (vein) (with gangrene)
434.1# Intracranial
326 Intracranial sinus (septic) late effect
325 Intracranial venous sinus (any)
437.6 Intracranial venous sinus nonpyogenic
593.81 Kidney (artery)
434.1# Meninges
5th digit: 433.8, 434.1
0. Without cerebral infarction
1. With cerebral infarction

557.0 Mesenteric (artery) (vein) (with gangrene)
444.9 Multiple NEC
0 Ophthalmic artery see 'Retinal Artery Occlusion'
444.9 Paradoxical NEC
607.82 Penis

E

EMBOLISM (continued)

444.22 Peripheral artery NEC
997.2 Peripheral vascular postoperative NEC
453.42 Peroneal vein deep
253.8 Pituitary
433.8# Pontine artery
444.22 Popliteal (artery)
453.41 Popliteal vein deep
452 Portal (vein)
433.8# Posterior communicating artery
997.2 Postoperative NEC
997.02 Postoperative cerebral artery NEC
997.71 Postoperative mesenteric artery
415.11 Postoperative pulmonary
415.12 Postoperative pulmonary septic
997.72 Postoperative renal artery
997.79 Postoperative other vessels
433.9# Precerebral artery NOS
433.3# Precerebral artery bilateral or multiple
433.8# Precerebral artery NEC

5th digit: 433.3, 8-9, 434.1
0. Without cerebral infarction
1. With cerebral infarction

415.11 Pulmonary (artery) (vein) iatrogenic
415.19 Pulmonary (artery) (vein) other and NOS
415.11 Pulmonary (artery) (vein) postoperative
415.12 Pulmonary (artery) (vein) septic
038.#(#) Pulmonary (artery) (vein) septic with septicemia [415.12]
415.12 Pulmonary (artery) (vein) (septic) postoperative
038.#(#) Pyemic (artery) (vein) septic with septicemia [415.12]

4th or 4th and 5th digit code for organism: 038
.9 NOS
.3 Anaerobic
.3 Bacteroides
.3 Clostridium
.42 E. coli
.49 Enterobacter aerogenes
.40 Gram negative
.49 Gram negative other
.41 Hemophilus influenzae
.2 Pneumococcal
.49 Proteus
.43 Pseudomonas
.44 Serratia
.10 Staphylococcal NOS
.11 Staphylococcal aureus
.19 Staphylococcal other
.0 Streptococcal (anaerobic)
.49 Yersinia enterocolitica
.8 Other specified

593.81 Renal artery
453.3 Renal vein
0 Retinal artery see 'Retinal Artery Occlusion'
444.0 Saddle aorta
0 Soap with abortion see 'Abortion', by type with embolism
0 Soap with ectopic or molar pregnancy see 'Ectopic Pregnancy' or 'Molar Pregnancy', by site or type with complication
444.89 Spinal artery
336.1 Spinal cord
324.1 Spinal cord septic or pyogenic
444.89 Spleen (artery)
453.41 Thigh vein deep
999.2 Thrombus following infusion, perfusion or transfusion
453.42 Tibial vein deep

EMBOLISM (continued)

444.21 Ulnar artery
453.9 Vein NOS
453.8 Vein lower extremity
453.4# Vein lower extremity deep

5th digit: 453.4
0. NOS
1. Proximal (femoral) (iliac) (popliteal) (thigh) (upper leg NOS)
2. Distal (calf) (peroneal) (tibial) (lower leg NOS)

453.8 Vein other specified site
0 Vein with inflammation or phlebitis see 'Thrombophlebitis'
453.2 Vena cava
433.2# Vertebral artery
433.3# Vertebral artery bilateral or multiple

5th digit: 433.2-3
0. Without cerebral infarction
1. With cerebral infarction

EMBOLISM COMPLICATING PREGNANCY

673.0# Air due to pregnancy
673.1# Amniotic fluid due to pregnancy
673.2# Blood-clot due to pregnancy
674.0# Brain due to pregnancy

When coding a maternal cardiovascular disease complicating pregnancy, 648.6#, use an additional code to identify the condition.

648.6# Cardiac current (co-existent)
674.0# Cerebral due to pregnancy
673.8# Fat due to pregnancy
671.5# Intracranial venous sinus nonpyogenic due to pregnancy
673.2# Pulmonary puerperal NOS due to pregnancy
673.8# Pulmonary other due to pregnancy
673.3# Septic (pyemic) due to pregnancy
671.5# Spinal due to pregnancy

648.9#: Use an additional code to identify the specific vascular or lymphatic embolus.

648.9# Vascular and lymphatic maternal current (co-existent) in pregnancy

When coding a maternal cardiovascular disease complicating pregnancy, 648.6#, use an additional code to identify the condition.

648.6# Other specified cardiovascular disease current (co-existent) in pregnancy

5th digit: 648.6, 9, 671.5, 673.0-3, 8, 674.0
0. Episode of care NOS or N/A
1. Delivered
2. Delivered with postpartum complication
3. Antepartum complication
4. Postpartum complication

186.9 EMBRYONAL CARCINOMA SITE NOS
0 EMBRYONAL CARCINOMA SITE SPECIFIED SEE 'CANCER', BY SITE M9070/3
752.41 EMBYRONIC CYST CERVIX VAGINA AND EXTERNAL FEMALE GENITALIA
270.2 EMBYRONIC FIXATION SYNDROME

E

787.03 EMESIS
787.01 EMESIS WITH NAUSEA

EMG

794.17 Abnormal
794.14 Eye abnormal
V72.83 Preoperative
V72.85 Screening

EMOTIONAL, EMOTIONALLY

309.29 Crisis NEC (see also 'Stress', 'Adjustment Reaction')
308.0 Crisis, acute reaction to stress
313.9 Disturbance of childhood or adolescence - unspecified
313.89 Disturbance of childhood or adolescence - other
301.3 Instability (excessive)
301.3 Pathological
V40.9 Problem
301.59 Unstable
300.9 Upset

EMPHYSEMA NONPULMONARY

958.7 Cellular tissue
908.6 Cellular tissue late effect
372.89 Conjunctiva
595.89 Emphysematous cystitis
376.89 Eye
374.85 Eyelid
416.9 Heart
958.7 Mediastinal tissue late effect
958.7 Mediastinal traumatic
908.6 Mediastinal traumatic late effect
376.89 Orbit
958.7 Subcutaneous traumatic
908.6 Subcutaneous traumatic late effect
998.81 Surgical resulting from a procedure
254.8 Thymus (congenital)

EMPHYSEMA PULMONARY

492.8 Unspecified
492.8 Atrophic
492.0 Bullous
492.8 Centriacinar
492.8 Centrilobular
518.2 Compensatory
770.2 Congenital
506.4 Due to fumes and vapors
492.0 Emphysematous bleb
492.0 Emphysematous bleb ruptured
518.1 Interstitial
770.2 Interstitial newborn
518.1 Mediastinal
770.2 Mediastinal in fetus or newborn
492.8 Obstructive
492.8 Panacinar
492.8 Panlobular
492.0 Ruptured emphysematous bleb
V81.3 Screening
492.8 Vesicular
491.2# With bronchitis (chronic)
5th digit: 491.2
0. NOS
1. With (acute) exacerbation
2. With acute bronchitis

492.0 EMPHYSEMATOUS BLEB
595.89 EMPHYSEMATOUS CYSTITIS
V62.1 EMPLOYMENT ADVERSE EFFECT OF ENVIRONMENT CAUSING ENCOUNTER
V62.2 EMPLOYMENT DISSATISFACTION CAUSING ENCOUNTER
253.8 EMPTY SELLA (TURCICA) SYNDROME

EMPYEMA NONPULMONARY

473.9 Accessory sinus
324.0 Brain
473.2 Ethmoid sinus
473.1 Frontal sinus
575.0 Gallbladder (see also 'Cholecystitis', acute)
383.00 Mastoid
526.4 Maxillary jaw
473.0 Maxillary sinus
473.9 Nasal sinus (chronic)
473.9 Nasal sinus accessory
473.3 Sphenoidal sinus
324.9 Subdural
593.89 Ureteral

EMPYEMA PULMONARY

510.9 Unspecified
510.9 Lung
513.0 Lung with abscess
510.0 Lung with fistula

ENAMEL HYPOPLASIA (TEETH)

520.4 Neonatal
520.4 Postnatal
520.4 Prenatal

ENCEPHALITIS

323.9 NOS
039.8 Actinomycosis [323.41]
136.9 Acute disseminated - infectious [323.61]
323.81 Acute disseminated - noninfectious
323.51 Acute disseminated - postimmunization or postvaccination
049.8 Acute inclusion body necrotizing
049.8 Acute necrotizing
136.2 Amebic (naegleria)
062.4 Australian
062.5 California virus
982.1 Carbon tetrachloride (solvent) [323.71]
078.3 Cat scratch disease [323.01]
063.2 Central european
046.2 Dawson's inclusion body
136.9 Due to infection classified elsewhere [323.41]
062.2 Eastern equine
049.8 Epidemic
323.51 Following immunization procedures
054.3 Herpes NOS
054.3 Herpes simplex
054.3 Herpes simian B
054.3 Herpesvirus human NOS
058.21 Herpesvirus human 6
058.29 Herpesvirus human other (7)
961.3 Hydroxyquinoline derivatives toxicity [323.71]
323.2 In protozoal diseases classified elsewhere
323.1 In rickettsial diseases classified elsewhere
323.01 In viral diseases classified elsewhere
062.8 Ilheus virus
487.8 Influenza [323.41]
046.1 Jakob Creutzfeldt with presenile dementia
062.0 Japanese
062.0 Japanese B
046.0 Kuru
062.5 La crosse
063.8 Langat

ENCEPHALITIS (continued)

326 Late effect
139.8 Late effect - due to infectious disease
326 Late effect - due to nervous system disease
139.0 Late effect - due to viral diseases
984.# Lead toxicity [323.71]
4th digit: 984
0. Inorganic compounds
1. Organic compounds
2. Other compounds
9. Unspecified

049.8 Lethargica
046.3 Leukoencephalopathy (multifocal) (progressive)
063.1 Louping ill
710.0 Lupus [323.81]
084.6 Malarial [323.2]
036.1 Meningococcal
985.0 Mercury toxicity [323.71]
075 Mononucleosis [323.01]
062.9 Mosquito borne viral
V73.5 Mosquito borne viral screening exam
072.2 Mumps
062.4 Murray valley
064 Negishi virus
073.7 Ornithosis [323.01]
323.81 Other causes
382.4 Otitic NEC [323.41]
123.9 Parasitic NEC [323.41]
341.1 Periaxialis (concentrica) (diffusa)
052.0 Post chickenpox
057.9 Postexanthematous NEC [323.62]
323.51 Postimmunization
136.9 Postinfectious [323.62]
055.0 Postmeasles
323.81 Posttraumatic
323.51 Postvaccinal (smallpox)
052.0 Postvaricella
079.99 Postviral NEC [323.62]
057.9 Postviral postexanthematous [323.62]
058.10 Postviral postexanthematous specified NEC [323.62]
063.8 Powassan
323.51 Prophylactic inoculation against smallpox
323.81 Rasmussen
083.9 Rickettsial [323.1]
049.8 Rio bravo
056.01 Rubella
063.0 Russian spring summer [taiga]
062.3 St Louis
984.9 Saturnine [323.71]
046.2 Subacute sclerosing
094.81 Syphilitic
090.41 Syphilitic congenital
985.8 Thallium toxicity [323.71]
V73.5 Tick borne screening exam
063.9 Tick borne viral
063.2 Tick borne viral central European
063.1 Tick borne viral louping ill
063.0 Tick borne viral Russian spring-summer
063.8 Tick borne viral other specified
117.5 Torula [323.41]
989.9 Toxic NEC [323.71]
130.0 Toxoplasmosis
771.2 Toxoplasmosis congenital [323.41]
124 Trichinosis [323.41]
086.0 Trypanosomal [323.2]

ENCEPHALITIS (continued)

013.6# Tuberculous
5th digit: 013.6
0. Unspecified
1. Lab not done
2. Lab pending
3. Microscopy positive (in sputum)
4. Culture positive - microscopy negative
5. Culture negative - microscopy positive
6. Culture and microscopy negative confirmed by other methods

081.9 Typhus (fever) [323.1]
323.51 Vaccination (smallpox))
V05.0 Vaccination (viral arthropod borne)
046.2 Van Bogaert's
066.2 Venezuelan equine
049.9 Viral
064 Viral arthropod borne vector unknown
139.0 Viral late effects
062.8 Viral other specified mosquito borne
063.8 Viral other specified tick borne
V73.5 Viral screening exam
063.9 Viral tick borne
066.41 West Nile
062.1 Western equine
323.81 Other specified cause

742.0 ENCEPHALOCELE CONGENITAL
376.81 ENCEPHALOCELE ORBITAL
759.6 ENCEPHALOCUTANEOUS ANGIOMATOSIS
742.0 ENCEPHALOCYSTOCELE CONGENITAL

ENCEPHALOMALACIA

434.9# NOS
431 Due to hemorrhage
435.9 Due to recurrent spasm of artery
434.1# Embolic
290.12 Subcorticalis chronicus arteriosclerotica
434.0# Thrombotic
5th digit: 434.0, 1, 9
0. Without cerebral infarction
1. With cerebral infarction

136.9 ENCEPHALOMYELITIS ACUTE DISSEMINATED (ADEM) – INFECTIOUS [323.61]
323.81 ENCEPHALOMYELITIS ACUTE DISSEMINATED (ADEM) - NONINFECTIOUS
323.51 ENCEPHALOMYELITIS POSTIMMUNIZATION OR POSTVACCINAL
326 ENCEPHALOMYELITIS POSTIMMUNIZATION OR POSTVACCINAL LATE EFFECT
0 ENCEPHALOMYELITIS SEE ALSO 'ENCEPHALITIS'

742.0 ENCEPHALOMYELOCELE CONGENITAL

ENCEPHALOPATHY

348.30 Unspecified
348.30 Acute
291.2 Alcohol induced
348.1 Anoxic
437.0 Arteriosclerotic
292.81 Drug induced
572.2 Hepatic
437.2 Hypertensive
251.2 Hypoglycemic

E

ENCEPHALOPATHY (continued)

768.7 Hypoxic – ischemic (HIE)
348.31 Metabolic
323.61 Necrotizing hemorrhagic
330.8 Necrotizing subacute
984.9 Saturnine [323.71]
348.31 Septic
349.82 Toxic metabolic
586 Uremia
348.39 Other specified type NEC

ENCEPHALOPATHY DUE TO OTHER CAUSES

774.7 Bilirubin perinatal
742.9 Congenital
294.8 Due to dialysis
293.9 Due to dialysis transient
265.2 Due to nicotine acid deficiency
310.2 Due to trauma (postconcussional)
323.51 Due to vaccination
251.2 Hypoglycemic
487.8 Influenza (due to)
984.9 Lead [323.71]
046.1 Spongiform subacute
094.81 Syphilitic
349.82 Toxic
086.9 Trypanosomal [323.2]
266.9 Vitamin B deficiency
265.1 Wernicke's (polioencephalitis)
0 With SIRS see 'SIRS' with encephalopathy

0 ENCEPHALORRHAGIA SEE 'HEMORRHAGE' BRAIN
756.4 ENCHONDROMATOSIS CONGENITAL
787.6 ENCOPRESIS
307.7 ENCOPRESIS PSYCHOGENIC

When using code V66.7, code the terminal illness first.

V66.7 END-OF-LIFE CARE ENCOUNTER
585.6 END STAGE RENAL DISEASE (ESRD)
585.6 END-STAGE RENAL FAILURE

ENDARTERITIS

447.6 Unspecified
414.0# Coronary Arteriosclerotic
414.0# Coronary arteriosclerotic with chronic complete or total occlusion [414.2]
5th digit: 414.0
0. Unspecified type of vessel, native or graft
1. Native coronary vessel
2. Autologous vein bypass graft
3. Nonautologous biological bypass graft
4. Autologous artery bypass graft (gastroepiploic) (internal mammary)
5. Unspecified type of bypass graft
6. Native vessel of transplanted heart
7. Bypass graft of transplanted heart

417.8 Pulmonary
362.18 Retinal
0 See also 'Arteritis'

0 ENDEMIC POLYARTHRITIS SEE 'KASCHIN-BECK DISEASE'

745.60 ENDOCARDIAL CUSHION DEFECT CONGENITAL
425.3 ENDOCARDIAL FIBROELASTOSIS
424.90 ENDOCARDIAL OBSTRUCTION
424.99 ENDOCARDIAL OBSTRUCTION ARTERIOSCLEROTIC
424.99 ENDOCARDIAL OBSTRUCTION SPECIFIED CAUSE, NONRHEUMATIC

ENDOCARDITIS

424.90 NOS
397.9 NOS - rheumatic inactive or quiescent (with chorea)
421.9 Acute (subacute)
391.1 Acute (subacute) - rheumatic
392.0 Acute (subacute) - rheumatic with chorea

AORTIC

424.1 NOS (arteriosclerotic) (hypertensive)
421.9 NOS acute (subacute)
746.89 Congenital
391.1 Rheumatic active (acute)
392.0 Rheumatic active (acute) - with chorea
396.9 Rheumatic active (acute) - with mitral disease
395.9 Rheumatic inactive (quiescent) (with chorea)
396.9 Rheumatic inactive (quiescent) with mitral disease (with chorea)
424.1 Other specified cause nonrheumatic

ENDOCARDITIS (continued)

424.90 Aseptic
421.0 Bacterial
424.90 Chronic valvular NOS
397.9 Chronic valvular NOS - rheumatic inactive or quiescent
425.3 Congenital
421.0 Constrictive
425.3 Fetal
996.61 Heart valve prosthesis complication - infection or inflammation
424.99 Hypertensive
421.0 Infectious or infective

When assigning code 449, use an additional code to identify the site of the embolism (433.0-433.9) (444.0-444.9).

449 Infectious or infective with septic arterial embolism
421.0 Lenta
421.0 Loffler's
421.0 Malignant

MITRAL

394.9 NOS (rheumatic)
391.1 Acute (active)
421.0 Acute (active) - bacterial
396.9 Acute (active) - with aortic disease
392.0 Acute (active) - with chorea
424.0 Arteriosclerotic
746.89 Congenital
424.0 Hypertensive
391.1 Rheumatic - acute (active)
392.0 Rheumatic - acute (active) with chorea
394.9 Rheumatic - inactive (quiescent) (with chorea)
396.9 Rheumatic - inactive (quiescent) with aortic valve disease (with chorea)

E

ENDOCARDITIS (continued)

PULMONARY

424.3 NOS (arteriosclerotic)
421.9 Acute or subacute
391.1 Acute or subacute - rheumatic (active)
392.0 Acute or subacute - rheumatic (active) with chorea
746.09 Congenital
424.3 Hypertensive
391.1 Rheumatic acute (active) (subacute)
392.0 Rheumatic acute (active) (subacute) with chorea
397.1 Rheumatic chronic (inactive)

ENDOCARDITIS (continued)

421.0 Purulent
391.1 Rheumatic active or acute valve NOS
392.0 Rheumatic active or acute valve NOS with chorea
397.9 Rheumatic chronic valve NOS
421.0 Septic
0 Subacute see 'Endocarditis', by site, acute
421.0 Suppurative
0 Toxic see 'Endocarditis', by site, acute

TRICUSPID

397.0 NOS
391.1 Active or acute
392.0 Active or acute with chorea
397.0 Chronic, inactive or quiescent
746.89 Congenital
424.2 Nonrheumatic (arteriosclerotic) (hypertensive)
421.9 Nonrheumatic acute or subacute
397.0 Rheumatic
391.1 Rheumatic active (acute)
392.0 Rheumatic active (acute) with chorea
397.0 Rheumatic inactive (chronic) (quiescent)

ENDOCARDITIS (continued)

421.0 Ulcerative
421.0 Vegetative

> ***The code in the left margin always sequences first. The additional code in brackets to the right of the description is sequenced second. Underlining shows the code number that corresponds to the underlined description. Underlining never implies correct sequencing.***

ENDOCARDITIS OTHER CAUSES

421.0 Acute bacterial due to streptococcal **[041.0#]**
5th digit: 041.0
0. NOS
1. Group A
2. Group B
3. Group C
4. Group D (enterococcus)
5. Group G
9. Other strep

424.99 Arteriosclerotic
116.0 Blastomycotic [421.1]
112.81 Candidal
996.61 Cardiac valve prosthesis
074.22 Coxsackie
098.84 Gonococcal
115.94 Histoplasma
115.04 Histoplasma capsulatum
115.14 Histoplasma duboisii
425.3 In endocardial fibroelastosis

ENDOCARDITIS OTHER CAUSES (continued)

710.0 Libman Sachs [424.91]
710.0 Lupus [424.91]
036.42 Meningococcal
112.81 Moniliasis
421.0 Mycotic
421.0 Pneumococcic [041.2]
083.0 Q fever (due to) [421.1]
421.0 Serratia marcescens
421.0 Subacute bacterial due to staphylococcal **[041.1#]**
5th digit: 041.1
0. Unspecified
1. Aureus
9. Other

093.20 Syphilitic NEC
093.22 Syphilitic aortic valve
093.21 Syphilitic mitral valve
093.24 Syphilitic pulmonic valve
093.23 Syphilitic tricuspid valve
017.9# Tuberculous [424.91]
5th digit: 017.9
0. Unspecified
1. Lab not done
2. Lab pending
3. Microscopy positive (in sputum)
4. Culture positive - microscopy negative
5. Culture negative - microscopy positive
6. Culture and microscopy negative confirmed by other methods

002.0 Typhoid [421.1]
996.61 Valve prosthesis
424.90 Valve unspecified cause unspecified
397.9 Valve unspecified cause rheumatic
424.99 Valve unspecified cause specified
710.0 Verrucous atypical [424.91]
425.3 With endocardial fibroelastosis
424.99 Other specified cause except rheumatic

616.0 ENDOCERVICITIS (NONOBSTETRICAL)

ENDOCRINE

258.0# Adenomatosis multiple polyglandular activity
5th digit: 258.01-3
1. Type I
2. Type IIA
3. Type IIB

259.9 Disorder
306.6 Disorder psychogenic
259.9 Disturbance
775.9 Disturbance fetus and newborn
775.89 Disturbance neonatal other transitory
794.6 Function study other abnormal
759.2 Gland NEC absence (congenital)
255.3 Hypertensive syndrome
306.6 Malfunction psychogenic
V18.11 Multiple neoplasia syndrome (MEN) family history
V84.81 Multiple neoplasia syndrome (MEN) susceptibility genetic
V77.99 Screening for disorder
259.8 Other specified disorder NEC

ENDODERMAL SINUS TUMOR

183.0 Female site unspecified
0 Female site specified see 'Cancer', by site M9071/3
186.9 Male site unspecified
0 Site specified see 'Cancer', by site M8931/1

526.6# ENDODONTIC TREATMENT WITH PERIRADICULAR PATHOLOGY
5th digit: 526.6
1. Perforation of root canal space
2. Endodontic overfill
3. Endodontic underfill
9. Other

236.0 ENDOLYMPHATIC STROMAL MYOSIS SITE NOS
0 ENDOLYMPHATIC STROMAL MYOSIS SITE SPECIFIED SEE 'NEOPLASM UNCERTAIN BEHAVIOR' BY SITE M8931/1
0 ENDOMETRIAL SEE 'ENDOMETRIUM, ENDOMETRIAL'
199.1 ENDOMETRIOID CARCINOMA SITE UNSPECIFIED
0 ENDOMETRIOID CARCINOMA SITE SPECIFIED SEE 'CANCER', BY SITE M8380/3

ENDOMETRIOSIS

617.9 NOS
617.5 Appendix
617.8 Bladder
617.3 Broad ligament
617.0 Cervix
617.5 Colon
617.3 Douglas cul de sac
617.2 Fallopian tube
617.8 Gallbladder
617.8 Genital organ NEC (female)
617.6 In scar of skin
617.0 Internal
617.5 Intestine
617.8 Lung
617.0 Myometrium
617.1 Ovary
617.3 Pelvic peritoneum
617.3 Peritoneal parametrium
617.4 Rectovaginal septum and vagina
617.5 Rectum
617.3 Round ligament
617.6 Skin
236.0 Stromal
617.8 Umbilicus
617.0 Uterus
617.4 Vagina
617.8 Vulva
617.8 Other specified site NEC

ENDOMETRITIS

615.9 NOS
615.0 Acute
760.8 Affecting fetus or newborn
616.0 Cervical (hyperplastic)
615.1 Chronic
098.16 Gonococcal acute
098.36 Gonococcal chronic
098.16 Blennorrhagic acute
098.36 Blennorrhagic chronic
639.0 Following ectopic molar or aborted pregnancy

ENDOMETRITIS (continued)

621.3# Hyperplastic
5th digit: 621.3
0. NOS
1. Simple
2. Complex
3. With atypia

616.0 Hyperplastic cervix
615.9 Senile (atrophic)
016.7# Tuberculous
5th digit: 016.7
0. Unspecified
1. Lab not done
2. Lab pending
3. Microscopy positive (in sputum)
4. Culture positive - microscopy negative
5. Culture negative - microscopy positive
6. Culture and microscopy negative confirmed by other methods

ENDOMETRITIS OBSTETRICAL

760.8 Affecting fetus
0 Associated with pregnancy see specific condition
670.0# Maternal due to pregnancy
5th digit: 670.0
0. Unspecified
2. Delivered with postpartum complication
4. Postpartum complication

639.0 Post abortion or ectopic/molar pregnancy

ENDOMETRIUM, ENDOMETRIAL

621.8 Atrophy (senile)
622.8 Atrophy (senile) cervix
617.1 Cystoma (ovarian)
621.3# Hyperplasia
5th digit: 621.3
0. NOS
1. Simple
2. Complex
3. With atypia

622.10 Hyperplasia cervix
621.8 Metaplasia squamous
621.0 Polyp
793.5 Thickened

425.2 ENDOMYOCARDIAL DISEASE, IDIOPATHIC MURAL
425.0 ENDOMYOCARDIAL FIBROSIS
425.2 ENDOMYOCARDIOPATHY SOUTH AFRICAN
0 ENDOMYOCARDITIS SEE 'ENDOCARDITIS'
0 ENDOMYOMETRITIS SEE 'ENDOMETRITIS'
425.0 ENDOMYOFIBROSIS
0 ENDOPERICARDITIS SEE 'ENDOCARDITIS'
362.18 ENDOPHLEBITIS RETINA
0 ENDOPHLEBITIS SEE 'THROMBOPHLEBITIS'
0 ENDOPHTHALMIA SEE 'ENDOPHTHALMITIS'

ENDOPHTHALMITIS

360.01 Acute
379.63 Bleb associated
360.03 Chronic
098.42 Gonorrheal
360.13 Parasitic

ENDOPHTHALMITIS (continued)

360.19 Phacoanaphylactic
360.00 Purulent
360.19 Specified type NEC
360.11 Sympathetic

236.2 ENDOSALPINGIOMA SITE UNSPECIFIED
0 ENDOSALPINGIOMA SITE SPECIFIED SEE 'NEOPLASM UNCERTAIN BEHAVIOR', BY SITE M9111/1
629.89 ENDOSALPINGIOSIS
287.8 ENDOTHELIOSIS
287.8 ENDOTHELIOSIS HEMORRHAGIC INFECTIONAL
0 ENDOTOXEMIA – CODE TO CONDITION

038.#(#) <u>ENDOTOXIC SHOCK INFECTIOUS 995.92</u> [785.52]

4th or 4th <u>and</u> 5th digit code for organism: 038

.9 NOS
.3 Anaerobic
.3 Bacteroides
.3 Clostridium
.42 E. coli
.49 Enterobacter aerogenes
.40 Gram negative
.49 Gram negative other
.41 Hemophilus influenzae
.2 Pneumococcal
.49 Proteus
.43 Pseudomonas
.44 Serratia
.10 Staphylococcal NOS
.11 Staphylococcal aureus
.19 Staphylococcal other
.0 Streptococcal (anaerobic)
.49 Yersinia enterocolitica
.8 Other specified

> ***When coding endotoxic shock, report first the underlying systemic infection (038.#(#)) or trauma. The SIRS code (995.92) would sequence next, followed by 785.52, endotoxic shock. Report also the initial localized infection if known, and any associated organ dysfunction.***

252.01 ENGEL-VON RECKLINGHAUSEN SYNDROME (OSTEITIS FIBROSA CYSTICA)
756.59 ENGELMANN'S DIAPHYSEAL SCLEROSIS
268.0 ENGLISH RICKETS
690.8 ENGMAN'S INFECTIOUS ECZEMATOID DERMATITIS
611.79 ENGORGEMENT BREAST NEC
778.7 ENGORGEMENT BREAST NEWBORN
362.37 ENGORGEMENT RETINAL VEIN
789.1 ENLARGEMENT OF LIVER UNSPECIFIED

ENOPHTHALMOS

376.50 NOS
376.51 Atrophic (of orbital tissue)
376.52 Traumatic or surgery

526.89 ENOSTOSIS
0 ENTAMOEBA HISTOLYTICA INFECTION SEE 'AMEBIC (AMEBIASIS)'
762.5 ENTANGLEMENT OF CORD AFFECTING FETUS OR NEWBORN

ENTERITIS COMMON TYPES

558.9 NOS
564.9 Adaptive
008.62 Adenovirus
558.3 Allergic
<u>558.3</u> <u>Allergic</u> due to ingested foods **[V15.0#]**

5th digit: V15.0
1. Peanuts
2. Milk products
3. Eggs
4. Seafood
5. Other foods

006.9 Amebic NOS
006.0 Amebic acute
006.1 Amebic chronic
004.9 Bacillary NEC
001.1 Cholera el tor
001.1 Choleriformis
007.4 Cryptosporidial
007.5 Cyclosporiasis
558.9 Dietary noninfectious
564.1 Due to irritable bowel syndrome
564.9 Due to membranous colitis
564.9 Due to mucous colitis
564.9 Due to myxomembranous colitis
564.9 Due to neurogenic colitis
564.9 Due to spasmodic colitis
564.9 Due to spastic colon
008.0# E. coli

5th digit: 008.0
0. E. coli
1. Enteropathogenic
2. Enterotoxigenic
3. Enteroinvasive
4. Enterohemorrhagic
9. Specified type NEC

008.67 Enterovirus NEC
009.0 Epidemic
009.0 Gangrenous
007.1 Giardial
009.0 Infectious NEC
009.0 Infectious (septic)
009.1 Infectious origin presumed
487.8 Influenzal
009.0 Necrotic
558.9 Noninfectious (other and unspecified)
008.63 Norwalk-like virus
008.63 Norwalk virus
007.# Protozoal

4th digit: 007
0. Balantidiasis
1. Giardiasis
2. Coccidiosis
3. Trichomoniasis
4. Cryptosporidiosis
5. Cyclosporiasis
8. Other specified
9. Unspecified

558.1 Radiation
003.0 Salmonella infection
003.0 Salmonellosis
009.0 Septic
004.9 Shigella
008.41 Staphylococcus
007.3 Trichomonal

E

ENTERITIS COMMON TYPES (continued)

556.9	Ulcerative (chronic)
008.69	Virus specified NEC
008.8	Virus
009.0	Zymotic

ENTERITIS COMPLETE LISTING

558.9	NOS
564.9	Adaptive
008.62	Adenovirus
008.2	Aerobacter aerogenes
558.3	Allergic
558.3	Allergic due to ingested foods [V15.0#]
	5th digit: V15.0
	1. Peanuts
	2. Milk products
	3. Eggs
	4. Seafood
	5. Other foods
006.9	Amebic NOS
006.0	Amebic acute
006.1	Amebic chronic
008.46	Anaerobic NEC (cocci) (gram-negative) (gram-positive) (mixed)
008.1	Arizona bacillus
008.66	Astrovirus
004.9	Bacillary NEC
008.5	Bacteria NEC
008.49	Bacteria other specified NEC
008.46	Bacteroides (fragilis) (melan in ogeniscus) (oralis)
007.0	Balantidial
008.46	Butyrivibrio (fibriosolvens)
008.65	Calcivirus
008.43	Camplyobacter
112.85	Candidal
007.8	Chilomastix
001.1	Choleriformis
008.45	Clostridium difficile
008.46	Clostridium haemolyticum
008.46	Clostridium novyi
008.43	Clostridium specified type NEC
008.46	Clostridium perfringens (C) (F)
007.2	Coccidial
008.64	Cockle agent
008.67	Coxsackie (virus)
007.4	Cryptosporidial
007.5	Cyclosporiasis
558.9	Dietary
008.64	Ditchling agent
564.1	Due to irritable bowel syndrome
564.9	Due to membranous colitis
564.9	Due to mucous colitis
564.9	Due to myxomembranous colitis
564.9	Due to neurogenic colitis
564.9	Due to spasmodic colitis
564.9	Due to spastic colon
008.0#	E. coli
	5th digit: 008.0
	0. E. Coli
	1. Enteropathogenic
	2. Enterotoxigenic
	3. Enteroinvasive
	4. Enterohemorrhagic
	9. Specified type NEC
008.67	Echo virus
001.1	El tor

ENTERITIS COMPLETE LISTING (continued)

007.8	Embadomonial
008.2	Enterobacter aerogenes
008.49	Enterococci
008.67	Enterovirus NEC
009.0	Epidemic
008.46	Eubacterium
558.9	Fermentative
008.46	Fusobacterium (nucleatum)
009.0	Gangrenous
007.1	Giardial
008.47	Gram-negative bacteria NEC
008.46	Gram-negative bacteria NEC anaerobic NEC
0	Granulomatous see 'Crohn's disease'
008.63	Hawaii agent
009.0	Infectious (septic)
009.0	Infectious NEC
009.1	Infectious origin presumed
487.8	Influenzal
558.9	Irritating foods (due to)
557.9	Ischemic NOS
557.0	Ischemic acute
557.1	Ischemic chronic
557.1	Ischemic due to mesenteric artery insufficiency
008.47	Klebsiella aerogenes
555.1	Large bowel noninfectious
555.2	Large bowel with small intestine noninfectious
008.66	Marin county agent
008.63	Montgomery county agent
009.0	Necrotic
005.2	Necroticans
555.9	Noninfectious site NOS
558.9	Noninfectious other and unspecified
008.63	Norwalk virus
008.63	Norwalk-like virus
008.63	Otofuke agent
008.1	Paracolobactrum arizonae
008.47	Paracolon bacillus NEC
008.64	Paramatta agent
002.9	Paratyphoid (fever)
008.46	Peptococcus
008.46	Peptostreptococcus
008.46	Proprionibacterium
008.3	Proteus (mirabilis) (morganii)
007.#	Protozoal
	4th digit: 007
	0. Balantidiasis
	1. Giardiasis
	2. Coccidiosis
	3. Trichomoniasis
	4. Cryptosporidiosis
	5. Cyclosporiasis
	8. Other specified
	9. Unspecified
008.42	Pseudomonas aeruginosa
558.1	Radiation
008.61	Rotavirus
003.0	Salmonella infection
003.0	Salmonellosis
008.63	Sapporo agent
555.9	Segmental
009.0	Septic
558.9	Simple

E

ENTERITIS COMPLETE LISTING (continued)

004.9 Shigella
004.2 Shigella boydii
004.0 Shigella dysenteriae
004.1 Shigella flexneri (group B)
004.3 Shigella sonei
004.8 Shigella other specified
555.0 Small intestine
008.64 Small round virus (SRV) NEC
008.63 Small round virus (SRV) NEC featureless NEC
008.63 Small round virus (SRV) NEC structured NEC
008.63 Snow mountain (SM) agent
008.49 Specified bacteria NEC
008.8 Specified organism, nonbacterial NEC
008.41 Staphylococcus
008.49 Streptococcus
008.46 Streptococcus anaerobic
008.63 Taunton agent
008.69 Torovirus
558.2 Toxic noninfectious
008.46 Treponema (denticola) (macrodentium)
007.3 Trichomonal
002.0 Typhosa
556.9 Ulcerative (chronic)
008.46 Veillonella
008.8 Virus
008.69 Virus specified NEC
008.64 Wollan (W) agent
008.44 Yersinia enterocolitica
009.0 Zymotic
0 See 'Amebic, Amebiasis'
0 See also 'Gastroenteritis'

099.3 ENTEROARTICULAR SYNDROME

099.3 ENTEROARTICULAR SYNDROME WITH ARTHROPATHY **[711.1#]**

5th digit: 711.1
- **0. Site NOS**
- **1. Shoulder region**
- **2. Upper arm (elbow) (humerus)**
- **3. Forearm (radius) (wrist) (ulna)**
- **4. Hand (carpal) (metacarpal) (fingers)**
- **5. Pelvic region and thigh (hip) (buttock) (femur)**
- **6. Lower leg (fibula) (knee) (patella) (tibia)**
- **7. Ankle and/or foot (metatarsals) (toes) (tarsals)**
- **8. Other (head) (neck) (rib) (skull) (trunk) (vertebrae)**
- **9. Multiple**

099.3 ENTEROARTICULAR SYNDROME WITH CONJUNCTIVITIS [372.33]

0 ENTEROBACTER AEROGENES SEE 'BACTERIAL INFECTION' OR SPECIFIED CONDITION

127.4 ENTEROBIASIS INFECTION

127.4 ENTEROBIUS VERMICULARIS INFECTION

618.6 ENTEROCELE VAGINAL (CONGENITAL OR ACQUIRED)

618.6 ENTEROCELE VAGINAL (CONGENITAL OR ACQUIRED) WITH STRESS INCONTINENCE [625.6]

618.6 ENTEROCELE VAGINAL (CONGENITAL OR ACQUIRED) WITH OTHER URINARY INCONTINENCE **[788.3#]**

5th digit: 788.3
- **1. Urge incontinence**
- **3. Mixed urge and stress**
- **4. Without sensory awareness**
- **5. Post-void dribbling**
- **6. Nocturnal enuresis**
- **7. Continuous leakage**
- **8. Overflow incontinence**
- **9. Other**

0 ENTEROCOCCUS SEE 'BACTERIAL INFECTION' OR SPECIFIED CONDITION

ENTEROCOLITIS

558.1 Due to radiation
777.5 Due to radiation in newborn
777.8 Fetus or newborn
777.5 Fetus or newborn necrotizing
557.0 Fulminant
555.2 Granulomatosis
557.0 Hemorrhagic acute
557.1 Hemorrhagic chronic
557.0 Necrotizing (acute membranous)
777.5 Necrotizing in fetus or newborn
008.45 Pseudomembranous
777.5 Pseudomembranous in newborn
008.41 Staphylococcal
556.0 Ulcerative

560.39 ENTEROLITH

ENTEROPATHY

569.9 NOS
579.8 Exudative
579.0 Gluten
557.0 Hemorrhagic terminal
579.8 Protein losing

569.89 ENTEROPTOSIS INTESTINE

564.9 ENTEROSPASM

ENTEROSTOMY

V53.5 Belt fitting and adjustment
V55.3 Care
V55.3 Catheter adjustment or repositioning
V55.3 Catheter removal or replacement
V55.3 Closure
569.60 Complication - NOS
569.62 Complication - mechanical
569.69 Complication - other
569.69 Fistula
569.69 Hernia

E

ENTEROSTOMY (continued)

When coding an infection of an ostomy, use an additional code to specify the organism. See 'Bacterial Infection'

569.61 Infection
569.61 Infection with cellulitis of abdomen [682.2]
569.61 Infection with septicemia [038.#(#)]

4th or 4th and 5th Digit Code for Organism: 038

.9 NOS
.3 Anaerobic
.3 Bacteroides
.3 Clostridium
.42 E. coli
.49 Enterobacter aerogenes
.40 Gram negative
.49 Gram negative other
.41 Hemophilus Influenzae
.2 Pneumococcal
.49 Proteus
.43 Pseudomonas
.44 Serratia
.10 Staphylococcal NOS
.11 Staphylococcal aureus
.19 Staphylococcal other
.0 Streptococcal (anaerobic)
.49 Yersinia enterocolitica
.8 Other specified

569.62 Malfunction
569.69 Prolapse
V44.3 Status
V55.3 Toilet stoma

078.89 ENTEROVIRUS DISEASE NEC
048 ENTEROVIRUS DISEASE CENTRAL NERVOUS SYSTEM NEC
008.67 ENTEROVIRUS GASTROENTERITIS
079.89 ENTEROVIRUS INFECTION IN DISEASES CLASSIFIED ELSEWHERE
077.4 ENTEROVIRUS TYPE 70 CONJUNCTIVITIS

ENTHESOPATHY

726.90 NOS
726.70 Ankle and tarsus
726.30 Elbow NOS
726.39 Elbow NEC
726.70 Foot
726.4 Hand
726.5 Hip
726.60 Knee NOS
726.69 Knee other specified
720.1 Spine
726.10 Shoulder (region)
726.0 Shoulder (region) adhesive
726.19 Shoulder (region) other specified
726.4 Wrist and carpus
726.8 Other peripheral

117.7 ENTOMOPHTHORA INFECTION
368.15 ENTOPTIC PHENOMENA
0 ENTRAPMENT SYNDROME SEE 'NEUROPATHY' ENTRAPMENT

ENTROPION (EYELID)

374.00 NOS
374.04 Cicatricial
743.62 Congenital

ENTROPION (EYELID) (continued)

374.02 Mechanical
374.02 Paralytic
374.01 Senile
374.03 Spastic
139.1 Trachoma late effect

871.3 ENUCLEATION TRAUMATIC

ENURESIS

788.30 NOS
788.36 Nocturnal
307.6 Psychogenic

277.6 ENZYMES DEFICIENCY
790.5 ENZYMES SERUM NEC ABNORMAL
277.9 ENZYMOPATHY
794.12 EOG ABNORMAL
288.59 EOSINOPENIA

EOSINOPHILIA

288.3 Allergic
288.3 Hereditary
288.3 Idiopathic
710.5 Myalgia syndrome
518.3 Pulmonary
288.3 Secondary
518.3 Tropical

277.89 EOSINOPHILIC GRANULOMA (BONE) (LUNG)

Carcinomas and neoplasms should be coded by site if possible. Code by cell type, "site NOS", only if a site is not specified in the diagnosis. Otherwise, refer to the appropriate category of neoplasm for a more specific code. See 'Cancer' 'Cancer Metastatic', 'Carcinoma In Situ', 'Neoplasm Uncertain Behavior', 'Neoplasm Unspecified Nature', or 'Benign Neoplasm'.

EPENDYMOMA

191.9 Site unspecified
0 Site specified see 'Cancer', by site M9391/3
191.9 Anaplastic type site unspecified
0 Anaplastic type site specified see 'Cancer', by site M9392/3
237.5 Myxopapillary site NOS
0 Myxopapillary site specified see 'Neoplasm Uncertain Behavior', by site M9394/1
237.5 Papillary site NOS
0 Papillary site specified see 'Neoplasm Uncertain Behavior', by site M9393/1

709.09 EPHELIDES
780.6 EPHEMERAL FEVER
743.62 EPIBLEPHARON CONGENITAL
743.63 EPICANTHUS (FOLD) (CONGENITAL)
726.32 EPICONDYLITIS LATERAL
726.31 EPICONDYLITIS MEDIAL

EPIDEMIC

078.89 Cervical myalgia
136.9 Disease NEC
077.4 Hemorrhagic conjunctivitis
078.6 Hemorrhagic fever
077.1 Keratoconjunctivitis
078.82 Vomiting syndrome

E

078.19 EPIDERMODYSPLASIA VERRUCIFORMIS

706.2 EPIDERMOID CYST

EPIDERMOLYSIS

757.39 Bullosa congenital
695.1 Combustiformis (toxica)
977.9 Drug induced

110.# EPIDERMOPHYTON INFECTIONS
4th digit: 110
0. Scalp and beard
1. Nail (unguium)
2. Hand (manuum)
3. Groin and perianal (cruris)
4. Foot (pedis)
5. Body (corporus)
6. Deep seated (granuloma trichophyticum)
8. Other specified site
9. Unspecified site

385.30 EPIDERMOSIS EAR (MIDDLE)

EPIDIDYMIS

V45.77 Absence acquired
752.89 Absence congenital
608.3 Atrophy
608.9 Disorder
752.89 Hypoplasia
959.14 Injury NOS
608.24 Torsion

EPIDIDYMITIS

604.90 NOS
604.0 And orchitis with abscess
604.90 And orchitis without abscess
032.89 Diphtheritic [604.91]
125.9 Filarial [604.91]
098.13 Gonococcal acute
098.33 Gonococcal chronic
604.0 With abscess
604.0 With orchitis and abscess
604.99 Other
095.8 Syphilitic [604.91]
016.4# Tuberculosis
5th digit: 016.4
0. Unspecified
1. Lab not done
2. Lab pending
3. Microscopy positive (in sputum)
4. Culture positive - microscopy negative
5. Culture negative - microscopy positive
6. Culture and microscopy negative confirmed by other methods

EPIDURAL

851.8# Contusion (with hemorrhage)
851.9# Contusion (with hemorrhage) with open intracranial wound
432.0 Hematoma
767.0 Hematoma fetus or newborn, birth trauma (intrapartum anoxia/hypoxia)
852.4# Hematoma traumatic
852.5# Hematoma traumatic with open intracranial wound
5th digit: 851.8-9, 852.4-5
0. Level of consciousness (LOC) NOS
1. No LOC
2. LOC < 1 HR
3. LOC 1 - 24 HRS
4. LOC > 24 HRS with return to prior level
5. LOC > 24 HRS without return to prior level: or death before regaining consciousness, regardless of duration of LOC
6. LOC duration unspecified
9. With concussion unspecified

767.0 Hemorrhage fetus or newborn, birth trauma (intrapartum anoxia/hypoxia)
674.0# Hemorrhage maternal due to pregnancy
5th digit: 674.0
0. Episode of care NOS or N/A
1. Delivered
2. Delivered with postpartum complication
3. Antepartum complication
4. Postpartum complication

852.4# Hemorrhage traumatic
852.5# Hemorrhage traumatic with open intracranial wound
5th digit: 852.4-5
0. Level of consciousness (LOC) NOS
1. No LOC
2. LOC < 1 HR
3. LOC 1 - 24 HRS
4. LOC > 24 HRS with return to prior level
5. LOC > 24 HRS without return to prior level: or death before regaining consciousness, regardless of duration of LOC
6. LOC duration unspecified
9. With concussion unspecified

536.9 EPIGASTRIC DISORDER FUNCTIONAL
306.4 EPIGASTRIC DISORDER FUNCTIONAL - PSYCHOGENIC
789.36 EPIGASTRIC MASS
789.06 EPIGASTRIC PAIN
959.12 EPIGASTRIC REGION INJURY
553.29 EPIGASTROCELE

E

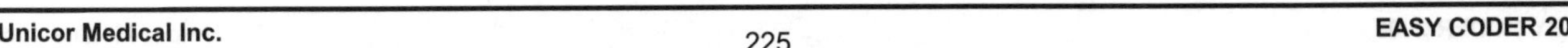

EPIGLOTTIS

748.3 Anomaly congenital
748.3 Atresia congenital
748.3 Fissure congenital
959.09 Injury

EPIGLOTTITIS

464.30 Acute
464.31 Acute with obstruction
464.30 Acute viral
464.31 Acute viral with obstruction
476.1 Chronic

759.4 EPIGNATHUS

Do not code epilepsy as intractable unless the physician states it is intractable. Recurrent seizures are not enough to indicate intractable epilepsy.

EPILEPSY, EPILEPTIC

345.9# NOS
345.0# Absence atonic
345.0# Absence typical
345.2 Absence status (petit mal status)
345.4# Automatism
345.5# Bravais-Jacksonian NOS
345.1# Clonic
293.0 Confusional state
345.9# Convulsion NOS
345.8# Cursive (running) (gelastic)

5th digit: 345.0, 1, 4, 5, 8, 9
0. Without mention of intractable epilepsy
1. With intractable epilepsy

345.## Dementia [294.1#]
345.## Deterioration [294.1#]

4th digit: 345
0. Generalized nonconvulsive
1. Generalized convulsive
4. Partial, with impairment of consciousness
5. Partial, without impairment of consciousness
6. Infantile spasms
7. Epilepsia partialis continua
8. Other forms
9. Unspecified, NOS

5th digit: 345
0. Without mention of intractable epilepsy
1. With intractable epilepsy

5th digit: 294.1
0. Without behavioral disturbance or NOS
1. With behavioral disturbance

V17.2 Family history
345.9# Fit NOS
345.5# Focal (motor)
345.7# Focal (motor) status

5th digit: 345.5, 7, 9
0. Without mention of intractable epilepsy
1. With intractable epilepsy

EPILEPSY, EPILEPTIC (continued)

345.1# Generalized convulsive
345.0# Generalized nonconvulsive
345.1# Grand mal
345.3 Grand mal status
345.6# Hypsarrhythmia
345.6# Infantile (spasms) (salaam) (lightning)
345.5# Jacksonian
345.4# Limbic system
345.4# Localization-related (focal) (partial) epilepsy and epileptic syndromes with complex partial seizures
345.5# Localization-related (focal) (partial) epilepsy and epileptic syndromes with simple partial seizures
345.1# Major (motor)

5th digit: 345.0-1, 4-6
0. Without mention of intractable epilepsy
1. With intractable epilepsy

Use an additional code to identify the specific maternal epilepsy. See 'Epilepsy, Epileptic'.

649.4# Maternal current (co-existent) in pregnancy

5th digit: 649.4
0. Episode of care unspecified or N/A
1. Delivered
2. Delivered with postpartum complication
3. Antepartum complication
4. Postpartum complication

345.0# Minor
345.1# Myoclonic
333.2 Myoclonic progressive
779.0 Newborn
345.5# Partial NOS
345.5# Partial motor
345.4# Partial psychosensory
345.4# Partial secondarily generalized
345.4# Partial with impairment of consciousness
345.5# Partial without impairment of consciousness
345.7# Partialis continua (Kojevnikov)
345.0# Petit mal
345.2 Petit mal status
345.4# Psychomotor
345.7# Psychomotor status

5th digit: 345.0-1, 4-5, 7
0. Without mention of intractable epilepsy
1. With intractable epilepsy

294.8 Psychosis [345.##]

4th digit: 345
0. Generalized nonconvulsive
1. Generalized convulsive
4. Partial, with impairment of consciousness
5. Partial, without impairment of consciousness
6. Infantile spasms
7. Epilepsia partialis continua
8. Other forms
9. Unspecified

5th digit: 345
0. Without mention of intractable epilepsy
1. With intractable epilepsy

E

EPILEPSY, EPILEPTIC (continued)

345.0# Pykno-epilepsy
345.9# Seizure NOS
345.0# Seizure akinetic
345.0# Seizure atonic
345.5# Sensory-induced
345.5# Somatomotor (somatosensory)
345.3 Status epilepticus (grand mal)
345.4# Temporal lobe (psychomotor)
345.7# Temporal lobe (psychomotor) status
345.1# Tonic (tonic-clonic)
293.0 Twilight state
345.5# Visceral
345.5# Visual
345.8# Other Specified
5th digit: 345.0-1, 4- 5, 7-9
0. Without mention of intractable epilepsy
1. With intractable epilepsy

780.39 EPILEPTIFORM ATTACK (CONVULSIONS) (SEIZURE)

301.3 EPILEPTOID PERSONALITY DISORDER

759.5 EPILOIA

259.3 EPINEPHRINE ECTOPIC SECRETION

EPIPHORA

375.21 Due to excess lacrimation
375.22 Due to insufficient drainage
375.20 Unspecified as to cause

0 EPIPHYSEAL SEE 'EPIPHYSIS, EPIPHYSEAL'

EPIPHYSIS, EPIPHYSEAL

733.91 Arrest
732.2 Arrest femoral head
756.56 Dysplasia multiple congenital
732.2 Femoral capital slipped nontraumatic
0 Slipped (traumatic) (old) see 'Osteochondritis', by site
0 Slipped (traumatic) current see 'Fracture', by site, closed
732.9 Slipped (postinfectional) (posttraumatic)

EPIPHYSITIS

732.9 NOS
732.6 Juvenile
732.6 Juvenile other site
732.5 Os calcis (juvenile)
732.0 Vertebral (juvenile)

EPISCLERITIS

379.00 NOS
274.89 Gouty [379.09]
379.09 NEC
379.02 Nodular
379.01 Periodica fugax
379.00 Staphylococcal
379.00 Suppurative
095.0 Syphilitic

EPISCLERITIS (continued)

017.3# Tuberculosis [379.09]
5th digit: 017.3
0. Unspecified
1. Lab not done
2. Lab pending
3. Microscopy positive (in sputum)
4. Culture positive - microscopy negative
5. Culture negative - microscopy positive
6. Culture and microscopy negative confirmed by other methods

674.3# EPISIOTOMY COMPLICATION (INFECTION) (OTHER)

674.2# EPISIOTOMY DISRUPTION (OF WOUND)
5th digit: 674.2-3
0. Episode of care unspecified or N/A
2. Delivered with postpartum complication
4. Postpartum complication

753.8 EPISPADIAS CONGENITAL - FEMALE

752.62 EPISPADIAS CONGENITAL - MALE

EPISTAXIS

784.7 NOS
448.0 Hereditary
784.7 Recurrent (chronic) (unspecified) (severe)
625.8 Vicarious menstruation

EPITHELIAL

364.61 Down growth eye (anterior chamber)
709.8 Hyperplasia
611.8 Hyperplasia - nipple
528.79 Hyperplasia - oral including tongue
709.8 Hyperplasia - skin
623.0 Hyperplasia - vaginal wall
229.9 Tumor benign site unspecified
0 Tumor benign site specified see 'Benign Neoplasm', by site M8010/0

> ***Carcinomas and neoplasms should be coded by site if possible. Code by cell type, "site NOS", only if a site is not specified in the diagnosis. Otherwise, refer to the appropriate category of neoplasm for a more specific code. See 'Cancer' 'Cancer Metastatic', 'Carcinoma In Situ', 'Neoplasm Uncertain Behavior', 'Neoplasm Unspecified Nature', or 'Benign Neoplasm'.***

EPITHELIOMA

229.9 Benign site unspecified
0 Benign site specified see 'Benign Neoplasm', by site M8011/0
216.# Intradermal
4th digit: 216
0. Lip
1. Eyelid including canthus
2. Ear external (auricle) (pinna)
3. Face (cheek) (nose)
4. Scalp, neck
5. Trunk, back, chest
6. Upper limb including shoulder
7. Lower limb including hip
8. Other specified sites
9. Skin unspecified
199.1 Malignant site unspecified
0 Malignant site specified see 'Cancer', by site M8011/3

E

363.15	EPITHELIOPATHY
757.5	EPONYCHIA
752.11	EPOOPHORON CYST CONGENITAL
332.1	EPS (EXTRAPYRAMIDAL SYNDROME)
075	EPSTEIN BARRE INFECTION (VIRAL)
780.79	EPSTEIN BARRE INFECTION (VIRAL) CHRONIC [139.8]
528.4	EPSTEIN'S PEARL (CYST MOUTH)
581.9	EPSTEIN'S SYNDROME
780.4	EQUILIBRIUM DISTURBANCE
024	EQUINIA
754.69	EQUINOVALGUS DEFORMITY CONGENITAL
754.51	EQUINOVARUS CONGENITAL
736.71	EQUINOVARUS DEFORMITY ACQUIRED
736.72	EQUINUS DEFORMITY OF FOOT ACQUIRED
767.6	ERB DUCHENNE PALSY OR PARALYSIS (BIRTH TRAUMA)
358.00	ERB (-OPPENHEIM) -GOLDFLAM SYNDROME
358.01	ERB (-OPPENHEIM) -GOLDFLAM SYNDROME WITH (ACUTE) EXACERBATION (CRISIS)
094.89	ERB'S DISEASE (SYPHILITIC)
359.1	ERB'S (-LANDOUZY) MUSCULAR DYSTROPHY
253.0	ERDHEIM'S SYNDROME (ACROMEGALIC MACROSPONDYLITIS)
607.84	ERECTILE DISORDER (DYSFUNCTION) MALE – NOS OR ORGANIC
302.72	ERECTILE DISORDER (DYSFUNCTION) MALE – PSYCHOSEXUAL OR NONORGANIC
607.3	ERECTION PAINFUL (PERSISTENT)
794.11	ERG ABNORMAL
349.82	ERGOTISM CORRECT SUBSTANCE (PROPERLY ADMINISTERED)
988.2	ERGOTISM DRUG THERAPY (MIGRAINE)
975.0	ERGOTISM OVERDOSE (WRONG SUBSTANCE)
300.16	ERICHSEN'S RAILWAY SPINE
732.4	ERLACHER BLOUNT SYNDROME (TIBIA VARA)

EROSION

447.2	Artery without rupture
535.4#	Gastric
535.4#	Pylorus
535.4#	Stomach

5th digit: 535.4
0. Without hemorrhage
1. With hemorrhage

302.89	EROTOMANIA
787.3	ERUCTATION
306.4	ERUCTATION NERVOUS OR PSYCHOGENIC

ERYSIPELAS

035	NOS
035	Ear (external) [380.13]
035	Pinna [380.13]
027.1	ERYSIPELOID OF ROSENBACH
027.1	ERYSIPELOTHRIX INFECTION

ERYTHEMA

695.9	NOS
695.0	Annulare (centrifugum) (rheumaticum)
695.1	Bullosum (gyratum)
088.81	Chronicum migrans
695.1	Conjunctiva
026.1	Epidemic arthritic
017.1#	Induratum

5th digit: 017.1
0. NOS
1. Lab not done
2. Lab pending
3. Microscopy positive (in sputum)
4. Culture positive - microscopy negative
5. Culture negative - microscopy positive
6. Culture and microscopy negative confirmed by other methods

057.0	Infectiosum
695.89	Intertrigo
695.1	Iris
695.1	Multiforme
695.2	Nodosum
017.1#	Nodosum, tuberculous

5th digit: 017.1
0. NOS
1. Lab not done
2. Lab pending
3. Microscopy positive (in sputum)
4. Culture positive - microscopy negative
5. Culture negative - microscopy positive
6. Culture and microscopy negative confirmed by other methods

991.5	Pernio
909.4	Pernio late effect
695.0	Scarlatiniform
0	Solare see 'Sunburn'
695.0	Toxic
695.0	Venenatum
443.82	ERYTHERMALGIA (PRIMARY)
443.82	ERYTHRALGIA
039.0	ERYTHRASMA
985.0	ERYTHREDEMA
985.0	ERYTHREDEMA POLYNEURITICA
985.0	ERYTHREDEMA POLYNEUROPATHY

ERYTHREMIA

207.0#	Acute site unspecified M9841/3
207.1#	Chronic M9842/3
207.0#	Myelosis M9841/3

5th digit: 207.0, 1
0. Without mention of remission
1. With mention of remission

284.89	ERYTHROBLASTOPENIA (ACQUIRED) (SECONDARY)
284.01	ERYTHROBLASTOPENIA CONGENITAL
284.01	ERYTHROBLASTOPHTHISIS
773.2	ERYTHROBLASTOSIS FETALIS
773.1	ERYTHROBLASTOSIS FETALIS DUE TO ABO ANITIBODIES
773.0	ERYTHROBLASTOSIS FETALIS DUE TO RH ANTIBODIES

443.89	ERYTHROCYANOSIS
284.9	ERYTHROCYTE ABSENCE
284.81	ERYTHROCYTE APLASIA
284.01	ERYTHROCYTE APLASIA CONGENITAL
283.19	ERYTHROCYTE FRAGMENTATION SYNDROME
285.9	ERYTHROCYTOPENIA

ERYTHRODERMA

695.89	Desquamativa (infants)
695.89	Exfoliative
757.1	Icthyosiform (congenital)
695.89	Infantum
696.2	Maculopapular
778.8	Neonatorum
696.1	Psoriatorum
695.9	Secondary

693.0	ERYTHRODYSESTHESIA, PALMAR PLANTAR (PPE)
284.09	ERYTHROGENESIS IMPERFECTA
289.89	ERYTHROID DYSPLASIA
289.9	ERYTHROID HYPERPLASIA
284.01	ERYTHROID HYPOPLASIA CONGENITAL
207.0#	ERYTHROLEUKEMIA M9840/3

5th digit: 207.0
0. Without mention of remission
1. With mention of remission

443.82	ERYTHROMELALGIA
701.8	ERYTHROMELIA
285.9	ERYTHROPENIA
289.9	ERYTHROPHAGOCYTOSIS
300.23	ERYTHROPHOBIA
528.79	ERYTHROPLAKIA ORAL (MOUTH) (TONGUE)
233.5	ERYTHROPLASIA SITE UNSPECIFIED
0	ERYTHROPLASIA SITE SPECIFIED SEE 'CARCINOMA IN SITU', BY SITE
284.81	ERYTHROPOIETIC, HYPOPLASIA CHRONIC ACQUIRED
284.9	ERYTHROPOIESIS ABSENCE
284.01	ERYTHROPOIESIS ABSENCE CONGENITAL
0	ESCHERICHIA COLI SEE 'BACTERIAL INFECTION' OR SPECIFIED CONDITION
530.89	ESOPHAGALGIA
0	ESOPHAGEAL SEE 'ESOPHAGUS, ESOPHAGEAL'
530.89	ESOPHAGECTASIS
530.0	ESOPHAGECTASIS CARDIOSPASM INDUCED
530.5	ESOPHAGISMUS

ESOPHAGITIS

530.10	NOS
530.12	Acute
530.10	Alkaline
112.84	Candidal
530.10	Chemical peptic
530.10	Chronic
530.10	Infectional
530.10	Necrotic
530.10	Postoperative
530.11	Reflux
530.19	Specified NEC

ESOPHAGITIS (continued)

017.8#	Tuberculous

5th digit: 017.8
0. Unspecified
1. Lab not done
2. Lab pending
3. Microscopy positive (in sputum)
4. Culture positive - microscopy negative
5. Culture negative - microscopy positive
6. Culture and microscopy negative confirmed by other methods

530.19	Ulcerative
530.89	ESOPHAGOBRONCHIAL FISTULA
750.3	ESOPHAGOBRONCHIAL FISTULA CONGENITAL
530.89	ESOPHAGOCUTANEOUS FISTULA
530.6	ESOPHAGOCELE ACQUIRED
530.89	ESOPHAGODYNIA
530.89	ESOPHAGOMALACIA
530.89	ESOPHAGOPLEUROCUTANEOUS FISTULA
530.89	ESOPHAGOPTOSIS
530.5	ESOPHAGOSPASM

ESOPHAGOSTOMY

530.86	Abscess
530.86	Cellulitis
530.87	Complication – mechanical
530.87	Dysfunction

> ***When coding an infection of an ostomy, use an additional code to specify the organism. See 'Bacterial Infection'***

530.86	Infection
530.87	Malfunction
530.84	ESOPHAGOTRACHEAL FISTULA
750.3	ESOPHAGOTRACHEAL FISTULA CONGENITAL

ESOPHAGUS, ESOPHAGEAL

530.19	Abscess
750.3	Absence (congenital)
530.89	Ampulla
530.0	Aperistalsis
530.85	Barrett's
530.3	Compression
530.5	Corkscrew
530.5	Curling
530.89	Cyst
530.89	Deformity (acquired)
530.89	Deviation (acquired)
530.89	Dilatation (acquired)
530.89	Displacement (acquired)
530.9	Disorder
530.5	Disorder functional
306.4	Disorder functional - psychogenic
530.89	Disorders other specified
530.6	Diverticulum acquired
530.5	Dyskinesia
530.89	Erosion
530.89	Esophagalgia
530.89	Fistula
530.82	Hemorrhage
530.89	Hypersensitive
530.10	Inflammation

E

ESOPHAGUS, ESOPHAGEAL (continued)

874.4 Injury cervical - traumatic
874.5 Injury cervical - traumatic with open wound
908.0 Injury late effect
862.22 Injury - traumatic
862.32 Injury - traumatic with open wound
530.89 Laceration
530.83 Leukoplakia
530.7 Mallory weiss tear
530.89 Necrosis
530.3 Obstruction
530.4 Perforation nontraumatic
787.24 Pharyngeal incoordination (newborn)
530.6 Pouch acquired
530.81 Reflux
530.4 Rupture nontraumatic
530.5 Spasm
530.3 Stricture and stenosis
530.84 Tracheoesophageal fistula
530.20 Ulcer
530.21 Ulcer with bleeding
530.20 Ulcer cardio-esophageal (peptic)
530.21 Ulcer cardio-esophageal (peptic) with bleeding
530.20 Ulcer due to ingestion of medicine/chemical agents
530.21 Ulcer due to ingestion of medicine/chemical agents with bleeding
530.20 Ulcer fungal
530.21 Ulcer fungal with bleeding
530.20 Ulcer infectional
530.21 Ulcer infectional with bleeding
456.1 Ulcer - varicose
456.0 Ulcer - varicose with bleeding

ESOPHAGUS, ESOPHAGEAL CONGENITAL ANOMALIES

750.3 Absence
750.3 Atresia
750.4 Dilatation
750.4 Displacement
750.4 Diverticulum
750.4 Duplication
750.4 Fistula
750.3 Fistula tracheoesophageal
750.4 Giant
750.6 Hernia (hiatal)
750.3 Imperforate
750.4 Pouch
750.3 Ring
750.3 Stenosis
750.3 Stricture
750.3 Webbed

ESOPHAGUS, ESOPHAGEAL VARICES

456.1 NOS
571.5 Due to cirrhosis (non alcoholic) [456.21]
572.3 Due to portal hypertension [456.21]
571.2 In alcoholic cirrhosis [456.21]
571.2 In alcoholic cirrhosis with bleeding [456.20]
571.6 In biliary cirrhosis [456.21]
571.6 In biliary cirrhosis with bleeding [456.20]
456.0 With bleeding
571.5 With bleeding due to cirrhosis [456.20]
572.3 With bleeding due to portal hypertension [456.20]

ESOPHORIA

378.41 Unspecified
378.84 Convergence excess
378.85 Divergence insufficiency

ESOTROPIA

378.0# NOS
378.35 Accommodative component
378.0# Convergent concomitant strabismus

5th digit: 378.0
0. Unspecified
1. Monocular unspecified
2. Monocular with A pattern
3. Monocular with V pattern
4. Monocular with other noncomitancies (X or Y pattern)
5. Alternating unspecified
6. Alternating with A pattern
7. Alternating with V pattern
8. Alternating with other noncomitancies (X or Y pattern)

378.20 Intermittent
378.22 Intermittent alternating
378.21 Intermittent monocular
378.00 Nonaccommodative

085.5 ESPUNDIA
790.1 ESR ABNORMAL
289.89 ESTERAPENIA
585.6 ESRD (END STAGE RENAL DISEASE)

Carcinomas and neoplasms should be coded by site if possible. Code by cell type, "site NOS", only if a site is not specified in the diagnosis. Otherwise, refer to the appropriate category of neoplasm for a more specific code. See 'Cancer' 'Cancer Metastatic', 'Carcinoma In Situ', 'Neoplasm Uncertain Behavior', 'Neoplasm Unspecified Nature', or 'Benign Neoplasm'.

160.0 ESTHESIONEUROBLASTOMA SITE UNSPECIFIED
0 ESTHESIONEUROBLASTOMA SITE SPECIFIED SEE 'CANCER', BY SITE M9522/3
160.0 ESTHESIONEUROCYTOMA SITE UNSPECIFIED
0 ESTHESIONEUROCYTOMA SITE SPECIFIED SEE 'CANCER', BY SITE M9521/3
160.0 ESTHESIONEUROEPITHELIOMA SITE UNSPECIFIED
0 ESTHESIONEUROEPITHELIOMA SITE SPECIFIED SEE 'CANCER', BY SITE M9523/3
099.1 ESTHIOMENE
V61.0 ESTRANGEMENT (REASON FOR ENCOUNTER)
256.39 ESTROGEN DECREASE
256.0 ESTROGEN HYPERSECRETION

Code first malignant neoplasm of breast see 'CANCER', breast

V86.1 ESTROGEN RECEPTOR NEGATIVE STATUS (ER-)
V86.0 ESTROGEN RECEPTOR POSITIVE STATUS (ER+)
0 ETHANOL SEE 'ALCOHOL'
270.8 ETHANOLAMINE METABOLISM DISORDERS
270.8 ETHANOLAMINURIA
0 ETHANOLISM SEE 'ALCOHOLISM'
461.2 ETHMOIDAL SINUS (ABSCESS) (INFECTION) (INFLAMMATION) ACUTE
478.19 ETHMOIDITIS INFLUENZAL

359.29 EULENBURG'S DISEASE (CONGENITAL PARAMYOTONIA)
257.2 EUNUCHOIDISM

EUSTACHIAN

744.24 Absence or atresia (congenital)
744.24 Anomalies specified congenital
744.24 Dilatation congenital
381.9 Disorder tube
381.89 Disorder other
381.81 Dysfunction
381.50 Infection
381.51 Infection - acute
381.52 Infection - chronic
959.09 Injury
381.60 Obstruction
381.63 Obstruction extrinsic cartilagenous (compression)
381.62 Obstruction intrinsic cartilagenous
381.61 Obstruction osseous (cholesteatoma) (polyp) (other lesion)
381.7 Patulous
381.81 Pressure
381.50 Salpingitis
381.51 Salpingitis acute
381.52 Salpingitis chronic
381.60 Stenosis (tube)
381.60 Stricture (tube)

790.94 EUTHYROID SICK SYNDROME

> ***V71 - V71.9 Are always sequenced first. They describe the evaluation and observation for suspected injury or illness. Example: Evaluation of a patient in a motor vehicle accident with no apparent injury.***

EVALUATION FOR SUSPECTED CONDITION (UNDIAGNOSED) (UNPROVEN) NOT FOUND

V71.9 Unspecified
V71.81 Abuse - child or adult
V71.6 Abuse - battery child or adult
V71.81 Abuse - neglect child or adult
V71.5 Abuse - rape child or adult
V71.3 Accident at work
V71.4 Accident NEC
V71.89 Acute abdomen
V71.82 Anthrax exposure
V71.01 Antisocial behavior - adult
V71.02 Antisocial behavior - child or adolescent
V71.6 Assault with no need for medical treatment
V71.89 Benign neoplasm
V71.83 Biological agent other exposure
V71.1 Cancer
V71.7 Cardiovascular disease
V71.4 Concussion - accidental
V71.6 Concussion - inflicted
V71.3 Concussion - work related
V71.89 CVA (cerebrovascular accident)
V71.82 Exposure anthrax
V71.83 Exposure SARS (severe acute respiratory syndrome)-associated corona-virus
V71.83 Exposure other biological agent
V71.89 Foreign body ingestion
V71.01 Gang activity adult with no manifest psychiatric disorder
V71.02 Gang activity child with no manifest psychiatric disorder
V71.89 Hemorrhage (non traumatic) (post op)

EVALUATION FOR SUSPECTED CONDITION (UNDIAGNOSED) (UNPROVEN) NOT FOUND (continued)

V71.89 Infectious disease not requiring isolation
V71.89 Ingestion of deleterious agent
V71.09 Mental condition
V71.4 MVA (motor vehicle accident) with no apparent injury
V71.7 Myocardial infarction

NEWBORN (28 DAYS OR LESS)

V29.9 Unspecified
V29.8 Cardiovascular disease
V29.8 Congenital abnormality
V29.3 Genetic condition
V29.8 Ingestion foreign object
V29.0 Infectious disease
V29.8 Injury
V29.3 Metabolic condition
V29.8 Neoplasm
V29.1 Neurological disease
V29.8 Poisoning
V29.2 Respiratory condition
V29.8 Specified NEC

EVALUATION FOR SUSPECTED CONDITION (UNDIAGNOSED) (UNPROVEN) NOT FOUND (continued)

V71.02 Psychiatric disorder - adolescent or child with antisocial behavior (gang activity)
V71.01 Psychiatric disorder - adult with antisocial behavior (gang activity)
V71.09 Psychiatric disorder other
V71.5 Rape (alleged)
V71.89 Rupture of membranes premature
V71.5 Seduction (alleged)
V71.89 Sepsis
V71.89 Stroke
V71.89 Suicide attempt (alleged)
V71.2 Tuberculosis
V71.4 Other accident
V71.6 Other inflicted injury
V71.89 Other specified suspected conditions

287.32 EVAN'S DISEASE OR SYNDROME (THROMBOCYTOPENIC PURPURA)

EVERSION

596.8 Bladder
616.0 Cervix with cervicitis
622.0 Cervix uteri
755.67 Foot congenital
736.79 Foot NEC
375.51 Lacrimal punctum
593.89 Ureter (meatus)
599.84 Urethra (meatus)
618.1 Uterus see also 'Uterus, Uterine Prolapse'

EVISCERATION

767.8 Birth trauma
674.1# C section wound
5th digit: 674.1
0. Episode of care NOS or N/A
2. Delivered with mention of postpartum complication
4. Postpartum condition or complication

553.29 Congenital

E

EVISCERATION (continued)

998.32 Operative wound
998.32 Operative wound external
998.31 Operative wound internal
674.2# Operative wound perineal obstetrical
674.1# Operative wound uterine obstetrical

5th digit: 674.1-2
0. Episode of care NOS or N/A
2. Delivered with mention of postpartum complication
4. Postpartum condition or complication

869.1 Traumatic
871.3 Traumatic - eye (globe)
908.2 Traumatic - late effect

EWING'S

170.# Angioendothelioma M9632/3
170.# Sarcoma M9632/3
170.# Tumor M9632/3

4th digit: 170
0. Skull and face
1. Mandible
2. Vertebral column
3. Ribs sternum clavicle
4. Scapula long bones upper limb
5. Short bones upper limb
6. Pelvic bones sacrum coccyx
7. Long bones lower limb
8. Short bones lower limb
9. Site unspecified

> ***V Codes are generally sequenced second, unless they are the reason for the encounter. (reason rule)***

EXAM

V72.9 NOS
V70.3 Administrative purposes (general)
V70.3 Admission to old age home (general) (administrative)
V70.3 Adoption (general) (administrative)
V72.7 Allergy
V70.0 Annual routine (health check-up)
V20.2 Annual routine (health check-up) infant or child (initial and subsequent routine newborn check)
V72.86 Blood typing
V70.3 Camp (general) (administrative)
V72.5 Chest x-ray (routine)
V72.2 Dental

> ***Use additional code(s) to identify: specific examination(s), screening and testing performed.***

V68.01 Disability
V70.8 Donor potential - organ or tissue
V70.3 Driving license (general) (administrative)
V70.3 Drug screening (general) (administrative)
V70.4 Drug test medicolegal
V72.19 Ears
V72.0 Eye

> ***Do not confuse follow up or routine aftercare with complications. Follow up exams and routine aftercare are planned visits that are part of the normal course of treatment. Complications are unexpected developments that require subsequent treatment.***

EXAM (continued)

FOLLOW-UP

V67.9 Unspecified
V67.2 Chemotherapy
V67.6 Combined treatment
V58.83 Drug monitoring therapeutic encounter
V58.83 Drug monitoring therapeutic encounter with long term drug use [V58.6#]

5th digit: V58.6
1. Anticoagulants
2. Antibiotics
3. Antiplatelets/antithrombotics
4. Anti-inflammatories non-steroidal (NSAID)
5. Steroids
6. Aspirin
7. Insulin
9. Other

V67.4 Fracture treatment - healed
0 Fracture treatment - healing or current see 'Aftercare', orthopedic

> ***Antibiotics, Coumadin, Digoxin, chemotherapy drugs, and any other drug with a risk of adverse reaction are considered high-risk medications.***

V58.83 High risk drug monitoring encounter
V58.83 High risk drug monitoring encounter with long term drug use [V58.6#]

5th digit: V58.6
1. Anticoagulants
2. Antibiotics
3. Antiplatelets/antithrombotics
4. Anti-inflammatories non-steroidal (NSAID)
5. Steroids
6. Aspirin
7. Insulin
9. Other

V67.51 High risk medication - completed therapy
V58.6# High risk medication - current therapy (long term)

5th digit: V58.6
1. Anticoagulants
2. Antibiotics
3. Antiplatelets/antithrombotics
4. Anti-inflammatories non-steroidal (NSAID)
5. Steroids
6. Aspirin
7. Insulin
9. Other

V76.47 Pap smear vaginal following hysterectomy [V45.77]
V76.47 Pap smear vaginal following hysterectomy for nonmalignant condition [V45.77]
V67.01 Pap smear vaginal following hysterectomy for cancer [V10.4#] [V45.77]

5th digit: V10.4
0. Genital organ unspecified
1. Cervix uteri
2. Other part of uterus
3. Ovary
4. Genital organ other

V67.3 Psychotherapy and other treatment
V67.1 Radiotherapy
V67.00 Surgery unspecified
V67.09 Surgery other
V67.59 Other treatment NEC

EXAM (continued)

V70.9 General (medical)
V72.31 Gynecological (routine)
V72.19 Hearing
V72.12 Hearing conservation and treatment
V72.11 Hearing following failed hearing screening
V70.3 Immigration and naturalization (general) (administrative)
V70.6 In population surveys (health)
V20.2 Infant/child annual routine (health check-up) (initial and subsequent newborn check)
0 Infant/newborn suspected condition (undiagnosed) (unproven) see 'Evaluation Newborn/Infant'
V70.3 Insurance certification (general) (administrative)
V72.6 Laboratory (routine)
V70.3 Marriage (general) (administrative)
V70.0 Medical (routine) (general)
V20.2 Newborn initial and subsequent check
0 Newborn/infant suspected condition (undiagnosed) (unproven) see 'Evaluation Newborn/Infant'
V70.5 Occupation (health)
V25.41 Oral contraception (routine)
0 Pap smear see 'Exam' routine, pap smear
V70.7 Participant or control in clinical research
V70.4 Paternity testing
V72.31 Pelvic (routine)
V70.5 Preemployment (health)

PREGNANCY

V25.41 For oral contraception (routine)
V72.41 Negative result
V72.42 Positive result
V72.40 Possible unconfirmed
V24.0 Postpartum (immediate)
V24.2 Postpartum routine follow up
V22.0 Prenatal first pregnancy
V22.1 Prenatal subsequent pregnancy
0 Prenatal see 'Supervision of Pregnancy'

EXAM (continued)

V70.3 Premarital (general) (administrative)

> ***V72.#, Preoperative examination, identifies the type of exam done rather than the type of surgery to be performed. The preoperative examination code should be listed first followed by the code for the condition necessitating the surgery. List also any codes for systemic disease substantiating medical necessity of the surgery.***

V72.8# Preoperative (pre-procedural)
5th digit: V72.8
1. Cardiovascular
2. Respiratory
3. Other specified preoperative exam
4. Preoperative exam unspecified

V70.3 Prison (general) (administrative)
V70.1 Psychiatric (general exam requested by authority)
V70.2 Psychiatric (general) other or unspecified
V72.5 Radiological NEC

ROUTINE

V72.9 NOS
V72.7 Allergy
V72.2 Dental
V72.19 Ears and/or hearing
V72.0 Eye
V72.31 Gynecological (routine)

EXAM (continued)

ROUTINE (continued)

V20.2 Health check infant or child
V72.6 Laboratory (routine)
V20.2 Newborn check initial and subsequent
0 Pap smear follow up to previous treatment with no recurrence see 'Exam' follow up
V72.31 Pap smear cervical and vaginal smears with GYN exam [V76.47]
V72.31 Pap smear cervical smear with GYN Exam
V72.32 Pap smear cervical to confirm findings of recent normal smear following initial abnormal smear
V76.2 Pap smear cervical without GYN exam
V71.1 Pap smear suspected neoplasm (unproven) (undiagnosed)
V76.47 Pap smear vaginal
V76.47 Pap smear vaginal following hysterectomy [V45.77]
V76.47 Pap smear vaginal following hysterectomy for nonmalignant condition [V45.77]
V67.01 Pap smear vaginal following hysterectomy for cancer **[V10.4#]** [V45.77]
5th digit: V10.4
0. Genital organ unspecified
1. Cervix uteri
2. Other part of uterus
3. Ovary
4. Genital organ other

V72.31 Pelvic (routine)
0 Pregnancy see 'Exam' pregnancy
V72.5 Radiological NEC
V72.2 Teeth
V20.2 Well baby
V65.5 Well-worried
V65.5 Worried-well
V72.0 Vision
V72.85 Other specified (specified type or reason NEC)

EXAM (continued)

V70.5 School (health)
V70.3 School admission (general) (administrative)
0 Screening see 'Screening'
V72.7 Skin hypersensitivity
V72.85 Special examination other (specified type or reason NEC)
V70.3 Sports competition (general) (administrative)
0 Suspected condition (undiagnosed) (unproven) see 'Evaluation'
0 Suspected condition infant/newborn (undiagnosed) (unproven) see 'Evaluation Newborn/Infant'
V72.2 Teeth
V72.0 Vision
0 With no illness or injury see 'Observation'
V65.5 Worried-well
V70.8 Other general medical
V72.85 Other specified special examination (specified type or reason NEC)

782.1 EXANTHEM
057.9 EXANTHEM VIRAL
058.10 EXANTHEMA SUBITUM (SIXTH DISEASE) NOS
058.11 EXANTHEMA SUBITUM (SIXTH DISEASE) DUE TO HUMAN HERPESVIRUS 6
058.12 EXANTHEMA SUBITUM (SIXTH DISEASE) DUE TO HUMAN HERPESVIRUS 7
255.0 EXCESS CORTISOL, IATROGENIC SYNDROME

E

EXCESSIVE

780.95 Crying child, adult, adolescent or NOS
780.92 Crying infant, baby or newborn
783.6 Eating
524.26 Horizontal overjet or overlap
524.37 Intermaxillary vertical dimension
527.7 Salivation
786.4 Sputum
780.8 Sweating
783.5 Thirst
701.5 Tissue granulation
278.02 Weight
783.1 Weight gain

> ***783.21 Use an additional code to identify body mass index (BMI), if known. See 'Body Mass Index'.***

783.21 Weight loss
278.02 Weight with body mass index 25 and above [**V85.#(#)**]

> ***V85.#(#): These codes are for use in persons over 20 years old.***

4th or 4th and 5th digit: V85
2#. 25-29
1. 25.0-25.9
2. 26.0-26.9
3. 27.0-27.9
4. 28.0-28.9
5. 29.0-29.9
3#. 30-39
0. 30.0-30.9
1. 31.0-31.9
2. 32.0-32.9
3. 33.0-33.9
4. 34.0-34.9
5. 35.0-35.9
6. 36.0-36.9
7. 37.0-37.9
8. 38.0-38.9
9. 39.0-39.9
4. 40 and over

298.1 EXCITATION REACTIVE (PSYCHOTIC)
698.4 EXCORIATION NEUROTIC
0 EXCORIATION (TRAUMATIC) SEE ANATOMICAL SITE, INJURY SUPERFICIAL

EXERCISE

V65.41 Counseling
V47.2 Intolerance cardiovascular (respiratory) at rest or ordinary activity
V69.0 Problem (lack of)

EXHAUSTION

991.8 Cold
994.5 Exertion excessive
909.4 Exertion excessive late effect
994.4 Exposure
909.4 Exposure late effect
779.89 Fetus or newborn
992.5 Heat
992.4 Heat - salt depletion
992.3 Heat - water depletion

EXHAUSTION (continued)

763.89 Maternal affecting fetus or newborn
669.8# Maternal complicating delivery
5th digit: 669.8
0. Episode of care NOS or N/A
1. Delivered
2. With postpartum complication
3. Antepartum complication
4. Postpartum complication

300.5 Mental
300.5 Nervous (psychogenic)
797 Old age (senile)
780.79 Physical NEC
780.79 Postinfectional
300.5 Syndrome

302.4 EXHIBITIONISM
756.79 EXOMPHALOS CONGENITAL

EXOPHORIA

378.42 NOS
378.83 Convergence insufficiency
378.85 Divergence excess

EXOPHTHALMOS

376.30 NOS
743.66 Congenital
376.31 Constant
376.33 Due to edema
376.32 Due to orbital hemorrhage
376.34 Intermittent
376.22 Ophthalmoplegia
376.35 Pulsating
242.## Thyrotoxic [376.21]
242.## Thyrotoxic with ophthalmoplegia [376.22]
4TH digit: 242
0 Diffuse
1. Uninodular
2. Multinodular
3. Nodular unspecified
4. Ectopic thyroid nodular
8. Other specified
9. Unspecified

5th digit: 242
0. Without mention of thyrotoxic crisis or storm
1. With mention of thyrotoxic crisis or storm

EXOSTOSIS

726.91 Site NOS
756.4 Site NOS congenital
380.81 Ear canal external
098.89 Gonococcal
726.5 Hip
733.3 Intracranial
526.81 Jaw
728.11 Luxurians
726.91 Nasal bones
376.42 Orbit
721.8 Spine
095.5 Syphilitic
726.4 Wrist

E

EXOTROPIA

378.1# NOS
378.1# Divergent noncomitant strabismus
5th digit: 378.1
0. Unspecified
1. Monocular unspecified
2. Monocular with A pattern
3. Monocular with V pattern
4. Monocular with other noncomitancies (X or Y pattern)
5. Alternating unspecified
6. Alternating with A pattern
7. Alternating with V pattern
8. Alternating with other noncomitancies (X or Y pattern)

378.20 Intermittent
378.24 Intermittent alternating
378.23 Intermittent monocular

V68.2 EXPERT EVIDENCE REQUEST
993.4 EXPLOSION EFFECTS OF AIR PRESSURE
909.4 EXPLOSION EFFECTS OF AIR PRESSURE LATE EFFECT
312.3# EXPLOSIVE DISORDER
5th digit: 312.3
4. Intermittent impulse control
5. Isolated impulse control

301.3 EXPLOSIVE PERSONALITY DISORDER

EXPOSURE

994.9 NOS
V01.9 NOS communicable disease
V01.79 AIDS
V01.81 Anthrax
V15.84 Asbestos history
V15.85 Body fluids - potentially hazardous history
V01.71 Chickenpox
V01.0 Cholera
V01.89 Coccidioidomycosis
V01.79 Coxsackie (CMV) (adenovirus)
V01.83 E. coli
V01.79 Echo (vacinnia) (herpes simplex)
V01.83 Escherichia coli
994.4 Exhaustion
909.4 Exhaustion late effect
V01.6 Gonorrhea
V01.89 H. influenza
V15.85 Hazardous body fluids history
V01.79 Hepatitis viral A/B or other
V01.6 Herpes genitalia
V01.89 Histoplasmosis
V01.79 HIV
V01.79 Influenza
V15.86 Lead history
V01.89 Lice
V01.79 Measles (rubeola)
V01.84 Meningococcus
V01.79 Mononucleosis
V01.79 Mumps

EXPOSURE (continued)

V01.89 Parasitic disease
V01.89 Pediculosis
V01.89 Pertussis
V01.89 Pneumococcus
V01.2 Poliomyelitis
V15.85 Potentially hazardous - body fluids history
V01.5 Rabies
V01.4 Rubella
V01.82 SARS (severe acute respiratory syndrome)-associated coronavirus
V01.82 Severe acute respiratory syndrome-associated coronavirus
V01.3 Smallpox
V01.89 Streptococcus
V01.6 Syphilis
V01.1 TB
V01.89 Trichomonas
V01.89 Tularemia
V01.71 Varicella
V01.6 VD
V01.6 Venereal disease
V01.79 Viral hepatitis A/B or other
V01.89 Other communicable disease
V01.79 Other viral diseases
0 See specified agent, i.e. rubella

772.0 EXSANGUINATION FETAL

EXTENSOR

883.2 Digiti minimi tendon laceration finger
882.2 Digiti minimi tendon laceration hand
891.2 Hallucis tendon laceration ankle
892.2 Hallucis tendon laceration foot
893.2 Hallucis tendon laceration toe
883.2 Indicus proprius laceration finger
882.2 Indicus proprius laceration hand
881.20 Pollicis longus laceration forearm
882.2 Pollicis longus laceration hand
883.2 Pollicis longus laceration thumb
881.22 Pollicis longus laceration wrist
883.2 Pollicis brevis laceration finger
882.2 Pollicis brevis laceration hand
727.63 Tendon hand and wrist rupture nontraumatic
891.2 Tendon toe laceration ankle
892.2 Tendon toe laceration foot
893.2 Tendon toe laceration toe

900.81 EXTERNAL JUGULAR VEIN INJURY
908.3 EXTERNAL JUGULAR VEIN INJURY LATE EFFECT
763.89 EXTRACTION FETAL MANUAL OR WITH HOOK AFFECTING FETUS OR NEWBORN
V15.87 EXTRACORPOREAL MEMBRANE OXYGENATION (ECMO) HISTORY
660.7# EXTRACTION FORCEPS OR VACUUM (FAILED)
5th digit: 660.7
0. Episode of care unspecified or N/A
1. Delivered
3. Antepartum complication

E

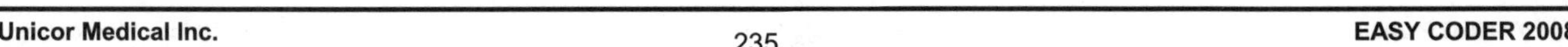

EXTRADURAL

851.8# Contusion (with hemorrhage)
851.9# Contusion (with hemorrhage) with open intracranial wound
432.0 Hematoma
767.0 Hematoma fetus or newborn, birth trauma (intrapartum anoxia/hypoxia)
852.4# Hematoma traumatic
852.5# Hematoma traumatic with open intracranial wound

5th digit: 851.8-9, 852.4-5
- **0. Level of consciousness (LOC) NOS**
- **1. No LOC**
- **2. LOC < 1 hr**
- **3. LOC 1 - 24 hrs**
- **4. LOC > 24 hrs with return to prior level**
- **5. LOC > 24 hrs without return to prior level: or death before regaining consciousness, regardless of duration of LOC**
- **6. LOC duration unspecified**
- **9. With concussion unspecified**

767.0 Hemorrhage fetus or newborn, birth trauma (intrapartum anoxia/hypoxia)
674.0# Hemorrhage maternal due to pregnancy

5th digit: 674.0
- **0. Episode of care NOS or N/A**
- **1. Delivered**
- **2. Delivered with postpartum complication**
- **3. Antepartum complication**
- **4. Postpartum complication**

852.4# Hemorrhage traumatic
852.5# Hemorrhage traumatic with open intracranial wound

5th digit: 852.4-5
- **0. Level of consciousness unspecified**
- **1. No LOC**
- **2. LOC < 1 hr**
- **3. LOC 1 - 24 hrs**
- **4. LOC > 24 hrs with return to prior level**
- **5. LOC > 24 hrs without return to prior level: or death before regaining consciousness, regardless of duration of LOC**
- **6. LOC duration unspecified**
- **9. With concussion unspecified**

333.90 EXTRAPYRAMIDAL DISEASE OR SYNDROME
781.0 EXTRAPYRAMIDAL SYMPTOMS

EXTRASYSTOLES

427.60 NOS
427.61 Atrial
997.1 Postoperative (during or resulting from a procedure)
427.69 Ventricular

EXTRAVASATION

459.0 Blood
457.8 Chyle into mesentery
788.8 Urine

EYE

743.00 Absence (congenital)
V45.78 Absence acquired
743.69 Absence adnexa (congenital)
743.69 Absence muscle extrinsic (congenital)

EYE (continued)

743.9 Anomaly (congenital)
743.48 Anomaly anterior segment multiple and combined (congenital)
743.49 Anomaly anterior segment other (congenital)
743.8 Anomaly other specified (congenital)
364.9 Anterior chamber disorder
360.42 Blind hypertensive
360.41 Blind hypotensive
374.43 Blinking
368.8 Blurred vision
379.93 Conjunctival redness
743.9 Deformity (congenital)
743.69 Deformity accessory muscles (congenital)
379.8 Deformity acquired
360.40 Degenerated
379.93 Discharge
379.90 Disorder unspecified
743.10 Dysplasia NOS (congenital)
743.11 Dysplasia simple (congenital)
743.12 Dysplasia with other anomalies of eye and adnexa (congenital)
364.61 Epithelial down growth

EXAM

V53.1 Fitting and adjustment (eyeglasses) (contact)
V72.0 Routine
V80.2 Screening for congenital anomaly
V80.2 Screening for other conditions

EYE (continued)

360.41 Eyeball atrophy
360.9 Eyeball disorder
379.24 Floaters
360.40 Globe degenerated
360.9 Globe disoders NOS
360.81 Globe luxation
743.10 Hypoplasia NOS (congenital)
743.11 Hypoplasia simple (congenital)
743.12 Hypoplasia with other anomalies of eye and adnexa (congenital)
364.3 Inflammatory

INJURIES

921.9 NOS
918.9 NOS superficial
871.3 Avulsion
767.8 Birth trauma damage
871.3 Enucleation traumatic
921.3 Eyeball
871.9 Eyeball open wound
871.5 Eyeball penetration with magnetic foreign body
871.6 Eyeball penetration with nonmagnetic foreign body
918.9 Eyeball superficial NOS
918.1 Eyeball superficial laceration/abrasion
871.4 Laceration unspecified
871.0 Laceration ocular
871.1 Laceration ocular with partial loss of intraocular tissue
996.59 Orbital implant prolapse
871.2 Rupture with partial loss of intraocular tissue

EYE (continued)

379.99 Itching
379.92 Mass
378.87 Movement dissociated deviation
378.9 Movement disorder NOS
379.58 Movement irregular deficiencies of smooth pursuit (see also by specific irregularity)
379.59 Movement irregularities other
743.69 Muscles deformity (congenital)
379.8 Muscles deformity acquired
379.91 Pain (in or around)
V41.1 Problems NEC

PROSTHESIS

V45.69 And adnexa surgery status
996.69 Complication - infection or inflammation
996.59 Complication - mechanical
996.79 Complication - other
V52.2 Fitting and adjustment (removal)
V43.0 Globe replacement (artificial) (prosthesis)

EYE (continued)

306.7 Psychogenic
379.93 Redness (conjunctiva)
378.71 Retraction syndrome
366.16 Sclerosis nuclear (senile)
378.87 Skew deviation
372.64 Socket contracture post enucleation
368.13 Strain
379.92 Swelling
360.89 Other (globe) disorders
379.99 Other ill-defined eye disorder
379.8 Other specified eye and adnexa disorder

959.09 EYEBROW INJURY

EYELID

374.89 Absence acquired
743.62 Absence congenital
743.62 Accessory congenital
743.69 Anomaly
743.63 Anomaly other specified
374.50 Atrophy (senile)
374.41 Contracture
374.84 Cyst
743.62 Deformities congenital
743.63 Deformity other specified congenital
0 Dermatitis see 'Dermatitis Eyelid'
373.34 Discoid lupus erythematosus
374.9 Disorder
374.43 Disorder abnormal innervation syndrome
374.50 Disorder degenerative
374.56 Disorder degenerative other
374.44 Disorder sensory
374.89 Disorder other
374.45 Disorder other sensorimotor
743.61 Drooping congenital
374.52 Dyspigmentation
374.82 Edema
373.13 Furuncle
374.82 Hyperemia
374.52 Hyperpigmentation
374.54 Hypertrichosis
374.53 Hypopigmentation
374.55 Hypotrichosis
373.9 Infection unspecified
373.9 Infiltrate
373.9 Inflammation
373.8 Inflammation other
921.1 Injury
918.0 Injury superficial
374.41 Lag or retraction (nervous)
374.55 Madarosis
756.0 Malar-mandible syndrome
373.11 Stye
374.85 Vascular anomalies
374.56 Other degenerative disorders of skin affecting eyelid
374.89 Other disorders

125.2 EYEWORM OF AFRICA

E

280.9 FABER'S ANEMIA (SYNDROME)
272.7 FABRY'S DISEASE OR SYNDROME (ANGIOKERATOMA CORPORIS DIFFUSUM)
272.7 FABRY'S DISEASE CEREBRAL DEGENERATION [330.2]

FACE, FACIAL

756.0 Absence - bones NEC congenital
744.89 Absence - specified part NEC congenital
744.9 Anomaly congenital
744.89 Anomaly specified NEC congenital
754.0 Asymmetry congenital
701.9 Atrophy (skin)
754.0 Compression congenital
738.19 Deformity
744.9 Deformity NOS congenital
781.94 Droop
438.83 Droop late effect of CVA
959.09 Injury
925.1 Injury crush
910.8 Injury other and unspecified (superficial)
910.9 Injury other and unspecified (superficial) infected
V50.1 Lift (elective) (for unacceptable cosmetic appearance)
351.8 Myokymia
351.8 Nerve (7th) atrophy
351.9 Nerve (7th) disorder
351.8 Nerve (7th) disorder other specified NEC
951.4 Nerve (7th) injury
767.5 Nerve (7th) injury newborn birth trauma
351.8 Nerve (7th) neuritis
351.8 Nerve (7th) pain
351.0 Nerve (7th) palsy
767.5 Nerve (7th) palsy newborn birth trauma
997.09 Nerve (7th) palsy postoperative
351.0 Nerve (7th) paralysis
784.0 Pain
350.2 Pain atypical
351.8 Pain nerve
374.43 Paradoxical movement
652.4# Presentation
660.0# Presentation obstructing labor **[652.4#]**
652.6# Presentation with multiple gestation
660.0# Presentation with multiple gestation obstructing labor **[652.6#]**
652.1# Presentation with version
660.0# Presentation with version obstructing labor **[652.1#]**

5th digit: 652.1, 4, 6, 660.0
- **0. Episode of care unspecified or N/A**
- **1. Delivered**
- **3. Antepartum complication**

781.94 Weakness
438.83 Weakness late effect of CVA

724.8 FACET SYNDROME
0 FACIAL SEE 'FACE, FACIAL'
300.19 FACTITIOUS DISORDER NOS
300.19 FACTITIOUS DISORDER WITH COMBINED PSYCHOLOGICAL AND PHYSICAL SIGNS AND SYMPTOMS
300.19 FACTITIOUS DISORDER WITH PREDOMINATELY PHYSICAL SIGNS AND SYMPTOMS
300.16 FACTITIOUS DISORDER WITH PREDOMINATELY PSYCHOLOGICAL SIGNS AND SYMPTOMS
300.19 FACTITIOUS DISORDER OTHER SPECIFIED
301.51 FACTITIOUS ILLNESS CHRONIC WITH PHYSICAL SYMPTOMS

FACTOR

286.3 I deficiency
286.3 II deficiency
286.3 V deficiency
289.81 V Leiden mutation
286.3 VII deficiency
286.0 VIII deficiency
286.0 VIII deficiency with functional defect
286.4 VIII deficiency with vascular defect
286.0 VIII disorder congenital
286.0 VIII (functional) deficiency
286.4 VIII with vascular defect
286.1 IX (functional) deficiency
286.1 IX disorder congenital
286.3 X deficiency
286.2 XI disorder congenital
286.3 XII deficiency
286.3 XIII deficiency
286.0 A deficiency
286.1 B deficiency
286.2 C deficiency

403.00 FAHR VOLHARD DISEASE (MALIGNANT NEPHROSCLEROSIS)
996.49 FAILED FUSION (JOINT) (SPINAL) **[V43.6#]**

5th digit: V43.6
- **0. Site unspecified**
- **1. Shoulder**
- **2. Elbow**
- **3. Wrist**
- **4. Hip**
- **5. Knee**
- **6. Ankle**
- **9. Other**

659.0# FAILED INDUCTION OF LABOR - MECHANICAL (VIA SURGICAL OR INSTRUMENTAL METHODS)
659.1# FAILED INDUCTION OF LABOR - MEDICAL (NOS OR VIA DRUGS)
660.6# FAILED TRIAL OF LABOR

5th digit: 659.0-1, 660.6
- **0. Episode of care or N/A**
- **1. Delivered**
- **3. Antepartum complication**

FAILURE

0 See specified site
661.2# To progress complicating labor and delivery

5th digit: 661.2
- **0. Episode of care or N/A**
- **1. Delivered**
- **3. Antepartum complication**

783.7 To thrive adult
783.41 To thrive child
996.8# Transplant organ

5th digit: 996.8
- **0. Organ unspecified**
- **1. Kidney**
- **2. Liver**
- **3. Heart**
- **4 lung**
- **5. Bone marrow**
- **6. Pancreas**
- **7. Intestine**
- **9. Other specified organ**

996.52 Transplant skin
996.55 Transplant skin - artificial
996.55 Transplant skin - decellularized allodermis

780.2 FAINTING
V15.88 FALL HEALTH HAZARD
V15.88 FALL HISTORY (AT RISK FOR FALLING)
734 FALLEN ARCHES

FALLOPIAN TUBE

V45.77	Absence acquired
752.19	Absence congenital
752.19	Accessory congenital
752.10	Anomaly congenital
752.19	Atresia congenital
620.3	Atrophy (senile)
620.8	Calcification
620.9	Disorder noninflammatory
620.8	Disorder noninflammatory other specified NEC
620.4	Displacement
752.19	Displacement congenital
620.8	Hematosalpinx
620.8	Infarction rupture cyst polyp
867.6	Injury traumatic
867.7	Injury traumatic with open wound into cavity
908.6	Injury traumatic late effect
V26.21	Insufflation
V26.22	Insufflation following sterilization reversal
752.19	Occlusion congenital
628.2	Occlusion (obstruction)
620.4	Prolapse (hernia)
0	Rupture - due to tubal pregnancy see 'Tubal', pregnancy
620.3	Senile involution
628.2	Stenosis
620.5	Torsion

745.2 FALLOT'S SYNDROME
746.09 FALLOT'S TRIAD
644.1# FALSE LABOR

5th digit: 644.1
0. Episode of care unspecified or N/A
3. Antepartum complication

FALSE POSITIVE BLOOD TEST

795.79	Hepatitis
795.6	Syphilis
795.5	TB

431 FALX SYNDROME

FAMILIAL

742.8	Dysautonomia
279.12	Eczema-thrombocytopenia syndrome
333.2	Essential myoclonus
288.4	Hemophagocytic lymphohistiocytosis
288.4	Hemophagocytic reticulosis
277.31	Mediterranean fever
277.31	Periodic amyloidosis
359.3	Periodic paralysis
211.3	Polyposis
190.5	Retinoblastoma syndrome

V61.9 FAMILY CIRCUMSTANCE NOS (REASON FOR ENCOUNTER)
V61.8 FAMILY CIRCUMSTANCE OTHER SPECIFIED (REASON FOR ENCOUNTER)
V61.0 FAMILY DISRUPTION (REASON FOR ENCOUNTER)

V codes explain circumstances such as why certain tests or studies were performed, such as a history of myocardial infarction, or family history of diabetes.

FAMILY HISTORY

V19.6	Allergy disorder
V18.2	Anemia
V17.7	Arthritis
V17.5	Asthma
V17.49	Atherosclerosis
V19.8	Baylor cretin syndrome
V19.0	Blindness
V18.3	Blood disorders other
V16.9	CA
V16.0	CA anorectal
V16.0	CA appendix
V16.52	CA bladder
V16.8	CA bone
V16.8	CA brain
V16.3	CA breast
V16.8	CA breast male
V16.1	CA bronchus
V16.49	CA cervix
V16.0	CA colon
V16.8	CA eye
V16.0	CA gallbladder
V16.0	CA gastrointestinal tract
V16.40	CA genital organs NOS
V16.49	CA genital organs other
V16.0	CA GI tract
V16.7	CA hematopoietic
V16.2	CA intrathoracic organs
V16.51	CA kidney
V16.2	CA larynx
V16.0	CA liver
V16.1	CA lung
V16.7	CA lymphatic and hematopoietic
V16.41	CA ovary, oviduct
V16.0	CA pancreas
V16.49	CA penis
V16.42	CA prostate
V16.2	CA respiratory
V16.0	CA stomach
V16.43	CA testis
V16.1	CA trachea
V16.59	CA urinary organs
V16.49	CA uterus
V16.49	CA vagina
V16.49	CA vulva
V16.8	CA other specified
V17.49	Cardiovascular diseases
V17.1	Cerebrovascular accident
V18.51	Colon polyp
V19.8	Conditions other
V19.5	Congenital anomalies
V19.7	Consanguinity
V17.3	Coronary artery disease
V17.1	CVA
V18.19	Cystic fibrosis
V19.2	Deafness
V18.0	Diabetes mellitus
V18.59	Digestive disorders
V19.5	Down's syndrome (mongolism)

FAMILY HISTORY (continued)

V19.3 Ear disorders (other)
V18.19 Endocrine and metabolic diseases
V17.2 Epilepsy
V19.1 Eye disorders other
V18.9 Genetic disease carrier
V18.7 Genitourinary diseases other
V18.69 Glomerulonephritis
V19.2 Hearing loss
V17.3 Heart disease (ischemic)
V16.7 Hodgkin's disease
V17.2 Huntington's chorea
V17.49 Hypertension
V18.8 Infectious diseases
V18.61 Kidney disease - polycystic
V18.69 Kidney disease - other
V16.6 Leukemia
V16.7 Lymphoma
V16.7 Lymphosarcoma
V18.11 MEN (multiple endocrine neoplasia syndrome)
V84.81 MEN (multiple endocrine neoplasia syndrome) susceptibility genetic
V18.4 Mental retardation
V18.19 Metabolic and endocrine disease
V18.11 Multiple endocrine neoplasia syndrome (MEN)
V84.81 Multiple endocrine neoplasia syndrome (MEN) susceptibility genetic
V17.89 Musculoskeletal diseases other
V17.3 Myocardial infarction
V17.2 Neurological disease other
V17.81 Osteoporosis
V18.8 Parasitic disease
V18.61 Polycystic kidney disease
V17.0 Psychiatric condition
V17.6 Respiratory conditions other chronic
V16.7 Reticulosarcoma
V19.4 Skin conditions
V17.1 Stroke
V17.41 Sudden cardiac death (SCD)
V19.0 Vision loss
V19.8 Other specified condition

V61.49 FAMILY MEMBER SICK OR HANDICAPPED (CARE OF) (PRESENCE OF)
V60.4 FAMILY MEMBER UNSUITED TO RENDER CARE (HANDICAPPED) (ILL) (OTHERWISE UNSUITED)
0 FAMILY PLANNING SEE 'COUNSELING' FAMILY PLANNING
994.2 FAMINE
909.4 FAMINE LATE EFFECT
301.0 FANATIC PERSONALITY DISORDER
270.0 FANCONI (-DE TONI) (-DEBRE) SYNDROME (CYSTINOSIS)
284.09 FANCONI'S ANEMIA (SYNDROME) (CONGENITAL PANCYTOPENIA)
367.0 FAR SIGHTEDNESS
272.8 FARBER UZMAN SYNDROME (DISSEMINATED LIPOGRANULOMATOSIS)
272.8 FARBER'S DISSEMINATED LIPOGRANULOMATOSIS
024 FARCY
495.0 FARMERS' LUNG
692.74 FARMERS' SKIN

FASCIA, FASCIAL

728.89 Calcification (contraction)
728.9 Disorder
728.89 Disorder other
728.89 Lata contraction (postural)
728.6 Palmar contracture
728.71 Plantar contracture

0 FASCIAL SEE 'FASCIA, FASCIAL'
728.11 FASCIALIS OSSIFICANS HYPERPLASIA (PROGRESSIVE)
781.0 FASCICULATION
377.32 FASCICULITIS OPTICA

When coding an infection, use an additional code, [041.#(#)], to identify the organism. See 'Bacterial Infection'.

FASCIITIS

729.4 NOS
728.89 Eosinophilic
728.86 Necrotizing
728.86 Necrotizing with gangrene [785.4]
728.79 Nodular
593.4 Perirenal
728.71 Plantar
728.79 Traumatic pseudosarcomatous

121.3 FASCIOLA GIGANTICA INFECTION
121.3 FASCIOLA HEPATICA INFECTION
121.3 FASCIOLA INFECTION
121.3 FASCIOLIASIS
121.4 FASCIOLOPSIASIS
121.4 FASCIOLOPSIS BUSKI INFECTION
359.1 FASCIOSCAPULOHUMERAL MUSCULAR DYSTROPHY

FAT

958.1 Embolism
908.2 Embolism late effect
673.8# Embolism maternal due to pregnancy

5th digit: 673.8

0. Episode of care unspecified or N/A
1. Delivered
2. Delivered with postpartum complication
3. Antepartum complication
4. Postpartum complication

677 Embolism obstetrical late effect
792.1 In stool
272.9 Metabolism disorder
611.3 Necrosis breast nonpuerperal
567.82 Necrosis peritoneal (mesentery) (omentum)
778.1 Necrosis subcutaneous neonatal
278.1 Pad
729.31 Pad knee hypertrophy

F

FATIGUE

780.79 NOS
308.9 Combat (see also 'Stress Reaction')
780.79 General
646.8# In pregnancy
5th digit: 646.8
0. Episode of care unspecified or N/A
1. Delivered with or without mention of antepartum condition
2. Delivered with postpartum complication
3. Antepartum complication
4. Postpartum complication
300.5 Psychogenic
797 Senile
780.71 Syndrome chronic
300.5 Syndrome NEC

277.85 FATTY ACID OXIDATION DISORDER
429.1 FATTY DEGENERATION HEART WITH ARTERIOSCLEROSIS [440.9]
571.8 FATTY LIVER
571.0 FATTY LIVER ALCOHOLIC
571.0 FATTY LIVER ALCOHOLIC WITH ESOPHAGEAL VARICES **[456.2#]**
5th digit: 456.2
0. With bleeding
1. Without bleeding

571.8 FATTY LIVER WITH ESOPHAGEAL VARICES **[456.2#]**
5th digit: 456.2
0. With bleeding
1. Without bleeding

254.8 FATTY THYMUS DEGENERATION
523.40 FAUCHARD'S DISEASE (PERIODONTITIS)
564.7 FAULTY BOWEL HABIT SYNDROME (IDIOPATHIC MEGACOLON)
282.2 FAVISM
099.1 FAVRE-DURAND-NICOLAS CLIMATIC BUBO
701.8 FAVRE-RACOUCHOT ELASTOIDOSIS CUTANEA NODULARIS
110.9 FAVUS
757.39 FDH SYNDROME (FOCAL DERMAL HYPOPLASIA)
780.31 FEBRILE SEIZURES NOS (CONVULSIONS) SIMPLE
780.32 FEBRILE SEIZURES (ATYPICAL OR COMPLICATED) COMPLEX
560.39 FECAL IMPACTION
787.6 FECAL INCONTINENCE
560.39 FECAL OBSTRUCTION
0 FECAL OBSTRUCTION WITH GANGRENOUS HERNIA SEE 'HERNIA', BY SITE, GANGRENOUS
0 FECAL OBSTRUCTION WITH HERNIA SEE 'HERNIA', BY SITE, INCARCERATED
560.39 FECAL RESERVOIR SYNDROME
0 FECAL RETENTION SEE 'CONSTIPATION'

FECALITH

560.39 NOS
543.9 Appendix
777.1 Congenital
0 With hernia, see 'Hernia', by site with obstruction
0 With hernia gangrenous, see 'Hernia', by site with gangrene

787.7 FECES ABNORMAL
529.0 FEDE'S DISEASE

FEEDING PROBLEM

783.3 NOS (elderly) (infant)
783.3 Difficulty adult, child or infant
307.59 Disorder of infancy or early childhood
307.59 Disorder of infancy or early childhood nonorganic
783.3 Elderly organic
307.59 Infantile psychogenic
783.3 Mismanagement
779.3 Neonatal
307.59 Psychogenic
779.3 Regulation newborn

784.99 FEELING OF FOREIGN BODY IN THROAT
985.0 FEER'S DISEASE
756.16 FEIL-KLIPPEL SYNDROME (BREVICOLLIS)
732.1 FELIX'S JUVENILE OSTEOCHONDROSIS, HIP
681.01 FELON (ANY DIGIT)
054.6 FELON HERPES SIMPLEX
714.1 FELTY'S SYNDROME (RHEUMATOID ARTHRITIS WITH SPLENOMEGALY AND LEUKOPENIA)
302.6 FEMINISM IN BOYS
0 FEMORAL SEE 'FEMUR, FEMORAL'

Injury of a blood vessel can be a laceration, A-V fistula, aneurysm, or hematoma. Use the injury code found by anatomical site (the name of the blood vessel).

FEMUR, FEMORAL

755.31 Agenesis NEC - with absence complete of distal elements
755.34 Agenesis NEC - with absence incomplete of distal elements
755.33 Agenesis NEC - with absence tibia and fibula incomplete
755.60 Anomaly NOS congenital
755.63 Anteversion (neck) congenital
442.3 Artery aneurysm (A-V fistula) (cirsoid) (false) (varicose) (ruptured)
440.2# Artery arteriosclerosis (degeneration)
440.2# Artery arteriosclerosis (degeneration) with chronic complete or total occlusion [440.4]
5th digit: 440.2
0. Unspecified
1. With intermittent claudication
2. With rest pain or rest pain and intermittent claudication
9. Other atherosclerosis extremities

F

FEMUR, FEMORAL (continued)

When coding arteriosclerosis of the extremities use an additional code, if applicable to identify chronic complete or total occlusion of the artery of the extremities (440.4).

440.24 Artery arteriosclerosis (degeneration) with ischemic gangrene or ischemic gangrene ulceration, or ulceration and intermittent claudication, rest pain [707.1#]
440.23 Artery arteriosclerosis (degeneration) with ulceration, or ulceration and intermittent claudication, rest pain [707.1#]

5th digit: 707.1
- **0. Unspecified**
- **1. Thigh**
- **2. Calf**
- **3. Ankle**
- **4. Heel and midfoot**
- **5. Other parts of foot, toes**
- **9. Other**

440.3# Artery bypass graft arteriosclerosis (extremities)
440.3# Artery bypass graft arteriosclerosis (extremities) with chronic complete or total occlusion [440.4]

5th digit: 440.3
- **0. Unspecified graft**
- **1. Autologous vein bypass graft**
- **2. Nonautologous biological bypass graft**

996.62 Artery bypass graft complication - infection or inflammation
996.1 Artery bypass graft complication - mechanical
996.74 Artery bypass graft complication - other
444.22 Artery embolism (thrombosis) (occlusion) (infarction)
904.0 Artery injury - above profunda origin
904.0 Artery injury - common
908.3 Artery injury - late effect
904.1 Artery injury - superficial
754.42 Bowing congenital
732.2 Epiphyseal separation
0 Epiphyseal separation traumatic see 'Fracture', femur
355.2 Nerve disorder
355.1 Nerve disorder (lateral cutaneous of thigh)
956.1 Nerve injury
907.5 Nerve injury late effect
355.2 Nerve neuritis
355.1 Nerve neuritis lateral cutaneous of thigh
355.2 Nerve other lesion
904.2 Vein injury
908.3 Vein injury late effect
904.2 Vein laceration (rupture) (hematoma) (avulsion) (aneurysm) traumatic
908.3 Vein laceration late effect
451.19 Vein phlebitis femoropopliteal
451.11 Vein phlebitis (deep) (superficial)

451.19 FEMOROPOPLITEAL VEIN PHLEBITIS
595.1 FENWICK ULCER
537.89 FENWICK'S GASTRIC ATROPHY
989.5 FER DE LANCE BITE
995.0 FER DE LANCE BITE WITH ANAPHYLAXIS [989.5]
441.9 FERNELS' AORTIC ANEURYSM
257.2 FERTILE EUNUCH SYNDROME

FERTILITY

V26.41 Counseling and advice using natural family planning
V26.49 Counseling and advice other

Use an additional code to identify the type of infertility.

V26.81 Encounter for assisted reproductive procedure cycle
V26.81 In vitro fertilization cycle encounter
V26.9 Management
V26.89 Management other specified
V26.21 Test

Fetal or newborn codes (760-779) sometimes require an additional code to further specify the cause of the condition, the infecting organism, or complicating diagnoses. Whenever appropriate, describe the patient's medical situation as clearly and concisely as possible using multiple codes.

FETAL - INFANT'S RECORD

768.2 Acidemia metabolic before onset of labor - liveborn infant
768.3 Acidemia metabolic first noted during labor and delivery - liveborn infant
768.4 Acidemia metabolic unspecified as to time - liveborn infant
768.9 Acidosis
760.71 Alcohol syndrome
760.71 Alcohol syndrome late effect

ANEMIA NEWBORN

773.2 Unspecified
776.5 Due to fetal blood loss
773.2 Due to isoimmunization - NOS
773.1 Due to isoimmunization - ABO
773.0 Due to isoimmunization - RH (rhesus), anti-D (RH)
773.2 Due to isoimmunization - other specified
773.5 Late due to isoimmunization
776.5 Posthemorrhagic
776.6 Prematurity neonatal

FETAL - INFANT'S RECORD (continued)

768.9 Anoxia NOS
770.81 Apnea essential
770.82 Apnea obstructive
770.81 Apnea primary
770.81 Apnea sleep
768.9 Asphyxia NOS
768.6 Asphyxia mild or moderate
768.5 Asphyxia severe
771.83 Bacteremia
779.89 Birth shock
773.# Blood (group) (type) incompatibility causing hemolytic disease
773.# Blood (group) (type) incompatibility causing hemolytic disease

4th digit: 773
- **0. RH (rhesus) isoimmunization**
- **1. ABO isoimmunization**
- **2. Other and NOS isoimmunization**

BLOOD LOSS

772.0 Unspecified
772.0 Cut end co-twin's cord
762.3 Due to placental transfusion [772.0]
772.0 Exsanguination
772.0 Mother's circulation

F

FETAL - INFANT'S RECORD (continued)

BLOOD LOSS (continued)

772.0 Placenta
772.0 Ruptured cord
772.0 Vasa previa

FETAL - INFANT'S RECORD (continued)

779.81 Bradycardia
779.85 Cardiac arrest
779.85 Cardiac failure
747.83 Circulation persistent
779.85 Circulatory failure
771.89 Clostridium infection intra-amniotic [041.84]
770.83 Cyanotic attacks

DEATH

779.9 NOS
768.0 Asphyxia or anoxia before labor
768.1 Asphyxia or anoxia during labor
779.6 Due to induced abortion
779.6 Due to termination of pregnancy
798.0 Infant syndrome (SIDS)
0 Infant syndrome (SIDS) near miss - code individual symptom(s)
779.9 Intrauterine NOS
798.9 Unattended (cause unknown)

DISTRESS

768.4 Liveborn - unspecified onset
768.2 Liveborn - before onset labor
768.3 Liveborn - during labor and delivery
768.0 Stillborn - before onset of labor
768.1 Stillborn - death during labor

FETAL - INFANT'S RECORD (continued)

760.70 Drug abuse maternal transmitted via placenta or breast milk affecting fetus/newborn
771.89 Escherichia coli (E. coli) infection intra-amniotic [041.4]

Fetal growth retardation: Use an additional code to specify the underlying cause of the growth retardation.

GROWTH RETARDATION

764.90 Unspecified (weight)
764.91 Less than 500 grams
764.92 500-749 grams
764.93 750-999 grams
764.94 1000-1249 grams
764.95 1250-1499 grams
764.96 1500-1749 grams
764.97 1750-1999 grams
764.98 2000-2499 grams
764.99 2500 grams and over

FETAL - INFANT'S RECORD (continued)

779.89 Heart failure fetus or newborn
763.81 Heart rate or rhythm abnormal - before onset of labor
763.82 Heart rate or rhythm abnormal - during labor
779.82 Heart rate or rhythm abnormal - fast (tachycardia)
779.81 Heart rate or rhythm abnormal - slow (bradycardia)
763.83 Heart rate or rhythm abnormal - unspecified as to time of onset

FETAL - INFANT'S RECORD (continued)

773.# Hemolytic disease due to isoimmunization
4th digit: 773
0. RH (rhesus) isoimmunization
1. ABO isoimmunization
2. Other and NOS isoimmunization

770.89 Hypercapnia
779.89 Hypotonia
768.9 Hypoxia
771.89 Infection intra-amniotic
779.89 Injury intrauterine
0 Jaundice see 'Jaundice Neonatal'

Fetal malnutrition: Use an additional code to further specify the cause of the malnutrition.

MALNUTRITION

764.20 Unspecified (weight)
764.21 Less than 500 grams
764.22 500-749 grams
764.23 750-999 grams
764.24 1000-1249 grams
764.25 1250-1499 grams
764.26 1500-1749 grams
764.27 1750-1999 grams
764.28 2000-2499 grams
764.29 2500 grams and over

FETAL - INFANT'S RECORD (continued)

779.89 Papyraceous
747.83 Persistent circulation
770.9 Respiratory condition
770.89 Respiratory depression
770.89 Respiratory distress
769 Respiratory distress syndrome
770.84 Respiratory failure
771.89 Salmonella infection [003.9]
771.81 Sepsis intrauterine
771.81 Septicemia
771.89 Streptococcal infection intra-amniotic (newborn) perinatal [041.0#]
5th digit: 041.0
0. NOS
1. Group A
2. Group B
3. Group C
4. Group D (enterococcus)
5. Group G
9. Other strep

779.82 Tachycardia
779.83 Umbilical cord separation delayed
771.82 UTI
763.89 Other specified complications of labor and delivery affecting fetus or newborn

F

FETAL - MOTHER'S RECORD

***Fetus abnormality affecting management of mother:* Use codes from this section only if the fetal condition causes a complication that affects the management of the mother. These can be an additional reason for observation, obstetrical care, or abortion. Use these codes only on the mother's record. Remember, do not use these codes if the fetal condition does not affect management of the mother.**

ABNORMALITY KNOWN/SUSPECT AFFECTING MANAGEMENT OF MOTHER

655.9# Unspecified
655.4# Alcoholism listeriosis toxoplasmosis
655.0# Anencephaly
655.1# Chromosome abnormality
655.0# CNS malformation
655.5# Damage from drugs
655.8# Exposure to toxins or IUD
655.8# Heart sounds inaudible
655.2# Hereditary familial
655.0# Hydrocephalus
655.4# Maternal disease damaging fetus
655.7# Movement decreased (lack of)
655.6# Radiation exposure
655.3# Rubella maternal
655.0# Spina bifida myelomeningocele
655.4# Toxoplasmosis maternal
655.3# Viral disease in mother
655.8# Other specified problems
5th digit: 655.0-9
0. Episode of care unspecified or N/A
1. Delivered
3. Antepartum complication

FETAL - MOTHER'S RECORD (continued)

656.8# Acid-base imbalance
656.8# Acidosis intrauterine
656.3# Acidemia metabolic fetal
653.7# Ascites (hydrops) (myelomeningocele) (teratoma) (neoplasm uncertain behavior) (conjoined twins)
660.1# Ascites (hydrops) (myelomeningocele) (teratoma) (neoplasm uncertain behavior) (conjoined twins) obstructing labor **[653.7#]**
5th digit: 653.7, 656.3, 8, 660.1
0. Episode of care unspecified or N/A
1. Delivered
3. Antepartum complication

656.2# Blood type incompatibility complicating pregnancy - ABO
656.1# Blood type incompatibility complicating pregnancy - anti-D antibodies (RH)
656.1# Blood type incompatibility complicating pregnancy - rhesus (RH)
5th digit: 656.1-2
0. Episode of care unspecified or N/A
1. Delivered
3. Antepartum complication

FETAL - MOTHER'S RECORD (continued)

656.2# Blood type incompatibility complicating pregnancy - other specified
659.7# Bradycardia
5th digit: 656.2, 659.7
0. Episode of care unspecified or N/A
1. Delivered
3. Antepartum complication

DEATH

656.4# After completion of 22 weeks' gestation
5th digit: 656.4
0. Episode of care unspecified or N/A
1. Delivered
3. Antepartum complication

632 Before completion of 22 weeks' gestation (retained)
669.9# During delivery
668.9# During delivery - anesthesia NEC
5th digit: 668.9, 669.9
0. Episode of care NOS or N/A
1. Delivered
2. Delivered with postpartum complication
4. Postpartum complication

DISPROPORTION

653.5# Unspecified fetal abnormality
660.1# Unspecified fetal abnormality obstructing labor **[653.5#]**
653.7# Other fetal abnormality causing disproportion
5th digit: 653.5, 7, 660.1
0. Episode of care unspecified or N/A
1. Delivered
3. Antepartum complication

0 See also 'Pregnancy Complications, Disproportion'

DISTRESS

656.8# NOS
656.3# Acidemia metabolic
5th digit: 656.3, 8
0. Episode of care unspecified or N/A
1. Delivered
3. Antepartum complication

GROWTH

656.6# Excessive
656.5# Poor, small or light-for-dates
5th digit: 656.5-6
0. Episode of care unspecified or N/A
1. Delivered
3. Antepartum complication

FETAL - MOTHER'S RECORD (continued)

659.7# Heart rate decelerations
659.7# Heart rate or rhythm abnormal
659.7# Heart tones depressed
653.6# Hydrocephalus causing disproportion
660.1# Hydrocephalus causing disproportion obstructing labor **[653.6#]**
655.0# Hydrocephalus known or suspected - concern for fetus
653.5# Large causing disproportion
659.8# Lung maturity evaluation
5th digit: 653.5-6, 659.7-8, 660.1
0. Episode of care unspecified or N/A
1. Delivered
3. Antepartum complication

FETAL - MOTHER'S RECORD (continued)

0 Malposition or malpresentation see 'Pregnancy Complications, Delivery Problems: Malpresentation/Malposition'
655.4# Maternal disease causing damage to fetus
656.0# Maternal hemorrhage
656.8# Meconium in liquor
659.7# Non-reassuring fetal heart rate or rhythm
646.0# Papyraceous
653.4# Pelvic disproportion
656.9# Problem unspecified
656.8# Problem other specified
656.1# RH incompatibility
659.7# Tachycardia

5th digit: 653.4, 655.4, 656.0-1, 8-9, 659.7
0. Episode of care unspecified or N/A
1. Delivered
3. Antepartum complication

302.81 FETISHISM
302.3 FETISHISM TRANSVESTIC

653.4# FETOPELVIC DISPROPORTION
646.0# FETUS PAPYRACEOUS

5th digit: 646.0, 653.4
0. Episode of care unspecified or N/A
1. Delivered
3. Antepartum complication

0 FETUS SEE 'FETAL'

FEVER

780.6 Unspecified
054.9 Blister
036.0 Cerebrospinal (meningococcal)
078.3 Due to cat scratch
277.31 Etiocholanolone
277.31 Familial Mediterranean
V73.5 Hemorrhagic screening exam
0 Hemorrhagic see 'Hemorrhagic Fever'
087.0 Louse-borne relapsing or recurrent
<u>**288.0#**</u> <u>Neutropenic</u> [780.6]

5th digit: 288.0
0. Unspecified
1. Congenital
2. Cyclic
3. Drug induced
4. Due to infection
9. Other

778.4 Newborn transitory
277.31 Periodic
998.89 Postoperative
998.59 Postoperative due to infection
672.0# Puerperal
670.0# Puerperal septic

5th digit: 670.0, 672.0
0. Unspecified
2. Delivered with postpartum complication
4. Postpartum complication

087.9 Relapsing or recurrent unspecified
082.0 Rocky mountain spotted
087.1 Tick-borne relapsing or recurrent
0 Undulant see 'Brucellosis'
780.6 Unknown etiology (origin)

FEVER (continued)

066.40 West Nile NOS
066.42 West Nile with cranial nerve disorder
066.41 West Nile with encephalitis

Use an additional code with 066.42 to specify the neurologic manifestation.

066.42 West Nile with neurologic manifestation other
066.42 West Nile with optic neuritis
066.42 West Nile with polyradiculitis

Use an additional code with 066.49 to specify the other condition.

066.49 West Nile with other complications
780.6 With chills
0 With leukemia – code first underlying leukemia
0 With sickle cell disease – code first underlying sickle cell disease
0 See also 'Pyrexia'

FIBRILLATION

427.31 Atrial (paroxysmal)
<u>997.1</u> Atrial (paroxysmal) <u>postoperative</u> [427.31]
427.32 Flutter syndrome
427.41 Ventricular
<u>997.1</u> Ventricular <u>postoperative</u> [427.41]

790.92 FIBRIN ABSENCE
286.6 FIBRINOGEN DEFICIENCY (TOTAL)
286.3 FIBRINOGEN DEFICIENCY CONGENITAL
790.92 FIBRINOGEN TITER ABNORMAL FINDINGS
286.6 FIBRINOGENOLYSIS HEMORRHAGIC

FIBRINOLYSIS

964.4 Affecting drugs
286.6 Pathologic
666.3# Postpartum

5th digit: 666.3
0. Unspecified
2. Delivered with postpartum complication
4. Postpartum complication

Carcinomas and neoplasms should be coded by site if possible. Code by cell type, "site NOS", only if a site is not specified in the diagnosis. Otherwise, refer to the appropriate category of neoplasm for a more specific code. See 'Cancer' 'Cancer Metastatic', 'Carcinoma In Situ', 'Neoplasm Uncertain Behavior', 'Neoplasm Unspecified Nature', or 'Benign Neoplasm'.

FIBROADENOMA

217 Site unspecified
0 Site specified see 'Benign Neoplasm', by site M9010/0

217 Cellular intracanalicular site unspecified
0 Cellular intracanalicular site specified see 'Benign Neoplasm', by site M9020/0

217 Intracanalicular site unspecified
0 Intracanalicular site specified see 'Benign Neoplasm', by site M9011/0

217 Juvenile site unspecified
0 Juvenile site specified see 'Benign Neoplasm', by site M9030/0

F

FIBROADENOMA (continued)

217 Pericanalicular site unspecified

0 Pericanalicular site specified see 'Benign Neoplasm', by site M9012/0

600.20 Prostate

> *See 'LUTS' or 'Lower Urinary Tract Symptoms' for the additional code to identify the specific lower urinary tract symptoms.*

600.21 Prostate with urinary obstruction, retention or other lower urinary tract symptoms

610.2 FIBROADENOSIS BREAST (CHRONIC) (CYSTIC) (DIFFUSE) (PERIODIC) (SEGMENTAL)

0 FIBROCASEOUS DISEASE OF LUNG SEE 'TUBERCULOSIS', PULMONARY

757.39 FIBROCUTANEOUS TAGS CONGENITAL (ANY AREA)

FIBROCYSTIC DISEASE

277.0# NOS

5th digit: 277.0
- **0. NOS**
- **1. With meconium ileus**
- **2. With pulmonary manifestations**
- **3. With gastrointestinal manifestations**
- **9. With other manifestations**

733.29 Bone

610.1 Breast

V83.81 Carrier (genetic)

526.2 Jaw bone

753.19 Kidney congenital

751.62 Liver

518.89 Lung

748.4 Lung congenital

277.01 Newborn

277.0# Pancreas

5th digit: 277.0
- **0. NOS**
- **1. With meconium ileus**
- **2. With pulmonary manifestations**
- **3. With gastrointestinal manifestations**
- **9. With other manifestations**

593.2 Renal acquired

753.19 Renal congenital

V77.6 Screening

FIBROID UTERINE

218.9 Unspecified

218.1 Intramural (interstitial)

654.1# Maternal complicating childbirth

660.2# Maternal obstructing labor [**654.1#**]

5th digit: 654.1
- **0. Episode of care unspecified or N/A**
- **1. Delivered**
- **2. Delivered with postpartum complication**
- **3. Antepartum complication**
- **4. Postpartum complication**

5th digit: 660.2
- **0. Episode of care NOS or N/A**
- **1. Delivered**
- **3. Antepartum complication**

FIBROID UTERINE (continued)

218.0 Submucous

218.2 Subserous

FIBROLIPOMA

214.# Spindle cell (intramuscular) M8851/0

4th digit: 214
- **0. Facial, skin and subcutaneous tissue**
- **1. Skin and subcutaneous tissue other**
- **2. Intrathoracic organs**
- **3. Intra-abdominal organs**
- **4. Spermatic cord**
- **8. Other specified sites**
- **9. Site unspecified**

FIBROMA

213.# Ameloblastic (upper jaw bone) M9330/0

4th digit: 213
- **0. Skull, face, upper jaw**
- **1. Lower jaw**

213.# Cementifying M9274/0

213.# Chondromyxoid M9241/0

4th digit: 213
- **0. Skull, face, upper jaw**
- **1. Lower jaw**
- **2. Spine**
- **3. Rib, sternum, clavicle**
- **4. Scapula, long bone of upper limb**
- **5. Short bone of upper limb**
- **6. Pelvis, sacrum, coccyx**
- **7. Long bone of lower limb**
- **8. Short bone of lower limb**
- **9. Site unspecified**

238.1 Desmoplastic site unspecified

0 Desmoplastic site specified see 'Neoplasm Uncertain Behavior', by site M8823/1

215.# Fascial M8813/0

4th digit: 215
- **0. Head, face, neck**
- **2. Upper limb including shoulder**
- **3. Lower limb including hip**
- **4. Thorax**
- **5. Abdomen (wall), gastric, gastrointestinal, intestine, stomach**
- **6. Pelvis, buttock, groin, inguinal region, perineum**
- **7. Trunk NOS, back NOS, flank NOS**
- **8. Other specified sites**
- **9. Site unspecified**

213.# Odontogenic M9321/0

4th digit: 213
- **0. Skull, face, upper jaw**
- **1. Lower jaw**

213.# Ossifying M9262/0

213.# Periosteal M8812/0

4th digit: 213
- **0. Skull, face, upper jaw**
- **1. Lower jaw**
- **2. Spine**
- **3. Rib, sternum, clavicle**
- **4. Scapula, Long bone of upper limb**
- **5. Short bone of upper limb**
- **6. Pelvis, sacrum, coccyx**
- **7. Long bone of lower limb**
- **8. Short bone of lower limb**
- **9. Site unspecified**

FIBROMA (continued)

600.20 Prostate

See 'LUTS' or 'Lower Urinary Tract Symptoms' for the additional code to identify the specific lower urinary tract symptoms.

600.21 Prostate with urinary obstruction, retention or other lower urinary tract symptoms

Carcinomas and neoplasms should be coded by site if possible. Code by cell type, "site NOS", only if a site is not specified in the diagnosis. Otherwise, refer to the appropriate category of neoplasm for a more specific code. See 'Cancer' 'Cancer Metastatic', 'Carcinoma In Situ', 'Neoplasm Uncertain Behavior', 'Neoplasm Unspecified Nature', or 'Benign Neoplasm'.

FIBROMATOSIS

728.79 NOS
238.1 Site unspecified
0 Site specified see 'Neoplasm Uncertain Behavior', by site
238.1 Abdominal site unspecified
0 Abdominal site specified see 'Neoplasm Uncertain Behavior', by site M8822/1
238.1 Aggressive site unspecified
0 Aggressive site specified see 'Neoplasm Uncertain Behavior', by site M8821/1
759.89 Congenital generalized (CGF)
728.6 Dupuytren's
523.8 Gingival
728.71 Plantar fascia
728.79 Proliferative
728.79 Pseudosarcomatous
728.79 Subcutaneous

447.8 FIBROMUSCULAR HYPERPLASIA OF ARTERY - NEC

447.3 FIBROMUSCULAR HYPERPLASIA OF ARTERY - RENAL

729.1 FIBROMYALGIA

FIBROMYOMA UTERINE

218.9 Unspecified
218.1 Intramural (interstitial)
218.0 Submucous
218.2 Subserous

729.1 FIBROMYOSITIS

214.# FIBROMYXOLIPOMA M8852/0
4th digit: 214
0. Facial skin and subcutaneous tissue
1. Other skin and subcutaneous tissue
2. Intrathoracic organs
3. Intra-abdominal organs
4. Spermatic cord
8. Other specified sites
9. Site unspecified

215.# FIBROMYXOMA M8811/0
171.# FIBROMYXOSARCOMA M8811/3
4th digit: 171, 215
0. Head, face, neck
2. Upper limb including shoulder
3. Lower limb including hip
4. Thorax
5. Abdomen (wall), gastric, gastrointestinal, intestine, stomach
6. Pelvis, buttock, groin, inguinal region, perineum
7. Trunk NOS, back NOS, flank NOS
8. Other specified sites
9. Site unspecified

213.# FIBRO-ODONTOMA AMELOBLASTIC M9290/0
4th digit: 213
0. Skull, face, upper jaw
1. Lower jaw unspecified

FIBROSARCOMA

171.# Unspecified M8810/3
4th digit: 171
0. Head face neck
2. Upper limb shoulder
3. Lower limb hip
4. Thorax
5. Abdomen (wall), gastric, gastrointestinal, intestine, stomach
6. Pelvis buttock groin inguinal region perineum
7. Trunk unspecified back unspecified flank unspecified
8. Other specified sites
9. Site unspecified

170.# Ameloblastic M9330/3
4th digit: 170
0. Skull and face
1. Jaw NOS, lower, inferior maxilla

171.# Fascial M8813/3
171.# Infantile M8814/3
4th digit: 171
0. Head face neck
2. Upper limb shoulder
3. Lower limb hip
4. Thorax
5. Abdomen (wall), gastric, gastrointestinal, intestine, stomach
6. Pelvis buttock groin inguinal region perineum
7. Trunk unspecified back unspecified flank unspecified
8. Other specified sites
9. Site unspecified

170.# Periosteal M8812/3
4th digit: 170
0. Skull and face
1. Mandible
2. Vertebral column
3. Ribs, sternum, clavicle
4. Scapula, long bones of upper limb
5. Short bones of upper limb
6. Pelvic bones, sacrum, coccyx
7. Long bones of lower limb
8. Short bones of lower limb
9. Site unspecified

159.1 Spleen

F

610.3 FIBROSCLEROSIS BREAST
710.8 FIBROSCLEROSIS MULTIFOCAL NEC
0 FIBROSCLEROSIS MYOCARDIOPATHY SEE 'CARDIOMYOPATHY'
607.89 FIBROSCLEROSIS PENIS, CORPORA CAVERNOSA

FIBROSIS

607.89 Corpus cavernosa
658.8# Chorion
5th digit: 658.8
0. Episode of care unspecified or N/A
1. Delivered
3. Antepartum complication

When coding an infection, use an additional code, [041.#(#)], to identify the organism. See 'Bacterial Infection'.

625.5 Congestion syndrome (pelvic)
277.0# Cystic
5th digit: 277.0
0. NOS
1. With meconium ileus
2. With pulmonary manifestations
3. With gastrointestinal manifestations
9. With other manifestations

V83.81 Cystic gene carrier status
V77.6 Cystic screening
0 Due to a device, implant or graft see 'Complication Of A Device, Implant Or Graft - Other Specified'
424.90 Endocardium
425.0 Endomyocardial
429.0 Heart see also 'Myocarditis'
519.3 Mediastinum
600.90 Median bar

See 'LUTS' or 'Lower Urinary Tract Symptoms' for the additional code to identify the specific lower urinary tract symptoms.

600.91 Median bar with urinary obstruction, retention or other lower urinary tract symptoms
349.2 Meninges
620.8 Ovary
620.8 Oviduct
577.8 Pancreas
277.0# Pancreas cystic
5th digit: 277.0
0. Without meconium ileus or NOS
1. With meconium ileus
2. With pulmonary manifestations
3. With gastrointestinal manifestations
9. With other manifestations

543.9 Periappendiceal
423.1 Pericardial
0 Perineum maternal see 'Vulva, Vulval Disorders Complicating Childbirth', Abnormality
511.0 Pleural
600.90 Prostate (chronic)

See 'LUTS' or 'Lower Urinary Tract Symptoms' for the additional code to identify the specific lower urinary tract symptoms.

600.91 Prostate (chronic) with urinary obstruction, retention or other lower urinary tract symptoms

FIBROSIS (continued)

515 Pulmonary chronic or unspecified
516.3 Pulmonary diffuse (interstitial)
503 Pulmonary due to bauxite
587 Renal
593.4 Retroperitoneal (idiopathic)
567.82 Sclerosing mesenteric (idiopathic)
528.8 Submucosal oral including tongue
621.8 Uterus
459.89 Vein

729.0 FIBROSITIS (SYNDROME)

FIBROUS

733.29 Dysplasia bone (monostotic)
733.29 Dysplasia bone or cartilage
756.54 Dysplasia bone polyostotic
756.59 Dysplasia diaphyseal progressive
526.89 Dysplasia jaw
0 Papule of the nose site specified see 'Benign Neoplasm', by site M8724/0

FIBROXANTHOMA

215.# Unspecified M8831/0
238.1 Atypical site unspecified
0 Atypical site specified see 'Neoplasm Uncertain Behavior', by site M8831/1
171.# Malignant M8831/3
4th digit: 171, 215
0. Head, face, neck
2. Upper limb including shoulder
3. Lower limb including hip
4. Thorax
5. Abdomen (wall), gastric, gastrointestinal, intestine, stomach
6. Pelvis, buttock, groin, inguinal region, perineum
7. Trunk NOS, back Nos, flank NOS
8. Other specified sites
9. Site unspecified

FIBULA, FIBULAR

755.31 Absence - with absence distal elements complete congenital
755.37 Absence - with absence distal elements incomplete congenital
755.35 Absence - with absence tibia congenital
755.33 Absence - with absence tibia with femur (incomplete) congenital

0 FIBULAR SEE 'FIBULA, FIBULAR'
100.0 FIEDLER'S LEPTOSPIRAL JAUNDICE
422.91 FIEDLER'S SYNDROME (ACUTE ISOLATED MYOCARDITIS)

099.3 FIESSINGER-LEROY (-REITER) SYNDROME
099.3 FIESSINGER-LEROY (-REITER) SYNDROME WITH ARTHROPATHY [711.1#]
5th digit: 711.1
0. Site NOS
1. Shoulder region
2. Upper arm (elbow) (humerus)
3. Forearm (radius) (wrist) (ulna)
4. Hand (carpal) (metacarpal) (fingers)
5. Pelvic region and thigh (hip) (buttock) (femur)
6. Lower leg (fibula) (knee) (patella) (tibia)
7. Ankle and/or foot (metatarsals) (toes) (tarsals)
8. Other (head) (neck) (rib) (skull) (trunk) (vertebrae)
9. Multiple
099.3 FIESSINGER-LEROY (-REITER) SYNDROME WITH CONJUNCTIVITIS [372.33]
695.1 FIESSINGER-RENDU SYNDROME (ERYTHEMA MULTIFORME EXUDATIVUM)
350.8 FIFTH CRANIAL NERVE (TRIGEMINAL) ATROPHY
350.9 FIFTH CRANIAL NERVE (TRIGEMINAL) DISORDER
951.2 FIFTH CRANIAL NERVE (TRIGEMINAL) INJURY
057.0 FIFTH DISEASE
0 FIFTH NERVE SEE 'TRIGEMINAL NERVE'
125.9 FILARIA WITH GENITAL DISEASE MALE [608.81]

FILARIASIS
125.9 Unspecified
125.0 Bancroftian
125.1 Malayan
125.5 Ozzardi infection
V75.6 Screening exam
125.6 Other specified

075 FILATOFF'S (FILATOV'S) INFECTIOUS MONONUCLEOSIS
984.9 FILE-CUTTER'S LEAD POISONING

FILLING DEFECT
793.3 Biliary tract
793.5 Bladder
793.3 Gallbladder
793.5 Kidney
793.4 Stomach
793.5 Ureter

078.89 FILTERABLE VIRUS DISEASE NEC
752.11 FIMBRIAL CYST CONGENITAL

FINGER
V49.62 Absence acquired
755.21 Absence (complete or partial) (all) or (transverse)
755.29 Absence congenital
755.29 Agenesis NEC
V49.62 Amputation status
736.29 Contraction acquired
755.59 Contraction congenital
718.44 Contraction joint

FINGER (continued)
736.20 Deformity (acquired)
736.29 Deformity (acquired) other
755.29 Deformity reduction congenital
736.29 Drop
959.5 Injury
915.8 Injury other and unspecified superficial
915.9 Injury other and unspecified superficial infected
718.94 Joint ligament relaxation
0 Joint ligament tear see 'Sprain'
718.14 Joint loose body
0 Joint see also 'Joint'
681.02 Nail abscess (infection)
703.8 Nail deformity (hypertrophy)
703.8 Nail discoloration
703.8 Nail disease other specified
681.01 Nail infection
703.0 Nail infection ingrown
703.0 Nail ingrown (infected)
959.5 Nail injury
703.8 Nail thickening
757.5 Nail thickening congenital

759.89 FINNISH TYPE NEPHROSIS (CONGENITAL)
989.5 FIRE ANT BITE
995.0 FIRE ANT BITE WITH ANAPHYLAXIS [989.5]

FIRST
756.0 Arch syndrome
426.11 Degree heart block AV
352.0 Nerve atrophy
352.0 Nerve disorders
951.8 Nerve injury

537.89 FISH HOOK STOMACH
495.8 FISH MEAL WORKERS' LUNG
270.8 FISH ODOR SYNDROME
701.1 FISH SKIN
757.1 FISH SKIN CONGENITAL
357.0 FISHER'S SYNDROME

FISSURE
756.79 Abdominal wall (congenital)
565.0 Anal
751.5 Anal congenital
863.89 Anal traumatic
863.99 Anal traumatic with open wound
908.1 Anal traumatic late effect
528.9 Buccal cavity
752.49 Clitoris (congenital)
744.29 Ear, lobule (congenital)
748.3 Epiglottis (congenital)
478.79 Larynx
748.3 Larynx congenital
528.5 Lip
0 Lip congenital see 'Cleft' lip
611.2 Nipple
676.1# Nipple puerperal, postpartum maternal due to pregnancy
5th digit: 676.1
0. Episode of care NOS or N/A
1. Delivered
2. Delivered with postpartum complication
3. Antepartum complication
4. Postpartum complication

0 Palate (congenital) see 'Cleft' palate

FISSURE (continued)

565.0 Postanal
565.0 Rectum
709.8 Skin
686.9 Skin streptococcal
0 Spine (congenital) see 'Spina Bifida'
756.3 Sternum (congenital)
529.5 Tongue
750.13 Tongue congenital

FISTULA

569.81 Abdominal wall
569.81 Abdominointestinal
569.81 Abdominorectal
569.81 Abdominosigmoidal
510.0 Abdominothoracic
619.2 Abdominouterine
752.3 Abdominouterine congenital
596.2 Abdominovesical
473.9 Accessory sinuses
0 Actinomycotic see 'Actinomycosis'
473.0 Alveolar antrum (see also 'Sinusitis' maxillary)
522.7 Alveolar process
565.1 Anal (to skin)
751.5 Anal congenital
565.1 Anorectal
619.1 Anovaginal
752.49 Anovaginal congenital
473.0 Antrobuccal (see also 'Sinusitis')
473.0 Antrum
747.29 Aortic sinus
447.2 Aortoduodenal
543.9 Appendix
447.0 Arteriovenous acquired
747.60 Arteriovenous vessel NOS (peripheral) congenital
0 Arteriovenous vessel specified congenital see 'Fistula', by site
747.69 Arteriovenous vessel other specified sites (peripheral) congenital
447.2 Artery
537.4 Astrocolic
383.81 Aural
744.49 Aural congenital
383.81 Auricle
744.49 Auricle congenital
619.8 Bartholin's gland
576.4 Bile duct
576.4 Biliary
751.69 Biliary congenital
596.2 Bladder
619.0 Bladder and female genital tract
733.99 Bone
348.8 Brain
437.3 Brain arteriovenous
747.81 Brain arteriovenous congenital
430 Brain arteriovenous with rupture
744.41 Branchial (cleft)
744.41 Branchiogenous
611.0 Breast
675.1# Breast maternal due to pregnancy

5th digit: 675.1

0. Episode of care NOS or N/A
1. Delivered
2. Delivered with postpartum complication
3. Antepartum complication
4. Postpartum complication

FISTULA (continued)

510.0 Bronchial
510.0 Bronchocutaneous
530.89 Bronchoesophageal
750.3 Bronchoesophageal congenital
510.0 Bronchomediastinal
510.0 Bronchopleural
510.0 Bronchovisceral
528.3 Buccal cavity (infective)
747.81 Carotid-cavernous congenital
430 Carotid-cavernous congenital with hemorrhage
447.0 Carotid-cavernous non-traumatic - acquired
430 Carotid-cavernous non-traumatic - acquired with hemorrhage
900.82 Carotid-cavernous traumatic
853.0# Carotid-cavernous traumatic with hemorrhage

5th digit: 853.0

0. Level of consciousness NOS
1. No LOC
2. LOC < 1 hr
3. LOC 1 - 24 hrs
4. LOC > 24 hrs with return to prior level
5. LOC > 24 hrs without return to prior level: or death before regaining consciousness, regardless of duration of LOC
6. LOC duration NOS
9. With concussion NOS

908.3 Carotid-cavernous traumatic late effect
569.81 Cecosigmoidal
569.69 Cecostomy
569.81 Cecum
349.81 Cerebrospinal (fluid)
744.41 Cervical lateral congenital
744.49 Cervicoaural congenital
619.1 Cervicosigmoid
619.0 Cervicovesical
619.8 Cervix
510.0 Chest wall
575.5 Cholecystocolic
575.5 Cholecystoduodenal
575.5 Cholecystoenteric
575.5 Cholecystogastric
575.5 Cholecystointestinal
576.4 Choledochoduodenal
685.1 Coccyx
685.0 Coccyx with abscess
569.81 Colon
569.69 Colostomy
619.1 Colovaginal
576.4 Common duct
360.32 Cornea, causing hypotony (postinflammatory) (post op) (posttraumatic)
414.19 Coronary arteriovenous
746.85 Coronary arteriovenous congenital
510.0 Costal region
619.8 Cul-de-sac (Douglas')
686.9 Cutaneous
575.5 Cystic duct
751.69 Cystic duct congenital
522.7 Dental
510.0 Diaphragm
V58.82 Drainage tube fitting
537.4 Duodenum
380.89 Ear canal
569.81 Enterocolic

FISTULA (continued)

569.81 Enterocutaneous
569.81 Enteroenteric
569.69 Enterostomy
619.1 Enterouterine
752.3 Enterouterine congenital
619.1 Enterovaginal
752.49 Enterovaginal congenital
596.1 Enterovesical
608.89 Epididymis
0 Epididymis due to TB see 'Tuberculosis', epididymis
530.89 Esophagobronchial
750.3 Esophagobronchial congenital
530.89 Esophagocutaneous
530.89 Esophagopleurocutaneous
530.84 Esophagotracheal
750.3 Esophagotracheal congenital
530.89 Esophagus
750.4 Esophagus congenital
473.2 Ethmoid sinus (see also 'Sinusitis', ethmoidal)
747.64 Extremity vessel (lower) arteriovenous congenital
747.63 Extremity vessel (upper) arteriovenous congenital
373.11 Eyelid
619.2 Fallopian tube (external)
473.1 Frontal sinus (see also 'Sinusitis', frontal)
575.5 Gallbladder
751.69 Gallbladder congenital
574.2# Gallbladder with calculus (see also 'Cholelithiasis')
5th digit: 574.2
0. Without obstruction
1. With obstruction
537.4 Gastric
537.4 Gastrocolic
750.7 Gastrocolic congenital
537.4 Gastroenterocolic
537.4 Gastroesophageal
747.61 Gastrointestinal vessel arteriovenous congenital
537.4 Gastrojejunal
537.4 Gastrojejunocolic
619.9 Genital tract female
619.1 Genital tract female - digestive to genital
619.2 Genital tract female - genital tract to skin
619.0 Genital tract female - urinary tract to genital
619.8 Genital tract female - other specified
608.89 Genital tract male
510.0 Hepatopleural
510.0 Hepatopulmonary
569.81 Ileorectal
569.81 Ileosigmoidal
569.69 Ileostomy
596.1 Ileovesical
569.81 Ileum
386.40 Inner ear
569.81 Intestine
569.81 Intestinocolonic (abdominal)
593.82 Intestinoureteral
619.1 Intestinouterine
619.1 Intestinovaginal
752.49 Intestinovaginal congenital
596.1 Intestinovesical
566 Ischiorectal
569.69 Jejunostomy
569.81 Jejunum

FISTULA (continued)

719.8# Joint
5th digit: 719.8
0. Site NOS
1. Shoulder region
2. Upper arm (elbow) (humerus)
3. Forearm (radius) (wrist) (ulna)
4. Hand (carpal) (metacarpal) (fingers)
5. Pelvic region (hip) (buttock) (femur) and thigh
6. Lower leg (fibula) (knee) (patella) (tibia)
7. Ankle and/or foot (metatarsals) (toes) (tarsals)
8. Other
9. Multiple
593.89 Kidney
619.8 Labium (majus) (minus)
386.40 Labyrinthine
386.42 Labyrinthine - oval window
386.41 Labyrinthine - round window
386.43 Labyrinthine - semicircular canal
386.48 Labyrinthine - combined sites
375.61 Lacrimal
748.3 Laryngotracheal
478.79 Larynx
528.5 Lip
750.25 Lip congenital
510.0 Lung
457.8 Lymphatic (node) (vessel)
611.0 Mamillary
611.0 Mammary gland
675.1# Mammary gland maternal due to pregnancy
5th digit: 675.1
0. Episode of care NOS or N/A
1. Delivered
2. Delivered with postpartum complication
3. Antepartum complication
4. Postpartum complication
383.1 Mastoid
473.0 Maxillary (see also 'Sinusitis', maxillary)
510.0 Mediastinal
510.0 Mediastinobronchial
510.0 Mediastinocutaneous
385.89 Middle ear
528.3 Mouth
478.19 Nasal (cavity) (septum)
0 Nasal sinus see 'Fistula', by specified sinus
478.29 Nasopharynx
478.19 Nose
360.32 Ocular causing hypotony (postinflammatory) (post op) (post traumatic)
528.3 Oral (cutaneous)
749.00 Oral nasal with cleft palate (see also 'Cleft', palate)
376.10 Orbit
473.0 Oroantral
473.0 Oromaxillary
386.42 Oval window
619.2 Oviduct (external)
526.89 Palate hard
528.9 Palate soft
577.8 Pancreatic
577.8 Pancreaticoduodenal
527.4 Parotid gland
528.3 Parotid region

FISTULA (continued)

569.81 Pelvoabdominointestinal
607.89 Penis
565.1 Perianal
423.8 Pericardium
569.81 Pericecal
569.81 Perineorectal
608.89 Perineo-urethroscrotal
599.1 Perineum perineal (with urethral involvement)
565.1 Perirectal
567.22 Peritoneum (see also 'Peritonitis')
599.1 Periurethral
478.29 Pharyngo-esophageal
478.29 Pharynx
744.41 Pharynx branchial cleft (congenital)
685.1 Pilonidal (infected) (rectum)
685.0 Pilonidal with abscess
510.0 Pleura pleurocutaneous
510.0 Pleurocutaneous
423.8 Pleuropericardial
510.0 Pleuroperitoneal
383.81 Postauricular
998.6 Postoperative (persistent)
744.46 Preauricular congenital
602.8 Prostate
510.0 Pulmonary
417.0 Pulmonary vessel arteriovenous
747.3 Pulmonary vessel arteriovenous congenital
510.0 Pulmonoperitoneal
565.1 Rectal (to skin)
619.1 Rectolabial
569.81 Rectosigmoid (intercommunicating)
593.82 Rectoureteral
599.1 Rectourethral
753.8 Rectourethral congenital
619.1 Rectouterine
752.3 Rectouterine congenital
619.1 Rectovaginal
752.49 Rectovaginal congenital
596.1 Rectovesical
753.8 Rectovesical congenital
619.1 Rectovesicovaginal
619.1 Rectovulval
752.49 Rectovulval congenital
593.89 Renal
747.62 Renal vessel arteriovenous congenital
743.58 Retinal vessel arteriovenous congenital
383.81 Retroauricular
386.41 Round window
527.4 Salivary gland
750.24 Salivary gland congenital
360.32 Sclera, causing hypotony (postinflammatory) (post op) (posttraumatic)
608.89 Scrotum
386.43 Semicircular canal
569.81 Sigmoid
596.1 Sigmoid vesicoabdominal
619.1 Sigmoidovaginal
752.49 Sigmoidovaginal congenital
747.29 Sinus of valsalva congenital
686.9 Skin (infected)
593.82 Skin - ureter
619.2 Skin - vagina
473.3 Sphenoidal sinus (see also 'Sinusitis', sphenoidal)
289.59 Splenocolic
747.82 Spinal vessel arteriovenous congenital

FISTULA (continued)

569.81 Stercoral
537.4 Stomach or duodenum
527.4 Sublingual gland
750.24 Sublingual gland congenital
527.4 Submaxillary gland
750.24 Submaxillary gland congenital
528.3 Submaxillary region
0 Surgically created arteriovenous dialysis catheter complication see 'Dialysis'
V45.1 Surgically created for dialysis (status)
457.8 Thoracic duct
510.0 Thoracic region
510.0 Thoracicoabdominal
510.0 Thoracicogastric
510.0 Thoracicointestinal
510.0 Thoracoabdominal
510.0 Thoracogastric
510.0 Thorax
759.2 Thyroglossal duct congenital
246.8 Thyroid
748.3 Trachea (congenital)
530.84 Tracheoesophageal
750.3 Tracheoesophageal congenital
519.09 Tracheoesophageal following tracheostomy
0 Traumatic arteriovenous see specified artery/vein injury
0 Traumatic brain arteriovenous see brain/cerebral injury by type
0 Tuberculous see 'Tuberculous'
002.0 Typhoid
759.89 Umbilical
753.8 Umbilico-urinary
753.7 Urachus congenital
593.82 Ureteral (to skin)
593.82 Ureteroabdominal
593.82 Ureterocervical
593.82 Ureterorectal
593.82 Ureterosigmoidoabdominal
619.0 Ureterovaginal
596.2 Ureterovesical
599.1 Urethral
753.8 Urethral congenital
599.1 Urethroperineal
596.2 Urethroperineovesical
599.1 Urethrorectal
753.8 Urethrorectal congenital
608.89 Urethroscrotal
619.0 Urethrovaginal
596.2 Urethrovesical
619.0 Urethrovesicovaginal
599.1 Urinary NOS (persistent) (recurrent)
619.0 Urinary genital tract female
619.2 Uteroabdominal (anterior wall)
752.3 Uteroabdominal (anterior wall) congenital
619.1 Uteroenteric
619.1 Uterointestinal
752.3 Uterointestinal congenital
619.1 Uterorectal
752.3 Uterorectal congenital
619.0 Uteroureteric
619.8 Uterovaginal
619.0 Uterovesical
752.3 Uterovesical congenital
619.2 Uterus to abdominal wall (skin)
619.8 Uterus other specified

F

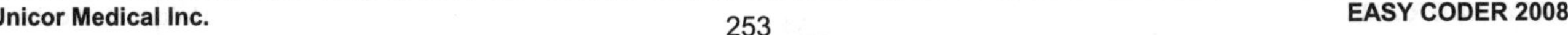

FISTULA (continued)

619.2 Vagina (to skin)
619.8 Vagina other specified
619.1 Vaginoileal
619.2 Vaginoperineal
596.2 Vesical female genital tract (between)
596.2 Vesical NEC (female)
596.2 Vesicoabdominal
619.0 Vesicocervicovaginal
596.1 Vesicocolic
596.2 Vesicocutaneous
596.1 Vesicoenteric
596.1 Vesicointestinal
619.1 Vesicometrorectal
596.2 Vesicoperineal
596.1 Vesicorectal
753.8 Vesicorectal congenital
596.1 Vesicosigmoidal
619.1 Vesicosigmoidovaginal
596.2 Vesicoureteral
619.0 Vesicoureterovaginal
596.2 Vesicourethral
596.1 Vesicourethrorectal
619.0 Vesicouterine
752.3 Vesicouterine congenital
619.0 Vesicovaginal
619.1 Vulvorectal
752.49 Vulvorectal congenital

780.39 FIT NOS
V68.09 FITNESS CERTIFICATE ISSUE
0 FITTING AND ADJUSTMENT SEE DEVICE OR SITE
V52.8 FITTING OTHER SPECIFIED PROSTHETIC DEVICE
099.56 FITZ-HUGH AND CURTIS SYNDROME DUE TO CHLAMYDIA TRACHOMATIS
098.86 FITZ-HUGH AND CURTIS SYNDROME DUE TO NEISSERIA GONORRHOEAE (GONOCOCCAL PERITONITIS)
577.0 FITZ'S SYNDROME (ACUTE HEMORRHAGIC PANCREATITIS)
736.79 FLACCID FOOT
736.09 FLACCID FOREARM
728.85 FLACCID MUSCLE PARALYTIC CONTRACTURE
750.26 FLACCID PALATE CONGENITAL
807.4 FLAIL CHEST
767.3 FLAIL CHEST NEWBORN (BIRTH TRAUMA)
718.8# FLAIL JOINT

5th digit: 718.8
- **0. Site NOS**
- **1. Shoulder region**
- **2. Upper arm (elbow) (humerus)**
- **3. Forearm (radius) (wrist) (ulna)**
- **4. Hand (carpal) (metacarpal) (fingers)**
- **5. Pelvic region and thigh (hip) (buttock) (femur)**
- **6. Lower leg (fibula) (knee) (patella) (tibia)**
- **7. Ankle and/or foot (metatarsals) (toes) (tarsals)**
- **8. Other**
- **9. Multiple**

242.0# FLAJANI (-BASEDOW) SYNDROME (EXOPHTHALMIC GOITER)

5th digit: 242.0
- **0. Without mention of thyrotoxic crisis or storm**
- **1. With mention of thyrotoxic crisis or storm**

FLANK

959.19 Injury
911.8 Injury other and unspecified superficial
911.9 Injury other and unspecified superficial infected
789.39 Mass
789.09 Pain
789.69 Tenderness

292.89 FLASHBACK DRUG INDUCED
734 FLAT FOOT ACQUIRED
754.61 FLAT FOOT CONGENITAL
754.61 FLAT FOOT RIGID (EVERTED) (SPASTIC)
341.1 FLATAU SCHILDER DISEASE
787.3 FLATULENCE
787.3 FLATUS
629.89 FLATUS VAGINALIS
504 FLAX DRESSERS' DISEASE
0 FLEA BITE SEE 'INSECT BITE NONVENOMOUS'
732.3 FLEISCHNER'S DISEASE
631 FLESHY MOLE
631 FLESHY MOLE WITH COMPLICATION DURING TREATMENT [639.#]
639.# FLESHY MOLE WITH COMPLICATION FOLLOWING TREATMENT

4th digit: 639
- **0. Genital tract and pelvic infection**
- **1. Delayed or excessive hemorrhage**
- **2. Damage to pelvic organs and tissue**
- **3. Renal failure**
- **4. Metabolic disorders**
- **5. Shock**
- **6. Embolism**
- **8. Other specified complication**
- **9. Unspecified complication**

300.11 FLEXIBILITAS CEREA
754.89 FLEXION CONTRACTURES OF LOWER LIMB JOINTS CONGENITAL
736.9 FLEXION DEFORMITY JOINT
004.1 FLEXNERI DYSENTERY - GROUP B SHIGELLA
004.1 FLEXNER'S BACILLUS DIARRHEA DYSENTERY

FLEXOR TENDON LACERATION

727.64 Tendon hand and wrist rupture nontraumatic
881.22 Carpi radialis
881.20 Carpi radialis proximal
881.22 Carpi ulnaris distal
881.20 Carpi ulnaris proximal
883.2 Digitorum profundus finger
882.2 Digitorum profundus hand
881.20 Digitorum profundus wrist
883.2 Digitorum superficialis finger
882.2 Digitorum superficialis hand
881.20 Digitorum superficialis wrist
891.2 Hallucis ankle
892.2 Hallucis foot
893.2 Hallucis toe
893.2 Toe
891.2 Toe ankle
892.2 Toe foot

502 FLINT DISEASE
424.1 FLINT MURMUR
379.24 FLOATERS VITREOUS
272.2 FLOATING-BETALIPOPROTEINEMIA
756.3 FLOATING RIB
781.99 FLOPPY INFANT SYNDROME
364.81 FLOPPY IRIS SYNDROME
424.0 FLOPPY VALVE SYNDROME (MITRAL)
571.2 FLORID CIRRHOSIS
571.2 FLORID CIRRHOSIS WITH ESOPHAGEAL VARICES [**456.2#**]
5th digit: 456.2
0. With bleeding
1. Without bleeding

FLU

487.# NOS
4th digit: 487
0. With pneumonia (any type)
1. Unspecified or with other respiratory manifestations
8. Other manifestations, (gastrointestinal)

487.1 Asian
008.8 Gastroenteritis viral NEC
487.8 Intestinal
760.2 Maternal affecting fetus or newborn
771.2 Maternal affecting fetus or newborn - manifested in newborn
487.1 Respiratory
487.0 Respiratory - with pneumonia
0 See also 'Influenza'
487.8 Stomach
V04.81 Vaccination
487.8 Other specified

FLUID

789.59 Abdomen
276.9 Disorder NEC
276.50 Loss (acute)
276.6 Overload
789.59 Overload causing ascites
782.3 Overload with localized edema
789.59 Peritoneal cavity
789.51 Peritoneal cavity malignant
276.6 Retention
782.3 Retention localized edema

FLUKE

120.9 Blood
121.9 Disease
121.3 Liver
121.0 Liver cat
121.1 Liver oriental
121.3 Liver sheep
121.2 Lung disease oriental

623.5 FLUOR
131.00 FLUOR (VAGINALIS) TRICHOMONAL
V07.31 FLUORIDE ADMINISTRATION PROPHYLACTIC
0 FLUOROQUINOLONES RESISTANT INFECTION SEE 'DRUG RESISTANCE'
V72.5 FLUOROSCOPY
520.3 FLUOROSIS
259.2 FLUSH SYNDROME
782.62 FLUSHING
627.2 FLUSHING MENOPAUSAL
627.4 FLUSHING MENOPAUSAL ARTIFICIAL

FLUTTER

427.32 Atrial
997.1 Atrial postoperative [427.32]
427.42 Ventricular
997.1 Ventricular postoperative [427.42]

009.0 FLUX
134.0 FLY LARVAE INFESTATION
694.4 FOGA SELVAGEN
336.1 FOIX-ALAJOUANINE (SYNDROME)
281.2 FOLATE-MALABSORPTION CONGENITAL
266.2 FOLIC ACID DEFICIENCY
281.2 FOLIC ACID DEFICIENCY ANEMIA
297.3 FOLIE A DEUX
253.4 FOLLICLE-STIMULATING HORMONE DEFICIENCY
253.1 FOLLICLE-STIMULATING HORMONE OVERPRODUCTION
620.0 FOLLICULAR CYST ATRESIA
620.0 FOLLICULAR CYST OVARIAN

FOLLICULITIS

704.8 Unspecified
704.8 Abscedens et suffodiens
704.09 Decalvans
706.1 Keloid (keloidalis)
704.8 Pustular
701.8 Ulerythematosa reticulata
704.8 Other specified diseases of hair

270.1 FOLLING'S PHENYLKETONURIA

Do not confuse follow up or routine aftercare with complications. Follow up exams and routine aftercare are planned visits that are part of the normal course of treatment. Complications are unexpected developments that require subsequent treatment.

FOLLOW-UP EXAM

V67.9 Unspecified
V67.2 Chemotherapy
V67.6 Combined treatment
V58.83 Drug monitoring therapeutic encounter
V58.83 Drug monitoring therapeutic encounter with long term drug use [**V58.6#**]
5th digit: V58.6
1. Anticoagulants
2. Antibiotics
3. Antiplatelets/antithrombotics
4. Anti-inflammatories non-steroidal (NSAID)
5. Steroids
6. Aspirin
7. Insulin
9. Other

V67.4 Fracture treatment - healed
0 Fracture treatment - healing or current see 'Aftercare', orthopedic

F

FOLLOW-UP EXAM (continued)

Coumadin, Digoxin, chemotherapy drugs, and any other drug with a risk of adverse reaction are considered high-risk medication. Code V67.51 is used to identify patients that have completed high risk medication therapy.

V58.6# High risk medication - current therapy (long term)
5th digit: V58.6
1. Anticoagulants
2. Antibiotics
3. Antiplatelets/antithrombotics
4. Anti-inflammatories non-steroidal (NSAID)
5. Steroids
6. Aspirin
7. Insulin
9. Other

V58.83 High risk medication drug monitoring encounter
V58.83 High risk medication drug monitoring encounter with long term drug use [V58.6#]
5th digit: V58.6
1. Anticoagulants
2. Antibiotics
3. Antiplatelets/antithrombotics
4. Anti-inflammatories non-steroidal (NSAID)
5. Steroids
6. Aspirin
7. Insulin
9. Other

V67.51 High risk medication therapy - completed
V76.47 Pap smear vaginal following hysterectomy [V45.77]
V76.47 Pap smear vaginal following hysterectomy for nonmalignant condition [V45.77]
V67.01 Pap smear vaginal following hysterectomy for cancer [V10.4#] [V45.77]
5th digit: V10.4
0. Genital organ unspecified
1. Cervix uteri
2. Other part of uterus
3. Ovary
4. Genital organ other

V67.3 Psychotherapy and other treatment
V67.1 Radiotherapy
V67.00 Surgery unspecified
V67.09 Surgery other
V67.59 Other treatment NEC

756.89 FONG'S SYNDROME (HEREDITARY OSTEO-ONYCHODYSPLASIA)

117.2 FONSECAEA COMPACTUM INFECTION

117.2 FONSECAEA PEDROSOI INFECTION

FOOD

693.1 Allergy dermatitis
V65.3 Allergy dietary counseling and surveillance
0 Allergy history see 'Allergy, Allergic History'
0 Anaphylactic shock see 'Anaphylaxis'
933.1 Asphyxiation (choking) (aspiration)
994.2 Deprivation
0 Intoxication see 'Food Poisoning'
995.7 Reaction adverse NEC
307.59 Refusal

FOOD POISONING

005.9 Unspecified
005.89 Bacillus cereus
005.1 Botulism
005.2 C welchii
005.2 Clostridia perfringens
005.3 Clostridium
005.1 Clostridium botulinum
989.7 Food contaminants
988.9 Noxious substance
005.89 Other bacterial
988.8 Other noxious
005.89 Other specified bacterium NEC
003.0 Salmonella - gastroenteritis
0 Salmonella - with other manifestations see 'Salmonella'
005.0 Staphylococcal toxemia
988.2 Toxic (berries) (plants)
988.0 Toxic fish shellfish
988.1 Toxic mushrooms
005.4 Vibrio
005.4 Vibrio parahaemolyticus
005.81 Vibrio vulnificus

FOOT

V49.73 Absence
755.31 Absence congenital
V49.73 Amputation status
078.4 And mouth disease
726.79 Bursa infection
736.74 Claw
755.67 Constriction band congenital

DEFORMITY

736.70 NOS (acquired)
754.70 NOS congenital
736.76 Calcaneus other
736.75 Cavovarus (acquired)
754.59 Cavovarus congenital
736.73 Cavus
736.72 Equinus
736.71 Equinovarus
736.79 Valgus (acquired)
754.60 Valgus congenital
754.69 Valgus congenital other NEC
736.79 Varus (acquired)
754.50 Varus congenital
754.59 Varus congenital other NEC
736.79 Other acquired NEC
754.79 Other congenital NEC

FOOT (continued)

736.79 Drop
959.7 Injury
917.8 Injury other and unspecified superficial
917.9 Injury other and unspecified superficial infected
719.87 Joint calcification
718.97 Joint ligament relaxation
0 Joint ligament tear see 'Sprain'
0 Joint see also 'Joint'
718.17 Loose body (joint)
581.3 Process disease
0 See 'Talipes'
845.10 Separation (rupture) (tear) (laceration) unspecified site
845.10 Strain (sprain) (avulsion) (hemarthrosis) unspecified site

F

348.4 FORAMEN MAGNUM SYNDROME
742.3 FORAMEN OF LUSCHKA ATRESIA
742.3 FORAMEN OF MAGENDIE ATRESIA
742.3 FORAMEN OF MUNRO OBSTRUCTION
741.0# FORAMEN OF MUNRO OBSTRUCTION WITH SPINA BIFIDA
5th digit: 741.0
0. Region NOS
1. Cervical region
2. Dorsal (thoracic) region
3. Lumbar region

745.5 FORAMEN OVALE PATENT CONGENITAL
253.1 FORBES-ALBRIGHT SYNDROME (NONPUERPERAL AMENORRHEA AND LACTATION ASSOCIATED WITH PITUITARY TUMOR)
271.0 FORBES' GLYCOGENOSIS III
763.89 FORCED BIRTH
763.2 FORCEPS DELIVERY AFFECTING FETUS OR NEWBORN
0 FORCEPS DELIVERY SEE 'DELIVERY', FORCEPS OR VACUUM
660.7# FORCEPS OR VACUUM EXTRACTOR FAILURE
5th digit: 660.7
0. Episode of care unspecified or N/A
1. Delivered
3. Antepartum complication

750.26 FORDYCE'S ECTOPIC SEBACEOUS GLANDS
705.82 FORDYCE-FOX APOCRINE MILIARIA

FOREARM

V49.65 Absence (acquired)
755.21 Absence congenital - including hand and fingers
755.25 Absence congenital - including incomplete absence distal elements
V49.65 Amputation status
736.00 Deformity acquired
736.09 Deformity acquired other
755.50 Deformity congenital
959.3 Injury
913.8 Injury other and unspecified superficial
913.9 Injury other and unspecified superficial infected
841.8 Separation (rupture) (tear) (laceration) other specified sites
841.8 Strain (sprain) (avulsion) (hemarthrosis)

738.19 FOREHEAD DEFORMITY
756.0 FOREHEAD DEFORMITY CONGENITAL
959.09 FOREHEAD INJURY

Foreign bodies can be superficial, such as a splinter. They can penetrate through an open wound, enter through an orifice, or be old or residual. Old or residual foreign bodies are found under 'Foreign Body', old. Granulomas from a retained foreign body are found under 'Foreign Body' granuloma and 'Granuloma'.

FOREIGN BODY

919.6 Site NOS superficial
919.7 Site NOS superficial infected
879.3 Abdominal wall (anterior) through open wound
879.5 Abdominal wall lateral through open wound
911.6 Abdominal wall superficial
911.7 Abdominal wall superficial infected
998.4 Accidentally left during a procedure
870.4 Adnexa (penetrating)

FOREIGN BODY (continued)

938 Alimentary tract NOS through orifice (swallowed)
916.6 Ankle superficial
916.7 Ankle superficial infected
891.1 Ankle through open wound
911.6 Anus superficial
911.7 Anus superficial infected
879.7 Anus through open wound
937 Anus through orifice
936 Appendix through orifice
912.6 Arm (upper) superficial
912.7 Arm (upper) superficial infected
880.13 Arm (upper) through open wound
884.1 Arm multiple through open wound
872.12 Auditory canal through open wound
931 Auditory canal through orifice
912.6 Axilla superficial
912.7 Axilla superficial infected
880.12 Axilla (area) through open wound
911.6 Back superficial
911.7 Back superficial infected
876.1 Back through open wound
939.0 Bladder through orifice
733.99 Bone - old
911.6 Breast superficial
911.7 Breast superficial infected
879.1 Breast through open wound
934.8 Bronchiole through orifice
934.1 Bronchus through orifice
873.71 Buccal mucosa through open wound
911.6 Buttock superficial
911.7 Buttock superficial infected
877.1 Buttock through open wound
916.6 Calf superficial
916.7 Calf superficial infected
891.1 Calf through open wound
930.1 Canthus (external) through orifice
936 Cecum through orifice
939.1 Cervix (canal) uterine through orifice
910.6 Cheek superficial
910.7 Cheek superficial infected
873.51 Cheek through open wound
935.0 Cheek through orifice
911.6 Chest wall superficial
911.7 Chest wall superficial infected
875.1 Chest wall through open wound
873.54 Chin through open wound
872.74 Cochlea through open wound
936 Colon through orifice
930.1 Conjunctiva (external) through orifice
930.0 Cornea (external) through orifice
875.1 Costal region through open wound
938 Digestive system NOS through orifice
936 Duodenum through orifice

EAR

872.9 NOS through open wound
931 NOS through orifice
872.12 Auditory canal through open wound
931 Auditory canal through orifice (external)
872.11 Auricle through open wound
931 Auricle through orifice (external)
872.71 Drum through open wound
872.10 External NOS through open wound
385.83 Middle (mastoid) retained
872.79 Multiple sites through open wound

F

FOREIGN BODY (continued)

EAR (continued)

872.11	Pinna through open wound
910.6	Superficial
910.7	Superficial infected
931	Through orifice NOS (external)
872.79	Other specified through open wound

FOREIGN BODY (continued)

881.11	Elbow
913.6	Elbow superficial
913.7	Elbow superficial infected
874.5	Esophagus cervical through open wound
935.1	Esophagus through orifice
872.73	Eustachian tube

EYE

930.1	Canthus (external) through orifice
930.1	Conjunctiva (external) through orifice
930.0	Cornea (external) through orifice
930.9	External through orifice
930.8	External through orifice other and combined sites
930.2	Lacrimal punctum (external)

EYE MAGNETIC

871.5	Acute eyeball current penetrating
360.51	Anterior chamber (old)
360.50	Globe (old)
360.50	Intraocular (old)
360.52	Iris or ciliary body (old)
360.53	Lens (old)
360.55	Posterior wall (old)
360.55	Retina (old)
360.54	Vitreous (old)
360.59	Other or multiple sites (old)

EYE NONMAGNETIC

871.6	Acute eyeball current penetrating
360.61	Anterior chamber (old)
360.60	Globe (old)
360.60	Intraocular (old)
360.62	Iris or ciliary body (old)
360.63	Lens (old)
360.65	Posterior wall (old)
360.65	Retina (old)
376.6	Retrobulbar (old)
360.64	Vitreous (old)
360.69	Other or multiple sites (old)

FOREIGN BODY (continued)

873.52	Eyebrow through open wound
930.1	Eyelid (external) through orifice
918.0	Eyelid and periocular area superficial
374.86	Eyelid retained
910.6	Face superficial
910.7	Face superficial infected
873.50	Face through open wound
873.59	Face other and multiple sites through open wound
784.99	Feeling of, in throat
883.1	Finger
915.6	Finger superficial
915.7	Finger superficial infected
879.5	Flank
911.6	Flank superficial
911.7	Flank superficial infected

F

FOREIGN BODY (continued)

892.1	Foot
917.6	Foot superficial
917.7	Foot superficial infected
881.10	Forearm
913.6	Forearm superficial
913.7	Forearm superficial infected
873.52	Forehead
878.9	Genitalia through open wound
939.9	Genitourinary tract NOS through orifice
938	GI tract through orifice
728.82	Granuloma - muscle
709.4	Granuloma - skin
728.82	Granuloma - soft tissue NEC
709.4	Granuloma - subcutaneous tissue
911.6	Groin superficial
911.7	Groin superficial infected
939.9	Gu tract site through orifice
910.6	Gum superficial
910.7	Gum superficial infected
873.72	Gum through open wound
935.0	Gum through orifice
914.6	Hand superficial
914.7	Hand superficial infected
882.1	Hand through open wound
873.9	Head through open wound
892.1	Heel
917.6	Heel superficial
917.7	Heel superficial infected
890.1	Hip
916.6	Hip superficial
916.7	Hip superficial infected
936	Ileum through orifice
938	Ingested
V71.89	Ingestion suspected (undiagnosed) (unproven)
0	Interphalangeal see 'Foreign Body', finger
911.6	Interscapular region superficial
911.7	Interscapular region superficial infected
936	Intestine through orifice
871.5	Intraocular penetration magnetic
871.6	Intraocular penetration nonmagnetic
934.8	Intrapulmonary through orifice
873.54	Jaw through open wound
916.6	Knee superficial
916.7	Knee superficial infected
891.1	Knee through open wound
911.6	Labia superficial
911.7	Labia superficial infected
878.5	Labia through open wound
930.2	Lacrimal punctum (external) through orifice
874.11	Larynx through open wound
933.1	Larynx through orifice
874.10	Larynx with trachea through open wound
908.5	Late effect in orifice
906.2	Late effect superficial
916.6	Leg superficial
916.7	Leg superficial infected
891.1	Leg through open wound
910.6	Lip superficial
910.7	Lip superficial infected
873.53	Lip through open wound
894.1	Lower limb multiple
934.8	Lung through orifice
0	Metacarpal see 'Foreign Body', hand

FOREIGN BODY (continued)

873.79	Mouth other and multiple sites through open wound
873.70	Mouth through open wound
935.0	Mouth through orifice
919.6	Multiple superficial
919.7	Multiple superficial infected
879.9	Multiple through open wound
729.6	Muscle - old
728.82	Muscle - old with granuloma
933.0	Nasopharynx through orifice
910.6	Neck superficial
910.7	Neck superficial infected
874.9	Neck through open wound
873.32	Nose (cavity) through open wound
873.39	Nose (multiple sites) through open wound
873.31	Nose (septum) through open wound complicated
873.33	Nose (sinus) through open wound
910.6	Nose superficial
910.7	Nose superficial infected
873.30	Nose through open wound
932	Nose through orifice
932	Nostril through orifice
870.4	Ocular adnexa (penetrating)
376.6	Ocular muscle old (residual)
733.99	Old bone - granuloma
733.99	Old bone - residual
0	Old eye see 'Foreign Body', eye
374.86	Old eyelid - residual
385.82	Old middle ear - granuloma
385.83	Old middle ear - residual
729.6	Old muscle
728.82	Old muscle - granuloma
376.6	Old ocular muscle
376.6	Old retrobulbar
729.6	Old skin
709.4	Old skin granuloma
729.6	Old soft tissue
728.82	Old soft tissue - granuloma muscle
709.4	Old soft tissue - granuloma skin subcutaneous tissue
729.6	Old subcutaneous
709.4	Old subcutaneous - granuloma
870.4	Orbit (penetrating)
376.6	Orbit retained/old (penetrating)
872.72	Ossicles (ear)
873.75	Palate through open wound
935.0	Palate through orifice
879.7	Pelvic area through open wound
911.6	Penis superficial
911.7	Penis superficial infected
878.1	Penis through open wound
939.3	Penis through orifice
911.6	Perineum superficial
911.7	Perineum superficial infected
933.0	Pharynx through orifice
874.5	Pharynx through open wound
872.11	Pinna through open wound
937	Rectosigmoid through orifice
937	Rectum through orifice
376.6	Ocular muscle old (residual)
733.99	Residual bone
374.86	Residual eyelid
385.83	Residual middle ear
729.6	Residual muscle
728.82	Residual muscle - granuloma
376.6	Residual retrobulbar

FOREIGN BODY (continued)

729.6	Residual skin
709.4	Residual skin - granuloma
729.6	Residual soft tissue
728.82	Residual soft tissue - granuloma muscle
709.4	Residual soft tissue - granuloma skin subcutaneous tissue
729.6	Residual subcutaneous
709.4	Residual subcutaneous - granuloma
934.8	Respiratory specified part NEC through orifice
934.9	Respiratory through orifice
376.6	Retrobulbar (penetrating) (old)
873.1	Scalp
910.6	Scalp superficial
910.7	Scalp superficial infected
880.11	Scapular area
912.6	Scapular region superficial
912.7	Scapular region superficial infected
911.6	Scrotum superficial
911.7	Scrotum superficial infected
878.3	Scrotum through open wound
880.10	Shoulder
880.19	Shoulder and arm multiple sites
912.6	Shoulder superficial
912.7	Shoulder superficial infected
932	Sinus (front) (max) (ethmoid) (nasal) through orifice
933.0	Sinus - pyriform through orifice
729.6	Skin - old
709.4	Skin - old with granuloma
729.6	Soft tissue - old (residual)
728.82	Soft tissue - old with granuloma muscle
709.4	Soft tissue - old with granuloma skin subcutaneous tissue
935.2	Stomach through orifice
729.6	Subcutaneous - old
709.4	Subcutaneous - old with granuloma
938	Swallowed
930.2	Tear ducts or glands
727.89	Tendon sheath (old) (residual)
911.6	Testis superficial
911.7	Testis superficial infected
890.1	Thigh
916.6	Thigh superficial
916.7	Thigh superficial infected
784.99	Throat, feeling of
910.6	Throat superficial
910.7	Throat superficial infected
933.0	Throat through orifice
883.1	Thumb
915.6	Thumb superficial
915.7	Thumb superficial infected
874.3	Thyroid gland through open wound
893.1	Toe
917.6	Toe superficial
917.7	Toe superficial infected
873.74	Tongue through open wound
935.0	Tongue through orifice
933.0	Tonsil through orifice
874.12	Trachea through open wound
934.0	Trachea through orifice
879.7	Trunk
911.6	Trunk superficial
911.7	Trunk superficial infected
872.71	Tympanic membrane

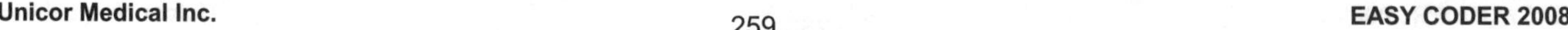

FOREIGN BODY (continued)

939.0 Ureter through orifice
939.0 Urethra through orifice
939.1 Uterus through orifice
911.6 Vagina superficial
911.7 Vagina superficial infected
878.7 Vagina through open wound
939.2 Vagina through orifice
911.6 Vulva superficial
911.7 Vulva superficial infected
878.5 Vulva through open wound
939.2 Vulva through orifice
881.12 Wrist
913.6 Wrist superficial
913.7 Wrist superficial infected
919.6 Other sites superficial
919.7 Other sites superficial infected

605 FORESKIN TIGHT
V20.2 FORMULA CHECK
100.89 FORT BRAGG FEVER
745.5 FOSSA OVALIS DEFECT CONGENITAL
V61.29 FOSTER CHILD PROBLEM (REASON FOR ENCOUNTER)
377.04 FOSTER KENNEDY SYNDROME
350.1 FOTHERGILL'S NEURALGIA
034.1 FOTHERGILL'S SCARLATINA ANGINOSA
V20.0 FOUNDLING SUPERVISION
079.81 FOUR CORNERS VIRUS
608.83 FOURNIER'S DISEASE
378.53 FOURTH CRANIAL NERVE DISORDER (ATROPHY) (PALSY)
951.1 FOURTH CRANIAL NERVE INJURY
664.3# FOURTH DEGREE LACERATION (PERINEAL)

5th digit: 664.3
0. Episode of care unspecified or N/A
1. Delivered
4. Postpartum complication

057.8 FOURTH DISEASE
743.55 FOVEA CENTRALIS ABSENCE
344.89 FOVILLE'S SYNDROME (PEDUNCULAR)
705.82 FOX FORDYCE APOCRINE MILIARIA
684 FOX'S IMPETIGO (CONTAGIOSA)

Compound fracture is a fracture (bone) open.

When you have a fracture/dislocation of a bone site, code only the fracture. Dislocation of the fracture site is included in the fracture code.

FRACTURE

829.0 Bone(s) NOS closed
829.1 Bone(s) NOS open
808.0 Acetabulum closed
808.1 Acetabulum open
811.01 Acromion closed
811.11 Acromion open

FRACTURE (continued)

AFTERCARE

V54.89 Change, checking or removal of an external device: (cast) (external fixation) (kirschner wire) (splint external) (traction device)
V54.01 Change, checking or removal of an internal device
V54.2# Pathological healing
V54.1# Traumatic healing

5th digit: V54.1-2
0. Arm
1. Arm upper
2. Arm lower
3. Hip
4. Leg
5. Leg upper
6. Leg lower
7. Vertebrae
9. Other (pelvis) (wrist) (ankle) (hand/foot) (fingers/toes)

FRACTURE (continued)

802.8 Alveolus closed
802.9 Alveolus open

ANKLE

824.8 NOS closed
824.9 NOS open
824.4 Bimalleolar closed
824.5 Bimalleolar open
825.21 Bone closed
825.31 Bone open
824.2 Lateral malleolus closed
824.3 Lateral malleolus open
824.0 Medial malleolus closed
824.1 Medial malleolus open
824.4 Pott's closed
824.5 Pott's open
824.6 Trimalleolar closed
824.7 Trimalleolar open

FRACTURE (continued)

0 Antrum see 'Fracture' skull basilar
818.0 Arm and forearm multiple sites closed
818.1 Arm and forearm multiple sites open
819.0 Arms both (any bones) closed
819.1 Arms both (any bones) open
812.20 Arm(s) upper NOS closed
812.30 Arm(s) upper NOS open
828.0 Arm(s) with leg(s) multiple closed
828.1 Arm(s) with leg(s) multiple open
819.0 Arm(s) with rib(s) and/or sternum closed
819.1 Arm(s) with rib(s) and/or sternum open
825.21 Astragalus closed
825.31 Astragalus open
0 Barton's see 'Fracture', radius distal
815.01 Bennett's closed
815.11 Bennett's open
824.4 Bimalleolar closed
824.5 Bimalleolar open
767.3 Bone (long bone) birth trauma
0 Bust see 'Fracture,' by site
0 Burst see 'Fracture,' by site
825.0 Calcaneus closed
825.1 Calcaneus open
814.07 Capitate closed
814.17 Capitate open

FRACTURE (continued)

812.49 Capitellum (humerus) closed
812.59 Capitellum (humerus) open
814.## Carpal
4th digit: 814
0. Closed
1. Open

5th digit: 814
0. Unspecified
1. Navicular (scaphoid)
2. Lunate (semilunar)
3. Triquetral (cuneiform)
4. Pisiform
5. Trapezium (larger multangular)
6. Trapezoid (smaller multangular)
7. Capitate (OS magnum)
8. Hammate (unciform)
9. Other

806.## Cervical with spinal cord injury
4th digit: 806
0. Closed
1. Open

5th digit: 806
0. C1-C4 with cord injury unspecified
1. C1-C4 with complete cord lesion
2. C1-C4 with anterior cord syndrome
3. C1-C4 with central cord lesion
4. C1-C4 with incomplete cord lesion unspecified or posterior cord syndrome
5. C5-C7 with cord injury unspecified
6. C5-C7 complete lesion of cord
7. C5-C7 with anterior cord syndrome
8. C5-C7 with central cord syndrome
9. C5-C7 with incomplete cord lesion unspecified or posterior cord syndrome

805.## Cervical without spinal cord injury
4th digit: 805
0. Closed
1. Open

5th digit: 805
0. Level unspecified
1. C1
2. C2
3. C3
4. C4
5. C5
6. C6
7. C7
8. Multiple

813.43 Chauffeur's closed
813.53 Chauffeur's open
810.## Clavicle
4th digit: 810
0. Closed
1. Open

5th digit: 810
0. Site unspecified
1. Sternal end
2. Shaft
3. Distal or acromial end

767.2 Clavicle birth trauma

FRACTURE (continued)

805.6 Coccyx closed
806.6# Coccyx closed with cord injury
5th digit: 806.6
0. Cord injury unspecified
1. Complete cauda equina injury
2. Other cauda equina injury
9. With other spinal cord injury

665.6# Coccyx obstetrical trauma
5th digit: 665.6
0. Episode of care unspecified or N/A
1. Delivered
4. Postpartum complication

805.7 Coccyx open
806.7# Coccyx open with cord injury
5th digit: 806.7
0. Cord injury unspecified
1. Complete cauda equina injury
2. Other cauda equina injury
9. With other spinal cord injury

0 Collar bone see 'Fracture', clavicle
813.41 Colles' closed
813.51 Colles' open

> ***Compound fracture is a fracture (bone) open.***

0 Compression see 'Fracture', by site or 'Fracture', pathological by site
756.9 Congenital
V66.4 Convalescence
811.02 Coracoid closed
811.12 Coracoid open
813.02 Coronoid (ulna) closed
813.12 Coronoid (ulna) open
959.13 Corpus cavernosum penis
0 Costochondral junction see 'Fracture' ribs
0 Costosternal junction see 'Fracture' ribs
807.5 Cricoid cartilage closed
807.6 Cricoid cartilage open
825.23 Cuboid closed
825.33 Cuboid open
825.24 Cuneiform foot closed
825.34 Cuneiform foot open
814.03 Cuneiform wrist closed
814.13 Cuneiform wrist open
525.73 Dental implant
525.64 Dental restoration material with loss of material
525.63 Dental restoration material without loss of material
0 Depressed see 'Fracture', by site closed or open
806.2# Dorsal or dorsolumbar with spinal cord injury closed
806.3# Dorsal or dorsolumbar with spinal cord injury open
5th digit: 806.2-3
0. T1-T6 with cord injury unspecified
1. T1-T6 with complete lesion of cord
2. T1-T6 with anterior cord syndrome
3. T1-T6 with central cord syndrome
4. T1-T6 with incomplete cord lesion unspecified or posterior cord syndrome
5. T7-T12 with cord injury unspecified
6. T7-T12 with complete lesion of cord
7. T7-T12 with anterior cord syndrome
8. T7-T12 with central cord syndrome
9. T7-T12 With spinal cord lesion unspecified or posterior cord syndrome

FRACTURE (continued)

805.2 Dorsal or dorsolumbar without spinal cord injury closed
805.3 Dorsal or dorsolumbar without spinal cord injury open

824.4 Dupuytren's ankle or fibula closed
824.5 Dupuytren's ankle or fibula open
813.42 Dupuytren's radius closed
813.52 Dupuytren's radius open

808.41 Duverney's closed
808.51 Duverney's open

812.40 Elbow closed
812.50 Elbow open

812.42 Epicondylar lateral (humerus) closed
812.52 Epicondylar lateral (humerus) open
812.43 Epicondylar medial (humerus) closed
812.53 Epicondylar medial (humerus) open

0 Ethmoid sinus see 'Fracture', skull basilar

804.## Facial bones multiple

4th digit: 804

0. Closed without intracranial injury
1. Closed with cerebral laceration and/or contusion
2. Closed with subarachnoid subdural extradural hemorrhage
3. Closed with other and unspecified intracranial hemorrhage
4. Closed with intracranial injury of other and unspecified nature
5. Open without mention of intracranial injury
6. Open with cerebral laceration and contusion
7. Open with subarachnoid subdural and extradural hemorrhage
8. Open with other and unspecified intracranial hemorrhage
9. Open with intracranial injury of other and unspecified

5th digit: 804

0. Level of consciousness unspecified
1. No LOC
2. LOC < 1 hr
3. LOC 1 - 24 hrs
4. LOC > 24 hrs with return to prior level
5. LOC > 24 hrs without return to prior level: or death before regaining consciousness, regardless of duration of LOC
6. LOC duration unspecified
9. With concussion unspecified

802.8 Facial bones other closed
802.9 Facial bones other open

FEMUR CLOSED

821.00 Unspecified
820.03 Cervicotrochanteric
821.21 Condyle
821.20 Distal
821.22 Distal epiphysis
821.29 Distal multiple
820.20 Extracapsular
820.09 Head
820.21 Intertrochanteric
820.00 Intracapsular
820.21 Intratrochanteric

FRACTURE (continued)

FEMUR CLOSED (continued)

820.02 Midcervical
820.8 Neck NOS
820.03 Neck base
820.09 Neck other area
820.20 Peritrochanteric
820.01 Proximal epiphysis
821.01 Shaft
820.09 Subcapital
820.22 Subtrochanteric
821.23 Supracondylar
820.02 Transcervical
820.01 Transepiphyseal
820.20 Trochanteric
821.21 T-shaped into knee joint

FEMUR OPEN

821.10 Unspecified
820.13 Cervicotrochanteric
821.31 Condyle
821.30 Distal
821.32 Distal epiphysis
821.39 Distal multiple
820.30 Extracapsular
820.19 Head
820.31 Intertrochanteric
820.10 Intracapsular
820.31 Intratrochanteric
820.12 Midcervical
820.9 Neck NOS
820.13 Neck base
820.19 Neck other area
820.30 Peritrochanteric
820.11 Proximal epiphysis
821.11 Shaft
820.19 Subcapital
820.32 Subtrochanteric
821.33 Supracondylar
820.12 Transcervical
820.11 Transepiphyseal
820.30 Trochanteric
821.31 T-shaped into knee joint

FRACTURE (continued)

823.## Fibula and/or tibia

4th digit: 823

0. Proximal (head) (plateau) closed
1. Proximal (head) (plateau) open
2. Shaft closed
3. Shaft open
4. Torus
8. Site unspecified closed
9. Site unspecified open

5th digit: 823

0. Tibia alone
1. Fibula alone
2. Tibia with fibula

824.8 Fibula distal end or epiphysis closed
824.9 Fibula distal end or epiphysis open
824.2 Fibula involving ankle closed
824.3 Fibula involving ankle open

823.4# Fibula torus

5th digit: 823.4

1. Fibula alone
2. With tibia

F

FRACTURE (continued)

816.## Finger or thumb
4th digit: 816
0. Closed
1. Open

5th digit: 816
0. Site unspecified
1. Middle or proximal
2. Distal
3. Multiple sites

817.0 Finger with metacarpal bones closed
817.1 Finger with metacarpal bones open
807.4 Flail chest
825.## Foot (except toes)
4th digit: 825
2. Closed
3. Open

5th digit: 825
0. Unspecified bone(s) of foot (except toes)
1. Astragalus
2. Navicular (scaphoid) foot
3. Cuboid
4. Cuneiform foot
5. Metatarsal bone(s)
9. Other

825.20 Foot instep closed
825.30 Foot instep open
827.0 Foot instep with toe(s) closed
827.1 Foot instep with toe(s) open
825.29 Foot sesamoid closed
825.39 Foot sesamoid open
813.80 Forearm NOS closed
813.90 Forearm NOS open
813.40 Forearm distal closed
813.50 Forearm distal open
813.## Forearm proximal (upper)
4th digit: 813
0. Closed
1. Open

5th digit: 813
0. Upper end of forearm unspecified
1. Olecranon process of ulna
2. Coronoid process of ulna
3. Monteggia's fracture
4. Other and unspecified fractures of proximal end of ulna (alone)
5. Head of radius
6. Neck of radius
7. Other and unspecified fractures of proximal end of radius (alone)
8. Radius with ulna upper end (any part)

813.20 Forearm shaft closed
813.30 Forearm shaft open
0 Fossa (anterior) (middle) (posterior) see 'Fracture', skull basilar

0 Frontal bone see 'Fracture', skull vault
0 Frontal sinus see 'Fracture', skull basilar

813.42 Galeazzi's closed
813.52 Galeazzi's open
811.03 Glenoid closed
811.13 Glenoid open
0 Gosselin's see 'Fracture', ankle
0 Greenstick see 'Fracture', by site

FRACTURE (continued)

812.21 Grenade-throwers' closed
812.31 Grenade-throwers' open
0 Gunshot (due to) see 'fracture', by site, open
814.08 Hamate closed
814.18 Hamate open
815.## Hand (except fingers)
4th digit: 815
0. Closed
1. Open

5th digit: 815
0. Site unspecified
1. Base of thumb
2. Base
3. Shaft
4. Neck
9. Multiple sites

817.0 Hand multiple bones with finger closed
817.1 Hand multiple bones with finger open
0 Healing see 'Fracture' aftercare
825.0 Heel bone closed
825.1 Heel bone open

HIP CLOSED

820.8 Unspecified
820.21 Intertrochanteric
820.22 Subtrochanteric
820.20 Trochanteric

HIP OPEN

820.9 Unspecified
820.31 Intertrochanteric
820.32 Subtrochanteric
820.30 Trochanteric

HUMERUS CLOSED

812.20 Site unspecified
812.02 Anatomical neck
812.44 Articular process or T-shaped
812.49 Capitellum
812.44 Condyle(s) or lower epiphysis
812.40 Distal
812.49 Distal multple
812.49 Distal other
812.42 External condyle
812.03 Greater tuberosity
812.09 Head or upper epiphysis
812.43 Internal epicondyle
812.42 Lateral condyle
812.09 Lesser tuberosity
812.43 Medial condyle
812.00 Proximal
812.21 Shaft
812.41 Supracondylar
812.01 Surgical neck
812.49 Trochlea

HUMERUS OPEN

812.30 Site unspecified
812.12 Anatomical neck
812.54 Articular process or T-shaped
812.59 Capitellum
812.54 Condyle(s) or lower epiphysis

F

FRACTURE (continued)

HUMERUS OPEN (continued)

812.50 Distal
812.59 Distal multiple
812.59 Distal other
812.52 External condyle
812.13 Greater tuberosity
812.19 Head or upper epiphysis
812.53 Internal epicondyle
812.52 Lateral condyle
812.19 Lesser tuberosity
812.53 Medial condyle
812.10 Proximal
812.31 Shaft
812.51 Supracondylar
812.11 Surgical neck
812.59 Trochlea

FRACTURE (continued)

807.5 Hyoid closed
807.6 Hyoid open
808.41 Ilium closed
808.51 Ilium open
0 Impacted see 'Fracture', by site closed or open
808.49 Innominate bone closed
808.59 Innominate bone open
825.20 Instep closed
825.30 Instep open
827.0 Instep with toe(s) closed
827.1 Instep with toe(s) open
0 Insufficiency see 'Fracture', pathologic, by site
808.42 Ischium closed
808.52 Ischium open
802.2# Jaw lower (bone) closed
802.3# Jaw lower (bone) open

5th digit: 802.2-3
0. Unspecified
1. Condylar process
2. Subcondylar
3. Coronoid process
4. Ramus unspecified
5. Angle of jaw
6. Symphysis of body
7. Alveolar border of body
8. Body other and unspecified
9. Multiple sites

802.4 Jaw upper (bone) closed
802.5 Jaw upper (bone) open
0 Knee cap see 'Fracture', patella
807.5 Larynx closed
807.6 Larynx open
905.4 Late effect lower extremities
905.5 Late effect multiple and unspecified bones
905.3 Late effect neck of femur
905.0 Late effect skull and face bones
905.1 Late effect spine and trunk no spinal cord lesion
905.2 Late effect upper extremities
812.42 Lateral condyle (humerus) closed
812.52 Lateral condyle (humerus) open
824.2 Lateral malleolus closed
824.3 Lateral malleolus open
0 Lefort's see 'Fracture', maxilla and 'Fracture' each other structure involved (ie., 'Fracture' facial bone(s), nasal cavity, orbit floor, and/or palate)

F

FRACTURE (continued)

827.0 Leg closed
827.1 Leg open
828.0 Leg closed bilateral
828.1 Leg open bilateral
823.8# Leg lower NOS closed
823.9# Leg lower NOS open

5th digit: 823.8-9
0. Tibia alone
1. Fibula alone
2. Tibia with fibula

828.0 Leg(s) with rib(s) or sternum closed
828.1 Leg(s) with rib(s) or sternum open
806.4 Lumbar spine with cord injury closed
806.5 Lumbar spine with cord injury open
805.4 Lumbar spine without cord injury closed
805.5 Lumbar spine without cord injury open
814.02 Lunate (wrist) closed
814.12 Lunate (wrist) open
802.4 Malar closed
802.5 Malar open
808.43 Malgaigne's closed
808.53 Malgaigne's open
824.8 Malleolus closed
824.9 Malleolus open
733.81 Malunion

733.81 Fracture malunion-means that healing has occurred but that the bone(s) or fracture fragments are in poor alignment.

802.## Mandible

4th digit: 802
2. Closed
3. Open

5th digit: 802
0. Unspecified
1. Condylar process
2. Subcondylar
3. Coronoid process
4. Ramus unspecified
5. Angle of jaw
6. Symphysis of body
7. Alveolar border of body
8. Body other and unspecified
9. Multiple sites

MARCH

733.95 NOS
733.94 Foot
733.93 Fibula
733.94 Metatarsals
733.93 Tibia
733.95 Other

FRACTURE (continued)

802.2# Maxilla inferior closed
802.3# Maxilla inferior open

5th digit: 802.2-3
0. Unspecified
1. Condylar process
2. Subcondylar
3. Coronoid process
4. Ramus unspecified
5. Angle of jaw
6. Symphysis of body
7. Alveolar border of body
8. Body other and unspecified
9. Multiple sites

802.4 Maxilla superior closed
802.5 Maxilla superior open
812.43 Medial condyle (humerus) closed
812.53 Medial condyle (humerus) open
824.0 Medial malleolus closed
824.1 Medial malleolus open
815.## Metacarpal

4th digit: 815
0. Closed
1. Open

5th digit: 815
0. Site unspecified
1. Base of thumb
2. Base
3. Shaft
4. Neck
9. Multiple sites

817.0 Metacarpal multiple with finger closed
817.1 Metacarpal multiple with finger open
825.25 Metatarsal(s) closed
825.35 Metatarsal(s) open
825.29 Metatarsal(s) with tarsal closed
825.39 Metatarsal(s) with tarsal open
813.03 Monteggia closed
813.13 Monteggia open
813.42 Moore's closed
813.52 Moore's open
814.05 Multangular bone larger closed
814.15 Multangular bone larger open
814.06 Multangular bone smaller closed
814.16 Multangular bone smaller open

FRACTURE (continued)

Multiple fractures should be sequenced by severity as listed below:

1. ***Skull and face with other bones***
2. ***Pelvis or vertebral column with other bones***
3. ***Multiple fracture both limb bones (lower), lower with upper, and lower limb with rib or sternum***
4. ***Multiple fractures both upper limbs, and upper limb with rib or sternum***
5. ***Fractures trunk (ill-defined)***

MULTIPLE BONES

829.0 NOS closed
829.1 NOS open
818.0 Arm NOS or multiple bones in same upper limb closed
818.1 Arm NOS or multiple bones in same upper limb open
819.0 Arm(s) with rib(s), sternum, or both upper limbs closed
819.1 Arm(s) with rib(s), sternum, or both upper limbs open
827.0 Leg NOS or multiple bones in same lower limb closed
827.1 Leg NOS or multiple bones in same lower limb open
828.0 Leg(s) with arm(s), rib(s), sternum or both lower limbs closed
828.1 Leg(s) with arm(s), rib(s), sternum or both lower limbs open
809.0 Trunk (ill defined) closed
809.1 Trunk (ill defined) open

FRACTURE (continued)

802.0 Nasal bones (septum) closed
802.1 Nasal bones (septum) open
0 Nasoethmoid bone see 'Fracture', skull basilar
825.22 Navicular foot closed
825.32 Navicular foot open
814.01 Navicular wrist closed
814.11 Navicular wrist open
0 Neural arch see 'Fracture', cervical, dorsal, lumbar, sacrum or coccyx

733.82, Fracture nonunion-means that no healing has occurred at the fracture site.

733.82 Nonunion
0 Occiput bone see 'Fracture', skull basilar
813.01 Olecranon closed
813.11 Olecranon open
802.8 Orbit closed
802.9 Orbit open
802.6 Orbit floor (blow out) closed
802.7 Orbit floor (blow out) open
0 Orbit roof see 'Fracture' skull basilar
825.0 Os calcis closed
825.1 Os calcis open

F

FRACTURE (continued)

802.8 Palate closed
802.9 Palate open
0 Parietal bone see 'Fracture' skull vault
822.0 Patella closed
822.1 Patella open

Pathological fracture (non traumatic),733.1#, are often found in bone weakened by disease such as osteoporosis, metastatic tumors, osteomyelitis, bone cysts, and Paget's disease. When the underlying condition is known, it should be reported also. Sequencing would depend on reason for encounter.

PATHOLOGICAL

733.1# Unspecified cause
733.1# Abscess bone **[730.2#]**
733.1# Abscess bone acute or subacute **[730.0#]**
733.1# Abscess bone chronic (old) **[730.1#]**
733.1# Abscess periosteum **[730.3#]**

5th digit: 733.1
- **0. Unspecified site**
- **1. Humerus**
- **2. Distal radius and ulna, wrist**
- **3. Vertebra**
- **4. Neck of femur, femur NOS, hip NOS**
- **5. Other specified part of femur**
- **6. Tibia or fibula, ankle**
- **9. Other specified site**

5th digit: 730.0-3
- **0. Site NOS**
- **1. Shoulder region**
- **2. Upper arm (elbow) (humerus)**
- **3. Forearm (radius) (wrist) (ulna)**
- **4. Hand (carpal) (metacarpal) (fingers)**
- **5. Pelvic region (hip) (buttock) (femur) and thigh**
- **6. Lower leg (fibula) (knee) (patella) (tibia)**
- **7. Ankle and or foot (metatarsals) (toes) (tarsals)**
- **8. Other (head) (neck) (rib) (skull) (trunk) (vertebrae)**
- **9. Multiple**

V54.2# Aftercare healing

5th digit: V54.2
- **0. Arm**
- **1. Arm upper**
- **2. Arm lower**
- **3. Hip**
- **4. Leg**
- **5. Leg upper**
- **6. Leg lower**
- **7. Vertebrae**
- **9. Other**

FRACTURE (continued)

PATHOLOGICAL (continued)

733.1# Algoneurodystrophy [733.7]
733.1# Arthritis hyperparathyroid **[252.0#]**

5th digit: 252.0
- **0. NOS**
- **1. Primary**
- **2. Secondary non-renal**
- **8. Other specified**

733.1# Busquet's disease **[730.1#]**
733.1# CA bone metastatic bone NOS [198.5]
733.1# CA bone or marrow metastatic [198.5]
733.1# Disuse atrophy of bone [733.7]
733.1# Granuloma bone **[730.1#]**
733.1# Hyperparathyroidism **[252.0#]**

5th digit: 252.0
- **0. NOS**
- **1. Primary**
- **2. Secondary non-renal**
- **8. Other specified**

733.1# Osteitis deformans with spine curvature abnormality [731.0]
733.1# Osteitis deformans without mention of bone tumor [731.0]
733.1# Osteitis fibrosa cystica generalisata [252.01]
733.1# Osteitis fibrosa cystica with kyphosis [252.01] [737.41]
733.1# Osteitis fibrosa cystica with lordosis [252.01] [737.42]
733.1# Osteitis fibrosa cystica with scoliosis [252.01] [737.43]
733.1# Osteitis fibrosa cystica with spine curvature abnormality NOS [252.01] [737.40]
733.1# Osteomyelitis acute **[730.0#]**
733.1# Osteomyelitis chronic **[730.1#]**

5th digit: 733.1
- **0. Unspecified site**
- **1. Humerus**
- **2. Distal radius and ulna, wrist**
- **3. Vertebra**
- **4. Neck of femur, femur NOS, hip NOS**
- **5. Other specified part of femur**
- **6. Tibia or fibula, ankle**
- **9. Other specified site**

5th digit: 730.0, 1
- **0. Site NOS**
- **1. Shoulder region**
- **2. Upper arm (elbow) (humerus)**
- **3. Forearm (radius) (wrist) (ulna)**
- **4. Hand (carpal) (metacarpal) (fingers)**
- **5. Pelvic region (hip) (buttock) (femur) and thigh**
- **6. Lower leg (fibula) (knee) (patella) (tibia)**
- **7. Ankle and or foot (metatarsals) (toes) (tarsals)**
- **8. Other (head) (neck) (rib) (skull) (trunk) (vertebrae)**
- **9. Multiple**

F

FRACTURE (continued)

PATHOLOGICAL (continued)

733.1# Osteoporosis [733.0#]

5th digit: 733.1
- **0. Unspecified site**
- **1. Humerus**
- **2. Distal radius and ulna, wrist**
- **3. Vertebra**
- **4. Neck of femur, femur NOS, hip NOS**
- **5. Other specified part of femur**
- **6. Tibia or fibula, ankle**
- **9. Other specified site**

5th digit: 733.0
- **0. NOS**
- **1. Postmenopausal**
- **1. Senile**
- **2. Idiopathic**
- **3. Disuse**
- **9. Drug induced**

733.1# Paget's disease of bone [731.0]

733.1# Parathyroid hyperplasia [252.0#]

5th digit: 252.0
- **0. NOS**
- **1. Primary**
- **2. Secondary non-renal**
- **8. Other specified**

733.1# Periostitis without osteomyelitIS [730.3#]

5th digit: 733.1
- **0. Unspecified site**
- **1. Humerus**
- **2. Distal radius and ulna, wrist**
- **3. Vertebra**
- **4. Neck of femur, femur NOS, hip NOS**
- **5. Other specified part of femur**
- **6. Tibia or fibula, ankle**
- **9. Other specified site**

5th digit: 730.3
- **0. Site NOS**
- **1. Shoulder region**
- **2. Upper arm (elbow) (humerus)**
- **3. Forearm (radius) (wrist) (ulna)**
- **4. Hand (carpal) (metacarpal) (fingers)**
- **5. Pelvic region (hip) (buttock) (femur) and thigh**
- **6. Lower leg (fibula) (knee) (patella) (tibia)**
- **7. Ankle and or foot (metatarsals) (toes) (tarsals)**
- **8. Other (head) (neck) (rib) (skull) (trunk) (vertebrae)**
- **9. Multiple**

733.1# Sudeck's atrophy (vertebra) [733.7]

5th digit: 733.1
- **0. Unspecified site**
- **1. Humerus**
- **2. Distal radius and ulna, wrist**
- **3. Vertebra**
- **4. Neck of femur, femur NOS, hip NOS**
- **5. Other specified part of femur**
- **6. Tibia or fibula, ankle**
- **9. Other specified site**

FRACTURE (continued)

PELVIS CLOSED

808.8 Unspecified closed
808.0 Acetabulum
808.41 Ilium
808.49 Innominate bone
808.42 Ischium
808.43 Multiple with disruption of pelvic circle
809.0 Multiple with other bones
808.2 Pubis
808.49 Rim

PELVIS OPEN

808.9 Unspecified open
808.1 Acetabulum
808.51 Ilium
808.59 Innominate bone
808.52 Ischium
808.53 Multiple with disruption of pelvic circle
809.1 Multiple with other bones
808.3 Pubis
808.59 Rim

FRACTURE (continued)

959.13 Penis corpus cavernosum
826.0 Phalanges foot closed
826.1 Phalanges foot open
816.00 Phalanges hand closed
816.10 Phalanges hand open
814.04 Pisiform closed
814.14 Pisiform open
824.4 Pott's closed
824.5 Pott's open
996.43 Prosthetic fixation device orthopedic internal – mechanical [V43.6#]

5th digit: V43.6
- **0. Site unspecified**
- **1. Shoulder**
- **2. Elbow**
- **3. Wrist**
- **4. Hip**
- **5. Knee**
- **6. Ankle**
- **9. Other**

996.44 Prosthetic - periprosthetic fixation device orthopedic internal – mechanical [V43.6#]

5th digit: V43.6
- **0. Site unspecified**
- **1. Shoulder**
- **2. Elbow**
- **3. Wrist**
- **4. Hip**
- **5. Knee**
- **6. Ankle**
- **9. Other**

808.2 Pubis closed
808.3 Pubis open
814.01 Quervain's closed
814.11 Quervain's open

FRACTURE (continued)

"With" means that both must be present. Fracture radius with ulna means that fractures of both bones must occur in order to use this code.

RADIUS CLOSED

813.81 NOS
813.83 NOS with ulna
813.42 Distal
813.44 Distal with ulna
813.05 Head or epiphysis
813.06 Neck
813.07 Proximal or multiple sites
813.08 Proximal or multiple sites with ulna
813.21 Shaft
813.23 Shaft with ulna
813.45 Torus

RADIUS OPEN

813.91 NOS
813.93 NOS with ulna
813.52 Distal
813.54 Distal with ulna
813.15 Head or epiphysis
813.16 Neck
813.17 Proximal or multiple sites
813.18 Proximal or multiple sites with ulna
813.31 Shaft
813.33 Shaft with ulna

FRACTURE (continued)

807.## Ribs
4th digit: 807
0. Closed
1. Open
5th digit: 807
0. Ribs unspecified
1. One rib
2. Two ribs
3. Three ribs
4. Four ribs
5. Five ribs
6. Six ribs
7. Seven ribs
8. Eight or more ribs
9. Multiple ribs unspecified

805.6 Sacrum and coccyx closed
805.7 Sacrum and coccyx open
806.6# Sacrum and coccyx with cord injury closed
806.7# Sacrum and coccyx with cord injury open
5th digit: 806.6-7
0. Cord injury unspecified
1. Complete cauda equina injury
2. Other cauda equina injury
9. With other spinal cord injury

A saltar fracture is a fracture involving a bone's epiphysis. Code as all other fractures; by bone (closed) (open).

825.22 Scaphoid foot closed
825.32 Scaphoid foot open
814.01 Scaphoid wrist closed
814.11 Scaphoid wrist open

FRACTURE (continued)

811.0# Scapula closed
811.1# Scapula open
5th digit: 811.0-1
0. Site unspecified
1. Acromion
2. Coracoid
3. Glenoid or neck
9. Body of scapula

0 Sesamoid see 'Fracture', by site
825.21 Shepherd's closed
825.31 Shepherd's open
0 Shoulder blade see 'Fracture', scapula
812.00 Shoulder closed
812.10 Shoulder open
813.42 Silverfork closed
813.52 Silverfork open
0 Sinus bones see 'Fracture', skull basilar
813.21 Skillern's closed
813.31 Skillern's open
803.## Skull
801.## Skull basilar
767.3 Skull birth trauma
803.## Skull multiple NOS
804.## Skull multiple with other bones of body
800.## Skull vault
4th digit: 800, 801, 803, 804
0. Closed without intracranial injury
1. Closed with cerebral laceration and/or contusion
2. Closed with subarachnoid subdural extradural and epidural hemorrhage
3. Closed with other and unspecified intracranial hemorrhage
4. Closed with intracranial injury of other and unspecified nature
5. Open without mention of intracranial injury
6. Open with cerebral laceration and contusion
7. Open with subarachnoid subdural epidural and extradural hemorrhage
8. Open with other and unspecified intracranial hemorrhage
9. Open with intracranial injury of other and unspecified
5th digit: 800, 801, 803, 804
0. Level of consciousness unspecified
1. No LOC
2. LOC < 1 hr
3. LOC 1 - 24 hrs
4. LOC > 24 hrs with return to prior level
5. LOC > 24 hrs without return to prior level: or death before regaining consciousness, regardless of duration of LOC
6. LOC duration unspecified
9. With concussion unspecified

813.41 Smith's closed
813.51 Smith's open
0 Sphenoid bone see 'Fracture', skull basilar
767.4 Spine or spinal cord birth trauma
0 Spine see 'Fracture', cervical, dorsal, lumbar, sacrum or coccyx
0 Spinous process see 'Fracture', cervical, dorsal, lumbar, sacrum or coccyx
0 Spontaneous see 'Fracture', pathological

FRACTURE (continued)

808.41 Sprinters' closed
808.51 Sprinters' open
807.2 Sternum closed
807.3 Sternum open
807.4 Sternum with flail chest open
821.20 Stieda's closed
821.30 Stieda's open

Stress fractures result from a crack in the bone caused by overexertion placed on a bone structure of the limb or metatarsal bone or from the pull of muscle on bone.

733.9# Stress
5th digit: 733.9
3. Tibia or fibula
4. Metatarsals
5. Other bone

815.02 Styloid process metacarpal closed
815.12 Styloid process metacarpal open
813.43 Styloid process ulna closed
813.53 Styloid process ulna open
813.44 Styloid process ulna with radius closed
813.54 Styloid process ulna with radius open
812.41 Supracondylar (humerus) closed
812.51 Supracondylar (humerus) open
0 Symphysis pubis see 'Fracture', pubis
825.21 Talus closed
825.31 Talus open
825.29 Tarsal with metatarsal(s) closed
825.39 Tarsal with metatarsal(s) open
0 Temporal bone see 'Fracture', skull basilar
805.2 Thoracic vertebra closed
805.3 Thoracic vertebra open
806.2# Thoracic vertebra with cord injury closed
806.3# Thoracic vertebra with cord injury open
5th digit: 806.2-3
0. T1-T6 with cord injury unspecified
1. T1-T6 with complete lesion of cord
2. T1-T6 with anterior cord syndrome
3. T1-T6 with central cord syndrome
4. T1-T6 with incomplete cord lesion unspecified or posterior cord syndrome
5. T7-T12 with cord injury unspecified
6. T7-T12 with complete lesion of cord
7. T7-T12 with anterior cord syndrome
8. T7-T12 with central cord syndrome
9. T7-T12 with spinal cord lesion unspecified or posterior cord syndrome

0 Thumb see 'Fracture', finger
807.5 Thyroid cartilage closed
807.6 Thyroid cartilage open
823.## Tibia and/or fibula
4th digit: 823
0. Proximal (head) (plateau) closed
1. Proximal (head) (plateau) open
2. Shaft closed
3. Shaft open
4. Torus
8. Site unspecified closed
9. Site unspecified open

5th digit: 823
0. Tibia alone
1. Fibula alone
2. Tibia with fibula

FRACTURE (continued)

824.8 Tibia distal end or epiphysis closed
824.9 Tibia distal end or epiphysis open
823.00 Tibia intercondylar spine/tuberosity closed
823.10 Tibia intercondylar spine/tuberosity open
824.0 Tibia involving ankle closed
824.1 Tibia involving ankle open
823.4# Tibia torus
5th digit: 823.4
0. Tibia alone
2. With fibula

823.00 Tibial plateau closed
823.10 Tibial plateau open
826.0 Toe(s) closed
826.1 Toe(s) open
873.63 Tooth
873.73 Tooth complicated
521.81 Tooth nontraumatic
823.4# Torus fibula
813.45 Torus radius
823.4# Torus tibia
5th digit: 823.4
0. Tibia alone
1. Fibula alone
2. Tibia with fibula

807.5 Trachea closed
807.6 Trachea open
0 Transverse process see 'Fracture', cervical, dorsal, lumbar, sacrum or coccyx
814.05 Trapezium closed
814.15 Trapezium open
814.06 Trapezoid closed
814.16 Trapezoid open
V67.4 Treatment follow up exam - healed
0 Treatment follow up exam - healing or current see 'Aftercare', orthopedic
824.6 Trimalleolar closed
824.7 Trimalleolar open
814.03 Triquetral closed
814.13 Triquetral open
812.49 Trochlea (humerus) closed
812.59 Trochlea (humerus) open

ULNA CLOSED

813.82 NOS
813.83 NOS with radius
813.43 Distal
813.44 Distal with radius
813.04 Proximal
813.04 Proximal multiple
813.08 Proximal with radius
813.22 Shaft
813.23 Shaft with radius

ULNA OPEN

813.92 NOS
813.93 NOS with radius
813.53 Distal
813.54 Distal with radius
813.14 Proximal
813.14 Proximal multiple
813.18 Proximal with radius
813.32 Shaft
813.33 Shaft with radius

F

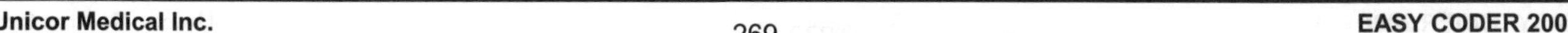

FRACTURE (continued)

814.08	Unciform closed
814.18	Unciform open
767.4	Vertebra birth trauma
733.13	Vertebra chronic
805.8	Vertebra closed
805.9	Vertebra open
809.0	Vertebra multiple closed
809.1	Vertebra multiple open
806.8	Vertebra with cord injury closed
806.9	Vertebra with cord injury open
802.0	Vomer closed
802.1	Vomer open
814.##	Wrist **4th digit: 814** **0. Closed** **1. Open** **5th digit: 814** **0. Unspecified** **1. Navicular (scaphoid)** **2. Lunate (semilunar)** **3. Triquetral (cuneiform)** **4. Pisiform** **5. Trapezium (larger multangular)** **6. Trapezoid (smaller multangular)** **7. Capitate (OS magnum)** **8. Hammate (unciform)** **9. Other**
802.4	Zygoma closed
802.5	Zygoma open

759.83	FRAGILE X SYNDROME
704.2	FRAGILITAS CRINIUM
756.51	FRAGILITAS OSSIUM
102.0	FRAMBESIA INITIAL OR PRIMARY
102.0	FRAMBESIA INITIAL ULCER
0	FRAMBESIA SEE ALSO 'YAWS'
102.4	FRAMBESIDE GUMMATOUS
102.2	FRAMBESIDE OF EARLY YAWS
102.1	FRAMBESIOMA
756.0	FRANCESCHETTI'S SYNDROME (MANDIBULOFACIAL DYSOSTOSIS)
021.9	FRANCIS' TULAREMIA
0	FRANCISELLA (PASTURELLA) TULARENSIS SEE 'TULAREMIA'
287.39	FRANK'S ESSENTIAL THROMBOCYTOPENIA
273.2	FRANKLIN'S HEAVY CHAIN DISEASE
759.89	FRASER'S SYNDROME
709.09	FRECKLE
272.3	FREDRICKSON TYPE I OR V HYPERLIPOPROTEINEMIA
272.0	FREDRICKSON TYPE IIA HYPERLIPOPROTEINEMIA
272.2	FREDRICKSON TYPE IIB OR III HYPERLIPOPROTEINEMIA
272.1	FREDRICKSON TYPE IV HYPERLIPOPROTEINEMIA
759.89	FREEMAN SHELDON SYNDROME
099.1	FREI'S CLIMATIC BUBO
732.5	FREIBERG'S FLATTENING METATARSAL
788.41	FREQUENCY (URINARY)
350.8	FREY'S AURICULOTEMPORAL SYNDROME
705.22	FREY'S SYNDROME (AURICULOTEMPORAL) (SECONDARY FOCAL HYPERHIDROSIS)

FRICTION RUB

786.7	Chest
785.3	Heart
786.7	Pleural

036.3	FRIDERICHSEN-WATERHOUSE SYNDROME
0	FRIEDLANDER'S BACILLUS SEE 'BACTERIAL INFECTION' OR SPECIFIED CONDITION
0	FRIEDLANDER'S ENDARTERITIS OBLITERANS SEE 'ARTERIOSCLEROSIS, ARTERIOSCLEROTIC'
334.0	FRIEDREICH'S ATAXIA
334.0	FRIEDREICH'S ATAXIA - CARDIOMYOPATHY [425.8]
756.0	FRIEDREICH'S FACIAL HEMIHYPERTROPHY
333.2	FRIEDREICH'S MYOCLONIA
757.39	FRIEDRICH-ERB-ARNOLD SYNDROME (ACROPACHYDERMA)
302.72	FRIGIDITY PSYCHOSEXUAL
253.8	FROHLICH'S ADIPOSOGENITAL DYSTROPHY (SYNDROME)
336.8	FROIN'S SYNDROME
676.6#	FROMMEL CHIARI SYNDROME MATERNAL DUE TO PREGNANCY **5th digit: 676.6** **0. Episode of care unspecified or N/A** **1. Delivered** **2. Delivered with postpartum complication** **3. Antepartum complication** **4. Postpartum complication**
738.19	FRONTAL BONE DEFORMITY
310.0	FRONTAL LOBE SYNDROME
461.1	FRONTAL SINUS (ABSCESS) (INFECTION) (INFLAMMATION) ACUTE
473.1	FRONTAL SINUS DISEASE CHRONIC

FROSTBITE

991.3	NOS
991.0	Face
991.2	Foot
991.1	Hand
909.4	Late effect
991.3	Other sites

302.89	FROTTEURISM
726.0	FROZEN SHOULDER
271.2	FRUCTOSE INTOLERANCE HEREDITARY
271.2	FRUCTOSEMIA METABOLISM DISORDER
271.2	FRUCTOSURIA ESSENTIAL BENIGN
371.57	FUCHS' ENDOTHELIAL DYSTROPHY
364.21	FUCHS' HETEROCHRONIC IRIDOCYCLITIS
271.8	FUCOSIDASE ABSENCE
271.8	FUCOSIDOSIS CARBOHYDRATE TRANSPORT DISORDERS
780.99	FUGUE
300.13	FUGUE DISSOCIATIVE
300.13	FUGUE HYSTERICAL (DISSOCIATIVE)
308.1	FUGUES REACTION (ACUTE) (STRESS)
277.87	FUKUHARA SYNDROME
756.59	FULLER ALBRIGHT'S SYNDROME (OSTEITIS FIBROSA DISSEMINATA)
502	FULLER'S EARTH DISEASE

987.9 FUMES INHALATION (NOXIOUS)

780.99 FUNCTIONAL ACTIVITY DECREASE
564.9 FUNCTIONAL BOWEL SYNDROME
752.89 FUNCTIONAL PREPUBERTAL CASTRATE SYNDROME
V62.89 FUNCTIONING BORDERLINE INTELLECTUAL
743.52 FUNDUS COLOBOMA CONGENITAL
362.76 FUNDUS FLAVIMACULATUS HEREDITARY
0 FUNGAL SEE 'FUNGUS, FUNGAL INFECTION'
117.9 FUNGEMIA

FUNGUS, FUNGAL INFECTION

117.9 NEC
0 Aspergillus see 'Aspergillosis'
110.0 Beard
110.5 Body
0 Candidal see 'Candidiasis'
0 Coccidioides (immitis) see 'Coccidioidomycosis'
117.8 Dematiacious
110.4 Foot
110.3 Groin
110.2 Hand
0 Histoplasma see 'Histoplasmosis'
110.1 Nail (finger) (toe)
118 Pathogenic to compromised host only
110.3 Perianal area
110.0 Scalp
110.8 Scrotum
111.9 Skin
110.4 Skin foot
110.2 Skin hand
0 Tinea see 'Tinea'
110.1 Toenail
117.9 Trachea
117.8 Other specified fungus

754.81 FUNNEL CHEST CONGENITAL
780.6 FUO (FEVER OF UNKNOWN ORIGIN)
690.18 FURFUR
495.8 FURRIERS' LUNG
373.13 FURUNCLE EYELID
0 FURUNCLE SEE 'CARBUNCLE'
118 FUSARIUM INFECTION TO COMPROMISED HOST ONLY
0 FUSIFORM CELL TYPE TUMOR MALIGNANT SITE SPECIFIED SEE 'CANCER', BY SITE M8004/3

FUSION, FUSED

756.9 Bone congenital
V45.4 Cervical arthrodesis status
746.5 Commissure mitral valve congenital
744.04 Ear ossicles (congenital)
996.49 Failed joint **[V43.6#]**
5th digit: V43.6
0. Site unspecified
1. Shoulder
2. Elbow
3. Wrist
4. Hip
5. Knee
6. Ankle
9. Other

FUSION, FUSED (continued)

718.54 Finger acquired
755.12 Finger (bone) congenital
718.57 Foot acquired
755.67 Foot talonavicular congenital
718.55 Hip acquired
718.5# Joint acquired (fibrous) (osseous)
5th digit: 718.5
0. Site NOS
1. Shoulder region
2. Upper arm (elbow) (humerus)
3. Forearm (radius) (wrist) (ulna)
4. Hand (carpal) (metacarpal) (fingers)
5. Pelvic region and thigh (hip) (buttock) (femur)
6. Lower leg (fibula) (knee) (patella) (tibia)
7. Ankle and/or foot (metatarsals) (toes) (tarsals)
8. Other except spine
9. Multiple

755.8 Joint congenital
996.49 Joint failed **[V43.6#]**
5th digit: V43.6
0. Site unspecified
1. Shoulder
2. Elbow
3. Wrist
4. Hip
5. Knee
6. Ankle
9. Other

718.56 Knee acquired
755.8 Limb congenital
755.69 Limb lower congenital
755.59 Limb upper congenital
724.6 Lumbosacral acquired (nonvertebral) (nondiscogenic)
V45.4 Lumbosacral arthrodesis status
756.15 Lumbosacral congenital
718.58 Neck acquired
718.58 Rib acquired
756.3 Rib congenital
724.6 Sacroiliac acquired (nonvertebral) (nondiscogenic)
755.69 Sacroiliac congenital
V45.4 Sacroiliac arthrodesis status
724.6 Sacrum acquired (nonvertebral) (nondiscogenic)
V45.4 Sacrum arthrodesis status
755.69 Sacrum congenital
724.9 Spine acquired (nonvertebral) (nondiscogenic)
756.15 Spine congenital
996.49 Spine failed [V43.69]
V45.4 Spine surgical status
755.67 Talonavicular congenital
V45.4 Thoracic arthrodesis status
718.57 Toes acquired
755.14 Toes congenital
368.33 Vision with defective stereopsis

780.91 FUSSY INFANT (BABY)

F

085.1 GAFSA BOIL
478.29 GAG REFLEX HYPERACTIVE
289.0 GAISBOCK'S DISEASE OR SYNDROME (POLYCYTHEMIA HYPERTONICA)
289.0 GAISBOCK'S POLYCYTHEMIA HYPERTONICA

GAIT

781.2 Abnormality (ataxic) (paralytic) (scissor) (spastic) (staggering)
719.7 Difficulty
719.7 Disorder
300.11 Disturbance hysterical
V57.81 Training in the use of artificial limbs

611.5 GALACTOCELE
676.8# GALACTOCELE PUERPERAL POSTPARTUM MATERNAL DUE TO PREGNANCY
5th digit: 676.8
0. Episode of care unspecified or N/A
1. Delivered
2. Delivered with postpartum complication
3. Antepartum complication
4. Postpartum complication

611.0 GALACTOPHORITIS
675.2# GALACTOPHORITIS PUERPERAL POSTPARTUM MATERNAL DUE TO PREGNANCY
5th digit: 675.2
0. Episode of care unspecified or N/A
1. Delivered
2. Delivered with postpartum complication
3. Antepartum complication
4. Postpartum complication

611.6 GALACTORRHEA
676.6# GALACTORRHEA MATERNAL DUE TO PREGNANCY
5th digit: 676.6
0. Episode of care unspecified or N/A
1. Delivered
2. Delivered with postpartum complication
3. Antepartum complication
4. Postpartum complication

271.1 GALACTOSE 1 PHOSPHATE URIDYL TRANSFERASE DEFICIENCY
271.1 GALACTOSEMIA
V77.4 GALACTOSEMIA SCREENING
271.1 GALACTOSEMIA WITH PERINATAL JAUNDICE [774.5]
271.1 GALACTOSURIA
791.1 GALACTURIA

GALLBLADDER

575.0 Abscess
0 Abscess with calculus see 'Cholecystitis', acute with cholelithiasis
V45.79 Absence acquired
751.69 Absence congenital
575.8 Adhesion
751.60 Anomaly NOS
751.69 Anomaly other specified
751.69 Atresia (congenital)
575.8 Atrophy

GALLBLADDER (continued)

575.8 Calcification
0 Calculus see 'Cholelithiasis'
575.6 Cholesterolosis
575.9 Disease NOS
646.8# Disease NOS complicating pregnancy **[574.2#]**
5th digit: 646.8
0. Episode of care unspecified or N/A
1. Delivered
2. Delivered with postpartum complication
3. Antepartum complication
4. Postpartum complication

5th digit: 574.2
0. Without obstruction
1. With obstruction

575.9 Disorder
575.8 Disorders other specified
793.3 Filling defect
793.3 Findings abnormal (nonvisualization)
575.5 Fistula
575.0 Gangrenous
0 Gangrenous with calculus see 'Cholecystitis'
575.3 Hydrops
575.8 Hypertrophy
868.02 Injury - unspecified
868.12 Injury - with open wound into cavity
908.1 Injury - late effect
575.8 Nonfunctioning
793.3 Nonvisualization
575.2 Obstruction or occlusion
0 Obstruction or occlusion with calculus see 'Cholecystitis'
575.4 Perforation
575.8 Ulcer

GALLBLADDER CONGENITAL ANOMALIES

751.69 Absence
751.60 Bile ducts and liver
751.60 Disorder
751.69 Duplication
751.69 Ectopic
751.69 Floating
751.69 Intrahepatic
751.69 Obstruction or occlusion
751.69 Obstruction or occlusion with jaundice [774.5]

0 GALLSTONE SEE 'CHOLELITHIASIS'
086.3 GAMBIAN SLEEPING SICKNESS
312.31 GAMBLING COMPULSIVE (PATHOLOGICAL)
V69.3 GAMBLING PROBLEM
842.13 GAMEKEEPER'S THUMB
279.00 GAMMA GLOBULIN ABSENCE
V07.2 GAMMA GLOBULIN ADMINISTRATION (PROPHYLACTIC)
277.39 GAMMALOIDOSIS
273.9 GAMMOPATHY
273.1 GAMMOPATHY MONOCLONAL
273.1 GAMMOPATHY MONOCLONAL ASSOCIATED WITH LYMPHOPLASMACYTIC DYSCRASIAS
289.51 GAMNA'S SIDEROTIC SPLENOMEGALY
754.71 GAMPSODACTYLIA CONGENITAL
359.3 GAMSTORP'S DISEASE

289.51 GANDY-NANTA SIDEROTIC SPLENOMEGALY
V71.01 GANG ACTIVITY EVALUATION - ADULT SUSPECTED PSYCHIATRIC DISORDER
V71.02 GANG ACTIVITY EVALUATION - CHILD OR ADOLESCENT SUSPECTED PSYCHIATRIC DISORDER
238.9 GANGLIOGLIOMA SITE UNSPECIFIED
0 GANGLIOGLIOMA SITE SPECIFIED SEE 'NEOPLASM UNCERTAIN BEHAVIOR', BY SITE M9505/1

GANGLION

727.43 Unspecified
351.1 Geniculi syndrome
727.41 Joint
333.90 Syndrome (basal, brain)
727.42 Tendon sheath

171.# GANGLIONEUROBLASTOMA M9490/3
215.# GANGLIONEUROMA M9490/0
215.# GANGLIONEUROMATOSIS M9491/0

4th digit: 171, 215
- **0. Head, face, neck**
- **2. Upper limb including shoulder**
- **3. Lower limb including hip**
- **4. Thorax**
- **5. Abdomen (wall), gastric, gastrointestinal, intestine, stomach**
- **6. Pelvis, buttock, groin, inguinal, region perineum**
- **7. Trunk NOS, back NOS, flank NOS**
- **8. Other specified sites**
- **9. Site NOS**

351.1 GANGLIONITIS GENICULATE UNSPECIFIED
330.1 GANGLIOSIDOSIS DISEASE

Gangrene, 785.4 should never be sequenced as the principal diagnosis if the cause is known. Always code the underlying disease first. For example, diabetic gangrene of the leg is coded with the diabetes first, 250.7.# and the gangrene second, 785.4.

GANGRENE

785.4 Unspecified
785.4 Abdomen (wall)
569.49 Anus

When coding arteriosclerosis of the extremities use an additional code, if applicable to identify chronic complete or total occlusion of the artery of the extremities (440.4).

440.24 Arteriosclerotic extremities (general) [707.#(#)]

4th or 4th and 5th digit: 707
- **1#. Lower limb except decubitus**
  - **10. Unspecified**
  - **11. Thigh**
  - **12. Calf**
  - **13. Ankle**
  - **14. Heel and midfoot**
  - **15. Other parts of foot, toes**
  - **19. Other**
- **8. Chronic of other specified site**
- **9. Chronic site NOS**

557.0 Bowel
785.4 Cellulitis
371.40 Cornea

GANGRENE (continued)

707.0# Decubital ulcer [785.4]

5th digit: 707.0
- **0. NOS**
- **1. Elbow**
- **2. Upper back (shoulder blades)**
- **3. Lower back (sacrum)**
- **4. Hip**
- **5. Buttock**
- **6. Ankle**
- **7. Heel**
- **9. Other site (head)**

250.7# Diabetic [785.4]

5th digit: 250.7
- **0. Type II, adult-onset, non-insulin dependent (even if requiring insulin), or unspecified; controlled**
- **1. Type I, juvenile-onset or insulin-dependent; controlled**
- **2. Type II, adult-onset, non-insulin dependent (even if requiring insulin); uncontrolled**
- **3. Type I, Juvenile-onset or insulin-dependent; uncontrolled**

443.0 Due to Raynaud's [785.4]
444.22 Embolus, thrombus arteries lower extremities [785.4]
444.21 Embolus,thrombus arteries upper extremities [785.4]
040.0 Emphysematous
988.2 Epidemic
785.4 Extremity
440.3# Extremity arteriosclerotic - bypass graft
440.3# Extremity arteriosclerotic - bypass graft with chronic, complete or total occlusion [440.4]

5th digit: 440.3
- **0. Unspecified graft**
- **1. Autologous vein bypass graft**
- **2. Nonautologous biological bypass graft**

When coding arteriosclerosis of the extremities use an additional code, if applicable to identify chronic complete or total occlusion of the artery of the extremities (440.4).

440.24 Extremity arteriosclerotic - native artery ischemic [707.#(#)]

4th or 4th and 5th digit: 707
- **1#. Lower limb except decubitus**
  - **10. Unspecified**
  - **11. Thigh**
  - **12. Calf**
  - **13. Ankle**
  - **14. Heel and midfoot**
  - **15. Other parts of foot, toes**
  - **19. Other**
- **8. Chronic of other specified site**
- **9. Chronic site NOS**

250.7# Extremity diabetic [785.4]

5th digit: 250.7
- **0. Type II, adult-onset, non-insulin dependent (even if requiring insulin), or unspecified; controlled**
- **1. Type I, juvenile-onset or insulin-dependent; controlled**
- **2. Type II, adult-onset, non-insulin dependent (even if requiring insulin); uncontrolled**
- **3. Type I, Juvenile-onset or insulin-dependent; uncontrolled**

GANGRENE (continued)

575.0 Gallbladder
0 Gallbladder with calculus see 'Cholecystitis', acute with cholelithiasis
040.0 Gas (bacillus)
523.8 Gingival
557.0 Intestinal

> *When coding arteriosclerosis of the extremities use an additional code, if applicable to identify chronic complete or total occlusion of the artery of the extremities (440.4).*

440.24 Ischemic arteriosclerotic extremities (general) [707.#(#)]
4th or 4th and 5th digit: 707
1#. Lower limb except decubitus
10. Unspecified
11. Thigh
12. Calf
13. Ankle
14. Heel and midfoot
15. Other parts of foot, toes
19. Other
8. Chronic of other specified site
9. Chronic site NOS

464.0# Laryngitis
5th digit: 464.0
0. Without mention of obstruction
1. With obstruction

573.8 Liver
513.0 Lung
104.8 Lung spirochetal
686.09 Meleney's (cutaneous)
034.0 Pharynx (septic)

> *When coding arteriosclerosis of the extremities use an additional code, if applicable to identify chronic complete or total occlusion of the artery of the extremities (440.4).*

440.24 Pott's ischemic [707.#(#)]
4th or 4th and 5th digit: 707
1#. Lower limb except decubitus
10. Unspecified
11. Thigh
12. Calf
13. Ankle
14. Heel and midfoot
15. Other parts of foot, toes
19. Other
8. Chronic of other specified site
9. Chronic site NOS

443.1 Presenile
513.0 Pulmonary
440.24 Senile ischemic [707.#(#)]
4th or 4th and 5th digit: 707
1#. Lower limb except decubitus
10. Unspecified
11. Thigh
12. Calf
13. Ankle
14. Heel and midfoot
15. Other parts of foot, toes
19. Other
8. Chronic of other specified site
9. Chronic site NOS

537.89 Stomach

502 GANNISTER DISEASE
300.16 GANSER'S SYNDROME HYSTERICAL
287.2 GARDNER-DIAMOND SYNDROME (AUTOERYTHROCYTE SENSITIZATION)
0 GARDNERELLA VAGINALIS SEE 'BACTERIAL INFECTION' OR SPECIFIED CONDITION
277.5 GARGOYLISM
0 GARRE'S SEE 'OSTEOMYELITIS'
728.79 GARROD'S OR KNUCKLE PADS
752.89 GARTNER'S DUCT ANOMALY
752.41 GARTNER'S DUCT CYST (PERSISTENT) CONGENITAL
040.0 GAS BACILLUS INFECTION
040.0 GAS GANGRENE
987.9 GAS INHALATION (NOXIOUS)
787.3 GAS PAIN
350.8 GASSERIAN GANGLION
134.0 GASTEROPHILUS (INTESTINALIS) INFESTATION
536.8 GASTRALGIA

GASTRIC

536.0 Anacidity
537.82 Antral vascular ectasia without hemorrhage
537.83 Antral vascular ectasia with hemorrhage
902.21 Artery injury traumatic (laceration) (rupture) (hematoma) (avulsion) (aneurysm)
908.4 Artery injury late effect
537.89 Atrophy
094.0 Crisis (tabetic)
536.1 Dilatation acute
536.8 Dilatation other specified
537.9 Disorder
536.9 Disorder functional unspecified
306.4 Disorder functional psychogenic
536.8 Disorder functional other specified (motility) (secretion)
536.1 Distention acute
537.1 Diverticulum
537.89 Duodenal rupture
535.4# Erosion
5th digit: 535.4
0. Without hemorrhage
1. With hemorrhage

537.89 Lesion
536.8 Motility disorder
537.89 Mucosa metaplasia
535.20 Mucosal hypertrophy
535.21 Mucosal hypertrophy with hemorrhage
537.0 Outlet obstruction
536.8 Pain
536.3 Paresis
537.89 Prolapse
536.8 Retention
537.89 Reflux
537.89 Rupture
536.8 Secretion disorder
536.3 Stasis
537.89 Stenosis

G

GASTRIC (continued)

531.## Ulcer
531.## Ulcer due to helicobacter pylori [041.86]
4th digit: 531
0. Acute with hemorrhage
1. Acute with perforation
2. Acute with hemorrhage and perforation
3. Acute
4. Chronic or unspecified with hemorrhage
5. Chronic or unspecified with perforation
6. Chronic or unspecified with hemorrhage and perforation
7. Chronic
9. Unspecified as acute or chronic
5th digit: 531
0. Without obstruction
1. Obstructed

902.39 Vein injury (laceration) (rupture) (hematoma) (avulsion) (aneurysm) traumatic
908.4 Vein injury late effect

251.5 GASTRIN SECRETION ABNORMALITY

Carcinomas and neoplasms should be coded by site if possible. Code by cell type, "site NOS", only if a site is not specified in the diagnosis. Otherwise, refer to the appropriate category of neoplasm for a more specific code. See 'Cancer' 'Cancer Metastatic', 'Carcinoma In Situ', 'Neoplasm Uncertain Behavior', 'Neoplasm Unspecified Nature', or 'Benign Neoplasm'.

GASTRINOMA

235.5 Site unspecified
0 Site specified see 'Neoplasm Uncertain Behavior', by site M8153/1
157.4 Malignant site unspecified M8153/3
0 Malignant site specified see 'Cancer', by site M8153/3

GASTRITIS

535.5# NOS
535.0# Acute
535.3# Alcoholic
535.4# Allergic
535.1# Atrophic
535.1# Atrophic (hyperplastic chronic)
535.4# Bile induced
535.0# Catarrhal
535.1# Chronic
535.4# Cirrhotic (sclerotic) (toxic)
269.9 Due to diet deficiency
535.4# Due to ingested substance
535.4# Eosinophilic (follicular) (glandular)
535.4# Erosive
535.4# Glandular
535.2# Hypertrophic
535.1# Infectious due to helicobacter pylori [041.86]
535.4# Irritant
306.4 Nervous (cyclical)
535.0# Phlegmonous
5th digit: 535.0-5
0. Without hemorrhage
1. With hemorrhage

GASTRITIS (continued)

535.4# Sclerotic
536.8 Spastic
535.0# Subacute
535.4# Superficial
535.4# Suppurative
535.4# Toxic
5th digit: 535.0-5
0. Without hemorrhage
1. With hemorrhage

121.8 GASTRODISCOIDES HOMINIS INFECTION
442.84 GASTRODUODENAL ARTERY (ANEURYSM) (A-V FISTULA) (CIRSOID) (FALSE) (VARICOSE)
535.5# GASTRODUODENITIS
5th digit: 535.5
0. Without hemorrhage
1. With hemorrhage

536.8 GASTRODYNIA

GASTROENTERITIS

558.9 NOS
008.62 Adenovirus
008.2 Aerobacter aerogenes
558.3 Allergic
558.3 Allergic due to ingested foods **[V15.0#]**
5th digit: V15.0
1. Peanuts
2. Milk products
3. Eggs
4. Seafood
5. Other foods

008.1 Arizona group of paracolon bacilli
008.66 Astrovirus
008.5 Bacterial
008.49 Bacterial other
008.46 Bacteroides (fragilis)
008.65 Calcivirus
558.9 Chronic
009.0 Colitis enteritis septic
009.1 Colitis enteritis of presumed infectious origin
558.9 Dietetic
008.0# E coli intestinal infection
5th digit: 008.0
0. Due to unspecified E. coli
1. Due to enteropathogenic E. coli
2. Due to enterotoxigenic E. coli
3. Due to enteroinvasive E. coli
4. Due to enterohemorrhagic E. coli
9. Due to other intestinal E. coli infections

008.67 Enterovirus NEC
009.0 Epidemic
009.0 Infectious (septic)
009.1 Infectious origin presumed
487.8 Influenza
008.63 Norwalk virus
008.3 Proteus mirabilis
008.42 Pseudomonas aeruginosa
558.1 Radiation
008.61 Rotavirus
003.0 Salmonella
008.41 Staphylococcus
558.2 Toxic

G

GASTROENTERITIS (continued)

008.8 Viral acute
008.69 Viral other specified
008.64 Virus other small round (SRV's)
558.9 Other and unspecified
0 See also 'Enteritis'

442.84 GASTROEPIPLOIC ARTERY (ANEURYSM) (A-V FISTULA) (CIRSOID) (FALSE) (VARICOSE)

530.89 GASTROESOPHAGEAL INSUFFICIENCY

530.0 GASTROESOPHAGEAL JUNCTION SYNDROME

530.7 GASTROESOPHAGEAL LACERATION-HEMORRHAGE SYNDROME

530.81 GASTROESOPHAGEAL REFLUX

530.19 GASTROESOPHAGITIS

GASTROINTESTINAL TRACT

793.4 Abnormal (x-ray) (ultrasound) (thermography)
V44.4 Artificial opening status other
569.89 Atrophy
578.9 Bleeding unspecified
277.39 Disorder amyloid
536.9 Disorder functional
777.9 Disorder perinatal
306.4 Disorder psychogenic
793.4 Filling defect
0 Infection see also 'Enteritis'
908.1 Injury late effect
863.80 Injury NOS site
863.90 Injury NOS site with open wound into cavity
863.89 Injury other specified site
863.99 Injury other specified site with open wound into cavity
0 Obstruction see 'Intestine, Intestinal', obstruction
787.99 Symptoms
306.4 Symptoms psychogenic

GASTROINTESTINAL TRACT ANOMALIES CONGENITAL

751.9 NOS
751.8 Agenesis NOS (complete) (partial)
751.2 Agenesis lower (large) (complete) (partial)
750.8 Agenesis upper (complete) (partial)
747.61 Anomaly artery peripheral vascular -(aberrant) (absence) (agenesis) (accessory) (aneurysm) (atresia) (deformity) (hypoplasia) (malposition)
751.9 Anomaly of fixation
750.8 Anomaly other specified (UGI)
751.8 Anomaly other specified anomaly of fixation
750.8 Anomaly upper other specified
750.9 Anomaly unspecified upper alimentary tract
747.61 Anomaly vein peripheral vascular- (aberrant) (absence) (agenesis) (accessory) (aneurysm) (deformity) (hypoplasia) (malposition)
751.2 Atresia lower (complete) (partial)
751.9 Deformity
750.9 Deformity upper alimentary tract
751.8 Duplication
751.8 Malposition

537.89 GASTROJEJUNAL LOOP OBSTRUCTION SYNDROME

534.## GASTROJEJUNAL ULCER

4th digit: 534
0. Acute with hemorrhage
1. Acute with perforation
2. Acute with hemorrhage and perforation
3. Acute
4. Chronic or unspecified with hemorrhage
5. Chronic or unspecified with perforation
6. Chronic or unspecified with hemorrhage and perforation
7. Chronic
9. Unspecified as acute or chronic

5th digit: 534
0. Without obstruction
1. Obstructed

537.89 GASTROLITHS

536.3 GASTROPARALYSIS

250.6# GASTROPARALYSIS DIABETIC [536.3]

5th digit: 250.6
0. Type II, adult-onset, non-insulin dependent (even if requiring insulin), or unspecified; controlled
1. Type I, juvenile-onset or insulin-dependent; controlled
2. Type II, adult-onset, non-insulin dependent (even if requiring insulin); uncontrolled
3. Type I, juvenile-onset or insulin-dependent; uncontrolled

536.3 GASTROPARESIS

250.6# GASTROPARESIS DIABETIC [536.3]

5th digit: 250.6
0. Type II, adult-onset, non-insulin dependent (even if requiring insulin), or unspecified; controlled
1. Type I, juvenile-onset or insulin-dependent; controlled
2. Type II, adult-onset, non-insulin dependent (even if requiring insulin); uncontrolled
3. Type I, juvenile-onset or insulin-dependent; uncontrolled

537.9 GASTROPATHY

537.89 GASTROPATHY CONGESTIVE PORTAL (HYPERTENSIVE)

535.5 GASTROPATHY ERYTHEMATOUS

579.8 GASTROPATHY, EXUDATIVE

537.89 GASTROPATHY PORTAL HYPERTENSIVE

537.5 GASTROPTOSIS

569.89 GASTROSCHISIS

756.79 GASTROSCHISIS CONGENITAL

578.0 GASTROSTAXIS

Malfunction or infection of a surgical procedure, implant, or artificial opening should be coded as a complication.

GASTROSTOMY

V55.1 Care
V55.1 Catheter adjustment or repositioning
V55.1 Catheter removal or replacement
V55.1 Closure
536.40 Complication NOS
536.42 Complication mechanical
536.49 Complication other
V53.5 Device fitting and adjustment

When coding an infection of an ostomy, use an additional code to specify the organism. See 'Bacterial Infection'

536.41 Infection
536.41 Infection with cellulitis of abdomen [682.2]
536.41 Infection with septicemia [**038.#(#)**]

4th or 4th and 5th digit code for organism: 038
.9 NOS
.3 Anaerobic
.3 Bacteroides
.3 Clostridium
.42 E. coli
.49 Enterobacter aerogenes
.40 Gram negative
.49 Gram negative other
.41 Hemophilus influenzae
.2 Pneumococcal
.49 Proteus
.43 Pseudomonas
.44 Serratia
.10 Staphylococcal NOS
.11 Staphylococcal aureus
.19 Staphylococcal other
.0 Streptococcal (anaerobic)
.49 Yersinia enterocolitica
.8 Other specified

536.42 Malfunction
V55.1 Removal or replacement
V44.1 Status
V55.1 Toilet stoma

272.7 GAUCHER'S CEREBRAL DEGENERATION [330.2]

272.7 GAUCHER'S DISEASE (CEREBROSIDE LIPIDOSIS)

538.82 GAVE (GASTRIC ANTRAL VASCULAR ESTASIA) NOS OR WITHOUT HEMORRHAGE

538.83 GAVE (GASTRIC ANTRAL VASCULAR ESTASIA) WITH HEMORRHAGE

265.1 GAYET-WERNICKE'S (SUPERIOR HEMORRHAGIC POLIOENCEPHALITIS)

265.1 GAYET'S SUPERIOR HEMORRHAGIC POLIOENCEPHALITIS

0 GC SEE 'GONORRHEA'

579.0 GEE (-HERTER) (-HEUBNER) (-THAYSEN) NONTROPICAL SPRUE

347.00 GELINEAU'S SYNDROME SEE ALSO 'NARCOLEPSY'

302.6 GENDER IDENTITY DISORDER NOS

302.85 GENDER IDENTITY DISORDER IN ADOLESCENTS WITH SEX REASSIGNMENT SURGERY [**302.5#**]

302.85 GENDER IDENTITY DISORDER IN ADULTS WITH SEX REASSIGNMENT SURGERY [**302.5#**]

5th digit: 302.5
0. With unspecified sexual history
1. With asexual history
2. With homosexual history
3. With heterosexual history

302.6 GENDER IDENTITY DISORDER IN CHILDREN

799.89 GENERAL CONGESTION

094.1 GENERAL PARESIS SYPHILIS

GENETIC

V83.81 Carrier status cystic fibrosis
V83.89 Carrier status other defect
V26.33 Counseling
V18.9 Disease carrier family history
V82.71 Disease carrier status screening - nonprocreative
V26.31 Female - carrier status testing for procreative management
V26.32 Female - other testing for procreative management

Use an additional code to identify habitual aborter, see 'Habitual Abortion'

V26.34 Male - carrier status testing for procreative management
V26.35 Male partner – carrier status testing of habitual aborter
V26.39 Male - other testing for procreative management
V82.71 Screening for disease carrier status
V82.79 Screening other - nonprocreative

SUSCEPTIBILITY

Code first any current malignant neoplasms. See 'Cancer', by site. Use an additional code, if applicable, for any personal history of malignant neoplasm. See 'History', CA, by site for those codes.

V84.0# Malignant neoplasm

5th digit: V84.0
1. Breast
2. Ovary
3. Prostate
4. Endometrium
9. Other site

Use an additional for any associated family history of the disease. See 'Family History.

V84.81 Mutilple endocrine neoplasia (MEN)
V84.81 Neoplasia multiple endocrine
V84.89 Specified disease

GENETIC (continued)

V26.31 Testing female - carrier status testing for procreative management
V26.32 Testing female - other testing for procreative management

G

GENETIC (continued)

V26.34 Testing male - carrier status testing for procreative management
V26.35 Testing male partner – carrier status testing of habitual aborter
V26.39 Testing male - other testing for procreative management
333.6 Torsion dystonia

351.1 GENICULATE GANGLIONITIS
053.11 GENICULATE GANGLIONITIS HERPETIC

GENITAL/GENITAL ORGAN

V45.77 Absence acquired (female) (male)
752.49 Absence female external (congenital)
752.89 Absence female internal NEC (congenital)
752.89 Absence male (congenital)
752.69 Absence male penis (congenital)
0 Absence see also specified organ
752.89 Accessory female internal NEC
752.89 Accessory male NEC (congenital)
752.9 Anomaly (congenital)
752.40 Anomaly female external (congenital)
752.49 Anomaly female other specified (congenital)
752.89 Anomaly male external (congenital)
752.81 Anomaly male scrotal transposition
752.89 Anomaly NEC
0 Anomaly see also specified organ
752.49 Atresia female external (congenital)
752.89 Atresia female internal (congenital)
752.89 Atresia male external (congenital)
752.89 Atresia male internal (congenital)
608.89 Atrophy male
629.89 Deformity female acquired
629.89 Disease female other specified
629.9 Disorder female
629.89 Disorder female other specified
608.9 Disorder male
752.89 Distortion female internal NEC
752.89 Distortion male NEC
054.10 Herpes
V13.29 History of genital system and obstetric disorder (non gravid)
629.89 Hyperplasia female
608.89 Hyperplasia male
752.89 Hypoplasia female internal
752.89 Hypoplasia male
959.14 Injury external
867.6 Injury internal NEC (traumatic)
867.7 Injury internal NEC (traumatic) with open wound
0 Injury see also specified organ
629.2# Mutilation (cutting) status female
660.8# Mutilation (cutting) status female causing obstructed labor and delivery [629.2#]

5th digit: 660.8
- **0. Episode of care unspecified or N/A**
- **1. Delivered**
- **3. Antepartum complication**

5th digit: 629.2
- **0. Unspecified**
- **1. Type I (clitorectomy)**
- **2. Type II (clitorectomy with excision of labia minora)**
- **3. Type III (infibulation)**
- **9. Type IV or other**

V47.5 Problem NEC

GENITAL/GENITAL ORGAN (continued)

618.9 Prolapse female
618.9 Prolapse female with stress incontinence [625.6]
618.9 Prolapse female with other urinary incontinence [788.3#]
618.8# Prolapse female - other specified
618.8# Prolapse female - other specified with stress incontinence [625.6]
618.8# Prolapse female - other specified with urinary incontinence [788.3#]

5th digit: 618.8
- **1. Pubocervical tissue incompetence (weakening)**
- **2. Rectovaginal tissue incompetence (weakening)**
- **3. Pelvic muscle wasting**
- **4. Cervical stump**
- **9. Other**

5th digit: 788.3
- **1. Urge incontinence**
- **3. Mixed urge and stress**
- **4. Without sensory awareness**
- **5. Post-void dribbling**
- **6. Nocturnal enuresis**
- **7. Continuous leakage**
- **8. Overflow incontinence**
- **9. Other**

625.9 Symptoms female unspecified
625.8 Symptoms female other specified
608.9 Symptoms male unspecified
608.89 Symptoms male other specified
760.8 Tract other localized maternal infection affecting fetus or newborn
078.19 Warts NOS, see also 'Warts', by type

099.1 GENITO-ANORECTAL SYNDROME

GENITOURINARY

793.5 Abnormality on x-ray
752.89 Absence organs NEC - congenital
752.89 Accessory organs NEC - congenital
752.89 Anomaly NEC
V18.7 Diseases other family history
306.50 Disorder (malfunction) psychogenic
599.89 Hemorrhage
599.0 Infection NEC
V81.6 Screening for other and unspecified conditons
306.59 Symptoms psychogenic other

GENU

736.5 Recurvatum acquired
754.40 Recurvatum congenital
736.41 Valgum acquired
755.64 Valgum congenital
736.42 Varum acquired
755.64 Varum congenital

529.1 GEOGRAPHIC TONGUE
307.52 GEOPHAGIA
117.9 GEOTRICHOSIS
300.29 GEPHYROPHOBIA
745.4 GERBODE DEFECT
530.81 GERD (GASTROESOPHAGEAL REFLUX DISEASE)
443.82 GERHARDT'S DISEASE (ERYTHROMELALGIA)
478.30 GERHARDT'S SYNDROME (VOCAL CORD PARALYSIS)

G

078.81 GERLIER'S EPIDEMIC VERTIGO

056.9 GERMAN MEASLES (RUBELLA)

0 GERMAN MEASLES WITH COMPLICATIONS SEE 'RUBELLA'

606.0 GERMINAL CELL APLASIA

606.1 GERMINAL CELL DESQUAMATION

199.1 GERMINOMA SITE UNSPECIFIED

0 GERMINOMA SITE SPECIFIED SEE 'CANCER', BY SITE M9064/3

371.41 GERONTOXON

784.69 GERSTMANN'S SYNDROME (FINGER AGNOSIA)

GESTATION

651.## Multiple

4th digit: 651
0. Twin
1. Triplet
2. Quadruplet
3. Twin with fetal loss
4. Triplet with fetal loss
5. Quadruplet with fetal loss
6. Other multiple pregnancy with fetal loss
7. Following (elective) fetal reduction
8. Other specified
9. Unspecified

5th digit: 651
0. Episode of care unspecified or N/A
1. Delivered
3. Antepartum complication

766.21 Prolonged syndrome over 40 completed weeks to 42 completed weeks

766.22 Prolonged syndrome over 42 completed weeks

0 See 'Pregnancy'

010.0# GHON TUBERCLE

5th digit: 010.0
0. Unspecified
1. Lab not done
2. Lab pending
3. Microscopy positive (in sputum)
4. Culture positive - microscopy negative
5. Culture negative - microscopy positive
6. Culture and microscopy negative confirmed by other methods

370.64 GHOST VESSELS CORNEAL

102.3 GHOUL HAND

578.9 GI BLEEDING

0 GI BLEEDING SEE SPECIFIC CAUSE AND SITE

536.9 GI DISORDER (FUNCTIONAL)

863.80 GI INJURY SITE NOS

863.90 GI INJURY SITE NOS WITH OPEN WOUND

0 GI TRACT SEE 'GASTROINTESTINAL TRACT'

057.8 GIANOTTI CROSTI SYNDROME DUE TO UNKNOWN VIRUS

0 GIANOTTI CROSTI SYNDROME DUE TO KNOWN VIRUS SEE SPECIFIED VIRUS

Carcinomas and neoplasms should be coded by site if possible. Code by cell type, "site NOS", only if a site is not specified in the diagnosis. Otherwise, refer to the appropriate category of neoplasm for a more specific code. See 'Cancer' 'Cancer Metastatic', 'Carcinoma In Situ', 'Neoplasm Uncertain Behavior', 'Neoplasm Unspecified Nature', or 'Benign Neoplasm'.

GIANT CELL

199.1 And spindle cell carcinoma site unspecified

0 And spindle cell carcinoma site specified see 'Cancer', by site M8030/3

446.5 Arteritis

648.9# Arteritis maternal current (co-existent) in pregnancy [446.5]

5th digit: 648.9
0. Episode of care unspecified or N/A
1. Delivered
2. Delivered with postpartum complication
3. Antepartum complication
4. Postpartum complication

199.1 Carcinoma site unspecified

0 Carcinoma site specified see 'Cancer', by site M8031/3

523.8 Epulis

245.1 Thyroiditis

238.0 Tumor bone NOS M9250/1

170.# Tumor bone (malignant) M9250/3

4th digit: 170
0. Skull and face
1. Mandible
2. Vertebral column
3. Ribs, sternum, clavicle
4. Scapula, long bones of upper limb
5. Short bones upper of limb
6. Pelvic bones, sacrum, coccyx
7. Long bones of lower limb
8. Short bones of lower limb
9. Site unspecified

523.8 Tumor gingiva

238.1 Tumor soft and connective tissue NOS

171.# Tumor soft and connective tissue malignant M9251/3

4th digit: 171
0. Head, face, neck
2. Upper limb including shoulder
3. Lower limb including hip
4. Thorax
5. Abdomen (wall), gastric, gastrointestinal, intestine, stomach
6. Pelvis, buttock, groin, inguinal region, perineum
7. Trunk NOS, back NOS, flank NOS,
8. Other specified sites
9. Site unspecified

727.02 Tumor synovial

727.02 Tumor tendon sheath

753.3 GIANT KIDNEY

007.1 GIARDIASIS (INTESTINAL)

696.3 GIBERT'S PITYRIASIS ROSEA

720.9 GIBNEY'S PERISPONDYLITIS

0 GIBRALTAR FEVER SEE 'BRUCELLOSIS'

780.4 GIDDINESS

271.0 GIERKE'S GLYCOGENOSIS I

213.# GIGANTIFORM CEMENTOMA
4th digit: 213
0. Skull, face, upper jaw
1. Lower jaw unspecified

253.0 GIGANTISM

989.5 GILA MONSTER BITE

995.0 GILA MONSTER BITE WITH ANAPHYLAXIS [989.5]

277.4 GILBERT'S SYNDROME (FAMILIAL NONHEMOLYTIC JAUNDICE)

116.0 GILCHRIST'S NORTH AMERICAN BLASTOMYCOSIS

259.8 GILFORD (-HUTCHINSON) SYNDROME (PROGERIA)

307.23 GILLES DE LA TOURETTE'S SYNDROME (MOTOR-VERBAL TIC)

759.89 GILLESPIE'S SYNDROME (DYSPLASIA OCULODENTODIGITALIS)

GINGIVAL

523.9 Disease NOS
523.8 Fibromatosis
523.8 Hyperplasia
0 Infection see 'Gingivitis'
523.10 Keratinization
523.8 Occlusion traumatic
523.2# Recession
5th digit: 523.2
0. Unspecified
1. Minimal
2. Moderate
3. Severe
4. Localized
5. Generalized

523.8 Ulcer

GINGIVITIS

523.10 NOS
523.0# Acute
101 Acute necrotizing (ulcerative)
523.00 Catarrhal
523.1# Chronic
523.1# Chronic nonherpetic
5th digit: 523.0, 1
0. Plaque induced or NOS
1. Non-plaque induced

523.10 Desquamative
523.40 Expulsive
054.2 Herpetic (simplex)
523.10 Hyperplastic
523.10 Marginal, simple
523.10 Ulcerative
101 Vincent's

523.40 GINGIVOPERICENTITIS
523.10 GINGIVOSIS
523.10 GINGIVOSTOMATITIS
054.2 GINGIVOSTOMATITIS HERPES
117.9 GIOVANNINI'S DISEASE
V09.8 GISA (GLYCOPEPTIDE INTERMEDIATE STAPHYLOCOCCUS AUREUS)
024 GLANDERS
289.3 GLANDULAR ATROPHY (LYMPH)
075 GLANDULAR FEVER
752.69 GLANS PENIS DIVISION

287.1 GLANZMANN'S HEREDITARY HEMORRHAGIC THROMBASTHENIA

527.1 GLASSBLOWERS' DISEASE

GLAUCOMA

365.9 NOS
365.9 NOS with glaucomatous flecks [366.31]
360.42 Absolute
365.22 Acute
365.2# Angle closure
365.2# Angle closure with glaucomatous flecks [366.31]
5th digit: 365.2
0. Primary unspecified
1. Intermittent (subacute)
2. Acute
3. Chronic
4. Residual stage

365.00 Borderline
365.01 Borderline open angle
365.01 Borderline open angle with glaucomatous flecks [366.31]
365.02 Borderline narrow angle
365.02 Borderline narrow angle with glaucomatous flecks [366.31]
365.04 Borderline ocular hypertension
365.04 Borderline ocular hypertension with glaucomatous flecks [366.31]
365.03 Borderline steroid responder
365.03 Borderline steroid responder with glaucomatous flecks [366.31]
365.00 Borderline with glaucomatous flecks [366.31]
365.14 Childhood or juvenile
365.14 Childhood or juvenile with glaucomatous flecks [366.31]
365.11 Chronic (simple) (noncongestive) (nonobstructive)
365.11 Chronic (simple) (noncongestive) (nonobstructive) with glaucomatous flecks [366.31]
743.20 Congenital infantile
743.21 Congenital infantile simple
365.3# Corticosteroid induced
365.3# Corticosteroid induced with glaucomatous flecks [366.31]
5th digit: 365.3
1. Glaucomatous stage
2. Residual stage

365.60 Hemorrhagic
365.60 Hemorrhagic with glaucomatous flecks [366.31]
365.81 Hypersecretion
365.81 Hypersecretion with glaucomatous flecks [366.31]
365.14 Infantile
365.14 Infantile with glaucomatous flecks [366.31]
365.14 Juvenile
365.14 Juvenile with glaucomatous flecks [366.31]
365.12 Low tension
365.12 Low tension with glaucomatous flecks [366.31]
365.83 Malignant
365.2# Narrow angle
365.2# Narrow angle with glaucomatous flecks [366.31]
5th digit: 365.2
0. Primary unspecified
1. Intermittent (subacute)
2. Acute
3. Chronic
4. Residual stage

365.60 Neovascular
743.20 Newborn
365.62 Ocular inflammation
365.62 Ocular inflammation with glaucomatous flecks [366.31]

GLAUCOMA (continued)

365.1# Open angle
365.1# Open angle with glaucomatous flecks [366.31]
5th digit: 365.1
0. Unspecified
1. Primary (chronic, simple)
2. Low tension
3. Pigmentary
4. Childhood (juvenile) (infantile)
5. Residual stage

365.01 Open angle with cupping of optic discs
365.01 Open angle with cupping of optic discs with glaucomatous flecks [366.31]
365.51 Phacolytic
365.51 Phacolytic with glaucomatous flecks [366.31]
365.13 Pigmentary
365.13 Pigmentary with glaucomatous flecks [366.31]
365.60 Postinfectious
365.60 Postinfectious with glaucomatous flecks [366.31]
365.52 Pseudoexfoliation
365.52 Pseudoexfoliation with glaucomatous flecks [366.31]
V80.1 Screening
365.60 Secondary
365.60 Secondary with glaucomatous flecks [366.31]
0 Suspect see 'Glaucoma', borderline
095.8 Syphilitic
365.10 Wide angle NOS
365.10 Wide angle NOS with glaucomatous flecks [366.31]
365.82 With episcleral venous pressure increased
365.82 With episcleral venous pressure increased with glaucomatous flecks [366.31]
365.89 Other specified
365.89 Other specified with glaucomatous flecks [366.31]

GLAUCOMA OTHER ETIOLOGIES

250.5# Diabetic [365.44]
5th digit: 250.5
0. Type II, adult-onset, non-insulin dependent (even if requiring insulin), or unspecified; controlled
1. Type I, juvenile-onset or insulin-dependent; controlled
2. Type II, adult-onset, non-insulin dependent (even if requiring insulin); uncontrolled
3. Type I, juvenile-onset or insulin-dependent; uncontrolled

365.65 Trauma (ocular) NEC
767.8 Trauma (ocular) birth trauma
921.3 Trauma (ocular) globe contusion [365.65]
365.65 Trauma (ocular) with glaucomatous flecks [366.31]
743.45 With aniridia [365.42]
743.44 With Axenfeld's anomaly [365.41]
379.33 With dislocation lens anterior [365.59]
379.34 With dislocation lens posterior [365.59]
364.61 With epithelial down growth [365.64]
364.22 With glaucomatocyclitic crisis [365.62]
366.18 With hypermature cataract [365.51]
364.41 With hyphema [365.63]
364.3 With iridocyclitis [365.62]
364.10 With iridocyclitis chronic [365.62]
743.46 With iris anomalies NEC [365.42]
364.51 With iris atrophica [365.42]
364.74 With iris bombe [365.61]
364.42 With iris rubeosis [365.63]
743.41 With microcornea [365.43]

GLAUCOMA OTHER ETIOLOGIES (continued)

224.# With neoplasm benign [365.64]
190.# With neoplasm malignant [365.64]
4th digit: 190, 224
0. Eye globe
1. Orbit
2. Lacrimal gland
3. Conjunctiva
4. Cornea
5. Retina
6. Choroid
7. Lacrimal duct
8. Other specified
9. Unspecified

237.70 With neurofibromatosis (multiple) [365.44]
237.71 With neurofibromatosis type I [365.44]
237.72 With neurofibromatosis type II [365.44]
365.60 With ocular disorder unspecified
365.59 With other lens disorders
365.61 With pupillary block
364.77 With recessed angle [365.65]
362.35 With retinal vein occlusion [365.63]
743.44 With Rieger's anomaly [365.41]
743.36 With spherophakia [365.59]
759.6 With Sturge Weber [365.44]
017.3# With tuberculosis [365.62]
5th digit: 017.3
0. NOS
1. Lab not done
2. Lab pending
3. Microscopy positive (in sputum)
4. Culture positive - microscopy negative
5. Culture negative - microscopy positive
6. Culture and microscopy negative confirmed by other methods

365.64 With tumors or cysts
365.63 With vascular disorders
237.71 With Von Recklinghausen's disease [365.44]

364.22 GLAUCOMATOCYCLITIC CRISES
364.22 GLAUCOMATOCYCLITIC PARS PLANA HYPERPLASIA
0 GLAUCOMATOUS FLECKS (SUBCAPSULAR) SEE 'GLAUCOMA'
569.89 GLENARD'S SYNDROME (ENTEROPTOSIS)
253.2 GLINSKI-SIMMONDS SYNDROME (PITUITARY CACHEXIA)

Carcinomas and neoplasms should be coded by site if possible. Code by cell type, "site NOS", only if a site is not specified in the diagnosis. Otherwise, refer to the appropriate category of neoplasm for a more specific code. See 'Cancer' 'Cancer Metastatic', 'Neoplasm Uncertain Behavior', 'Neoplasm Unspecified Nature', or 'Benign Neoplasm'.

GLIOBLASTOMA

191.9 Site unspecified
0 Site specified see 'Cancer', by site M9440/3
191.9 Giant cell site unspecified
0 Giant cell site specified see 'Cancer', by site M9441/3
191.9 With sarcomatous component site unspecified
0 With sarcomatous component site specified see 'Cancer', by site M9442/3

GLIOMA

191.9 Malignant site unspecified
0 Malignant site specified see 'Cancer', by site M9380/3
191.9 Mixed site unspecified
0 Mixed site specified see 'Cancer', by site M9382/3
237.5 Subependymal site unspecified
0 Subependymal site specified see 'Neoplasm Uncertain Behavior', by site M9383/1

191.9 GLIOMATOSIS CEREBRI SITE UNSPECIFIED
0 GLIOMATOSIS CEREBRI SITE SPECIFIED SEE 'CANCER', BY SITE M9381/3
349.89 GLIOSIS CEREBRAL
336.0 GLIOSIS SPINAL
268.0 GLISSON'S DISEASE (SEE ALSO 'RICKETS')

GLOBE

360.41 Atrophy
360.40 Degeneration
360.20 Degenerative disorder
360.29 Degenerative disorder other
360.9 Disorder
360.89 Disorders other (eye)
376.36 Displacement lateral
360.81 Luxation
0 Protrusion see 'Exophthalmos'

526.1 GLOBULOMAXILLARY CYST
306.4 GLOBUS
300.11 GLOBUS HYSTERICUS
228.0# GLOMANGIOMA M8712/0
5th digit: 228.0
0. Site unspecified
1. Skin and subcutaneous tissue
2. Intracranial structures
3. Retina
4. Intra abdominal structures
9. Other sites

171.# GLOMANGIOSARCOMA M8710/3
4th digit: 171
0. Head, face, neck
2. Upper limb including shoulder
3. Lower limb including hip
4. Thorax
5. Abdomen (wall), gastric, gastrointestinal, intestine, stomach
6. Pelvis, buttock, groin, inguinal region, perineum
7. Trunk NOS, back NOS, flank NOS
8. Other specified sites
9. Site NOS

581.1 GLOMERULAR DISEASE MEMBRANOUS IDIOPATHIC
581.3 GLOMERULAR DISEASE MINIMAL CHANGE
581.3 GLOMERULITIS MINIMAL CHANGE
583.4 GLOMERULITIS PROGRESSIVE OR NECROTIZING

GLOMERULONEPHRITIS

583.# NOS
4th digit: 583
0. Proliferative (diffuse)
1. Membranous
2. Membranoproliferative hypocomplementemic persistent, lobular, mesangiocapillary, mixed membranous and proliferative
4. Rapidly progressive, necrotizing, extracapillary with epithelial crescents
6. With cortical necrosis
7. With medullary (papillary) necrosis
9. Unspecified lesion in kidney

580.# Acute
4th digit: 580
0. Proliferative or post streptococcal
4. Rapidly progressive necrotizing, extracapillary with epithelial crescents
9. Unspecified or hemorrhagic

582.# Chronic
4th digit: 582
0. Proliferative (diffuse)
1. Membranous, sclerosing, focal, segmental hyalinosis
2. Membranoproliferative, endothelial, hypocomplementemic persistent, lobular, mesangiocapillary, mixed membranous and proliferative
4. Rapidly progressive, necrotizing, extracapillary with epithelial crescents
9. Unspecified or hemorrhagic

581.# With nephrotic syndrome
4th digit: 581
0. Proliferative
1. Membranous, epimembranous, focal, sclerosing, segmental hyalinosis
2. Membranoproliferative, lobular, endothelial, hypocomplementemic persistent, lobular, mesangiocapillary, mixed membranous and proliferative
3. Minimal change, foot process, lipoid
9. Unspecified lesion in kidney

The code in the left margin always sequences first. The additional code in brackets to the right of the description is sequenced second. Underlining shows the code number that corresponds to the underlined description. Underlining never implies correct sequencing.

GLOMERULONEPHRITIS DUE TO OTHER CAUSES

277.39 Amyloid [583.81]
277.39 Amyloid chronic [582.81]
277.39 Amyloid with nephrotic syndrome [581.81]
0 Arteriolar see 'Hypertensive', chronic kidney disease
0 Arteriosclerotic see 'Hypertensive', chronic kidney disease
0 Ascending see 'Pyelonephritis'
421.0 Bacterial endocarditis subacute [580.81]
583.89 Basement membrane NEC

G

GLOMERULONEPHRITIS DUE TO OTHER CAUSES (continued)

446.21 Basement membrane with pulmonary hemorrhage (Goodpasture's syndrome) [583.81]
582.89 Chronic (exudative) (focal) (interstitial)
587 Cirrhotic
250.4# Diabetic [583.81]

5th digit: 250.4
0. Type II, adult-onset, non-insulin dependent (even if requiring insulin), or unspecified; controlled
1. Type I, juvenile-onset or insulin-dependent; controlled
2. Type II, adult-onset, non-insulin dependent (even if requiring insulin); uncontrolled
3. Type I, juvenile-onset or insulin-dependent; uncontrolled

032.89 Diphtheria [580.81]
421.0 Endocarditis bacterial subacute [580.81]
581.9 Edema see also 'Nephrosis'
583.89 Exudative NEC
580.89 Exudative acute
582.89 Exudative chronic
583.9 Focal see also 'Nephritis'
098.19 Gonococcal infection acute [583.81]
098.39 Gonococcal infection chronic or lasting 2 or more months [583.81]
582.89 Granular
582.89 Granulomatous
070.9 Hepatitis (infectious) [580.81]
070.6 Hepatitis (infectious) with hepatic coma [580.81]
070.1 Hepatitis viral A (infectious) [580.81]
070.0 Hepatitis viral A (infectious) with hepatic coma [580.81]
070.3# Hepatitis viral B (Australian antigen) [580.81]
070.2# Hepatitis viral B (Australian antigen) with hepatic coma [580.81]

5th digit: 070.2-3
0. Acute or unspecified
1. Acute or unspecified with delta
2. Chronic
3. Chronic with delta

070.70 Hepatitis viral C NOS [580.81]
070.71 Hepatitis viral C NOS with hepatic coma [580.81]
070.5# Hepatitis viral C [580.81]
070.4# Hepatitis viral C with hepatic coma [580.81]

5th digit: 070.4, 5
1. Acute
4. Chronic

070.5# Hepatitis viral other specified (D) (E) [580.81]
070.4# Hepatitis viral other specified (D) (E) with hepatic coma [580.81]

5th digit: 070.4, 5
2. Delta, or delta with B carrier state
3. Hepatitis E
9. Other specified viral

581.9 Hydremic see also 'Nephrosis'
583.89 Immune complex NEC
590.80 Infective see also 'Pyelonephritis'
583.89 Interstitial nephritis (diffuse) (focal) NEC
580.89 Interstitial nephritis (diffuse) (focal) acute
582.89 Interstitial nephritis (diffuse) (focal) chronic
581.89 Interstitial nephritis (diffuse) (focal) with nephrotic syndrome
582.9 Latent or quiescent

GLOMERULONEPHRITIS DUE TO OTHER CAUSES (continued)

710.0 Lupus [583.81]
710.0 Lupus (chronic) (due to) [582.81]
084.9 Malarial [581.81]
072.79 Mumps (due to) [580.81]
581.89 Parenchymatous
590.80 Purulent see also 'Pyelonephritis'
590.80 Septic see also 'Pyelonephritis'
583.89 Specified pathology or lesion NEC
580.89 Specified pathology or lesion acute
582.89 Specified pathology or lesion chronic
581.89 Specified pathology or lesion with nephrotic syndrome
590.80 Suppurative (acute) (disseminated) see also 'Pyelonephritis'
039.8 Streptotrichosis [583.81]
095.4 Syphilis (late)
090.5 Syphilis congenital [583.81]
091.69 Syphilis early [583.81]
016.0# TB [583.81]

5th digit: 016.0
0. Unspecified
1. Lab not done
2. Lab pending
3. Microscopy positive (in sputum)
4. Culture positive - microscopy negative
5. Culture negative - microscopy positive
6. Culture and microscopy negative confirmed by other methods

002.0 Typhoid [580.81]
581.89 With nephrotic syndrome (exudative)
277.39 With nephrotic syndrome amyloid [581.81]

Type I (insulin - dependent) diabetics cannot produce enough insulin to sustain life. Type II (non-insulin dependent) diabetics produce insulin, but have problems utilizing it. Though they may be taking insulin on a day - to - day basis, they are still considered to be non-insulin dependent and therefore, type II diabetics. The physician must document the type for the record to be coded. Use the additional code, V58.67 long-term (current) insulin use for Type II diabetics that take insulin on a day – to – day basis.

250.4# With nephrotic syndrome diabetic [581.81]

5th digit: 250.4
0. Type II, adult-onset, non-insulin dependent (even if requiring insulin), or unspecified; controlled
1. Type I, juvenile-onset or insulin-dependent; controlled
2. Type II, adult-onset, non-insulin dependent (even if requiring insulin); uncontrolled
3. Type I, juvenile-onset or insulin-dependent; uncontrolled

710.0 With nephrotic syndrome lupus [581.81]
084.9 With nephrotic syndrome malarial [581.81]
446.0 With nephrotic syndrome polyarteritis [581.81]

G

Type I (insulin - dependent) diabetics cannot produce enough insulin to sustain life. Type II (non-insulin dependent) diabetics produce insulin, but have problems utilizing it. Though they may be taking insulin on a day - to - day basis, they are still considered to be non-insulin dependent and therefore, type II diabetics. The physician must document the type for the record to be coded. Use the additional code, V58.67 long-term (current) insulin use for Type II diabetics that take insulin on a day – to – day basis.

250.4# GLOMERULOSCLEROSIS DIABETIC [583.81]

5th digit: 250.4

0. Type II, adult-onset, non-insulin dependent (even if requiring insulin), or unspecified; controlled
1. Type I, juvenile-onset or insulin-dependent; controlled
2. Type II, adult-onset, non-insulin dependent (even if requiring insulin); uncontrolled
3. Type I, juvenile-onset or insulin-dependent; uncontrolled

237.3 GLOMUS JUGULARE TUMOR SITE UNSPECIFIED

0 GLOMUS JUGULARE TUMOR SITE SPECIFIED SEE 'NEOPLASM UNCERTAIN BEHAVIOR', BY SITE M8690/1

228.0# GLOMUS TUMOR M8711/0

5th digit: 228.0

0. Site unspecified
1. Skin and subcutaneous tissue
2. Intracranial structures
3. Retina
4. Intrabdominal structures
9. Other sites

GLOSSITIS

529.0 NOS
529.1 Areata exfoliativa
529.4 Atrophic
529.1 Benign migratory
529.0 Gangrenous
529.4 Hunter's (Moeller's)
529.2 Median rhomboid
529.4 Moeller's
265.2 Pellagrous
529.0 Tongue

529.8 GLOSSOCELE

529.6 GLOSSODYNIA

529.4 GLOSSODYNIA EXFOLIATIVA

GLOSSOPHARYNGEAL

352.2 Nerve atrophy
352.2 Nerve disorders (NEC)
951.8 Nerve injury
352.1 Neuralgia
352.1 Neuritis

529.3 GLOSSOPHYTIA

529.8 GLOSSOPTOSIS

529.6 GLOSSOPYROSIS

529.3 GLOSSOTRICHIA

0 GLOTTIC SEE 'GLOTTIS, GLOTTIC'

GLOTTIS, GLOTTIC

748.3 Atresia (absence) congenital
478.6 Edema
478.79 Obstruction
478.30 Paralysis
748.2 Webbing of larynx congenital

251.4 GLUCAGON EXCESS WITH HYPERPLASIA OF PANCREATIC SLIT ALPHA CELLS

251.4 GLUCAGON SECRETION ABNORMALITY

Carcinomas and neoplasms should be coded by site if possible. Code by cell type, "site NOS", only if a site is not specified in the diagnosis. Otherwise, refer to the appropriate category of neoplasm for a more specific code. See 'Cancer' 'Cancer Metastatic', 'Neoplasm Uncertain Behavior', 'Neoplasm Unspecified Nature', or 'Benign Neoplasm'.

211.7 GLUCAGONOMA SITE UNSPECIFIED

0 GLUCAGONOMA SITE SPECIFIED SEE 'BENIGN NEOPLASM', BY SITE M8152/0

157.4 GLUCAGONOMA MALIGNANT SITE UNSPECIFIED

0 GLUCAGONOMA MALIGNANT SITE SPECIFIED SEE 'CANCER', BY SITE M8152/3

270.7 GLUCOGLYCINURIA

255.41 GLUCOCORTICOID COMBINED WITH MINERALOCORTICOID DEFIECIENCY

255.41 GLUCOCORTICOID DEFICIENCY

GLUCOSE

271.0 6 phosphatase deficiency
790.29 Abnormal test NOS
790.21 Abnormal test fasting

Use an additional code, if applicable, for associated insulin use (V58.67), when using code 648.8#.

648.8# Abnormal test of pregnancy (fasting, non-fasting, tolerance test)

5th digit: 648.8

0. Episode of care unspecified or N/A
1. Delivered
2. Delivered with postpartum complication
3. Antepartum complication
4. Postpartum complication

790.22 Abnormal tolerance test
271.3 Galactose intolerance or malabsorption

277.4 GLUCURONYL TRANSFERASE DEFICIENCY

277.4 GLUCURONYL TRANSFERASE SYNDROME

381.20 GLUE EAR SYNDROME

305.9# GLUE SNIFFING ABUSE (NONDEPENDENT)

304.6# GLUE SNIFFING ADDICTION (DEPENDENT)

5th digit: 304.6, 305.9

0. Unspecified
1. Continuous
2. Episodic
3. In remission

270.7 GLUTAMINE METABOLISM DISTURBANCES

270.7 GLUTARIC ACIDURIA TYPE I

277.85 GLUTARIC ACIDURIA TYPE II (TYPE IIA, IIB, IIC)

277.86 GLUTARIC ACIDURIA TYPE III

G

726.5 GLUTEAL TENDINITIS
579.0 GLUTEN ENTEROPATHY
270.7 GLYCINE METABOLISM DISTURBANCES
270.7 GLYCINEMIA
270.0 GLYCINURIA (RENAL)
271.0 GLYCOGEN STORAGE METABOLISM DISORDER (NEC) - CARDIAC [425.7]
271.0 GLYCOGEN STORAGE METABOLISM DISORDER (NEC) - GENERALIZED
271.0 GLYCOGEN STORAGE METABOLISM DISORDER (NEC) – HEPATORENAL
271.0 GLYCOGEN SYNTHETASE DEFICIENCY
271.0 GLYCOGENOSIS CARDIAC - CARDIOMYOPATHY [425.7]
271.0 GLYCOGENOSIS CORI TYPES I-VII
271.0 GLYCOGENOSIS MYOPHOSPHORLASE DEFICIENCY
271.8 GLYCOLIC ACIDURIA CARBOHYDRATE TRANSPORT DISORDERS
V09.8 GLYCOPEPTIDE INTERMEDIATE STAPHYLOCOCCUS AUREUS (GISA)
V09.8 GLYCOPEPTIDE RESISTANT ENTEROCOCCUS OR STAPHYLOCOCCUS AUREUS (GRSA)
270.8 GLYCOPROLINURIA

GLYCOSURIA

791.5 Unspecified
250.4# Diabetic

5th digit: 250.4

0. Type II, adult-onset, non-insulin dependent (even if requiring insulin), or unspecified; controlled

1. Type I, juvenile-onset or insulin-dependent; controlled

2. Type II, adult-onset, non-insulin dependent (even if requiring insulin); uncontrolled

3. Type I, juvenile-onset or insulin-dependent; uncontrolled

271.4 Renal
128.1 GNATHOSTOMA SPINIGERUM INFECTION
128.1 GNATHOSTOMIASIS

GOITER

240.9 Unspecified
241.9 Adenomatous
246.1 Congenital (dyshormonogenic)
240.9 Diffuse colloid
246.1 Due to enzyme defect in synthesis of thyroid hormone
246.1 Dyshormonogenic
240.9 Endemic
0 Exophthalmic see 'Thyrotoxicosis'
0 Goiter thyrotoxic see 'Thyrotoxicosis'
240.9 Hyperplastic
245.2 Lymphadenoid
240.9 Nontoxic diffuse
241.1 Nontoxic multinodular
241.9 Nontoxic nodular
241.0 Nontoxic uninodular
240.9 Parenchymatous
240.0 Simple
240.9 Sporadic
0 Toxic or with hyperthyroidism see 'Thyrotoxicosis'

259.5 GOLDBERG (-MAXWELL) (-MORRIS) SYNDROME (TESTICULAR FEMINIZATION)
440.1 GOLDBLATT'S HYPERTENSION DUE TO RENAL ARTERY OBSTRUCTION
756.0 GOLDENHAR'S SYNDROME (OCULOAURICULOVERTEBRAL DYSPLASIA)
358.00 GOLDFLAM -ERB DISEASE OR SYNDROME
358.01 GOLDFLAM -ERB DISEASE OR SYNDROME WITH (ACUTE) EXACERBATION (CRISIS)
757.39 GOLDSCHEIDER'S EPIDERMOLYSIS BULLOSA
448.0 GOLDSTEIN'S FAMILIAL HEMORRHAGIC TELANGIECTASIA
726.32 GOLFER'S ELBOW
757.39 GOLTZ-GORLIN SYNDROME (DERMAL HYPOPLASIA)

GONADAL

752.7 Dysgenesis (congenital) (pure)
758.6 Dysgenesis (ovarian) (X O syndrome)

GONADOBLASTOMA

236.2 Female site unspecified
0 Female site specified see 'Neoplasm Uncertain Behavior', by site M8710/3
236.4 Male site unspecified
0 Male site specified see 'Neoplasm Uncertain Behavior', by site M8710/3

125.6 GONGYLONEMIASIS
364.73 GONIOSYNECHIAE

GONOCOCCAL

098.0 NOS
098.7 Anusitis
098.7 Anus infection
098.50 Arthritis
098.52 Bursitis
098.35 Cervicitis chronic
098.2 Chronic NEC
098.84 Endocarditis
098.36 Endometritis chronic
098.42 Endophthalmia
098.13 Epididymo-orchitis acute
098.33 Epididymo-orchitis chronic
098.40 Eye (newborn)
098.49 Eye infection other
098.37 Fallopian tube (chronic)
098.17 Fallopian tube acute
0 Genitourinary see 'Gonorrhea'
098.89 Gonococcemia other
098.85 Heart disease other
098.41 Iridocyclitis
098.50 Joint NOS
098.59 Joint other
098.43 Keratitis
098.81 Keratoderma
098.81 Keratosis (blennorrhagica)
098.89 Lymphatic (gland) (node)
098.82 Meningitis
098.13 Orchitis acute
098.33 Orchitis chronic
098.19 Pelvis (acute)
098.39 Pelvis chronic
098.83 Pericarditis
098.86 Peritonitis
098.6 Pharyngitis
098.6 Pharynx infection

G

GONOCOCCAL (continued)

098.7 Proctitis
098.12 Prostatitis acute
098.32 Prostatitis chronic
098.37 Pyosalpinx (chronic)
098.17 Pyosalpinx acute
098.7 Rectum infection
098.59 Rheumatism
098.17 Salpingitis acute
098.37 Salpingitis chronic
098.14 Seminal vesiculitis acute
098.34 Seminal vesiculitis chronic
098.89 Septicemia
098.89 Skin
098.53 Spondylitis
098.51 Synovitis
098.51 Tenosynovitis
098.6 Throat
0 Urethra see 'Gonorrhea'
0 Vulva see 'Gonorrhea'
098.89 Other

Acute sequences before chronic.

098.89 GONOCOCCEMIA

GONORRHEA

098.0 Acute
098.50 Arthritis
098.11 Bladder acute
098.31 Bladder chronic
098.52 Bursitis
V02.7 Carrier
098.35 Cervicitis chronic
098.15 Cervix (acute)
098.2 Chronic (lower GU tract)
098.30 Chronic upper tract
098.39 Chronic other site
098.40 Conjunctivitis (neonatorum)
V65.45 Counseling
098.31 Cystitis chronic
098.36 Endometritis chronic
098.33 Epididymo-orchitis chronic
V01.6 Exposure
098.89 Gonococcemia other
098.10 Infection (acute) upper genitourinary tract site unspecified
098.59 Infection of joint other
098.19 Infection other acute
655.4# Maternal (with known/suspected damage to fetus)
5th digit: 655.4
0. Episode of care unspecified or N/A
1. Delivered
3. Antepartum complication

647.1#, Use an additional code to identify the maternal gonorrhea.

647.1# Maternal current (co-existent) in pregnancy
5th digit: 647.1
0. Episode of care unspecified or N/A
1. Delivered
2. Delivered with postpartum complication
3. Antepartum complication
4. Postpartum complication

GONORRHEA (continued)

098.6 Pharyngitis
098.32 Prostatitis chronic
098.59 Rheumatism
098.17 Salpingitis acute
098.37 Salpingitis chronic
098.14 Seminal vesiculitis acute
098.34 Seminal vesiculitis chronic
098.53 Spondylitis
098.51 Synovitis
098.51 Tenosynovitis
098.16 Uterus (acute)
098.36 Uterus chronic
098.89 Other specified site
098.59 Other

279.06 GOOD'S SYNDROME
078.82 GOODALL'S EPIDEMIC VOMITING
446.21 GOODPASTURE'S SYNDROME (PNEUMORENAL)
648.9# GOODPASTURE'S SYNDROME MATERNAL CURRENT (CO-EXISTENT) IN PREGNANCY [446.21]
5th digit: 648.9
0. Episode of NOS or N/A
1. Delivered
2. Delivered with postpartum complication
3. Antepartum complication
4. Postpartum complication

446.21 GOODPASTURE'S SYNDROME WITH NEPHRITIS [583.81]
266.2 GOPALAN'S SYNDROME (BURNING FEET)
579.8 GORDON'S EXUDATIVE ENTEROPATHY
709.1 GOUGEROT BLUM DERMATITIS
701.8 GOUGEROT CARTEAUD SYNDROME OR DISEASE (CONFLUENT RETICULATE PAPILLOMATOSIS)
757.39 GOUGEROT-HAILEY-HAILEY DISEASE (BENIGN FAMILIAL CHRONIC PEMPHIGUS)
710.2 GOUGEROT (-HOUWER) -SJOGREN SYNDROME (KERATOCONJUNCTIVITIS SICCA)
423.2 GOULEY'S SYNDROME (CONSTRICTIVE PERICARDITIS)
102.6 GOUNDOU

GOUT

274.9 Unspecified
274.0 Arthritis
274.89 Other manifestations
V77.5 Screening
274.0 Synovitis
095.8 Syphilitic [274.9]

GOUTY

274.89 Neuritis [357.4]
274.10 Neuropathy
274.19 Neuropathy other
274.81 Tophi ear
274.82 Tophi heart
274.82 Tophi other sites

359.1 GOWER'S MUSCULAR DYSTROPHY
377.04 GOWERS PATON KENNEDY SYNDROME
780.2 GOWER'S VASOVAGAL SYNDROME
620.0 GRAAFIAN FOLLICLE CYST
383.02 GRADENIGO'S SYNDROME

G

GRAFT

440.3# Bypass arteriosclerosis extremities
440.3# Bypass arteriosclerosis extremities with chronic complete or total occlusion [440.4]
5th digit: 440.3
0. Unspecified graft
1. Autologous vein bypass graft
2. Nonautologous biological bypass graft

414.0# Bypass coronary arteriosclerosis
414.0# Bypass coronary arteriosclerosis with chronic complete or total occlusion [414.2]
5th digit: 414.0
2. Autologous vein bypass graft
3. Nonautologous biological bypass graft
4. Autologous artery bypass graft (gastroepiploic) (internal mammary)
5. Unspecified type of bypass graft
7. Bypass graft of transplanted heart

996.61 Bypass coronary artery - infection or inflammation
996.03 Bypass coronary artery - mechanical complication
996.72 Bypass coronary artery - other complication
V45.81 Bypass coronary status
V45.3 Bypass intestinal status
996.52 Complication other tissue NEC mechanical
996.69 Corneal - infection or inflammation
996.51 Corneal - mechanical complication
996.79 Corneal - other complication
996.55 Skin artificial failure or rejection (dislodgement) (displacement) (non-adherence) (poor incorporation) (shearing)
996.55 Skin decellularized allodermis failure or rejection (dislodgement) (displacement) (non-adherence) (poor incorporation) (shearing)
996.52 Skin failure or rejection
996.69 Skin infection inflammation
996.79 Skin other complication
996.85 Versus host disease (bone marrow)

424.3 GRAHAM STEELL'S MURMUR
495.8 GRAIN HANDLERS' DISEASE OR LUNG
0 GRAM NEGATIVE SEE 'BACTERIAL INFECTION' OR SPECIFIED CONDITION
0 GRANCHER'S SPLENOPNEUMONIA SEE 'PNEUMONIA'

GRAND MAL EPILEPSY

345.10 NOS
345.11 With intractable epilepsy
345.3 With status

659.4# GRAND MULTIPARITY
5th digit: 659.4
0. Episode of care unspecified or N/A
1. Delivered
3. Antepartum complication

GRANULAR CELL

0 Carcinoma site specified see 'Cancer', by site M8320/3
215.# Tumor benign M9580/0
171.# Tumor malignant M9580/3
4th digit: 171, 215
0. Head, face, neck
2. Upper limb including shoulder
3. Lower limb including hip
4. Thorax
5. Abdomen (wall), gastric, gastrointestinal, intestine, stomach
6. Pelvis, buttock, groin, inguinal region, perineum
7. Trunk unspecified, back unspecified, flank unspecified
8. Other specified sites
9. Site unspecified

701.5 GRANULATION EXCESSIVE
701.5 GRANULATION TISSUE POSTOPERATIVE
288.69 GRANULOCYTIC HYPERPLASIA
288.00 GRANULOCYTOPENIA (PRIMARY)
288.09 GRANULOCYTOPENIA MALIGNANT

GRANULOMA

568.89 Abdomen wall
695.89 Annulare
569.49 Anus
522.6 Apical
543.9 Appendix
380.23 Aural
503 Beryllium lung
709.4 Beryllium skin
730.1# Bone
5th digit: 730.1
0. Site unspecified
1. Shoulder region
2. Upper arm (elbow) (humerus)
3. Forearm (radius) (wrist) (ulna)
4. Hand (carpal) (metacarpal) (fingers)
5. Pelvic thigh (hip) (buttock) (femur)
6. Lower leg (fibula) (knee) (patella) (tibia)
7. Ankle and/or foot (metatarsals) (toes) (tarsals)
8. Other (head) (neck) (rib) (skull) (trunk) (vertebrae)
9. Multiple

277.89 Bone - eosinophilic
526.3 Bone jaw
733.99 Bone residual foreign body
348.8 Cerebral
375.81 Canaliculus lacrimalis
385.82 Cholesterin mastoid
385.82 Cholesterin middle ear
114.3 Coccidioidal (progressive)
114.4 Coccidioidal lung chronic
114.0 Coccidioidal lung primary
114.2 Coccidioidal meninges
569.89 Colon
372.61 Conjunctiva
522.6 Dental
385.82 Ear (middle) and mastoid (cholesterin)
0 Ear with otitis media see 'Otitis Media'

G

GRANULOMA (continued)

277.89 Eosinophilic
277.89 Eosinophilic - bone
277.89 Eosinophilic - lung
528.9 Eosinophilic - oral mucosa
374.89 Eyelid
701.8 Faciale
523.8 Fissuratum (gum)
686.1 Foot NEC (pyogenic)
733.99 Foreign body - bone
728.82 Foreign body - muscle
709.4 Foreign body - skin and subcutaneous tissue
728.82 Foreign body - soft tissue
0 Fungoides see 'Mycosis Fungoides'
446.3 Gangraenescens
526.3 Giant cell - central
523.8 Giant cell - gingiva
523.8 Giant cell - gum
526.3 Giant cell - jaw
523.8 Giant cell - peripheral
0 Hodgkin's see 'Hodgkin's Disease', granuloma
523.8 Gum (giant cell)
569.89 Ileum
136.9 Infectious NEC
099.2 Inguinale
569.89 Intestine
364.10 Iridocyclitis
590.9 Kidney
375.81 Lacrimal passages
478.79 Larynx
446.3 Lethal midline
277.89 Lipid
277.89 Lipoid
572.8 Liver
515 Lung NOS or chronic
114.4 Lung - coccidioidal
515 Lung - due to inorganic dust
277.89 Lung - eosinophilic (infectious)
289.3 Lymph gland
110.6 Majocchi's
446.3 Malignant (face)
526.3 Mandible
519.3 Mediastinum
112.3 Monilial (of skin and nails)
728.82 Muscle
473.9 Nasal sinus (see also 'Sinusitis')
998.59 Operation wound
528.9 Oral mucosa (eosinophilic) (pyogenic)
376.11 Orbital
116.1 Paracoccidioidal
099.2 Penis venereal
568.89 Peritoneal
383.33 Postmastoidectomy cavity
998.59 Postoperative wound
601.8 Prostate
099.2 Pudendi (ulcerating)
522.6 Pyogenic - maxillary alveolar ridge
528.9 Pyogenic - oral mucosa
686.1 Pyogenic - skin
569.49 Rectal sphincter
277.89 Reticulohistiocytic
705.89 Rubrum nasi
135 Sarcoid
686.1 Septic (skin)
709.4 Silica skin

GRANULOMA (continued)

709.4 Skin from foreign body
686.1 Skin pyogenic
686.1 Skin septic
686.1 Skin suppurative
094.89 Spine syphilitic (epidural)
015.0# Spine tuberculous [730.88]

5th digit: 015.0
- **0. NOS**
- **1. Lab not done**
- **2. Lab pending**
- **3. Microscopy positive (in sputum)**
- **4. Culture positive - microscopy negative**
- **5. Culture negative - microscopy positive**
- **6. Culture and microscopy negative confirmed by other methods**

998.89 Stitch postoperative - external
998.89 Stitch postoperative - internal
686.1 Suppurative (skin)
998.89 Suture postoperative - external
998.89 Suture postoperative - internal
031.1 Swimming pool
728.82 Talc
998.7 Talc in operation wound
686.1 Telangiectaticum (skin)
521.49 Tooth pulp (internal)
519.09 Tracheostomy
110.6 Trichophyticum
102.4 Tropicum
686.1 Umbilicus
771.4 Umbilicus newborn
599.84 Urethral
364.10 Uveitis
099.2 Vagina (venereum)
099.2 Venereum
478.5 Vocal cords
446.4 Wegener's (necrotizing respiratory granulomatosis)

277.89 GRANULOMATOSIS LIPOID
446.4 GRANULOMATOSIS RESPIRATORY NECROTIZING
686.1 GRANULOMATOSIS NEC
288.1 GRANULOMATOUS DISEASE CHRONIC (CHILDHOOD)

Carcinomas and neoplasms should be coded by site if possible. Code by cell type, "site NOS", only if a site is not specified in the diagnosis. Otherwise, refer to the appropriate category of neoplasm for a more specific code. See 'Cancer' 'Cancer Metastatic', 'Carcinoma In Situ', 'Neoplasm Uncertain Behavior', 'Neoplasm Unspecified Nature', or 'Benign Neoplasm'.

GRANULOSA CELL

236.2 Theca cell tumor site unspecified
0 Theca cell tumor site specified see 'Neoplasm Uncertain Behavior', by site M8621/1
183.0 Tumor malignant site unspecified
0 Tumor malignant site specified see 'Cancer', by site M8620/3
236.2 Tumor site unspecified
0 Tumor site specified see 'Neoplasm Uncertain Behavior', by site M8620/1

705.89 GRANULOSIS RUBRA NASI

503 GRAPHITE LUNG DISEASE
242.00 GRAVES DISEASE (EXOPHTHALMIC GOITER)
242.01 GRAVES DISEASE (EXOPHTHALMIC GOITER) WITH CRISIS OR STORM
994.9 GRAVITATIONAL EFFECTS ABNORMAL
909.4 GRAVITATIONAL EFFECTS ABNORMAL LATE EFFECT
779.4 GRAY OR GREY SYNDROME (CHLORAMPHENICOL) (NEWBORN)
0 GREASE GUN INJURY SEE 'OPEN WOUND', BY SITE, COMPLICATED
078.89 GREEN MONKEY DISEASE
330.0 GREENFIELD'S DISEASE
309.0 GRIEF REACTION
756.0 GRIEG'S SYNDROME (HYPERTELORISM)
126.9 GRIESINGER'S DISEASE (SEE ALSO 'ANCYLOSTOMA, ANCYCLOSOMIASIS')
502 GRINDERS' DISEASE
723.5 GRISEL'S DISEASE

GROIN

959.19 Injury
911.8 Injury superficial
911.9 Injury superficial infected
848.8 Sprain

GROWTH

253.3 Hormone deficiency
253.0 Hormone overproduction
783.43 Failure childhood
783.43 Lack childhood
V21.0 Rapid in childhood
783.43 Retardation childhood
0 Retardation fetal see 'Fetal - Infant's Record', growth retardation

V09.8 GRSA (GLYCOPEPTIDE RESISTANT STAPHYLOCOCCUS AUREUS)
110.0 GRUBY'S DISEASE (TINEA TONSURANS)
0 GSW SEE 'OPEN WOUND', BY SITE OR ANATOMICAL INJURY
599.0 GU INFECTION NEC

646.6#: Specify the type of maternal GU infection with an additional code.

646.6# GU INFECTION COMPLICATING PREGNANCY
5th digit: 646.6
0. Episode of care unspecified or N/A
1. Delivered
2. Delivered with postpartum complication
3. Antepartum complication
4. Postpartum complication

066.3 GUAMA FEVER (VIRAL)
344.89 GUBLER (-MILLARD) PARALYSIS (SYNDROME)
754.89 GUERIN-STERN SYNDROME (ATHROGRYPOSIS MULTPLEX CONGENITA)
049.8 GUERTIN'S DISEASE (ELECTRIC CHOREA)

357.0 GUILLAIN-BARRE (-STROHL) SYNDROME ACUTE INFECTIVE POLYNEURITIS
125.7 GUINEA WORM INFECTION
307.23 GUINON'S DISEASE (MOTOR-VERBAL TIC)
750.3 GULLET ATRESIA (CONGENITAL)
244.# GULL'S DISEASE (THYROID ATROPHY WITH MYXEDEMA)
4th digit: 244
0. Postsurgical
1. Postablative (irradiation)
2. Iodine ingestion
3. PAS, phenylbut, resorcinol
8. Secondary NEC
9. NOS

GUM

523.2# Atrophy (attrition)
5th digit: 523.2
0. Unspecified
1. Minimal
2. Moderate
3. Severe
4. Localized
5. Generalized

523.9 Disease NEC
523.8 Hyperplasia
523.8 Hypertrophy
959.09 Injury
910.8 Injury superficial
910.9 Injury superficial infected
523.30 Suppuration
0 See also 'Alveolar' or 'Gingival'

102.6 GUMMA, BONE OF YAWS (LATE)
090.5 GUMMA DUE TO CONGENITAL SYPHILIS MANIFEST 2 YRS. OR MORE AFTER BIRTH
0 GUMMA SEE 'SYPHILIS'
102.6 GUMMATOUS OSTEITIS OR PERIOSTEITIS OF YAWS (LATE)
0 GUN SHOT WOUND SEE 'OPEN WOUND', BY SITE OR ANATOMICAL INJURY
742.8 GUNN'S SYNDROME (JAW-WINKING SYNDROME)
277.1 GUNTHER'S DISEASE OR SYNDROME (CONGENITAL ERYTHROPOIETIC PORPHYRIA)
350.8 GUSTATORY SWEATING SYNDROME
752.7 GYNANDRISM CONGENITAL

GYNANDROBLASTOMA

236.2 Female site unspecified
0 Female site specified see 'Neoplasm Uncertain Behavior', by site M8632/1
236.4 Male site unspecified
0 Male site specified see 'Neoplasm Uncertain Behavior', by site M8632/1

738.6 GYNECOID PELVIS MALE
629.9 GYNECOLOGICAL DISEASE
629.89 GYNECOLOGICAL DISEASE SPECIFIED NEC
V72.31 GYNECOLOGICAL EXAM (ROUTINE)
611.1 GYNECOMASTIA NONPUERPERAL
300.29 GYNEPHOBIA

759.81 H 30 SYNDROME
270.0 H DISEASE
0 H. INFLUENZA SEE 'BACTERIAL INFECTION' OR SPECIFIED CONDITION
0 H. PYLORI INFECTION SEE 'BACTERIAL INFECTION' OR SPECIFIED CONDITION
732.3 HAAS' DISEASE
696.2 HABERMANN'S DISEASE (ACUTE PARAPSORIASIS VARIOLIFORMIS)
629.81 HABITUAL ABORTER
V26.35 HABITUAL ABORTER ENCOUNTER FOR TESTING OF MALE PARTNER
646.3# HABITUAL ABORTER CURRENT PREGNANCY
5th digit: 646.3
0. Episode of care NOS OR N/A
1. Delivered
3. Antepartum complication

634.## HABITUAL ABORTER WITH CURRENT ABORTION
4th digit: 634
0. With infection
1. Delayed or excessive hemorrhage
2. Damage to pelvic organs or tissue
3. Renal failure
4. Metabolic disorder
5. Shock
6. Embolism
7. Other specified complications
8. Unspecified complication
9. Uncomplicated
5th digit: 634
0. NOS
1. Incomplete
2. Complete

577.8 HADFIELD CLARKE SYNDROME PANCREATIC INFANTILISM
985.1 HAFF DISEASE
286.3 HAGEMAN FACTOR II DEFICIENCY
717.89 HAGLUND-LAWEN-FRUND SYNDROME
732.5 HAGLUND'S DISEASE (OSTEOCHONDROSIS OS TIBIALE EXTERNUM)
731.2 HAGNER'S DISEASE (HYPERTROPHIC PULMONARY OSTEOARTHROPATHY)
757.39 HAILEY-HAILEY DISEASE (BENIGN FAMILIAL CHRONIC PEMPHIGUS)

HAIR
757.4 Absence (congenital)
704.9 And hair follicles disease
704.8 And hair follicles disease specified NEC
704.2 Atrophic
704.3 Canities (premature)
704.3 Circumscripta acquired
704.3 Color variation
704.3 Grayness (premature)
704.1 Growth excessive (unusual location)
704.3 Heterochromia
704.00 Loss
307.9 Plucking
704.00 Thinning
915.8 Tourniquet syndrome fingers
915.9 Tourniquet syndrome fingers infected
911.8 Tourniquet syndrome penis
911.9 Tourniquet syndrome penis infected
917.8 Tourniquet syndrome toe
917.9 Tourniquet syndrome toe infected
V50.0 Transplant (elective)

257.8 HAIRLESS WOMEN SYNDROME
202.4# HAIRY CELL LEUKEMIA M9940/3
5th digit: 202.4
0. NOS
1. Lymph nodes of head, face, neck
2. Lymph nodes intrathoracic
3. Lymph nodes abdominal
4. Lymph nodes axilla and upper limb
5. Lymph nodes inguinal region and lower limb
6. Lymph nodes intrapelvic
7. Spleen
8. Lymph nodes multiple sites

784.99 HALITOSIS
756.0 HALLERMANN STREIFF SYNDROME
333.0 HALLERVORDEN SPATZ DISEASE
696.1 HALLOPEAU'S ACRODERMATITIS
701.0 HALLOPEAU'S DISEASE (LICHEN SCLEROSUS ET ATROPHICUS)

HALLUCINATION
780.1 NOS (auditory) (gustatory) (olfactory) (tactile)
291.3 Alcoholic (acute) (psychotic)
305.3# Drug induced (bad trip)
5th digit: 305.3
0. NOS
1. Continuous
2. Episodic
3. In remission

292.12 Drug induced (nonhallucinogenic drug)
780.1 Nonpsychotic nonorganic
293.82 Transient psychotic disorder in conditions classified elsewhere
368.16 Visual

305.3# HALLUCINOGEN ABUSE (NONDEPENDENT)
304.5# HALLUCINOGEN ADDICTION (DEPENDENT)
5th digit: 304.5, 305.3
0. NOS
1. Continuous
2. Episodic
3. In remission

760.73 HALLUCINOGENIC TRANSMITTED VIA PLACENTA OR BREAST MILK AFFECTING FETUS OR NEWBORN

HALLUX
735.9 Deformity acquired
735.8 Limitus
735.3 Malleus
735.2 Rigidus
735.0 Valgus acquired
755.66 Valgus congenital
735.1 Varus acquired
755.66 Varus congenital

368.15 HALO VISUAL
757.32 HAMARTOMAS VASCULAR CONGENITAL
759.6 HAMARTOSES OTHER SPECIFIED NEC CONGENITAL
516.3 HAMMAN RICH SYNDROME
518.1 HAMMAN'S SYNDROME (SPONTANEOUS MEDIASTINAL EMPHYSEMA)
735.4 HAMMER TOE ACQUIRED
755.66 HAMMER TOE CONGENITAL

H

728.89 HAMSTRING CONTRACTURE NOS
728.85 HAMSTRING CONTRACTURE MUSCLE
727.81 HAMSTRING CONTRACTURE TENDON
843.8 HAMSTRING SPRAIN

HAND

755.21 Absence (complete) (partial) (congenital)
V49.63 Absence acquired
755.28 Agenesis
V49.63 Amputation status
726.4 Bone spur
736.00 Deformity acquired
074.3 Foot and mouth disease
693.0 Foot syndrome
959.4 Injury - NOS (except finger)
914.8 Injury - other and NOS superficial
914.9 Injury - other and NOS superficial infected
719.84 Joint calcification
842.10 Separation (rupture) (tear) (laceration) site NOS
842.10 Strain (sprain) (avulsion) (hemarthrosis) site NOS

277.89 HAND - SCHULLER - CHRISTIAN DISEASE (CHRONIC HISTIOCYTOSIS X)
V61.49 HANDICAPPED PERSON (CARE) (PRESENCE) (PROBLEM) (IN FAMILY) (IN HOUSEHOLD)
V60.4 HANDICAPPED PERSON (FAMILY MEMBER) UNSUITED TO RENDER CARE
305.0# HANGOVER
5th digit: 305.0
0. NOS
1. Continuous
2. Episodic
3. In remission

275.0 HANOT-CHAUFFARD (-TROISIER) (BRONZE DIABETES) SYNDROME
0 HANOT'S DISEASE SEE 'CIRRHOSIS', BILIARY
0 HANSEN'S DISEASE SEE 'LEPROSY'
079.81 HANTAAN PUUMALA VIRUS
079.81 HANTAVIRUS INFECTION
757.39 HAR HAILEY SYNDROME
363.22 HARADA'S DISEASE OR SYNDROME
749.1# HARE LIP
5th digit: 749.1
0. NOS
1. Unilateral complete
2. Unilateral incomplete
3. Bilateral complete
4. Bilateral incomplete

162.3 HARE'S SYNDROME (CARCINOMA, PULMONARY APEX) M8010/3
446.0 HARKAVY'S SYNDROME
779.89 HARLEQUIN COLOR CHANGE SYNDROME
757.1 HARLEQUIN FETUS
283.2 HARLEY'S DISEASE (INTERMITTENT HEMOGLOBINURIA)
251.1 HARRIS' SYNDROME (ORGANIC HYPERINSULISM)
575.8 HARTMANN'S POUCH
V55.3 HARTMANN'S POUCH OF INTESTINE ATTENTION TO
V44.3 HARTMANN'S POUCH OF INTESTINE STATUS
270.0 HARTNUP DISEASE

270.0 HART'S SYNDROME (PELLAGRA-CEREBELLAR ATAXIA-RENAL AMINOACIDURIA)
304.3# HASHISH ADDICTION (DEPENDENT)
5th digit: 304.3
0. NOS
1. Continuous
2. Episodic
3. In remission

245.2 HASHIMOTO'S THYROIDITIS (STRUMA LYMPHOMATOSA)
371.41 HASSALL HENLE BODIES
026.1 HAVERHILL FEVER

HAY FEVER

477.9 Unspecified
477.2 Due to dander, animal (cat) (dog)
477.1 Due to food
477.2 Due to hair, animal (cat) (dog)
477.0 Due to pollen
477.8 Due to other allergen

280.9 HAYEM-FABER SYNDROME (ACHLORHYDRIC ANEMIA)
283.9 HAYEM-WIDAL SYNDROME (ACQUIRED HEMOLYTIC JAUNDICE)
715.04 HAYGARTH'S NODULE
282.5 HB AS GENOTYPE
282.49 HB BART'S DISEASE
282.5 HB S
790.09 HCT ABNORMAL
790.01 HCT DROP (PRECIPITOUS)
272.5 HDL DEFICIENCY (HIGH DENSITY LIPOID)

HEAD

307.3 Banging
900.9 Blood vessel NOS injury
0 Blood vessel NEC injury - intracranial see 'Intracranial Injury'
900.82 Blood vessel NEC injury - multiple
900.89 Blood vessel NEC injury - specified NEC
V48.0 Deficiency
738.1# Deformity other acquired
5th digit: 738.1
0. Unspecified
1. Zygomatic hyperplasia
2. Zygomatic hypoplasia
9. Other specified

V48.6 Disfigurement
959.01 Injury NOS
0 Injury with concussion see 'Concussion'
0 Injury with intracranial injury see specified intracranial injury
132.0 Lice
781.0 Movements abnormal
784.0 Pain
V48.9 Problem
V48.2 Problem mechanical and motor
V48.8 Problem other
V48.4 Problem sensory
739.0 Region segmental or somatic dysfunction
784.2 Swelling mass or lump
784.99 Symptom other

HEADACHE

784.0 NOS
346.2# Allergic
784.0 Analgesic rebound
346.2# Cluster
346.2# Histamine
349.0 Lumbar puncture (due to)
627.2 Menopausal
627.4 Menopausal artificial
0 Migraine see 'Migraine'
625.4 Premenstrual
307.81 Psychogenic or of inorganic origin
349.0 Saddle block (due to)
346.1# Sick
5th digit: 346.1-2
0. Without mention intractable migraine
1. With intractable migraine
668.8# Spinal complicating labor and delivery
5th digit: 668.8
0. Episode of care NOS
1. Delivered with or without mention of antepartum condition
2. Delivered with mention of postpartum complication
3. Antepartum condition
4. Postpartum complication
349.0 Spinal fluid loss (due to)
668.8# Spinal postpartum
5th digit: 668.8
0. Episode of care NOS
1. Delivered with or without mention of antepartum condition
2. Delivered with mention of postpartum complication
3. Antepartum condition
4. Postpartum complication
307.81 Tension
784.0 Vascular
346.9# Vasomotor
5th digit: 346.9
0. Without mention intractable migraine
1. With intractable migraine

0 HEALTH CHECK TYPE SEE 'EXAM'
0 HEALTH COUNSELING SEE 'COUNSELING'
V65.0 HEALTHY PERSON ACCOMPANYING SICK PERSON

HEARING

V53.2 Aid fitting and adjustment
V72.12 Conservation and treatment
V72.19 Exam
V72.11 Exam following failed hearing screening
V20.2 Exam infant

Code first hearing and/or visual impairment.

V49.85 Impairment dual (blindness with deafness) (combined visual hearing impairment)
V41.2 Problem
0 See 'Auditory'

HEARING LOSS

389.9 NOS
389.14 Central

HEARING LOSS (continued)

CONDUCTIVE

389.00 NOS
389.06 Bilateral
389.08 Combined types
389.01 External ear
389.04 Inner ear
389.03 Middle ear
389.02 Tympanic membrane
389.05 Unilateral

HEARING LOSS (continued)

V19.2 Family history of hearing loss
389.8 High frequency
389.8 Low frequency
389.20 Mixed conductive and sensorineural
389.22 Mixed conductive and sensorineural bilateral
389.21 Mixed conductive and sensorineural unilateral
389.12 Nerve bilateral
389.13 Nerve unilateral
389.12 Neural bilateral
389.13 Neural unilateral
388.12 Noise induced bilateral
307.6 Psychogenic

SENSORINEURAL

389.10 NOS
389.16 Asymmetrical
389.18 Bilateral
389.14 Central
389.12 Nerve bilateral
389.13 Nerve unilateral
389.12 Neural bilateral
389.13 Neural unilateral
389.11 Sensory bilateral
389.17 Sensory unilateral
389.15 Unilateral

HEARING LOSS (continued)

388.2 Sudden
388.02 Transient ischemic
951.5 Traumatic
389.8 Other specified forms

HEART

746.87 Abdominal congenital
785.3 Abnormal heart sounds
759.89 Absence congenital
746.87 And cardiac apex malposition congenital
746.9 Anomaly congenital
746.84 Anomaly obstructive congenital NEC
V43.21 Assist device status
429.1 Atrophy (see also 'Myocardial', degeneration)
785.1 Beat awareness
785.0 Beat rapid
779.82 Beat rapid neonatal
0 Block see 'Heart Block'
429.89 Clot without myocardial infarction
426.9 Conduction defect
861.01 Contusion
861.11 Contusion with open wound into thorax
908.0 Contusion late effect
0 Crisis see 'Heart Failure'
277.39 Degeneration amyloid [425.7]
0 Disease see 'Heart Disease'
746.89 Diverticulum congenital

H

HEART (continued)

V59.8 Donor
0 Dysrhythmia see 'Dysrhythmias'
0 Failure see 'Heart Failure'
429.1 Fatty degeneration of heart or myocardium with mention of arteriosclerosis [440.9]
785.3 Friction rub or fremitus
746.7 Hypoplastic left (syndrome) congenital
861.00 Injury NOS
908.0 Injury NOS late effect
861.10 Injury NOS with open wound into thorax
861.0# Laceration
908.0 Laceration late effect
861.1# Laceration with open wound into thorax
5th digit: 861.0-1
2. Without penetration of heart chambers
3. With penetration of heart chambers

0 Leaky see 'Endocarditis'
746.87 Malposition congenital
785.2 Murmur
785.1 Palpitations
V43.22 Replacement status (artificial) (prosthesis) (fully implantable)
793.2 Shadow abnormal (CXR)
785.3 Sounds abnormal
785.3 Sounds increased decreased
V15.1 Surgery history
423.3 Tamponade
996.83 Transplant rejection (failure)
V42.1 Transplant (status)
746.89 Valve atresia NEC (congenital)
996.61 Valve prosthesis complication - infection or inflammation
996.02 Valve prosthesis complication - mechanical (leakage) (obstruction) (displacement)
996.71 Valve prosthesis complication - other non-mechanical (embolism) (fibrosis) (hemorrhage) (pain) (stenosis) (thrombus)
V43.3 Valve replacement status (artificial) (prosthesis)
V42.2 Valve transplant status
428.9 Weak

HEART BLOCK

426.9 NOS
426.10 Atrioventricular block (incomplete) (partial)
426.0 Atrioventricular complete
426.10 AV block (incomplete) (partial)
426.0 AV block complete
0 Bundle branch see 'Heart Block - Bundle Branch'
746.86 Congenital
426.11 First degree AV
426.6 Intraventricular NOS
426.13 Mobitz (type) I (Wenckeback's)
426.12 Mobitz (type) II AV
426.13 Second degree - mobitz (type) I (Wenckeback's)
426.12 Second degree - mobitz (type) II AV
426.13 Second degree AV - other
426.6 Sinoatrial
426.6 Sinoauricular
426.0 Third degree atrioventricular block
426.13 Wenckebach's

HEART BLOCK - BUNDLE BRANCH

426.50 NOS
426.53 Bifascicular NOS
426.53 Bilateral NOS
426.3 Left NOS
426.2 Left anterior fascicular
426.3 Left anterior with left posterior
426.3 Left complete
426.2 Left hemiblock
426.2 Left posterior fascicular
0 Left with right see 'Heart Block - Bundle Branch', right with left
426.4 Right NOS
426.53 Right with left NOS (incomplete) (main stem)
426.52 Right with left anterior fascicular
426.51 Right with left posterior fascicular
426.54 Right with left anterior with left posterior
426.54 Trifascicular block

HEART DISEASE

429.9 NOS
277.39 Amyloid [425.7]
424.1 Aortic valve NOS (see also 'Aorta, Aortic')
395.# Aortic valve rheumatic (see also 'Aorta, Aortic')
4th digit: 395
0. Stenosis
1. Insufficiency
2. Stenosis with insufficiency
9. Other and unpecified aortic disease

414.0# Arteriosclerotic
414.0# Arteriosclerotic with chronic complete or total occlusion [414.2]
5th digit: 414.0
0. Unspecified type of vessel, native or graft
1. Native coronary vessel
2. Autologous vein bypass graft
3. Nonautologous biological bypass graft
4. Autologous artery bypass graft (gastroepiploic) (internal mammary)
5. Unspecified type of bypass graft
6. Native vessel of transplanted heart
7. Bypass graft of transplanted heart

0 Cardiomyopathy see 'Cardiomyopathy'

When coding a maternal cardiovascular disease complicating pregnancy, 648.6#, use an additional code to identify the condition.

648.6# Complicating pregnancy current (co-existent)
5th digit: 648.6
0. Episode of care NOS or N/A
1. Delivered
2. Delivered with postpartum complication
3. Antepartum complication
4. Postpartum complication

746.9 Congenital NOS
760.3 Congenital maternal affecting fetus or newborn
746.89 Congenital specified type NEC
428.0 Congestive (see also 'CHF (Congestive Heart Failure)')
414.9 Coronary (ischemic)
429.9 Cryptogenic
359.21 Due to mytonia atrophica [425.8]
V17.3 Family history
098.85 Gonococcal NEC
274.82 Gouty

HEART DISEASE (continued)

429.82 Hyperkinetic
402.#0 Hypertensive
4th digit: 402.#0
0. Malignant
1. Benign
9. NOS
402.#1 Hypertensive with heart failure [428.#(#)]
4th digit: 402
0. Malignant
1. Benign
9. NOS
4th digit: 428
0. Congestive
1. Left
2#. Systolic
3#. Diastolic
4#. Combined systolic and diastolic
9. NOS
5th digit: 428.2-4
0. Nos
1. Acute
2. Chronic
3. Acute on chronic
414.9 Ischemic
0 Ischemic acute - with myocardial infarction see 'MI acute'
411.89 Ischemic acute - without MI
411.81 Ischemic acute - without MI with coronary occlusion
414.9 Ischemic chronic
414.1# Ischemic chronic - aneurysm
5th digit: 414.1
0. Heart wall
1. Coronary vessels (arteriovenous)
2. Coronary artery dissection
9. Other
414.0# Ischemic chronic - arteriosclerotic
414.0# Ischemic chronic – arteriosclerotic with chronic complete or total occlusion [414.2]
5th digit: 414.0
0. Unspecified type of vessel, native or graft
1. Native coronary vessel
2. Autologous vein bypass graft
3. Nonautologous biological bypass graft
4. Autologous artery bypass graft (gastroepiploic) (internal mammary)
5. Unspecified type of bypass graft
6. Native vessel of transplanted heart
7. Bypass graft of transplanted heart
414.8 Ischemic chronic - other
416.1 Kyphoscoliotic
394.9 Mitral NOS (see also 'Mitral Insufficiency' and 'Mitral Regurgitation')
396.# Mitral and aortic valve (non rheumatic) (rheumatic)
4th digit: 396
0. Mitral stenosis and aortic stenosis
1. Mitral stenosis and aortic insufficiency
2. Mitral insufficiency and aortic stenosis
3. Mitral insufficiency and aortic insufficiency
8. Multiple involvement mitral and aortic
9. Unspecified

HEART DISEASE (continued)

394.# Mitral rheumatic (see also 'Mitral Insufficiency' and 'Mitral Regurgitation')
4th digit: 394
0. Stenosis
1. Insufficiency
2. Stenosis with insufficiency
9. Other and unspecified mitral disease
306.2 Psychogenic
415.0 Pulmonary acute (acute cor pulmonale)
416.9 Pulmonary chronic unspecified (chronic cor pulmonale)
416.0 Pulmonary hypertension primary
416.8 Pulmonary hypertension secondary
416.8 Pulmonary other chronic
424.3 Pulmonary valve
746.00 Pulmonary valve congenital
397.1 Pulmonary valve rheumatic
398.90 Rheumatic acute
392.0 Rheumatic acute - with chorea
391.8 Rheumatic acute - specified NEC
398.90 Rheumatic chronic
V81.0 Screening for ischemic heart disease
429.0 Senile arteriosclerotic [440.9]
093.89 Syphilitic
093.1 Syphilitic aortitis
090.5 Syphilitic aortitis congenital
424.2 Tricuspid NOS (see also 'Tricuspid')
397.0 Tricuspid rheumatic (see also 'Tricuspid')
424.90 Valvular cause unspecified
746.9 Valvular NOS congenital
746.89 Valvular specified NEC congenital
429.89 Other specified NEC

For coding purposes, CHF and right ventricular failure are considered to be synonymous. Both are assigned a 4th digit of "0". Left ventricular failure is not the same as CHF. Left ventricular failure is assigned a 4th digit of "1".

HEART FAILURE

428.9 NOS
428.4# Combined diastolic and systolic
5th digit: 428.4
0. NOS
1. Acute
2. Chronic
3. Acute on chronic
428.0 Compensated
0 Complicating abortion see 'Abortion', by type with other specified complication
0 Complicating pregnancy, labor, or delivery, see 'Heart Failure Obstetrical'
428.0 Congestive see also 'CHF'
429.1 Degenerative with arteriosclerosis [440.9]
428.3# Diastolic
428.4# Diastolic and systolic
5th digit: 428.3-4
0. NOS
1. Acute
2. Chronic
3. Acute on chronic
997.1 During a procedure
0 Hypertensive see 'Hypertensive', cardiovascular disease

H

HEART FAILURE (continued)

428.1 Left
428.1 Left (ventricular failure)
428.0 Left (ventricular failure) with congestion
428.1 Left (ventricular failure) with pulmonary edema
779.89 Newborn
997.1 Postoperative - (resulting from a procedure)
429.4 Postoperative - due to cardiac prosthesis
997.1 Postoperative heart surgery - immediate
429.4 Postoperative heart surgery - late
398.91 Rheumatic
391.8 Rheumatic acute or active
398.91 Rheumatic chronic or inactive (with chorea)
428.2# Systolic
428.4# Systolic and diastolic
5th digit: 428.2-4
0. NOS
1. Acute
2. Chronic
3. Acute on chronic

When coding a maternal cardiovascular disease complicating pregnancy, 648.6#, use an additional code to identify the condition.

HEART FAILURE OBSTETRICAL

779.89 Affecting fetus or newborn
0 Maternal complicating abortion see 'Abortion', by type with other specified complication
669.4# Maternal complicating labor and delivery
648.6# Maternal current (co-existent) in pregnancy
668.1# Maternal due to anesthesia or other sedation in L&D
5th digit: 648.6, 668.1, 669.4
0. Episode of care NOS
1. Delivered with or without mention of antepartum condition
2. Delivered with mention of postpartum complication
3. Antepartum condition
4. Postpartum complication

639.8 Maternal following abortion, ectopic, or molar pregnancy

787.1 HEARTBURN

HEAT

992.1 Collapse
992.2 Cramps
992.7 Edema
992.9 Effects NOS
992.8 Effects other specified
992.5 Exhaustion
992.4 Exhaustion - salt (and water) depletion
992.3 Exhaustion - water depletion
992.6 Fatigue transient
992.9 Injury
V60.1 Lack (inadequate housing)
909.4 Late effect
0 Prostration see 'Heat', exhaustion
992.0 Pyrexia
705.1 Rash
782.0 Sense absence
992.0 Stroke
992.1 Syncope

304.5# HEAVENLY BLUE ADDICTION
5th digit: 304.5
0. NOS
1. Continuous
2. Episodic
3. In remission

273.2 HEAVY CHAIN (GAMMA G) DISEASE
766.1 HEAVY FOR DATES INFANT
796.0 HEAVY METAL ABNORMAL TOXICOLOGY
V82.5 HEAVY METAL POISONING SCREENING
626.2 HEAVY PERIODS
626.3 HEAVY PERIODS PUBERTAL
295.1# HEBEPHRENIA
5th digit: 295.1
0. NOS
1. Subchronic
2. Chronic
3. Subchronic with acute exacerbation
4. Chronic with acute
5. In remission

715.04 HEBERDEN'S NODES (OSTEOARTHRITIS)
413.9 HEBERDEN'S SYNDROME (ANGINA PECTORIS)

HEBRA'S

695.89 Dermatitis exfoliativa
695.1 Erythema multiforme exudativum
696.3 Pityriasis maculata et circinata
695.89 Pityriasis rubra
696.4 Pityriasis rubra pilaris
698.2 Prurigo

259.2 HEDINGER'S SYNDROME (MALIGNANT CARCINOID)
135 HEERFORDT'S DISEASE (UVEOPAROTITIS)
288.2 HEGGLIN'S SYNDROME
290.1# HEIDENHAIN'S DISEASE
5th digit: 290.1
0. Uncomplicated
1. With delirium
2. With delusional features
3. With depressive features

781.91 HEIGHT LOSS
207.1# HEILMEYER SCHONER DISEASE
5th digit: 207.1
0. Without mention of remission
1. In remission

045.9 HEINE-MEDIN DISEASE (SEE ALSO 'POLIOMYELITIS')
282.7 HEINZ-BODY ANEMIA, CONGENITAL
0 HELICOBACTER PYLORI SEE 'BACTERIAL INFECTION' OR SPECIFIED CONDITION
093.1 HELLER-DOHLE DISEASE (SYPHILITIC AORTITIS)
299.1# HELLER'S DISEASE OR SYNDROME (SEE ALSO 'PSYCHOSIS CHILDHOOD')
5th digit: 299.1
0. Active state
1. Residual state

642.5# HELLP (SYNDROME)
5th digit: 642.5
0. Episode of care NOS or N/A
1. Delivered
2. Delivered with postpartum complications
3. Antepartum complication
4. Postpartum complications

0 HELMINTH INFECTION NOS SEE 'HELMINTHIASIS'

HELMINTHIASIS

128.9 NOS
126.9 Ancylostoma
126.2 Ancylostoma braziliense
126.3 Ancylostoma ceylanicum
126.0 Ancylostoma duodenale
126.8 Ancylostoma other type
128.8 Angiostrongylus cantonensis
127.1 Anisakis
127.0 Ascarid
127.5 Capillaria
128.1 Gnathostoma spinigerum
127.9 Intestinal
127.7 Intestinal other specified
V75.7 Intestinal screening exam
127.8 Mixed intestinal
126.9 Necator
126.1 Necator americanus
127.4 Oxyuris vermicularis (pin worm)
127.2 Strongyloid
128.0 Toxocara (dog)
127.3 Trichuris
128.8 Other specified

238.1 HEMANGIOBLASTOMA SITE NOS

0 HEMANGIOBLASTOMA SITE SPECIFIED SEE 'NEOPLASM UNCERTAIN BEHAVIOR', BY SITE M9161/1

HEMANGIOENDOTHELIOMA

238.9 Site NOS
0 Site specified see 'Neoplasm Uncertain Behavior', by site M9130/1
228.0# Benign M9130/0
5th digit: 228.0
0. Site NOS
1. Skin and subcutaneous tissue
2. Intracranial structures
3. Retina
4. Intra abdominal structures
9. Other sites

0 Bone (diffuse) malignant see 'Cancer', bone by site
171.# Malignant
4th digit: 171
0. Head, face, neck
2. Upper limb including shoulder
3. Lower limb including hip
4. Thorax
5. Abdomen (wall), gastric, gastrointestinal, intestine, stomach
6. Pelvis, buttock, groin, inguinal region, perineum
7. Trunk NOS, back NOS, flank NOS
8. Other specified sites
9. Site NOS

228.09 Nervous system M9130/0

HEMANGIOMA

228.0# Unspecified M9120/0
228.0# Capillary M9131/0
228.0# Cavernous M9121/0
5th digit: 228.0
0. Site NOS
1. Skin and subcutaneous tissue
2. Intracranial structures
3. Retina
4. Intra abdominal structures
9. Other sites

228.09 Choroid
228.09 CNS
228.09 Heart
228.0# Intramuscular M9132/0
5th digit: 228.0
0. Site NOS
1. Skin and subcutaneous tissue
2. Intracranial structures
3. Retina
4. Intra abdominal structures
9. Other sites

228.09 Iris
228.04 Peritoneum
228.00 Racemose
228.03 Retina
228.04 Retroperitoneal tissue
228.09 Spinal cord
228.09 Subglottic
228.0# Venous M9122/0
228.0# Verrucous keratotic M9142/0
5th digit: 228.0
0. Site NOS
1. Skin and subcutaneous tissue
2. Intracranial structures
3. Retina
4. Intra abdominal structures
9. Other sites

238.1 HEMANGIOPERICYTOMA NOS M9150/1
215.# HEMANGIOPERICYTOMA BENIGN M9150/0
171.# HEMANGIOPERICYTOMA MALIGNANT M9150/3
171.# HEMANGIOSARCOMA M9120/3
4th digit: 171, 215
0. Head, face, neck
2. Upper limb including shoulder
3. Lower limb including hip
4. Thorax
5. Abdomen (wall), gastric, gastrointestinal, intestine, stomach
6. Pelvis, buttock, groin, inguinal region, perineum
7. Trunk NOS, back NOS, flank NOS
8. Other specified sites
9. Site NOS

0 HEMARTHROSIS - CURRENT INJURY SEE 'SPRAIN', BY SITE
719.1# HEMARTHROSIS - OLD (NONTRAUMATIC)
5th digit: 719.1
0. Site NOS
1. Shoulder region
2. Upper arm (elbow) (humerus)
3. Forearm (radius) (wrist) (ulna)
4. Hand (carpal) (metacarpal) (fingers)
5. Pelvic region and thigh (hip) (buttock) (femur)
6. Lower leg (fibula) (knee) (patella) (tibia)
7. Ankle and/or foot (metatarsals) (toes) (tarsals)
8. Other
9. Multiple

HEMATEMESIS

578.0 NOS
777.3 Due to swallowed maternal blood
0 With ulcer see 'Ulcer'

705.89 HEMATIDROSIS
791.2 HEMATINURIA
576.8 HEMATOBILIA

HEMATOCELE

620.7 Broad ligament
629.0 Canal of nuck
608.83 Cord male
620.8 Fallopian tube
629.0 Female
569.89 Ischiorectal
608.83 Male genitalia
629.0 Ovary
629.0 Pelvis female
0 Pelvis female with ectopic pregnancy see 'Ectopic Pregnancy'
629.0 Periuterine
629.0 Retrouterine
608.83 Scrotum
608.83 Spermatic cord
608.84 Testis
608.83 Tunica vaginalis
621.4 Uterus
623.6 Vagina
624.5 Vulva

578.1 HEMATOCHEZIA
0 HEMATOCHEZIA WITH ULCER SEE 'ULCER'
275.0 HEMATOCHROMATOSIS
371.12 HEMATOCORNEA

HEMATOCRIT

790.09 Abnormal
790.01 Drop (precipitous)
282.7 Elevated abnormal findings
285.9 Low abnormal findings

776.9 HEMATOLOGICAL DISORDER PERINATALTRANSIENT
776.8 HEMATOLOGICAL DISORDER NEONATAL TRANSIENT OTHER SPECIFIED

A hematoma is a localized collection of blood in an organ space or tissue. In ICD-9 coding, hematomas are classified as traumatic or nontraumatic. Hematomas unspecified as to traumatic or nontraumatic should be coded as traumatic hematomas, except those of the genital organs, or the eye. Unspecified hematomas of the genital organs or eye should be coded as non-traumatic hematomas. Hematomas that complicate pregnancy or delivery should be coded as pregnancy or labor and delivery complications.

HEMATOMA - NONTRAUMATIC

658.8# Amnion
5th digit: 658.8
0. Episode of care NOS or N/A
1. Delivered
3. Antepartum complication

441.0# Aorta dissecting
5th digit: 441.0
0. Unspecified site
1. Thoracic
2. Abdominal
3. Thoracoabdominal

430 Arachnoid
772.2 Arachnoid fetus or newborn
380.31 Auricle (ear)
431 Brain
772.9 Brain newborn NOS
772.8 Brain newborn NEC
611.8 Breast
620.7 Broad ligament
431 Cerebral
772.9 Cerebral newborn NOS
772.8 Cerebral newborn NEC
674.3# Cesarean section wound NOS
5th digit: 674.3
0. Episode of care unspecified or N/A
2. Delivered with postpartum complication
4. Postpartum complication

656.7# Chorion (obstetrical)
5th digit: 656.7
0. Episode of care NOS or N/A
1. Delivered
3. Antepartum complication

998.12 Complicating a procedure
607.82 Corpus cavernosum
620.1 Corpus luteum
432.1 Dura (mater)
767.0 Dura (mater) fetus or newborn
380.31 Ear external
608.83 Epididymis
432.0 Epidural
767.0 Epidural fetus or newborn
674.3# Episiotomy
5th digit: 674.3
0. Episode of care NOS or N/A
2. Delivered with postpartum complication
4. Postpartum complication

432.0 Extradural
767.0 Extradural fetus or newborn
374.81 Eyelid
620.8 Fallopian tube
629.89 Genital organ female NEC
608.83 Genital organ male NEC

HEMATOMA - NONTRAUMATIC (continued)

620.0 Graafian follicle (ruptured)
432.9 Intracranial
767.0 Intracranial fetus or newborn
593.81 Kidney cystic
624.5 Labia
573.8 Liver (subcapsular)
430 Meninges brain
772.2 Meninges brain fetus or newborn
620.8 Mesosalpinx
674.3# Obstetrical surgical wound
5th digit: 674.3
0. Episode of care NOS or N/A
2. Delivered with postpartum complication
4. Postpartum complication

377.42 Optic nerve sheaths
376.32 Orbit
620.1 Ovary
629.89 Pelvis female
608.83 Pelvis male
607.82 Penis
674.3# Perineal wound (obstetrical)
5th digit: 674.3
0. Episode of care NOS or N/A
2. Delivered with postpartum complication
4. Postpartum complication

593.81 Perirenal cystic
380.31 Pinna or auricle
656.7# Placental (obstetrical)
5th digit: 656.7
0. Episode of care NOS or N/A
1. Delivered
3. Antepartum complication

998.12 Postoperative
568.81 Retroperitoneal
568.81 Retropubic male
608.83 Scrotum
608.83 Seminal vesicle
608.83 Spermatic cord
336.1 Spinal cord
430 Subarachnoid
772.2 Subarachnoid fetus or newborn
372.72 Subconjunctival
432.1 Subdural
767.0 Subdural fetus or newborn
267 Subperiosteal (syndrome)
772.6 Superficial fetus or newborn
656.7# Syncytium
608.83 Testis
0 Traumatic see 'Hematoma - Traumatic'
608.83 Tunica vaginalis
663.6# Umbilical cord maternal
5th digit: 656.7, 663.6
0. Episode of care NOS or N/A
1. Delivered
3. Antepartum complication

762.6 Umbilical cord affecting fetus or newborn
620.7 Uterine ligament
621.4 Uterus
623.6 Vaginal
608.83 Vas deferens
379.23 Vitreous
624.5 Vulva

Do not code traumatic hematomas when they accompany a fracture, dislocation, laceration, or a crush injury. They are considered to be incidental to these injuries and only a code for the specific injury is required.

For traumatic hematomas of sites not listed below, use the injury code found by anatomical site.

HEMATOMA - TRAUMATIC

924.9 NOS
922.2 Abdomen wall or muscle
868.00 Abdominal organ unspecified
868.10 Abdominal organ unspecified with open wound
868.09 Abdominal organ other or multiple
868.19 Abdominal organ other or multiple with open wound
921.9 Adnexa eye
868.01 Adrenal gland
868.11 Adrenal gland with open wound
924.21 Ankle
924.20 Ankle and foot
902.0 Aorta abdominal
901.0 Aorta thoracic
852.0# Arachnoid
852.1# Arachnoid with open intracranial wound
5th digit: 852.0-1
0. Level of consciousness NOS
1. No LOC
2. LOC < 1 hr
3. LOC 1 - 24 hrs
4. LOC > 24 hrs with return to prior level
5. LOC > 24 hrs without return to prior level: or death before regaining consciousness, regardless of duration of LOC
6. LOC duration NOS
9. With concussion NOS

772.2 Arachnoid fetus or newborn
923.9 Arm
923.09 Arm and shoulder
923.10 Arm lower
923.03 Arm upper
923.8 Arm multiple sites
0 Artery see specific artery injury
920 Auditory canal (external) (meatus)
920 Auricle ear
923.02 Axillary region
923.09 Axillary region and shoulder
923.09 Axillary region and upper arm
922.31 Back
868.02 Bile duct
868.12 Bile duct with open wound
767.8 Birth injury other specified
0 Blood vessel see specific blood vessel injury
924.9 Bone unspecified

H

HEMATOMA - TRAUMATIC (continued)

853.0# Brain
853.1# Brain with open intracranial wound
5th digit: 853.0-1
0. Level of consciousness NOS
1. No LOC
2. LOC < 1 hr
3. LOC 1 - 24 hrs
4. LOC > 24 hrs with return to prior level
5. LOC > 24 hrs without return to prior level: or death before regaining consciousness, regardless of duration of LOC
6. LOC duration NOS
9. With concussion NOS

767.0 Brain fetus or newborn
0 Brain with contusion see 'Cerebral Contusion'
922.0 Breast
867.6 Broad ligament
867.7 Broad ligament with open wound
665.7# Broad ligament (obstetrcal trauma)
5th digit: 665.7
0. Episode of care NOS or N/A
1. Delivered
2. Delivered with postpartum complication
4. Postpartum complication

920 Brow
922.32 Buttock
959.9 Calcified unspecified site
921.1 Canthus
920 Capitis
767.19 Capitis due to birth injury
767.19 Capitis newborn
861.01 Cardiac
861.11 Cardiac with open wound into thorax
952.4 Cauda equina (spine)
853.0# Cerebral
853.1# Cerebral with open intracranial wound
5th digit: 853.0-1
0. Level of consciousness NOS
1. No LOC
2. LOC < 1 hr
3. LOC 1 - 24 hrs
4. LOC > 24 hrs with return to prior level
5. LOC > 24 hrs without return to prior level: or death before regaining consciousness, regardless of duration of LOC
6. LOC duration NOS
9. With concussion NOS

767.0 Cerebral fetus or newborn
0 Cerebral with contusion see 'Cerebral Contusion'
920 Cheek
922.1 Chest (wall)
920 Chin
922.4 Clitoris
998.12 Complicating a procedure
664.5# Complicating delivery perineum or vulva (obstetrical trauma)
5th digit: 664.5
0. Episode of care NOS or N/A
1. Delivered
4. Postpartum complication

HEMATOMA - TRAUMATIC (continued)

665.7# Complicating delivery pelvic or vagina (obstetrical trauma)
5th digit: 665.7
0. Episode of care NOS or N/A
1. Delivered
2. Delivered with postpartum complication
4. Postpartum complication

921.1 Conjunctiva
952.4 Conus medullaris (spine)
921.3 Cornea
922.4 Corpus cavernosum
922.1 Costal region
852.2# Dura (mater)
852.3# Dura (mater) with open intracranial wound
5th digit: 852.2-3
0. Level of consciousness NOS
1. No LOC
2. LOC < 1 hr
3: LOC 1 - 24 hrs
4. LOC > 24 hrs with return to prior level
5. LOC > 24 hrs without return to prior level: or death before regaining consciousness, regardless of duration of LOC
6. LOC duration NOS
9. With concussion NOS

767.0 Dura (mater) fetus or newborn
920 Ear (auricle)
923.11 Elbow
923.10 Elbow with forearm
922.4 Epididymis
852.4# Epidural
852.5# Epidural with open intracranial wound
767.0 Epidural fetus or newborn
922.2 Epigastric region
852.4# Extradural
852.5# Extradural with open intracranial wound
5th digit: 852.4-5
0. Level of consciousness NOS
1. No LOC
2. LOC < 1 hr
3. LOC 1 - 24 hrs
4. LOC > 24 hrs with return to prior level
5. LOC > 24 hrs without return to prior level: or death before regaining consciousness, regardless of duration of LOC
6. LOC duration NOS
9. With concussion NOS

767.0 Extradural fetus or newborn
924.5 Extremity lower
924.4 Extremity lower multiple sites
923.9 Extremity upper
923.8 Extremity upper multiple sites
921.9 Eye
921.0 Eye and adnexa (black eye)
921.3 Eyeball
921.1 Eyelid
920 Face
767.19 Face except eye due to birth injury
922.2 Femoral triangle
772.6 Fetus or newborn superficial
923.3 Finger
923.3 Fingernail
922.2 Flank

HEMATOMA - TRAUMATIC (continued)

924.20	Foot
924.20	Foot and ankle
923.10	Forearm
923.10	Forearm and elbow
920	Forehead
868.02	Gallbladder
868.12	Gallbladder with open wound
922.4	Genital organs external
921.3	Globe (eye)
922.2	Groin
920	Gum
923.20	Hand
920	Head
861.01	Heart
861.11	Heart with open wound of thorax
924.20	Heel
924.01	Hip
924.00	Hip with thigh
922.2	Iliac region
922.2	Inguinal region
0	Internal organs see also specific organ, injury
922.33	Interscapular region
853.##	Intracranial
	4th digit: 853
	0. Without open intracranial wound
	1. With open intracranial wound
	5th digit: 853
	0. Level of consciousness NOS
	1. No LOC
	2. LOC < 1 hr
	3. LOC 1 - 24 hrs
	4. LOC > 24 hrs with return to prior level
	5. LOC > 24 hrs without return to prior level: or death before regaining consciousness, regardless of duration of LOC
	6. LOC duration NOS
	9. With concussion NOS
767.0	Intracranial fetus or newborn
921.3	Iris (eye)
866.01	Kidney
866.11	Kidney with open wound into cavity
924.11	Knee
924.10	Knee with lower leg
922.4	Labia
921.1	Lacrimal apparatus, gland or sac
920	Larynx
0	Late effect see 'Late Effect'
924.5	Leg
924.10	Leg lower
924.4	Leg multiple sites
921.3	Lens
920	Lingual
920	Lip
864.01	Liver
864.11	Liver with open wound
767.8	Liver fetus or newborn (subcapsular)
922.31	Lumbar region
861.21	Lung
861.31	Lung with open wound
920	Malar region
920	Mandibular joint area
920	Mastoid region

HEMATOMA - TRAUMATIC (continued)

852.0#	Meningeal brain
852.1#	Meningeal brain with open intracranial wound
	5th digit: 852.0-1
	0. Level of consciousness NOS
	1. No LOC
	2. LOC < 1 hr
	3. LOC 1 - 24 hrs
	4. LOC > 24 hrs with return to prior level
	5. LOC > 24 hrs without return to prior level: or death before regaining consciousness, regardless of duration of LOC
	6. LOC duration NOS
	9. With concussion NOS
772.2	Meningeal brain fetus or newborn
922.1	Midthoracic region
920	Mouth
924.8	Multiple sites
924.4	Multiple sites lower limb
922.8	Multiple sites trunk
923.8	Multiple sites upper limb
924.9	Muscle site unspecified
861.01	Myocardial
861.11	Myocardial with open wound of thorax
920	Nasal (septum)
920	Neck
767.19	Neck due to birth injury
920	Nose
920	Occipital region
921.2	Orbital area
867.6	Ovary
867.7	Ovary with open wound
920	Palate
920	Parietal region
665.7#	Pelvic complication delivery (obstetrical trauma)
	5th digit: 665.7
	0. Episode of care NOS or N/A
	1. Delivered
	2. Delivered with postpartum complication
	4. Postpartum complication
922.9	Pelvis
922.4	Penis
861.01	Pericardium
861.11	Pericardium with open wound of thorax
920	Pericranial
767.19	Pericranial due to birth injury
664.5#	Perineal wound complicating delivery (obstetrical trauma)
	5th digit: 664.5
	0. Episode of care NOS or N/A
	1. Delivered
	4. Postpartum complication
922.4	Perineum
921.1	Periocular
921.2	Periorbital
868.03	Peritoneum
868.13	Peritoneum with open wound
920	Pharynx
924.11	Popliteal space

HEMATOMA - TRAUMATIC (continued)

998.12 Postoperative
674.3# Postoperative obstetrical
5th digit: 674.3
0. Episode of care unspecified or N/A
2. Delivered with postpartum complication
4. Postpartum complication

922.4 Prepuce
922.4 Pubic region
922.4 Pudenda
861.21 Pulmonary
861.31 Pulmonary with open wound
924.00 Quadriceps femoralis
866.01 Renal
866.11 Renal with open wound into cavity
921.2 Retrobulbar
868.04 Retroperitoneum
868.14 Retroperitoneum with open wound
922.1 Rib
922.31 Sacral region
920 Salivary ducts or gland
920 Scalp
767.19 Scalp due to birth injury
923.01 Scapula
923.09 Scapula and shoulder
923.01 Scapular region
921.3 Sclera (eye)
922.4 Scrotum
923.00 Shoulder
923.09 Shoulder and arm multiple sites
923.00 Shoulder region
924.9 Skin unspecified site
920 Skull
767.19 Skull due to birth injury
922.4 Spermatic cord
952.4 Spinal cord cauda equina
952.4 Spinal cord conus medullaris
767.4 Spinal cord fetus or newborn
865.01 Spleen
865.11 Spleen with open wound into cavity
922.1 Sternal region
767.8 Sternocleidomastoid birth injury
767.8 Sternomastoid birth injury
852.0# Subarachnoid
852.1# Subarachnoid with open intracranial wound
772.2 Subarachnoid fetus or newborn
921.1 Subconjunctival
924.9 Subcutaneous unspecified site
852.2# Subdural
852.3# Subdural with open intracranial wound
5th digit: 852.0-3
0. Level of consciousness NOS
1. No LOC
2. LOC < 1 hr
3. LOC 1 - 24 hrs
4. LOC > 24 hrs with return to prior level
5. LOC > 24 hrs without return to prior level: or death before regaining consciousness, regardless of duration of LOC
6. LOC duration NOS
9. With concussion NOS

767.0 Subdural fetus or newborn
920 Submaxillary region
920 Submental region

HEMATOMA - TRAUMATIC (continued)

924.9 Subperiosteal
923.3 Subungual fingernail or thumbnail
924.3 Subungual toenail
772.6 Superficial fetus or newborn
920 Supraclavicular fossa
920 Supraorbital
920 Temple
922.4 Testis
767.8 Testis birth injury
924.00 Thigh
924.00 Thigh and hip
922.1 Thorax
920 Throat
923.3 Thumb
923.3 Thumbnail
924.3 Toe
924.3 Toenail
920 Tongue
922.9 Trunk
922.8 Trunk multiple sites
922.4 Tunica vaginalis
920 Tympanum
920 Uvula
922.4 Vagina
665.7# Vaginal complicating delivery (obstetrical trauma)
5th digit: 665.7
0. Episode of care NOS or N/A
1. Delivered
2. Delivered with postpartum complication
4. Postpartum complication

0 Vein see specific vein, injury
920 Vocal cord
922.4 Vulva
767.8 Vulva birth trauma fetus or newborn
664.5# Vulva complicating delivery (obstetrical trauma)
5th digit: 664.5
0. Episode of care NOS or N/A
1. Delivered
4. Postpartum complication

923.21 Wrist
923.20 Wrist and hand

621.4 HEMATOMETRA
752.3 HEMATOMETRA CONGENITAL
752.2 HEMATOMETRA CONGENITAL WITH DOUBLING OF CERVIX AND VAGINA
336.1 HEMATOMYELIA
288.02 HEMATOPOIESIS CYCLIC
289.9 HEMATOPOIETIC ORGAN DISORDER
277.1 HEMATOPORPHYRIA
277.1 HEMATOPORPHYRINURIA
620.8 HEMATOSALPINX OVARY OR FALLOPIAN TUBE
608.82 HEMATOSPERMIA
599.7 HEMATURIA BENIGN (ESSENTIAL)
368.10 HEMERALOPIA
781.8 HEMI-AKINESIA
781.8 HEMI-INATTENTION
799.89 HEMIABIOTROPHY
740.0 HEMIANENCEPHALY CONGENITAL

HEMIANOPSIA

368.46 Altitudinal
368.47 Binasal
368.47 Bitemporal
368.47 Heteronymous
368.46 Homonymous
095.8 Syphilitic

307.9 HEMIASOMATOGNOSIA

799.89 HEMIATROPHY

HEMIAZYGOS

901.89 Vein injury
908.4 Vein injury late effect
901.89 Vein laceration (rupture) (hematoma) (avulsion) (aneurysm) traumatic
908.4 Vein laceration late effect

333.5 HEMIBALLISM

306.8 HEMIC DISORDER PSYCHOGENIC

740.0 HEMICEPHALY CONGENITAL

754.0 HEMIFACIAL ATROPHY

759.89 HEMIHYPERTROPHY (CONGENITAL)

756.0 HEMIHYPERTROPHY CRANIAL

HEMIMELIA

755.4 NOS
755.30 Lower limb
755.31 Lower limb transverse
755.20 Upper limb
755.21 Upper limb transverse

0 HEMIPARESIS SEE 'HEMIPLEGIA'

HEMIPLEGIA

342.## Acquired (old) (cause other or NOS)
434.91 Acquired due to CVA acute **[342.##]**

4th digit: 342
0. Flaccid
1. Spastic
8. Other specified
9. Unspecified

5th digit: 342
0. Unspecified side
1. Dominant side
2. Nondominant side

344.89 Alternans facialis
437.0 Arteriosclerotic
344.89 Ascending (spinal) NEC
343.4 Birth injury late effect
437.8 Cerebral (current episode)
343.1 Congenital
300.11 Conversion disorder (hysterical)
434.1# Embolic (current)

5th digit: 434.1
0. Without cerebral infarction
1. With cerebral infarction

342.0# Flaccid acquired (old) (cause other or NOS)
437.8 Hypertensive (current episode)
300.11 Hysterical
343.4 Infantile
438.2# Late effect cerebrovascular disease

5th digit: 342.0, 438.2
0. Unspecified side
1. Dominant side
2. Nondominant side

HEMIPLEGIA (continued)

342.## Late effect viral encephalitis [139.0]

4th digit: 342
0. Flaccid
1. Spastic
8. Other specified
9. Unspecified

5th digit: 342
0. Unspecified side
1. Dominant side
2. Nondominant side

344.89 Middle alternating NEC
767.0 Newborn NEC
436 Seizure acute (current)
342.1# Spastic acquired (old) (cause other or NOS)

5th digit: 342.1
0. Unspecified side
1. Dominant side
2. Nondominant side

434.0# Thrombotic

5th digit: 434.0
0. Without cerebral infarction
1. With cerebral infarction

342.## Viral encephalitic (late) [139.0]

4th digit: 342
0. Flaccid
1. Spastic
8. Other specified
9. Unspecified

5th digit: 342
0. Unspecified side
1. Dominant side
2. Nondominant side

781.8 HEMISPATIAL NEGLECT

117.9 HEMISPOROSIS

756.14 HEMIVERTEBRA CONGENITAL

576.8 HEMOBILIA

792.1 HEMOCCULT POSITIVE STOOL

575.8 HEMOCHOLECYST

275.0 HEMOCHROMATOSIS

238.72 HEMOCHROMATOSIS WITH REFRACTORY ANEMIA

HEMOGLOBIN

282.7 Disease
289.89 Dysfunction
282.7 Elevated abnormal findings
282.7 Fetal hereditary HPFH
282.7 Hb disease
282.7 Hemolytic disease unstable
282.49 Lepore
285.9 Low abnormal findings
289.7 M (HB-M) disease
289.7 Pathies
0 Sickle cell see 'Sickle Cell'
282.7 Trait abnormal
282.49 Trait abnormal with thalassemia
282.49 Trait lepore
0 With thalassemia see 'Thalassemia'

H

HEMOGLOBINOPATHY
282.7 NOS
282.7 C HB-C
282.7 D
282.7 D HB-D
282.7 E
282.7 E HB-E
289.6 Familial
289.6 Familial polycythemia
289.7 HBM disease
289.0 High oxygen affinity
282.7 Other NOS
V78.3 Other screening
289.0 Polycythemia
282.7 Stockholm HBD
282.7 Zurich HB-zurich
0 With sickle cell see 'Sickle Cell'
282.49 With thalassemia see also 'Thalassemia'

HEMOGLOBINURIA
791.2 NOS
283.2 Acute intravascular hemolysis
283.2 Due to hemolysis from external causes
283.2 Exertional
283.2 Intermittent
283.2 March
283.2 Paroxysmal (cold) (nocturnal)

084.8 HEMOGLOBINURIC FEVER (BILIOUS)
999.8 HEMOLYSIS TRANSFUSION
228.1 HEMOLYMPHANGIOMA SITE NOS
0 HEMOLYMPHANGIOMA SITE SPECIFIED SEE 'BENIGN NEOPLASM', BY SITE M9175/0

HEMOLYTIC
773.2 Blood type reaction perinatal - unspecified
773.1 Blood type reaction perinatal - ABO
773.0 Blood type reaction perinatal - RH
773.2 Blood type reaction perinatal - other
773.2 Disease fetus or newborn
283.0 Disease fetus or newborn - autoimmune (cold type) (warm type)
283.11 Uremic syndrome (adult) (child)

621.4 HEMOMETRA
752.3 HEMOMETRA CONGENITAL

HEMOPERICARDIUM
423.0 NOS
772.8 Newborn
423.0 Rheumatic
860.2 Traumatic
908.0 Traumatic late effect
860.3 Traumatic with open wound

HEMOPERITONEUM
568.81 NOS
567.29 Infectional
868.03 Traumatic
908.1 Traumatic late effect
868.13 Traumatic with open wound

288.4 HEMOPHAGOCYTIC LYMPHOHISTIOCYTOSIS, FAMILIAL
288.4 HEMOPHAGOCYTIC RETICULOSIS, FAMILIAL
288.4 HEMOPHAGOCYTIC SYNDROME (INFECTION-ASSOCIATED)

HEMOPHILIA
286.0 NOS
286.0 A
286.5 Acquired
286.1 B
286.2 C
V83.01 Carrier status
V83.02 Carrier status - symptomatic
286.0 Classical
286.0 Familial
286.0 Hereditary
286.7 Nonfamilial
286.5 Secondary
286.4 Vascular

0 HEMOPHILUS INFLUENZAE (H. INFLUENZAE) SEE 'BACTERIAL INFECTION' OR SPECIFIED CONDITION

360.43 HEMOPHTHALMOS EXCEPT CURRENT INJURY

HEMOPNEUMOTHORAX
511.8 Nontraumatic
860.4 Traumatic
908.0 Traumatic late effect
860.5 Traumatic with open wound

786.3 HEMOPTYSIS

When you code a hemorrhagic disorder or hemorrhage due a circulating anti-coagulant such as coumadin or heparin, assign it to hemorrhage by site with an additional E-code from the table of drugs and chemicals (therapeutic use) to identify the specific substance causing the adverse effect. For example, 578.9, hemorrhage gastrointestinal due to an adverse effect of coumadin [E934.2].

HEMORRHAGE
459.0 NOS nontraumatic
459.0 Abdomen
641.2# Abruptio placenta
5th digit: 641.2
0. Episode of care NOS or N/A
1. Delivered
3. Antepartum complication
762.1 Abruptio placenta affecting fetus or newborn
474.8 Adenoid
255.41 Adrenal (capsule) (gland) (medulla)
772.5 Adrenal perinatal
770.3 Alveolar (lung) perinatal
525.8 Alveolar process
998.11 Amputation stump (surgical)
997.69 Amputation stump secondary or delayed
569.3 Anus
0 Arachnoid see 'Hemorrhage' subarachnoid
459.0 Artery NEC
431 Artery brain (basilar) (bulbar)
431 Basilar artery
596.8 Bladder
596.7 Bladder wall
578.9 Bowel

HEMORRHAGE (continued)

BRAIN

When assigning a code for nontraumatic brain hemorrhage (430-432.#), use an additional code to identify the presence of hypertension.

431 NOS
767.0 NOS fetus or newborn birth trauma (intrapartum hypoxia/anoxia)
674.0# NOS maternal due to pregnancy
5th digit: 674.0
0. Episode of care NOS or N/A
1. Delivered
2. Delivered with postpartum complication
3. Antepartum complication
4. Postpartum complication

094.89 NOS syphilitic
853.0# NOS traumatic
853.1# NOS traumatic with open intracranial wound
5th digit: 853.0-1
0. Level of consciousness NOS
1. No LOC
2. LOC < 1 hr
3. LOC 1 - 24 hrs
4. LOC > 24 hrs with return to prior level
5. LOC > 24 hrs without return to prior level: or death before regaining consciousness, regardless of duration of LOC
6. LOC duration NOS
9. With concussion NOS

430 Aneurysm ruptured (congenital)
431 Artery (basilar) (bulbar)
431 Blood vessel
431 Cerebellar
431 Cerebral
853.0# Cerebral traumatic
853.1# Cerebral traumatic with open intracranial wound
431 Cerebromeningeal
431 Cortex (cortical)
432.0 Epidural
852.4# Epidural traumatic
852.5# Epidural traumatic with open intracranial wound
432.0 Extradural
852.4# Extradural traumatic
852.5# Extradural traumatic with open intracranial wound
5th digit: 853.0-1, 852.4-5
0. Level of consciousness (LOC) NOS
1. No LOC
2. LOC < 1 hr
3. LOC 1 - 24 hrs
4. LOC > 24 hrs with return to prior level
5. LOC > 24 hrs without return to prior level: or death before regaining consciousness, regardless of duration of LOC
6. LOC duration NOS
9. With concussion NOS

HEMORRHAGE (continued)

BRAIN (continued)

767.0 Fetus or newborn - birth trauma (intrapartum hypoxia/anoxia) (cerebral) (subdural)
767.11 Fetus or newborn - birth trauma epicranial subaponeurotic (massive)
772.1# Fetus or newborn - intraventricular
5th digit: 772.1
0. Unspecified
1. Grade I (bleeding into germinal matrix)
2. Grade II (bleeding into ventricle)
3. Grade III (bleeding with enlargement of ventricle)
4. Grade IV (bleeding into cerebral cortex)

772.2 Fetus or newborn - subarachnoid (arachnoid) (menigeal)
V12.54 History without residual
997.02 Iatrogenic
431 Internal capsule
431 Intracerebral
432.9 Intracranial NOS
853.0# Intracranial traumatic
853.1# Intracranial traumatic with open intracranial wound
5th digit: 853.0-1
0. Level of consciousness (LOC) NOS
1. No LOC
2. LOC < 1 hr
3. LOC 1 - 24 hrs
4. LOC > 24 hrs with return to prior level
5. LOC > 24 hrs without return to prior level: or death before regaining consciousness, regardless of duration of LOC
6. LOC duration NOS
9. With concussion NOS

431 Intrapontine
674.0# Maternal due to pregnancy
5th digit: 674.0
0. Episode of care NOS or N/A
1. Delivered
2. Delivered with postpartum complication
3. Antepartum complication
4. Postpartum complication

430 Meningeal
852.0# Meningeal middle traumatic
852.1# Meningeal middle traumatic with open intracranial wound
0 Nontraumatic by site, see 'Hemorrhage', specified brain site
0 Old with residual see 'Late Effect', cerebrovascular disease
431 Pontine
997.02 Postoperative
430 Subarachnoid

HEMORRHAGE (continued)

BRAIN (continued)

852.0# Subarachnoid traumatic
852.1# Subarachnoid traumatic with open intracranial wound
431 Subcortical
432.1 Subdural
852.2# Subdural traumatic
852.3# Subdural traumatic with open intracranial wound

5th digit: 852.0-3
0. Level of consciousness NOS
1. No LOC
2. LOC < 1 hr
3. LOC 1 - 24 hrs
4. LOC > 24 hrs with return to prior level
5. LOC > 24 hrs without return to prior level: or death before regaining consciousness, regardless of duration of LOC
6. LOC duration NOS
9. With concussion NOS

0 Traumatic by site see also 'Hemorrhage', specified brain site
431 Ventricular
431 Other specified
767.0 Other specified fetus or newborn birth trauma (intrapartum hypoxia/anoxia)
674.0# Other specified maternal due to pregnancy

5th digit: 674.0
0. Episode of care NOS or N/A
1. Delivered
2. Delivered with postpartum complication
3. Antepartum complication
4. Postpartum complication

853.0# Other specified traumatic
853.1# Other specified traumatic with open intracranial wound

5th digit: 853.0-1
0. Level of consciousness NOS
1. No LOC
2. LOC < 1 hr
3. LOC 1 - 24 hrs
4. LOC > 24 hrs with return to prior level
5. LOC > 24 hrs without return to prior level: or death before regaining consciousness, regardless of duration of LOC
6. LOC duration NOS
9. With concussion NOS

0 See also 'Hemorrhage', by specified brain site

HEMORRHAGE (continued)

611.79 Breast
786.3 Bronchus (cause unknown)
431 Bulbar artery
727.89 Bursa
448.9 Capillary
429.89 Cardiovascular
431 Cerebellar

HEMORRHAGE (continued)

431 Cerebral
767.0 Cerebral fetus or newborn due to birth trauma (intrapartum hypoxia/anoxia)
853.0# Cerebral traumatic
853.1# Cerebral traumatic with open intracranial wound

5th digit: 853.0-1,
0. Level of consciousness (LOC) NOS
1. No LOC
2. LOC < 1 hr
3. LOC 1 - 24 hrs
4. LOC > 24 hrs with return to prior level
5. LOC > 24 hrs without return to prior level: or death before regaining consciousness, regardless of duration of LOC
6. LOC duration NOS
9. With concussion NOS

431 Cerebromeningeal
431 Cerebrospinal
622.8 Cervix
674.3# Cesarean section wound

5th digit: 674.3
0. Episode of care unspecified or N/A
2. Delivered with postpartum complication
4. Postpartum complication

363.61 Choroid
363.62 Choroid expulsive
386.8 Cochlea
578.9 Colon NOS
562.13 Colon due to diverticulitis
562.12 Colon due to diverticulosis
998.11 Complicating a procedure
641.9# Complicating pregnancy, antepartum NOS
640.9# Complicating pregnancy, antepartum (<22 weeks) NOS
640.8# Complicating pregnancy, antepartum (<22 weeks) other specified

5th digit: 640.8-9, 641.9
0. Episode of care NOS or N/A
1. Delivered
3. Antepartum complication

762.1 Complicating pregnancy, antepartum affecting fetus or newborn
641.3# Complicating pregnancy, antepartum associated with coagulation defects
641.8# Complicating pregnancy, antepartum , intrapartum - other (trauma, uterine leiomyoma)

5th digit: 641.3, 8
0. Episode of care NOS or N/A
1. Delivered
3. Antepartum complication

372.72 Conjunctiva
772.8 Conjunctiva newborn
607.82 Corpus cavernosum
620.1 Corpus luteum cyst
431 Corpus luysii

HEMORRHAGE (continued)

431 Cortex (cortical)

853.0# Cortex (cortical) traumatic

853.1# Cortex (cortical) traumatic with open intracranial wound

5th digit: 853.0-1,

- **0. Level of consciousness (LOC) NOS**
- **1. No LOC**
- **2. LOC < 1 hr**
- **3. LOC 1 - 24 hrs**
- **4. LOC > 24 hrs with return to prior level**
- **5. LOC > 24 hrs without return to prior level: or death before regaining consciousness, regardless of duration of LOC**
- **6. LOC duration NOS**
- **9. With concussion NOS**

782.7 Cutaneous

772.6 Cutaneous perinatal

639.1 Due to abortion

286.5 Due to antithrombinemia

286.5 Due to antithromboplastinemia

286.5 Due to antithromboplastinogenemia

0 Due to esophageal varices see 'Esophagus, Esophageal Varices'

0 Due to gastroduodenitis see 'Gastritis'

286.5 Due to hyperheparinemia

286.5 Due to increase in anti-viiia

286.5 Due to intrinsic circulating anticoagulant

0 Due to ulcer see 'Ulcer'

537.83 Duodenum due to angiodysplasia

562.03 Duodenum due to diverticulitis

562.02 Duodenum due to diverticulosis

388.69 Ear

767.11 Epicranial subaponeurotic (massive) birth trauma

432.0 Epidural

852.4# Epidural traumatic

852.5# Epidural traumatic with open intracranial wound

5th digit: 852.4-5

- **0. Level of consciousness (LOC) NOS**
- **1. No LOC**
- **2. LOC < 1 hr**
- **3. LOC 1 - 24 hrs**
- **4. LOC > 24 hrs with return to prior level**
- **5. LOC > 24 hrs without return to prior level: or death before regaining consciousness, regardless of duration of LOC**
- **6. LOC duration NOS**
- **9. With concussion NOS**

530.82 Esophagus

456.0 Esophagus variceal

530.7 Esophagus Weiss syndrome

432.0 Extradural

767.0 Extradural - fetus or newborn due to birth injury (intrapartum hypoxia/anoxia) (traumatic)

674.0# Extradural - maternal due to pregnancy

5th digit: 674.0

- **0. Episode of care NOS or N/A**
- **1. Delivered**
- **2. Delivered with postpartum complication**
- **3. Antepartum complication**
- **4. Postpartum complication**

HEMORRHAGE (continued)

852.4# Extradural traumatic

852.5# Extradural traumatic with open intracranial wound

5th digit: 852.4-5

- **0. Level of consciousness (LOC) NOS**
- **1. No LOC**
- **2. LOC < 1 hr**
- **3. LOC 1 - 24 hrs**
- **4. LOC > 24 hrs with return to prior level**
- **5. LOC > 24 hrs without return to prior level: or death before regaining consciousness, regardless of duration of LOC**
- **6. LOC duration NOS**
- **9. With concussion NOS**

360.43 Eye

364.41 Eye - ciliary body

372.72 Eye - conjunctiva

362.81 Eye - fundus

360.43 Eye - intraocular

364.41 Eye - iris (postinfectional) (postinflammatory) (toxic)

362.81 Eye - retinal (periretinal) (subretinal)

376.89 Eye - retrobulbar

374.81 Eyelid

921.0 Eyelid - black eye NOS

620.8 Fallopian tube

656.0# Fetal-maternal affecting management of mother

5th digit: 656.0

- **0. Episode of care NOS or N/A**
- **1. Delivered**
- **3. Antepartum complication**

772.0 Fetomaternal

772.9 Fetus or newborn - NOS

772.5 Fetus or newborn - adrenal

767.0 Fetus or newborn - cerebral birth trauma (intrapartum anoxia/hypoxia)

772.8 Fetus or newborn - conjunctival

772.6 Fetus or newborn - cutaneous

767.11 Fetus or newborn - epicranial subaponeurotic (massive) due to birth trauma

772.0 Fetus or newborn - exsanguination

772.1# Fetus or newborn - intraventricular

5th digit: 772.1

- **0. Unspecified**
- **1. Grade I (bleeding into germinal matrix)**
- **2. Grade II (bleeding into ventricle)**
- **3. Grade III (bleeding with enlargement of ventricle)**
- **4. Grade IV (bleeding into cerebral cortex)**

772.2 Fetus or newborn - subarachnoid

767.0 Fetus or newborn - subdural birth trauma (intrapartum anoxia/hypoxia)

772.3 Fetus or newborn - umbilical after birth

772.8 Fetus or newborn - other specified

V73.5 Fever screening exam

286.6 Fibrinolytic acquired

703.8 Fingernail

767.19 Fontanel due to birth trauma

578.9 Gastric (see also 'Hemorrhage', gastrointestinal)

578.9 Gastrointestinal unspecified

772.4 Gastrointestinal perinatal

0 Gastrointestinal with ulcer see 'Ulcer'

599.89 Genitourinary

0 Genitourinary with incontinence see 'Urethra, Urethral Disorders With Incontinence'

H

HEMORRHAGE (continued)

562.03 Ileum due to diverticulitis
562.02 Ileum due to diverticulosis
626.6 Intermenstrual - irregular
626.5 Intermenstrual - regular
431 Internal capsule (brain)
578.9 Intestine
569.85 Intestine due to angiodysplasia
562.03 Intestine small due to diverticulitis
562.02 Intestine small due to diverticulosis
431 Intracerebral
432.9 Intracranial NOS
853.0# Intracranial traumatic
853.1# Intracranial traumatic with open intracranial wound

5th digit: 853.0-1
0. Level of consciousness (LOC) NOS
1. No LOC
2. LOC < 1 hr
3. LOC 1 - 24 hrs
4. LOC > 24 hrs with return to prior level
5. LOC > 24 hrs without return to prior level: or death before regaining consciousness, regardless of duration of LOC
6. LOC duration NOS
9. With concussion NOS

998.11 Intraoperative
629.89 Intrapelvic female
431 Intrapontine
431 Intraventricular
772.1# Intraventricular (perinatal) fetus or newborn

5th digit: 772.1
0. Unspecified
1. Grade I (bleeding into germinal matrix)
2. Grade II (bleeding into ventricle)
3. Grade III (bleeding with enlargement of ventricle)
4. Grade IV (bleeding into cerebral cortex)

578.9 Jejunum unspecified
562.03 Jejunum due to diverticulitis
562.02 Jejunum due to diverticulosis
0 Joint see 'Hemarthrosis'
459.0 Leg NEC
573.8 Liver
786.3 Lung
770.3 Lung alveolar perinatal
762.1 Maternal affecting fetus or newborn

648.9#: Use an additional code to identify the specific hemorrhage.

648.9# Maternal current (co-existent) in pregnancy

5th digit: 648.9
0. Episode of care unspecified or N/A
1. Delivered
2. Delivered with postpartum complication
3. Antepartum complication
4. Postpartum complication

763.89 Maternal due to coagulation defect affecting fetus or newborn
786.3 Mediastinum
431 Medulla

HEMORRHAGE (continued)

430 Meningeal
852.0# Meningeal middle traumatic
852.1# Meningeal middle traumatic with open intracranial wound

5th digit: 852.0-1
0. Level of consciousness (LOC) NOS
1. No LOC
2. LOC < 1 hr
3. LOC 1 - 24 hrs
4. LOC > 24 hrs with return to prior level
5. LOC > 24 hrs without return to prior level: or death before regaining consciousness, regardless of duration of LOC
6. LOC duration NOS
9. With concussion NOS

0 Menstrual see 'Bleeding' menstrual
568.81 Mesentery
431 Midbrain
528.9 Mouth
728.89 Muscle
784.7 Nasal
0 Newborn see 'Hemorrhage', fetus or newborn
611.79 Nipple
568.89 Omentum
377.42 Optic nerve sheaths
376.32 Orbital
620.1 Ovary due to corpus lutem cyst ruptured
577.8 Pancreas
252.8 Parathyroid gland
607.82 Penis
423.0 Pericardium
674.3# Perineal wound obstetrical surgery

5th digit: 674.3
0. Episode of care unspecified or N/A
2. Delivered with postpartum complication
4. Postpartum complication

474.8 Peritonsillar tissue
998.11 Peritonsillar tissue post tonsillectomy
253.8 Pituitary gland
641.9# Placenta NOS
641.8# Placenta from surgical or instrument damage
762.1 Placenta affecting fetus or newborn
641.1# Placenta previa

5th digit: 641.1, 8-9
0. Episode of care NOS or N/A
1. Delivered
3. Antepartum complication

762.0 Placenta previa affecting fetus or newborn
666.0# Placenta retained

5th digit: 666.0
0. Episode of care unspecified or N/A
2. Delivered with postpartum complication
4. Postpartum complication

511.8 Pleurisy
431 Pons
431 Pontine

H

HEMORRHAGE (continued)

998.11 Postoperative
997.02 Postoperative brain
674.3# Postoperative obstetrical
666.1# Postpartum atonic
666.2# Postpartum secondary or delayed
666.0# Postpartum third stage
5th digit: 666.0-2, 674.3
0. Episode of care unspecified or N/A
2. Delivered with postpartum complication
4. Postpartum complication

V23.49 Previous pregnancy, affecting management of current pregnancy
602.1 Prostate
786.3 Pulmonary
770.3 Pulmonary perinatal
446.21 Pulmonary renal syndrome
569.3 Rectum and anus (not gi bleeding)
958.2 Recurrent due to trauma
593.81 Renal (artery)
362.81 Retinal (periretinal) (deep) (subretinal)
767.19 Scalp due to birth trauma
608.83 Scrotum
782.7 Skin
608.83 Spermatic cord
459.0 Spontaneous NEC
782.7 Spontaneous petechial
431 Stem brain
578.9 Stomach
537.83 Stomach due to angiodysplasia
767.11 Subaponeurotic (massive) due to birth trauma
430 Subarachnoid
772.2 Subarachnoid fetus or newborn
674.0# Subarachnoid maternal due to pregnancy
5th digit: 674.0
0. Episode of care NOS or N/A
1. Delivered
2. Delivered with postpartum complication
3. Antepartum complication
4. Postpartum complication

772.2 Subarachnoid perinatal (fetus or newborn) (any cause)
094.87 Subarachnoid syphilitic
852.0# Subarachnoid traumatic
852.1# Subarachnoid traumatic with open intracranial wound
5th digit: 852.0-1
0. Level of consciousness (LOC) NOS
1. No LOC
2. LOC < 1 hr
3. LOC 1 - 24 hrs
4. LOC > 24 hrs with return to prior level
5. LOC > 24 hrs without return to prior level: or death before regaining consciousness, regardless of duration of LOC
6. LOC duration NOS
9. With concussion NOS

372.72 Subconjunctival
431 Subcortical
432.1 Subdural
767.0 Subdural fetus or newborn due to birth trauma (intrapartum hypoxia/anoxia)

HEMORRHAGE (continued)

674.0# Subdural maternal due to pregnancy
5th digit: 674.0
0. Episode of care NOS or N/A
1. Delivered
2. Delivered with postpartum complication
3. Antepartum complication
4. Postpartum complication

852.2# Subdural traumatic
852.3# Subdural traumatic with open intracranial wound
5th digit: 852.2-3,
0. Level of consciousness (LOC) NOS
1. No LOC
2. LOC < 1 hr
3. LOC 1 - 24 hrs
4. LOC > 24 hrs with return to prior level
5. LOC > 24 hrs without return to prior level: or death before regaining consciousness, regardless of duration of LOC
6. LOC duration NOS
9. With concussion NOS

767.11 Subgaleal fetus or newborn due to birth trauma
608.83 Testis
784.8 Throat
238.71 Thrombocythemia
246.3 Thyroid
703.8 Toenail
519.09 Tracheostomy stoma
958.2 Traumatic secondary and recurrent
608.83 Tunica vaginalis
0 Ulcer (due to) see 'Ulcer'
663.8# Umbilical cord complicating delivery
5th digit: 663.8
0. Episode of care NOS or N/A
1. Delivered
3. Antepartum complication

772.0 Umbilical cord complication affecting fetus or newborn
772.3 Umbilical cord stump
772.3 Umbilical fetus or newborn after birth
599.84 Urethral (nontraumatic)
626.9 Uterine (abnormal)
996.76 Uterine - intrauterine contraceptive device
996.32 Uterine - intrauterine contraceptive device perforating uterus
608.83 Vas deferens
663.5# Vasa previa
5th digit: 663.5
0. Episode of care NOS or N/A
1. Delivered
3. Antepartum complication

772.0 Vasa previa affecting fetus or newborn
431 Ventricular
379.23 Vitreous
624.8 Vulva

HEMORRHAGIC

287.9 Diathesis (familial)
776.0 Diathesis of newborn
287.9 Disease NEC
286.9 Disease caused by coagulation defects
776.0 Disease of newborn
287.9 Disorder NEC
286.5 Disorder due to intrinsic circulating anticoagulant
287.8 Disorder other specified

H

HEMORRHAGIC (continued)

286.6 Fibrinogenolysis
078.6 Nephrosonephritis
0 Ulcer see 'Ulcer'

HEMORRHAGIC FEVER

065.9 Arbovirus
078.7 Arenaviral
078.7 Argentine
065.9 Arthropod borne
065.8 Arthropod borne other specified
078.7 Bolivian
065.0 Central asian
065.4 Chikungunya
065.0 Crimean
065.4 Dengue
065.8 Ebola
078.6 Epidemic
078.7 Junin virus
078.6 Korean
078.7 Machupos virus
065.8 Mite borne
065.4 Mosquito borne
065.1 Omsk
065.3 Other tick borne
078.6 Russian
078.6 With renal syndrome

HEMORRHOIDS

UNSPECIFIED

455.6 NOS
455.8 Bleeding

> ***648.9#: Use an additional code to identify the specific type of hemorrhoids.***

648.9# Maternal current (co-existent) in pregnancy
671.8# Maternal due to pregnancy
5th digit: 648.9, 671.8
0. Episode of care NOS or N/A
1. Delivered
2. Delivered with postpartum complication
3. Antepartum complication
4. Postpartum complication

455.8 Prolapsed
455.9 Skin tags
455.8 Strangulated
455.7 Thrombosed
455.8 Ulcerated
455.6 Without complication

EXTERNAL

455.3 NOS
455.5 Bleeding
455.5 Prolapsed
455.5 Strangulated
455.4 Thrombosed
455.5 Ulcerated
455.3 Without complication

INTERNAL

455.0 NOS
455.2 Bleeding
455.2 Prolapsed
455.2 Strangulated

HEMORRHOIDS (continued)

INTERNAL (continued)

455.1 Thrombosed
455.2 Ulcerated
455.0 Without complication

371.11 HEMOSIDERIN DEPOSITS OF CORNEAL SCAR
275.0 HEMOSIDEROSIS
275.0 HEMOSIDEROSIS IDIOPATHIC PULMONARY [516.1]
608.82 HEMOSPERMIA
286.9 HEMOSTASIS DISORDER

HEMOTHORAX

511.8 Nontraumatic
511.1 Pneumococcal
998.11 Postoperative
998.11 Postoperative complicating a procedure [511.8]
511.1 Staphylococcal
511.1 Streptococcal
860.2 Traumatic
908.0 Traumatic late effect
860.3 Traumatic with open wound into thorax
012.0# Tuberculous pleuritic
5th digit: 012.0
0. NOS
1. Lab not done
2. Lab pending
3. Microscopy positive (in sputum)
4. Culture positive - microscopy negative
5. Culture negative - microscopy positive
6. Culture and microscopy negative confirmed by other methods

511.1 Other bacterial

385.89 HEMOTYMPANUM
304.3# HEMP ADDICTION (DEPENDENT)
5th digit: 304.3
0. NOS
1. Continuous
2. Episodic
3. In remission

719.3# HENCH ROSENBERG SYNDROME (PALINDROMIC ARTHRITIS)
5th digit: 719.3
0. Site NOS
1. Shoulder region
2. Upper arm (elbow) (humerus)
3. Forearm (radius) (wrist) (ulna)
4. Hand (carpal) (metacarpal) (fingers)
5. Pelvic region and thigh (hip) (buttock) (femur)
6. Lower leg (fibula) (knee) (patella) (tibia)
7. Ankle and/or foot (metatarsals) (toes) (tarsals)
8. Other
9. Multiple

371.41 HENLE'S WARTS
287.0 HENOCH GLOSSITIS
287.0 HENOCH-SCHONLEIN (SYNDROME) (ALLERGIC PURPURA)
102.6 HENPUE

HEPATIC

442.84 Artery (aneurysm) (A-V fistula) (cirsoid) (false) (varicose) (ruptured)
902.22 Artery injury
908.4 Artery injury late effect
902.22 Artery laceration (rupture) (hematoma) (avulsion) (aneurysm) traumatic
908.4 Artery laceration late effect
572.2 Coma
751.69 Duct accessory congenital
576.2 Duct obstruction (see also 'Bile Duct', obstruction)
751.61 Duct obstruction congenital
572.2 Encephalopathy
570 Failure
570 Failure acute (noninfective) (acquired)
997.4 Failure specified as due to a procedure
569.89 Flexure syndrome
573.4 Infarction
573.8 Insufficiency
573.8 Obstruction
902.11 Vein injury
908.4 Vein injury late effect
902.11 Vein laceration (rupture) (hematoma) (avulsion) (aneurysm) traumatic
908.4 Vein laceration late effect
453.0 Vein thrombosis

HEPATITIS INFECTIOUS OR VIRAL

V02.60 Carrier (suspected) NOS
V02.61 Carrier (suspected) viral B (HAA) (serum)
V02.62 Carrier (suspected) viral C
V02.69 Carrier (suspected) viral other
V01.79 Exposure
795.79 False positive serological test
V12.09 History (B) (C)
070.1 Infectious
070.3# Serum (Australian antigen)
070.2# Serum (Australian antigen) with hepatic coma
5th digit: 070.2-3
0. Acute or unspecified
1. Acute or unspecified with delta
2. Chronic
3. Chronic with delta

V02.61 Serum (Australian antigen) carrier
V05.3 Vaccination and inoculation (prophylactic)
070.9 Viral
070.6 Viral with hepatic coma
070.1 Viral A (infectious)
070.0 Viral A (infectious) with hepatic coma
070.3# Viral B (Australian antigen)
070.2# Viral B (Australian antigen) with hepatic coma
5th digit: 070.2-3
0. Acute or unspecified
1. Acute or unspecified with delta
2. Chronic
3. Chronic with delta

V02.61 Viral B carrier
V02.62 Viral C carrier
070.54 Viral C in remission
070.70 Viral C NOS
070.71 Viral C NOS with hepatic coma
070.5# Viral C
070.4# Viral C with hepatic coma
5th digit: 070.4, 5
1. Acute
4. Chronic

HEPATITIS INFECTIOUS OR VIRAL (continued)

760.8 Viral maternal affecting fetus or newborn

> ***647.6#: Use an additional code to identify the specific viral hepatitis.***

647.6# Viral maternal current (co-existent) in pregnancy
5th digit: 647.6
0. Episode of care unspecified or N/A
1. Delivered
2. Delivered with postpartum complication
3. Antepartum complication
4. Postpartum complication

070.5# Viral other specified (D) (E)
070.4# Viral other specified with hepatic coma (D) (E)
5th digit: 070.4, 5
2. Delta, or delta with B carrier state
3. Hepatitis E
9. Other specified viral

HEPATITIS NON-INFECTIOUS

573.3 NOS
571.1 Acute alcoholic
571.1 Acute alcoholic with esophageal varices [**456.2#**]
570 Acute non infective
571.1 Alcoholic
571.1 Alcoholic with esophageal varices [**456.2#**]
571.49 Autoimmune
573.3 Chemical
573.8 Cholangiolitic
573.8 Cholestatic
571.40 Chronic
571.40 Chronic with esophageal varices [**456.2#**]
571.49 Chronic active
571.49 Chronic active with esophageal varices [**456.2#**]
571.41 Chronic persistent
571.41 Chronic persistent with esophageal varices [**456.2#**]
771.2 Congenital (active)
573.3 Diffuse
573.3 Drug induced
795.79 False positive serological test
774.4 Giant cell (neonatal)
573.8 Hemorrhagic
571.49 Hypertrophic chronic
571.49 Hypertrophic chronic with esophageal varices [**456.2#**]
571.49 Interstitial chronic
571.49 Interstitial chronic with esophageal varices [**456.2#**]
710.0 Lupoid [571.49]
571.49 Lupoid lung hepatization chronic
571.49 Lupoid lung hepatization chronic with esophageal varices [**456.2#**]
5th digit: 456.2
0. With bleeding
1. Without bleeding

760.8 Maternal affecting newborn or fetus
646.7# Maternal complicating pregnancy
5th digit: 646.7
0. Episode of care NOS or N/A
1. Delivered
3. Antepartum complication

H

HEPATITIS (OTHER TYPES)

573.3 NOS
277.39 Amyloid
074.8 Coxsackie virus disease (due to) [573.1]
078.5 CMV [573.1]
078.5 Cytomegaloviral disease (due to) [573.1]
795.79 False positive serological test
774.4 Fetus or newborn
571.49 Fibrous (chronic)
0 Fulminant see 'Hepatitis Infectious Or Viral'
084.9 Malarial [573.2]
075 Mononucleosis [573.1]
072.71 Mumps
573.3 Noninfectious
573.3 Peliosis
571.49 Plasma cell
571.49 Plasma cell with esophageal varices **[456.2#]**
997.4 Postoperative acute
571.49 Recurrent
571.49 Recurrent with esophageal varices **[456.2#]**

5th digit: 456.2
0. With bleeding
1. Without bleeding

572.0 Suppurative
091.62 Syphilis secondary
095.3 Syphilitic late
130.5 Toxoplasmosis
017.9# Tuberculosis

5th digit: 017.9
0. NOS
1. Lab not done
2. Lab pending
3. Microscopy positive (in sputum)
4. Culture positive - microscopy negative
5. Culture negative - microscopy positive
6. Culture and microscopy negative confirmed by other methods

155.0 HEPATOBLASTOMA SITE NOS
0 HEPATOBLASTOMA SITE SPECIFIED SEE 'CANCER', BY SITE M8970/3

HEPATOCELLULAR

155.0 Carcinoma site NOS
0 Carcinoma site specified see 'Cancer', by site M8170/3
155.0 Cholangiocarcinoma combined site NOS
0 Cholangiocarcinoma combined site specified see 'Cancer', by site M8180/3

572.2 HEPATOCEREBRAL INTOXICATION
211.5 HEPATOCHOLANGIOMA BENIGN SITE NOS
0 HEPATOCHOLANGIOMA BENIGN SITE SPECIFIED SEE 'BENIGN NEOPLASM', BY SITE M8180/0
573.8 HEPATOCHOLANGITIS
575.1# HEPATOCYSTITIS (SEE ALSO 'CHOLECYSTITIS')

5th digit: 575.1
0. NOS
1. Chronic
2. Acute and chronic

570 HEPATODYSTROPHY

275.1 HEPATOLENTICULAR DEGENERATION
275.1 HEPATOLENTICULAR DEGENERATION WITH DEMENTIA **[294.1#]**

5th digit: 294.1
0. Without behavioral disturbance or NOS
1. With behavioral disturbance

0 HEPATOLITHIASIS SEE 'CHOLEDOCHOLITHIASIS'

HEPATOMA

211.5 Benign M8170/0
155.0 Congenital M8970/3
155.0 Embryonal M8970/3
155.0 Malignant M8170/3

271.0 HEPATOMEGALIA GLYCOGENIA DIFFUSA
789.1 HEPATOMEGALY
751.69 HEPATOMEGALY CONGENITAL
573.8 HEPATOPTOSIS
572.4 HEPATORENAL SYNDROME
674.8# HEPATORENAL SYNDROME MATERNAL DUE TO PREGNANCY

5th digit: 674.8
0. NOS
2. Delivered with postpartum complication
4. Postpartum complication

997.4 HEPATORENAL SYNDROME SPECIFIED AS DUE TO A PROCEDURE [572.4]
573.8 HEPATORRHEXIS
571.8 HEPATOSPLENOMEGALY
571.8 HEPATOSPLENOMEGALY WITH ESOPHAGEAL VARICES **[456.2#]**

5th digit: 456.2
0. With bleeding
1. Without bleeding

572.4 HEPATOUROLOGIC SYNDROME

HEREDITARY

363.55 Choroideremia
277.1 Coproporphyria
448.0 Hemorrhagic telangiectasia
282.49 Leptocytosis
356.0 Peripheral neuropathy
356.2 Sensory neuropathy
334.1 Spastic paraplegia
282.0 Spherocytosis with anemia
757.0 Trophedema congenital

330.9 HEREDODEGENERATION
331.89 HEREDODEGENERATIVE DISEASE NEC - BRAIN
331.89 HEREDODEGENERATIVE DISEASE NEC – BRAIN WITH DEMENTIA **[294.1#]**

5th digit: 294.1
0. Without behavioral disturbance or NOS
1. With behavioral disturbance

336.8 HEREDODEGENERATIVE DISEASE NEC - SPINAL CORD
356.3 HEREDOPATHIA ATACTICA POLYNEURITIFORMIS
752.7 HERMAPHRODITISM CONGENITAL

HERNIA

553.9	NOS
551.9	Gangrenous NOS (obstructed)
552.9	Incarcerated NOS (obstructed) (strangulated) (irreducible)
	ABDOMINAL (WALL)
553.20	NOS
551.20	Gangrenous (obstructed)
552.20	Incarcerated (obstructed) (strangulated) (irreducible)
553.21	Recurrent
551.21	Recurrent gangrenous (obstructed)
552.21	Recurrent incarcerated (obstructed) (strangulated) (irreducible)
	BLADDER
756.71	Congenital (female) (male)
0	Female see 'Cystocele', female
596.8	Male

HERNIA (continued)

569.69	Cecostomy
364.89	Ciliary body
569.69	Colostomy
	DIAPHRAGMATIC
553.3	NOS
756.6	Congenital
551.3	Gangrenous (obstructed)
552.3	Incarcerated (obstructed) (strangulated) (irreducible)
0	Traumatic see 'Diaphragm', injury

HERNIA (continued)

0	Disc (intervertebral) see 'Herniated Disc'
569.69	Enterostomy
	EPIGASTRIC
553.29	NOS
551.29	Gangrenous (obstructed)
552.29	Incarcerated (obstructed) (strangulated) (irreducible)
	ESOPHAGEAL
553.3	NOS
750.6	Congenital
551.3	Gangrenous (obstructed)
552.3	Incarcerated (obstructed) (strangulated) (irreducible)
	FEMORAL
553.0#	NOS
551.0#	Gangrenous (obstructed)
552.0#	Incarcerated (obstructed) (strangulated) (irreducible)

5th digit: 551.0, 552.0, 553.0
0. Unilateral NOS
1. Unilateral or NOS recurrent
2. Bilateral NOS
3. Bilateral recurrent

	HIATAL
553.3	NOS
750.6	Congenital
551.3	Gangrenous (obstructed)
552.3	Incarcerated (obstructed) (strangulated) (irreducible)

HERNIA (continued)

569.69	Ileostomy

HERNIA (continued)

	INCISIONAL
553.21	NOS
551.21	Gangrenous (obstructed)
552.21	Incarcerated (obstructed) (strangulated) (irreducible)
553.21	Recurrent
	INGUINAL
550.9#	NOS
550.0#	Gangrenous (obstructed)
550.1#	Incarcerated

5th digit: 550.0-1, 9
0. Unilateral NOS
1. Unilateral or NOS recurrent
2. Bilateral NOS
3. Bilateral recurrent

HERNIA (continued)

364.89	Iris
	ISCHIATIC
553.8	NOS
560.81	Due to adhesion with obstruction
551.8	Gangrenous (obstructed)
552.8	Incarcerated (obstructed) (strangulated) (irreducible)
	ISCHIORECTAL
553.8	NOS
560.81	Due to adhesion with obstruction
551.8	Gangrenous (obstructed)
552.8	Incarcerated

HERNIA (continued)

569.69	Jejunostomy
	LUMBAR
553.8	NOS
560.81	Due to adhesion with obstruction
551.8	Gangrenous (obstructed)
552.8	Incarcerated (obstructed) (strangulated) (irreducible)
	LUNG
518.89	NOS
748.69	Congenital
	OBTURATOR
553.8	NOS
560.81	Due to adhesion with obstruction
551.8	Gangrenous (obstructed)
552.8	Incarcerated (obstructed) (strangulated) (irreducible)
	PARAESOPHAGEAL
553.3	NOS
750.6	Congenital
551.3	Gangrenous (obstructed)
552.3	Incarcerated (obstructed) (strangulated) (irreducible)
	PARUMBILICAL
553.1	NOS
551.1	Gangrenous (obstructed)
552.1	Incarcerated (obstructed) (strangulated) (irreducible)

HERNIA (continued)

PUDENDAL

553.8 NOS
560.81 Due to adhesion with obstruction
551.8 Gangrenous (obstructed)
552.8 Incarcerated (obstructed) (strangulated) (irreducible)

RETROPERITONEAL

553.8 NOS
560.81 Due to adhesion with obstruction
551.8 Gangrenous (obstructed)
552.8 Incarcerated (obstructed) (strangulated) (irreducible)

SCIATIC

553.8 NOS
560.81 Due to adhesion with obstruction
551.8 Gangrenous (obstructed)
552.8 Incarcerated (obstructed) (strangulated) (irreducible)

SCROTAL

550.9# NOS
550.0# Gangrenous (obstructed)
550.1# Incarcerated (obstructed) (strangulated) (irreducible)

5th digit: 550.0-1, 9
0. Unilateral NOS
1. Unilateral or NOS recurrent
2. Bilateral NOS
3. Bilateral recurrent

SPIGELIAN

553.29 NOS
551.29 Gangrenous (obstructed)
552.29 Incarcerated (obstructed) (strangulated) (irreducible)

TESTICULAR

550.9# NOS
550.0# Gangrenous (obstructed)
550.1# Incarcerated (obstructed) (strangulated) (irreducible)
550.9# Scrotal hernia

5th digit: 550.0-1, 9
0. Unilateral NOS
1. Unilateral or NOS recurrent
2. Bilateral NOS
3. Bilateral recurrent

095.8 Syphilis late

THORACIC STOMACH

553.3 NOS
750.6 Congenital
551.3 Gangrenous (obstructed)
552.3 Incarcerated (obstructed) (strangulated) (irreducible)

HERNIA (continued)

752.89 Tunica vaginalis

UMBILICAL

553.1 NOS
551.1 Gangrenous (obstructed)
552.1 Incarcerated (obstructed) (strangulated) (irreducible)

HERNIA (continued)

VENTRAL

553.20 NOS
551.20 Gangrenous (obstructed)
552.20 Incarcerated (obstructed) (strangulated) (irreducible)
553.21 Recurrent
551.21 Recurrent gangrenous (obstructed)
552.21 Recurrent incarcerated (obstructed) (strangulated) (irreducible)

OTHER TYPES

756.6 Foramen of morgagni congenital
519.3 Mediastinum
553.8 NOS
560.81 Due to adhesion with obstruction
551.8 Gangrenous (obstructed)
552.8 Incarcerated (obstructed) (strangulated) (irreducible)

When coding back disorders due to degeneration, displacement or HNP of the intervertebral disc, it is important to distinguish whether these conditions are with or without myelopathy. Myelopathy refers to functional disturbances and/or pathological changes in the spinal cord that result from compression.

HERNIATED DISC (HNP)

722.2 Site unspecified
722.70 Site unspecified with myelopathy
722.0 Cervical
722.71 Cervical with myelopathy
722.10 Lumbar
722.73 Lumbar with myelopathy
722.11 Thoracic
722.72 Thoracic with myelopathy

304.0# HEROIN ADDICTION

5th digit: 304.0
0. NOS
1. Continous
2. Episodic
3. In remission

074.0 HERPANGINA

HERPES

110.5 Circinatus
694.5 Circinatus bullosus
771.2 Congenital or perinatal
054.0 Eczema herpeticum
V01.79 Exposure
054.6 Felon
054.10 Genital NOS
054.19 Genital other specified sites NEC (scrotum)
646.8# Gestationis

5th digit: 646.8
0. Episode of care NOS or N/A
1. Delivered
2. Delivered with postpartum complication
3. Antepartum complication
4. Postpartum complication

054.2 Gingivostomatitis
058.81 Infection human 6
058.82 Infection human 7
058.89 Infection human 8
058.89 Infection human NEC
695.1 Iris

HERPES (continued)

058.89 Kaposi's sarcoma-associated
054.43 Keratoconjunctivitis simplex
054.3 Meningoencephalitis
054.40 Ophthalmic complication NOS
054.49 Ophthalmic complication other specified
054.13 Penile infection
054.10 Progenitalis
054.2 Stomatitis
054.12 Vulval ulceration
054.11 Vulvovaginitis
054.6 Whitlow
054.8 Other specified complication

HERPES SIMPLEX

054.9 NOS
054.8 With complication NOS
054.19 Anus
771.2 Congenital or perinatal
054.43 Conjunctivitis
054.43 Cornea
054.43 Cornea disciform
054.41 Dermatitis of eyelid
054.0 Eczema herpeticum
054.3 Encephalitis
054.6 Felon
0 Genital see 'Herpes'
054.2 Gingivostomatitis
054.44 Iridocyclitis
054.42 Keratitis dendritic
054.43 Keratitis disciform
054.9 Lip
054.72 Meningitis
054.3 Meningoencephalitis
054.74 Myelitis
054.40 Ophthalmic complication NOS
054.49 Ophthalmic complication other specified
054.73 Otitis externa
054.5 Septicemia
054.71 Visceral
054.6 Whitlow
054.79 Other complication

HERPES ZOSTER

053.9 NOS
053.8 With complication NOS
053.21 Conjunctivitis
053.21 Cornea
053.20 Dermatitis eyelid
053.11 Geniculate
053.11 Geniculate ganglionitis
053.22 Iridocyclitis
053.21 Keratoconjunctivitis
053.0 Meningitis
053.14 Myelitis
053.10 Nervous system complication unspecified
053.19 Nervous system complication other specified
053.29 Ophthalmic complication other specified
053.20 Ophthalmicus
053.71 Otitis externa
053.13 Polyneuropathy post herpetic
053.12 Trigeminal neuralgia postherpetic
053.79 Other specified complication

053.11 HERPETIC GENICULATE GANGLIONITIS

HERPETIC KERATITIS

090.3 Congenital syphilis interstitial
054.42 Dendritic herpes simplex
054.43 Disciform herpes simplex
053.21 Herpes zoster

0 HERRICK'S ANEMIA SYNDROME WITH CRISIS SEE 'SICKLE CELL'

271.0 HERS' DISEASE (GLYCOGENOSIS VI)

579.0 HERTER (-GEE) DISEASE OR SYNDROME (NONTROPICAL SPRUE)

579.0 HERTER'S INFANTILISM

701.8 HERXHEIMER'S DISEASE (DIFFUSE IDIOPATHIC CUTANEOUS ATROPHY)

995.0 HERXHEIMER'S REACTION

909.9 HERXHEIMER'S REACTION LATE EFFECT

788.64 HESITANCY URINARY

364.53 HETEROCHROMIA IRIS (ACQUIRED)

HETEROPHORIA

378.40 NOS
378.45 Alternating hyperphoria
378.44 Cyclophoria
378.41 Esophoria
378.42 Exophoria
378.43 Vertical

121.6 HETEROPHYIASIS INFECTION

368.8 HETEROPSIA

742.4 HETEROTOPIA CEREBRALIS

742.59 HETEROTOPIA SPINALIS

728.13 HETEROTOPIC CALCIFICATION POSTOPERATIVE

HETEROTROPIA

378.2# Intermittent
5th digit: 378.2
0. NOS
1. Esotropic monocular
2. Esotropic alternating
3. Exotropic monocular
4. Exotropic alternating

378.3# Other or unspecified
5th digit: 378.3
0. NOS
1. Vertical
2. Hypotropic
3. Cyclotropic
4. Microtropic (monofixation)
5. Accommodative esotropic

579.0 HEUBNER HERTER DISEASE OR SYNDROME (NONTROPICAL SPRUE)

094.89 HEUBNER'S DISEASE

755.00 HEXADACTYLISM

572.4 HEYD'S SYNDROME (HEPATORENAL)

795.04 HGSIL CERVIX (HIGH GRADE SQUAMOUS INTRAEPITHELIAL LESION) (CYTOLOGIC FINDING) (PAP SMEAR FINDING)

759.81 HHHO SYNDROME

0 HIATAL HERNIA SEE 'HERNIA', HIATAL

V03.81 HIB VACCINATION

214.# HIBERNOMA M8880/0
4th digit: 214
0. Face skin and subcutaneous tissue
1. Skin and subcutaneous tissue other
2. Intrathoracic organs
3. Intra abdominal organs
4. Spermatic cord
8. Other specified sites
9. Unspecified site

786.8 HICCOUGH

306.1 HICCOUGH PSYCHOGENIC

644.1# HICKS (BRAXTON) CONTRACTIONS
5th digit: 644.1
0. Episode of care NOS or N/A
3. Antepartum complication

752.65 HIDDEN PENIS CONGENITAL

705.83 HIDRADENITIS

705.83 HIDRADENITIS SUPPURATIVA

0 HIDROCYSTOMA SEE 'BENIGN NEOPLASM', SKIN BY SITE M8404/0

768.7 HIE (HYPOXIC-ISCHEMIC ENCEPHALOPATHY)

786.8 HIGH COMPLIANCE BLADDER

272.5 HIGH DENSITY LIPOID DEFICIENCY

282.49 HIGH FETAL GENE DISEASE

238.73 HIGH GRADE MYELODYSPLASTIC SYNDROME

238.73 HIGH GRADE MYELODYSPLASTIC WITH 5Q DELETION SYNDROME

HIGH HEAD

652.5# At term
652.6# At term with multiple gestation
<u>660.0#</u> At term with multiple gestation <u>obstructing</u> <u>labor</u> **[652.6#]**
5th digit: 652.5-6, 660.0
0. Episode of care NOS or N/A
1. Delivered
3. Antepartum complication

> ***Coumadin, Digoxin, chemotherapy drugs, and any other drug with a risk of adverse reactions are considered to be high-risk medication. Code V67.51 is to be used to identify patients that have completed high risk medication therapy.***

V58.83 HIGH RISK MEDICATION DRUG MONITORING ENCOUNTER

V58.83 HIGH RISK MEDICATION DRUG MONITORING ENCOUNTER WITH <u>LONG TERM</u> <u>DRUG</u> <u>USE</u> **<u>[V58.6#]</u>**
5th digit: V58.6
1. Anticoagulants
2. Antibiotics
3. Antiplatelets/antithrombotics
4. Anti-inflammatories non-steroidal (NSAID)
5. Steroids
6. Aspirin
7. Insulin
9. Other

V67.51 HIGH RISK MEDICATION FOLLOW UP - COMPLETED THERAPY

V58.6# HIGH RISK MEDICATION MANAGEMENT - CURRENT THERAPY (LONG TERM)
5th digit: V58.6
1. Anticoagulants
2. Antibiotics
3. Antiplatelets/antithrombotics
4. Anti-inflammatories non-steroidal (NSAID)
5. Steroids
6. Aspirin
7. Insulin
9. Other

0 HIGH RISK PREGNANCY SUPERVISION SEE 'PREGNANCY SUPERVISION', HIGH RISK

220 HILAR CELL TUMOR SITE NOS

0 HILAR CELL TUMOR SITE SPECIFIED SEE 'BENIGN NEOPLASM', BY SITE M8660/0

081.9 HILDENBRAND'S DISEASE (TYPHUS)

337.0 HILGER'S SYNDROME

579.1 HILL DIARRHEA

017.0# HILLIARD'S LUPUS
5th digit: 017.0
0. NOS
1. Lab not done
2. Lab pending
3. Microscopy positive (in sputum)
4. Culture positive - microscopy negative
5. Culture negative - microscopy positive
6. Culture and microscopy negative confirmed by other ethods

744.29 HILLOCK EAR CONGENITAL

HIP

V49.77 Amputation status
726.5 Capsulitis
736.30 Deformity - acquired
736.39 Deformity - acquired other NEC
755.63 Deformity - congenital other (see also 'Hip', joint disorder congenital)
754.32 Flexion deformity congenital
959.6 Injury
916.8 Injury other and NOS superficial
916.9 Injury other and NOS superficial infected
719.85 Joint calcification
0 Joint disorder see also 'Joint'
719.95 Joint disorder
755.63 Joint disorder - congenital
754.3# Joint disorder - congenital dislocation or subluxation
5th digit: 754.3
0. Dislocation unilateral or unspecified
1. Dislocation bilateral
2. Subluxation unilateral
3. Subluxation bilateral
5. Dislocation one hip, subluxation other hip
V82.3 Joint disorder - congenital dislocation or subluxation screening
711.05 Joint disorder - suppurative (pyogenic)

H

HIP (continued)

015.1# Joint disorder - tuberculous [730.85]
5th digit: 015.1
0. NOS
1. Lab not done
2. Lab pending
3. Microscopy positive (in sputum)
4. Culture positive - microscopy negative
5. Culture negative - microscopy positive
6. Culture and microscopy negative confirmed by other methods

718.85 Joint instability (old)
718.15 Joint loose body
718.95 Joint ligament relaxation
0 Joint ligament tear see 'Sprain'
0 Joint see also 'Joint'
754.32 Predislocation status at birth
754.32 Preluxation congenital
739.5 Region segmental or somatic dysfunction
V54.81 Replacement aftercare [V43.64]
V43.64 Replacement status
V82.3 Screening for congenital dislocation or subluxation
843.9 Separation (rupture) (tear) (laceration) site NOS
843.8 Separation (rupture) (tear) (laceration) other specified sites
843.9 Strain (sprain) (avulsion) (hemarthrosis) site NOS
843.8 Strain (sprain) (avulsion) (hemarthrosis) other specified sites

759.6 HIPPEL'S DISEASE (RETINOCEREBRAL ANGIOMATOSIS)

379.49 HIPPUS DYSFUNCTION (PUPIL)

250.0# HIRSCHFELD'S DISEASE (ACUTE DIABETES MELLITUS)
5th digit: 250.0
0. Type II, adult-onset, non-insulin dependent (even if requiring insulin), or unspecified; controlled
1. Type I, juvenile-onset or insulin-dependent; controlled
2. Type II, adult-onset, non-insulin dependent (even if requiring insulin); uncontrolled
3. Type I, juvenile-onset or insulin-dependent; uncontrolled

751.3 HIRSCHSPRUNG'S DISEASE (CONGENITAL MEGACOLON)

704.1 HIRSUTISM

134.2 HIRUDINIASIS

134.2 HIRUDINIASIS EXTERNAL INTERNAL

083.1 HIS-WERNER DISEASE (TRENCH FEVER)

004.1 HISS RUSSELL DYSENTERY

270.5 HISTIDINE METABOLISM DISTURBANCES
270.5 HISTIDINEMIA
270.5 HISTIDINURIA

HISTIOCYTIC

202.3# Medullary reticulosis M9721/3
5th digit: 202.3
0. NOS
1. Lymph nodes of head, face, neck
2. Lymph nodes intrathoracic
3. Lymph nodes abdominal
4. Lymph nodes axilla and upper limb
5. Lymph nodes inguinal region and lower limb
6. Lymph nodes intrapelvic
7. Spleen
8. Lymph nodes multiple sites

288.4 Syndrome

HISTIOCYTOMA

216.# Fibrous atypical M8830/1
4th digit: 216
0. Lip skin
1. Eyelid including canthus
2. Ear external (auricle) (pinna)
3. Face (cheek) (nose) (temple) (eyebrow)
4. Scalp, neck
5. Trunk and back except scrotum
6. Upper limb including shoulder
7. Lower limb including hip
8. Other specified sites
9. Skin NOS

171.# Fibrous malignant M8830/3
4th digit: 171
0. Head, face, neck
2. Upper limb including shoulder
3. Lower limb including hip
4. Thorax
5. Abdomen (wall), gastric, gastrointestinal, intestine, stomach
6. Pelvis, buttock, groin, inguinal region, perineum
7. Trunk NOS, back NOS, flank NOS
8. Other specified sites
9. Site NOS

HISTIOCYTOSIS

277.89 Acute
277.89 Cholesterol
277.89 Chronic (subacute)
202.5# Differentiated progressive acute M9722/3
277.89 Essential
202.3# Malignant M9720/3
202.5# X acute (progressive) M9722/3
5th digit: 202.3, 5
0. NOS
1. Lymph nodes of head, face, neck
2. Lymph nodes intrathoracic
3. Lymph nodes abdominal
4. Lymph nodes axilla and upper limb
5. Lymph nodes inguinal region and lower limb
6. Lymph nodes intrapelvic
7. Spleen
8. Lymph nodes multiple sites

277.89 X (chronic)

795.4 HISTOLOGICAL FINDINGS OTHER NOS ABNORMAL

115.9# HISTOPLASMOSIS
115.0# HISTOPLASMOSIS CAPSULATUM (AMERICAN) (SMALL FORM)
115.1# HISTOPLASMOSIS DUBOISII (AFRICAN) (LARGE FORM)

5th digit: 115.0-1, 9
0. Unspecified
1. Meningitis
2. Retinitis
3. Pericarditis
4. Endocarditis
5. Pneumonia
9. Other site

> ***The V-codes for history are not assigned if the condition is still present or being treated. They are further explanatory, however, as additional codes in showing the medical complexity of a patient.***

HISTORY

V15.4# Abuse (emotional) (physical)

5th digit: V15.4
1. Physical abuse, rape, sexual
2. Emotional abuse, neglect
9. Other

V11.8 Addiction to drugs
V11.8 Adjustment reaction
V11.1 Affective disorders
V11.1 Affective disorder (not in remission)
V11.3 Alcoholism
V14.6 Allergy analgesic agent
V14.4 Allergy anesthetic agent
V15.06 Allergy bugs
V14.5 Allergy codeine
V15.08 Allergy contrast media used for x-rays
V15.09 Allergy diathesis
V15.03 Allergy eggs
V15.05 Allergy food additives
V15.06 Allergy insects (bites and stings)
V15.07 Allergy latex
V14.9 Allergy medicinal agent
V15.02 Allergy milk products
V14.5 Allergy narcotic
V15.05 Allergy nuts other than peanuts
V14.1 Allergy other antibiotic agent
V14.3 Allergy other anti-infective agent
V15.01 Allergy peanuts
V14.0 Allergy penicillin
V15.08 Allergy radiographic dye
V15.04 Allergy seafood (octopus) (squid) ink
V14.7 Allergy serum
V15.04 Allergy shellfish
V15.06 Allergy spiders (spider bites)
V14.2 Allergy sulfa
V14.7 Allergy vaccine
V15.05 Allergy other food
V14.8 Allergy other specified medicinal agents
V15.09 Allergy other than to medicinal agents
V12.3 Anemia
V13.4 Arthritis
V15.84 Asbestos exposure
V11.8 Autism
V12.41 Benign neoplasm brain
V11.1 Bipolar psychosis
V12.3 Blood disorder
V12.3 Blood forming organ disorder

HISTORY (continued)

V15.85 Body fluids exposure (potentially hazardous)
V10.9 Cancer
V10.22 Cancer accessory sinus
V10.88 Cancer adrenal
V10.06 Cancer anus
V10.09 Cancer bile duct
V10.51 Cancer bladder
V10.81 Cancer bone
V10.85 Cancer brain
V10.3 Cancer breast
V10.11 Cancer bronchus and lung
V10.05 Cancer cecum
V10.41 Cancer cervix
V10.05 Cancer colon
V10.89 Cancer connective tissue
V10.00 Cancer digestive system
V10.22 Cancer ear (middle)
V10.88 Cancer endocrine glands (other specified glands)
V10.48 Cancer epididymis
V10.03 Cancer esophagus
V10.84 Cancer eye
V10.09 Cancer gallbladder
V10.00 Cancer gastrointestinal
V10.09 Cancer gastrointestinal other specified sites
V10.40 Cancer genital organ female
V10.44 Cancer genital organ female other specified
V10.45 Cancer genital organ male
V10.49 Cancer genital organ male other specified
V10.00 Cancer GI tract
V10.09 Cancer GI tract other specified sites
V10.02 Cancer gum
V10.20 Cancer intrathoracic
V10.52 Cancer kidney
V10.05 Cancer large intestine
V10.21 Cancer larynx
V10.02 Cancer lip
V10.07 Cancer liver
V10.11 Cancer lung and bronchus
V10.79 Cancer lymphatic and hematopoietic other
V10.29 Cancer mediastinum
V10.82 Cancer melanoma skin (malignant)
V10.02 Cancer mouth
V10.22 Cancer nasal cavities middle ear accessory
V10.86 Cancer nervous system other parts
V10.02 Cancer oral cavity including lip
V10.43 Cancer ovary
V10.09 Cancer pancreas
V10.88 Cancer parathyroid
V10.09 Cancer penis
V10.02 Cancer pharynx
V10.88 Cancer pineal pituitary
V10.29 Cancer pleura
V10.46 Cancer prostate
V10.06 Cancer rectum (rectosigmoid junction) (anus)
V10.53 Cancer renal pelvis
V10.29 Cancer respiratory and intrathoracic organs
V10.20 Cancer respiratory organ
V10.02 Cancer salivary gland
V10.83 Cancer skin
V10.82 Cancer skin - melanoma
V10.09 Cancer small intestine
V10.89 Cancer soft tissue
V10.04 Cancer stomach
V10.47 Cancer testis
V10.87 Cancer thyroid

HISTORY (continued)

V10.29 Cancer thymus
V10.01 Cancer tongue
V10.12 Cancer trachea
V10.50 Cancer urinary tract
V10.59 Cancer urinary tract other specified
V10.42 Cancer uterus (excluding cervix)
V10.89 Cancer other sites
V10.09 Cancer other specified sites
V12.53 Cardiac arrest (successfully resuscitated)
V12.50 Cardiovascular disease unspecified
V12.59 Cardiovascular disease other specified
V12.42 Central nervous system disease
V13.22 Cervical dysplasia
V12.50 Circulatory disease unspecified
V12.59 Circulatory disease other specified
V12.59 Circulatory system specified NEC
V14.5 Codeine allergy
V12.72 Colon polyps
V13.61 Congenital malformation - hypospadias
V13.69 Congenital malformation - other
V15.7 Contraception
V12.59 Coronary artery disease
V12.54 CVA
V11.8 Dementia
V11.1 Depressive psychosis
V15.42 Desertion
V15.09 Diathesis
V12.70 Digestive system disease
V12.79 Digestive system disease other specified
V13.8 Disease other specified
V13.9 Disease unspecified
V11.8 Drug abuse
V13.22 Dysplasia cervical
V15.87 ECMO (extracorporeal membrane oxygenation)
V12.51 Embolism (pulmonary) (venous)
V15.42 Emotional abuse
V12.42 Encephalitis
V12.2 Endocrine disorder
V12.49 Epilepsy
V15.84 Exposure asbestos
V15.85 Exposure body fluids - potentially hazardous
V15.9 Exposure health hazard NOS
V15.89 Exposure health hazard other
V15.86 Exposure lead
V15.87 Extracorporeal membrane oxygenation (ECMO)
V15.88 Fall (at risk for falling)

FAMILY

V19.6 Allergy disorder
V18.2 Anemia
V17.7 Arthritis
V17.5 Asthma
V17.49 Atherosclerosis
V19.8 Baylor cretin syndrome
V19.0 Blindness
V18.3 Blood disorders other
V16.9 CA
V16.0 CA anorectal
V16.0 CA appendix
V16.52 CA bladder
V16.8 CA bone
V16.8 CA brain
V16.3 CA breast
V16.8 CA breast male
V16.1 CA bronchus

HISTORY (continued)

FAMILY (continued)

V16.49 CA cervix
V16.0 CA colon
V16.8 CA eye
V16.0 CA gallbladder
V16.0 CA gastrointestinal tract
V16.40 CA genital organs NOS
V16.49 CA genital organs other
V16.0 CA GI tract
V16.7 CA hematopoietic
V16.2 CA intrathoracic organs
V16.51 CA kidney
V16.2 CA larynx
V16.0 CA liver
V16.1 CA lung
V16.7 CA lymphatic and hematopoietic
V16.41 CA ovary, oviduct
V16.0 CA pancreas
V16.49 CA penis
V16.42 CA prostate
V16.2 CA respiratory
V16.0 CA stomach
V16.43 CA testis
V16.1 CA trachea
V16.59 CA urinary organs
V16.49 CA uterus
V16.49 CA vagina
V16.49 CA vulva
V16.8 CA other specified
V17.49 Cardiovascular diseases
V17.1 Cerebrovascular accident
V18.51 Colon polyps
V19.8 Conditions other
V19.5 Congenital anomalies
V19.7 Consanguinity
V17.3 Coronary artery disease
V17.1 CVA
V18.19 Cystic fibrosis
V19.2 Deafness
V18.0 Diabetes mellitus
V18.59 Digestive disorders
V19.5 Down's syndrome (mongolism)
V19.3 Ear disorders other
V18.19 Endocrine and metabolic diseases
V17.2 Epilepsy
V19.1 Eye disorders other
V18.9 Genetic disease carrier
V18.7 Genitourinary diseases other
V18.69 Glomerulonephritis
V18.19 Gout
V19.2 Hearing loss
V17.3 Heart disease (ischemic)
V16.7 Hodgkin's disease
V17.2 Huntington's chorea
V17.49 Hypertension
V17.3 Infarction myocardial
V18.8 Infectious diseases
V18.61 Kidney disease - polycystic
V18.69 Kidney disease - other
V16.6 Leukemia
V16.7 Lymphoma
V16.7 Lymphosarcoma
V18.11 MEN (multiple endocrine neoplasia syndrome)
V84.81 MEN (multiple endocrine neoplasia syndrome) susceptibility genetic

H

HISTORY (continued)

FAMILY (continued)

V18.4 Mental retardation
V18.19 Metabolic and endocrine disease
V18.11 Multiple endocrine neoplasia syndrome (MEN)
V84.81 Multiple endocrine neoplasia syndrome (MEN) susceptibility genetic
V16.7 Multiple myeloma
V17.89 Musculoskeletal diseases other
V17.3 Myocardial infarction
V17.2 Neurological disease other
V17.81 Osteoporosis
V18.8 Parasitic disease
V17.0 Psychiatric condition
V17.6 Respiratory conditions other chronic
V16.7 Reticulosarcoma
V17.41 SCD (Sudden cardiac death)
V19.4 Skin conditions
V17.1 Stroke
V17.41 Sudden cardiac death (SCD)
V19.0 Vision loss
V19.8 Other specified condition

HISTORY (continued)

V13.29 Genital system disorder
V15.9 Health hazards
V15.89 Health hazards other specified
V15.1 Heart and/or great vessels surgery
V15.1 Heart surgery
V12.09 Hepatits (B) (C)
V23.89 High risk pregnancy other (see also 'Pregnancy Supervision', high risk)
V10.72 Hodgkin's disease
V23.1 Hydatidiform mole affecting pregnancy supervision
V12.59 Hypertension
V13.61 Hypospadias
V12.2 Immunity disorder
V12.54 Infarction, cerebral, without residual deficits
V12.00 Infectious and parasitic disease unspecified other
V12.09 Infectious and parasitic disease other specified
V15.5 Injury
V15.86 Lead exposure
V10.60 Leukemia
V10.61 Leukemia lymphoid
V10.63 Leukemia monocytic
V10.62 Leukemia myeloid
V10.69 Leukemia other type
V21.3# Low birth weight status
5th digit: V21.3
0. Unspecified
1. Less than 500 grams
2. 500-999 grams
3. 1000-1499 grams
4. 1500-1999 grams
5. 2000-2500 grams
V10.61 Lymphoid leukemia
V10.71 Lymphosarcoma not in remission
V10.71 Lymphosarcoma and reticulosarcoma not in remission
V12.03 Malaria
0 Maternal affecting management of pregnancy see 'Pregnancy Supervision'
V10.82 Melanoma skin (malignant)
V12.42 Meningitis

HISTORY (continued)

V11.# Mental disorder (not in remission)
4th digit: V11
0. Schizophrenia
1. Affective disorder
2. Neurosis
8. Other mental disorders
9. Mental disorder NOS
V23.89 Mental disorder maternal affecting supervision of pregnancy
V12.2 Metabolic disorder
V10.63 Monocytic leukemia
V13.5 Musculoskeletal disorder
V10.62 Myeloid leukemia
412 Myocardial infarction
V15.42 Neglect (abuse)
V13.03 Nephrotic Syndrome
V12.40 Nervous system disorder NOS
V12.49 Nervous system disorder other
V11.2 Neurosis
V15.81 Noncompliance with medical treatment
V12.1 Nutritional deficiency
V13.29 Obstetric disorder
V13.21 Obstetric disorder pre-term labor
V13.29 Obstetric poor
0 Obstetric disorder affecting management of current pregnancy see 'Pregnancy Supervision', high risk
V12.00 Parasitic disease unspecified other
V12.09 Parasitic disease other specified
V12.71 Peptic ulcer
V13.7 Perinatal problems
V21.3# Perinatal problems - low birthweight status
5th digit: V21.3
0. Unspecified
1. Less than 500 grams
2. 500-999 grams
3. 1000-1499 grams
4. 1500-1999 grams
5. 2000-2500 grams
V15.41 Physical abuse
V12.61 Pneumonia (recurrent)
V15.6 Poisoning
V12.02 Poliomyelitis
V12.72 Polyps colon
V13.21 Pre-term labor
V12.54 Prolonged reversible ischemic neurologic deficit (PRIND)
V15.4# Psychological trauma
5th digit: V15.4
1. Physical abuse, rape, sexual
2. Emotional abuse, neglect
9. Other
V11.8 Psychosis
V12.51 Pulmonary embolism
V15.3 Radiation exposure
V15.41 Rape
V13.01 Renal calculus
V13.00 Renal disease
V12.60 Respiratory disease NOS
V12.69 Respiratory disease other specified
V10.71 Reticulosarcoma not in remission
V12.54 Reversible ischemic neurologic deficit (RIND)
V11.0 Schizophrenia
V12.40 Sense organ disorder NOS
V12.49 Sense organ disorder other
V14.7 Serum allergy

HISTORY (continued)

V13.3 Skin disease
V12.54 Stroke
V12.53 Sudden cardiac arrest (successfully resuscitated)
V14.2 Sulfa allergy
V14.2 Sulfonamides allergy
V15.2 Surgery major organs other specified
V12.54 TIA
V15.82 Tobacco use
V12.52 Thrombophlebitis
V12.51 Thrombosis
V13.1 Trophoblastic disease (nongravid)
V12.01 Tuberculosis
V13.01 Urinary calculi
V13.03 Urinary nephrotic syndrome
V13.00 Urinary system disorder
V13.09 Urinary system disorder other specified
V13.02 Urinary (tract) infection
V14.7 Vaccine allergy
V12.51 Venous embolism or thrombosis

301.50 HISTRIONIC PERSONALITY DISORDER

> ***AIDS, ARC and symptomatic HIV infection are all reported with 042. This code should be sequenced as the principal diagnosis with an additional code for any manifestation. Exception: If the encounter is for an unrelated condition such as a trauma, sequence the trauma as the principal diagnosis, followed by the 042 code, and then the additional codes for any manifestations.***

HIV

V08 Asymptomatic
V08 Carrier with confirmed HIV positive status (no HIV symptoms present)
V65.44 Counseling (advice) (education) (instruction on prevention)
V01.79 Exposure
079.51 HTLV I
079.52 HTLV II
V08 Infection asymptomatic
647.6# Infection asymptomatic - maternal current (co-existent) in pregnancy [V08]
042 Infection symptomatic
647.6# Infection symptomatic - maternal current (co-existent) in pregnancy [042]

5th digit: 647.6
- **0. Episode of care unspecified or N/A**
- **1. Delivered**
- **2. Delivered with postpartum complication**
- **3. Antepartum complication**
- **4. Postpartum complication**

042 Infection due to HIV II [079.53]
795.71 Nonspecific serologic evidence
V08 Positive (asymptomatic)
V08 Status (asymptomatic)
V73.89 Test
V73.89 Test high risk group individual [V69.8]
V65.44 Test results encounter - negative test

708.9 HIVES
995.7 HIVES DUE TO ADVERSE FOOD REACTION NEC [708.0]

> ***When coding back disorders due to degeneration, displacement or HNP of the intervertebral disc, it is important to distinguish whether these conditions are with or without myelopathy. Myelopathy refers to functional disturbances and/or pathological changes in the spinal cord that result from compression.***

HNP

722.2 Site unspecified
722.70 Site unspecified with myelopathy
722.0 Cervical
722.71 Cervical with myelopathy
722.10 Lumbar
722.73 Lumbar with myelopathy
722.11 Thoracic
722.72 Thoracic with myelopathy

784.49 HOARSENESS VOICE
V60.0 HOBO (HOMELESS PERSON)

HODGKIN'S DISEASE

201.9# NOS M9650/3
201.1# Granuloma M9661/3
201.7# Lymphocytic depletion M9653/3
201.7# Lymphocytic depletion diffuse fibrosis M9654/3
201.7# Lymphocytic depletion reticular type M9655/3
201.4# Lymphocytic predominance M9651/3
201.9# Lymphogranuloma M9650/3
201.9# Lymphoma M9650/3
201.6# Mixed cellularity M9652/3
201.5# Nodular sclerosis M9656/3
201.5# Nodular sclerosis cellular phase M9657/3
201.0# Paragranuloma M9660/3
201.2# Sarcoma M9662/3

5th digit: 201.0-2, 4-7, 9
- **0. Unspecified site, extranodal and solid organ sites**
- **1. Lymph nodes of head, face, neck**
- **2. Lymph nodes intrathoracic**
- **3. Lymph nodes abdominal**
- **4. Lymph nodes axilla and upper limb**
- **5. Lymph nodes inguinal region and lower limb**
- **6. Lymph nodes intrapelvic**
- **7. Spleen**
- **8. Lymph nodes multiple sites**

V76.89 Screening

784.49 HOARSENESS VOICE
441.9 HODGSON'S DISEASE
441.5 HODGSON'S DISEASE - RUPTURED
272.8 HOFFA'S (-KASTERT) DISEASE OR SYNDROME (LIPOSYNOVITIS PREPATELLARIS)
244.9 HOFFMANN'S SYNDROME (MYXEDEMA WITH MYOPATHY) [359.5]
427.2 HOFFMANN-BOUVERET SYNDROME (PAROXYSMAL TACHYCARDIA)
335.0 HOFFMANN-WERDNIG SYNDROME
V60.5 HOLIDAY RELIEF CARE
282.0 HOLLA DISEASE (SEE ALSO 'SPHEROCYTOSIS')
272.6 HOLLANDER-SIMONS SYNDROME (PROGRESSIVE LIPODYSTROHY)
362.33 HOLLENHORST PLAQUE
736.73 HOLLOW FOOT
754.71 HOLLOW FOOT CONGENITAL

379.46 HOLMES-ADIE SYNDROME
368.16 HOLMES' SYNDROME (VISUAL DISORIENTATION)
742.2 HOLOPROSENCEPHALY CONGENITAL
V60.4 HOME CARE INADEQUATE DUE TO HOUSEHOLD MEMBER UNABLE TO RENDER CARE
V60.1 HOME INADEQUATE FOR CARE DUE TO TECHNICAL DEFECTS
V60.0 HOMELESS PERSON
270.4 HOMOCYSTINE METABOLISM DISTURBANCES
270.4 HOMOCYSTINURIA
270.2 HOMOGENTISIC ACID DEFECTS
302.0 HOMOSEXUAL CONFLICT DISORDER
302.2 HOMOSEXUAL PEDOPHILIA
302.0 HOMOSEXUALITY
282.61 HOMOZYGOUS - HB-S DISEASE
0 HOMOZYGOUS - HB-S DISEASE WITH CRISIS SEE 'SICKLE CELL'
518.89 HONEYCOMB LUNG
748.4 HONEYCOMB LUNG CONGENITAL
117.3 HONG KONG EAR
752.49 HOODED CLITORIS
752.69 HOODED PENIS CONGENITAL
078.4 HOOF AND MOUTH DISEASE
126.9 HOOKWORM
358.00 HOPPE GOLDFLAM SYNDROME
358.01 HOPPE GOLDFLAM SYNDROME WITH (ACUTE) EXACERBATION (CRISIS)

HORDEOLUM

373.11 NOS
373.11 Externum
373.12 Internum

259.9 HORMONE ABNORMAL FINDINGS
259.9 HORMONE DISORDER (DISTURBANCE)
259.8 HORMONE DISORDER (DISTURBANCE) - OTHER SPECIFIED
V07.4 HORMONE REPLACEMENT THERAPY (POSTMENOPAUSAL)
259.2 HORMONE SECRETION BY CARCINOID TUMORS
702.8 HORN CUTANEOUS

HORNER'S

337.2# Syndrome
5th digit: 337.2
0. Unspecified
1. Upper limb
2. Lower limb
9. Other specified site
954.0 Syndrome traumatic
520.4 Teeth

753.3 HORSESHOE KIDNEY
361.32 HORSESHOE TEAR RETINAL DEFECT WITHOUT DETACHMENT
446.5 HORTON'S DISEASE (TEMPORAL ARTERITIS)
346.2# HORTON'S NEURALGIA
5th digit: 346.2
0. Without mention intractable migraine
1. With intractable migraine

When using code V66.7, code the terminal illness first.

V66.7 HOSPICE CARE ENCOUNTER
301.51 HOSPITAL ADDICTION SYNDROME
309.83 HOSPITALISM

HOST-VERSUS-GRAFT REJECTION (IMMUNE) (NON-IMMUNE)

996.80 Organ unspecified
996.85 Bone marrow
996.51 Cornea
996.55 Decellularized allodermis
996.83 Heart
996.87 Intestines
996.81 Kidney
996.82 Liver
996.84 Lung
996.86 Pancreas
996.52 Skin
996.55 Skin - artificial
996.89 Other specified NEC

627.2 HOT FLASHES (MENOPAUSAL)
627.4 HOT FLASHES MENOPAUSAL ARTIFICIAL
537.6 HOURGLASS STRICTURE STOMACH

HOUSING

V60.9 Circumstance
V60.8 Circumstance other specified
V60.0 Homeless
V60.1 Inadequate
V60.0 Lack of

282.7 HPFH (HEREDITARY PERSISTENCE FETAL HEMOGLOBIN)
079.4 HPV
V73.81 HPV (HUMAN PAPILLOMAVIRUS) SCREENING
078.1# HPV (HUMAN PAPILLOMAVIRUS) WART
5th digit: 078.1
0. Unspecified, condyloma NOS, verruca NOS, verruca vulgaris, warts (infectious)
1. Condyloma acuminatum
9. Other specified viral, genital NOS, verruca: plana, plantaris

079.51 HTLV I
079.52 HTLV II
0 HTLV III SEE 'HIV' INFECTION
0 HTN (HYPERTENSION) SEE 'HYPERTENSION'
401.9 HUCHARD'S DISEASE (CONTINUED ARTERIAL HYPERTENSION)
371.11 HUDSON STAHLI LINES
218.9 HUGUIER'S DISEASE (UTERINE FIBROMA)
0 HUMAN BITE SEE 'OPEN WOUND', BY SITE, COMPLICATED
253.3 HUMAN GROWTH HORMONE DEFICIENCY
253.0 HUMAN GROWTH HORMONE OVERPRODUCTION
0 HUMAN IMMUNODEFICIENCY VIRUS SEE 'HIV' INFECTION

795.05 HUMAN PAPILLOMAVIRUS (HPV) DNA TEST POSITIVE CERVIX HIGH RISK [079.4]

795.09 HUMAN PAPILLOMAVIRUS (HPV) DNA TEST POSITIVE CERVIX LOW RISK [079.4]

079.4 HUMAN PAPILLOMAVIRUS (HPV) INFECTION

V73.81 HUMAN PAPILLOMAVIRUS (HPV) SCREENING

078.1# HUMAN PAPILLOMAVIRUS (HPV) WART

5th digit: 078.1

0. Unspecified, condyloma NOS, verruca NOS, verruca vulgaris, warts (infectious)

1. Condyloma acuminatum

9. Other specified viral, genital NOS, verruca: plana, plantaris

079.83 HUMAN PARVOVIRUS

755.21 HUMERUS ABSENCE WITH ABSENCE COMPLETE DISTAL ELEMENTS - CONGENITAL

755.24 HUMERUS ABSENCE WITH ABSENCE INCOMPLETE DISTAL ELEMENTS - CONGENITAL

755.23 HUMERUS ABSENCE WITH ABSENCE RADIUS AND ULNA (INCOMPLETE) - CONGENITAL

736.89 HUMERUS DEFORMITY

755.50 HUMERUS DEFORMITY CONGENITAL

737.9 HUNCHBACK ACQUIRED

994.2 HUNGER

909.4 HUNGER LATE EFFECT

595.1 HUNNER'S ULCER

334.2 HUNT'S DISEASE (DYSSYNERGIA CEREBELLARIS MYOCLONICA)

053.11 HUNT'S SYNDROME (HERPETIC GENICULATE GANGLIONITIS)

529.4 HUNTERIAN GLOSSITIS SYNDROME

HUNTER'S

277.5 Cerebral degeneration disease of childhood [330.3]

529.4 Glossitis

277.5 Syndrome (mucopolysaccharidosis I)

333.4 HUNTINGTON'S CHOREA

333.4 HUNTINGTON'S CHOREA WITH DEMENTIA **[294.1#]**

5th digit: 294.1

0. Without behavioral disturbance or NOS

1. With behavioral disturbance

V17.2 HUNTINGTON'S CHOREA FAMILY HISTORY

203.0# HUPPERT'S DISEASE (MULTIPLE MYELOMA) M9730/3

5th digit: 203.0

0. Without mention of remission

1. In remission

277.5 HURLER'S SYNDROME (MUCOPOLYSACCHARIDOSIS I)

HUTCHINSON'S

709.1 Angioma serpeginosum

705.81 Cheiropompholyx

090.5 Incisors or teeth syndrome

HUTCHINSON'S (continued)

173.# Melanotic freckle malignant M8742/2

4TH digit: 173

0. Skin of lip

1. Eyelid including canthus

2. Skin of ear, auricular, canal external, external meatus pinna

3. Skin of unspecified parts of face, cheek external, chin, eyebrow, forehead, nose

4. Scalp and skin of neck

5. All skin trunk, axillary fold, perianal, abdominal wall, anus, back, breast (or mastectomy site), buttock

6. All skin upper limb, shoulder, arm, finger, forearm, hand

7. All skin lower limb, hip, ankle, foot, heel, knee, leg, thigh, toe, popiteal area

8. Other specified skin sites, contiguous overlapping sites, undetermined point of origin

9. Site unspecified

692.72 Prurigo estivalis (acute)

692.72 Summer eruption (acute)

090.5 Teeth manifest 2 yrs. or more after birth

135 HUTCHINSON-BOECK SYNDROME (SARCOIDOSIS)

259.8 HUTCHINSON-GILFORD DISEASE OR SYNDROME (PROGERIA)

728.9 HYALINE DISEASE (DIFFUSE) (GENERALIZED)

371.49 HYALINE FORMATION CORNEA

769 HYALINE MEMBRANE DISEASE (PULMONARY) NEWBORN

581.1 HYALINOSIS SEGMENTAL

379.22 HYALITIS (ASTEROID)

0 HYDATID DISEASE SEE 'ECHINOCOCCUS'

752.89 HYDATID OF MORGAGNI ANOMALY (CONGENITAL)

HYDATIDIFORM MOLE

236.1 NOS M9100/1

630 Benign

630 Benign with complication during treatment **[639.#]**

639.# Benign with complication following treatment

630 Complicating pregnancy (delivery) (undelivered)

630 Complicating pregnancy (delivery) (undelivered) with complication during treatment **[639.#]**

639.# Complicating pregnancy (delivery) (undelivered) with complication following treatment

4th digit: 639

0. Genital tract and pelvic infection

1. Delayed or excessive hemorrhage

2. Damage to pelvic organs and tissue

3. Renal failure

4. Metabolic disorders

5. Shock

6. Embolism

8. Other specified complication

9. Unspecified complication

V23.1 History affecting pregnancy supervision

236.1 Invasive M9100/1

186.9 Male choriocarcinoma

236.1 Malignant M9100/1

0 HYDATIDOSIS SEE 'ECHINOCOCCUS'

698.3 HYDE'S DISEASE (PRURIGO NODULARIS)

HYDRAMNIOS

761.3 Acute (chronic) affecting fetus or newborn
657.0# Hydramnios
5th digit: 657.0
0. Episode of care NOS or N/A
1. Delivered
3. Antepartum complication

0 See 'Polyhydramnios'

742.3 HYDRANENCEPHALY
102.6 HYDRARTHROSIS OF YAWS, (EARLY) (LATE)
868.00 HYDRAULIC CONCUSSION SYNDROME (ABDOMEN)
285.9 HYDREMIA

HYDROA

694.0 NOS
692.72 Aestivale
646.8# Gestationis
5th digit: 646.8
0. Episode of care NOS or N/A
1. Delivered
2. Delivered with postpartum complication
3. Antepartum complication
4. Postpartum complication
694.0 Herpetiformis
694.0 Pruriginosa
692.72 Vacciniforme

0 HYDROADENITIS SEE 'HIDRADENITIS'

719.0# HYDROARTHROSIS
719.3# HYDROARTHROSIS INTERMITTENT
5th digit: 719.0, 3
0. Site NOS
1. Shoulder region
2. Upper arm (elbow) (humerus)
3. Forearm (radius) (wrist) (ulna)
4. Hand (carpal) (metacarpal) (fingers)
5. Pelvic region and thigh (hip) (buttock) (femur)
6. Lower leg (fibula) (knee) (patella) (tibia)
7. Ankle and/or foot (metatarsals) (toes) (tarsals)
8. Other
9. Multiple

591 HYDROCALYCOSIS
753.29 HYDROCALYCOSIS CONGENITAL

HYDROCELE

603.9 NOS
629.1 Canal of nuck
752.41 Canal of nuck congenital
778.6 Congenital
603.0 Encysted (testes) (tunica) (spermatic cord)
629.89 Female NEC
603.1 Infected (testes) (tunica) (spermatic cord)
603.1 Infected E. coli [041.4]
603.1 Infected H. flu [041.5]
603.1 Infected klebsiella [041.3]
603.1 Infected pneumococcus [041.2]
603.1 Infected pneumoniae [041.89]
603.1 Infected proteus [041.6]

HYDROCELE (continued)

603.1 Infected staph **[041.1#]**
5th digit: 041.1
0. NOS
1. Aureus
9. Other staph

603.1 Infected strep **[041.0#]**
5th digit: 041.0
0. NOS
1. Group A
2. Group B
3. Group C
4. Group D (enterococcus)
5. Group G
9. Other strep

603.1 Infected other specified **[041.8#]**
5th digit: 041.8
1. Mycoplasma, Eaton's agent, PPLO
2. Bacteroides fragilis
3. Clostridium perfringens
4. Other anaerobes
5. Aerobacter aerogenes, mima polymorpha, serratia, (other gram-negative)
9. Other specified bacteria

629.89 Round ligament
603.9 Testes (tunica) (spermatic cord)
603.8 Other specified types male genital

HYDROCEPHALUS

331.4 NOS
331.4 NOS with dementia **[294.1#]**
331.4 Acquired
331.4 Acquired with dementia **[294.1#]**
5th digit: 294.1
0. Without behavioral disturbance or NOS
1. With behavioral disturbance

742.3 Cerebral degeneration (congenital) [331.7]
741.0# Cerebral degeneration (congenital) (spina bifida) [331.7]
5th digit: 741.0
0. Region NOS
1. Cervical region
2. Dorsal (thoracic) region
3. Lumbar region

331.3 Communicating (acquired)
331.3 Communicating (acquired) **[294.1#]**
5th digit: 294.1
0. Without behavioral disturbance or NOS
1. With behavioral disturbance

742.3 Congenital
742.3 Due to aqueduct sylvius anomaly (congenital)
742.3 Due to atresia foramina of magendie and luschka (congenital)
771.2 Due to toxoplasmosis (congenital)
655.0# Fetalis affecting pregnancy management
653.6# Fetalis causing disproportion
660.1# Fetalis causing disproportion and obstructing labor **[653.6#]**
5th digit: 653.6, 655.0, 660.1
0. Episode of care NOS or N/A
1. Delivered
3. Antepartum complication

HYDROCEPHALUS (continued)

742.3 Newborn congenital
331.5 Normal pressure (idiopathic) (INPH)
331.5 Normal pressure (idiopathic) (INPH) with dementia [294.1#]
331.3 Normal pressure secondary
331.3 Normal pressure secondary with dementia [294.1#]
331.4 Obstructive
331.4 Obstructive with dementia [294.1#]

5th digit: 294.1
- **0. Without behavioral disturbance or NOS**
- **1. With behavioral disturbance**

348.2 Otitic
741.0# With spina bifida

5th digit: 741.0
- **0. Region NOS**
- **1. Cervical region**
- **2. Dorsal (thoracic) region**
- **3. Lumbar region**

623.8 HYDROCOLPOS CONGENITAL
216.# HYDROCYSTOMA M8404/0

4th digit: 216
- **0. Lip (skin of)**
- **1. Eyelid including canthus**
- **2. Ear (external) (auricle) (pinna)**
- **3. Face (cheek) (nose) (eyebrow) (temple)**
- **4. Scalp, neck, trunk except scrotum**
- **5. Trunk, back**
- **6. Upper limb including shoulder**
- **7. Lower limb including hip**
- **8. Other specified sites**
- **9. Skin NOS**

742.0 HYDROENCEPHALOCELE CONGENITAL

HYDROMENINGOCELE

741.91 Cervical spinal region congenital
741.01 Cervical spinal region congenital with hydrocephalus congenital
742.0 Cranial congenital
741.92 Dorsal (thoracic) region congenital
741.02 Dorsal (thoracic) region congenital with hydrocephalus
741.93 Lumbar region congenital
741.03 Lumbar region congenital with hydrocephalus
741.90 Spinal region congenital
741.00 Spinal region congenital with hydrocephalus

621.8 HYDROMETRA
742.1 HYDROMICROCEPHALY CONGENITAL
742.53 HYDROMYELIA SPINAL CORD CONGENITAL

HYDROMYELOCELE

741.91 Cervical spinal region congenital
741.01 Cervical spinal region congenital with hydrocephalus congenital
741.92 Dorsal (thoracic) region congenital
741.02 Dorsal (thoracic) region congenital with hydrocephalus
741.93 Lumbar region congenital
741.03 Lumbar region congenital with hydrocephalus
741.90 Spinal region congenital
741.00 Spinal region congenital with hydrocephalus

591 HYDRONEPHROSIS
753.29 HYDRONEPHROSIS CONGENITAL
789.59 HYDROPERITONEUM
071 HYDROPHOBIA
511.8 HYDROPNEUMOTHORAX
782.3 HYDROPS
789.59 HYDROPS ABDOMINIS
773.3 HYDROPS FETALIS DUE TO BLOOD TYPE REACTION [773.#]

4th digit: 773
- **0. RH (rhesus) isoimmunization**
- **1. ABO isoimmunization**
- **2. Other and NOS isoimmunization**

778.0 HYDROPS FETALIS IDIOPATHIC
575.3 HYDROPS GALLBLADDER
742.53 HYDRORHACHIS SPINAL CORD CONGENITAL
478.19 HYDRORRHEA (NASAL)
614.1 HYDROSALPINX
511.8 HYDROTHORAX
593.5 HYDROURETER
753.22 HYDROURETER CONGENITAL
591 HYDROURETERONEPHROSIS
599.84 HYDROURETHRA
270.2 HYDROXYKYNURENINURIA
255.2 HYDROXYLASE 21 DEFICIENCY
270.8 HYDROXYPROLINEMIA
255.2 HYDROXYSTEROID 18 DEHYDROGENASE DEFICIENCY
228.1 HYGROMA CYSTIC
727.3 HYGROMA PREPATELLAR
0 HYGROMA SUBDURAL SEE 'HEMATOMA', SUBDURAL

HYMEN

752.49 Absence (congenital)
752.49 Accessory (congenital)
623.3 Atresia (postinfective)
752.42 Atresia congenital
752.49 Division
752.49 Hyperplasia congenital
752.42 Imperforate congenital
959.14 Injury
623.3 Occlusion
752.42 Occlusion congenital
0 Persistent maternal see 'Vulva, Vulval Disorders Complicating Childbirth'
623.3 Rigid acquired or congenital
623.3 Tight acquired or congenital

123.6 HYMENOLEPIASIS
123.6 HYMENOLEPIS DIMINUTA NANA INFECTION
782.0 HYPALGESIA
447.8 HYPERABDUCTION SYNDROME
536.8 HYPERACIDITY STOMACH
596.51 HYPERACTIVE BLADDER
0 HYPERACTIVE BLADDER WITH INCONTINENCE SEE 'BLADDER DISORDERS WITH INCONTINENCE'
787.5 HYPERACTIVE BOWEL SOUNDS
564.9 HYPERACTIVE BOWEL (SYNDROME)
314.01 HYPERACTIVITY (ADULT) (CHILD)
388.42 HYPERACUSIS

HYPERALDOSTERONISM

255.10 NOS
255.10 Atypical
255.13 Bartter's syndrome
255.10 Congenital

H

HYPERALDOSTERONISM (continued)

255.12 Conn's syndrome
255.11 Familial aldosteronism type I
255.11 Glucocorticoid-remediable
255.10 Hyperplastic
255.10 Normoaldosteronal
255.10 Normotensive
255.10 Primary
255.13 Secondary with juxtaglomerular hyperplasia (Bartter's)
255.14 Secondary other
255.13 With hypokalemic alkalosis (syndrome)

783.6 HYPERALIMENTATION ORGANIC
278.8 HYPERALIMENTATION OTHER (EXCESSIVE INTAKE)

270.6 HYPERAMMONEMIA
780.93 HYPERAMNESIA
791.9 HYPERAZOTEMIA
V46.8 HYPERBARIC CHAMBER DEPENDENCE
272.0 HYPERBETALIPOPROTEINEMIA
272.2 HYPERBETALIPOPROTEINEMIA WITH PREBETALIPOPROTEINEMIA

HYPERBILIRUBINEMIA

782.4 NOS
277.4 Congenital
277.4 Disorders of bilirubin excretion
774.6 Neonatal NOS (transient)
774.1 Neonatal birth trauma
774.30 Neonatal delayed conjugation NOS
774.39 Neonatal delayed conjugation disease other
774.4 Neonatal due to liver damage
277.4 Neonatal Gilbert's syndrome [774.31]
774.1 Neonatal hemolytic
282.# Neonatal hereditary hemolytic [774.0]

4th or 4th and 5th digit: 282
- **0. Spherocytic**
- **1. Elliptocytotic**
- **2. G6PD (glutathione reductase)**
- **3. Hexokinase (PK) (TPI) deficiency nonspherocytotic type II**
- **4#. Thalassemias**
  - **41. Sickle cell without crisis (NOS) (Hb-S)**
  - **42. Sickle cell with crisis (vaso-occlusive pain) (Hb-S)**
  - **49. Other (Mediterranean) (Cooley's)**
- **5. Sickle cell trait**
- **6#. Sickle cell disease**
  - **60. NOS (anemia)**
  - **61. Hb-SS without crisis**
  - **62. Hb-SS with crisis (vaso-occlusive pain)**
  - **63. Sickle cell/ Hb-C without crisis**
  - **64. Sickle cell/ Hb-C with crisis (vaso-occlusive pain)**
  - **68. Other without crisis (Hb-S/Hb-D) (Hb-S/Hb-E) (Hb-SS/Hb-D) (Hb-SS/Hb-E)**
  - **69. Other with crisis (Hb-S/Hb-D) (Hb-S/Hb-E) (Hb-SS/Hb-D) (Hb-SS/Hb-E) (vaso-occlusive pain)**
- **7. Hemoglobinopathy NOS (HB-C) (HB-D) (HB-E) (fetal)**
- **8. Other specified (stomatocytosis)**
- **9. NOS**

HYPERBILIRUBINEMIA (continued)

243 Neonatal hypothyroidism congenital [774.31]
774.2 Neonatal prematurity
0 See also 'Jaundice'

275.42 HYPERCALCEMIA DISORDER OR SYNDROME
588.89 HYPERCALCEMIC NEPHROPATHY
275.40 HYPERCALCINURIA
786.09 HYPERCAPNIA
770.89 HYPERCAPNIA FETAL
276.4 HYPERCAPNIA WITH MIXED ACID-BASE DISORDER
278.3 HYPERCAROTINEMIA
276.9 HYPERCHLOREMIA

HYPERCHOLESTEROLEMIA

272.0 NOS
272.2 And hyperglyceridemia

V65.3 Use an additional code to identify body mass index (BMI), if known. See 'Body Mass Index'.

V65.3 Dietary counseling and surveillance
V77.91 Screening

272.3 HYPERCHYLOMICRONEMIA
289.81 HYPERCOAGULATION SYNDROME PRIMARY
289.82 HYPERCOAGULATION SYNDROME SECONDARY
289.89 HYPERCOAGULATION SYNDROME NEC
289.81 HYPERCOAGULABLE STATE (PRIMARY)
289.82 HYPERCOAGULABLE STATE SECONDARY
759.89 HYPEREKPLEXIA
536.2 HYPEREMESIS
643.0# HYPEREMESIS GRAVIDARUM MILD
643.1# HYPEREMESIS GRAVIDARUM WITH METABOLIC DISTURBANCE

5th digit: 643.0-1
- **0. Episode of care NOS or N/A**
- **1. Delivered**
- **3. Antepartum complication**

780.99 HYPEREMIA
374.82 HYPEREMIA EYELID
780.99 HYPEREMIA PASSIVE
362.89 HYPEREMIA RETINA
288.3 HYPEREOSINOPHILIC SYNDROME (IDIOPATHIC)
782.0 HYPERESTHESIA SKIN
256.0 HYPERESTROGENISM
759.89 HYPEREXPLEXIA
718.8# HYPEREXTENSION OF JOINT

5th digit: 718.8
- **0. Site NOS**
- **1. Shoulder region**
- **2. Upper arm (elbow) (humerus)**
- **3. Forearm (radius) (wrist) (ulna)**
- **4. Hand (carpal) (metacarpal) (fingers)**
- **5. Pelvic region and thigh (hip) (buttock) (femur)**
- **6. Lower leg (fibula) (knee) (patella) (tibia)**
- **7. Ankle and/or foot (metatarsals) (toes) (tarsals)**
- **8. Other**
- **9. Multiple**

256.0 HYPERFUNCTION OVARY ESTROGEN

256.1 HYPERFUNCTION OVARY OTHER

HYPERGAMMAGLOBULINEMIA

289.89 NOS
273.1 Benign monoclonal (BMH)
273.0 Benign primary
273.0 Polyclonal Waldenstrom's

273.8 HYPERGLOBULINEMIA

HYPERGLYCEMIA

790.29 NOS
0 Due to diabetes see 'Diabetes, Diabetic'
251.3 Postpancreatectomy

272.3 HYPERGLYCERIDEMIA MIXED

272.1 HYPERGLYCERIDEMIA PURE

270.7 HYPERGLYCINEMIA

286.5 HYPERHEPARINEMIA HEMORRHAGIC DUE TO INTRINSIC CIRCULATING ANTICOAGULANTS

HYPERHIDROSIS

705.21 NOS
705.21 Focal (localized) - NOS
705.21 Focal (localized) - primary
705.22 Focal (localized) - secondary
780.8 Generalized
306.3 Psychogenic
780.8 Secondary

270.5 HYPERHISTIDINEMIA

251.1 HYPERINSULIN ECTOPIC (FUNCTIONAL)

775.0 HYPERINSULIN INFANTILE (OF DIABETIC MOTHER)

775.6 HYPERINSULIN NEONATAL CAUSING HYPOGLYCEMIA

HYPERINSULINISM

251.1 NOS
251.1 Ectopic (functional)
251.1 Hyperplasia pancreatic islet beta cells
251.0 Iatrogenic
775.0 Infantile (of diabetic mother)

276.9 HYPERIODEMIA

276.7 HYPERKALEMIA (HYPERKALEMIC SYNDROME)

701.1 HYPERKERATOSIS (FOLLICULARIS) (PALMOPLANTARIS)

622.2 HYPERKERATOSIS CERVIX

371.89 HYPERKERATOSIS CORNEA (LIMBIC)

702.0 HYPERKERATOSIS SENILE

624.09 HYPERKERATOSIS VULVA

HYPERKINETIC

314.2 Conduct disorder
314.1 Conduct disorder with development delay
314.9 Syndrome - NOS
429.82 Syndrome - heart
314.00 Syndrome - with attention deficit
314.01 Syndrome - with attention deficit and hyperactivity
314.1 Syndrome - with developmental delay
314.8 Syndrome - with other specified manifestations

375.20 HYPERLACRIMATION

571.1 HYPERLIPEMIA-HEMOLYTIC ANEMIA-ICTERUS SYNDROME

HYPERLIPIDEMIA

272.4 NOS
272.4 Combined
272.1 Endogenous
272.0 Group A
272.1 Group B
272.3 Group D
272.2 Mixed
V77.91 Screening
272.4 Other specified

272.7 HYPERLIPIDOSIS

HYPERLIPOPROTEINEMIA

272.4 NOS
272.3 Fredrickson type I or V
272.0 Fredrickson type IIA
272.2 Fredrickson type IIB or III
272.1 Fredrickson type IV
272.0 LDL
272.1 VLDL
272.4 Other specified

492.8 HYPERLUCENT LUNG UNILATERAL

491.2# HYPERLUCENT LUNG WITH (CHRONIC) BRONCHITIS

5th digit: 491.2
0. NOS
1. With (acute) exacerbation
2. With acute bronchitis

256.1 HYPERLUTEINIZATION

270.7 HYPERLYSINEMIA

275.2 HYPERMAGNESEMIA

275.2 HYPERMAGNESEMIA METABOLISM DISORDERS

775.5 HYPERMAGNESEMIA NEONATAL

766.21 HYPERMATURITY INFANT OR FETUS POST TERM >40 COMPLETED WEEKS TO 42 COMPLETED WEEKS

766.22 HYPERMATURITY INFANT OR FETUS PROLONGED GESTATION >42 COMPLETED WEEKS

626.2 HYPERMENORRHEA

627.0 HYPERMENORRHEA PREMENOPAUSAL

626.3 HYPERMENORRHEA PUBERTY

794.7 HYPERMETABOLISM

270.4 HYPERMETHIONINEMIA

367.0 HYPERMETROPIA

HYPERMOBILITY

564.9 Cecum
724.71 Coccyx
564.9 Colon
306.4 Colon psychogenic
564.89 Ileum
564.89 Intestinal

H

HYPERMOBILITY (continued)

718.8# Joint (acquired)
5th digit: 718.8
0. Site
1. Shoulder region
2. Upper arm (elbow) (humerus)
3. Forearm (radius) (wrist) (ulna)
4. Hand (carpal) (metacarpal) (fingers)
5. Pelvic region (hip) (buttock) (femur)
6. Lower leg (fibula) (knee) (patella) (tibia)
7. Ankle and/or foot (metatarsals) (toes) (tarsals)
8. Other
9. Multiple

753.3 Kidney, congenital
717.5 Knee meniscus
718.81 Scapula
536.8 Stomach
306.4 Stomach psychogenic
728.5 Syndrome
752.52 Testis congenital
599.81 Urethral

784.49 HYPERNASALITY
276.0 HYPERNATREMIA (SYNDROME)
238.9 HYPERNEPHROID TUMOR SITE NOS
0 HYPERNEPHROID TUMOR SITE SPECIFIED SEE 'NEOPLASM UNCERTAIN BEHAVIOR', BY SITE M8311/1
367.0 HYPEROPIA
270.6 HYPERORNITHINEMIA
276.0 HYPEROSMOLALITY
276.0 HYPEROSMOLALITY SODIUM [NA] EXCESS
276.0 HYPEROSMOLARITY SYNDROME
733.99 HYPEROSTEOGENESIS

HYPEROSTOSIS

733.90 NOS
733.3 Calvarial
733.3 Cortical
756.59 Cortical infantile
733.3 Frontal, internal of skull
733.3 Interna frontalis
733.99 Monomelic
733.3 Skull
756.0 Skull congenital
721.8 Vertebral
721.6 Vertebral ankylosing

271.8 HYPEROXALURIA (PRIMARY) CARBOHYDRATE TRANSPORT DISORDERS
987.8 HYPEROXIA
252.0# HYPERPARATHYROIDISM
5th digit: 252.0
0. NOS
1. Primary
2. Secondary non-renal
8. Other specified (tertiary)

259.3 HYPERPARATHYROIDISM ECTOPIC HORMONE SECRETION
588.81 HYPERPARATHYROIDISM SECONDARY (RENAL)
997.01 HYPERPERFUSION SYNDROME
787.4 HYPERPERISTALSIS
270.1 HYPERPHENYLALANINEMIA
378.45 HYPERPHORIA ALTERNATING
275.3 HYPERPHOSPHATEMIA
709.00 HYPERPIGMENTATION
374.52 HYPERPIGMENTATION OF EYELID
0 HYPERPLASIA / HYPERPLASTIC SEE ANATOMICAL SITE
276.7 HYPERPOTASSEMIA
272.1 HYPERPREBETALIPOPROTEINEMIA
272.3 HYPERPREBETALIPOPROTEINEMIA WITH CHYLOMICRONEMIA
272.1 HYPERPREBETALIPOPROTEINEMIA FAMILIAL
253.1 HYPERPROLACTINEMIA
270.8 HYPERPROLINEMIA
273.8 HYPERPROTEINEMIA
289.89 HYPERPROTHROMBINEMIA
780.6 HYPERPYREXIA
995.86 HYPERPYREXIA MALIGNANT DUE TO ANESTHESIA
909.9 HYPERPYREXIA MALIGNANT DUE TO ANESTHESIA - LATE EFFECT
344.61 HYPERREFLEXIA DETRUSOR
0 HYPERREFLEXIA DETRUSOR WITH INCONTINENCE SEE 'BLADDER DISORDERS WITH INCONTINENCE'
527.7 HYPERSALIVATION
270.8 HYPERSARCOSINEMIA
288.2 HYPERSEGMENTATION LEUKOCYTES HEREDITARY

HYPERSENSITIVITY

995.3 NOS
995.27 NOS due to drug
909.9 Late effect
478.8 Reaction upper respiratory
V72.7 Screening exam

HYPERSOMNIA

780.54 Unspecified
291.82 Alcohol induced
307.43 Associated with acute or intermittent emotional reactions or conflicts
307.44 Associated with depression
349.89 Bulimia syndrome
292.85 Drug induced
327.11 Idiopathic with long sleep time
327.12 Idiopathic without long sleep time
327.13 Kleine-Levin syndrome
327.13 Menstrual related
307.43 Nonorganic
307.44 Nonorganic persistent (primary)
307.43 Nonorganic transient
327.10 Organic NOS
327.19 Organic other

327.14-327.15: Code first the underlying medical or mental disorder.

327.14 Organic due to medical condition
327.15 Organic due to mental disorder
307.44 Persistent
307.44 Primary
327.13 Recurrent
307.43 Transient
780.53 With sleep apnea unspecified

289.4 HYPERSPLENIC SYNDROME
289.4 HYPERSPLENISM
289.53 HYPERSPLENISM PRIMARY NEUTROPENIA
0 HYPERSYMPATHETIC SYNDROME SEE 'NEUROPATHY PERIPHERAL', AUTONOMIC
246.8 HYPER-TBG-NEMIA
756.0 HYPERTELORISM CONGENITAL
376.41 HYPERTELORISM ORBIT
756.0 HYPERTELORISM ORBIT CONGENITAL

> ***Hypertension and heart disease: Unless the cause of the heart disease is stated as "due to hypertension", "hypertensive heart disease", or "hypertensive cardioviascular disease" do not assume a cause and effect relationship. Code the conditions separately. Example: CHF - 428.0, hypertension - 401.9.***

HYPERTENSION

401.9 NOS
401.0 Accelerated
401.1 Benign
401.# Essential
4th digit: 401
0. Malignant, accelerated
1. Benign
9. NOS

440.1 Goldblatt's
V12.59 History
348.2 Intracranial (benign)
401.# Labile
4th digit: 401
0. Malignant, accelerated
1. Benign
9. NOS

401.0 Malignant
760.0 Maternal affecting fetus or newborn
0 Maternal complicating pregnancy see 'Hypertension Complicating Pregnancy'
365.04 Ocular
572.3 Portal
572.3 Portal with esophageal varices **[456.2#]**
5th digit: 456.2
0. With bleeding
1. Without bleeding

997.91 Postoperative (due to a procedure)
306.2 Psychogenic
416.0 Pulmonary chronic primary
416.0 Pulmonary chronic primary idiopathic
416.8 Pulmonary chronic secondary
747.83 Pulmonary persistent congenital
747.83 Pulmonary primary of newborn
405.91 Renovascular secondary
405.11 Renovascular secondary - benign
405.01 Renovascular secondary - malignant
V81.1 Screening

HYPERTENSION (continued)

405.## Secondary
4th digit: 405
0. Malignant, accelerated
1. Benign
9. NOS

5th digit: 405
1. Renovascular
9. Other

796.2 Transient
459.3# Venous chronic
5th digit: 459.3
0. NOS
1. With ulcer
2. With inflammation
3. With ulcer and inflammation
9. With other complication

459.30 Venous chronic asymptomatic
459.1# Venous chronic due to deep vein thrombosis
5th digit: 459.1
0. NOS
1. With ulcer
2. With inflammation
3. With ulcer and inflammation
9. With other complication

HYPERTENSION COMPLICATING PREGNANCY

642.9# Unspecified
642.0# Benign
642.2# Malignant
642.6# Eclampsia
642.7# Eclampsia or pre-eclampsia with pre-existing hypertension
642.0# Essential - NOS or benign
642.7# Essential - NOS or benign with superimposed pre-eclampsia or eclampsia
642.3# Gestational - NOS
642.0# Pre-existing (chronic) - NOS
642.0# Pre-existing (chronic) - benign
642.2# Pre-existing (chronic) - malignant
642.7# Pre-existing (chronic) - with superimposed pre-eclampsia or eclampsia
642.1# Secondary to renal disease
642.7# Secondary to renal disease with superimposed pre-eclampsia or eclampsia
642.3# Transient - NOS
642.2# With chronic kidney and/or heart disease
642.4# With edema and/or albuminuria - mild
642.5# With edema and/or albuminuria - severe
5th digit: 642
0. Episode of care NOS or N/A
1. Delivered
2. Delivered with postpartum complications
3. Antepartum complication
4. Postpartum complications

H

HYPERTENSIVE

360.42 Blind eye
402.#0 Cardiovascular disease
402.#1 Cardiovascular disease with heart failure NOS [428.9]
402.#1 Cardiovascular disease with heart failure congestive [428.0]
402.#1 Cardiovascular disease with heart failure diastolic **[428.3#]**
402.#1 Cardiovascular disease with heart failure diastolic and systolic **[428.4#]**
402.#1 Cardiovascular disease with heart failure left [428.1]
402.#1 Cardiovascular disease with heart failure systolic **[428.2#]**
402.#1 Cardiovascular disease with heart failure systolic and diastolic **[428.4#]**

4th digit: 402.#0, 402.#1
0. Malignant
1. Benign
9. NOS

5th digit: 428.2-4
0. NOS
1. Acute
2. Chronic
3. Acute on chronic

403.#0 Chronic kidney disease stage I through IV or NOS **[585.#]**

4th digit: 403
0. Malignant
1. Benign
9. NOS

4th digit: 585
1. Stage I
2. Stage II (mild)
3. Stage III (moderate)
4. Stage IV (severe)
9. Unspecified stage

403.#1 Chronic kidney disease stage V or end stage renal disease **[585.#]**

4th digit: 403
0. Malignant
1. Benign
9. NOS

5th digit: 585
5. Stage V
6. End stage

0 Crisis see 'Hypertension'
760.0 Disorder affecting fetus or newborn
437.2 Encephalopathy
404.#0 Heart and chronic kidney disease stage I through stage IV or NOS **[585.#]**

4th digit: 404
0. Malignant
1. Benign
9. NOS

4th digit: 585
1. Stage I
2. Stage II (mild)
3. Stage III (moderate)
4. Stage IV (severe)
9. Unspecified stage

HYPERTENSIVE (continued)

404.#2 Heart and chronic kidney disease stage V or end stage renal disease **[585.#]**

4th digit: 404
0. Malignant
1. Benign
9. NOS

5th digit: 585
5. Stage V
6. End stage

404.#1 Heart and chronic kidney disease with heart failure and chronic kidney disease stage I through IV or NOS **[428.#(#)]** **[585.#]**

4th digit: 404.#1
0. Malignant
1. Benign
9. NOS

4th digit: 428
0. Congestive
1. Left
2#. Systolic
3#. Diastolic
4#. Combined systolic and diastolic
9. NOS

5th digit: 428.2-4
0. NOS
1. Acute
2. Chronic
3. Acute on chronic

4th digit: 585
1. Stage I
2. Stage II (mild)
3. Stage III (moderate)
4. Stage IV (severe)
9. Unspecified stage

404.#3 Heart and chronic kidney disease with heart failure and chronic kidney disease stage V or end stage renal disease **[428.#(#)]** **[585.#]**

4th digit: 404.#3
0. Malignant
1. Benign
9. NOS

4th digit: 428
0. Congestive
1. Left
2#. Systolic
3#. Diastolic
4#. Combined systolic and diastolic
9. NOS

5th digit: 428.2-4
0. NOS
1. Acute
2. Chronic
3. Acute on chronic

4th digit: 585
5. Stage V
6. End stage

362.11 Retinopathy

780.6 HYPERTHERMIA NOS
995.86 HYPERTHERMIA MALIGNANT (DUE TO ANESTHESIA)
909.9 HYPERTHERMIA MALIGNANT DUE TO ANESTHESIA - LATE EFFECT
778.4 HYPERTHERMIA NEWBORN
301.11 HYPERTHYMIC PERSONALITY DISORDER
254.8 HYPERTHYMISM
242.## HYPERTHYROIDISM

4th digit: 242

0. Diffuse
1. Uninodular
2. Multinodular
3. Nodular unspecified
4. Ectopic thyroid nodular
8. Other specified
9. NOS

5th digit: 242

0. Without mention of thyrotoxic crisis or storm
1. With mention of thyrotoxic crisis or storm

775.3 HYPERTHYROIDISM NEONATAL
763.7 HYPERTONIC LABOR AFFECTING FETUS OR NEWBORN
661.4# HYPERTONIC UTERINE CONTRACTIONS (INCOORDINATE) OR (PROLONGED)

5th digit: 661.4

0. Episode of care NOS or N/A
1. Delivered
3. Antepartum complication

596.51 HYPERTONICITY BLADDER
0 HYPERTONICITY BLADDER WITH INCONTINENCE SEE 'BLADDER DISORDERS WITH INCONTINENCE'
779.89 HYPERTONICITY INFANT
779.89 HYPERTONICITY INFANT DUE TO ELECTROLYTE IMBALANCE
728.85 HYPERTONICITY MUSCLE
779.89 HYPERTONICITY NEWBORN
776.4 HYPERTRANSFUSION SYNDROME, NEWBORN

HYPERTRICHOSIS

704.1 NOS
757.4 Congenital
374.54 Eyelid

272.1 HYPERTRIGLYCERIDEMIA, ESSENTIAL
701.4 HYPERTROPHIC SCAR
569.49 HYPERTROPHY ANAL PAPILLAE
729.31 HYPERTROPHY FAT PAD KNEE
599.89 HYPERTROPHY VERUMONTANUM
270.2 HYPERTYROSINEMIA AMINO ACID METABOLISM (AROMATIC) DISTURBANCES
790.6 HYPERURICEMIA
270.3 HYPERVALINEMIA

HYPERVENTILATION

786.01 NOS
306.1 Psychogenic
306.1 Syndrome, psychogenic

273.3 HYPERVISCOSITY SYNDROME (OF SERUM)
289.0 HYPERVISCOSITY SYNDROME (OF SERUM) POLYCYTHEMIC
282.8 HYPERVISCOSITY SYNDROME (OF SERUM) SCLEROTHYMIC

HYPERVITAMINOSIS

278.2 A
963.5 A due to poisoning
278.4 D
963.5 D due to poisoning
278.8 NEC

276.6 HYPERVOLEMIA
364.41 HYPHEMA
305.4# HYPNOTIC ABUSE
304.1# HYPNOTIC ADDICTION (DEPENDENT)

5th digit: 304.1, 305.4

0. NOS
1. Continuous
2. Episodic
3. In remission

255.41 HYPOADRENALISM
255.41 HYPOADRENOCORTICISM
273.8 HYPOALBUMINEMIA
255.42 HYPOALDOSTERONISM
272.5 HYPOALPHALIPOPROTEINEMIA
993.2 HYPOBAROPATHY
909.4 HYPOBAROPATHY LATE EFFECT
272.5 HYPOBETALIPOPROTEINEMIA (FAMILIAL)

HYPOCALCEMIA

275.41 NOS
775.4 Cow's milk newborn
269.3 Dietary
775.4 Newborn
775.4 Phosphate - loading neonatal

276.9 HYPOCHLOREMIA
536.8 HYPOCHLORHYDRIA STOMACH
300.7 HYPOCHONDRIASIS
286.9 HYPOCOAGULABILITY SEE ALSO 'COAGULATION'
288.59 HYPOEOSINOPHILIA
782.0 HYPOESTHESIA
256.39 HYPOESTRINISM
256.39 HYPOESTRINISM WITH <u>NATURAL</u> <u>MENOPAUSE</u> <u>[627.2]</u>
256.39 HYPOESTROGENISM WITH <u>ARTIFICIAL</u> <u>MENOPAUSE</u> <u>[627.4]</u>
256.39 HYPOESTROGENISM
280.9 HYPOFERREMIA
280.0 HYPOFERREMIA DUE TO BLOOD LOSS CHRONIC
286.6 HYPOFIBRINOGENEMIA
286.3 HYPOFIBRINOGENEMIA CONGENITAL

HYPOGAMMAGLOBULINEMIA

279.00 Unspecified
279.06 Acquired primary
279.06 Congenital
279.04 Congenital sex-linked
279.09 Infancy transient
279.06 Sporadic

H

HYPOGASTRIC

902.51 Artery injury
908.4 Artery injury late effect
902.51 Artery laceration (rupture) (hematoma) (avulsion) (aneurysm) traumatic
908.4 Artery laceration late effect
908.4 Blood vessels other injury late effect
902.52 Vein injury
908.4 Vein injury late effect

752.89 HYPOGENITALISM (CONGENITAL) (MALE) (FEMALE)
352.5 HYPOGLOSSAL NERVE ATROPHY
352.5 HYPOGLOSSAL NERVE DISORDERS
951.7 HYPOGLOSSAL NERVE INJURY

HYPOGLYCEMIA

251.2 NOS
251.0 Administered insulin or oral agent
250.8# Diabetic
250.3# Diabetic coma

5th digit: 250.3, 8

0. Type II, adult-onset, non-insulin dependent (even if requiring insulin), or unspecified; controlled
1. Type I, juvenile-onset or insulin-dependent; controlled
2. Type II, adult-onset, non-insulin dependent (even if requiring insulin); uncontrolled
3. Type I, juvenile-onset or insulin-dependent; uncontrolled

> *V65.3 Use an additional code to identify body mass index (BMI), if known. See 'Body Mass Index'.*

V65.3 Dietary counseling and surveillance
251.2 Familial idiopathic
579.3 Following GI surgery
251.1 Hyperinsulinism (ectopic) (functional)
251.1 Hyperplastic pancreatic islet beta cells
251.0 Iatrogenic
270.3 Leucine induced
775.6 Neonatal
775.0 Neonatal caused by maternal diabetes
251.2 Reactive
251.2 Reactive spontaneous or due to diabetes treatment
251.2 Syndrome (familial) (neonatal)
251.1 Syndrome functional (familial) (neonatal)
962.3 Therapeutic misadventure
251.0 With coma (iatrogenic)
251.2 With polyneuropathy [357.4]
251.1 Other specified NEC

HYPOGONADISM

256.39 Female
256.39 Female with natural menopause [627.2]
253.4 Gonadotropic (isolated)
253.4 Hypogonadotropic with anosmia
257.2 Male
259.5 Male hereditary familial
256.39 Ovarian (primary)
256.39 Ovarian (primary) with natural menopause [627.2]
253.4 Pituitary (secondary)
257.2 Testicular

705.0 HYPOHIDROSIS
251.3 HYPOINSULINEMIA POSTSURGICAL
276.8 HYPOKALEMIA (SYNDROME)
588.89 HYPOKALEMIA RENAL
359.3 HYPOKALEMIC PERIODIC PARALYSIS
588.89 HYPOKALEMIC NEPHROPATHY
780.99 HYPOKINESIA
288.50 HYPOLEUKOCYTOSIS
272.5 HYPOLIPOPROTEINEMIA
275.2 HYPOMAGNESEMIA
775.4 HYPOMAGNESEMIA NEWBORN

HYPOMANIA

296.4# Circular, current or most recent episode manic
301.11 Hypomanic personality disorder chronic
296.0# Mild
296.0# Single episode
296.1# Recurrent

5th digit: 296.0, 1, 4

1. Mild
2. Moderate
3. Severe without mention of psychotic behavior
4. Severe specified as with psychotic behavior
5. In partial or NOS remission
6. In full remission

626.1 HYPOMENORRHEA
783.9 HYPOMETABOLISM
784.49 HYPONASALITY
276.1 HYPONATREMIA SODIUM [NA] DEFICIENCY
256.39 HYPO-OVARIANISM
256.39 HYPO-OVARIANISM WITH NATURAL MENOPAUSE [627.2]
252.1 HYPOPARATHYROIDISM
775.4 HYPOPARATHYROIDISM TRANSIENT NEONATAL
275.3 HYPOPHOSPHATASIA
275.3 HYPOPHOSPHATEMIA FAMILIAL
433.8# HYPOPHYSEAL ARTERY OBSTRUCTION OR OCCLUSION (THROMBOSIS)

5th digit: 433.8

0. Without cerebral infarction
1. With cerebral infarction

253.8 HYPOPHYSEAL SYNDROME
253.8 HYPOPHYSEOTHALAMIC SYNDROME
253.9 HYPOPHYSIS DISORDER
253.1 HYPOPHYSIS HYPERFUNCTION
253.2 HYPOPHYSIS HYPOFUNCTION
709.00 HYPOPIGMENTATION
374.53 HYPOPIGMENTATION OF EYELID

HYPOPITUITARISM

253.2 NOS
253.7 Hormone induced
253.7 Hypophysectomy-induced
253.7 Postablative
253.7 Postsurgical
253.7 Radiotherapy induced
253.2 Syndrome

H

0 HYPOPLASIA/HYPOPLASTIC SEE ANATOMICAL SITE
746.7 HYPOPLASTIC LEFT HEART SYNDROME
276.8 HYPOPOTASSEMIA SYNDROME
286.3 HYPOPROCONVERTINEMIA
273.8 HYPOPROTEINEMIA
286.7 HYPOPROTHROMBINEMIA ACQUIRED
364.05 HYPOPYON
370.04 HYPOPYON ULCER (CORNEAL)
780.99 HYPOPYREXIA
790.99 HYPORENINEMIA EXTREME
255.10 HYPORENINEMIA PRIMARY ALDOSTERONISM
790.99 HYPORENINISM EXTREME
780.09 HYPORESPONSIVE EPISODE
288.2 HYPOSEGMENTATION LEUKOCYTES HEREDITARY
780.52 HYPOSOMNIA UNSPECIFIED SEE ALSO 'INSOMNIA'
307.42 HYPOSOMNIA PERSISTENT ASSOCIATED WITH ANXIETY, DEPRESSION OR PSYCHOSIS
307.41 HYPOSOMNIA TRANSIENT DUE TO EMOTIONAL CONFLICT/ REACTION
780.51 HYPOSOMNIA WITH SLEEP APNEA UNSPECIFIED
276.1 HYPOSOMOLALITY AND/OR HYPONATREMIA (SYNDROME)
753.8 HYPOSPADIAS CONGENITAL - FEMALE
V13.61 HYPOSPADIAS CONGENITAL - HISTORY
752.61 HYPOSPADIAS CONGENITAL - MALE
606.1 HYPOSPERMATOGENESIS
372.72 HYPOSPHAGMA
255.41 HYPOSUPRARENALISM
246.8 HYPO-TBG-NEMIA

HYPOTENSION

458.9 NOS
458.1 Chronic
458.21 Hemodialysis (due to)
458.29 Iatrogenic
458.21 Iatrogenic due to hemodialysis

> ***648.9#: Use an additional code to identify the specific type of hypotension.***

648.9# Maternal current (co-existent) in pregnancy
669.2# Maternal syndrome

5th digit: 648.9, 669.2
- **0. Episode of care NOS or N/A**
- **1. Delivered**
- **2. Delivered with postpartum complication**
- **3. Antepartum complication**
- **4. Postpartum complication**

458.0 Orthostatic
333.0 Orthostatic with Parkinsonian syndrome idiopathic
333.0 Orthostatic with Parkinsonian syndrome symptomatic
458.1 Permanent idiopathic
458.29 Postoperative
458.0 Postural
458.8 Other specified

443.89 HYPOTHENAR HAMMER SYNDROME

HYPOTHERMIA

991.6 NOS
991.6 Accidental
909.4 Accidental late effect
995.89 Due to anesthesia
909.9 Due to anesthesia late effect
778.3 Newborn other
780.99 Not associated with low environmental temperature

HYPOTHYROIDISM

244.9 NOS
244.8 Acquired other specified
243 Congenital
246.1 Congenital dyshormonogenic goiter
244.3 Iatrogenic
244.0 Postsurgical
244.0 Postsurgical with myopathy [359.5]
244.1 Post irradiation
244.2 Resulting from administration or ingestion of iodide
244.8 Secondary NEC

301.12 HYPOTHYMIC PERSONALITY DISORDER
781.3 HYPOTONIA
779.89 HYPOTONIA AFFECTING FETUS OR NEWBORN
759.81 HYPOTONIA-HYPOMENTIA-HYPOGONADISM-OBESITY SYNDROME
728.9 HYPOTONIA MUSCLE

HYPOTONIC UTERINE DYSFUNCTION

763.7 Affecting fetus or newborn
661.0# Primary
661.1# Secondary
661.2# Other and unspecified

5th digit: 661.0-2
- **0. Episode of care NOS or N/A**
- **1. Delivered**
- **3. Antepartum complication**

HYPOTONY EYE

360.30 NOS (postinflammatory) (post op) (posttraumatic)
360.34 Anterior chamber flat (postinflammatory) (post op) (posttraumatic)
360.33 Associated with other ocular disorders
360.32 Due to ocular fistula (postinflammatory) (post op) (posttraumatic)
360.32 Following loss of aqueous or vitreous
360.31 Primary (postinflammatory) (post op) (posttraumatic)

704.09 HYPOTRICHOSIS
704.09 HYPOTRICHOSIS POSTINFECTION
378.32 HYPOTROPIA
786.09 HYPOVENTILATION
327.25 HYPOVENTILATION CONGENITAL CENTRAL ALVEOLAR SYNDROME
327.24 HYPOVENTILATION IDIOPATHIC SLEEP RELATED NONOBSTRUCTIVE ALVEOLAR

327.26: Code first the underlying medical or mental disorder.

327.26	HYPOVENTILATION IN CONDITIONS CLASSIFIED ELSEWHERE
264.9	HYPOVITAMINOSIS A NOS

HYPOVOLEMIA

276.52	NOS
998.0	Postoperative
958.4	Traumatic
908.6	Traumatic late effect

277.2	HYPOXANTHINE GUANINE PHOSPHORIBOSYLTRANSFERASE DEFICIENCY (HG PRT DEFICIENCY)
799.02	HYPOXEMIA

327.26: Code first the underlying medical or mental disorder.

327.26	HYPOXEMIA IN CONDITIONS CLASSIFIED ELSEWHERE
770.88	HYPOXEMIA NEWBORN

HYPOXIA

799.02	NOS
768.9	Birth - unspecified
768.6	Birth - mild
768.6	Birth - moderate
768.5	Birth - severe
768.5	Birth - severe with neurologic involvement
348.1	Cerebral
770.88	Cerebral newborn
997.01	Cerebral resulting from a procedure
770.88	Fetal
993.2	High altitude
909.4	High altitude late effect
0	Intrauterine see 'Fetal', distress
768.7	Ischemic encephalopathy (HIE)
411.89	Myocardial see also 'Coronary Insufficiency'
770.88	Newborn
327.24	Sleep related

768.7	HYPOXIC-ISCHEMIC ENCEPHALOPATHY (HIE)
V45.89	HYSTERECTOMY STATUS
300.10	HYSTERIA
300.11	HYSTERIA CONVERSION
301.50	HYSTERICAL PERSONALITY
300.11	HYSTERICAL TETANY

272.7 I CELL DISEASE
255.0 IATROGENIC SYNDROME OF EXCESS CORTISOL
049.8 ICELAND DISEASE (EPIDEMIC NEUROMYASTHENIA)
286.6 ICF SYNDROME (INTRAVASCULAR COAGULATION-FIBRINOLYSIS)
701.1 ICHTHYOSIS
757.1 ICHTHYOSIS CONGENITAL

ICTERUS

782.4 NOS
646.7# Gravis of pregnancy
5th digit: 646.7
0. Episode of care NOS or N/A
1. Delivered
3. Antepartum complication

774.6 Neonatorum
576.8 Obstruction
751.61 Obstruction congenital

992.0 ICTUS SOLARIS
909.4 ICTUS SOLARIS LATE EFFECT
692.89 ID REACTION
0 IDDM (INSULIN DEPENDENT DIABETES MELLITUS) SEE 'DIABETES'
0 IDENTITY CRISIS SEE 'IDENTITY DISORDER'

IDENTITY DISORDER

313.82 NOS
300.14 Dissociative
313.82 Emotional disturbance childhood or adolescence
302.6 Gender - NOS
302.85 Gender - adolescent
302.85 Gender - adult
302.6 Gender - childhood
302.6 Psychosexual - NOS
302.85 Psychosexual - adolescent
302.85 Psychosexual - adult
302.6 Psychosexual - childhood

IDIOPATHIC

769 Cardiorespiratory distress syndrome, newborn
516.3 Fibrosing alveolitis
425.1 Hypertrophic subaortic stenosis
425.2 Mural cardiomyopathy
425.2 Mural endomyocardial disease
581.9 Nephrotic syndrome (infantile)
331.5 Normal pressure hydrocephalus (INPH)
331.5 Normal pressure hydrocephalus (INPH) with dementia [294.1#]
5th digit: 294.1
0. Without behavioral disturbance or NOS
1. With behavioral disturbance

337.0 Peripheral autonomic neuropathy
356.4 Progressive polyneuropathy
275.0 Pulmonary hemosiderosis [516.1]
769 Respiratory distress syndrome newborn
593.4 Retroperitoneal fibrosis
579.0 Steatorrhea
238.71 Thrombocythemia (hemorrhagic)
0 Thrombocythemia site specified see 'Neoplasm Uncertain Behavior', by site M9962/1
0 See also specified condition

318.2 IDIOT IQ LESS THAN 20

310.8 IEED (INVOLUNTARY EMOTIONAL EXPRESSION DISORDER)
790.21 IFG (IMPAIRED FASTING GLUCOSE) (ELEVATED)
364.81 IFIS (INTRAOPERATIVE FLOPPY IRIS SYNDROME)
279.01 IGA SELECTIVE IMMUNODEFICIENCY
279.03 IGG OTHER SELECTIVE IMMUNOGLOBULIN DEFICIENCY
279.02 IGM IMMUNODEFICIENCY SELECTIVE
279.05 IGM INCREASED IMMUNODEFICIENCY

IHD (ISCHEMIC HEART DISEASE)

414.9 NOS
0 Acute, with MI see 'MI Acute'
411.89 Acute, without MI
411.81 Acute, without MI, with coronary (artery) occlusion
411.89 Acute subendocardial
414.10 Aneurysm (mural) (ventricular)
414.12 Aneurysm coronary dissecting
414.11 Aneurysm coronary vessels
414.19 Aneurysm other
414.0# Arteriosclerotic
414.0# Arteriosclerotic with chronic complete or total occlusion [414.2]
5th digit: 414.0
0. Unspecified type of vessel, native or graft
1. Native coronary vessel
2. Autologous vein bypass graft
3. Nonautologous biological bypass graft
4. Autologous artery bypass graft (gastroepiploic) (internal mammary)
5. Unspecified type of bypass graft
6. Native vessel of transplanted heart
7. Bypass graft of transplanted heart

414.9 Chronic
414.1# Chronic - aneurysm
5th digit: 414.1
0. Heart wall
1. Coronary vessels (arteriovenous)
2. Coronary artery dissecting
9. Other

414.0# Chronic - arteriosclerotic
414.0# Chronic – arteriosclerotic with chronic complete or total occlusion [414.2]
5th digit: 414.0
0. Unspecified type of vessel, native or graft
1. Native coronary vessel
2. Autologous vein bypass graft
3. Nonautologous biological bypass graft
4. Autologous artery bypass graft (gastroepiploic) (internal mammary)
5. Unspecified type of bypass graft
6. Native vessel of transplanted heart
7. Bypass graft of transplanted heart

414.8 Chronic - myocardial
414.8 Chronic - other
411.89 Coronary insufficiency acute
V17.3 Family history
411.89 Subacute
411.89 Other specified - acute
414.8 Other specified - chronic

425.1	IHSS (IDIOPATHIC HYPERTROPHIC SUBAORTIC STENOSIS)
	ILEITIS
558.9	NOS (chronic)
558.3	Allergic
<u>558.3</u>	<u>Allergic</u> due to ingested foods **[V15.0#]**
	5th digit: V15.0
	1. Peanuts
	2. Milk products
	3. Eggs
	4. Seafood
	5. Other foods
558.9	Dietetic
009.0	Infectious
558.9	Noninfectious NOS
555.0	Regional (segmental) (terminal)
555.2	Regional (segmental) (terminal) with large intestine
0	See also 'Enteritis'
560.9	ILEOCECAL COIL OBSTRUCTION (SEE ALSO 'INTESTINE, INTESTINAL', OBSTRUCTION)
564.89	ILEOCECAL COIL STASIS
902.26	ILEO-COLIC ARTERY INJURY
908.4	ILEO-COLIC ARTERY INJURY LATE EFFECT
902.31	ILEO-COLIC VEIN INJURY
908.4	ILEO-COLIC VEIN INJURY LATE EFFECT
556.1	ILEOCOLITIS ULCERATIVE (CHRONIC)
	ILEOSTOMY
V53.5	Belt fitting and adjustment
V55.2	Care
V55.2	Catheter adjustment or repositioning
V55.2	Catheter removal or replacement
V55.2	Closure
569.60	Complication - NOS
569.62	Complication - mechanical
569.69	Complication - other
569.69	Fistula
569.69	Hernia

When coding an infection of an ostomy, use an additional code to specify the organism. See 'Bacterial Infection'

569.61	Infection
<u>569.61</u>	<u>Infection</u> with cellulitis of abdomen [682.2]
<u>569.61</u>	<u>Infection</u> with septicemia **[038.#(#)]**
	4th or 4th <u>and</u> 5th digit code for organism: 038
	.9 NOS
	.3 Anaerobic
	.3 Bacteroides
	.3 Clostridium
	.42 E. coli
	.49 Enterobacter aerogenes
	.40 Gram negative
	.49 Gram negative other
	.41 Hemophilus influenzae
	.2 Pneumococcal
	.49 Proteus
	.43 Pseudomonas
	.44 Serratia
	.10 Staphylococcal NOS
	.11 Staphylococcal aureus
	.19 Staphylococcal other
	.0 Streptococcal (anaerobic)
	.49 Yersinia enterocolitica
	.8 Other specified

ILEOSTOMY (continued)

569.62	Malfunction
569.69	Prolapse
V44.2	Status
V55.3	Toilet stoma
569.62	Valve malfunction
	ILEUM, ILEAL
V45.72	Absence postsurgical
751.1	Atresia (absence) congenital
564.89	Dilatation
306.4	Dilatation psychogenic
562.00	Diverticula
863.29	Injury (traumatic)
863.29	Injury (traumatic) with open wound
564.89	Irritability
560.9	Obstruction see also 'Intestine, Intestinal', obstruction
569.83	Perforation
211.3	Polyp
564.89	Stasis
	ILEUS
560.1	Adynamic
537.2	Chronic duodenal
560.31	Gallstone
751.3	Hirschsprung's
777.1	Meconium
277.01	Meconium due to cystic fibrosis
564.89	Myxedema
777.4	Newborn transitory
560.1	Paralytic
997.2	Postoperative
062.8	ILHEUS VIRAL ENCEPHALITIS

Injury of a blood vessel can be a laceration, A-V fistula, aneurysm, or hematoma. Use the injury code, found by anatomical site (the name of the blood vessel).

	ILIAC
442.2	Aneurysm
902.53	Aneurysm traumatic
	ARTERY
444.81	Embolism
443.22	Dissection
444.81	Infarction
902.53	Injury
902.59	Injury specified branch NEC
908.4	Injury or laceration late effect
902.53	Laceration traumatic (rupture) (hematoma) (avulsion) (aneurysm)
444.81	Occlusion
444.81	Thrombosis

ILIAC (continued)

908.4	Blood vessel injury - late effect
902.50	Blood vessel injury - unspecified vessel (traumatic) (aneurysm)
902.59	Blood vessel injury - other specified vessel
726.5	Bone spur
959.19	Region injury
902.54	Vein injury (traumatic)
908.4	Vein injury or laceration late effect
902.54	Vein laceration traumatic (rupture) (hematoma) (avulsion) (aneurysm)

444.81	ILIOFEMORAL ARTERY OBSTRUCTION
843.0	ILIOFEMORAL STRAIN (SPRAIN) (AVULSION) (HEMARTHROSIS) (SEPARATION)
335.79	ILIOHYPOGASTRIC MONONEUROPATHY
355.79	ILIOHYPOGASTRIC NERVE COMPRESSION (ENTRAPMENT)
355.79	ILIOHYPOGASTRIC NERVE DISORDER (LESION)
335.79	ILIOINGUINAL MONONEUROPATHY
355.79	ILIOINGUINAL NERVE COMPRESSION (ENTRAPMENT)
355.79	ILIOINGUINAL NERVE DISORDER (LESION)
355.79	ILIOINGUINAL NEURITIS
728.89	ILIOTIBIAL BAND FRICTION SYNDROME
799.89	ILL-DEFINED DISEASE
V61.6	ILLEGITIMACY CAUSING FAMILY PROBLEM (REASON FOR ENCOUNTER)
318.0	IMBECILE
281.1	IMERSLUND GRASBECK SYNDROME (ANEMIA DUE TO FAMILIAL SELECTIVE VITAMIN B-12 MALABSORPTION)
270.5	IMIDAZOLE AMINO ACID DISORDER
270.8	IMIDOGLYCINURIA FAMILIAL
270.8	IMINOACIDOPATHY
301.89	IMMATURE PERSONALITY DISORDER
994.1	IMMERSION (NON FATAL DROWNING)
909.4	IMMERSION (NON FATAL DROWNING) LATE EFFECT
991.4	IMMERSION FOOT
728.3	IMMOBILITY SYNDROME

IMMUNE

279.3	Deficiency
279.10	Disorder cell mediated deficiency unspecified
279.19	Disorder cell mediated deficiency other specified NEC
V12.2	Disorder history
V77.99	Disorders screening
279.9	Mechanism disorder
279.8	Mechanism disorder specified NEC
V07.2	Sera [gamma globulin] prophylactic administration
760.79	Sera transmitted via placenta or breast milk affecting fetus or newborn
287.31	Thrombocytopenic purpura (ITP)

279.2	IMMUNITY DEFICIENCY SYNDROME, COMBINED
0	IMMUNIZATION SEE 'VACCINATION'

IMMUNODEFICIENCY

279.3	NOS
279.2	Agammaglobulinemia autosomal recessive
279.04	Agammaglobulinemia Bruton's type
279.2	Agammaglobulinemia Swiss-type
279.04	Agammaglobulinemia X-linked
279.2	Agammaglobulinemia X-linked recessive
279.2	Aplasia or dysplasia
334.8	Ataxia telangiectasia (Louis-Bar)
279.2	Autosomal recessive Swiss-type
279.00	B-cell
279.13	Cellular with abnormal immunoglobulin deficiency
279.2	Combined severe
279.06	Common variable (CVID)
279.8	Complement C1-C9 deficiency
279.06	Dysgammaglobulinemia acquired (congenital) (primary)
0	Human virus see 'HIV' infection

IMMUNODEFICIENCY (continued)

279.00	Hypogammaglobulinemia
279.06	Hypogammaglobulinemia acquired primary
279.06	Hypogammaglobulinemia congenital
279.04	Hypogammaglobulinemia congenital sex-linked
279.09	Hypogammaglobulinemia infancy transient
279.06	Hypogammaglobulinemia sporadic
279.01	IGA selective
279.03	IGG
279.05	IGM increased
279.02	IGM selective
279.9	Immune mechanism disorder
279.19	Other cell mediated deficiency
334.8	Other cell mediated deficiency causing ataxia telangiectasia
279.2	Syndrome combined
279.10	T-Cell
279.2	Thymic
279.05	With hyper IGM autosomal recessive
279.05	With hyper IGM X-linked

795.79	IMMUNOGLOBULINS ELEVATED
795.79	IMMUNOLOGICAL FINDINGS ABNORMAL OTHER AND UNSPECIFIED
203.8#	IMMUNOPROLIFERATIVE NEOPLASM OTHER
203.1#	IMMUNOPROLIFERATIVE PLASMA CELL LEUKEMIA

5th digit: 203.1, 8
- **0. Without mention of remission**
- **1. In remission**

V58.12	IMMUNOTHERAPY ANTINEOPLASTIC ENCOUNTER (MAINTENANCE)
V07.2	IMMUNOTHERAPY PROPHYLACTIC
380.4	IMPACTED CERUMEN
560.30	IMPACTION COLON
560.39	IMPACTION FECAL
560.30	IMPACTION INTESTINE
411.1	IMPENDING CORONARY SYNDROME
752.42	IMPERFORATE HYMEN CONGENITAL

IMPETIGO

684	NOS
684	Bullous
684	Circinate
684	Ear (external) [380.13]
684	Eyelid [373.5]
694.3	Herpetiformis
684	Neonatorum
684	Pinna [380.13]
684	Simplex
686.8	Ulcerative
684	Vulgaris

726.2	IMPINGEMENT SHOULDER SYNDROME
524.89	IMPINGEMENT SOFT TISSUE BETWEEN TEETH - NOS
524.81	IMPINGEMENT SOFT TISSUE BETWEEN TEETH - ANTERIOR
524.82	IMPINGEMENT SOFT TISSUE BETWEEN TEETH - POSTERIOR
724.4	IMPINGEMENT VERTEBRAL BODIES SYNDROME

IMPOTENCE

607.84 NOS
250.6# Diabetic (due to peripheral neuropathy) [607.84]
250.7# Diabetic peripheral (due to vascular disease) [607.84]
5th digit: 250.6-7
0. Type II, adult onset, non-insulin dependent (even if requiring insulin), or unspecified; controlled
1. Type I, juvenile onset or insulin-dependent; controlled
2. Type II, adult onset, non-insulin dependent (even if requiring insulin); uncontrolled
3. Type I, juvenile onset or insulin-dependent; uncontrolled

607.84 Organic
997.99 Organic postprostatectomy [607.84]
302.72 Psychosexual

V62.5 IMPRISONMENT
312.3# IMPULSE CONTROL DISORDER
5th digit: 312.3
0. Unspecified
1. Pathological gambling
2. Kleptomania
3. Pyromania
4. Intermittent explosive
5. Isolated explosive
6. Other

INANITION

263.9 NOS
994.2 Due to deprivation of food
263.9 Due to malnutrition
780.6 Fever

253.6 INAPPROPRIATE ADH (SYNDROME)
V68.09 INCAPACITY CERTIFICATE ISSUE
654.3# INCARCERATED UTERUS RETROVERTED COMPLICATING CHILDBIRTH
5th digit: 654.3
0. Episode of care NOS or N/A
1. Delivered
2. Delivered with postpartum complication
3. Antepartum complication
4. Postpartum complication

526.1 INCISOR CANAL CYST
077.0 INCLUSION CONJUNCTIVITIS
078.5 INCLUSION DISEASE
078.5 INCLUSION DISEASE SALIVARY GLAND
761.0 INCOMPETENT CERVIX AFFECTING FETUS OR NEWBORN
756.0 INCOMPLETE MANDIBULOFACIAL SYNDROME

When coding urinary incontinence, code the underlying cause of the incontinence, such as the cystocele, rectocele, prostatitis, or bladder disorders. The cause would be sequenced first. The incontinence would be sequenced second.

INCONTINENCE

787.6 Fecal
787.6 Sphincter ani
599.84 Urethral sphincter

INCONTINENCE (continued)

URINE

788.30 NOS
788.37 Continuous leakage
788.30 Male NOS
788.39 Neurogenic
788.36 Nocturnal enuresis
788.38 Overflow
788.39 Paradoxical
788.35 Post-void dribbling
625.6 Stress, female
788.32 Stress, male
788.33 Urge and stress mixed (male) (female)
788.31 Urge incontinence
788.34 Without sensory awareness
788.39 Specified NEC
788.39 Other

INCONTINENCE (continued)

0 With bladder disorders see 'Bladder Disorders With Incontinence'

757.33 INCONTINENTIA PIGMENTI
781.3 INCOORDINATION MUSCULAR
385.24 INCUS ABSENCE
744.04 INCUS ABSENCE CONGENITAL
082.1 INDIAN TICK TYPHUS
270.2 INDICANURIA AMINO ACID METABOLISM AROMATIC DISTURBANCES
536.8 INDIGESTION
791.9 INDOLACETIC ACID ABNORMAL URINARY EVALUATION (ELEVATION)
099.8 INDOLENT BUBO
763.89 INDUCTION OF LABOR (MEDICAL) AFFECTING FETUS OR NEWBORN
607.81 INDURATIO PENIS PLASTICA
782.8 INDURATION SKIN
305.0# INEBRIETY NOS
5th digit: 305.0
0. NOS
1. Continuous
2. Episodic
3. In remission

INFANT

780.92 Crying excessive
798.0 Death sudden syndrome (SIDS)
0 Death sudden syndrome (SIDS) near miss - code individual symptom(s)
0 Evaluation for suspected condition not found see 'Observation Newborn / Infant Suspected Condition (Undiagnosed) (Unproven) not found'
780.91 Fussy
766.1 Heavy for dates
766.0 Large exceptionally (birthweight > 4500 grams)
766.1 Large for dates other (regardless of gestation)
0 Light for dates see 'Light For Dates'
255.2 Hercules syndrome
766.22 Postmaturity NOS (>42 completed weeks)
766.21 Post term (>40 to 42 completed weeks)

INFANT (continued)

765.##: Use an additional code if necessary, to further specify the condition of the premature infant.

PREMATURE

765.10 Weight unspecified weeks gestation [765.2#]
765.14 1000-1249 grams weeks gestation [765.2#]
765.15 1250-1499 grams weeks gestation [765.2#]
765.16 1500-1749 grams weeks gestation [765.2#]
765.17 1750-1999 grams weeks gestation [765.2#]
765.18 2000-2499 grams weeks gestation [765.2#]
765.19 2500 grams and over weeks gestation [765.2#]
765.00 Weight unspecified weeks gestation [765.2#]
765.01 Less than 500 grams weeks gestation [765.2#]
765.02 500-749 grams weeks gestation [765.2#]
765.03 750-999 grams weeks gestation [765.2#]

5th digit: 765.2
0. Unspecified
1. Less than 24 completed
2. 24 completed
3. 25 - 26 completed
4. 27 - 28 completed
5. 29 - 30 completed
6. 31 - 32 completed
7. 33 - 34 completed
8. 35 - 36 completed
9. 37 or more completed

INFANT (continued)

766.22 Prolonged gestation (>42 completed weeks)
995.55 Shaken syndrome
271.8 Sialic acid storage disorder
798.0 SIDS (sudden infant death syndrome)
0 SIDS near miss (sudden infant death syndrome) - code individual symptom(s)
775.0 Syndrome of diabetic mother

INFANTILE

261 Atrophy (malnutrition severe)
288.01 Genetic agranulocytosis
330.8 Necrotizing encephalomyelopathy
345.6# Spasms

5th digit: 345.6
0. Without mention of intractable epilepsy
1. With intractable epilepsy

335.0 Spinal muscular atrophy

259.9 INFANTILISM

253.3 INFANTILISM SYNDROME

INFARCTION

0 See also specified organ
255.41 Adrenal (capsule) (gland)
557.0 Appendices epiploicae
410.8# Atrial

5th digit: 410.8
0. Episode NOS
1. Initial episode
2. Subsequent episode

557.0 Bowel

INFARCTION (continued)

434.91 Brain stem
434.11 Brain stem embolic
V12.54 Brain stem history without residual
997.02 Brain stem iatrogenic
997.02 Brain stem postoperative
434.01 Brain stem thrombotic
0 Brain stem with residual see 'Late Effect', cerebrovascular disease
611.8 Breast
434.91 Cerebellum
434.11 Cerebellum embolic
434.01 Cerebellum thrombotic
434.91 Cerebral
434.91 Cerebral aborted
434.11 Cerebral embolic
997.02 Cerebral postoperative
434.01 Cerebral thrombotic
434.91 Cortical
620.8 Fallopian tube
575.8 Gallbladder
573.4 Hepatic
415.19 Lung
415.12 Lung (artery) (vein) septic
415.11 Lung iatrogenic
415.11 Lung postoperative
457.8 Lymphatic
557.0 Mesenteric
0 Myocardial see 'Myocardial Infarction Acute'
620.8 Ovary
577.8 Pancreas
252.8 Parathyroid
253.8 Pituitary
762.2 Placenta affecting fetus or newborn
656.7# Placenta affecting management of mother

5th digit: 656.7
0. Episode of care NOS or N/A
1. Delivered
3. Antepartum Complication

602.8 Prostate
415.19 Pulmonary
415.12 Pulmonary (artery) (vein) (postoperative) septic
415.11 Pulmonary iatrogenic
415.11 Pulmonary postoperative
038.#(#) Pulmonary septic with septicemia [415.12]

4th or 4th and 5th digit code for organism: 038
.9 NOS
.3 Anaerobic
.3 Bacteroides
.3 Clostridium
.42 E. coli
.49 Enterobacter aerogenes
.40 Gram negative
.49 Gram negative other
.41 Hemophilus influenzae
.2 Pneumococcal
.49 Proteus
.43 Pseudomonas
.44 Serratia
.10 Staphylococcal NOS
.11 Staphylococcal aureus
.19 Staphylococcal other
.0 Streptococcal (anaerobic)
.49 Yersinia enterocolitica
.8 Other specified

593.81 Renal

I-J-K

INFARCTION (continued)

362.84 Retinal
336.1 Spinal cord
289.59 Spleen
608.83 Testicular
246.3 Thyroid

When coding an infection, use an additional code, [041.#], to identify the organism. See 'Bacterial Infection'.

INFECTION

997.62 Amputation stump (chronic)
0 Amputation stump original admission see 'Amputation', by site, 'Traumatic Complicated'
0 Bacteria see 'Bacterial Infection'
996.64 Catheter (indwelling) (urinary)

999.31 Other infection - Use an additional code to identify the specified infection such as septicemia, (038.#(#)).

999.31 Catheter-related blood stream (CRBSI)
999.31 Catheter central venous
997.62 Chronic of stump following amputation
0 Complication of internal prosthesis implant or graft see 'Complication Of An Internal Prosthesis Implant Or Graft - Infection Or Inflammation' by specified device

999.39 Other infection - Use an additional code to identify the specified infection such as septicemia, (038.#(#)).

999.39 Following infusion injection transfusion or vaccination
659.3# Labor generalized
5th digit: 659.3
0. Episode of care NOS or N/A
1. Delivered
3. Antepartum complication
760.2 Maternal affecting fetus or newborn not manifested in fetus or newborn
647.9# Maternal current (co-existent) in pregnancy NOS
646.6# Maternal genitourinary complicating pregnancy
5th digit: 646.6, 647.9
0. Episode of care NOS or N/A
1. Delivered
2. Delivered with postpartum complication
3. Antepartum complication
4. Postpartum complication

760.1 Maternal renal or urinary affecting fetus or newborn
647.6# Maternal viral current (co-existent) in pregnancy
647.8# Maternal other specified current (co-existent) in pregnancy
5th digit: 647.6, 8
0. Episode of care NOS or N/A
1. Delivered
2. Delivered with postpartum complication
3. Antepartum complication
4. Postpartum complication

771.4 Navel cord or perinatal
771.89 Newborn generalized
0 Ostomy see specified ostomy
771.89 Perinatal Other

INFECTION (continued)

998.59 Postoperative
674.3# Postoperative obstetrical
5th digit: 674.3
0. Episode of care unspecified or N/A
2. Delivered with postpartum complication
4. Postpartum complication
998.51 Postoperative seroma
771.4 Umbilical stump
079.#(#) Viral and chlamydial in conditions classified elsewhere, site NOS
4th or 4th and 5th digit: 079
0. Adenovirus
1. Echo virus
2. Coxsackie virus
3. Rhinovirus
6. Respiratory syncytial virus (RSV)
8#. Other specified viral and chlamydial
88. Other specified chlamydial
89. Other specified viral
9#. Unspecified viral and chlamydial
98. Unspecified chlamydial
99. Unspecified viral
958.3 Wound, posttraumatic NEC following trauma
908.6 Wound, posttraumatic NEC following trauma late effect
0 See also 'Open Wound' or 'Laceration', complicated

INFECTIOUS

136.9 And parasitic disease unspecified
139.8 And parasitic disease late effects

647.8#: Use an additional code to identify the maternal infection or parasitic disease.

647.8# And parasitic diseases maternal current (co-existent) in pregnancy other specified
5th digit: 647.8
0. Episode of care NOS or N/A
1. Delivered
2. Delivered with postpartum complication
3. Antepartum complication
4. Postpartum complication
462 Angina throat
136.9 Disease unspecified
V12.00 Disease unspecified history
V12.09 Disease other history
V75.9 Disease screening exam
0 See also specified organ

INFERIOR MESENTERIC

954.1 Plexus injury
902.32 Vein injury
908.4 Vein injury late effect
902.32 Vein laceration (rupture) (hematoma) (avulsion) (aneurysm) traumatic
908.4 Vein laceration late effect

INFERIOR VENA CAVA

747.40 Anomaly
902.10 Injury
908.4 Injury late effect
902.19 Injury other site
459.2 Obstruction
453.2 Occlusion
459.2 Syndrome
453.2 Thrombosis

Code V26.21 is to be used for couples undergoing fertility testing. V26.21 is assigned for both the male and female. Assign the code for the cause of the infertility as a secondary code on the infertile partner's record. Remember, do not use a male diagnosis code on a female's record or a female diagnosis code on a male's record.

INFERTILITY FEMALE

628.9 Unspecified
628.8 Age related
628.0 Associated with annovulation
628.4 Associated with anomaly of cervical mucus
628.4 Associated with congenital structural anomaly
628.4 Cervical or vaginal origin
628.4 Dysmucorrhea
V23.0 History affecting pregnancy supervision
V26.21 Investigation, management and testing
V26.29 Investigation, management and testing other
628.3 Non implantation
628.1 Pituitary-hypothalamic origin
628.2 Tubal origin (block) (stenosis) (occlusion)
628.3 Uterine origin
628.8 Other specified origin

INFERTILITY FEMALE DUE TO OTHER CAUSES

253.0 Acromegaly [628.1]
253.8 Adiposogenital dystrophy [628.1]
253.1 Forbes-Albright [628.1]
256.39 Ovarian failure [628.0]
253.2 Panhypopituitarism [628.1]
614.6 Peritubular adhesions (postoperative) (postinfection) [628.2]
253.3 Pituitary dwarfism [628.1]
253.4 Prolactin deficiency [628.1]
256.4 Stein Leventhal [628.0]

Code V26.21 is to be used for couples undergoing fertility testing. V26.21 is assigned for both the male and female. Assign the code for the cause of the infertility as a secondary code on the infertile partner's record. Remember, do not use a male diagnosis code on a female's record or a female diagnosis code on a male's record.

INFERTILITY MALE

606.9 Unspecified
606.0 Azoospermia
606.8 Due to infection (radiation) (drugs) (disease)
606.8 Extratesticular causes (drugs, disease, infection, radiation)
606.0 Germinal cell aplasia
606.1 Germinal cell desquamation
606.1 Hypospermatogenesis
V26.21 Investigation, management and testing
V26.29 Investigation, management and testing other
606.8 Obstruction efferent ducts
606.1 Oligospermia
606.0 Spermatogenic arrest complete
606.1 Spermatogenic arrest incomplete
606.8 Systemic disease

134.9 INFESTATION (SKIN) NOS

Use an additional code to identify estrogen receptor status. V86.0 Estrogen receptor positive status (ER+) or V86.1 Estrogen receptor negative status (ER-).

INFILTRATING

174.9 Duct carcinoma site NOS
0 Duct carcinoma site specified see 'Cancer', by site M8500/3
174.9 Ductular carcinoma site NOS
0 Ductular carcinoma site specified see 'Cancer', by site M8521/3

799.89 INFIRMITY
996.60 INFLAMMATION COMPLICATION OF INTERNAL PROSTHESIS IMPLANT OR GRAFT
199.0 INFLAMMATORY CARCINOMA SITE NOS
0 INFLAMMATORY CARCINOMA SITE SPECIFIED SEE 'CANCER', BY SITE M8530/3

In order to correctly code influenza with pneumonia (487.0), use an additional code from the pneumonia category to identify the type of pneumonia, if known. Ie., Influenza with e. coli pneumonia 487.0 and 482.82.

INFLUENZA

487.1 NOS
487.1 Asian
488 Avian virus
487.8 Encephalitis
487.8 Gastroenteritis
487.8 Gastrointestinal involvement
487.1 Laryngitis
487.8 Myocarditis
487.8 Otitis media [382.02]
487.1 Pharyngitis
487.0 Pneumonia
487.1 Respiratory involvement
487.0 Respiratory involvement - with pneumonia
487.1 Sinusitis
487.1 Syndrome
V04.81 Vaccination

524.34 INFRAERUPTION TEETH
726.69 INFRAPATELLAR BURSITIS
840.3 INFRASPINATUS SEPARATION (RUPTURE) (TEAR) (LACERATION)
840.3 INFRASPINATUS STRAIN (SPRAIN) (AVULSION) (HEMARTHROSIS)
746.83 INFUNDIBULAR PULMONIC STENOSIS CONGENITAL
996.62 INFUSION PUMP COMPLICATION - INFECTION OR INFLAMMATION
996.1 INFUSION PUMP COMPLICATION - MECHANICAL
996.74 INFUSION PUMP COMPLICATION - OTHER
703.0 INGROWN FINGERNAIL (WITH INFECTION)
703.0 INGROWN TOENAIL (WITH INFECTION)
305.9# INHALANT ABUSE
304.6# INHALANT ADDICTION (DEPENDENT)

5th digit: 304.6, 305.9
0. NOS
1. Continuous
2. Episodic
3. In remission

0 INHALATION FLAME SEE 'BURN', INTERNAL ORGANS

I-J-K

740.2 INIENCEPHALY CONGENITAL

Injury to internal organs, such as the lung, spleen, liver, or kidney, can be a contusion, laceration, tear, or rupture. You may find the code under the type of injury or the anatomical site.

INJURY

959.9 Site NOS
919.8 Site NOS superficial
919.9 Site NOS superficial infected
0 Blood vessel see specified blood vessel, anatomical site or 'Blood Vessel Injury'
0 Diffuse axonal see 'Intracranial', injury
V71.3 Evaluation work related with no apparent injury
V15.5 History
0 Internal - for specific injury see anatomical site
869.0 Internal - unspecified or ill-defined organs
869.1 Internal - unspecified or ill-defined organs with open wound into cavity
868.00 Internal - intraabdominal unspecified organ
868.10 Internal - intraabdominal unspecified organ with open wound into cavity
868.09 Internal - intraabdominal other and/or multiple organ(s)
868.19 Internal - intraabdominal other and/or multiple organ(s) with open wound into cavity
908.0 Internal - late effect (chest)
908.1 Internal - late effect (intra abdominal organs)
908.2 Internal - late effect (other internal organs)
908.9 Late effect (NOS)
760.5 Maternal affecting fetus or newborn
648.9# Maternal non-obstetrical current (co-existent) in pregnancy
5th digit: 648.9
0. Episode of care unspecified or N/A
1. Delivered
2. Delivered with postpartum complication
3. Antepartum complication
4. Postpartum complication
V71.4 MVA, evaluation with no apparent injury
V65.43 Prevention counseling
959.8 Other specified site including multiple
0 See also anatomical site injured or type of injury

V61.3 IN-LAW PROBLEM

653.2# INLET CONTRACTION PELVIS

660.1# INLET CONTRACTION PELVIS OBSTRUCTING LABOR [653.2#]
5th digit: 653.2, 660.1
0. Episode of care NOS or N/A
1. Delivered
3. Antepartum complication

Injury of a blood vessel can be a laceration, A-V fistula, aneurysm, or hematoma. Use the injury code found by anatomical site (the name of the blood vessel).

INNOMINATE

747.69 Artery origin anomaly (aberrant) (absence) (agenesis) (accessory) (aneurysm) (deformity) (hypoplasia) (malposition)
901.1 Artery injury
908.4 Artery injury late effect
901.1 Artery laceration (rupture) (hematoma) (avulsion) (aneurysm) traumatic
908.4 Artery laceration late effect

INNOMINATE (continued)

901.3 Vein injury
908.4 Vein injury late effect
901.3 Vein laceration (rupture) (hematoma) (avulsion) (aneurysm) traumatic
908.4 Vein laceration late effect

0 INOCULATION SEE 'VACCINATION (NEED FOR)'

331.5 INPH (IDIOPATHIC NORMAL PRESSURE HYDROCEPHALUS)

331.5 INPH (IDIOPATHIC NORMAL PRESSURE HYDROCEPHALUS) WITH DEMENTIA [**294.1#**]
5th digit: 294.1
0. Without behavioral disturbance or NOS
1. With behavioral disturbance

When coding for an insect bite or sting, the important distinction to be made is whether the insect is venomous or nonvenomous, rather than if the contact is a bite or sting. Below are the nonvenomous codes. Venomous codes are listed under 'Sting Venomous'.

INSECT BITE NONVENOMOUS

919.4 NOS
919.5 NOS infected
911.4 Abdominal wall
911.5 Abdominal wall infected
V15.06 Allergy history
916.4 Ankle
916.5 Ankle infected
911.4 Anus
911.5 Anus infected
912.4 Arm (upper)
912.5 Arm (upper) infected
912.4 Axilla
912.5 Axilla infected
911.4 Back
911.5 Back infected
911.4 Breast
911.5 Breast infected
911.4 Buttock
911.5 Buttock infected
916.4 Calf
916.5 Calf infected
910.4 Cheek
910.5 Cheek infected
911.4 Chest wall
911.5 Chest wall infected
910.4 Ear
910.5 Ear Infected
913.4 Elbow
913.5 Elbow infected
918.0 Eyelid and periocular area
919.5 Eyelid and periocular area infected
910.4 Face
910.5 Face infected
915.4 Finger
915.5 Finger infected
911.4 Flank
911.5 Flank infected
917.4 Foot
917.5 Foot Infected
913.4 Forearm
913.5 Forearm infected

INSECT BITE NONVENOMOUS (continued)

911.4 Groin
911.5 Groin infected
910.4 Gum
910.5 Gum infected
914.4 Hand
914.5 Hand infected
917.4 Heel
917.5 Heel infected
916.4 Hip
916.5 Hip infected
911.4 Interscapular region
911.5 Interscapular region infected
916.4 Knee
916.5 Knee infected
911.4 Labia
911.5 Labia infected
906.2 Late effect
916.4 Leg
916.5 Leg infected
910.4 Lip
910.5 Lip infected
919.4 Multiple
919.5 Multiple infected
910.4 Neck
910.5 Neck infected
910.4 Nose
910.5 Nose infected
911.4 Penis
911.5 Penis infected
911.4 Perineum
911.5 Perineum infected
910.4 Scalp
910.5 Scalp infected
912.4 Scapular region
912.5 Scapular region infected
911.4 Scrotum
911.5 Scrotum infected
912.4 Shoulder
912.5 Shoulder infected
911.4 Testis
911.5 Testis infected
916.4 Thigh
916.5 Thigh infected
910.4 Throat
910.5 Throat infected
915.4 Thumb
915.5 Thumb infected
917.4 Toe
917.5 Toe infected
911.4 Trunk
911.5 Trunk infected
911.4 Vagina
911.5 Vagina infected
911.4 Vulva
911.5 Vulva infected
913.4 Wrist
913.5 Wrist infected
919.4 Other sites
919.5 Other sites infected

989.5 INSECT BITE VENOMOUS (SPIDER)
134.9 INSECT INFESTATION
134.8 INSECT INFESTATION OTHER SPECIFIED
V26.1 INSEMINATION ARTIFICIAL

INSOMNIA

780.52 Unspecified
307.41 Adjustment
291.82 Alcohol induced
V69.5 Behavioral of childhood
292.85 Drug induced
307.42 Idiopathic
627.2 Menopausal
627.4 Menopausal artificial
307.41 Nonorganic origin
307.42 Nonorganic persistent (primary)
307.41 Nonorganic transient
327.00 Organic NOS

> ***327.01-327.02: Code first the underlying medical or mental disorder.***

327.01 Organic due to medical condition
327.02 Organic due to mental disorder
327.09 Organic other
307.42 Paradoxical
307.42 Persistent associated with anxiety/depression/psychosis
307.42 Persistent psychogenic
307.42 Primary
307.42 Psychophysiological
307.49 Subjective complaint
307.41 Transient psychogenic
780.51 With sleep apnea unspecified
780.52 Other
0 See also 'Sleep Disorder/Disturbance'

774.4 INSPISSATED BILE SYNDROME, NEWBORN

INSTABILITY

596.59 Detrusor
0 Detrusor with incontinence see 'Bladder Disorders With Incontinence'
718.8# Joint (old) (posttraumatic)
5th digit: 718.8
0. Site NOS
1. Shoulder region
2. Upper arm, elbow
3. Forearm, wrist
4. Hand
5. Pelvic region, thigh, and hip
6. Lower leg, knee
7. Ankle and/or foot
8. Other
9. Multiple

724.6 Joint - lumbosacral
724.6 Joint - sacroiliac
599.83 Urethral

307.44 INSUFFICIENT SLEEP SYNDROME
251.0 INSULIN COMA
250.3# INSULIN COMA DIABETIC
5th digit: 250.3
0. Type II, adult-onset, non-insulin dependent (even if requiring insulin), or unspecified; controlled
1. Type I, juvenile-onset or insulin-dependent; controlled
2. Type II, adult-onset, non-insulin dependent (even if requiring insulin); uncontrolled
3. Type I, juvenile-onset or insulin-dependent; uncontrolled

I-J-K

I-J-K

251.3 INSULIN DEFICIENCY POSTSURGICAL
V67.51 INSULIN DRUG FOLLOW UP EXAM - COMPLETED THERAPY
V58.67 INSULIN DRUG FOLLOW UP EXAM - CURRENT THERAPY
V58.83 INSULIN DRUG MONITORING ENCOUNTER
V58.83 INSULIN DRUG MONITORING ENCOUNTER WITH LONG TERM USE [V58.67]

Underdose of insulin due to insulin pump failure should be coded 996.57, mechanical complication due to insulin pump, as the principal diagnosis followed by the appropriate diabetes code. Overdose of insulin due to insulin pump failure should be coded 996.57, mechanical complication due to insulin pump, as the principal followed by code 962.3, poisoning by insulins and antidiabetic agents, and the appropriate diabetes mellitus code.

INSULIN PUMP

996.69 Complication – infection (inflammation)
996.57 Complication - mechanical
996.79 Complication - other specified
V53.91 Fitting and adjustment
V45.85 Status
V53.91 Titration
V65.46 Training

995.23 INSULIN REACTION ADVERSE EFFECT OF DRUG, MEDICINAL AND BIOLOGICAL SUBSTANCE
277.7 INSULIN RESISTANCE

INSULINOMA

211.7 Site NOS
0 Site specified see 'Benign Neoplasm', by site M8151/0
157.4 Malignant site NOS
0 Malignant site specified see 'Cancer', by site M8151/3

INTEGUMENT

757.9 Anomaly congenital
757.8 Anomalies other specified congenital
778.9 Condition NOS involving temperature regulation (perinatal)

0 INTERACTIONAL (CHILDHOOD) DISORDER PSYCHOTIC SEE 'PSYCHOSIS CHILDHOOD'

INTERCOSTAL

901.81 Artery injury
908.4 Artery injury late effect
901.81 Artery laceration traumatic (rupture) (hematoma) (avulsion) (aneurysm)
908.4 Artery laceration late effect
786.59 Muscle pain
353.8 Nerve disorder (lesion)
901.81 Vein Injury
908.4 Vein Injury late effect
908.4 Vein laceration late effect
901.81 Vein laceration traumatic (rupture) (hematoma) (avulsion) (aneurysm)

524.56 INTERFERENCE BALANCING SIDE (NON-WORKING SIDE)
279.4 INTERFERON DEFICIENCY
411.1 INTERMEDIATE CORONARY (ARTERY) SYNDROME

626.6 INTERMENSTRUAL BLEEDING IRREGULAR
626.5 INTERMENSTRUAL BLEEDING REGULAR

625.2 INTERMENSTRUAL PAIN
443.9 INTERMITTENT CLAUDICATION NOS
453.8 INTERMITTENT CLAUDICATION VENOUS
431 INTERNAL CAPSULE HEMORRHAGE (CEREBRAL)
433.1# INTERNAL CAROTID ARTERY SYNDROME
5th digit: 433.1
0. Without cerebral infarction
1. With cerebral infarction

INTERNAL FIXATION DEVICE ORTHOPEDIC

996.67 Complication (pin) (rod) (screw) - infection or inflammation
996.4# Complication (pin) (rod) (screw) - mechanical complication [V43.6#]
5th digit: 996.4
0. Unspecified device, implant or graft
Internal fixation nail, rod or plate
1. Loosening prosthetic joint
Aseptic loosening
2. Dislocation prosthetic joint
Instability, subluxation
3. Implant failure prosthetic joint
Breakage, fracture
4. Periprosthetic fracture around prosthetic joint
5. Periprosthetic osteolysis
6. Articular bearing surface wear prosthetic joint
Breakage, fracture
7. Other mechanical complication of prosthetic joint
9. Other mechanical complication of other device implant or graft
Bone graft
Cartilage graft
External fixation with internal components
Muscle graft
Tendon graft
5th digit: V43.6
0. Site unspecified
1. Shoulder
2. Elbow
3. Wrist
4. Hip
5. Knee
6. Ankle
9. Other
996.78 Complication (pin) (rod) (screw) - other specified complication
V54.02 Growth rod adjustment/lengthening
V54.01 Growth rod removal
V54.01 Removal
V54.09 Other aftercare

INTERNAL INJURY

0 For specific injury see anatomical site
869.0 Unspecified or ill-defined organs
869.1 Unspecified or ill-defined organs with open wound into cavity
868.00 Intra-abdominal unspecified organ
868.10 Intra-abdominal unspecified organ with open wound into cavity
868.09 Intra-abdominal other and/or multiple organ(s)
868.19 Intra-abdominal other and/or multiple organ(s) with open wound into cavity
908.0 Late effect chest
908.1 Late effect intra-abdominal organs
908.2 Late effect other internal organs

900.1 INTERNAL JUGULAR VEIN INJURY
908.3 INTERNAL JUGULAR VEIN INJURY LATE EFFECT

901.82 INTERNAL MAMMARY ARTERY OR VEIN INJURY
908.4 INTERNAL MAMMARY ARTERY OR VEIN INJURY LATE EFFECT
V47.9 INTERNAL ORGAN PROBLEM
V47.0 INTERNAL ORGANS DEFICIENCIES
V47.1 INTERNAL ORGANS MECHANICAL AND MOTOR PROBLEM

INTERPHALANGEAL

842.13 Hand separation (rupture) (tear) (laceration)
842.13 Hand strain (sprain) (avulsion) (hemarthrosis)
845.13 Foot separation (rupture) (tear) (laceration)
845.13 Foot strain (sprain) (avulsion) (hemarthrosis)

INTERSCAPULAR REGION

959.19 Injury
911.8 Injury other and NOS superficial
911.9 Injury other and NOS superficial infected

724.8 INTERSPINOUS LIGAMENT SYNDROME
253.4 INTERSTITIAL CELL-STIMULATING HORMONE DEFICIENCY
253.1 INTERSTITIAL CELL-STIMULATING HORMONE OVERPRODUCTION
695.89 INTERTRIGO
112.3 INTERTRIGO CANDIDAL
0 INTERTRIGO MYCOTIC SEE SPECIFIC MYCOSIS
745.4 INTERVENTRICULAR SEPTAL DEFECT (CONGENITAL)
429.71 INTERVENTRICULAR SEPTAL DEFECT ACQUIRED

When coding back disorders due to degeneration, displacement or HNP of the intervertebral disc, it is important to distinguish whether these conditions are with or without myelopathy. Myelopathy refers to functional disturbances and/or pathological changes in the spinal cord that result from compression.

INTERVERTEBRAL DISC

CALCIFICATION OR DISCITIS

722.90 NOS
722.91 Cervical
722.93 Lumbar (lumbosacral)
722.92 Thoracic (thoracolumbar)

DEGENERATIVE DISEASE (DEGENERATION)

722.6 Site NOS
722.70 Site NOS with myelopathy
722.4 Cervical
722.71 Cervical with myelopathy
722.52 Lumbar (lumbosacral)
722.73 Lumbar (lumbosacral) with myelopathy
722.51 Thoracic (thoracolumbar)
722.72 Thoracic (thoracolumbar) with myelopathy

DISORDER

722.90 Unspecified
722.70 Unspecified with myelopathy

DISPLACEMENT (RUPTURE)

722.2 Site NOS
722.70 Site NOS with myelopathy
722.0 Cervical
722.71 Cervical with myelopathy

INTERVERTEBRAL DISC (continued)

DISPLACEMENT (RUPTURE) (continued)

722.10 Lumbar
722.73 Lumbar with myelopathy
722.11 Thoracic
722.72 Thoracic with myelopathy

HERNIATION

722.2 Site NOS
722.70 Site NOS with myelopathy
722.0 Cervical
722.71 Cervical with myelopathy
722.10 Lumbar
722.73 Lumbar with myelopathy
722.11 Thoracic
722.72 Thoracic with myelopathy

INTERVERTEBRAL DISC (continued)

959.19 Injury

INTESTINE, INTESTINAL

751.2 Absence congenital - large
751.1 Absence congenital - small
V45.72 Absence postsurgical - large or small
V45.3 Anastomosis status
557.1 Angina
V53.5 Appliance or device other fitting and adjustment
564.89 Atony
751.2 Atresia large (congenital)
751.1 Atresia small (congenital)
569.89 Atrophy
V45.3 Bypass status
V76.50 Cancer screening - NOS
V76.51 Cancer screening - large
V76.52 Cancer screening - small
259.2 Carcinoid syndrome
560.39 Concretion
789.0# Cramp

5th digit: 789.0

0. Unspecified site
1. Upper right quadrant
2. Upper left quadrant
3. Lower right quadrant
4. Lower left quadrant
5. Periumbilic
6. Epigastric
7. Generalized
9. Other specified site (multiple)

306.4 Cramp psychogenic
277.39 Degeneration amyloid lardaceous
123.4 Diphyllobothriasis
569.9 Disorder
564.9 Disorder functional
751.3 Disorder functional - congenital
564.81 Disorder functional - neurogenic
564.4 Disorder functional - postoperative
306.4 Disorder functional - psychogenic
564.89 Disorder functional - other specified
277.39 Disorder lardaceous
562.10 Diverticulum (large)
562.00 Diverticulum small
751.5 Diverticulum congenital (small) (large)
751.5 Duplication congenital
569.89 Enteroptosis
793.4 Filling defect
557.0 Gangrene
787.3 Gas syndrome

I-J-K

INTESTINE, INTESTINAL (continued)

569.89 Granuloma
V44.3 Hartmann's pouch care, closure, removal, replacement
V44.3 Hartmann's pouch status
564.9 Hyperactive
564.89 Hypermobility
564.9 Hypermotility
569.89 Hyperplasia lymphoid
564.89 Hypofunction
564.89 Hypomotility
564.89 Immobility
560.30 Impaction
560.39 Impaction by calculus
560.31 Impaction by gallstone
0 Infection see 'Gastroenteritis'
863.89 Injury NOS
863.99 Injury NOS with open wound into cavity
863.4# Injury - large intestine (traumatic)
863.5# Injury - large intestine (traumatic) with open wound

5th digit: 863.4, 5

0. Large unspecified site
1. Ascending (right) colon
2. Transverse colon
3. Descending (left) colon
4. Sigmoid colon
5. Rectum
6. Multiple sites in colon and rectum
9. Other

908.1 Injury - late effect
863.2# Injury - small intestine (traumatic)
863.3# Injury - small intestine (traumatic) with open wound

5th digit: 863.2-3

0. Unspecified site
1. Duodenum
9. Other specified site

560.0 Invagination
564.9 Irritation
557.1 Ischemia
560.2 Knot syndrome
569.89 Lesion
040.2 Lipodystrophy
751.4 Malrotation congenital
557.0 Necrosis

OBSTRUCTION/ OCCLUSION (DUE TO)

560.9 NOS
560.1 Adynamic
560.81 Adhesions (postoperative)
127.0 Ascaris lumbricoides
560.81 Band
560.39 Calculus
560.30 Colon impaction
751.2 Congenital - large
751.1 Congenital - small
997.4 Due to a procedure
997.5 Due to a procedure involving urinary tract
560.39 Fecal impaction
560.31 Gallstones

INTESTINE, INTESTINAL (continued)

OBSTRUCTION/ OCCLUSION (DUE TO) (continued)

0 Hernia see 'Hernia', by site, incarcerated
0 Hernia gangrenous see 'Hernia', by site, gangrenous
751.2 Infantile - large
751.1 Infantile - small
560.89 Mural thickening
777.2 Newborn due to inspissated milk perinatal
777.1 Newborn due to meconium
277.01 Newborn due to meconium in mucoviscidosis
777.4 Newborn transitory
560.81 Postoperative (due to adhesions)
560.2 Volvulus
560.89 Other specified cause

INTESTINE, INTESTINAL (continued)

569.83 Perforation
569.89 Pericolitis
569.89 Perisigmoiditis
569.89 Prolapse
560.89 Pseudo-obstruction acute
564.9 Spasm
306.4 Spasm psychogenic
564.89 Stasis
560.2 Torsion (volvulus) (strangulation)
996.87 Transplant rejection (failure)
V42.84 Transplant status
751.5 Transposition congenital
557.9 Vascular insufficiency NOS
557.0 Vascular insufficiency acute
557.1 Vascular insufficiency chronic
569.89 Visceroptosis

IN-TOEING (DUE TO)

755.64 Bowleg (genu varum)
755.63 Femoral anteversion
754.53 Metatarsus varus
755.69 Tibia torsion, internal

303.0# INTOXICATION ALCOHOL ACUTE - DEPENDENT
305.0# INTOXICATION ALCOHOL ACUTE - NON DEPENDENT

5th digit: 303.0, 305.0

0. NOS
1. Continuous
2. Episodic
3. In remission

291.4 INTOXICATION ALCOHOL ACUTE - PATHOLOGIC (IDIOSYNCRATIC)
291.0 INTOXICATION DELIRIUM ALCOHOL
292.81 INTOXICATION DELIRIUM DRUG
0 INTOXICATION DRUG SEE 'DRUG', ABUSE
292.81 INTOXICATION DRUG WITH DELIRIUM
0 INTOXICATION NON FOODBORNE DUE TO TOXINS OF CLOSTRIDIUM BOTULINUM [C.BOTULINUM]-SEE BOTULISM

431 INTRACEREBRAL HEMORRHAGE (RUPTURED ANEURYSM)

853.## INTRACEREBRAL HEMORRHAGE TRAUMATIC

4th digit: 853
- **0. Without mention of open intracranial wound**
- **1. With open intracranial wound**

5th digit: 853
- **0. Level of consciousness NOS**
- **1. No LOC**
- **2. LOC < 1 hr**
- **3. LOC 1 - 24 hrs**
- **4. LOC > 24 hrs with return to prior level of consciousness**
- **5. LOC > 24 hrs without return to prior level: or death before regaining consciousness, regardless of duration of LOC**
- **6. LOC duration NOS**
- **9. With concussion NOS**

907.0 INTRACEREBRAL INJURY LATE EFFECT

905.0 INTRACEREBRAL INJURY LATE EFFECT WITH MENTION OF SKULL FRACTURE

INTRACRANIAL

432.9 Hemorrhage

853.0# Hemorrhage traumatic

853.1# Hemorrhage traumatic with open wound

5th digit: 853.0-1
- **0. Level of consciousness (LOC) NOS**
- **1. No LOC**
- **2. LOC < 1 hr**
- **3. LOC 1 - 24 hrs**
- **4. LOC > 24 hrs with return to prior level**
- **5. LOC > 24 hrs without return to prior level: or death before regaining consciousness, regardless of duration of LOC**
- **6. LOC duration NOS**
- **9. With concussion NOS**

907.0 Injury late effect

905.0 Injury late effect with mention of skull fracture

854.## Injury traumatic

4th digit: 854
- **0. Without mention of open intracranial wound**
- **1. With mention of open intracranial wound**

5th digit: 854
- **0. Level of consciousness NOS**
- **1. No LOC**
- **2. LOC < 1 hr**
- **3. LOC 1 - 24 hrs**
- **4. LOC > 24 hrs with return to prior level of consciousness**
- **5. LOC > 24 hrs without return to prior level: or death before regaining consciousness, regardless of duration of LOC**
- **6. LOC duration NOS**
- **9. With concussion NOS**

781.99 Pressure increased

348.2 Pressure increased due to benign intracranial hypertension

0 Pressure increased due to hydrocephalus see 'Hydrocephalus'

767.8 Pressure increased due to injury at birth

INTRADUCTAL CARCINOMA IN SITU

233.0 Noninfiltrating site NOS

0 Noninfiltrating site specified see 'Carcinoma In Situ', by site M8500/2

216.# INTRAEPIDERMAL EPITHELIOMA OF JODASSOHN M8096/0

4th digit: 216
- **0. Lip skin**
- **1. Eyelid including canthus**
- **2. Ear external (auricle) (pinna)**
- **3. Face (cheek) (nose) (eyebrow) (temple)**
- **4. Scalp, neck**
- **5. Trunk and back except scrotum**
- **6. Upper limb including shoulder**
- **7. Lower limb including hip**
- **8. Other specified sites**
- **9. Skin NOS**

365.00 INTRAOCULAR PRESSURE INCREASED

364.81 INTRAOPERATIVE FLOPPY IRIS SYNDROME (IFIS)

V53.09 INTRATHECAL INFUSION PUMP DEVICE FITTING AND ADJUSTMENT

862.8 INTRATHORACIC ORGANS INJURY MULTIPLE OR UNSPECIFIED

862.9 INTRATHORACIC ORGANS INJURY MULTIPLE OR UNSPECIFIED WITH OPEN WOUND

862.2# INTRATHORACIC ORGANS INJURY OTHER SPECIFIED

862.3# INTRATHORACIC ORGANS INJURY OTHER SPECIFIED WITH OPEN WOUND INTO CAVITY

5th digit: 862.2-3
- **1. Bronchus**
- **2. Esophagus**
- **9. Other**

908.0 INTRATHORACIC ORGANS INJURY LATE EFFECT

779.89 INTRAUTERINE ACCIDENT

0 INTRAUTERINE CONTRACEPTIVE DEVICE SEE 'IUD'

286.6 INTRAVASCULAR COAGULATION-FIBRINOLYSIS SYNDROME (ICF)

286.6 INTRAVASCULAR COAGULOPATHY SYNDROME (ICF)

639.1 INTRAVASCULAR HEMOLYSIS POST ABORTION OR ECTOPIC/MOLAR PREGNANCY

426.6 INTRAVENTRICULAR BLOCK NOS (HEART)

313.22 INTROVERSION OF CHILDHOOD

313.22 INTROVERTED DISORDER OF CHILDHOOD OR ADOLESCENCE

301.21 INTROVERTED PERSONALITY

INTUSSUSCEPTION

543.9 Appendix

560.0 Colon any part

620.8 Fallopian tube

560.0 Intestine any part

751.5 Intestine congenital

560.0 Rectum

593.4 Ureter (with obstruction)

560.0 INVAGINATION COLON

560.0 INVAGINATION INTESTINE

799.89 INVALID (SINCE BIRTH)

799.89 INVALIDISM (CHRONIC)

759.89 INVERTED MARFAN'S SYNDROME

310.8	INVOLUNTARY EMOTIONAL EXPRESSION DISORDER (IEED)
296.2#	INVOLUTIONAL MELANCHOLIA (PSYCHOSIS)
296.3#	INVOLUTIONAL MELANCHOLIA (PSYCHOSIS) RECURRENT
	5th digit: 296.2-3 **0. NOS** **1. Mild** **2. Moderate** **3. Severe without mention of psychotic behavior** **4. Severe with psychotic behavior** **5. In partial or NOS remission** **6. In full remission**
269.3	IODINE DEFICIENCY (DIETARY)
0	IODINE THERAPY RADIOACTIVE, CODE THE UNDERLYING DISEASE

IQ

318.2	<20 (profound retardation)
318.1	20-34 (severe retardation)
318.0	35-49 (moderate retardation)
317	50-70 (mild retardation)
769	IRDS NEWBORN (IDIOPATHIC RESPIRATORY DISTRESS)

IRIDOCYCLITIS

364.3	NOS
364.00	Acute subacute
364.04	Allergic
364.10	Chronic
098.41	Gonococcal
364.23	Lens induced
363.21	Posterior (cyclitis)
364.01	Primary
364.02	Recurrent
364.04	Secondary
364.03	Secondary infectious
054.44	Herpes simplex
053.22	Herpes zoster

IRIDOCYCLITIS ASSOCIATED WITH OTHER DISORDERS

135	Chronic due to sarcoid [364.11]
017.3#	Chronic due to TB [364.11]
364.21	Fuchs' heterochromic
360.11	Sympathetic (uveitis)
091.52	Syphilitic secondary
017.3#	Tuberculous [364.11]
	5th digit: 017.3 **0. NOS** **1. Lab not done** **2. Lab pending** **3. Microscopy positive (in sputum)** **4. Culture positive - microscopy negative** **5. Culture negative - microscopy positive** **6. Culture and microscopy negative confirmed by other methods**
0	See also 'Iritis'
364.76	IRIDODIALYSIS
364.89	IRIDODONESIS
379.49	IRIDOPLEGIA (COMPLETE) (PARTIAL) (REFLEX)
364.52	IRIDOSCHISIS

IRIS

743.45	Absence (congenital)
364.70	Adhesions
364.9	And ciliary body disorder NOS
364.77	And ciliary body recession of chamber angle
743.20	Atresia, filtration angle
364.59	Atrophy (generalized) (sector shaped)
364.51	Atrophy essential or progressive
364.51	Atrophy essential or progressive with congenital glaucoma [365.42]
364.54	Atrophy sphincter
364.74	Bombe
365.62	Bombe with glaucoma [364.22]
743.46	Coloboma congenital
364.56	Degeneration chamber angle
364.57	Degeneration changes of ciliary body
364.53	Degeneration pigmentary
364.54	Degeneration pupillary margin
364.9	Disorder
364.89	Disorder NEC
364.54	Ectropion of pigment epithelium
364.89	Edema
364.81	Floppy syndrome
364.41	Hemorrhage
364.89	Hernia
364.53	Heterochromia acquired
364.81	Intraoperative floppy iris syndrome (IFIS)
364.42	Neovascularization
364.53	Pigment dispersion syndrome
364.89	Prolapse NOS
871.1	Prolapse traumatic
364.53	Translucency

IRITIS

364.3	NOS
364.01	Acute primary
364.02	Acute recurrent
364.00	Acute subacute
364.04	Secondary
364.03	Secondary infectious
091.52	Syphilitic (secondary)
0	See also 'Iridocyclitis'
0	See also 'Uveitis'

IRITIS OTHER

098.41	Gonococcal
274.89	Gouty [364.11]
054.44	Herpes simplex
053.22	Herpes zoster
364.10	Rheumatic
790.6	IRON ABNORMAL BLOOD LEVEL
V46.1#	IRON LUNG DEPENDENCE
	5th digit: V46.1 **1. Status** **2. Encounter during power failure** **3. Encounter for weaning from** **4. Mechanical complication**
285.0	IRON METABOLIC DISORDERS SIDEROBLASTIC ANEMIA
275.0	IRON METABOLISM DISORDERS
799.2	IRRITABILITY
564.1	IRRITABLE BOWEL SYNDROME
316	IRRITABLE COLON PSYCHOGENIC [564.1]
306.2	IRRITABLE HEART SYNDROME
300.5	IRRITABLE WEAKNESS SYNDROME

0 ISAMBERT'S DISEASE SEE 'TUBERCULOSIS', LARYNGITIS

435.9 ISCHEMIC ATTACK CEREBRAL TRANSIENT (TIA)

557.9 ISCHEMIC BOWEL SYNDROME (TRANSIENT)

557.1 ISCHEMIC BOWEL SYNDROME CHRONIC

557.1 ISCHEMIC BOWEL SYNDROME DUE TO MESENTERIC ARTERY SYNDROME

ISCHEMIC HEART DISEASE (IHD)

414.9 NOS
411.89 Acute
411.89 Acute subendocardial
411.81 Acute with coronary occlusion (artery)
0 Acute with MI see 'MI (Myocardial Infarction) Acute'
414.10 Aneurysm (mural) (ventricular)
414.12 Aneurysm coronary artery dissecting
414.11 Aneurysm coronary vessels
414.19 Aneurysm other
414.0# Arteriosclerotic
414.0# Arteriosclerotic with chronic complete or total occlusion [414.2]

5th digit: 414.0
0. Unspecified type of vessel, native or graft
1. Native coronary vessel
2. Autologous vein bypass graft
3. Nonautologous biological bypass graft
4. Autologous artery bypass graft (gastroepiploic) (internal mammary)
5. Unspecified type of bypass graft
6. Native vessel of transplanted heart
7. Bypass graft of transplanted heart

414.9 Chronic
414.1# Chronic - aneurysm

5th digit: 414.1
0. Heart wall
1. Coronary vessels (arteriovenous)
2. Coronary artery dissecting
9. Other

414.0# Chronic - arteriosclerotic
414.0# Chronic – arteriosclerotic with chronic complete or total occlusion [414.2]

5th digit: 414.0
0. Unspecified type of vessel, native or graft
1. Native coronary vessel
2. Autologous vein bypass graft
3. Nonautologous biological bypass graft
4. Autologous artery bypass graft (gastroepiploic) (internal mammary)
5. Unspecified type of bypass graft
6. Native vessel of transplanted heart
7. Bypass graft of transplanted heart

414.8 Chronic - myocardial
414.8 Chronic - other
411.89 Coronary insufficiency acute
V17.3 Family history
411.89 Subacute
411.89 Other specified - acute
414.8 Other specified - chronic

553.8 ISCHIATIC HERNIA

843.1 ISCHIOCAPSULAR SEPARATION (RUPTURE) (TEAR) (LACERATION)

843.1 ISCHIOCAPSULAR STRAIN (SPRAIN) (AVULSION) (HEMARTHROSIS)

732.1 ISCHIOPUBIC SYNCHONDROSIS (OF VAN NECK) HIP AND PELVIS JUVENILE

553.8 ISCHIORECTAL HERNIA

599.82 ISD - INTRINSIC (URETHRAL) SPHINCTER DEFICIENCY

732.5 ISELIN'S DISEASE (OSTEOCHONDROSIS FIFTH METATARSAL)

081.2 ISLAND DISEASE (SCRUB TYPHUS)

251.1 ISLANDS OF LANGERHANS HYPERPLASIA

157.4 ISLET CELL CARCINOMA SITE NOS

0 ISLET CELL CARCINOMA SITE SPECIFIED SEE 'CANCER', BY SITE M8150/3

251.9 ISLET CELL (PANCREATIC) HYPERPLASIA

251.5 ISLET CELL (PANCREATIC) HYPERPLASIA - ALPHA CELLS WITH EXCESS GASTRIN

251.4 ISLET CELL (PANCREATIC) HYPERPLASIA - ALPHA CELLS WITH EXCESS GLUCAGON

251.1 ISLET CELL (PANCREATIC) HYPERPLASIA - BETA CELLS

V28.5 ISOIMMUNIZATION SCREENING ANTENATAL

0 ISOIMMUNIZATION SEE 'BLOOD', TYPE

253.3 ISOLATED DEFICIENCY HGH

253.3 ISOLATED DEFICIENCY OF HUMAN GROWTH HORMONE [HGH]

V07.0 ISOLATION (FOR INFECTION PROPHYLAXIS)

V62.4 ISOLATION SOCIAL

270.3 ISOLEUCINE METABOLISM DISTURBANCES

256.4 ISOSEXUAL VIRILIZATION

007.2 ISOSPORA (BELLI) (HOMINIS) INTESTINAL INFECTION

007.2 ISOSPORIASIS

985.5 ITAI-ITAI DISEASE

ITCH

698.9 Unspecified
698.0 Anus
110.3 Dhobie
698.9 Ear
379.99 Eye
698.1 Genital organs
110.3 Jock
306.3 Psychogenic
V61.10 Seven-year
698.8 Uremic
698.8 Other specified
0 See also 'Pruritus'

287.31 ITP - IDIOPATHIC THROMBOCYTOPENIC PURPURA

255.0 ITSENKO-CUSHING SYNDROME (PITUITARY BASOPHILISM)

IUD

996.65 Complication - infection
996.32 Complication - mechanical (embedded) (displaced) (perforation)
996.76 Complication - other
V25.1 Insertion
V25.02 Prescription
V25.42 Prescription repeat

I-J-K

IUD (continued)

V25.42 Reinsertion checking
V25.42 Removal
V25.42 Routine care
V45.51 Status

286.6 IVC SYNDROME (INTRAVASCULAR COAGULOPATHY)
759.0 IVEMARK'S SYNDROME (ASPLENIA WITH CONGENITAL HEART DISEASE)
362.62 IWANOFF'S CYSTS

I-J-K

714.4 JACCOUD'S SYNDROME
751.4 JACKSON'S MEMBRANE
344.89 JACKSON'S PARALYSIS (SYNDROME)
751.4 JACKSON'S MEMBRANE (COLON) CONGENITAL
757.5 JADASSOHN-LEWANDOWSKI SYNDROME (PACHYONYCHIA CONGENITA)
701.3 JADASSOHN-PELLIZARI'S DISEASE (ANETODERMA)
252.01 JAFFE-LICHTENSTEIN (-UEHLINGER) SYNDROME
759.6 JAHNKE'S SYNDROME (ENCEPHALOCUTANEOUS ANGIOMATOSIS)
046.1 JAKOB CREUTZFELDT (NEW VARIANT) DISEASE OR SYNDROME
046.1 JAKOB CREUTZFELDT (NEW VARIANT) DISEASE OR SYNDROME WITH DEMENTIA **[294.1#]**

5th digit: 294.1
0. Without behavioral disturbance or NOS
1. With behavioral disturbance

285.8 JAKSCH (-LUZET) (-HAYEM) DISEASE OR SYNDROME (PSEUDOLEUKEMIA INFANTUM)
300.89 JANET'S DISEASE
330.1 JANSKY BIELSCHOWSKY DISEASE
062.0 JAPANESE ENCEPHALITIS
321.8 JAPANESE MENINGITIS
081.2 JAPANESE RIVER FEVER
100.89 JAPANESE SEVEN DAY FEVER

JAUNDICE

782.4 NOS
277.4 Bilirubin excretion disorders
282.0 Familial acholuric
100.0 Leptospiral (hemorrhagic)
0 Neonatal see 'Jaundice Neonatal'
576.8 Obstructive
100.0 Spirochetal (hemorrhagic)

JAUNDICE NEONATAL

774.6 NOS
774.2 NOS associated with preterm delivery
773.1 ABO reaction perinatal
774.1 Bruising perinatal
774.30 Conjugation delayed NOS
774.39 Conjugation delayed breast milk inhibitors
774.39 Conjugation delayed developmental
774.2 Conjugation delayed pre-term delivery
774.39 Conjugation other
774.2 Delivery pre-term

JAUNDICE NEONATAL (continued)

774.1 Drugs transmitted from mother
774.1 Hemolytic perinatal
774.1 Infection
773.# Isoimmunization maternal (due to)

4th digit: 773
0. RH (Rhesus) isoimmunization
1. ABO isoimmunization
2. Other and NOS isoimmunization

774.4 Liver damage
773.0 RH reaction perinatal
774.1 Swallowed maternal blood
774.1 Toxins transmitted from mother

JAUNDICE NEONATAL OTHER

282.# Anemia hemolytic hereditary [774.0]

4th or 4th and 5th digit: 282
0. Spherocytic
1. Elliptocytotic
2. G6PD (glutathione reductase)
3. Hexokinase (PK) (TPI) deficiency nonspherocytotic type II
4#. Thalassemias
41. Sickle cell without crisis (NOS) (Hb-S)
42. Sickle cell with crisis (vaso-occlusive pain) (Hb-S)
49. Other (Mediterranean) (Cooley's)
5. Sickle cell trait
6#. Sickle cell disease
60. NOS (anemia)
61. Hb-SS without crisis
62. Hb-SS with crisis (vaso-occlusive pain)
63. Sickle cell/ Hb-C without crisis
64. Sickle cell/ Hb-C with crisis (vaso-occlusive pain)
68. Other without crisis (Hb-S/Hb-D) (Hb-S/Hb-E) (Hb-SS/Hb-D) (Hb-SS/Hb-E)
69. Other with crisis (Hb-S/Hb-D) (Hb-S/Hb-E) (Hb-SS/Hb-D) (Hb-SS/Hb-E) (vaso-occlusive pain)
7. Hemoglobinopathy NOS (HB-C) (HB-D) (HB-E) (fetal)
8. Other specified (stomatocytosis)
9. NOS

751.61 Bile duct obstruction (congenital) [774.5]
277.4 Crigler Najjar [774.31]
277.00 Cystic fibrosis [774.5]
277.03 Cystic fibrosis with gastrointestinal manifestations [774.5]
277.01 Cystic fibrosis with meconium ileus [774.5]
277.02 Cystic fibrosis with pulmonary manifestations [774.5]
277.09 Cystic fibrosis with other manifestations [774.5]
271.1 Galactosemic [774.5]
277.4 Gilbert's [774.31]
243 Hypothyroid (congenital) [774.31]
277.01 Mucoviscidosis [774.5]

JAW

0 Anomaly see 'Jaw Anomalies'
374.43 Blinking
524.51 Closure abnormal

JAW (continued)

526.9 Disease NEC
526.2 Disease fibrocystic
526.89 Disease other specified
524.89 Distortion
524.07 Excessive tuberosity
526.89 Fibrous dysplasia
524.09 Hypoplasia
959.09 Injury
848.1 Separation (rupture) (tear) (laceration)
848.1 Strain (sprain) (avulsion) (hemarthrosis)
742.8 Winking syndrome
0 See also 'Mandible, Mandibular'
0 See also 'Maxilla, Maxillary'

JAW ANOMALIES

524.7# Dentoalveolar
5th digit: 524.7
0. Unspecified (mandible) (maxilla)
1. Maxillary hyperplasia
2. Mandibular hyperplasia
3. Maxillary hypoplasia
4. Mandibular hypoplasia
5. Vertical displacement
6. Occlusal plane deviation
9. Other specified

524.1# Jaw relationship to cranial base
5th digit: 524.1
0. Unspecified anomaly
1. Maxillary asymmetry
2. Other jaw asymmetry
9. Other specified anomaly

524.0# Jaw size (major anomalies)
5th digit: 524.0
0. Unspecified anomaly
1. Maxillary hyperplasia
2. Mandibular hyperplasia
3. Maxillary hypoplasia
4. Mandibular hypoplasia
5. Macrogenia
6. Microgenia
7. Excessive tuberosity
9. Other specified anomaly

291.5 JEALOUSY ALCOHOLIC PSYCHOTIC
313.3 JEALOUSY SIBLING
0 JEJUNAL SEE 'JEJUNUM, JEJUNAL'

JEJUNITIS

558.9 NOS
558.3 Allergic
<u>558.3</u> <u>Allergic</u> due to ingested foods **[V15.0#]**
5th digit: V15.0
1. Peanuts
2. Milk products
3. Eggs
4. Seafood
5. Other foods

558.9 Dietetic
558.9 Noninfectious
0 See also 'Enteritis'

JEJUNOSTOMY

V53.5 Belt fitting and adjustment
V55.3 Care
V55.3 Catheter adjustment or repositioning
V55.3 Catheter removal or replacement

JEJUNOSTOMY (continued)

V55.3 Closure
569.60 Complication - NOS
569.62 Complication - mechanical
569.69 Complication - other
569.69 Fistula
569.69 Hernia

> ***When coding an infection of an ostomy, use an additional code to specify the organism. See 'Bacterial Infection'***

569.61 Infection
<u>569.61</u> <u>Infection</u> with cellulitis of abdomen [682.2]
<u>569.61</u> <u>Infection</u> with septicemia **[038.#(#)]**
4th or 4th <u>and</u> 5th digit code for organism:
<u>038</u>
.9 NOS
.3 Anaerobic
.3 Bacteroides
.3 Clostridium
.42 E. coli
.49 Enterobacter aerogenes
.40 Gram negative
.49 Gram negative other
.41 Hemophilus influenzae
.2 Pneumococcal
.49 Proteus
.43 Pseudomonas
.44 Serratia
.10 Staphylococcal NOS
.11 Staphylococcal aureus
.19 Staphylococcal other
.0 Streptococcal (anaerobic)
.49 Yersinia enterocolitica
.8 Other specified

569.62 Malfunction
569.69 Prolapse
V44.4 Status
V55.3 Toilet stoma

JEJUNUM, JEJUNAL

751.1 Absence congenital
V45.72 Absence postsurgical
751.1 Atresia (congenital)
564.89 Dilatation
306.4 Dilatation psychogenic
562.00 Diverticulum
751.1 Imperforate congenital
863.29 Injury traumatic
863.39 Injury traumatic with open wound
564.89 Irritability
560.9 Obstruction (see also 'Intestine, Intestinal', obstruction)
564.89 Stasis
564.2 Syndrome

363.05 JENSEN'S DISEASE
426.82 JERVELL-LANGE NIELSEN SYNDROME
327.35 JET LAG SYNDROME
756.4 JEUNE'S DISEASE OR SYNDROME CONGENITAL (ASPHYXIATING THORACIC DYSTROPHY)
134.1 JIGGER DISEASE
779.5 JITTERY BABY
V62.2 JOB DISSATISFACTION
288.1 JOB'S SYNDROME (CHRONIC GRANULOMATOUS DISEASE)
110.3 JOCK ITCH

695.1 JOHNSON-STEVENS DISEASE (ERYTHEMA MULTIFORME EXUDATIVUM)

JOINT

755.8 Absence NEC congenital
718.5# Ankylosis
719.8# Calcification
718.4# Contracture
754.32 Contracture congenital hip
754.89 Contracture congenital generalized (lower limb) (multiple)
755.59 Contracture congenital upper limb (shoulder)
719.6# Crepitus

5th digit: 718.4, 5, 719.6, 8
0. Site NOS
1. Shoulder region
2. Upper arm (elbow) (humerus)
3. Forearm (radius) (wrist) (ulna)
4. Hand (carpal) (metacarpal) (fingers)
5. Pelvic region and thigh (hip) (buttock) (femur)
6. Lower leg (fibula) (knee) (patella) (tibia)
7. Ankle and/or foot (metatarsals) (toes) (tarsals)
8. Other
9. Multiple

718.9# Derangement (Old)
717.9 Derangement (old) - knee
724.9 Derangement (old) - spine
718.3# Derangement (old) - recurrent
724.9 Derangement (old) - recurrent spine
718.8# Derangement (old) - other NEC
0 Dislocation see 'Dislocation'
719.9# Disorder
306.0 Disorder psychogenic (articulation disorder)
724.9 Disorder spine
719.0# Effusion
719.3# Effusion intermittent
719.8# Fistula
718.8# Flail
719.1# Hemarthrosis
0 Hemarthrosis current injury see 'Sprain'
719.1# Hemorrhage (nontraumatic)
719.0# Hydrarthrosis
719.3# Hydrarthrosis intermittent
718.8# Hyperextension (old)
0 Hyperextension traumatic - see 'Sprain', by site

5th digit: 718.3, 8, 9, 719.0-1, 3, 8-9
0. Site NOS
1. Shoulder region
2. Upper arm (elbow) (humerus)
3. Forearm (radius) (wrist) (ulna)
4. Hand (carpal) (metacarpal) (fingers)
5. Pelvic region and thigh (hip) (buttock) (femur)
7. Ankle and/or foot (metatarsals) (toes) (tarsals)
8. Other
9. Multiple

JOINT (continued)

716.9# Inflammation
718.8# Instability (old)

5th digit: 716.9, 718.8
0. Site NOS
1. Shoulder region
2. Upper arm (elbow) (humerus)
3. Forearm (radius) (wrist) (ulna)
4. Hand (carpal) (metacarpal) (fingers)
5. Pelvic region and thigh (hip) (buttock) (femur)
7. Ankle and/or foot (metatarsals) (toes) (tarsals)
8. Other
9. Multiple

724.6 Instability lumbosacral (old) - (nonvertebral) (nondiscogenic)
724.6 Instability sacroiliac (old) - (nonvertebral) (nondiscogenic)
719.9# Ligament relaxation
717.9 Ligament relaxation - knee
0 Ligament tear see 'Sprain'
0 Meniscus tear see 'Meniscus'
718.1# Mice

5th digit: 718.1, 719.9
0. Site NOS
1. Shoulder region
2. Upper arm (elbow) (humerus)
3. Forearm (radius) (wrist) (ulna)
4. Hand (carpal) (metacarpal) (fingers)
5. Pelvic region and thigh (hip) (buttock) (femur)
6. Lower leg (fibula) (knee) (patella) (tibia)
7. Ankle and/or foot (metatarsals) (toes) (tarsals)
8. Other
9. Multiple

717.6 Mice knee
724.9 Mice vertebral (facet)
719.4# Pain

5th digit: 719.4
0. Site NOS
1. Shoulder region
2. Upper arm (elbow) (humerus)
3. Forearm (radius) (wrist) (ulna)
4. Hand (carpal) (metacarpal) (fingers)
5. Pelvic region and thigh (hip) (buttock) (femur)
6. Lower leg (fibula) (knee) (patella) (tibia)
7. Ankle and/or foot (metatarsals) (toes) (tarsals)
8. Other
9. Multiple

0 Prosthesis complication see complication
996.66 Prosthesis infection or inflammation
V54.81 Replacement aftercare [**V43.6#**]

5th digit: V43.6
0. Site unspecified
1. Shoulder
2. Elbow
3. Wrist
4. Hip
5. Knee
6. Ankle
9. Other

JOINT (continued)

V43.60 Replacement status
V43.66 Replacement status - ankle
V43.62 Replacement status - elbow
V43.69 Replacement status - finger
V43.64 Replacement status - hip
V43.65 Replacement status - knee
V43.61 Replacement status - shoulder
V43.63 Replacement status - wrist
V43.69 Replacement status - other
719.6# Snapping
727.05 Snapping finger or thumb
524.69 Snapping jaw
524.64 Snapping jaw temporomandibular joint sounds on opening and closing
717.9 Snapping knee
0 Sprain or strain see 'Sprain'
719.5# Stiffness
724.6 Stiffness lumbosacral
724.6 Stiffness sacroiliac
719.0# Swelling
0 Tear see 'Sprain'
719.6# Other symptoms referable to joint
719.8# Other disorders of joint

5th digit: 719.0, 5-6, 8

0. Site NOS
1. Shoulder region
2. Upper arm (elbow) (humerus)
3. Forearm (radius) (wrist) (ulna)
4. Hand (carpal) (metacarpal) (fingers)
5. Pelvic region and thigh (hip) (buttock) (femur)
6. Lower leg (fibula) (knee) (patella) (tibia)
7. Ankle and/or foot (metatarsals) (toes) (tarsals)
8. Other
9. Multiple

288.2 JORDAN'S SYNDROME
284.01 JOSEPH-DIAMOND-BLACKFAN SYNDROME (CONGENITAL HYPOPLASTIC ANEMIA)
759.89 JOUBERT SYNDROME
523.00 JOURDAIN'S DISEASE (ACUTE GINGIVITIS)

JUGULAR VEIN

352.6 Foramen syndrome
900.81 Vein injury - site NOS
900.81 Vein injury - external
900.1 Vein injury - internal
908.3 Vein injury - late effect
451.89 Phlebitis

727.2 JUMPER'S KNEE
427.60 JUNCTIONAL PREMATURE CONTRACTION
135 JUNGLING'S DISEASE (SARCOIDOSIS)
286.4 JURGENS' DISEASE
174.9 JUVENILE BREAST CARCINOMA SITE NOS
0 JUVENILE BREAST CARCINOMA SITE SPECIFIED SEE 'CANCER', BY SITE M8502/3
312.9 JUVENILE DELINQUENCY
090.40 JUVENILE GENERAL PARESIS
102.7 JUXTA-ARTICULAR NODULE
593.89 JUXTAGLOMERULAR HYPERPLASIA (COMPLEX) (KIDNEY)
236.91 JUXTAGLOMERULAR TUMOR SITE NOS
0 JUXTAGLOMERULAR TUMOR SITE SPECIFIED SEE 'NEOPLASM UNCERTAIN BEHAVIOR', BY SITE M8361/1

759.89 KABUKI SYNDROME
203.0# KAHLER'S DISEASE OR SYNDROME (MULTIPLE MYELOMA)

5th digit: 203.0

0. Without mention of remission
1. In remission

759.6 KALISCHER'S DISEASE OR SYNDROME (ENCEPHALOCUTANEOUS ANGIOMATOSIS)
253.4 KALLMANN'S SYNDROME (HYPOGONADOTROPIC HYPOGONADISM WITH ANOSMIA)
299.0# KANNER'S SYNDROME (AUTISTIC DISORDER)

5th digit: 299.0

0. Active
1. Residual

KAPOSI'S

058.89 Associated herpesvirus infection
757.33 Disease congenital
697.8 Lichen ruber
696.4 Lichen ruber acuminatus
697.8 Lichen ruber moniliformis
176.# Sarcoma M9140/3

4th digit: 176

0. Skin
1. Soft tissue
2. Soft palate
3. Gastrointestinal
4. Lung
5. Lymph nodes
8. Other specified sites (external genitalia) (scrotum) (vulva)
9. Site unspecified

054.0 Varicelliform eruption herpes simplex
757.33 Xeroderma pigmentosum

759.3 KARTAGENER'S SYNDROME (SINUSITIS, BRONCHIECTASIS, SITUS INVERSUS)
795.2 KARYOTYPE ABNORMAL
287.39 KASABACH-MERRITT SYNDROME (CAPILLARY HEMANGIOMA ASSOCIATED WITH THROMBOCYTOPENIC PURPURA)
716.0# KASCHIN BECK DISEASE (ENDEMIC POLYARTHRITIS)

5th digit: 716.0

0. Site NOS
1. Shoulder region
2. Upper arm (elbow) (humerus)
3. Forearm (radius) (wrist) (ulna)
4. Hand (carpal) (metacarpal) (fingers)
5. Pelvic region and thigh (hip) (buttock) (femur)
6. Lower leg (fibula) (knee) (patella) (tibia)
7. Ankle and/or foot (metatarsals) (toe) (tarsals)
8. Other (head) (neck) (rib) (skull) ((trunk) (vertebrae)
9. Multiple

756.4 KAST'S SYNDROME (DYSCHONDROPLASIA WITH HEMANGIOMA)
120.2 KATAYAMA DISEASE OR FEVER
446.1 KAWASAKI DISEASE
275.1 KAYSER FLEISCHER RING (CORNEA) DUE TO COPPER METABOLISM DISORDER [371.14]
284.01 KAZNELSON'S SYNDROME (CONGENITAL HYPOPLASTIC ANEMIA)
277.87 KEARNS-SAYRE SYNDROME
081.2 KEDANI FEVER (SCRUB TYPHUS)
280.8 KELLY'S SYNDROME (SIDEROPENIC DYSPHAGIA)
701.4 KELOID
371.00 KELOID CORNEA
066.1 KEMEROVO TICK BORNE FEVER
335.11 KENNEDY SYNDROME
082.1 KENYA TICK TYPHUS
706.2 KERATIN CYST

KERATITIS

370.9 NOS
370.24 Actinic
370.22 Areolar
370.23 Filamentary
370.50 Interstitial
370.52 Interstitial diffuse
370.59 Interstitial other
370.22 Macular
370.22 Nummular
370.21 Punctate
370.54 Sclerosing
370.22 Stellate
370.22 Striate
370.20 Superficial
370.40 Superficial with conjunctivitis
370.00 Ulcerated
370.24 Welders'
370.8 Other forms

KERATITIS OTHER

054.42 Arborescens
054.42 Dendritic
052.7 Disciform varicella [370.44]
372.13 Epithelialis vernalis [370.32]
098.43 Gonococcal
055.71 Measles (rubeola mobilli)
055.71 Rubeola
050.9 Smallpox [370.44]
090.3 Syphilitic
017.3# Tuberculous interstitial [370.59]

5th digit: 017.3

0. NOS
1. Lab not done
2. Lab pending
3. Microscopy positive (in sputum)
4. Culture positive - microscopy negative
5. Culture negative - microscopy positive
6. Culture and microscopy negative confirmed by other methods

0 See also 'Keratoconjunctivitis'

238.2 KERATOACANTHOMA

KERATOCONJUNCTIVITIS

370.40 NOS
052.7 Chickenpox [370.44]
051.0 Cowpox [370.44]
077.1 Epidemic
370.34 Exposure (due to)
054.42 Herpes simplex dendritic
054.43 Herpes simplex disciform
053.21 Herpetic (zoster)
372.13 Limbar and corneal involvement in vernal conjunctivitis [370.32]
055.71 Measles (rubeola mobilli)
370.35 Neurotrophic
370.31 Phlyctenular
055.71 Rubeola
370.33 Sicca
710.2 Sicca (Sjogrens)
050.9 Smallpox [370.44]
372.13 Vernal with corneal involvement [370.32]
370.49 Other

KERATOCONJUNCTIVITIS OTHER TYPES

017.3# TB [370.31]

5th digit: 017.3

0. NOS
1. Lab not done
2. Lab pending
3. Microscopy positive (in sputum)
4. Culture positive - microscopy negative
5. Culture negative - microscopy positive
6. Culture and microscopy negative confirmed by other methods

052.8 Varicella (due to)
053.21 Zoster (due to)

KERATOCONUS

371.60 NOS
371.62 Acute hydrops
371.61 Stable condition

KERATODERMA

701.1 Acquired
701.1 Climactericum
757.39 Congenital
701.1 Palmaris Et Plantaris
701.1 Tylodes progressive

695.89 KERATOLYSIS EXFOLIATIVA
757.39 KERATOLYSIS EXFOLIATIVA CONGENITAL, NEONATORUM

KERATOMA

701.1 NOS
757.39 Congenital
757.1 Malignum congenitale
702.0 Senile

KERATOMALACIA

371.45 NOS
264.4 Vitamin A deficiency

111.1 KERATOMYCOSIS NIGRICANS

KERATOPATHY

371.43 Band-shaped
371.40 Degenerative
371.49 Discrete colliquative
371.50 Hereditary

KERATOSIS

701.1 NOS
702.0 Actinic
702.0 Actinic solar
692.4 Arsenical
701.1 Blennorrhagica
098.81 Blennorrhagica gonococcal
757.39 Congenital (any type)
264.8 Follicular due to vitamin A deficiency
701.1 Follicularis acquired
757.39 Follicularis congenital
264.8 Follicularis due to vitamin A deficiency
757.39 Follicularis spinulosa
629.89 Genitalia female (external)
608.89 Genitalia male external
607.89 Genitalia male penile
098.81 Gonococcal
701.2 Nigricans
380.21 Obturans of external ear (canal)
528.72 Oral epithelium residual ridge mucosa excessive
528.71 Oral epithelium residual ridge mucosa minimal
757.39 Palmaris Et Plantaris
607.89 Penile
757.39 Pilaris
701.1 Pilaris acquired
701.1 Punctata
608.89 Scrotal
702.1# Seborrheic

5th digit: 702.1
1. Inflamed
9. Other

702.0 Senile
702.0 Solar
757.39 Spinulosa decalvans
757.39 Suprafollicularis
478.29 Tonsillaris
623.1 Vagina
757.39 Vegetans

110.0 KERION

KERNICTERUS

773.4 Due to blood type reaction perinatal **[773.#]**

4th digit: 773
0. RH (Rhesus) isoimmunization
1. ABO isoimmunization
2. Other and NOS isoimmunization

774.7 Newborn
774.7 Not due to isoimmunization perinatal

276.2 KETOACIDOSIS
0 KETOACIDOSIS DIABETIC SEE 'DIABETES, DIABETIC', KETOACIDOSIS
791.6 KETONURIA
270.3 KETONURIA BRANCHED CHAIN
791.9 KETOSTEROIDS (17) ELEVATED

KIDNEY

V45.73 Absence postsurgical
593.89 Adhesions
587 Atrophy (contraction) (cirrhosis) (fibrosis)
593.89 Calcification
592.0 Calculus
788.0 Colic
0 Congenital disorder see 'Kidney Congenital'
587 Contracted
866.01 Contusion
866.11 Contusion with open wound into cavity
908.1 Contusion late effect
277.39 Degeneration amyloid lardaceous waxy [583.81]
593.89 Dilatation
593.9 Disease acute or NOS
585.# Disease chronic

4th digit: 585
1. Stage I
2. Stage II (mild)
3. Stage III (moderate)
4. Stage IV (severe)
5. Stage V
6. End stage
9. Unspecified stage

585.6 Disease chronic stage V requiring chronic dialysis
V18.61 Disease family history - polycystic
V18.69 Disease family history - other
593.9 Disorder (chronic)
593.81 Disorder vascular
593.89 Disorder other specified
588.9 Disorder functional
588.89 Disorder functional other specified
593.89 Diverticulum
V59.4 Donor non-autogenous
654.4# Ectopic complicating pregnancy
660.2# Ectopic obstructing labor **[654.4#]**

5th digit: 654.4
0. Episode of care unspecified or N/A
1. Delivered
2. Delivered with postpartum complication
3. Antepartum complication
4. Postpartum complication

5th digit: 660.2
0. Episode of care unspecified or N/A
1. Delivered
3. Antepartum complication

0 Failure see 'Renal Failure'
793.5 Filling defect
593.0 Floating
794.4 Function study abnormal
593.89 Hyperplasia
593.1 Hypertrophy
590.9 Infection
866.## Injury

4th digit: 866
0. Closed
1. With open wound into cavity

5th digit: 866
0. Injury NOS
1. Contusion/Hematoma
2. Laceration
3. Rupture

908.1 Injury late effect
593.9 Insufficiency (acute) (chronic)

I-J-K

KIDNEY (continued)

866.02 Laceration
866.12 Laceration with open wound into cavity
908.1 Laceration late effect
593.89 Obstruction
593.89 Occlusion
0 Renal cyst see 'Cyst', renal
794.4 Scan abnormal
584.5 Shock syndrome
958.5 Shock syndrome following crush injury
908.6 Shock syndrome following crush injury late effect
589.9 Small
589.1 Small bilateral
589.0 Small unilateral
592.0 Staghorn calculus
592.0 Stone
274.11 Stone uric acid
996.81 Transplant rejection (failure)
V42.0 Transplant (status)
589.9 Undersized
589.1 Undersized bilateral
589.0 Undersized unilateral

KIDNEY CONGENITAL

753.0 Absence
753.3 Accessory
753.3 Atresia
753.0 Atrophy
753.0 Atrophy infantile
753.3 Calculus
753.3 Contracted
753.11 Cyst
753.11 Cyst single
753.10 Cystic disease
753.19 Cystic disease other specified
753.3 Discoid
753.3 Displaced
753.3 Double with double pelvis
753.15 Dysplasia
753.3 Ectopic
753.19 Fibrocystic
753.3 Fusion
753.3 Giant
753.3 Horseshoe
753.3 Hyperplasia
753.0 Hypoplasia
753.3 Lobulation
753.3 Malrotation
753.16 Medullary cystic
753.17 Medullary sponge
753.19 Multicystic
753.12 Polycystic (disease of)
753.13 Polycystic autosomal dominant
753.14 Polycystic autosomal recessive
753.12 Polycystic type unspecified
753.17 Spongiform
0 See also 'Renal'

732.3 KIENBOCK'S DISEASE (CARPAL LUNATE) (WRIST)
289.3 KIKUCHI DISEASE

250.4# KIMMELSTIEL WILSON SYNDROME DIABETIC [581.81]

5th digit: 250.4

0. Type II, adult onset, non-insulin dependent (even if requiring insulin), or unspecified; controlled
1. Type I, juvenile onset or insulin-dependent; controlled
2. Type II, adult onset, non-insulin dependent (even if requiring insulin); uncontrolled
3. Type I, juvenile onset or insulin-dependent; uncontrolled

275.1 KINNIER WILSON'S DISEASE (HEPATOLENTICULAR DEGENERATION)
798.1 KIROSHI SYNDROME
V54.89 KIRSCHNER WIRE REMOVAL
075 KISSING DISEASE
721.5 KISSING SPINE
695.1 KLAUDER'S SYNDROME (ERYTHEMA MULTIFORME EXUDATIVUM)
583.9 KLEBS DISEASE
0 KLEBSIELLA PNEUMONIAE SEE 'BACTERIAL INFECTION' OR SPECIFIED CONDITION
270.2 KLEIN-WAARDENBURG SYNDROME (PTOSIS-EPICANTHUS)
327.13 KLEINE LEVIN SYNDROME
312.32 KLEPTOMANIA
758.7 KLINEFELTER'S SYNDROME
446.4 KLINGER'S DISEASE
756.16 KLIPPEL - FEIL SYNDROME (BREVICOLLIS)
759.89 KLIPPEL TRENAUNAY SYNDROME
723.8 KLIPPEL'S DISEASE (CERVICAL)
767.6 KLUMPKE DEJERINE PALSY, PARALYSIS OR SYNDROME (INJURY TO BRACHIAL PLEXUS AT BIRTH)
310.0 KLUVER-BUCY (-TERZIAN) SYNDROME

KNEE

736.5 Back (genu recurvatum)
719.86 Calcification
0 Cap see 'Patella, Patellar'
726.60 Capsulitis
844.0 Collateral ligaments sprain - lateral
844.1 Collateral ligaments sprain - medial
717.89 Collateral ligaments sprain old - NOS
717.81 Collateral ligaments sprain old - lateral
717.82 Collateral ligaments sprain old - medial
718.46 Contracture
719.66 Crepitus
844.2 Cruciate ligament sprain - acute
717.89 Cruciate ligament sprain - NOS old
717.83 Cruciate ligament sprain - anterior old
717.84 Cruciate ligament sprain - posterior old
736.6 Deformity acquired
755.64 Deformity (joint) congenital
736.6 Deformity other (acquired)
717.9 Derangement internal (old)
717.89 Derangement internal (old) - other
719.06 Effusion
719.36 Effusion intermittent

KNEE (continued)

719.86 Fistula
718.86 Flail
719.16 Hemarthrosis
0 Hemarthrosis current injury see 'Sprain'
719.06 Hydrarthrosis
719.36 Hydrarthrosis intermittent
718.86 Hyperextension (old)
716.96 Inflammation
959.7 Injury
916.8 Injury other and unspecified superficial
916.9 Injury other and unspecified superficial infected
718.86 Instability (old)
719.86 Joint calcification
736.41 Knock
755.64 Knock congenital

836.1 Lateral meniscus tear acute
717.41 Lateral meniscus tear bucket handle (old)
717.40 Lateral meniscus derangement (old)
717.42 Lateral meniscus derangement anterior horn (old)
717.43 Lateral meniscus derangement posterior horn (old)
717.49 Lateral meniscus derangement other (old)

717.89 Ligament disruption (old)
717.85 Ligament disruption (old) - capsular
717.83 Ligament disruption (old) - cruciate anterior
717.84 Ligament disruption (old) - cruciate posterior
717.81 Ligament disruption (old) - lateral collateral
717.82 Ligament disruption (old) - medial collateral
717.85 Ligament disruption (old) - other ligament
717.89 Ligament relaxation
0 Ligament sprain see 'Sprain', knee

717.6 Loose body old

836.0 Medial meniscus - tear acute
836.0 Medial meniscus - bucket handle tear acute
717.0 Medial meniscus - bucket handle tear old
717.3 Medial meniscus derangement - unspecified (old)
717.1 Medial meniscus derangement - anterior horn (old)
717.2 Medial meniscus derangement - posterior horn (old)
717.3 Medial meniscus derangement - other (old)

844.8 Patellar sprain
717.89 Patellar sprain - old
727.83 Plica
V54.81 Replacement aftercare [V43.65]
V43.65 Replacement status
717.9 Snapping
0 Sprain see 'Sprain', knee
719.56 Stiffness
719.06 Swelling
0 Tear see 'Sprain'
719.66 Other symptoms referable to joint
719.86 Other disorders of joint

911.1 KNIGHT'S DISEASE (INFECTED ABRASION)
736.41 KNOCK KNEE
755.64 KNOCK KNEE CONGENITAL

794.19 KOBAYASHI ABNORMAL FUNCTION STUDY
757.39 KOBNER'S DISEASE (EPIDERMYLOSIS BULLOSA)
694.4 KOENIG-WICHMANN DISEASE (PEMPHIGUS)

KOHLER

732.4 Disease patellar
732.5 Disease tarsal navicular (bone) (osteoarthrosis juvenilis)
732.5 Freiberg disease (infraction metatarsal head)
732.5 Mouchet disease (osteoarthrosis juvenilis)
726.62 Pellegrini-Stieda syndrome (calcification knee joint)

703.8 KOILONYCHIA
757.5 KOILONYCHIA CONGENITAL
345.7# KOJEVNIKOV'S EPILEPSY

5th digit: 345.7
0. Without mention of intractable epilepsy
1. With intractable epilepsy

759.89 KOK DISEASE
747.21 KOMMERELL'S DIVERTICULUM CONGENITAL
732.7 KONIG'S DISEASE (OSTEOCHONDRITIS DISSECANS)
564.89 KONIG'S SYNDROME
294.0 KORSAKOFF'S (-WERNICKE) PSYCHOSIS OR SYNDROME
291.1 KORSAKOFF'S (-WERNICKE) PSYCHOSIS OR SYNDROME ALCOHOLIC
288.01 KOSTMANN'S SYNDROME (INFANTILE GENETIC AGRANULOCYTOSIS)

KRABBE'S

756.89 Congenital muscle hypoplasia (syndrome)
759.6 Cutaneocerebral angioma (syndrome)
330.0 Disease

0 KRAEPELIN-MOREL DISEASE SEE 'SCHIZOPHRENIA'
759.6 KRAFT-WEBER-DIMITRI DISEASE
607.0 KRAUROSIS PENIS
371.13 KRUKENBERG SPINDLE
198.6 KRUKENBERG'S TUMOR OVARY M8490/6
793.5 KUB ABNORMAL
330.1 KUFS' DISEASE
335.11 KUGELBERG WELANDER DISEASE
362.52 KUHNT JUNIUS DEGENERATION
721.7 KUMMELL'S (-VERNEUIL) (SPONDYLITIS) DISEASE
0 KUNDRAT'S DISEASE SEE 'LYMPHOSARCOMA'
571.49 KUNKEL SYNDROME (LUPOID HEPATITIS)
046.0 KURU
446.0 KUSSMAUL (-MEIER) DISEASE (POLYARTERITIS NODOSA)
V82.89 KVEIM TEST
260 KWASHIORKOR
065.2 KYASANUR FOREST DISEASE
270.2 KYNURENINASE DEFECTS

I-J-K

I-J-K

KYPHOSCOLIOSIS, KYPHOSCOLIOTIC

737.30 Acquired
737.30 And scoliosis idiopathic
756.19 Congenital
737.33 Due to radiation
737.30 Idiopathic
737.32 Idiopathic - infantile progressive
737.31 Idiopathic - infantile resolving
416.1 Heart disease
268.1 Late effect of ricket's [737.43]
737.34 Thoracogenic
015.0# Tuberculous [737.43]
5th digit: 015.0
0. Unspecified
1. Lab not done
2. Lab pending
3. Microscopy positive (in sputum)
4. Culture positive - microscopy negative
5. Culture negative - microscopy positive
6. Culture and microscopy negative confirmed by other methods
737.39 Other specified NEC

KYPHOSIS, KYPHOTIC

737.10 Acquired (postural)
737.19 Acquired other
737.0 Adolescent postural
737.41 Associated with other conditions
356.1 Charcot Marie tooth [737.41]
756.19 Congenital
737.11 Due to radiation
277.5 Mucopolysaccharidosis [737.41]
237.7# Neurofibromatosis [737.41]
5th digit: 237.7
0. Unspecified
1. Type I
2. Type II

731.0 Osteitis deformans [737.41]
252.01 Osteitis fibrosa cystica [737.41]
733.0# Osteoporotic [737.41]
5th digit: 733.0
0. Unspecified
1. Senile
2. Idiopathic
3. Disuse
9. Drug induced

KYPHOSIS, KYPHOTIC (continued)

045.## Poliomyelitis [737.41]
4th Dgit: 045
0. Acute bulbar paralytic
1. Acute with other paralysis
2. Acute non paralytic
9. Acute unspecified

5th dgit: 045
0. Poliovirus unspecified
1. Poliovirus type I
2. Poliovirus type II
3. Poliovirus type III

138 Poliomyelitis late effect [737.41]
737.12 Postlaminectomy
737.11 Radiation
015.0# Tuberculous [737.41]
5th digit: 015.0
0. Unspecified
1. Lab not done
2. Lab pending
3. Microscopy positive (in sputum)
4. Culture positive - microscopy negative
5. Culture negative - microscopy positive
6. Culture and microscopy negative confirmed by other methods

237.7# Von Recklinghausen's disease [737.41]
5th digit: 237.7
0. Unspecified or multiple
1. Type I
2. Type II

737.19 Other specified cause NEC

701.1 KYRLE'S DISEASE (HYPERKERATOSIS FOLLICULARIS IN CUTEM PENETRANS)

307.23 LA TOURETTE'S DISORDER
796.2 LABILE BLOOD PRESSURE
301.59 LABILE PERSONALITY DISORDER

LABIUM, LABIAL (MAJUS) (MINUS)

752.49 Absence congenital
624.4 Adherent (minus)
752.49 Adhesion congenital
624.8 Cyst
616.10 Disease inflammatory
624.9 Disease noninflammatory
624.8 Disease noninflammatory - other NEC
616.10 Disorder inflammatory
624.9 Disorder noninflammatory
624.8 Disorder noninflammatory - other NEC
624.8 Edema
752.49 Fusion congenital
624.3 Hypertrophy
959.14 Injury
911.8 Injury other and unspecified superficial
911.9 Injury other and unspecified superficial - infected
749.1# Leporinum
5th digit: 749.1
0. Cleft unspecified
1. Cleft unilateral complete
2. Cleft unilateral incomplete
3. Cleft bilateral complete
4. Cleft bilateral incomplete

752.49 Minora division congenital
624.6 Polyp
624.4 Scarring

LABOR ABNORMALITIES

661.9# Unspecified
5th digit: 661.9
0. Episode of care unspecified or N/A
1. Delivered
3. Antepartum complication

669.9# Complication unspecified
669.4# Complication other of obstetrical surgery and procedures
669.8# Complication other specified
5th digit: 669.4, 8-9
0. Episode of care unspecified or N/A
1. Delivered
2. Delivered with postpartum complication
3. Antepartum complication
4. Postpartum complication

LABOR ABNORMALITIES (continued)

0 Desultory see 'Uterus, Uterine Disorders Complicating Pregnancy', inertia other
661.4# Dyscoordinate
659.1# Failed induction NOS (drugs)
659.0# Failed induction mechanical
660.6# Failed trial
5th digit: 659.0-1, 660.6, 661.4
0. Episode of care unspecified or N/A
1. Delivered
3. Antepartum complication

644.1# False >37 weeks
644.0# False >22 and <37 weeks
5th digit: 644.0-1
0. Episode of care unspecified or N/A
3. Antepartum complication

0 Irregular see 'Uterus, Uterine Disorders Complicating Pregnancy', inertia other
661.3# Precipitate
5th digit: 661.3
0. Episode of care unspecified or N/A
1. Delivered
3. Antepartum complication

644.2# Premature with onset of delivery <37 weeks
5th digit: 644.2
0. Episode of care unspecified or N/A
1. Delivered

644.0# Premature without delivery >22 and <37 weeks
5th digit: 644.0
0. Episode of care unspecified or N/A
3. Antepartum complication

662.1# Prolonged
662.0# Prolonged first stage
662.2# Prolonged second stage
5th digit: 662.0-2
0. Episode of care unspecified or N/A
1. Delivered
3. Antepartum complication

644.1# Threatened >37 weeks
644.0# Threatened >22 and <37 weeks (due to irritable uterus)
5th digit: 644.0-1
0. Episode of care unspecified or N/A
3. Antepartum complication

0 See also 'Uterus, Uterine Disorders Complicating Pregnancy', inertia

L

LABOR AND DELIVERY COMPLICATIONS
ABNORMALITIES OF PELVIC ORGANS OR TISSUE OBSTRUCTING LABOR

660.9# Obstructed labor NOS
660.2# Bladder dilatation obstructing labor **[654.4#]**
660.2# Cervical incompetence obstructing labor **[654.5#]**
660.2# Cervical polyp obstructing labor **[654.6#]**
660.2# Cervical stenosis obstructing labor **[654.6#]**
660.2# Cervix abnormality obstructing labor **[654.6#]**
660.2# Cervix cicatrix obstructing labor **[654.6#]**
660.2# Cervix rigid obstructing labor **[654.6#]**
660.2# Cervix tumor obstructing labor **[654.6#]**
660.2# Cesarean section (previous) obstructing labor **[654.2#]**
660.2# Cystocele obstructing labor **[654.4#]**
660.9# Dystocia NOS obstructing labor
660.8# Genital mutiliation obstructing labor **[648.9#]**
660.2# Kidney ectopic obstructing labor **[654.4#]**
660.5# Locked twins obstructing labor **[652.6#]**
660.0# Malposition of fetus at onset obstructing labor **[652.9#]**
660.2# Pelvic or soft tissue obstructing labor **[654.9#]**
660.2# Perineal fibrosis obstructing labor **[654.8#]**
660.2# Persistent hymen obstructing labor **[654.8#]**
660.2# Previous C section obstructing labor **[654.2#]**
660.2# Previous surgery to rectum obstructing labor **[654.8#]**
660.2# Rectocele obstructing labor **[654.4#]**
660.2# Septate vagina obstructing labor **[654.7#]**
660.2# Shirodkar suture obstructing labor **[654.5#]**
660.0# Shoulder dystocia obstructing labor **[652.8#]**
660.4# Shoulder girdle dystocia obstructing labor
660.3# Transverse and persistent occipito-posterior position obstructing labor **[652.8#]**
660.2# Uterine abnormality congenital obstructing labor **[654.0#]**
660.2# Uterine fibroid obstructing labor **[654.1#]**
660.2# Uterine sacculation obstructing labor **[654.4#]**
660.2# Uterus prolapse obstructing labor **[654.4#]**
660.2# Uterus retroverted (incarcerated) obstructing labor **[654.3#]**
660.2# Uterus bicornis obstructing labor **[654.0#]**
660.2# Vagina abnormality obstructing labor **[654.7#]**
660.2# Vaginal prolapse obstructing labor **[654.7#]**
660.2# Vaginal stenosis obstructing labor **[654.7#]**
660.2# Vaginal tumor obstructing labor **[654.7#]**
660.2# Vulva abnormality obstructing labor **[654.8#]**
660.2# Vulva tumor obstructing labor **[654.8#]**
660.2# Vulva varicose veins obstructing labor **[671.1#]**

When coding other obstructed labor (660.8#), use an additional code to identify the specific condition.

660.8# Other obstructed labor

5th digit: 652.6, 8 -9, 654.2, 660.0-9
- **0. Episode of care unspecified or N/A**
- **1. Delivered**
- **3. Antepartum complication**

5th digit: 648.9, 654.0-1, 3-9, 671.1
- **0. Episode of care unspecified or N/A**
- **1. Delivered**
- **2. Delivered with postpartum complication**
- **3. Antepartum complication**
- **4. Postpartum complication**

LABOR AND DELIVERY COMPLICATIONS
DISPROPORTIONS

653.9# Disproportion unspecified
660.1# Disproportion unspecified obstructing labor **[653.9#]**
653.0# Bony pelvis abnormality NOS
660.1# Bony pelvis abnormality NOS obstructing labor **[653.0#]**
655.0# Cephalopelvic disproportion due to anencephaly, hydrocephaly, spina bifida (suspected/known) affecting management of mother
653.4# Cephalopelvic disproportion NOS
660.1# Cephalopelvic disproportion NOS obstructing labor **[653.4#]**
653.7# Conjoined twins
660.1# Conjoined twins obstructing labor **[653.7#]**
653.7# Fetal ascites
660.1# Fetal ascites obstructing labor **[653.7#]**
655.0# Fetal CNS malformation (suspected/known) affecting management of mother
653.5# Fetal disproportion NOS
660.1# Fetal disproportion NOS obstructing labor **[653.5#]**
656.6# Fetal growth excessive
653.6# Fetal hydrocephalus
660.1# Fetal hydrocephalus obstructing labor **[653.6#]**
653.7# Fetal hydrops
660.1# Fetal hydrops obstructing labor **[653.7#]**
653.7# Fetal myelomeningocele
660.1# Fetal myelomeningocele obstructing labor **[653.7#]**
653.7# Fetal sacral tumor
660.1# Fetal sacral tumor obstructing labor **[653.7#]**
653.7# Fetal tumor
660.1# Fetal tumor obstructing labor **[653.7#]**
653.4# Fetopelvic disproportion
660.1# Fetopelvic disproportion obstructing labor **[653.4#]**
655.0# Fetopelvic disproportion due to anencephaly, hydrocephaly, spina bifida (suspected/known) affecting management of mother
653.5# Fetus unusually large
660.1# Fetus unusually large obstructing labor **[653.5#]**
653.2# Inlet contraction (pelvis)
660.1# Inlet contraction (pelvis) obstructing labor **[653.2#]**
656.6# Large for dates
653.0# Pelvic deformity NOS
660.1# Pelvic deformity NOS obstructing labor **[653.0#]**
653.1# Pelvis contracted
660.1# Pelvis contracted obstructing labor **[653.1#]**
660.4# Shoulder (girdle) dystocia
653.8# Disproportion other
660.1# Disproportion other obstructing labor **[653.8#]**

5th digit: 653.0-2, 4-9, 655.0, 656.6, 660.1, 4
- **0. Episode of care unspecified or N/A**
- **1. Delivered**
- **3. Antepartum complication**

LABOR AND DELIVERY COMPLICATIONS
FETAL ABNORMALITY (KNOWN/SUSPECTED) AFFECTING MANAGEMENT OF MOTHER

655.9# Abnormality unspecified
655.4# Alcohol addiction maternal
655.0# Anencephaly
655.1# Chromosomal abnormality
655.5# Drug damage
655.8# Environmental toxins
655.8# Heart sounds inaudible
655.2# Hereditary disease in family
655.0# Hydrocephalus
655.8# IUD
655.4# Maternal
655.7# Movement (absent) (decreased)
655.8# Other abnormality NEC
655.6# Radiation
655.3# Rubella maternal
655.0# Spina bifida (with myelomeningocele)
655.4# Toxoplasmosis maternal
655.3# Viral disease maternal
655.8# Other specified fetal abnormality

5th digit: 655.0-9
0. Episode of care unspecified or N/A
1. Delivered
3. Antepartum complication

LABOR AND DELIVERY COMPLICATIONS
FETAL AND PLACENTAL PROBLEMS AFFECTING MANAGEMENT OF MOTHER

656.2# ABO isoimmunization
0 Abortion missed see 'Abortion', missed
656.1# Anti-D (RH) antibodies
656.2# Anti-E isoimmunization
659.7# Depressed fetal heart tones
656.8# Fetal acid-base balance abnormal
656.9# Fetal and placental problem unspecified
656.0# Fetal blood leakage into maternal circulation
659.7# Fetal brady/tachycardia
0 Fetal death < 22 weeks see 'Abortion', missed
656.4# Fetal death >22 weeks
656.4# Fetal death, intrauterine
656.3# Fetal distress - NOS
656.3# Fetal distress - metabolic acidemia
659.7# Fetal heart rate or rhythm deceleration
656.0# Fetal-maternal hemorrhage
656.3# Fetal metabolic acidemia
656.8# Intrauterine acidosis
656.2# Isoimmunization anti-E
656.6# Large for dates
656.5# Light for dates
656.8# Lithopedian
656.8# Meconium in liquor
659.7# Non-reassuring fetal heart rate or rhythm
656.7# Placenta abnormal
656.7# Placental condition other
656.7# Placental infarct
656.5# Placental insufficiency

5th digit: 656.0-9, 659.7
0. Episode of care unspecified or N/A
1. Delivered
3. Antepartum complication

LABOR AND DELIVERY COMPLICATIONS
FETAL AND PLACENTAL PROBLEMS AFFECTING MANAGEMENT OF MOTHER (continued)

674.4# Placental polyp

5th digit: 674.4
0. Episode of care unspecified or N/A
2. Delivered with postpartum complication
4. Postpartum complication

658.4# Placentitis
656.1# RH incompatibility
656.1# Rhesus isoimmunization
656.5# Small for dates
656.8# Placenta and fetal problems other specified

5th digit: 656.1, 5, 8, 658.4
0. Episode of care unspecified or N/A
1. Delivered
3. Antepartum complication

LABOR AND DELIVERY COMPLICATIONS
MALPOSITION / MALPRESENTATION

652.9# NOS of fetus at onset
660.0# NOS of fetus at onset obstructing labor **[652.9#]**
652.2# Breech delivery
660.0# Breech delivery obstructing labor **[652.2#]**
652.1# Breech presentation with version
660.0# Breech presentation with version obstructing labor **[652.1#]**
652.2# Breech presentation
660.0# Breech presentation obstructing labor **[652.2#]**
652.6# Breech presentation with multiple gestation
660.0# Breech presentation with multiple gestation obstructing labor **[652.6#]**
652.4# Brow presentation
660.0# Brow presentation obstructing labor **[652.4#]**
652.2# Buttocks presentation
660.0# Buttocks presentation obstructing labor **[652.2#]**
652.1# Cephalic version
660.0# Cephalic version obstructing labor **[652.1#]**
652.4# Chin presentation
660.0# Chin presentation obstructing labor **[652.4#]**
652.2# Complete breech presentation
660.0# Complete breech presentation obstructing labor **[652.2#]**
652.8# Compound presentation
660.0# Compound presentation obstructing labor **[652.8#]**
652.4# Extended head presentation
660.0# Extended head presentation obstructing labor **[652.4#]**
652.4# Face presentation
660.0# Face presentation obstructing labor **[652.4#]**
652.8# Face to pubes presentation
660.0# Face to pubes presentation obstructing labor **[652.8#]**
652.8# Footling presentation
660.0# Footling presentation obstructing labor **[652.8#]**
652.2# Frank breech presentation
660.0# Frank breech presentation obstructing labor **[652.2#]**

5th digit: 652.1-2, 4-6, 8-9, 660.0
0. Episode of care unspecified or N/A
1. Delivered
3. Antepartum complication

L

LABOR AND DELIVERY COMPLICATIONS MALPOSITION / MALPRESENTATION (continued)

652.5# High head at term
652.6# High head at term with multiple gestation
660.0# High head at term with multiple gestation obstructing labor [652.6#]
652.8# Incomplete breech presentation
660.0# Incomplete breech presentation obstructing labor [652.8#]
652.6# Locked twins
660.0# Locked twins obstructing labor [652.6#]
652.8# Malpresentation other specified
660.0# Malpresentation other specified obstructing labor [652.8#]
652.6# Malpresentation with multiple gestation
660.0# Malpresentation with multiple gestation obstructing labor [652.6#]
652.1# Malpresentation with version
660.0# Malpresentation with version obstructing labor [652.1#]
652.3# Oblique lie
660.0# Oblique lie obstructing labor [652.3#]
652.6# Oblique lie with multiple gestation
660.0# Oblique lie with multiple gestation obstructing labor [652.6#]
652.7# Prolapse arm
660.0# Prolapse arm obstructing labor [652.7#]
652.6# Prolapse arm with multiple gestation
660.0# Prolapse arm with multiple gestation obstructing labor [652.6#]
652.8# Prolapse foot
660.0# Prolapse foot obstructing labor [652.8#]
652.8# Prolapse leg
660.0# Prolapse leg obstructing labor [652.8#]
660.3# Transverse arrest of fetal head
652.3# Transverse and persistent occipito-posterior position
660.0# Transverse and persistent occipito-posterior position obstructing labor [652.3#]
652.3# Transverse lie
660.0# Transverse lie obstructing labor [652.3#]
652.6# Transverse lie with multiple gestation
660.0# Transverse lie with multiple gestation obstructing labor [652.6#]
652.0# Unstable lie
660.0# Unstable lie obstructing labor [652.0#]
652.6# Unstable lie with multiple gestation
660.0# Unstable lie with multiple gestation obstructing labor [652.6#]

5th digit: 652.0-1, 3, 6-8, 660.0, 3
0. Episode of care unspecified or N/A
1. Delivered
3. Antepartum complication

LABOR AND DELIVERY COMPLICATIONS MATERNAL DISORDERS AFFECTING FETUS OR NEWBORN

In order to use the following codes, the medical record must specify that the maternal condition is a cause of morbidity or mortality in the fetus or newborn and the condition originated in the perinatal period, which is before birth through the first 28 days after birth.. The fact that the condition existed in the mother or complicated the pregnancy does not warrant the use of these codes on the newborn's record. Remember, codes 760-763 apply only to the infant and are never assigned to the mother's record. Conversely, never code the mother's condition with these fetal/newborn codes.

762.9 Unspecified abnormalities of chorion and amnion
761.9 Unspecified complications - due to current pregnancy
760.9 Unspecified conditions - unrelated to current pregnancy
762.6 Unspecified conditions of umbilical cord
763.9 Unspecified disorder - due to labor and delivery
761.4 Abdominal pregnancy
763.1 Abnormality bony
763.89 Abnormality soft tissues
761.8 Abortion spontaneous
762.1 Abruptio placentae
760.79 Adrenogenital iatrogenic syndrome affecting fetus or newborn
760.71 Alcohol transmitted via placenta or breast milk
762.1 Amniocentesis damage to placenta
762.8 Amnion adhesion to fetus
762.7 Amnionitis
763.5 Analgesics administered during labor and delivery
763.5 Anesthetics administered during labor and delivery
760.74 Antibiotics (anti-infectives) transmitted via placenta or breast milk
760.77 Anticonvulsants transmitted via placenta or breast milk
760.74 Antifungals transmitted via placenta or breast milk
760.78 Antimetabolic agents transmitted via placenta or breast milk
760.1 Bacteriuria
763.1 Bladder dilatation
762.1 Blood loss maternal
763.0 Breech delivery and extraction
761.7 Breech malpresentation before labor and delivery
760.77 Carbamazepine transmitted via placenta or breast milk
760.8 Cervicitis
763.89 Cervix abnormality
761.0 Cervix incompetent
763.89 Cervix scar
763.1 Cervix scar obstructing labor
763.89 Cervix stenosis/stricture
763.1 Cervix stenosis/stricture obstructing labor
763.4 Cesarean delivery
763.89 Cesarean scar previous
762.1 Cesarean section damage (separation) (hemorrhage) to placenta
762.7 Chorioamnionitis
762.9 Chorion and amnion abnormality
762.8 Chorion and amnion abnormalities other specified
760.3 Circulatory disease maternal chronic
763.89 Cleidotomy fetal
760.75 Cocaine transmitted via placenta or breast milk

LABOR AND DELIVERY COMPLICATIONS MATERNAL DISORDERS AFFECTING FETUS OR NEWBORN (continued)

> *In order to use the following codes, the medical record must specify that the maternal condition is a cause of morbidity or mortality in the fetus or newborn and the condition originated in the perinatal period, which is before birth through the first 28 days after birth.. The fact that the condition existed in the mother or complicated the pregnancy does not warrant the use of these codes on the newborn's record. Remember, codes 760-763 apply only to the infant and are never assigned to the mother's record. Conversely, never code the mother's condition with these fetal/newborn codes.*

763.7	Contraction ring
760.75	Crack (cocaine) transmitted via placenta or breast milk
763.89	Cranioclasis, fetal
763.89	Craniotomy, fetal
763.89	Cystocele
763.1	Cystocele obstructing labor
761.6	Death (maternal)
763.89	Delayed birth or delivery NEC
763.89	Delayed birth or delivery second twin, triplet etc.
763.0	Delivery and extraction
763.6	Delivery rapid second stage
760.76	DES (diethylstilbestrol) transmitted via placenta or breast milk
763.89	Destructive operation or procedure on live fetus to facilitate delivery
775.0	Diabetes causing fetal hypoglycemia
760.76	Diethylstilbestrol (DES) transmitted via placenta or breast milk
760.70	Drug abuse maternal transmitted via placenta or breast milk affecting fetus/newborn
763.5	Drug reaction maternal
761.4	Ectopic pregnancy
763.89	Endocervical OS stenosis/stricture
763.1	Endocervical OS stenosis/stricture obstructing labor
760.8	Endometritis
763.89	Exhaustion maternal
761.7	External version malpresentation before labor and delivery
763.89	Extraction fetal manual or with hook
762.3	Fetal blood loss due to placental transfusion [772.0]
763.89	Forced birth
763.2	Forceps delivery
760.73	Hallucinogenic transmitted via placenta or breast milk
762.1	Hemorrhage complicating pregnancy, antepartum
763.89	Hemorrhage due to coagulation defect
760.8	Hepatitis maternal
761.3	Hydramnios acute (chronic)
760.0	Hypertensive disorders maternal
760.79	Immune sera transmitted via placenta or breast milk
763.89	Induction of labor (medical)
760.8	Infection genital tract other localized maternal
760.2	Infection maternal not manifested in fetus or newborn
760.1	Infection urinary tract
760.2	Influenza
763.89	Injury due to obstetrical trauma
760.5	Injury maternal
761.4	Intraperitoneal pregnancy
760.1	Kidney necrosis
760.8	Liver necrosis

LABOR AND DELIVERY COMPLICATIONS MATERNAL DISORDERS AFFECTING FETUS OR NEWBORN (continued)

761.7	Malpresentation/malposition before labor
763.1	Malpresentation/malposition during labor
761.6	Maternal death
760.79	Medicinal agents NEC transmitted via placenta or breast milk
762.7	Membranitis
760.78	Methotrexate transmitted via placenta or breast milk
763.89	Multiparity
761.5	Multiple pregnancy
763.5	Narcosis due to drug (correctly administered)
763.5	Narcotic reaction (intoxication) maternal during L&D
760.72	Narcotic transmitted via placenta or breast milk
760.70	Noxious substance unspecified transmitted via placenta or breast milk
760.79	Noxious substance other specified transmitted via placenta or breast milk
760.4	Nutritional deficiency disorders maternal
761.7	Oblique lie before labor and delivery
761.2	Oligohydramnios
763.5	Opiate reaction (intoxication) maternal during L&D
763.89	Os uteri stricture
763.1	Os uteri stricture obstructing labor
763.89	Ovarian cyst
763.1	Ovarian cyst obstructing labor
763.1	Pelvis bony
763.1	Pelvis contracted
763.89	Pelvis cyst
763.1	Pelvis cyst obstructing labor
763.89	Pelvis deformity
760.8	Pelvis inflammatory disease
763.89	Pelvis organs or soft tissue abnormality
763.89	Pelvis organs surgery previous
763.1	Pelvis Robert's
763.89	Pendulous abdomen
761.4	Peritoneal pregnancy
763.1	Persistent occipitoposterior position
760.77	Phenobarbital transmitted via placenta or breast milk
760.77	Phenytoin transmitted via placenta or breast milk
762.1	Placenta damage
762.2	Placenta infarction
762.0	Placenta previa
762.3	Placenta transfusion syndromes
762.7	Placentitis
762.3	Polycythemia neonatorum placental transfusion [776.4]
761.3	Polyhydramnios
763.6	Precipitate delivery
760.0	Pre-eclampsia
761.1	Premature rupture of membranes
760.3	Respiratory disease maternal chronic
760.78	Retinoic acid transmitted via placenta or breast milk
762.1	Rupture marginal sinus
760.8	Salpingitis
763.1	Shoulder dystocia
763.1	Shoulder presentation
763.1	Spondylolisthesis
763.1	Spondylolysis
760.78	Statins transmitted via placenta or breast milk
760.6	Surgery maternal
762.1	Surgical induction with damage to placenta

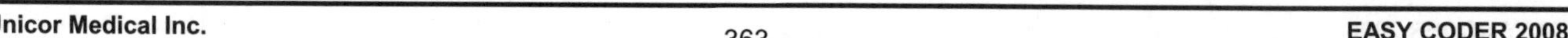

LABOR AND DELIVERY COMPLICATIONS
MATERNAL DISORDERS AFFECTING FETUS OR NEWBORN (continued)

760.70 Toxic substance NOS transmitted via placenta or breast milk
760.79 Toxic substance NEC transmitted via placenta or breast milk
763.5 Tranquilizer reaction (maternal)
761.7 Transverse lie before labor and delivery
763.1 Transverse lie-presentation during labor and delivery
761.5 Triplet pregnancy
761.4 Tubal pregnancy
761.5 Twin pregnancy
762.5 Umbilical cord entanglement (cord around neck, knot, torsion)
762.4 Umbilical cord prolapse (presentation)
762.6 Umbilical cord other and unspecified conditions
761.7 Unstable lie before labor and delivery
760.1 Urinary tract diseases maternal
763.89 Uterus abnormality
763.89 Uterus abscess (to abdominal wall)
763.89 Uterus adhesion
763.89 Uterus bicornis/double
763.89 Uterus body polyp (corpus) (mucous)
763.7 Uterus contractions abnormal
763.7 Uterus hypertonic/hypotonic
763.7 Uterus inertia-dysfunction
763.89 Uterus perforation with obstetrical trauma
763.1 Uterus prolapse
763.89 Uterus rupture
763.1 Uterus sacculation
763.89 Uterus shape abnormality
763.89 Uterus surgery previous
763.89 Uterus version
763.3 Vacuum extractor delivery
763.3 Vacuum rupture
763.89 Vagina abnormality
763.89 Vagina stenosis/stricture
763.1 Vagina stenosis/stricture obstructing labor
760.8 Vaginitis
760.77 Valproic acid transmitted via placenta or breast milk
763.89 Vulva abnormality
762.8 Other specified abnormalities of chorion and amnion
761.8 Other specified complications - due to current pregnancy
760.8 Other specified conditions - unrelated to current pregnancy
762.6 Other specified conditions of umbilical cord
763.89 Other specified disorder - due to labor and delivery

LABOR AND DELIVERY COMPLICATIONS
TRAUMA OBSTETRICAL

665.9# NOS
654.8# Anal sphincter tear (healed) (old)

5th digit: 665.9
0. Episode of care NOS or N/A
1. Delivered
2. Delivered with postpartum complication
3. Antepartum complication
4. Postpartum complication

664.6# Anal sphincter tear during delivery not associated with third-degree perineal laceration

5th digit: 664.6
0. Episode of care NOS or N/A
1. Delivered
4. Postpartum complication

LABOR AND DELIVERY COMPLICATIONS
TRAUMA OBSTETRICAL (continued)

664.4# Perineal laceration unspecified (delivery)
664.0# Perineal laceration first degree (delivery)
664.1# Perineal laceration second degree (delivery)
664.2# Perineal laceration third degree (delivery)
664.3# Perineal laceration fourth degree (delivery)
664.5# Vulva and perineum hematoma, (delivery)
664.9# Vulva and perineum trauma unspecified, (delivery)
664.8# Vulva and perineum trauma other specified (delivery)

5th digit: 664.0-5, 8-9
0. Episode of care unspecified or N/A
1. Delivered
4. Postpartum complication

665.1# Uterine rupture
665.0# Uterine rupture before onset

5th digit: 665.0, 1
0. Episode of care unspecified or N/A
1. Delivered
3. Antepartum complication

665.1# Uterine rupture during labor

5th digit: 665.1
0. Episode of care unspecified or N/A
1. Delivered

665.8# Other

5th digit: 665.8
0. Episode of care NOS or N/A
1. Delivered
2. Delivered with postpartum complication
3. Antepartum complication
4. Postpartum complication

LABOR AND DELIVERY COMPLICATIONS
OTHER COMPLICATIONS

Elderly multigravida is the second or more pregnancy in a woman who will be 35 years of age or older at the expected date of delivery.

659.6# Age advanced maternal - elderly multigravida

Elderly primigravida is the first pregnancy in a woman who will be 35 years of age or older at the expected date of delivery.

659.5# Age advanced maternal - elderly primigravida

Young maternal age is a pregnancy in female who is less than 16 years old at the expected date of delivery.

659.8# Age young maternal complicating labor and delivery
659.3# Bacteremia during labor

5th digit: 659.3, 5-6, 8
0. Episode of care NOS or N/A
1. Delivered
3. Antepartum complication

644.0# False labor >22 and <37 weeks
644.1# False labor >37 weeks

5th digit: 644.0-1
0. Episode of care unspecified or N/A
3. Antepartum complication

L

LABOR AND DELIVERY COMPLICATIONS

OTHER COMPLICATIONS (continued)

659.3# Infection generalized
5th digit: 659.3
0. Episode of care NOS or N/A
1. Delivered
3. Antepartum complication

> *648.9#: Use an additional code to identify the specific nonobstetrical trauma.*

648.9# Injury-trauma non-obstetrical current (co-existent) in pregnancy
669.9# Labor and delivery complication
669.4# Labor and delivery complication other of obstetrical surgery and procedures
669.8# Labor and delivery complication other specified
5th digit: 648.9, 669.4, 8-9
0. Episode of care unspecified or N/A
1. Delivered
2. Delivered with postpartum complication
3. Antepartum complication
4. Postpartum complication

677 Late effect

> *Elderly multigravida is the second or more pregnancy in a woman who will be 35 years of age or older at the expected date of delivery.*

659.6# Multigravida elderly
5th digit: 659.6
0. Episode of care NOS or N/A
1. Delivered
3. Antepartum complication

644.2# Premature labor with onset of delivery <37 weeks
5th digit: 644.2
0. Episode of care unspecified or N/A
1. Delivered

644.0# Premature labor without delivery >22 and <37 weeks
5th digit: 644.0
0. Episode of care unspecified or N/A
3. Antepartum complication

> *Elderly primigravida is the first pregnancy in a woman who will be 35 years of age or older at the expected date of delivery.*

659.5# Primigravida elderly
659.2# Pyrexia or fever during labor
5th digit: 659.2, 5
0. Episode of care unspecified or N/A
1. Delivered
3. Antepartum complication

669.1# Shock during labor and delivery
5th digit: 669.1
0. Episode of care NOS or N/A
1. Delivered
2. Delivered with postpartum complication
3. Antepartum complication
4. Postpartum complication

LABOR AND DELIVERY COMPLICATIONS

OTHER COMPLICATIONS (continued)

644.0# Threatened labor >22 and <37 weeks (due to irritable uterus)
644.1# Threatened labor >37 weeks
5th digit: 644.0-1
0. Episode of care unspecified or N/A
3. Antepartum complication

> *648.9#: Use an additional code to identify the specific nonobstetrical trauma.*

648.9# Trauma-injury non-obstetrical current (co-existent) in pregnancy
665.9# Trauma-injury obstetrical
5th digit: 648.9, 665.9
0. Episode of care NOS or N/A
1. Delivered
2. Delivered with postpartum complication
3. Antepartum complication
4. Postpartum complication
663.0# Umbilical cord prolapse
659.9# Unspecified indication for care or intervention of L&D
659.8# Unspecified indication for care or intervention of L&D other specified
5th digit: 659.8-9, 663.0
0. Episode of care unspecified or N/A
1. Delivered
3. Antepartum complication

V72.6 LABORATORY EXAM OR TEST (ROUTINE)

LABYRINTH, LABYRINTHINE

744.05 Absence congenital
386.9 Disorder
386.8 Disorder other
386.50 Dysfunction
386.58 Dysfunction other forms and combinations
386.52 Hyperactive bilateral
386.51 Hyperactive unilateral
386.54 Hypoactive bilateral
386.53 Hypoactive unilateral
959.09 Injury
386.56 Loss of reactivity bilateral
386.55 Loss of reactivity unilateral
386.50 Syndrome
386.9 Vertiginous syndromes

LABYRINTHITIS

386.30 Unspecified
386.31 Diffuse
386.31 Serous
386.32 Circumscribed
386.32 Focal
386.33 Purulent
386.33 Suppurative
386.34 Toxic
386.35 Viral

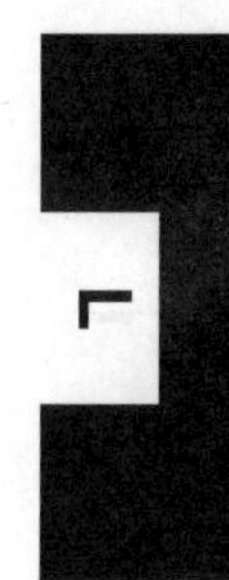

When an open wound or laceration is accompanied by cellulitis, two codes are needed. Use the code for the complicated open wound or laceration and a code for the cellulitis. Sequencing depends on which diagnosis required the major work and effort. Use additional code from 041.## to identify the specific baterial infection.

LACERATION

0 See also 'Open Wound', by site

879.8 NOS
879.9 NOS complicated

879.2 Abdomen wall anterior
879.3 Abdomen wall anterior complicated

879.4 Abdomen wall lateral
879.5 Abdomen wall lateral complicated

998.2 Accidental during a procedure
892.2 Achilles tendon (open)
V58.3# Aftercare
5TH digit: V58.3
0. NOS or nonsurgical wound dressing removal or change
1. Surgical wound dressing removal or change
2. Removal of sutures or staples

873.62 Alveolar (gum)
873.72 Alveolar (gum) complicated

891.0 Ankle
891.1 Ankle complicated
891.2 Ankle with tendon involvement

879.6 Anus (sphincter)
879.7 Anus (sphincter) complicated
569.43 Anus nontraumatic
664.2# Anus obstetrical (during delivery)
664.3# Anus obstetrical (during delivery) including mucosa (anal) (rectal)
5th digit: 664.2-3
0. Episode of care unspecified or N/A
1. Delivered
4. Postpartum complication

884.0 Arm NOS
884.1 Arm NOS complicated
884.2 Arm NOS with tendon involvement

0 Arm lower see 'Laceration', forearm

A complicated laceration or open wound is defined as that which is infected, contains a foreign body, grossly contaminated, or with mention of delayed healing. Use additional code to identify the specific infection.

884.0 Arm multiple sites
884.1 Arm multiple sites complicated
884.0 Arm multiple sites of one upper limb
884.2 Arm multiple sites with tendon involvement

880.03 Arm upper
880.13 Arm upper complicated
880.23 Arm upper with tendon involvement

0 Artery see specific artery

872.02 Auditory canal
872.12 Auditory canal complicated

LACERATION (continued)

872.01 Auricle (pinna)
872.11 Auricle (pinna) complicated

880.02 Axilla
880.12 Axilla complicated
880.22 Axilla with tendon involvement

880.09 Axilla with other sites of upper arm
880.19 Axilla with other sites of upper arm complicated
880.29 Axilla with other sites of upper arm with tendon involvement

876.0 Back
876.1 Back complicated

0 Blood vessel see 'Blood Vessel Injury', by site

665.5# Bowel obstetrical
5th digit: 665.5
0. Episode of care unspecified or N/A
1. Delivered
4. Postpartum complication

BRAIN

851.8# NOS (with hemorrhage)
851.9# NOS with open intracranial wound (with hemorrhage)
851.6# Cerebellum (with hemorrhage)
851.7# Cerebellum with open intracranial wound (with hemorrhage)
851.2# Cerebral cortex (with hemorrhage)
851.3# Cerebral cortex with open intracranial wound (with hemorrhage)
851.8# Cerebral other (with hemorrhage)
851.9# Cerebral other with open intracranial wound (with hemorrhage)
851.2# Cortex (with hemorrhage)
851.3# Cortex with open intracranial wound (with hemorrhage)
851.6# Stem (with hemorrhage)
851.7# Stem with open intracranial wound (with hemorrhage)
851.8# Other (with hemorrhage)
851.9# Other with open intracranial wound (with hemorrhage)
5th digit: 851.2-3, 6-9
0. Level of consciousness (LOC) NOS
1. No LOC
2. LOC < 1 hr
3. LOC 1 - 24 hrs
4. LOC > 24 hrs with return to prior level of consciousness
5. LOC > 24 hrs without return to prior level: or death before regaining consciousness, regardless of duration of LOC
6. LOC duration NOS
9. With concussion NOS

LACERATION (continued)

879.0 Breast
879.1 Breast complicated

620.6 Broad ligament syndrome

0 Brow see 'Laceration', eyebrow

873.61 Buccal mucosa
873.71 Buccal mucosa complicated

LACERATION (continued)

877.0 Buttock
877.1 Buttock complicated

> ***When an open wound or laceration is accompanied by cellulitis, two codes are needed. Use the code for the complicated open wound or laceration and a code for the cellulitis. Sequencing depends on which diagnosis required the major work and effort. Use additional code from 041.## to identify the specific baterial infection.***

891.0 Calf
891.1 Calf complicated
891.2 Calf with tendon involvement

870.8 Canaliculus lacrimalis
870.2 Canaliculus lacrimalis with laceration of eyelid

870.8 Canthus, eye

851.6# Cerebellum (with hemorrhage)
851.7# Cerebellum with open intracranial wound (with hemorrhage)
851.2# Cerebral cortex (with hemorrhage)
851.3# Cerebral cortex with open intracranial wound (with hemorrhage)
851.8# Cerebral other (with hemorrhage)
851.9# Cerebral other with open intracranial wound (with hemorrhage)

5th digit: 851.2-3, 6-9
- **0. Level of consciousness (LOC) NOS**
- **1. No LOC**
- **2. LOC < 1 hr**
- **3. LOC 1 - 24 hrs**
- **4. LOC > 24 hrs with return to prior level of consciousness**
- **5. LOC > 24 hrs without return to prior level: or death before regaining consciousness, regardless of duration of LOC**
- **6. LOC duration NOS**
- **9. With concussion NOS**

622.3 Cervix nonpuerperal nontraumatic
665.3# Cervix obstetrical

5th digit: 665.3
- **0. Episode of care unspecified or N/A**
- **1. Delivered**
- **4. Postpartum complication**

873.41 Cheek external
873.51 Cheek external complicated

873.61 Cheek internal
873.71 Cheek internal complicated

875.0 Chest wall
875.1 Chest wall complicated

873.44 Chin
873.54 Chin complicated

429.5 Chordae heart
363.63 Choroid

878.8 Clitoris
878.9 Clitoris complicated

LACERATION (continued)

> ***A complicated laceration or open wound is defined as that which is infected, contains a foreign body, is grossly contaminated, or with mention of delayed healing. Use additional code to identify the specific infection.***

872.64 Cochlea
872.74 Cochlea complicated

871.9 Conjunctiva (alone)
0 Cornea see 'Laceration', eyeball

851.2# Cortex brain (with hemorrhage)
851.3# Cortex brain with open intracranial wound (with hemorrhage)

5th digit: 851.2-3
- **0. Level of consciousness (LOC) NOS**
- **1. No LOC**
- **2. LOC < 1 hr**
- **3. LOC 1 - 24 hrs**
- **4. LOC > 24 hrs with return to prior level of consciousness**
- **5. LOC > 24 hrs without return to prior level: or death before regaining consciousness, regardless of duration of LOC**
- **6. LOC duration NOS**
- **9. With concussion NOS**

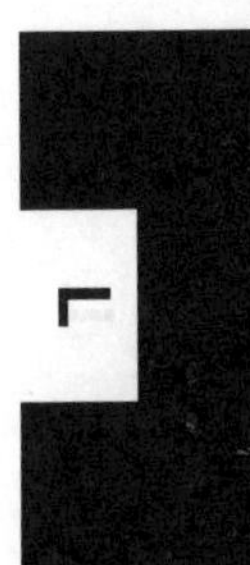

875.0 Costal region
875.1 Costal region complicated

0 Descemet's membrane see 'Laceration', eyeball

862.0 Diaphragm
862.1 Diaphragm with open wound into cavity
908.0 Diaphragm late effect

872.8 Ear
872.9 Ear complicated

872.01 Ear auricle (pinna)
872.11 Ear auricle (pinna) complicated

872.02 Ear canal
872.12 Ear canal complicated

872.61 Ear drum
872.71 Ear drum complicated

872.00 Ear external NOS
872.10 Ear external NOS complicated

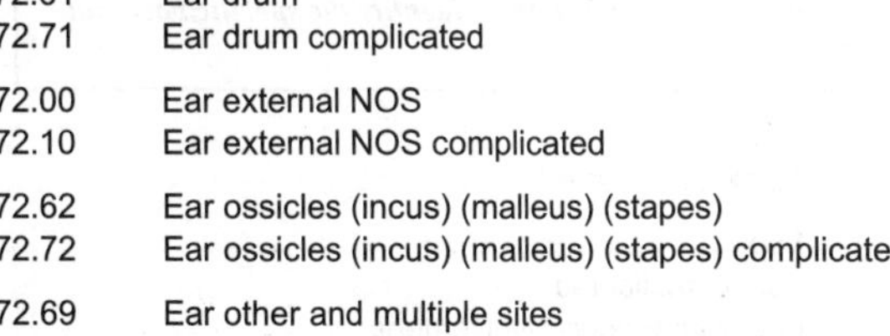

872.62 Ear ossicles (incus) (malleus) (stapes)
872.72 Ear ossicles (incus) (malleus) (stapes) complicated

872.69 Ear other and multiple sites
872.79 Ear other and multiple sites complicated

881.01 Elbow
881.11 Elbow complicated
881.21 Elbow with tendon involvement

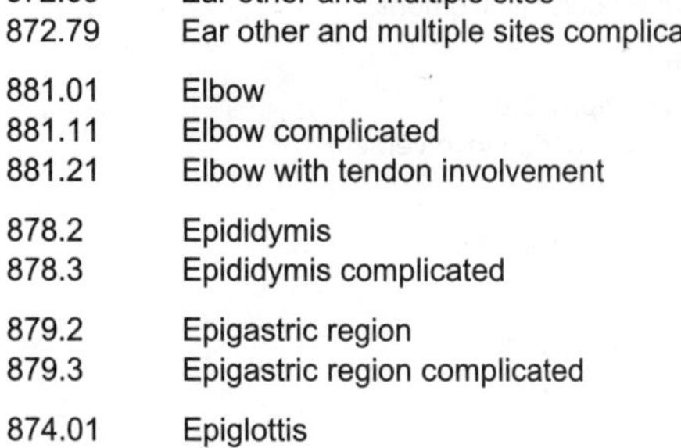

878.2 Epididymis
878.3 Epididymis complicated

879.2 Epigastric region
879.3 Epigastric region complicated

874.01 Epiglottis
874.11 Epiglottis complicated

LACERATION (continued)

874.4 Esophagus cervical
874.5 Esophagus cervical complicated

862.22 Esophagus thoracic
862.32 Esophagus thoracic with open wound into cavity
908.0 Esophagus thoracic late effect
530.7 Esophagus Mallory Weiss tear

872.63 Eustachian tube
872.73 Eustachian tube complicated

871.4 Eye
870.9 Eye ocular adnexa
870.8 Eye (ocular adnexa) other specified
870.3 Eye (orbit) penetrating
0 Eye with foreign body see 'Foreign Body', eye

871.4 Eyeball NOS
871.7 Eyeball penetrating NOS
871.2 Eyeball with partial loss of intraocular tissue
0 Eyeball with foreign body see 'Foreign Body', eye
871.1 Eyeball with prolapse of intraocular tissue
871.0 Eyeball without prolapse of intraocular tissue

873.42 Eyebrow
873.52 Eyebrow complicated

870.8 Eyelid NEC
870.0 Eyelid and periocular area
870.1 Eyelid full thickness
870.2 Eyelid involving lacrimal passages

873.40 Face
873.50 Face complicated

873.49 Face other and multiple sites
873.59 Face other and multiple sites complicated

883.0 Finger (nail)
883.1 Finger (nail) complicated
883.2 Finger (nail) with tendon involvement

When an open wound or laceration is accompanied by cellulitis, two codes are needed. Use the code for the complicated open wound or laceration and a code for the cellulitis. Sequencing depends on which diagnosis required the major work and effort. Use additional code from 041.## to identify the specific bacterial infection.

879.4 Flank
879.5 Flank complicated

892.0 Foot
892.1 Foot complicated
892.2 Foot with tendon involvement

881.00 Forearm
881.10 Forearm complicated
881.20 Forearm with tendon involvement

873.42 Forehead
873.52 Forehead complicated

878.8 Genitalia
878.9 Genitalia complicated

873.62 Gingiva
873.72 Gingiva complicated

0 Globe see 'Laceration', eyeball

LACERATION (continued)

879.4 Groin
879.5 Groin complicated

873.62 Gum
873.72 Gum complicated

882.0 Hand
882.1 Hand complicated
882.2 Hand with tendon involvement

873.8 Head
873.9 Head complicated

861.02 Heart
861.03 Heart with penetration of chamber
861.12 Heart with open wound into thorax
861.13 Heart with open wound into thorax and penetration of chamber
908.0 Heart late effect

0 Heel see 'Laceration', foot

890.0 Hip
890.1 Hip complicated
890.2 Hip with tendon involvement

878.6 Hymen
878.7 Hymen complicated

664.0# Hymen obstetrical
5th digit: 664.0
0. Episode of care unspecified or N/A
1. Delivered
4. Postpartum complication

879.4 Hypochondrium
879.5 Hypochondrium complicated

879.2 Hypogastric region
879.3 Hypogastric region complicated

879.4 Iliac region
879.5 Iliac region complicated

879.4 Inguinal region
879.5 Inguinal region complicated

892.0 Instep
892.1 Instep complicated
892.2 Instep with tendon involvement

0 Internal organ see specific organ

876.0 Interscapular region
876.1 Interscapular region complicated

0 Iris see 'Laceration', eyeball

873.44 Jaw
873.54 Jaw complicated

866.02 Kidney
866.03 Kidney with complete disruption of parenchyma
866.13 Kidney with complete disruption of parenchyma and open wound into cavity
866.12 Kidney with open wound into cavity
908.1 Kidney late effect

891.0 Knee
891.1 Knee complicated
891.2 Knee with tendon involvement

LACERATION (continued)

878.4 Labia
878.5 Labia complicated
664.0# Labia obstetrical (during delivery)

5th digit: 664.0
- **0. Episode of care unspecified or N/A**
- **1. Delivered**
- **4. Postpartum complication**

870.8 Lacrimal apparatus, gland or sac
870.2 Lacrimal apparatus, gland or sac with laceration of eyelid

> ***A complicated laceration or open wound is defined as that which is infected, contains a foreign body, grossly contaminated, or with mention of delayed healing. Use additional code to identify any specific infection.***

874.## Larynx

4th digit: 874
- **0. Unspecified**
- **1. Complicated**

5th digit: 874
- **0. Larynx with trachea**
- **1. Larynx**

908.0 Late effect diaphragm
908.0 Late effect esophagus
906.1 Late effect extremities
906.0 Late effect head, neck or trunk
908.0 Late effect heart
908.1 Late effect kidney
908.1 Late effect liver
908.0 Late effect lung
908.0 Late effect myocardium
908.0 Late effect pulmonary
908.1 Late effect renal
908.1 Late effect spleen
908.2 Late effect urethra
905.8 Late effect with tendon involvement

891.0 Leg NOS or lower
891.1 Leg NOS or lower complicated
891.2 Leg NOS or lower with tendon involvement

890.0 Leg upper
890.1 Leg upper complicated
890.2 Leg upper with tendon involvement

894.0 Limb lower NOS or multiple sites
894.1 Limb lower NOS or multiple sites complicated
894.2 Limb lower NOS or multiple sites with tendon involvement
884.0 Limb upper NOS or multiple sites
884.1 Limb upper NOS or multiple sites complicated
884.2 Limb upper NOS or multiple sites with tendon involvement

873.43 Lip
873.53 Lip complicated

LACERATION (continued)

864.0# Liver
864.1# Liver with open wound into cavity

5th digit: 864.0-1
- **0. Injury unspecified**
- **1. Hematoma, contusion**
- **2. Minor (< 1 cm. Deep)**
- **3. Moderate (< 10 cm. long - < 3 cm. deep)**
- **4. Major (10 cm. long - 3 cm. deep, multiple moderates or stellate)**
- **5. Laceration unspecified**
- **9. Other**

908.1 Liver late effect

> ***When an open wound or laceration is accompanied by cellulitis, two codes are needed. Use the code for the complicated open wound or laceration and a code for the cellulitis. Sequencing depends on which diagnosis required the major work and effort. Use additional code from 041.## to identify the specific bacterial infection.***

876.0 Loin
876.1 Loin complicated

876.0 Lumbar region
876.1 Lumbar region complicated

861.22 Lung
861.32 Lung with open wound
908.0 Lung late effect

873.41 Malar
873.51 Malar complicated

873.44 Mandible
873.54 Mandible complicated

873.49 Mastoid
873.59 Mastoid complicated

851.8# Meninges (with hemorrhage)
851.9# Meninges with open intracranial wound (with hemorrhage)

5th digit: 851.8, 9
- **0. Level of consciousness (LOC) NOS**
- **1. No LOC**
- **2. LOC < 1 hr**
- **3. LOC 1 - 24 hrs**
- **4. LOC > 24 hrs with return to prior level of consciousness**
- **5. LOC > 24 hrs without return to prior level: or death before regaining consciousness, regardless of duration of LOC**
- **6. LOC duration NOS**
- **9. With concussion NOS**

0 Meniscus see 'Meniscus' tear

875.0 Midthoracic region
875.1 Midthoracic region complicated

873.60 Mouth
873.70 Mouth complicated

873.64 Mouth floor
873.74 Mouth floor complicated

873.69 Mouth other and multiple sites
873.79 Mouth other and multiple sites complicated

LACERATION (continued)

879.8 Multiple
879.9 Multiple complicated

894.0 Multiple lower limb
894.1 Multiple lower limb complicated
894.2 Multiple lower limb with tendon involvement

A complicated laceration or open wound is defined as that which is infected, contains a foreign body, grossly contaminated, or with mention of delayed healing. Use additional code to identify any specific infection.

884.0 Multiple upper limb
884.1 Multiple upper limb complicated
884.2 Multiple upper limb with tendon involvement

618.7 Muscles pelvic floor (old)
618.7 Muscles pelvic floor (old) with stress incontinence [625.6]
618.7 Muscles pelvic floor (old) with other urinary incontinence [788.3#]

5th digit: 788.3
1. Urge incontinence
3. Mixed urge and stress
4. Without sensory awareness
5. Post-void dribbling
6. Nocturnal enuresis
7. Continuous leakage
8. Overflow incontinence
9. Other

664.1# Muscles vaginal obstetrical

5th digit: 664.1
0. Episode of care unspecified or N/A
1. Delivered
4. Postpartum complication

861.02 Myocardium
908.0 Myocardium late effect
861.03 Myocardium with penetration of chamber
861.12 Myocardium with open wound into thorax
861.13 Myocardium with open wound into thorax and penetration of chamber

0 Nail see 'Laceration', finger, thumb or toe

0 Nasal see 'Laceration', nose

873.22 Nasopharynx
873.32 Nasopharynx complicated

874.8 Neck
874.9 Neck complicated

874.8 Neck nape
874.9 Neck nape complicated

874.8 Neck other and unspecified
874.9 Neck other and unspecified complicated

NERVE

957.9 Unspecified
956.4 Cutaneous sensory lower limb
955.5 Cutaneous sensory upper limb
957.0 Head and neck superficial
957.8 Multiple unspecified
956.8 Pelvic girdle and lower limb multiple
956.5 Pelvic girdle and lower limb other specified
956.9 Pelvic girdle and lower limb unspecified

LACERATION (continued)

NERVE (continued)

907.3 Root injury late effect
953.8 Root injury multiple sites
953.9 Root injury site unspecified
955.8 Shoulder girdle and upper limb multiple injury
955.7 Shoulder girdle and upper limb other specified
955.9 Shoulder girdle and upper limb unspecified
954.9 Trunk unspecified
954.8 Trunk other specified
957.1 Other specified
0 See also 'Nerve Injury'

LACERATION (continued)

873.20 Nose
873.30 Nose complicated

873.22 Nose cavity
873.32 Nose cavity complicated

873.29 Nose multiple sites
873.39 Nose multiple sites complicated

873.21 Nose septum
873.31 Nose septum complicated

873.23 Nose sinus
873.33 Nose sinus complicated

851.8# Occipital lobe (with hemorrhage)
851.9# Occipital lobe with open intracranial wound (with hemorrhage)

5th digit: 851.8, 9
0. Level of consciousness (LOC) NOS
1. No LOC
2. LOC < 1 hr
3. LOC 1 - 24 hrs
4. LOC > 24 hrs with return to prior level of consciousness
5. LOC > 24 hrs without return to prior level: or death before regaining consciousness, regardless of duration of LOC
6. LOC duration NOS
9. With concussion NOS

870.8 Orbit
870.3 Orbit penetrating
870.4 Orbit penetrating with foreign body
870.9 Orbital region

0 Organ internal see specific organ

872.62 Ossicles ear
872.72 Ossicles ear complicated

873.65 Palate
873.75 Palate complicated

0 Palm see 'Laceration', hand

A complicated laceration or open wound is defined as that which is infected, contains a foreign body, grossly contaminated, or with mention of delayed healing. Use additional code to identify any specific infection.

874.2 Parathyroid gland
874.3 Parathyroid gland complicated

0 Parietal region see 'Laceration', scalp

LACERATION (continued)

879.6 Pelvic region
879.7 Pelvic region complicated

618.7 Pelvic floor muscles (old)
618.7 Pelvic floor muscles (old) with stress incontinence [625.6]
618.7 Pelvic floor muscles (old) with other urinary incontinence **[788.3#]**
5th digit: 788.3
1. Urge incontinence
3. Mixed urge and stress
4. Without sensory awareness
5. Post-void dribbling
6. Nocturnal enuresis
7. Continuous leakage
8. Overflow incontinence
9. Other

664.1# Pelvic floor muscles obstetrical (during delivery)
5th digit: 664.1
0. Episode of care unspecified or N/A
1. Delivered
4. Postpartum complication

878.0 Penis
878.1 Penis complicated

0 Perineal (old) (postpartal) see 'Laceration', pelvic floor muscles
664.4# Perineal obstetrical NOS
664.0# Perineal 1st degree obstetrical involving : (fourchette) (hymen) (labia) (skin) (vagina) (vulva)
664.1# Perineal 2nd degree obstetrical involving : (pelvic floor) (perineal muscles) (vaginal muscles)
664.2# Perineal 3rd degree obstetrical Involving : (anal sphincter) (rectovaginal septum) (sphincter NOS)
664.3# Perineal 4th degree obstetrical involving: 3rd degree and (anal mucosa) (rectal mucosa)
5th digit: 664.0-4
0. Episode of care unspecified or N/A
1. Delivered
4. Postpartum complication

879.6 Perineum
879.7 Perineum complicated

870.8 Periocular area
870.0 Periocular area with laceration of skin

665.5# Peritoneum obstetrical (during delivery)
665.5# Periurethral obstetrical (during delivery)
5th digit: 665.5
0. Episode of care unspecified or N/A
1. Delivered
4. Postpartum complication

874.4 Pharynx
874.5 Pharynx complicated

872.01 Pinna
872.11 Pinna complicated

891.0 Popliteal
891.1 Popliteal complicated
891.2 Popliteal with tendon involvement

0 Prepuce see 'Laceration', penis

LACERATION (continued)

879.2 Pubic region
879.3 Pubic region complicated

878.8 Pudenda
878.9 Pudenda complicated

861.22 Pulmonary
861.32 Pulmonary with open wound of thorax
908.0 Pulmonary late effect

878.8 Rectovaginal (septum)
878.9 Rectovaginal (septum) complicated
665.4# Rectovaginal (septum) obstetrical
5th digit: 665.4
0. Episode of care unspecified or N/A
1. Delivered
4. Postpartum complication

623.4 Rectovaginal (septum) old

866.02 Renal
866.12 Renal with open wound into cavity
908.1 Renal late effect

877.0 Sacral region
877.1 Sacral region complicated

0 Sacroiliac region see 'Laceration', sacral region

873.69 Salivary (ducts) (gland)
873.79 Salivary (ducts) (gland) complicated

When an open wound or laceration is accompanied by cellulitis, two codes are needed. Use the code for the complicated open wound or laceration and a code for the cellulitis. Sequencing depends on which diagnosis required the major work and effort. Use additional code from 041.## to identify the specific bacterial infection.

873.0 Scalp
873.1 Scalp complicated

880.01 Scapular
880.11 Scapular area complicated
880.21 Scapular with tendon involvement

871.9 Sclera

878.2 Scrotum
878.3 Scrotum complicated

891.0 Shin
891.1 Shin complicated
891.2 Shin with tendon involvement

880.00 Shoulder
880.10 Shoulder complicated
880.20 Shoulder with tendon involvement

880.09 Shoulder and arm multiple sites
880.19 Shoulder and arm multiple sites complicated
880.29 Shoulder and arm multiple sites with tendon involvement
879.8 Skin NOS
879.9 Skin NOS complicated

0 Spermatic cord (scrotal) see 'Laceration', scrotum

0 Spinal cord see 'Spinal Cord', injury, by site
767.4 Spine or spinal cord due to birth trauma

L

LACERATION (continued)

865.09 Spleen
865.04 Spleen with disruption of parenchyma
865.14 Spleen with disruption of parenchyma with open wound into cavity
865.19 Spleen with open wound into cavity
908.1 Spleen late effect

A complicated laceration or open wound is defined as that which is infected, contains a foreign body, grossly contaminated, or with mention of delayed healing. Use additional code to identify any specific infection.

865.02 Spleen capsule
865.12 Spleen capsule with open wound into cavity
908.1 Spleen capsule late effect

865.03 Spleen into parenchyma
865.13 Spleen into parenchyma with open wound into cavity
908.1 Spleen into parenchyma late effect

875.0 Sternal region
875.1 Sternal region complicated

0 Submaxillary region see 'Laceration', jaw
0 Submental region see 'Laceration', jaw

0 Subungual see 'Laceration', finger, thumb or toe

874.8 Supraclavicular region
874.9 Supraclavicular region complicated

0 Supraorbital see 'Laceration', forehead

873.49 Temple
873.59 Temple complicated

0 Temporal region see 'Laceration', temple

TENDON

881.20 Abductor pollicis forearm
882.2 Abductor pollicis hand
883.2 Abductor pollicis thumb
881.22 Abductor pollicis wrist
845.09 Achilles
892.2 Achilles with open wound
881.20 Biceps distal
891.2 Biceps femoris
880.23 Biceps proximal
883.2 Extensor digiti minimumi finger
882.2 Extensor digiti minimumi hand
891.2 Extensor hallucis ankle
892.2 Extensor hallucis foot
893.2 Extensor hallucis toe
883.2 Extensor indicus proprius finger
882.2 Extensor indicus proprius hand
882.2 Extensor pollicis brevis hand
883.2 Extensor pollicis brevis thumb
881.20 Extensor pollicis longus forearm
882.2 Extensor pollicis longus hand
883.2 Extensor pollicis longus thumb
881.22 Extensor pollicis longus wrist
893.2 Extensor toe
891.2 Extensor toe ankle
892.2 Extensor toe foot
881.22 Flexor carpi radialis distal
881.20 Flexor carpi radialis proximal

LACERATION (continued)

TENDON (continued)

881.22 Flexor carpi ulnaris distal
881.20 Flexor carpi ulnaris proximal

When an open wound or laceration is accompanied by cellulitis, two codes are needed. Use the code for the complicated open wound or laceration and a code for the cellulitis. Sequencing depends on which diagnosis required the major work and effort. Use additional code from 041.## to identify the specific bacterial infection.

883.2 Flexor digitorum profundus finger
882.2 Flexor digitorum profundus hand
881.22 Flexor digitorum profundus wrist
883.2 Flexor digitorum superficialis finger
882.2 Flexor digitorum superficialis hand
881.22 Flexor digitorum superficialis wrist
891.2 Flexor hallucis ankle
892.2 Flexor hallucis foot
893.2 Flexor hallucis toe
893.2 Flexor toe
891.2 Flexor toe ankle
892.2 Flexor toe foot
905.8 Late effect
844.9 Lower limb NEC
894.2 Lower limb with open wound
891.2 Patellar
890.2 Quadriceps
891.2 Quadriceps in knee
881.20 Triceps distal
880.21 Triceps proximal
840.9 Upper limb NEC
884.2 Upper limb with open wound

LACERATION (continued)

878.2 Testis
878.3 Testis complicated

890.0 Thigh
890.1 Thigh complicated
890.2 Thigh with tendon involvement

875.0 Thorax external
875.1 Thorax external complicated

874.8 Throat
874.9 Throat complicated

883.0 Thumb (nail)
883.1 Thumb (nail) complicated
883.2 Thumb (nail) with tendon involvement

874.2 Thyroid gland
874.3 Thyroid gland complicated

893.0 Toe (nail)
893.1 Toe (nail) complicated
893.2 Toe (nail) with tendon involvement

873.64 Tongue
873.74 Tongue complicated

873.64 Tongue and floor of mouth
873.74 Tongue and floor of mouth complicated

LACERATION (continued)

874.## Trachea
4th digit: 874
0. Unspecified
1. Complicated
5th digit: 874
0. Larynx with trachea
2. Trachea

879.6 Trunk
879.7 Trunk complicated

878.2 Tunica vaginalis
878.3 Tunica vaginalis complicated

872.61 Tympanic membrane
872.71 Tympanic membrane complicated

> ***When an open wound or laceration is accompanied by cellulitis, two codes are needed. Use the code for the complicated open wound or laceration and a code for the cellulitis. Sequencing depends on which diagnosis required the major work and effort. Use additional code from 041.## to identify the specific bacterial infection.***

879.2 Umbilical region
879.3 Umbilical region complicated

599.84 Urethra nontraumatic
665.5# Urethra obstetrical (during delivery)
5th digit: 665.5
0. Episode of care unspecified or N/A
1. Delivered
4. Postpartum complication

867.0 Urethra traumatic
908.2 Urethra traumatic late effect
867.1 Urethra traumatic with open wound into cavity

665.1# Uterus obstetrical NEC during labor
5th digit: 665.1
0. Episode of care unspecified or N/A
1. Delivered

665.5# Uterus obstetrical trauma other specified
5th digit: 665.5
0. Episode of care unspecified or N/A
1. Delivered
2. Delivered with postpartum complication
3. Antepartum complication
4. Postpartum complication

621.8 Uterus old (postpartum)

873.69 Uvula
873.79 Uvula complicated

878.6 Vagina
878.7 Vagina complicated
664.1# Vagina muscles obstetrical
665.4# Vagina obstetrical
5th digit: 664.1, 665.4
0. Episode of care unspecified or N/A
1. Delivered
4. Postpartum complication

LACERATION (continued)

623.4 Vagina old
618.7 Vagina old involving muscles
618.7 Vagina old involving muscles with stress incontinence [625.6]
618.7 Vagina old involving muscles with other urinary incontinence **[788.3#]**
5th digit: 788.3
1. Urge incontinence
3. Mixed urge and stress
4. Without sensory awareness
5. Post-void dribbling
6. Nocturnal enuresis
7. Continuous leakage
8. Overflow incontinence
9. Other

0 Vein see specific vein, injury
871.2 Vitreous (humor)

878.4 Vulva
878.5 Vulva complicated
664.0# Vulva obstetrical (during delivery)
5th digit: 664.0
0. Episode of care unspecified or N/A
1. Delivered
4. Postpartum complication

624.4 Vulva old or scarring

881.02 Wrist
881.12 Wrist complicated
881.22 Wrist with tendon involvement

524.36 LACK OF ADEQUATE INTERMAXILLARY VERTICAL DIMENSION
783.40 LACK OF DEVELOPMENT IN CHILDHOOD
783.43 LACK OF GROWTH IN CHILDHOOD
799.89 LACK OF MEDICAL ATTENTION
783.40 LACK OF NORMAL PHYSIOLOGICAL DEVELOPMENT IN CHILDHOOD NOS

LACRIMAL

743.65 Anomalies (apparatus) (passages) (specified) congenital
743.65 Atresia (congenital)
375.13 Atrophy primary
375.14 Atrophy secondary
375.53 Canaliculi obstruction or occlusion
375.53 Canaliculi stenosis
375.31 Canaliculitis acute
375.61 Fistula
743.64 Gland anomalies (specified) congenital
375.12 Gland cystic degeneration
375.16 Gland dislocation
375.00 Gland disorder
375.03 Gland enlargement chronic
375.89 Gland disorder - other
375.81 Granuloma (passages)
375.43 Mucocele
743.65 Obstruction or occlusion congenital
375.69 Passages changes other
375.51 Punctum eversion
375.52 Punctum obstruction or occlusion
375.52 Punctum stenosis
375.54 Sac obstruction or occlusion
375.54 Stenosis (sac)
375.9 System disorder
375.89 System disorders other

LACTATION

676.9# Disorder (lactating) maternal due to pregnancy
676.8# Disorders other specified maternal due to pregnancy
611.6 Excessive
676.6# Excessive maternal due to pregnancy
676.4# Failure maternal due to pregnancy
676.5# Suppressed maternal due to pregnancy
5th digit: 676.4, 5, 6, 8, 9
0. Episode of care unspecified or N/A
1. Delivered
2. Delivered with postpartum complication
3. Antepartum complication
4. Postpartum complication

579.2 LACTEAL OBSTRUCTION WITH STEATORRHEA
790.4 LACTIC ACID DEHYDROGENASE ABNORMAL BLOOD LEVEL
271.3 LACTOSE (INTOLERANCE) (MALABSORPTION) (METABOLISM DISORDER)
434.91 LACUNAR INFARCT
571.2 LAENNEC'S CIRRHOSIS (LIVER)
571.5 LAENNEC'S CIRRHOSIS (LIVER) WITH ESOPHAGEAL VARICES [**456.2#**]
5th digit: 456.2
0. With bleeding
1. Without bleeding

333.2 LAFORA'S DISEASE
759.6 LAGLEYZE-VON HIPPEL DISEASE CONGENITAL

LAGOPHTHALMOS

374.20 Unspecified
374.23 Cicatricial
374.22 Mechanical
374.21 Paralytic

286.3 LAKI LORAND DEFICIENCY
307.9 LALLING
007.1 LAMBLIASIS
704.1 LANUGINOSA ACQUIRED
100.0 LANCERAUX-MATHIEU DISEASE (LEPTOSPIRAL JAUNDICE)
359.1 LANDOUZY DEJERINE MUSCULAR DYSTROPHY
357.0 LANDRY'S DISEASE
569.89 LANE'S DISEASE
063.8 LANGAT ENCEPHALITIS
758.0 LANGDON DOWN SYNDROME (MONGOLISM)

LANGUAGE

Use an additional code to indentify the type of hearing loss. See 'HEARING LOSS'

315.34 Developmental delay due to hearing loss
315.31 Disorder developmental - expressive
315.32 Disorder developmental - mixed receptive-expressive
438.1# Disorder late effect of cerebrovascular disease
5th digit: 438.1
0. Unspecified
1. Aphasia
2. Dysphasia
9. Other

757.4 LANUGO PERSISTENT CONGENITAL

V64.41 LAPAROSCOPIC SURGICAL PROCEDURE CONVERTED TO OPEN PROCEDURE
277.39 LARDACEOUS DEGENERATION OR DISEASE (ANY SITE)
766.0 LARGE BABY EXCEPTIONALLY (BIRTHWEIGHT >4500 GRAMS)
199.1 LARGE CELL CARCINOMA SITE NOS
0 LARGE CELL CARCINOMA SITE SPECIFIED SEE 'CANCER', BY SITE M8012/3
656.6# LARGE FOR DATES AFFECTING MANAGEMENT OF MOTHER
5th digit: 656.6
0. Episode of care unspecified or N/A
1. Delivered
3. Antepartum complication

766.1 LARGE FOR DATES INFANT (REGARDLESS OF GESTATION PERIOD)
115.1# LARGE FORM HISTOPLASMOSIS
5th digit: 115.1
0. Without mention of manifestation
1. Meningitis
2. Retinitis
3. Pericarditis
4. Endocarditis
5. Pneumonia
9. Other

751.2 LARGE INTESTINE (ABSENCE) (ATRESIA) (STENOSIS) (OBSTRUCTION) CONGENITAL
783.9 LARGE STATURE
100.0 LARREY-WEIL DISEASE (LEPTOSPIRAL JAUNDICE)
732.4 LARSEN (-JOHANSSON) DISEASE (JUVENILE OSTEOPATHIA PATELLAE)
755.8 LARSEN'S SYNDROME (FLATTENED FACIES AND MULTIPLE CONGENITAL DISLOCATIONS)
126.9 LARVA MIGRANS CUTANEOUS
128.0 LARVA MIGRANS VISCERALIS INFECTION

0 LARYNGEAL SEE 'LARYNX, LARYNGEAL'

LARYNGITIS

464.0# Acute
464.0# Acute H. flu
487.1 Acute influenzal
464.0# Acute pneumococcal
5th digit: 464.0
0. Without mention of obstruction
1. With obstruction

034.0 Acute streptococcal
476.0 Catarrhal
476.0 Chronic
476.0 Chronic atrophic
476.1 Chronic with tracheitis
476.0 Hypertrophic
487.1 Influenza
464.01 Obstructive
476.0 Sicca
478.75 Spasmodic
464.0# Spasmodic acute
464.0# Ulcerative
5th digit: 464.0
0. Without mention of obstruction
1. With obstruction

748.3 LARYNGOCELE CONGENITAL
465.0 LARYNGOPHARYNGITIS ACUTE
478.30 LARYNGOPLEGIA
478.75 LARYNGOSPASM

LARYNGOTRACHEITIS

464.20 Acute
464.21 Acute with obstruction
476.1 Chronic
032.3 Diphtheritic

LARYNX, LARYNGEAL

478.79 Abscess
748.3 Absence or agenesis congenital
748.3 Atresia congenital
478.79 Atrophy
478.79 Calcification
478.71 Cellulitis and perichondritis
925.2 Crushing injury
478.70 Disease
478.6 Edema
478.79 Granuloma
959.09 Injury
478.79 Leukoplakia
478.79 Necrosis
352.3 Nerve disorder recurrent
478.79 Nodule
478.79 Obstruction
748.3 Obstruction congenital
478.79 Pachyderma
478.30 Paralysis
478.34 Paralysis bilateral complete
478.33 Paralysis bilateral partial
478.32 Paralysis unilateral complete
478.31 Paralysis unilateral partial
478.4 Polyp
212.1 Polyp adenomatous
0 Polyp malignant see 'Cancer', larynx
V43.81 Replacement (prosthesis) status
478.75 Spasm
478.74 Stenosis
748.3 Stenosis congenital
748.3 Stridor congenital
748.2 Subglottic congenital
478.79 Ulcer
748.2 Web
748.2 Web glottic

297.9 LASEGUE'S DISEASE (PERSECUTION MANIA)
780.79 LASSITUDE

> *Late effects are recognized to be those residual problems stemming from an old injury or disorder (such as paralysis from an old stroke).*

LATE EFFECT

326 Abscess intracranial or intraspinal
909.5 Adverse effect of drug, medicinal or biological substance
909.9 Allergic reaction
997.6# Amputation postoperative stump
5th digit: 997.6
0. NOS
1. Neuroma of stump
2. Infection (chronic)
9. Other

905.9 Amputation traumatic

LATE EFFECT (continued)

909.5 Biological substance adverse effect
906.9 Burn - site NOS
906.5 Burn - eye, face, head and neck
906.6 Burn - wrist and hand
906.7 Burn - other extremities
906.8 Burn - other specified sites

> *When the late effect or residual condition is not identified in the 438.## code, use an additional code to specify that condition. For example codes 438.5 and 438.89.*

CEREBROVASCULAR DISEASE

438.9 Unspecified
438.81 Apraxia
438.84 Ataxia
438.0 Cognitive defect
438.82 Dysphagia [787.2#]
5th digit: 787.2
0. Unspecified
1. Oral phase
2. Oropharyngeal phase
3. Pharyngeal phase
4. Pharyngoesophageal phase
9. Other

438.83 Facial droop
438.83 Facial weakness
438.2# Paralytic - hemiplegia or hemiparesis
438.4# Paralytic - monoplegia lower limb
438.3# Paralytic - monoplegia upper limb
5th digit: 438.2-4
0. Unspecified side
1. Dominant side
2. Nondominant side

438.5# Paralytic - other syndrome
5th digit: 438.5
0. Unspecified side
1. Dominant side
2. Nondominant side
3. Bilateral

> *Use an additional code to identify the altered sensation.*

438.6 Sensation alteration
438.1# Speech and language deficit
5th digit: 438.1
0. Unspecified
1. Aphasia
2. Dysphasia
9. Other

438.85 Vertigo

> *Use an additional code to identify the visual disturbance.*

438.7 Vision disturbance
438.89 Other specified

LATE EFFECT (continued)

677 Complications childbirth, delivery, pregnancy or puerperium
909.3 Complications of surgical and medical care
908.6 Complications early of trauma other specified
906.3 Contusion
906.4 Crush injury

L

LATE EFFECT (continued)

0 CVA see 'Late Effect', cerebrovascular disease
677 Delivery complication
905.6 Dislocation (any site)
909.5 Drug adverse effect
326 Encephalitis NOS and NEC
326 Encephalitis postimmunization
139.0 Encephalitis viral
326 Encephalomyelitis postimmunization
909.4 Environmental causes
780.79 Epstein Barre infection (viral) chronic [139.8]
908.5 Foreign body in orifice
905.0 Fracture face and skull bones
905.4 Fracture of lower extremities
905.5 Fracture of multiple and unspecified bones
905.3 Fracture of neck of femur
905.2 Fracture of upper extremities
905.0 Fracture skull and face bones
905.1 Fracture spine and trunk without spinal cord lesion
907.2 Fracture spine and trunk with spinal cord lesion
906.3 Hematoma traumatic
326 Infection intracranial pyogenic
139.8 Infectious and parasitic disease
908.9 Injury unspecified
908.3 Injury blood vessel of head, neck and extremities
908.4 Injury blood vessel of thorax, abdomen and pelvis
908.6 Injury certain complications of trauma
908.1 Injury internal abdominal organs
908.0 Injury internal chest
908.2 Injury internal other organs
907.0 Injury intracranial
905.0 Injury intracranial with skull fracture
907.1 Injury nerve cranial
907.5 Injury nerve of pelvic girdle and lower limb peripheral
907.4 Injury nerve of shoulder girdle and upper limb peripheral
907.3 Injury nerve root(s) spinal plexus(es) and other nerves of trunk
907.9 Injury nerve other and unspecified
907.2 Injury spinal cord
907.3 Injury spinal nerve root and plexus(es)
906.2 Injury superficial
905.8 Injury tendon
909.5 Medicine adverse effect
139.8 Measles
326 Myelitis
905.8 Open wound of extremities with tendon injury
906.1 Open wound of extremities without tendon injury
906.0 Open wound of head, neck and trunk
139.8 Parasitic disease
326 Phlebitis of intracranial venous sinuses
138 Poliomyelitis
909.0 Poisoning due to drug, medicinal or biological substance
677 Pregnancy, childbirth or puerperal complication
326 Pyogenic intracranial infection
909.2 Radiation
268.1 Rickets
905.7 Sprain and strain
905.8 Sprain and strain with tendon injury
0 Stroke see 'Late Effect', cerebrovascular disease
326 Thrombophlebitis of intracranial venous sinuses
137.0 TB (respiratory or NOS)
137.3 TB bones and joints
137.1 TB central nervous system
137.2 TB genitourinary
137.4 TB other organs

LATE EFFECT (continued)

909.0 Toxic effects of drugs, medicinal or biological substances
909.1 Toxic effects of nonmedical substances
139.1 Trachoma
909.9 Other and unspecified external causes
909.4 Other external environmental causes

766.21 LATE INFANT POST TERM >40 COMPLETED WEEKS TO 42 COMPLETED WEEKS

766.22 LATE INFANT PROLONGED GESTATION >42 COMPLETED WEEKS

645.1# LATE PREGNANCY – POST-TERM (> 40 COMPLETED WEEKS TO 42 COMPLETED WEEKS GESTATION)

645.2# LATE PREGNANCY - PROLONGED (> 42 COMPLETED WEEKS GESTATION)

5th digit: 645.1-2
0. Episode of care unspecified or N/A
1. Delivered
3. Antepartum complication

783.42 LATE TALKER

783.42 LATE WALKER

LATERAL

717.81 Collateral ligament disruption (old)
717.9 Collateral ligament relaxation
844.0 Collateral ligament sprain, strain or tear
355.1 Cutaneous nerve of thigh syndrome
726.32 Epicondylitis
355.1 Femoral cutaneous nerve (thigh) (compression) (syndrome)
436 Medullary syndrome
717.40 Meniscus derangement (knee) (old)
717.42 Meniscus derangement (knee) anterior horn (old)
717.43 Meniscus derangement (knee) posterior horn (old)
717.49 Meniscus derangement (knee) other (old)
836.1 Meniscus tear (knee) acute
717.41 Meniscus tear bucket handle (knee) (old)

V15.07 LATEX ALLERGY OR SENSITIVITY HISTORY

989.82 LATEX POISONING OR REACTION

362.63 LATTICE DEGENERATION RETINAL

272.8 LAUNOIS BENSAUDE'S LIPOMATOSIS

253.8 LAUNOIS-CLERET SYNDROME (ADIPOSOGENITAL DYSTROPHY)

253.0 LAUNOIS' SYNDROME (PITUITARY GIGANTISM)

759.89 LAURENCE-MOON (-BARDET) -BIEDL SYNDROME (OBESITY, POLYDACTYLY AND MENTAL RETARDATION)

0 LAV (LYMPHADENOPATHY- ASSOCIATED VIRUS) SEE 'HIV' INFECTION

759.6 LAWFORD'S SYNDROME (ENCEPHALOCUTANEOUS ANGIOMATOSIS)

305.9# LAXATIVE ABUSE NONDEPENDENT

5th digit: 305.9
0. Unspecified
1. Continuous
2. Episodic
3. In remission

288.09 LAZY LEUKOCYTE SYNDROME

728.3 LAZY POSTURE SYNDROME

426.3 LBBB (LEFT BUNDLE BRANCH BLOCK)

277.85 LCAD, VLCAD (LONG CHAIN/VERY LONG CHAIN ACYL COA DEHYDROGENASE DEFICIENCY)
277.85 LCHAD (LONG CHAIN 3-HYDROXYACYL COA DEHYDROGENASE DEFICIENCY)
790.4 LDH ELEVATED
272.0 LDL ELEVATED (LOW DENSITY LIPIDS)
790.6 LEAD ABNORMAL BLOOD LEVEL
V82.5 LEAD, HEAVY METAL SCREENING
V15.86 LEAD EXPOSURE HISTORY
371.15 LEAD INCRUSTATION CORNEA
0 LEAKY HEART SEE 'ENDOCARDITIS'
0 LEARNING DIFFICULTIES (DELAY IN DEVELOPMENT) SEE 'DEVELOPMENTAL DISORDER'
V40.0 LEARNING PROBLEM
377.16 LEBER'S OPTIC ATROPHY
283.19 LEDERER-BRILL SYNDROME (ACQUIRED INFECTIOUS HEMOLYTIC ANEMIA)
283.19 LEDERER'S ANEMIA OR DISEASE (ACQUIRED INFECTIOUS HEMOLYTIC ANEMIA)
134.2 LEECHE INFESTATION (AQUATIC) (LAND)
802.4 LEFORT'S FRACTURE CLOSED
802.5 LEFORT'S FRACTURE OPEN
781.8 LEFT SIDED NEGLECT

LEFT VENTRICLE, VENTRICULAR

746.89 Diverticulum congenital
428.1 Failure
391.8 Failure rheumatic - acute
392.0 Failure rheumatic - acute with chorea
398.91 Failure rheumatic - chronic
398.91 Failure rheumatic - chronic with chorea
429.3 Hypertrophy
745.4 Right atrial communication congenital

LEG

V49.70 Absence acquired NOS
V49.76 Absence acquired above the knee
V49.75 Absence acquired below the knee
755.31 Absence congenital - with complete absence of distal elements (foot and toes)
755.35 Absence congenital - with incomplete absence of distal elements
0 Amputation status see 'Amputation' status - lower limb
904.8 Blood vessel NEC injury
904.7 Blood vessel NEC injury multiple
904.7 Blood vessel injury specified NEC
736.42 Bowing acquired
754.44 Bowing long bones congenital
732.1 Calve perthes
736.89 Deformity (acquired) NEC
959.7 Injury
916.8 Injury superficial NOS
916.9 Injury superficial NOS infected
916.8 Injury superficial other specified
916.9 Injury superficial other specified infected
736.81 Length discrepancy (acquired)
755.30 Length discrepancy congenital
V52.1 Prosthesis (fitting and adjustment) (removal)
755.30 Shortening congenital

V62.5 LEGAL PROBLEM (REASON FOR ENCOUNTER)
732.1 LEGG (-CALVE) (-PERTHES) DISEASE (CAPITAL FEMORAL OSTEOCHONDROSIS)

482.84 LEGIONNAIRES' DISEASE
757.0 LEGS HEREDITARY EDEMA CONGENITAL
330.8 LEIGH'S DISEASE
695.89 LEINER'S DISEASE (EXFOLIATIVE DERMATITIS)

LEIOMYOMA

215.9 Site NOS
0 Site specified see 'Benign Neoplasm', connective tissue (soft tissue) by site M8890/0
215.# Bizarre M8893/0

4th digit: 215
- **0. Head, face, neck**
- **2. Upper limb including shoulder**
- **3. Lower limb including hip**
- **4. Thorax**
- **5. Abdomen (wall), gastric, gastrointestinal, intestine, stomach**
- **6. Pelvis, buttock, groin, inguinal region, perineum**
- **7. Trunk NOS, back NOS, flank NOS**
- **8. Other specified sites**
- **9. Site unspecified**

238.1 Cellular site NOS
0 Cellular site specified see 'Neoplasm Uncertain Behavior', by site M8892/1
238.1 Epithelioid site NOS
0 Epithelioid site specified see 'Neoplasm Uncertain Behavior', by site M8891/1
600.20 Prostate (polypoid)

See 'LUTS' or 'Lower Urinary Tract Symptoms' for the additional code to identify the specific lower urinary tract symptoms.

600.21 Prostate (polypoid) with urinary obstruction, retention or other lower urinary tract symptoms
218.9 Uterine
218.1 Uterine intramural (interstitial)
0 Uterine see 'Fibroid Uterine'
218.0 Uterine submucous
218.2 Uterine subperitoneal
218.2 Uterine subserous

238.1 LEIOMYOMATOSIS INTRAVASCULAR SITE NOS
0 LEIOMYOMATOSIS INTRAVASCULAR SITE SPECIFIED SEE 'NEOPLASM UNCERTAIN BEHAVIOR', BY SITE M8890/1

LEIOMYOSARCOMA

171.# Unspecified M8890/3
171.# Epithelioid M8891/3

4th digit: 171
- **0. Head, face, neck**
- **2. Upper limb including shoulder**
- **3. Lower limb including hip**
- **4. Thorax**
- **5. Abdomen (wall), gastric, gastrointestinal, intestine, stomach**
- **6. Pelvis, buttock, groin, inguinal region, perineum**
- **7. Trunk NOS, back NOS, flank NOS**
- **8. Other specified sites**
- **9. Site NOS**

L

LEISHMANIASIS

085.9 Unspecified

CUTANEOUS

085.2 Acute necrotizing
085.4 American
085.2 Asian desert
085.3 Diffuse
085.1 Dry form
085.3 Ethiopian
085.1 Late
085.3 Lepromatous
085.1 Recurrent
085.2 Rural
085.1 Ulcerating
085.1 Urban
085.2 Wet form
085.2 Zoonotic form

LEISHMANIASIS (continued)

085.0 Dermal, post-Kala-Azar
085.5 Eyelid [373.6]
085.5 Leishmania Braziliensis
085.0 Leishmania donovani
085.3 Leishmania Ethiopica
085.0 Leishmania infantum
085.4 Leishmania Mexicana
085.1 Leishmania tropica (minor)
085.2 Leishmania tropica major
085.0 Mediterranean
085.5 Mucocutaneous (American) conjunctivitis [372.15]
V75.2 Screening exam
085.4 Tegumentaria diffusa
V05.2 Vaccination
085.0 Visceral (Kala-Azar) (Indian)

695.4 LELOIR'S DISEASE (LUPUS ERYTHEMATOSUS)

451.89 LEMIERE SYNDROME

426.0 LENEGRE'S DISEASE

345.0# LENNOX-GASTAUT SYNDROME

345.0# LENNOX'S SYNDROME (SEE ALSO 'EPILEPSY, EPILEPTIC')

5th digit: 345.0
0. Without mention of intractable epilepsy
1. With intractable epilepsy

LENS

379.31 Absence
743.35 Absence congenital
V45.61 Absence status post cataract extraction
743.9 Anomaly
743.36 Anomaly - shape
743.39 Anomaly - specified NEC
366.8 Calcification
743.36 Defect (shape) congenital
743.37 Ectopic congenital
379.39 Other disorders nonsurgical
996.53 Prolapse (ocular)
V43.1 Replacement (artificial) (prosthesis) (mechanical)
V45.61 Replacement status (artificial) (prosthesis) following cataract extraction [V43.1]

275.1 LENTICULAR SYNDROME

709.09 LENTIGO (JUVENILE) (SENILE)

0 LENTIGO MALIGNA SEE 'MELANOMA'

733.3 LEONTIASIS OSSIUM

242.9# LEOPOLD-LEVI'S SYNDROME (PAROXYSMAL THYROID INSTABILITY)

5th digit: 242.9
0. Without mention of thyrotoxic crisis or storm
1. With mention of thyrotoxic crisis or storm

282.49 LEPORE HEMOGLOBIN SYNDROME (TRAIT)

LEPROSY

030.9 Unspecified
030.3 Borderline (group B)
030.9 Cornea [371.89]
030.3 Dimorphous
030.0 Eyelid [373.4]
030.2 Indeterminate (group I)
030.0 Lepromatous (type L)
030.1 Tuberculoid (type T)
030.8 Other specified
V74.2 Screening exam

282.49 LEPTOCYTOSIS HEREDITARY

322.9 LEPTOMENINGITIS NOS (SEE ALSO 'MENINGITIS')

LEPTOSPIROSIS

100.9 Unspecified
100.89 Australis
100.89 Bataviae
100.0 Icterohemorrhagica
100.81 Meningitis
100.89 Pyrogenes
V74.8 Screening exam

756.59 LERI WEILL SYNDROME

444.0 LERICHE'S SYNDROME (AORTIC OCCLUSION)

733.7 LERICHE'S DISEASE (POSTTRAUMATIC OSTEOPOROSIS)

386.00 LERMOYEZ'S SYNDROME

302.0 LESBIANISM

277.2 LESCH-NYHAN SYNDROME (HYPOXANTHINE-GUANINE PHOSPHOROIBOSYLTRANSFERASE DEFICIENCY)

> ***To code a lesion of a site not listed below, see the specified anatomical site, or proper name.***

LESION

378.54 Abducens nerve
103.2 Achromic of pinta
525.8 Alveolar process
569.49 Anorectal
0 Aortic (valve) see 'Endocarditis', aortic
388.5 Auditory nerve
333.90 Basal ganglion
576.8 Bile duct
596.9 Bladder
733.90 Bone
353.0 Brachial plexus
348.8 Brain
742.9 Brain congenital
0 Brain vascular see 'Lesion' cerebrovascular
528.9 Buccal
373.9 Canthus
0 Carate see 'Pinta'

LESION (continued)

537.89 Cardia
0 Cardiac see 'Heart Disease'
103.2 Cardiovascular of pinta
344.60 Cauda equina
344.61 Cauda equina with neurogenic bladder
569.89 Cecum

CEREBROVASCULAR

437.9 NOS
437.1 Degenerative
V12.54 Healed
0 Healed with residual see 'Late Effect', cerebrovascular disease
437.2 Hypertensive
437.8 Specified type NEC

LESION (continued)

353.2 Cervical root (nerve) NEC
377.54 Chiasmal
377.52 Chiasmal neoplasm NEC
377.51 Chiasmal neoplasm pituitary
377.51 Chiasmal pituitary disorder
377.53 Chiasmal vascular disorder
377.54 Chiasmal with inflammatory disorder

> ***To code a lesion of a site not listed below, see the specified anatomical site, or proper name.***

351.8 Chorda tympani
103.2 Cicatricial of pinta
793.1 Coin, lung
569.89 Colon
372.9 Conjunctiva
0 Coronary artery see 'CAD (Coronary Artery Disease)'

CRANIAL NERVE

352.9 NOS
352.0 First
377.49 Second
378.51 Third partial
378.52 Third total
378.53 Fourth
350.9 Fifth
378.54 Sixth
351.9 Seventh
388.5 Eighth
352.2 Ninth
352.3 Tenth
352.4 Eleventh
352.5 Twelfth

LESION (continued)

0 Cystic see 'Cyst', by site
709.9 Dermal (skin)
537.84 Dieulafoy (hemorrhagic) duodenum
569.86 Dieulafoy (hemorrhagic) intestine
537.84 Dieulafoy (hemorrhagic) stomach
537.89 Duodenum
537.84 Duodenum dieulafoy (hemorrhagic)
537.3 Duodenum with obstruction
103.2 Dyschromic of pinta
373.9 Eyelid
350.8 Gasserian ganglion
537.89 Gastric
537.89 Gastroduodenal

LESION (continued)

569.89 Gastrointestinal
352.2 Glossopharyngeal nerve
0 Heart (organic) see 'Heart Disease'
0 Heart vascular see 'Cardiovascular Disease'
709.9 Helix (ear)
103.1 Hyperchromic, due to pinta (carate)
701.1 Hyperkeratotic see also 'Keratosis'
352.5 Hypoglossal nerve
478.29 Hypopharynx
253.9 Hypothalamic
569.89 Ileocecal coil
569.89 Ileum
355.79 Iliohypogastric nerve
355.79 Ilioinguinal nerve
0 Incontinuity see 'Nerve Injury', by site
569.89 Intestine
569.86 Intestine dieulafoy (hemorrhagic)
0 Intracerebral see 'Lesion' cerebrovascular
0 Intrachiasmal see 'Lesion' chiasmal
784.2 Intracranial, space-occupying NEC
0 Joint see 'Joint', disorder
701.1 Keratotic see also 'Keratosis'
593.9 Kidney NOS
352.3 Laryngeal nerve (recurrent)
030.0 Leonine
528.5 Lip
573.8 Liver
353.1 Lumbosacral plexus
250.6# Lumbosacral plexus with diabetes [353.1]

5th digit: 250

0. Type II, adult-onset, non-insulin dependent (even if requiring insulin), or unspecified; controlled
1. Type I, juvenile-onset or insulin-dependent; controlled
2. Type II, adult-onset, non-insulin dependent (even if requiring insulin); uncontrolled
3. Type I, juvenile-onset or insulin-dependent; uncontrolled

353.4 Lumbosacral root (nerve) NEC
518.89 Lung
793.1 Lung coin
473.0 Maxillary sinus
0 Mitral see 'Endocarditis', mitral
348.8 Motor cortex
238.73 Myelodysplastic high grade syndrome
238.72 Myelodysplastic low grade syndrome
0 Nerve see specified nerve by site, disorder
349.9 Nervous system
742.9 Nervous system, congenital

> ***To code a lesion of a site not listed below, see the specified anatomical site, or proper name.***

NONALLOPATHIC

739.9 Abdomen
739.7 Acromioclavicular
739.1 Cervical, cervicothoracic
739.8 Costochondral
739.8 Costovertebral
739.6 Extremity, lower
739.7 Extremity, upper
739.0 Head
739.5 Hip

L

LESION (continued)

NONALLOPATHIC (continued)

739.6 Lower extremity
739.3 Lumbar, lumbosacral
739.0 Occipitocervical
739.5 Pelvic
739.5 Pubic
739.8 Rib cage
739.4 Sacral, sacrococcygeal, sacroiliac
739.8 Sternochondral
739.7 Sternoclavicular
739.2 Thoracic, thoracolumbar
739.7 Upper extremity

LESION (continued)

478.19 Nose (internal)
0 Obstructive see 'Obstruction', by site
355.79 Obturator nerve
0 Occlusive artery see 'Embolism', by site
0 Organ or site NEC see organ by site, disease
733.90 Osteolytic
620.8 Ovary
363.32 Paramacular of retina
537.89 Peptic
523.8 Periodontal, due to traumatic occlusion
569.49 Perirectal
568.89 Peritoneum (granulomatous)
709.00 Pigmented (skin)
0 Pinta see 'Pinta'
0 Polypoid see 'Polyp', by site
0 Prechiasmal see 'Lesion' chiasmal
0 Primary see 'Syphilis Primary'
103.0 Primary carate
103.0 Primary pinta
102.0 Primary yaws
518.89 Pulmonary
793.1 Pulmonary coin
537.89 Pylorus
990 Radiation NEC
990 Radium NEC
569.89 Rectosigmoid
0 Retina, retinal see 'Retinopathy'
362.17 Retina vascular
568.89 Retroperitoneal
720.1 Romanus
724.6 Sacroiliac (joint)
527.8 Salivary gland
527.8 Salivary gland benign lymphoepithelial
355.79 Saphenous nerve
0 Secondary syphilis see 'Syphilis Secondary'
569.89 Sigmoid
473.9 Sinus (accessory) (nasal) see also 'Sinusitis'
709.9 Skin
686.00 Skin suppurative
840.7 SLAP (superior glenoid labrum lesion)
784.2 Space-occupying, intracranial NEC
336.9 Spinal cord
742.9 Spinal cord congenital
0 Spinal cord, traumatic see 'Spinal Cord', injury, by site
289.50 Spleen
537.89 Stomach
537.84 Stomach dieulafoy (hemorrhagic)

LESION (continued)

To code a lesion of a site not listed below, see the specified anatomical site, or proper name.

0 Syphilitic see 'Syphilis'
0 Tertiary see 'Syphilis Tertiary'
353.3 Thoracic root (nerve)
474.9 Tonsillar fossa
525.8 Tooth, teeth
521.01 Tooth, teeth white spot
0 Tricuspid see 'Endocarditis', tricuspid
350.9 Trigeminal nerve
0 Ulcerated or ulcerative see 'Ulcer', by site
621.9 Uterus NEC
623.8 Vagina
352.3 Vagus nerve
424.90 Valvular NOS

VASCULAR

459.9 NOS
0 Affecting central nervous system see 'Lesion' cerebrovascular
904.9 Following trauma see also specified blood vessel, injury
362.17 Retina
663.6# Umbilical cord
5th digit: 663.6
0. Episode of care NOS or N/A
1. Delivered
3. Antepartum complication

762.6 Umbilical cord affecting fetus or newborn

LESION (continued)

377.73 Visual cortex NEC
377.63 Visual pathway NEC
0 Warty see 'Verruca'
990 X-ray NEC - effects of
0 X-ray findings - see 'Lesion', anatomical site

446.3 LETHAL MIDLINE GRANULOMA
648.9# LETHAL MIDLINE GRANULOMA MATERNAL CURRENT (CO-EXISTENT) IN PREGNANCY [446.3]
5th digit: 648.9
0. Episode of NOS or N/A
1. Delivered
2. Delivered with postpartum complication
3. Antepartum complication
4. Postpartum complication

780.79 LETHARGY
202.5# LETTERER SIWE DISEASE M9722/3
5th digit: 202.5
0. Unspecified
1. Lymph nodes of head, face, neck
2. Lymph nodes intrathoracic
3. Lymph nodes abdominal
4. Lymph nodes axilla and upper limb
5. Lymph nodes inguinal region and lower limb
6. Lymph nodes intrapelvic
7. Spleen
8. Lymph nodes multiple sites

270.3 LEUCINE METABOLISM DISTURBANCES
270.3 LEUCINOSIS

360.44	LEUCOCORIA EYE
371.04	LEUCOMA ADHERENT (CORNEA)

LEUKEMIA QUICK REFERENCE

208.9#	NOS M9800/3
208.0#	Acute NOS M9801/3
208.0#	Aleukemic NOS M9804/3
205.1#	Basophilic M9870/3
208.0#	Blast cell M9801/3
208.1#	Chronic NOS M9803/3
207.8#	Compound M9810/3
205.1#	Eosinophilic M9880/3
207.0#	Erythremia acute M9841/3
207.1#	Erythremia chronic M9842/3
207.0#	Erythremia erythroleukemia acute M9801/3
202.4#	Hairy cell M9940/3
204.9#	Lymphoid NOS M9820/3
204.0#	Lymphoid acute M9821/3
204.8#	Lymphoid aleukemic M9824/3
204.1#	Lymphoid chronic M9823/3
204.2#	Lymphoid subacute M9822/3
207.8#	Lymphosarcoma cell M9850/3
207.8#	Mast cell M9900/3
207.2#	Megakaryocytic M9910/3
206.9#	Monocytic NOS M9890/3
206.0#	Monocytic acute M9891/3
206.8#	Monocytic aleukemic M9894/3
206.1#	Monocytic chronic M9893/3
206.2#	Monocytic subacute M9892/3
205.9#	Myeloid NOS M9860/3
205.0#	Myeloid acute M9861/3
205.8#	Myeloid aleukemic subleukemic M9864/3
205.1#	Myeloid chronic M9863/3
205.2#	Myeloid subacute M9862/3
205.1#	Naegeli-type monocytic M9863/3
205.1#	Neutrophilic M9865/3
203.1#	Plasma cell M9830/3
204.9#	Prolymphocytic site NOS M9825/3
0	Prolymphocytic site specified see 'Leukemia Quick Reference', lymphoid
205.0#	Promyelocytic acute M9866/3
0	Schilling type monocytic see 'Leukemia Quick Reference', monocytic
208.0#	Stem cell M9801/3
208.2#	Subacute NOS M9802/3
208.8#	Subleukemic NEC M9804/3
207.2#	Thrombocytic M9910/3
208.0#	Undifferentiated M9801/3

5th digit: 202, 203, 204, 205, 206, 207, 208
0. Without mention of remission
1. In remission

LEUKEMIA

208.##	NOS cell type **4th digit: 208** **0. Acute M9801/3** **1. Chronic (acute exacerbation of chronic) M9803/3** **2. Subacute M9802/3** **8. Other leukemia of unspecified cell type M9800/3** **9. Unspecified M9800/3** **5th digit: 208** **0. Without mention of remission** **1. In remission**

LEUKEMIA (continued)

V16.6	Family history
205.##	Granulocytic (myeloid) **4th digit: 205** **0. Acute M9800/3** **1. Chronic (acute exacerbation of chronic) M9863/3** **2. Subacute M9862/3** **8. Aleukemic leukemia (granulocytic) myelogenous myeloid myelosis M9864/3** **9. Unspecified M9860/3** **5th digit: 205** **0. Without mention of remission** **1. In remission**
206.9#	Histiocytic M9890/3 **5th digit: 206.9** **0. Without mention of remission** **1. In remission**
V10.60	History
V10.63	History monocytic
V10.69	History other type
204.##	Lymphatic
204.0#	Lymphoblastic M9821/3
204.##	Lymphocytic
204.##	Lymphogenous
204.##	Lymphoid **4th digit: 204** **0. Acute (blastic) M9821/3** **1. Chronic M9823/3** **2. Subacute M9822/3** **8. Aleukemic leukemia M9824/3** **9. Unspecified M9820/3** **5th digit: 204** **0. Without mention of remission** **1. In remission**
207.8#	Lymphosarcoma cell M9850/3
207.8#	Mast cell M9900/3
207.2#	Megakaryocytic M9910/3 **5th digit: 207.2, 8** **0. Without mention of remission** **1. In remission**
206.0#	Monoblastic M9891/3
206.##	Monocytic
206.##	Monocytoid **4th digit: 206** **0. Acute M9891/3** **1. Chronic (acute exacerbation of chronic) M9893/3** **2. Subacute M9892/3** **8. Aleukemic leukemia (monocytic monocytoid) M9894/3** **9. Unspecified M9890/3** **5th digit: 206** **0. Without mention of remission** **1. In remission**

LEUKEMIA (continued)

205.0# Myeloblastic (myeloid) M9861/3
205.## Myelocytic (myeloid)
205.## Myelogenous (myeloid)
205.## Myeloid
205.3# Myeloid sarcoma M9930/3
205.## Myelomonocytic (myeloid)
205.## Myelosclerotic (myeloid)
205.## Myelosis (myeloid)

4th digit: 205
0. Acute M9861/3
1. Chronic (acute exacerbation of chronic) M9863/3
2. Subacute M9862/3
3. Myeloid sarcoma M9930/3
8. Aleukemic leukemia (granulocytic) myelogenous myeloid, aleukemic myelosis M9864/3
9. Unspecified M9860/3

5th digit: 205
0. Without mention of remission
1. In remission

L

203.1# Plasma cell M9830/3

5th digit: 203.1
0. Without mention of remission
1. In remission

202.4# LEUKEMIC RETICULOENDOTHELIOSIS M9940/3

5th digit: 202.4
0. Unspecified
1. Lymph nodes of head, face, neck
2. Lymph nodes intrathoracic
3. Lymph nodes abdominal
4. Lymph nodes axilla and upper limb
5. Lymph nodes inguinal region and lower limb
6. Lymph nodes intrapelvic
7. Spleen
8. Lymph nodes multiple sites

288.62 LEUKEMOID REACTION (BASOPHILIC) (LYMPHOCYTIC) (MONOCYTIC) (MYELOCYTIC) (NEUTROPHILIC)
446.29 LEUKOCLASTIC VASCULITIS
288.50 LEUKOCYTE DECREASE
288.60 LEUKOCYTE ELEVATED
288.2 LEUKOCYTIC ANOMALY HEREDITARY
288.50 LEUKOCYTOPENIA
288.60 LEUKOCYTOSIS
288.3 LEUKOCYTOSIS EOSINOPHILIC
709.09 LEUKODERMA

LEUKODYSTROPHY

330.0 Unspecified
330.0 Globoid cell
330.0 Lipidosis
330.0 Metachromatic
330.0 Sudanophilic

528.79 LEUKOEDEMA ORAL (MOUTH) (TONGUE)
136.9 <u>LEUKOENCEPHALITIS</u> <u>ACUTE</u> <u>HEMORRHAGIC</u> (POSTINFECTIOUS) NEC <u>[323.61]</u>
323.51 LEUKOENCEPHALITIS ACUTE HEMORRHAGIC (POSTINFECTIOUS) POSTIMMUNIZATION OR POSTVACCINAL
323.9 LEUKOENCEPHALOPATHY (SEE ALSO 'ENCEPHALITIS')
136.9 <u>LEUKOENCEPHALOPATHY</u> <u>ACUTE</u> <u>NECROTIZING</u> <u>HEMORRHAGIC</u> (POSTINFECTIOUS) NEC <u>[323.61]</u>
323.51 LEUKOENCEPHALOPATHY ACUTE NECROTIZING HEMORRHAGIC (POSTINFECTIOUS) POSTIMMUNIZ OR POSTVACCINAL
046.3 LEUKOENCEPHALOPATHY MULTIFOCAL
289.9 LEUKOERYTHROBLASTOSIS
702.8 LEUKOKERATOSIS NEC
528.79 LEUKOKERATOSIS NICOTINA PALATI
528.6 LEUKOKERATOSIS ORAL MUCOSA
779.7 LEUKOMALACIA PERIVENTRICULAR PERINATAL
288.2 LEUKOMELANOPATHY HEREDITARY
703.8 LEUKONYCHIA (PUNCTATA) (STRIATA)
757.5 LEUKONYCHIA CONGENITAL

LEUKOPENIA

288.50 NOS
288.59 Basophilic
288.01 Congenital (nontransient)
288.02 Cyclic
288.59 Eosinophilic
288.59 Familial
288.09 Malignant
776.7 Neonatal transitory
288.02 Periodic

LEUKOPLAKIA

569.49 Anus
622.2 Cervix
530.83 Esophagus
528.6 Gingiva
478.79 Larynx
528.6 Lips
528.6 Oral mucosa including tongue
607.0 Penis
702.8 Skin NEC
528.6 Tongue
478.29 Tonsil
599.84 Urethra (post infectional)
621.8 Uterus
623.1 Vagina
596.8 Vesical
0 Vesical with incontinence see 'Bladder Disorders With Incontinence'
478.5 Vocal cord
624.09 Vulva

LEUKORRHEA

623.5 NOS
623.5 Noninfective
131.00 Trichomonal

426.0 LEV'S HEART BLOCK (SYNDROME)
253.3 LEVI'S DWARFISM (SYNDROME)
746.87 LEVOCARDIA (ISOLATED)
334.3 LEVY-ROUSSY SYNDROME

078.19 LEWANDOWSKI-LUTZ DISEASE

017.0# LEWANDOWSKI'S DISEASE (TUBERCULOSIS)
5th digit: 017.0
0. Unspecified
1. Lab not done
2. Lab pending
3. Microscopy positive (in sputum)
4. Culture positive - microscopy negative
5. Culture negative - microscopy positive
6. Culture and microscopy negative confirmed by other methods

331.82 LEWY BODY DISEASE WITH DEMENTIA [**294.1#**]
5th digit: 294.1
0. Without behavioral disturbance or NOS
1. With behavioral disturbance

536.2 LEYDEN'S DISEASE (PERIODIC VOMITING)

257.2 LEYDIG'S CELL FAILURE (ADULT)

LEYDIG CELL TUMOR

236.2 Female site NOS
0 Female site specified see 'Neoplasm Uncertain Behavior', by site M8650/1
236.4 Male site NOS
0 Male site specified see 'Neoplasm Uncertain Behavior', by site M8650/1

220 Benign female site NOS
0 Benign female site specified see 'Benign Neoplasm', by site M8650/0
222.0 Benign male site NOS
0 Benign male site specified see 'Benign Neoplasm', by site M8650/0
183.0 Malignant female site NOS
0 Malignant female site specified see 'Cancer', by site M8630/3
186.9 Malignant male site NOS
0 Malignant male site specified see 'Cancer', by site M8650/3

795.03 LGSIL CERVIX (LOW GRADE SQUAMOUS INTRAEPITHELIAL LESION)

099.1 LGV

647.2# LGV MATERNAL CURRENT (CO-EXISTENT) IN PREGNANCY
5th digit: 647.2
0. Episode of care unspecified or N/A
1. Delivered
2. Delivered with postpartum complication
3. Antepartum complication
4. Postpartum complication

V84.01 LI FRAUMENI CANCER SYNDROME

799.81 LIBIDO DECREASED

710.0 LIBMAN SACKS DISEASE (VERRUCOUS ENDOCARDITIS) [424.91]

LICE

132.9 Unspecified
132.0 Head
132.1 Body
132.2 Pubic
0 See 'Pediculosis'

LICHEN

697.9 NOS
698.3 Lichenification
697.1 Nitidus
698.3 Obtusus corneus
757.39 Pilaris (congenital)
697.0 Planopilaris (ruber planus)
697.0 Planus
696.4 Ruber acuminatus
697.8 Ruber moniliforme striata
701.0 Sclerosus et atrophicus
017.0# Scrofulosus (tuberculous)
5th digit: 017.0
0. Unspecified
1. Lab not done
2. Lab pending
3. Microscopy positive (in sputum)
4. Culture positive - microscopy negative
5. Culture negative - microscopy positive
6. Culture and microscopy negative confirmed by other methods
698.3 Simplex chronicus
757.39 Spinulosus (congenital)
697.8 Striata
698.2 Urticatus
697.8 Other

281.0 LICHTHEIM'S DISEASE OR SYNDROME (SUBACUTE COMBINED SCLEROSIS WITH PERNICIOUS ANEMIA) [336.2]

374.41 LID RETRACTION OR LAG

289.59 LIEN MIGRANS

0 LIENTERY SEE 'DIARRHEA'

Lifestyle problems, V69.#, may be used to identify risk factors such as lack of physical exercise or high risk sexual behavior. These codes should be assigned as additional diagnoses when the physician documents the presence of risk factors in the medical record. These codes are clinically important because they show the presence of risk factors that require surveillance and prevention programs. These codes, however, should not be used as the principal diagnosis when the reason for encounter is for counseling of the risk factors.

LIFESTYLE PROBLEM

V69.9 NOS
V69.1 Diet and eating habits inappropriate
V69.3 Gambling and betting
V69.0 Physical exercise (lack of)
V69.8 Self-damaging behavior
V69.2 Sexual behavior high risk
V69.8 Other

LIGAMENT

728.89 Calcification
717.89 Calcification knee (medial collateral)
728.89 Contraction
756.89 Contraction congenital
728.9 Disorder
728.89 Disorder other
0 Division see 'Sprain', by site
0 Division with open wound see 'Laceration'
728.4 Laxity
728.89 Ossification

LIGAMENT (continued)

718.9# Relaxation joint
5th digit: 718.9
0. Site NOS
1. Shoulder region
2. Upper arm (elbow) (humerus)
3. Forearm (radius) (wrist) (ulna)
4. Hand (carpal) (metacarpal) (fingers)
5. Pelvic region and thigh (hip) (buttock) (femur)
7. Ankle and/or foot (metatarsals) (toes) (tarsals)
8. Other
9. Multiple

717.9 Relaxation joint - knee
724.6 Relaxation joint - lumbosacral
724.6 Relaxation joint - sacroiliac

203.0# LIGHT CHAIN DISEASE
5th digit: 203.0
0. Without mention of remission
1. In remission

LIGHT FOR DATES

656.5# Affecting management of mother
5th digit: 656.5
0. Episode of care unspecified or N/A
1. Delivered
3. Antepartum complication

WITH FETAL MALNUTRITION

764.10 Weight unspecified
764.11 < 500 grams
764.12 500 - 749 grams
764.13 750 - 999 grams
764.14 1000 - 1249 grams
764.15 1250 - 1499 grams
764.16 1500 - 1749 grams
764.17 1750 - 1999 grams
764.18 2000-2499 grams
764.19 2500 grams and over

WITHOUT MENTION OF FETAL MALNUTRITION

764.00 Weight unspecified
764.01 < 500 grams
764.02 500 - 749 grams
764.03 750 - 999 grams
764.04 1000 - 1249 grams
764.05 1250 - 1499 grams
764.06 1500 - 1749 grams
764.07 1750 - 1999 grams
764.08 2000- 2499 grams
764.09 2500 grams and over

780.4 LIGHT HEADEDNESS
362.13 LIGHT REFLEX INCREASED RETINA
994.0 LIGHTNING (STRUCK BY)
909.4 LIGHTNING (STRUCK BY) LATE EFFECT
0 LIGHTNING BURN SEE 'BURN'
588.89 LIGHTWOOD'S DISEASE OR SYNDROME (RENAL TUBULAR ACIDOSIS)
270.0 LIGNAC'S (-DE TONI) (-FANCONI) (-DEBRE) DISEASE OR SYNDROME (CYSTINOSIS)
413.9 LIKOFF'S SYNDROME (ANGINA IN MENOPAUSAL WOMEN)

LIMB

755.4 Absence - NOS (complete) (partial) - congenital
755.30 Absence lower - NOS congenital (acquired)
755.31 Absence lower - complete/transverse congenital (acquired)
755.32 Absence lower - incomplete congenital (acquired)
755.20 Absence upper - NOS congenital (acquired)
755.21 Absence upper - complete/transverse congenital (acquired)
755.22 Absence upper - incomplete congenital (acquired)
0 Amputation (absence) status see 'Amputation', status
755.9 Anomaly congenital - limb unspecified
755.60 Anomaly congenital - lower limb
755.50 Anomaly congenital - upper limb
755.8 Anomaly other specified congenital - limb unspecified
V49.0 Deficiency
736.9 Deformity acquired site NOS
736.89 Deformity acquired NEC, arm, leg, shoulder
V49.4 Disfigurement
780.58 Disorder – movement sleep related unspecified
327.51 Disorder – movement periodic
729.89 Disorder - musculoskeletal
306.0 Disorder - psychogenic (musculoskeletal)
729.9 Disorder - soft tissue
754.89 Flexion contractures of joints (lower limb) congenital
359.1 Girdle muscular dystrophy
729.5 Pain
V49.9 Problem
V49.1 Problem mechanical
V49.2 Problem motor
V49.3 Problem sensory
V49.5 Problem other
V43.7 Replacement status (artificial) (prosthesis)
729.81 Swelling
747.64 Vessel lower atresia
747.63 Vessel upper atresia

759.6 LINDAU'S DISEASE (RETINOCEREBRAL ANGIOMATOSIS)
529.3 LINGUA VILLOSA NIGRA
151.9 LINITIS PLASTICA SITE NOS
0 LINITIS PLASTICA SITE SPECIFIED SEE 'CANCER', BY SITE M8142/3

LIP

528.5 Abscess
750.26 Absence congenital
528.5 Atrophy
528.9 Biting
528.5 Cyst
528.5 Disease NEC
054.9 Fever blister
749.1# Fissure (congenital)
5th digit: 749.1
0. Cleft unspecified
1. Cleft unilateral complete
2. Cleft unilateral incomplete
3. Cleft bilateral complete
4. Cleft bilateral incomplete

528.5 Fistula
750.25 Fistula congenital
528.5 Hypertrophy
744.81 Hypertrophy congenital
959.09 Injury
910.8 Injury other and unspecified (superficial)
910.9 Injury other and unspecified (superficial) infected
750.25 Pits (mucus) congenital

LIP (continued)

709.2 Scar
528.5 Ulcer

790.5 LIPASE ABNORMAL BLOOD LEVEL

272.3 LIPEMIA RETINALIS

LIPID, LIPOID

272.9 Abnormal findings NEC
220 Cell tumor of ovary
272.8 Dermatoarthritis [713.0]
272.9 Disorder (metabolism) - NOS
272.7 Disorder (metabolism) - storage
272.8 Disorder (metabolism) - specified NEC
V77.91 Disorder screening
272.5 High-density deficiency
272.9 Metabolism disorder - NOS
272.7 Metabolism disorder - storage
272.8 Metabolism disorder - other specified NEC
581.3 Nephrosis
507.1 Pneumonia
516.8 Pneumonia endogenous
507.1 Pneumonia exogenous
272.7 Storage disease

LIPIDOSIS

272.7 NOS
330.1 Cerebral (Tay Sach's)
272.7 Chemically induced
330.0 Sulfatide

229.9 LIPOADENOMA SITE NOS

0 LIPOADENOMA SITE SPECIFIED SEE 'BENIGN NEOPLASM', BY SITE M8324/0

229.9 LIPOBLASTOMATOSIS SITE NOS

0 LIPOBLASTOMATOSIS SITE SPECIFIED SEE 'BENIGN NEOPLASM', BY SITE M8881/0

277.5 LIPOCHONDRODYSTROPHY

288.1 LIPOCHROME HISTIOCYTOSIS (FAMILIAL)

LIPODYSTROPHY

272.6 NOS
040.2 Intestinal
567.82 Mesenteric
272.6 Progressive

272.8 LIPOGRANULOMATOSIS DISSEMINATED

0 LIPOID SEE 'LIPID, LIPOID'

LIPOMA

214.# NOS M8850/0
214.# Intramuscular M8856/0
214.# Spindle cell M8857/0

4th digit: 214
0. Facial skin and subcutaneous tissue
1. Skin and subcutaneous tissue other
2. Intrathoracic organs
3. Intra-abdominal organs
4. Spermatic cord
8. Other specified sites muscle, fascia M8856/0
9. Unspecified site M8850/0

LIPOMATOSIS (DOLOROSA)

272.8 NOS
214.8 Epidural
0 Fetal see 'Lipoma', by site
272.8 Launois-Bensaude's

289.89 LIPOPHAGOCYTOSIS

272.8 LIPOPROTEIN A LEVEL ELEVATED

272.5 LIPOPROTEIN DISORDER (DEFICIENCY) (METABOLISM)

LIPOSARCOMA

171.# Unspecified M8850/3
171.# Mixed type M8855/3
171.# Myxoid M8855/3
171.# Pleomorphic M8854/3
171.# Round cell M8853/3
171.# Well differentiated type M8851/3

4th digit: 171
0. Head, face, neck
2. Upper limb including shoulder
3. Lower limb including hip
4. Thorax
5. Abdomen (wall), gastric, gastrointestinal, intestine, stomach
6. Pelvis, buttock, groin, inguinal region, perineum
7. Trunk NOS, back NOS, flank NOS
8. Other specified sites
9. Site unspecified

272.8 LIPOSYNOVITIS PREPATELLARIS

616.50 LIPSCHUTZ'S DISEASE OR ULCER

307.9 LISPING

027.0 LISTERIA MONOCYTOGENES INFECTION (SEPTICEMIA)

027.0 LISTERIOSIS

771.2 LISTERIOSIS CONGENITAL OR PERINATAL

655.4# LISTERIOSIS MATERNAL WITH SUSPECTED DAMAGE TO FETUS

5th digit: 655.4
0. Episode of care unspecified or N/A
1. Delivered
3. Antepartum complication

780.79 LISTLESSNESS

790.6 LITHIUM ABNORMAL BLOOD LEVEL

656.8# LITHOPEDIAN FETUS AFFECTING MOTHER

5th digit: 656.8
0. Episode of care unspecified or N/A
1. Delivered
3. Antepartum complication

V62.5 LITIGATION PROBLEM (REASON FOR ENCOUNTER)

718.82 LITTLE LEAGUERS ELBOW

718.81 LITTLE LEAGUERS SHOULDER

0 LITTLE'S DISEASE SEE 'CEREBRAL PALSY'

782.61 LIVEDO (ANNULARIS) (RACEMORE) (RETICULARIS)

LIVER

0 See also 'Hepatic'
751.69 Absence (lobe) congenital
751.69 Accessory congenital
571.0 Alcoholic fatty
277.39 Amyloid degeneration
751.60 Anomaly NOS
751.69 Anomaly other specified
570 Atrophy (see also 'Necrosis', liver)
639.8 Atrophy post abortive (ectopic) (molar) pregnancy

L

LIVER (continued)

571.2 Cirrhosis alcoholic
571.5 Cirrhosis obstructive (see also 'Cirrhosis', liver)
573.0 Congestion, chronic passive
0 Contusion see 'Liver Trauma', contusion
573.8 Cyst
751.62 Cyst congenital
122.8 Cyst echinococcal
122.0 Cyst echinococcal granulosis
127.4 Cyst oxyuris vermicularis
570 Degeneration (parenchymatous)
571.3 Disease alcoholic
571.1 Disease alcoholic - acute
571.3 Disease alcoholic - chronic
571.9 Disease chronic
571.3 Disease chronic alcoholic
571.8 Disease chronic nonalcoholic other
572.8 Disease chronic other sequelae
573.3 Disease drug induced
572.8 Disease end stage
573.9 Disorder

646.7#: Specify the maternal liver disorder with an additional code.

646.7# Disorder in pregnancy
5th digit: 646.7
0. Episode of care unspecified or N/A
1. Delivered
3. Antepartum complication

573.8 Disorders other specified
V59.6 Donor non-autogenous
751.69 Duplication of, congenital
573.9 End stage disease
573.9 Engorgement
789.1 Enlargement
570 Failure acute
997.4 Failure due to a procedure
572.8 Failure sequelae of other disease
571.0 Fatty alcoholic
571.8 Fatty nonalcoholic
272.8 Flap
751.69 Floating congenital
121.3 Fluke
121.0 Fluke cat
121.1 Fluke chinese (oriental)
794.8 Function study abnormal - radiologic
790.6 Function test (LFT)
790.5 Function test (LFT) - alkaline phosphatase
790.4 Function test (LFT) - aminotransferase
782.4 Function test (LFT) - bilirubin
790.5 Function test (LFT) - hepatic enzyme NEC
790.4 Function test (LFT) - lactate dehydrogenase
271.0 Glycogen infiltration
271.0 Glycogenosis
0 Hematoma traumatic see 'Liver Trauma', hematoma
572.4 Hepatorenal syndrome
674.8# Hepatorenal syndrome maternal due to pregnancy
5th digit: 674.8
0. Unspecified
2. Delivered with postpartum complication
4. Postpartum complication

LIVER (continued)

751.69 Hyperplasia (congenital)
0 Injury traumatic see 'Liver Trauma'
572.4 Kidney syndrome
0 Laceration see 'Liver Trauma', laceration
277.39 Lardaceous degeneration
277.39 Large waxy degeneration
570 Necrosis acute subacute massive

646.7#: Specify the maternal necrosis with an additional code.

646.7# Necrosis of pregnancy
5th digit: 646.7
0. Episode of care unspecified or N/A
1. Delivered
3. Antepartum complication

639.8 Necrosis post abortive (ectopic) (molar) pregnancy
573.8 Obstruction
751.62 Polycystic disease congenital
573.8 Prolapse
573.8 Ptosis
767.8 Rupture - birth trauma fetus
573.8 Rupture - nontraumatic
0 Rupture - traumatic see 'Liver Trauma', rupture
794.8 Scan abnormal
709.09 Spots
V42.7 Transplant (status)
996.82 Transplant rejection (failure)
277.39 Waxy degeneration

Injury to internal organs, such as lung, spleen, liver, or kidney can be a contusion, laceration, tear, or rupture. You may find the code under the type of injury or the anatomical site.

LIVER TRAUMA

864.00 Unspecified
864.10 Unspecified with open wound into cavity
864.01 Contusion
864.11 Contusion with open wound into cavity
864.01 Hematoma
864.11 Hematoma with open wound into cavity
864.00 Injury
864.## Laceration
4th digit: 864
0. Closed
1. With open wound into cavity

5th digit: 864
2. Minor (< 1cm. Deep)
3. Moderate (<10 cm long - <3 cm deep)
4. Major 10 cm. long - 3 cm deep, multiple, moderate or stellate)
5. Unspecified

908.1 Late effect
864.04 Rupture
864.14 Rupture with open wound into cavity
864.09 Other
864.19 Other with open wound into cavity

989.5 LIZARD BITE
995.0 LIZARD BITE WITH ANAPHYLAXIS [989.5]
258.1 LLOYD'S SYNDROME
125.2 LOA LOA INFECTION
V45.89 LOBECTOMY STATUS
116.2 LOBO'S DISEASE (KELOID BLASTOMYCOSIS)

116.2 LOBOA (BLASTOMYCES) LOBOI INFECTION
116.2 LOBOMYCOSIS
310.0 LOBOTOMY SYNDROME
756.51 LOBSTEIN'S DISEASE (BRITTLE BONES AND BLUE SCLERA)

755.58 LOBSTER-CLAW HAND CONGENITAL

LOBULAR

174.9 Carcinoma site NOS
0 Carcinoma site specified see 'Cancer', by site M8520/3

233.0 Carcinoma in situ site NOS
0 Carcinoma in situ site specified see 'CA In Situ', by site M8520/2

0 LOCKED BOWEL SEE 'BOWEL', OBSTRUCTION
344.81 LOCKED IN STATE
438.53 LOCKED IN STATE LATE EFFECT OF CEREBROVASCULAR DISEASE [344.81]
652.6# LOCKED TWINS COMPLICATING PREGNANCY
660.5# LOCKED TWINS OBSTRUCTING LABOR **[652.6#]**
5th digit: 652.6, 660.5
0. Episode of care unspecified or N/A
1. Delivered
3. Antepartum complication

334.9 LOCOMOTOR SYSTEM DISEASE
421.0 LOFFLER'S ENDOCARDITIS
518.3 LOFFLER'S SYNDROME (EOSINOPHILIC PNEUMONITIS)
135 LOFGREN'S SYNDROME (SARCOIDOSIS)
125.2 LOIASIS BANCROFTIAN
125.2 LOIASIS EYELID [373.6]
082.8 LONE STAR FEVER
758.39 LONG ARM 18 OR 21 DELETION SYNDROME
277.85 LONG CHAIN 3-HYDROXYACYL COA DEHYDROGENASE DEFICIENCY (LCHAD)
277.85 LONG CHAIN/VERY LONG CHAIN ACYL COA DEHYDROGENASE DEFICIENCY (LCAD, VLCAD)
754.0 LONG FACE SYNDROME
426.82 LONG QT SYNDROME
0 LOOSE BODY JOINT SEE 'JOINT', MICE
525.8 LOOSE TEETH
268.2 LOOSER (-DEBRAY) - MILKMAN SYNDROME (OSTEOMALACIA WITH PSEUDOFRACTURES)
253.3 LORAIN LEVI SYNDROME (PITUITARY DWARFISM)

The code in the left margin always sequences first. The additional code in brackets to the right of the description is sequenced second. Underlining shows the code number that corresponds to the underlined description. Underlining never implies correct sequencing.

LORDOSIS

737.20 Acquired (postural)
737.29 Acquired other
737.22 Acquired other postsurgical
737.42 Associated with other conditions
356.1 Charcot Marie tooth [737.42]
277.5 Mucopolysaccharidosis [737.42]

LORDOSIS (continued)

237.7# Neurofibromatosis [737.42]
5th digit: 237.7
0. Unspecified
1. Type I
2. Type II

252.01 Osteitis fibrosa cystica [737.42]
733.0# Osteoporotic [737.42]
5th digit: 733.0
0. Unspecified
1. Senile
2. Idiopathic
3. Disuse
9. Other

045.## Poliomyelitis [737.42]
4th dgit: 045
0. Acute bulbar paralytic
1. Acute with other paralysis
2. Acute non paralytic
9. Acute unspecified

5th digit: 045
0. Unspecified
1. Type I
2. Type II
3. Type III

138 Poliomyelitis late effect [737.42]
737.21 Postlaminectomy
754.2 Postural congenital
237.7# Von Recklinghausen's disease [737.42]
5th digit: 237.7
0. Unspecified
1. Type I
2. Type II

0 LOSS OF APPETITE SEE 'APPETITE'
729.89 LOSS OF FUNCTION MUSCULOSKELETAL NEC
781.91 LOSS OF HEIGHT
0 LOSS OF HEIGHT DUE TO OSTEOPOROSIS SEE 'OSTEOPOROSIS'
780.93 LOSS OF MEMORY
335.20 LOU GEHRIG'S DISEASE
334.8 LOUIS-BAR SYNDROME (ATAXIA-TELANGIECTASIA)
993.2 LOW ATMOSPHERIC PRESSURE SYNDROME
724.2 LOW BACK PAIN SYNDROME (NONVERTEBRAL) (NONDISCOGENIC)
306.0 LOW BACK PAIN SYNDROME PSYCHOGENIC
V21.3# LOW BIRTH WEIGHT STATUS
5th digit: V21.3
0. Unspecified
1. Less than 500 grams
2. 500-999 grams
3. 1000-1499 grams
4. 1500-1999 grams
5. 2000-2500 grams

596.52 LOW COMPLIANCE BLADDER
0 LOW COMPLIANCE BLADDER WITH INCONTINENCE SEE 'BLADDER DISORDERS WITH INCONTINENCE'
428.9 LOW OUTPUT SYNDROME (CARDIAC)
270.8 LOWE'S SYNDROME (OCULOCEREBRORENAL DYSTROPHY)
270.8 LOWE-TERREY-MCLACHLAN SYNDROME (OCULOCEREBRORENAL DYSTROPHY)

L

739.6	LOWER EXTREMITIES SEGMENTAL OR SOMATIC DYSFUNCTION
755.31	LOWER LIMB ABSENCE CONGENITAL
755.60	LOWER LIMB ANOMALY NOS CONGENITAL
767.4	LOWER RADICULAR SYNDROME, NEWBORN

LOWER URINARY TRACT SYMPTOMS (LUTS)

788.6#	Abnormalities other
	5th digit: 788.6
	2. Slowing of urinary stream
	3. Urgency
	4. Hesitancy
	5. Straining
788.4#	Frequency
	5th digit: 788.4
	1. Frequency
	3. Nocturia
788.3#	Incontinence
	5th digit: 788.3
	0. Unspecified
	1. Urge incontinence
	2. Stress, male
	3. Mixed urge and stress
	4. Without sensory awareness
	5. Post-void dribbling
	6. Nocturnal enuresis
	7. Continuous leakage
	8. Overflow incontinence
	9. Other
599.69	Obstruction
788.2#	Retention
	5th digit: 788.2
	0. Unspecified
	1. Incomplete bladder emptying

426.81	LOWN (-GANONG) - LEVINE SYNDROME (SHORT P-R INTERVAL, NORMAL QRS COMPLEX AND SUPRAVENTRICULAR TACHYCARDIA)
305.3#	LSD ABUSE (NONDEPENDENT)
304.5#	LSD ADDICTION (DEPENDENT)
	5th digit: 304.5, 305.3
	0. Unspecified
	1. Continuous
	2. Episodic
	3. In remission
466.0	LUCAS-CHAMPIONNIERE DISEASE (FIBRINOUS BRONCHITIS)
774.30	LUCEY-DRISCOLL SYNDROME (JAUNDICE DUE TO DELAYED CONJUGATION)
528.3	LUDORICI ANGINA
528.3	LUDWIG'S ANGINA
528.3	LUDWIG'S DISEASE (SUBMAXILLARY CELLULITIS)
0	LUETIC DISEASE SEE 'SYPHILIS'
276.51	LUETSCHER'S DEHYDRATION SYNDROME
724.2	LUMBAGO NONVERTEBRAL (NONDISCOGENIC)
724.2	LUMBALGIA

> ***When coding back disorders due to degeneration, displacement or HNP of the intervertebral disc, it is important to distinguish whether these conditions are with or without myelopathy. Myelopathy refers to functional disturbances and/or pathological changes in the spinal cord that result from compression.***

LUMBAR

756.13	Absence (congenital) (vertebra)
756.11	Absence (congenital) (vertebra) - isthmus
756.11	Absence (congenital) (vertebra) - pars articularis
721.3	Arthritis
722.93	Disc calcification or discitis
722.52	Disc disease/degeneration
722.73	Disc disease/degeneration - with myelopathy
722.93	Disc disorder
722.73	Disc disorder with myelopathy
722.10	Disc displacement
722.73	Disc displacement with myelopathy
722.10	Disc herniation
722.73	Disc herniation with myelopathy
722.73	Disc syndrome
553.8	Hernia
722.10	Nerve compression - discogenic
722.73	Nerve compression - discogenic with myelopathy
724.4	Nerve compression - root (by scar tissue) NEC
722.83	Nerve compression - root postoperative
721.3	Osteoarthritis
997.09	Puncture fluid leakage
349.0	Puncture reaction (headache)
724.4	Radiculitis (nonvertebral) (nondiscogenic)
959.19	Region injury
739.3	Region segmental or somatic dysfunction
953.2	Root injury (nerve)
847.2	Separation (rupture) (tear) (laceration)
724.02	Stenosis
847.2	Strain (sprain) (avulsion) (hemarthrosis)
721.3	Spondylarthritis
721.3	Spondylosis
721.42	Spondylosis with myelopathy (cord compression)
721.3	Spondylosis with osteoporosis **[733.0#]**
721.7	Spondylosis traumatic with osteoporosis **[733.0#]**
	5th digit: 733.0
	0. Unspecified
	1. Senile
	2. Idiopathic
	3. Disuse
	9. Drug induced
724.4	Vertebral syndrome

LUMBOSACRAL

724.6	Ankylosis (nonvertebral) (nondiscogenic)
724.6	Disorder (nonvertebral) (nondiscogenic)
0	Disorder discogenic see 'Intervertebral Disc'
724.6	Instability (nonvertebral) (nondiscogenic)
353.1	Plexus disorder (lesion) (nondiscogenic)

LUMBOSACRAL (continued)

953.5 Plexus injury (nerve)

250.6# Plexus disorder (lesion) (nondiscogenic with diabetes [353.1])

5th digit: 250.6

- **0. Type II, adult-onset, non-insulin dependent (even if requiring insulin), or unspecified; controlled**
- **1. Type I, juvenile-onset or insulin-dependent; controlled**
- **2. Type II, adult-onset, non-insulin dependent (even if requiring insulin); uncontrolled**
- **3. Type I, juvenile-onset or insulin-dependent; uncontrolled**

959.19 Region injury

739.3 Region segmental or somatic dysfunction

353.4 Root (nerve) disorder (lesion) NEC (nondiscogenic)

846.0 Separation (rupture) (tear) (laceration)

721.3 Spondylosis

721.42 Spondylosis with myelopathy (cord compression)

721.3 Spondylosis with osteoporosis **[733.0#]**

721.7 Spondylosis traumatic with osteoporosis **[733.0#]**

5th digit: 733.0

- **0. Unspecified**
- **1. Senile**
- **2. Idiopathic**
- **3. Disuse**
- **9. Drug induced**

846.0 Strain (sprain) (avulsion) (hemarthrosis)

724.6 Strain (sprain) chronic (nonvertebral) (nondiscogenic)

LUNG

V45.76 Absence acquired (any part)

748.5 Absence congenital (bilateral) (unilateral) (lobe)

748.5 Agenesis, hypoplasia or dysplasia congenital

748.60 Anomaly congenital

748.69 Anomaly congenital other

748.5 Atresia (congenital)

518.89 Atrophy (senile)

748.69 Atrophy congenital

748.69 Azygos lobe (fissure) congenital

503 Barium disease

492.0 Bleb

770.5 Bleb congenital

518.89 Calcification

515 Cirrhosis

518.0 Collapse, see also 'Atelectasis'

786.9 Congestion

460 Congestion due to common cold

514 Congestion due hypostatic pneumonia

861.21 Contusion

861.31 Contusion with open wound into cavity

908.0 Contusion late effect

518.89 Cystic acquired

748.4 Cystic congenital

518.89 Disease NEC

277.39 Disease in amyloidosis [517.8]

748.60 Disease congenital

748.4 Disease congenital cystic (polycystic)

518.89 Disease restrictive

508.0 Disorders due to radiation acute

508.1 Disorders due to radiation chronic

508.8 Disorders due to other external agents

508.9 Disorders due to unspecified external agents

V59.8 Donor non-autogenous

LUNG (continued)

748.5 Dysplasia congenital

518.4 Edema

515 Fibrosis (atrophic) (massive) (confluent) (peribronchial) (perialveolar)

121.2 Fluke (oriental)

518.89 Hernia

748.5 Hypoplasia congenital

515 Induration

415.19 Infarction

415.11 Infarction iatrogenic

415.11 Infarction postoperative

415.12 Infarction septic

038.#(#) Infarction septic with septicemia [415.12]

4th or 4th and 5th digit code for organism: 038

- **.9 NOS**
- **.3 Anaerobic**
- **.3 Bacteroides**
- **.3 Clostridium**
- **.42 E. coli**
- **.49 Enterobacter aerogenes**
- **.40 Gram negative**
- **.49 Gram negative other**
- **.41 Hemophilus influenzae**
- **.2 Pneumococcal**
- **.49 Proteus**
- **.43 Pseudomonas**
- **.44 Serratia**
- **.10 Staphylococcal NOS**
- **.11 Staphylococcal aureus**
- **.19 Staphylococcal other**
- **.0 Streptococcal (anaerobic)**
- **.49 Yersinia enterocolitica**
- **.8 Other specified**

518.3 Infiltrate

793.1 Infiltrate x-ray finding

861.20 Injury NOS

861.30 Injury NOS with open wound into thorax

908.0 Injury NOS late effect

518.7 Injury acute transfusion related (TRALI)

515 Interstitial lung disease chronic

277.39 Involvement amyloidosis [517.8]

135 Involvement sarcoid [517.8]

095.1 Involvement syphilitic

710.1 Involvement systemic sclerosis [517.2]

861.22 Laceration

861.32 Laceration with open wound into thorax

908.0 Laceration late effect

518.89 Lesion

793.1 Lesion coin

748.69 Lobe accessory congenital

518.0 Middle lobe syndrome

492.8 Nodule emphysematous

518.89 Nodule solitary

518.89 Obstruction or occlusion NOS

496 Obstruction airway chronic

0 Obstruction chronic see 'COPD'

0 Obstruction with asthma see 'Asthma'

491.2# Obstruction with bronchitis (chronic)

5th digit: 491.2

- **0. NOS**
- **1. With (acute) exacerbation**
- **2. With acute bronchitis**

492.8 Obstruction with emphysema

L

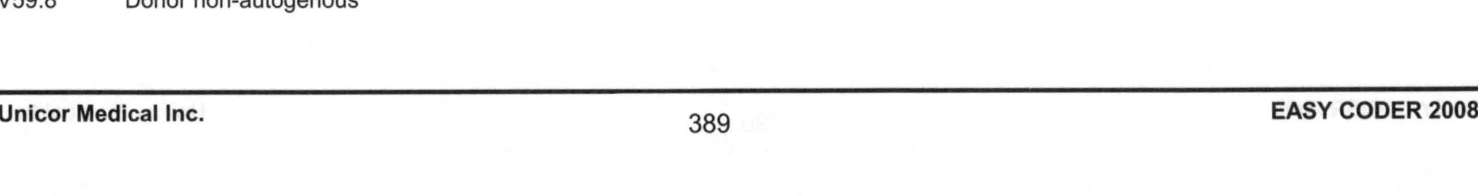

LUNG (continued)

518.89 Polycystic
493.2# Polycystic asthma
5th digit: 493.2
0. NOS
1. With status asthmaticus
2. With (acute) exacerbation

748.4 Polycystic congenital
518.89 Pseudocyst
513.0 Purulent (cavitary)
V45.89 Resection status
518.89 Restrictive (disease)
714.81 Rheumatoid
794.2 Scan abnormal
748.5 Sequestration congenital
793.1 Shadow (radiological finding)
V42.6 Transplant (status)
996.84 Transplant rejection (failure)
492.0 Vanishing

135 LUPOID OF BOECK (MILIARY)

LUPUS

710.0 NOS
289.81 Anticoagulant
695.4 Discoid (local)
695.4 Erythematosus
373.34 Erythematosus (discoid) (local) eyelid
710.0 Erythematosus disseminated
710.0 Erythematosus disseminated polyneuropathy [357.1]
710.0 Erythematosus endocarditis [424.91]
286.5 Erythematosus inhibitor
710.0 Erythematosus nephritis [583.81]
710.0 Erythematosus nephritis acute [580.81]
710.0 Erythematosus nephritis chronic [582.81]
710.0 Erythematosus nephrotic syndrome [581.81]
710.0 Erythematosus renal disease [583.81]
710.0 Erythematosus systemic
286.5 Erythematosus systemic [SLE] inhibitor increase
710.0 Erythematosus systemic with encephalitis [323.81]
017.0# Exedens tuberculous
017.0# Hilliard's tuberculous
017.0# Miliaris disseminatus faciei tuberculous
135 Pernio (besnier)
017.0# Vulgaris tuberculous
017.0# Vulgaris tuberculous eyelid dermatitis [373.4]
5th digit: 017.0
0. Unspecified
1. Lab not done
2. Lab pending
3. Microscopy positive (in sputum)
4. Culture positive - microscopy negative
5. Culture negative - microscopy positive
6. Culture and microscopy negative confirmed by other methods

620.1 LUTEIN CYST
253.4 LUTEINIZING HORMONE DEFICIENCY
253.1 LUTEINIZING HORMONE OVERPRODUCTION
745.5 LUTEMBACHER'S SYNDROME (ATRIAL SEPTAL DEFECT WITH MITRAL STENOSIS)
220 LUTEOMA SITE NOS
0 LUTEOMA SITE SPECIFIED SEE 'BENIGN NEOPLASM', BY SITE M8610/0

620.1 LUTEUM CORPUS RUPTURE (INFECTED) (OVARY)

LUTS (LOWER URINARY TRACT SYMPTOMS)

788.6# Abnormalities other
5th digit: 788.6
2. Slowing of urinary stream
3. Urgency
4. Hesitancy
5. Straining

788.4# Frequency
5th digit: 788.4
1. Frequency
3. Nocturia

788.3# Incontinence
5th digit: 788.3
0. Unspecified
1. Urge incontinence
2. Stress, male
3. Mixed urge and stress
4. Without sensory awareness
5. Post-void dribbling
6. Nocturnal enuresis
7. Continuous leakage
8. Overflow incontinence
9. Other

599.69 Obstruction
788.2# Retention
5th digit: 788.2
0. Unspecified
1. Incomplete bladder emptying

701.1 LUTZ MIESCHER DISEASE (ELASTOSIS PERFORANS SERPIGINOSA)
116.1 LUTZ- SPLENDORE-DE ALMEIDA DISEASE (BRAZILIAN BLASTOMYCOSIS)
360.81 LUXATION EYE (GLOBE)
429.3 LVH (LEFT VENTRICULAR HYPERTROPHY)
695.1 LYELL'S SYNDROME (TOXIC EPIDERMAL NECROLYSIS) DUE TO DRUG PROPERLY ADMINISTERED
977.9 LYELL'S SYNDROME (TOXIC EPIDERMAL NECROLYSIS) DUE TO OVERDOSE (WRONG DRUG GIVEN OR TAKEN)

LYME DISEASE

088.81 NOS
088.81 With arthritis [711.8#]
5th digit: 711.8
0. Site unspecified
1. Shoulder region
2. Upper arm
3. Forearm
4. Hand
5. Pelvic region and thigh
6. Lower leg
7. Ankle and foot
8. Other specified sites
9. Multiple sites

088.81 With meningioencephalitis [320.7]
088.81 With meningitis [320.7]
088.81 With myocarditis [422.0]

LYMPH, LYMPHATIC

> *648.9#: Use an additional code to identify lymphatic channel disorder.*

648.9# Channels disorder maternal current (co-existent) in pregnancy
5th digit: 648.9
0. Episode of NOS or N/A
1. Delivered
2. Delivered with postpartum complication
3. Antepartum complication
4. Postpartum complication

457.9 Channels disorder noninfectious
457.8 Channels noninfectious disorder other
457.1 Channels obstruction
277.39 Gland (system) degeneration lardaceous
289.9 Gland (system) disorder
306.8 Gland (system) disorder psychogenic
289.3 Node - calcification
785.6 Node - enlargement
457.8 Node - fistula
785.6 Node - hyperplasia
457.8 Node - infarction
228.1 Node - lymphangioma
457.8 Node - rupture
457.1 Obstruction
457.1 Occlusion
289.9 System (gland) disorder
306.8 System (gland) disorder psychogenic
457.9 Vessel - disorder noninfectious
457.8 Vessel - disorder noninfectious other specified
457.8 Vessel - fistula
457.8 Vessel - infarction
457.1 Vessel - obstruction
457.8 Vessel - rupture

LYMPHADENITIS

289.3 Unspecified
683 Acute
289.2 Acute mesenteric
616.89 Bartholin's gland
675.2# Breast maternal due to pregnancy
5th digit: 675.2
0. Episode of NOS or N/A
1. Delivered
2. Delivered with postpartum complication
3. Antepartum complication
4. Postpartum complication

289.3 Cervical
099.0 Chancroidal
289.1 Chronic
289.2 Chronic mesenteric
695.89 Dermatopathic
500 Due to anthracosis (occupational)
125.1 Due to brugia (Wuchereria) malayi
032.89 Due to diphtheria (toxin)
099.1 Due to lymphogranuloma venereum
125.0 Due to Wuchereria Bancrofti
289.3 Generalized
098.89 Gonorrheal
289.1 Granulomatous
683 Infectional (purulent) (pyogenic) (streptococcal)

LYMPHADENITIS (continued)

289.2 Mesenteric acute, chronic or subacute
002.0 Mesenteric due bacillus typhi
027.2 Mesenteric due pasteurella multocida
078.3 Regional
683 Septic
289.1 Subacute
289.2 Subacute mesenteric
683 Suppurative
091.4 Syphilitic (early) (secondary)
095.8 Syphilitic late
0 TB see 'Tuberculosis', lymph nodes
099.1 Venereal

LYMPHADENOPATHY

785.6 NOS
0 -Associated virus (LAV) see 'HIV' infection
785.6 Unknown etiology

LYMPHANGIECTASIS

457.1 NOS
372.89 Conjunctiva
457.1 Postinfectional
457.1 Scrotum

LYMPHANGIOMA

228.1 NOS M9170/0
228.1 Any site
228.1 Capillary any site M9171/0
228.1 Cavernous nevus any site M9172/0
228.1 Congenital any site M9170/0
228.1 Cystic any site M9173/0

228.1 LYMPHANGIOMYOMA M9174/0
238.1 LYMPHANGIOMYOMATOSIS SITE NOS
0 LYMPHANGIOMYOMATOSIS SITE SPECIFIED SEE 'NEOPLASM UNCERTAIN BEHAVIOR' BY SITE M9174/1

171.# LYMPHANGIOSARCOMA M9170/3
4th digit: 171
0. Head, face, neck
2. Upper limb including shoulder
3. Lower limb including hip
4. Thorax
5. Abdomen (wall), gastric, gastrointestinal, intestine, stomach
6. Pelvis, buttock, groin, inguinal region, perineum
7. Trunk NOS, back NOS, flank NOS
8. Other specified sites
9. Site NOS

LYMPHANGITIS

457.2 NOS
682.9 Acute
0 Acute see 'Cellulitis'
682.3 Acute arm and forearm, maxilla, shoulder
682.5 Acute buttock (gluteal)
682.0 Acute face, nose, submandibular
682.7 Acute foot (except toes)
682.4 Acute hand (except fingers)
682.8 Acute head and scalp
682.1 Acute neck
682.9 Acute site unspecified
682.6 Acute thigh (leg), ankle
682.2 Acute trunk and groin

L

LYMPHANGITIS (continued)

675.2# Breast due to pregnancy
5th digit: 675.2
0. Episode of care unspecified or N/A
1. Delivered
2. Delivered with postpartum complication
3. Antepartum complication
4. Postpartum complication

457.2 Chronic (subacute)
125.1 Due to Brugia (Wuchereria) malayi
125.0 Due to Wuchereria Bancrofti
682.2 Groin

648.9#: Use an additional code to identify lymphangitis.

648.9# Maternal current (co-existent) in pregnancy
5th digit: 648.9
0. Episode of NOS or N/A
1. Delivered
2. Delivered with postpartum complication
3. Antepartum complication
4. Postpartum complication

0 LYMPHATIC SEE 'LYMPH, LYMPHATIC'

LYMPHEDEMA

457.1 Acquired (praecox) (secondary) (obliterans) NOS

648.9#: Use an additional code to identify lymphedema acquired.

648.9# Acquired (praecox) (secondary) (obliterans) maternal current (co-existent) in pregnancy
5th digit: 648.9
0. Episode of NOS or N/A
1. Delivered
2. Delivered with postpartum complication
3. Antepartum complication
4. Postpartum complication

997.99 Acquired (praecox) (secondary) (obliterans) surgical NEC
757.0 Congenital
457.0 Postmastectomy syndrome

200.1# LYMPHOBLASTOMA M9630/3
5th digit: 200.1
0. Unspecified site, extranodal and solid organ sites
1. Lymph nodes of head, face, neck
2. Lymph nodes intrathoracic
3. Lymph nodes abdominal
4. Lymph nodes axilla and upper limb
5. Lymph nodes inguinal region and lower limb
6. Lymph nodes intrapelvic
7. Spleen
8. Lymph nodes multiple sites

457.8 LYMPHOCELE
V59.8 LYMPHOCYTE DONOR NON-AUTOGENOUS
288.51 LYMPHOCYTES DECREASED
288.61 LYMPHOCYTES ELEVATED
288.51 LYMPHOCYTHEMIA
049.0 LYMPHOCYTIC CHORIOMENINGITIS

201.4# LYMPHOCYTIC HISTIOCYTIC PREDOMINANCE HODGKINS M9651/3

200.1# LYMPHOCYTOMA
5th digit: 200.1, 201.4
0. Unspecified site, extranodal and solid organ sites
1. Lymph nodes of head, face, neck
2. Lymph nodes intrathoracic
3. Lymph nodes abdominal
4. Lymph nodes axilla and upper limb
5. Lymph nodes inguinal region and lower limb
6. Lymph nodes intrapelvic
7. Spleen
8. Lymph nodes multiple sites

288.51 LYMPHOCYTOPENIA
288.61 LYMPHOCYTOSIS (SYMPTOMATIC)
199.1 LYMPHOEPITHELIAL CARCINOMA SITE NOS
0 LYMPHOEPITHELIAL CARCINOMA SITE SPECIFIED SEE 'CANCER', BY SITE M8082/3
099.1 LYMPHOGRANULOMA INGUINALE

201.9# LYMPHOGRANULOMA MALIGNANT M9650/3
5th digit: 201.9
0. Unspecified site, extranodal and solid organ sites
1. Lymph nodes of head, face, neck
2. Lymph nodes intrathoracic
3. Lymph nodes abdominal
4. Lymph nodes axilla and upper limb
5. Lymph nodes inguinal region and lower limb
6. Lymph nodes intrapelvic
7. Spleen
8. Lymph nodes multiple sites

099.1 LYMPHOGRANULOMA VENEREUM

647.2# LYMPHOGRANULOMA VENEREUM MATERNAL CURRENT (CO-EXISTENT) IN PREGNANCY [099.1]
5th digit: 647.2
0. Episode of care unspecified or N/A
1. Delivered
2. Delivered with postpartum complication
3. Antepartum complication
4. Postpartum complication

655.4# LYMPHOGRANULOMA VENEREUM MATERNAL WITH KNOWN/SUSPECTED FETAL DAMAGE
5th digit: 655.4
0. Episode of care unspecified or N/A
1. Delivered
3. Antepartum complication

135 LYMPHOGRANULOMATOSIS BENIGN (SCHAUMANN'S) M9650/3

201.9# LYMPHOGRANULOMATOSIS MALIGNANT M9650/3
5th digit: 201.9
0. Unspecified site, extranodal and solid organ sites
1. Lymph nodes of head, face, neck
2. Lymph nodes intrathoracic
3. Lymph nodes abdominal
4. Lymph nodes axilla and upper limb
5. Lymph nodes inguinal region and lower limb
6. Lymph nodes intrapelvic
7. Spleen
8. Lymph nodes multiple sites

288.4 LYMPHOHISTIOCYTOSIS, FAMILIAL HEMOPHAGOCYTIC

V10.61 LYMPHOID LEUKEMIA HISTORY

LYMPHOMA

202.8# NOS (malignant) M9590/3
200.6# Anaplastic large cell
0 Benign see 'Benign Neoplasm', by site M9590/0
200.2# Burkitt's lymphoma M9750/3
202.0# Centroblastic type follicular malignant M9697/3
202.8# Centroblastic type malignant M9632/3
202.8# Centroblastic-centrocytic diffuse malignant M9614/3
202.8# Centrocytic malignant M9622/3
202.8# Convoluted cell type malignant M9602/3
202.8# Diffuse NEC (large B cell) M9590/3
202.0# Follicular (giant) M9690/3
202.0# Follicular center cell cleaved M9695/3
202.8# Follicular center cell cleaved malignant M9623/3
202.0# Follicular center cell noncleaved M9698/3
202.8# Follicular center cell noncleaved malignant M9633/3
202.8# Follicular center cell malignant M9615/3
202.0# Follicular centroblastic-centrocytic malignant M9692/3
202.0# Follicular lymphocytic intermediate differentiation M9694/3
200.0# Histiocytic (diffuse) M9640/3
200.0# Histiocytic (diffuse) nodular M9642/3
200.0# Histiocytic (diffuse) pleomorphic cell type M9641/3
200.8# Immunoblastic type malignant M9612/3
200.7# Large cell M9640/3
200.6# Large cell anaplastic
200.1# Lymphoblastic (diffuse) M9630/3
200.1# Lymphocytic intermediate M9621/3
202.0# Lymphocytic intermediate differentiation nodular malignant M9694/3
202.0# Lymphocytic, nodular M9690/3
202.0# Lymphocytic poorly differentiated M9696/3
202.0# Lymphocytic poorly differentiated nodular malignant M9696/3
200.1# Lymphocytic poorly differentiated malignant M9630/3
200.1# Lymphocytic well differentiated malignant M9620/3
202.0# Lymphocytic well differentiated nodular malignant M9693/3
202.8# Lymphocytic-histiocytic mixed malignant M9613/3
200.8# Lymphoplasmacytoid type malignant M9611/3
200.1# Lymphosarcoma type M9610/3
202.8# Malignant NOS M9590/3
200.4# Mantle cell
200.3# Marginal zone (extranodal, nodal, and splenic B-cell)
200.8# Mixed lymphocytic-histiocytic (diffuse) M9613/3
202.0# Mixed lymphocytic-histiocytic nodular malignant M9691/3
200.3# Mucosa associated lymphoid tissue (MALT)
202.0# Nodular malignant M9690/3

5th digit: 200.0-8, 202.0, 8
0. Unspecified site, extranodal and solid organ sites
1. Lymph nodes of head, face, neck
2. Lymph nodes intrathoracic
3. Lymph nodes abdominal
4. Lymph nodes axilla and upper limb
5. Lymph nodes inguinal region and lower limb
6. Lymph nodes intrapelvic
7. Spleen
8. Lymph nodes multiple sites

LYMPHOMA (continued)

202.8# Non Hodgkin's type malignant M9591/3
202.7# Peripheral T cell
200.5# Primary central nervous system
200.0# Reticulum cell type M9640/3
202.8# Stem cell type malignant M9601/3
202.1# T cell
202.7# T-cell peripheral
202.8# Undifferentiated cell type malignant M9600/3

5th digit: 200.5, 202.1, 7, 8
0. Unspecified site, extranodal and solid organ sites
1. Lymph nodes of head, face, neck
2. Lymph nodes intrathoracic
3. Lymph nodes abdominal
4. Lymph nodes axilla and upper limb
5. Lymph nodes inguinal region and lower limb
6. Lymph nodes intrapelvic
7. Spleen
8. Lymph nodes multiple sites

229.9 LYMPHOMATOUS TUMOR BENIGN SITE NOS
0 LYMPHOMATOUS TUMOR BENIGN SITE SPECIFIED SEE 'BENIGN NEOPLASM', BY SITE M9590/0
288.51 LYMPHOPENIA

LYMPHOPROLIFERATIVE

238.79 Disease (chronic) NOS
0 Disease chronic site specified see 'Neoplasm Uncertain Behavior', by site M9970/1

078.3 LYMPHORETICULOSIS BENIGN (OF INOCULATION)

LYMPHOSARCOMA

200.1# Lymphosarcoma M9610/3
200.2# Burkitt's tumor lymphoma M9750/3
200.1# Diffuse NOS M9610/3
202.0# Follicular (giant) M9690/3
V10.71 History
200.1# Lymphoblastic (diffuse) M9630/3
200.1# Lymphocytic (diffuse) M9610/3
200.8# Mixed (diffuse) M9613/3
202.0# Nodular M9690/3
200.1# Prolymphocytic M9631/3

5th digit: 200.1, 2, 8, 202.0
0. Unspecified site, extranodal and solid organ sites
1. Lymph nodes of head, face, neck
2. Lymph nodes intrathoracic
3. Lymph nodes abdominal
4. Lymph nodes axilla and upper limb
5. Lymph nodes inguinal region and lower limb
6. Lymph nodes intrapelvic
7. Spleen
8. Lymph nodes multiple sites

270.7 LYSINE METABOLISM DISTURBANCES
071 LYSSA

L

031.2 MAC BACTEREMIA (MYCOBACTERIUM AVIUM-INTRACELLULARE COMPLEX)
334.8 MACHADO-JOSEPH DISEASE
V46.9 MACHINE DEPENDENCE

MACLEOD'S SYNDROME

492.8 NOS
491.2# With bronchitis (chronic)
5th digit: 491.2
0. NOS
1. With (acute) exacerbation
2. With acute bronchitis

756.0 MACROCEPHALY
744.81 MACROCHEILIA CONGENITAL
751.3 MACROCOLON CONGENITAL
289.89 MACROCYTOSIS (MACROCYTHEMIA)
755.57 MACRODACTYLIA FINGERS
755.65 MACRODACTYLIA TOES
520.2 MACRODONTIA
742.4 MACROENCEPHALY CONGENITAL
524.05 MACROGENIA
259.8 MACROGENITOSOMIA PRAECOX (SYNDROME)
255.2 MACROGENITOSOMIA PRAECOX MALE
273.3 MACROGLOBULINEMIA (SYNDROME)
750.15 MACROGLOSSIA CONGENITAL

MACROGNATHIA

524.00 Unspecified
524.02 Mandibular
524.72 Mandibular alveolar
524.01 Maxillary
524.71 Maxillary alveolar

742.4 MACROGYRIA CONGENITAL
V09.2 MACROLIDES RESISTANT INFECTION (SEE 'DRUG RESISTANCE')
288.4 MACROPHAGE ACTIVATION SYNDROME
368.14 MACROPSIA
744.83 MACROSTOMIA CONGENITAL
744.22 MACROTIA CONGENITAL

MACULAR

743.55 Changes congenital
362.83 Edema
362.53 Edema cystoid
250.5# Edema diabetic with retinopathy [**362.0#**] [362.07]
5th digit: 250.5
0. Type II, adult-onset, non-insulin dependent (even if requiring insulin), or unspecified; controlled
1. Type I, juvenile-onset or insulin-dependent; controlled
2. Type II, adult-onset, non-insulin dependent (even if requiring insulin); uncontrolled
3. Type I, Juvenile-onset or insulin-dependent; uncontrolled

4th digit: 362.0
1. Background or NOS
2. Proliferative
3. Nonproliferative NOS
4. Nonproliferative mild
5. Nonproliferative moderate
6. Nonproliferative severe

MACULAR (continued)

362.56 Puckering
363.32 Scar (other)
V80.2 Senile lesions (screening for)
362.55 Toxic maculopathy

MACULAR DEGENERATION

362.50 Unspecified
362.75 Congenital
362.54 Cyst
362.53 Cystoid
362.52 Exudative (senile)
362.54 Hole (pseudohole)
362.75 Juvenile
362.54 Pseudohole
362.50 Senile
362.51 Senile atrophic dry
362.52 Senile disciform wet
362.52 Senile exudative
362.51 Senile nonexudative
362.55 Toxic

362.55 MACULOPATHY TOXIC
374.55 MADAROSIS EYELID
755.54 MADELUNG'S DEFORMITY
272.8 MADELUNG'S DISEASE (LIPOMATOSIS)

MADURA

117.4 Foot
039.4 Foot actinomycotic

117.4 MADURELLA GRISEA INFECTION
117.4 MADURELLA MYCETOMII INFECTION
039.9 MADUROMYCOSIS NOS (SEE ALSO 'ACTINOMYCOSIS')
117.4 MADUROMYCOSIS MYCOTIC INFECTION
756.4 MAFFUCCI'S SYNDROME (DYSCHONDROPLASIA WITH HEMANGIOMAS)
306.4 MAGENBLASE SYNDROME
134.0 MAGGOT INFECTION ORBIT (EYE) [376.13]
134.0 MAGGOT INFESTATION
526.4 MAGITOT'S DISEASE
790.6 MAGNESIUM ABNORMAL BLOOD LEVEL
781.7 MAGNESIUM DEFICIENCY SYNDROME
275.2 MAGNESIUM METABOLISM DISORDER
031.0 MAI (MYCOBACTERIUM AVIUM INTRACELLULARE)
709.1 MAJOCCHI'S DISEASE (PURPURA ANNULARIS TELANGIECTODES)
110.6 MAJOCCHI'S GRANULOMA
780.4 MAL DE DEBARQUEMENT SYNDROME
707.15 MAL PERFORANT

MALABSORPTION

579.8 Calcium
579.8 Carbohydrate
579.8 Drug induced
579.8 Due to bacterial overgrowth
579.8 Fat
579.9 Intestinal
271.3 Lactose
579.3 Postsurgical syndrome
579.8 Protein

M

MALABSORPTION (continued)

331.3 Spinal fluid syndrome
331.3 Spinal fluid syndrome with dementia [294.1#]
5th digit: 294.1
0. Without behavioral disturbance or NOS
1. With behavioral disturbance
579.9 Syndrome

MALACOPLAKIA

596.8 Bladder
0 Bladder with incontinence see 'Bladder Disorders With Incontinence'
569.89 Colon
593.89 Pelvis (kidney)
593.89 Ureter
599.84 Urethra

V62.4 MALADJUSTMENT SOCIAL (REASON FOR ENCOUNTER)
780.79 MALAISE

MALARIA

084.6 NOS
084.9 Algid
084.9 Cardiac
V02.9 Carrier (suspected)
084.9 Cerebral
771.2 Congenital or perinatal
084.0 Falciparum [malignant tertian]
084.6 Fever NOS
084.5 Fever by more than one parasite
084.0 Fever by plasmodium falciparum
084.2 Fever by plasmodium malariae
084.3 Fever by plasmodium ovale
084.1 Fever by plasmodium vivax
084.8 Hemoglobinuric
084.9 Hepatitis [573.2]
V12.03 History
084.7 Induced (therapeutically)
084.2 Malariae
655.4# Maternal with known/suspected damage to fetus
5th digit: 655.4
0. Episode of care unspecified or N/A
1. Delivered
3. Antepartum complication

647.4#: Use an additional code to identify the maternal malaria.

647.4# Maternal current (co-existent) in pregnancy
5th digit: 647.4
0. Episode of care unspecified or N/A
1. Delivered
2. Delivered with postpartum complication
3. Antepartum complication
4. Postpartum complication

084.5 Mixed
084.4 Monkey
084.9 Nephrotic syndrome [581.81]
084.3 Ovale
084.2 Quartan
V75.1 Screening
084.0 Subtertian
084.1 Vivax (benign tertian)

608.89 MALASSEZ'S DISEASE (CYSTIC)
111.0 MALASSEZIA (PITYROSPORUM) FURFUR INFECTION
607.84 MALE ERECTILE DISORDER ORGANIC
302.72 MALE ERECTILE DISORDER PSYCHOSEXUAL
608.9 MALE GENITAL ORGAN DISORDER
919.8 MALIBU DISEASE
919.9 MALIBU DISEASE INFECTED
259.2 MALIGNANT CARCINOID SYNDROME
0 MALIGNANT NEOPLASM SEE 'CANCER', BY SITE
199.0 MALIGNANT NEOPLASM UNSPECIFIED SITE
0 MALIGNANT SEE SPECIFIED CONDITION
V65.2 MALINGERER
024 MALLEOMYCES MALLEI INFECTION
025 MALLEOMYCES PSEUDOMALLEI
736.1 MALLET FINGER
024 MALLEUS
385.21 MALLEUS IMPAIRED MOBILITY
530.7 MALLORY WEISS SYNDROME

MALNUTRITION

263.9 NOS (calorie)
263.9 Calorie
261 Calorie deficiency severe
269.9 Deficiency unspecified
995.84 Due to neglect - adult
995.52 Due to neglect - child
269.9 Due to nutritional deficiency
263.9 Dystrophy
579.3 Following GI surgery
263.2 Physical retardation
263.9 Protein-calorie
263.1 Protein-calorie mild
263.0 Protein-calorie moderate
263.8 Protein calorie weight for age
263.8 Protein-calorie other
262 Protein-calorie other severe
V77.2 Screening
263.9 Weight for age

MALNUTRITION FETAL

764.20 Weight unspecified
764.21 <500 grams
764.22 500-749 grams
764.23 750-999 grams
764.24 1000-1249 grams
764.25 1250-1499 grams
764.26 1500-1749 grams
764.27 1750-1999 grams
764.28 2000-2499 grams
764.29 2500 grams

MALNUTRITION FETAL - LIGHT FOR DATES

764.10 Weight unspecified
764.11 < 500 grams
764.12 500 - 749 grams
764.13 750 - 999 grams
764.14 1000 - 1249 grams
764.15 1250 - 1499 grams
764.16 1500 - 1749 grams
764.17 1750 - 1999 grams
764.18 2000-2499 grams
764.19 2500 grams and over

MALOCCLUSION

524.4 NOS (top and bottom teeth)
524.59 Abnormal swallowing
524.31 Accessory teeth (causing crowding)
524.2# Dental arch anomaly (angle's)
5th digit: 524.2
1. Class I
2. Class II
3. Class III

524.89 Dentofacial abnormality
520.6 Impacted teeth
524.30 Missing teeth
524.59 Mouth breathing
524.59 Sleep postures
524.31 Supernumerary teeth (causing crowding)
524.59 Thumb sucking
524.69 Temporomandibular
524.59 Tongue, lip or finger habits

MALOCCLUSION DUE TO JAW ANOMALIES

524.7# Dentoalveolar
5th digit: 524.7
0. Unspecified (mandible) (maxilla)
1. Maxillary hyperplasia
2. Mandibular hyperplasia
3. Maxillary hypoplasia
4. Mandibular hypoplasia
5. Vertical displacement
6. Occlusal plane deviation
9. Other specified

524.1# Jaw relationship to cranial base
5th digit: 524.1
0. Unspecified anomaly
1. Maxillary asymmetry
2. Other jaw asymmetry
9. Other specified anomaly

524.0# Jaw size
5th digit: 524.0
0. Unspecified anomaly
1. Maxillary hyperplasia
2. Mandibular hyperplasia
3. Maxillary hypoplasia
4. Mandibular hypoplasia
5. Macrogenia
6. Microgenia
7. Excessive tuberosity
9. Other specified anomaly

MALPOSITION/MALPRESENTATION

652.9# NOS
660.0# NOS obstructing labor **[652.9#]**
761.7 Affecting fetus or newborn before labor
763.1 Affecting fetus or newborn during labor
652.4# Brow presentation
652.2# Buttocks presentation
660.0# Buttocks presentation obstructing labor **[652.2#]**
652.4# Chin presentation
660.0# Chin presentation obstructing labor **[652.4#]**
652.2# Complete breech presentation
660.0# Complete breech presentation obstructing labor **[652.2#]**
652.8# Compound presentation
660.0# Compound presentation obstructing labor **[652.8#]**
5th digit: 652.2, 4, 8, 9, 660.0
0. Episode of care unspecified or N/A
1. Delivered
3. Antepartum complication

MALPOSITION/MALPRESENTATION (continued)

652.4# Extended head presentation
660.0# Extended head presentation obstructing labor **[652.4#]**
652.4# Face presentation
660.0# Face presentation obstructing labor **[652.4#]**
652.8# Face to pubes presentation
660.0# Face to pubes presentation obstructing labor **[652.8#]**
652.8# Footling presentation
660.0# Footling presentation obstructing labor **[652.8#]**
652.2# Frank breech presentation
660.0# Frank breech presentation obstructing labor **[652.2#]**
652.5# High head at term
652.8# Incomplete breech presentation
660.0# Incomplete breech presentation obstructing labor **[652.8#]**
652.9# Malposition of fetus at onset complicating pregnancy
660.0# Malposition of fetus at onset obstructing labor **[652.9#]**
652.7# Prolapsed arm
660.0# Prolapsed arm obstructing labor **[652.7#]**
0 See also 'Pregnancy Complications, Delivery Problems: Malpresentation/Malposition'
652.3# Transverse lie (oblique lie)
660.0# Transverse lie (oblique lie) obstructing labor **[652.3#]**
652.0# Unstable lie
660.0# Unstable lie obstructing labor **[652.0#]**
652.6# With multiple gestation
660.0# With multiple gestation obstructing labor **[652.6#]**
652.1# With version
660.0# With version obstructing labor **[652.1#]**
652.8# Other specified
660.0# Other specified obstructing labor **[652.8#]**
5th digit: 652.0-9, 660.0
0. Episode of care unspecified or N/A
1. Delivered
3. Antepartum complication

200.3# MALT (MUCOSA ASSOCIATED LYMPHOID TISSUE)
5th digit: 200.3
0. Unspecified site, extranodal and solid organ sites
1. Lymph nodes of head, face, neck
2. Lymph nodes intrathoracic
3. Lymph nodes abdominal
4. Lymph nodes axilla and upper limb
5. Lymph nodes inguinal region and lower limb
6. Lymph nodes intrapelvic
7. Spleen
8. Lymph nodes multiple sites

495.4 MALT WORKERS' LUNG
0 MALTA FEVER SEE 'BRUCELLA'

> ***733.81 Fracture malunion-means that healing has occurred but that the bone(s) or fracture fragments are in poor alignment.***

733.81 MALUNION FRACTURE

MAMMARY

901.82 Artery internal injury
908.4 Artery internal injury late effect
901.82 Artery internal laceration traumatic (rupture) (hematoma) (avulsion) (aneurysm)
908.4 Artery internal laceration late effect
610.4 Duct ectasia
611.8 Duct occlusion

M

MAMMARY (continued)

610.9 Dysplasia benign
611.1 Gland hypertrophy (enlargement)
901.82 Vein internal injury
908.4 Vein internal injury late effect
901.82 Vein internal laceration traumatic (rupture) (hematoma) (avulsion) (aneurysm)
908.4 Vein internal laceration late effect

MAMMOGRAM

793.8# Abnormal finding
5th digit: 793.8
0. Unspecified
1. Mammographic microcalcification
9. Other abnormal findings (calcification) (calculus)

V71.1 Evaluation suspected malignant neoplasm, none found
V72.5 Routine exam
V76.11 Screening breast cancer for high risk patient
V76.12 Screening breast cancer other

MANDIBLE, MANDIBULAR

526.4 Abscess (osteitis) (periostitis) acute suppurative
524.09 Absence (congenital)
524.72 Alveolar hyperplasia
524.74 Alveolar hypoplasia
526.89 Condylar unilateral hyperplasia
524.53 Deviation opening and closing
526.89 Disease (other specified)
524.02 Hyperplasia
524.04 Hypoplasia
524.52 Limited range of motion
526.4 Necrosis
524.29 Teeth posterior lingual occlusion

756.0 MANDIBULOFACIAL DYSOSTOSIS SYNDROME

MANIC DEPRESSIVE PSYCHOSIS BIPOLAR

296.7 Circular (alternating) - current or most recent episode NOS
296.5# Circular (alternating) - current or most recent episode depressed
296.4# Circular (alternating) - current or most recent episode manic
296.6# Circular (alternating) - current or most recent episode mixed
296.7 Type I - current or most recent episode NOS
296.5# Type I - current or most recent episode depressed
296.4# Type I - current or most recent episode manic
296.6# Type I - current or most recent episode mixed
296.0# Type I - single manic episode
5th digit: 296.0, 4-6
0. Unspecified
1. Mild
2. Moderate
3. Severe without mention of psychotic behavior
4. Severe specified as with psychotic behavior
5. In partial or unspecified remission
6. In full remission

296.89 Type II
296.8# Other and unspecified
5th digit: 296.8
0. Unspecified
1. Atypical manic
2. Atypical depressive
9. Other (mixed)

MANIC DEPRESSIVE PSYCHOSIS MONOPOLAR

296.0# Hypomanic single episode or unspecified
296.1# Hypomanic recurrent
296.0# Manic single episode or unspecified
296.1# Manic recurrent
296.2# Depressed single episode or unspecified
296.3# Depressed recurrent
5th digit: 296.0-3
0. Unspecified
1. Mild
2. Moderate
3. Severe without mention of psychotic behavior
4. Severe specified as with psychotic behavior
5. In partial or unspecified remission
6. In full remission

731.2 MANKOWSKY'S FAMILIAL DYSPLASTIC OSTEOPATHY (SYNDROME)
271.8 MANNOSIDOSIS CARBOHYDRATE TRANSPORT DISORDERS
125.5 MANSONELLA OZZARDI INFECTION
120.1 MANSON'S DISEASE (SCHISTOSOMA)
V74.1 MANTOUX TEST (TB)
795.5 MANTOUX TEST ABNORMAL
495.6 MAPLE BARK STRIPPERS' LUNG
270.3 MAPLE SYRUP (URINE) DISEASE OR SYNDROME
447.4 MARABLE'S SYNDROME (CELIAC ARTERY COMPRESSION)
261 MARASMUS
078.89 MARBURG DISEASE
759.89 MARCHESANI WEILL BRADYMORPHISM ECTOPIA LENTIS (SYNDROME)
341.8 MARCHIAFAVA BIGNAMI DISEASE OR SYNDROME
283.2 MARCHIAFAVA-MICHELI SYNDROME (PAROXYSMAL NOCTURNAL HEMOGLOBINURIA)
742.8 MARCUS GUNN'S SYNDROME (JAW-WINKING SYNDROME)
759.82 MARFAN'S SYNDROME (ARACHNODACTYLY)
090.49 MARFAN'S SYNDROME, CONGENITAL SYPHILIS
090.49 MARFAN'S SYNDROME, CONGENITAL SYPHILIS WITH LUXATION OF LENS [379.32]
731.2 MARIE-BAMBERGER DISEASE (HYPERTROPHIC PULMONARY OSTEOARTHROPATHY)
757.39 MARIE-BAMBERGER DISEASE PRIMARY (ACROPACHYDERMA)
720.0 MARIE STRUMPELL SPONDYLITIS
334.2 MARIE'S CEREBELLAR ATAXIA
253.0 MARIE'S SYNDROME (ACROMEGALY)
757.39 MARIE'S SYNDROME PRIMARY OR IDIOPATHIC (ACROPACHYDERMA)
731.2 MARIE'S SYNDROME SECONDARY (HYPERTROPHIC PULMONARY OSTEOARTHROPATHY)

305.2# MARIJUANA ABUSE (NONDEPENDENT)
304.3# MARIJUANA ADDICTION (DEPENDENT)

5th digit: 304.3, 305.2
0. Unspecified
1. Continuous
2. Episodic
3. In remission

379.46 MARKUS-ADIE SYNDROME
596 MARION'S DISEASE (BLADDER NECK OBSTRUCTION)
0 MARION'S DISEASE (BLADDER NECK OBSTRUCTION)
V61.10 MARITAL PROBLEMS
277.5 MAROTEAUX LAMY SYNDROME (MUCOPOLYSACCHARIDOSIS VI)
277.5 MARQUIO BRAILSFORD DISEASE
082.1 MARSEILLES FEVER
242.0# MARSH'S DISEASE (EXOPHTHALMIC GOITER)

5th digit: 242.0
0. Without mention of thyrotoxic crisis or storm
1. With mention of thyrotoxic crisis or storm

715.27 MARTIN'S DISEASE SYNDROME (OSTEOARTHRITIS)
275.49 MARTIN-ALBRIGHT SYNDROME (PSEUDOHYPOPARATHYROIDISM)
446.7 MARTORELL-FABRE SYNDROME (PULSELESS DISEASE)
302.83 MASOCHISM SEXUAL
301.89 MASOCHISTIC PERSONALITY DISORDER

To code a mass of a site not listed below, see disorder or disease by anatomical site.

MASS

789.3# Abdomen

5th digit: 789.3
0. Unspecified site
1. Upper right quadrant
2. Upper left quadrant
3. Lower right quadrant
4. Lower left quadrant
5. Periumbilic
6. Epigastric
7. Generalized
9. Other specified site (multiple)

787.99 Anal
733.90 Bone
348.8 Brain
611.72 Breast
784.2 Cheek
786.6 Chest
569.89 Colon
0 Cystic see 'Cyst'
388.8 Ear
789.36 Epigastric
379.92 Eye

MASS (continued)

625.8 Genital organs female
784.2 Gum
784.2 Head
784.2 Intracranial
719.6# Joint

5th digit: 719.6
0. Site NOS
1. Shoulder region
2. Upper arm (elbow) (humerus)
3. Forearm (radius) (wrist) (ulna)
4. Hand (carpal) (metacarpal) (fingers)
5. Pelvic region and thigh (hip) (buttock) (femur)
6. Lower leg (fibula) (knee) (patella) (tibia)
7. Ankle and/or foot (metatarsals) (toes) (tarsals)
8. Other
9. Multiple

593.9 Kidney
786.6 Lung
785.6 Lymph node
786.6 Mediastinum
784.2 Mouth
729.89 Muscle (limb)
784.2 Nasal sinus
784.2 Neck
784.2 Nose
784.2 Palate
789.39 Pelvic
607.89 Penis
625.8 Perineum
789.35 Periumbilic
787.99 Rectal
593.9 Renal
789.39 Retroperitoneal
608.89 Scrotum
782.2 Skin
729.9 Soft tissue
789.2 Spleen
782.2 Subcutaneous
786.6 Substernal
240.9 Substernal thyroid
782.2 Superficial localized
608.89 Testes
784.2 Throat
784.2 Tongue
789.35 Umbilicus
625.8 Uterus
625.8 Vagina
625.8 Vulva

For codes 770.12, 770.18, use an additional code to identify any secondary pulmonary hypertension (416.8), if applicable.

770.12 MASSIVE ASPIRATION MECONIUM OF NEWBORN SYNDROME
770.18 MASSIVE ASPIRATION OF NEWBORN SYNDROME

M

MAST CELL

757.33 Disease congenital
202.6# Sarcoma M9740/3
202.6# Systemic tissue mast cell disease M9741/3
202.6# Tumor malignant M9740/3
5th digit: 202.6
0. Unspecified site, extranodal and solid organ sites
1. Lymph nodes of head, face, neck
2. Lymph nodes intrathoracic
3. Lymph nodes abdominal
4. Lymph nodes axilla and upper limb
5. Lymph nodes inguinal region and lower limb
6. Lymph nodes intrapelvic
7. Spleen
8. Lymph nodes multiple sites

238.5 Tumor uncertain behavior site NOS M9740/1

620.6 MASTERS ALLEN SYNDROME

V41.6 MASTICATION PROBLEM

MASTITIS

611.0 Acute
610.1 Chronic cystic
771.5 Neonatal infective
778.7 Neonatal noninfective
610.4 Periductal
610.4 Plasma cell
611.0 Retromammary
611.0 Submammary

MASTITIS OBSTETRICAL

675.2# Maternal due to pregnancy NOS (interstitial) (parenchymatous)
675.1# Maternal due to pregnancy - purulent (retromammary) (submammary)
5th digit: 675.1-2
0. Episode of care unspecified or N/A
1. Delivered
2. Delivered with postpartum complication
3. Antepartum complication
4. Postpartum complication

238.5 MASTOCYTOMA SITE NOS

0 MASTOCYTOMA SITE SPECIFIED SEE 'NEOPLASM UNCERTAIN BEHAVIOR', BY SITE M9740/1

202.6# MASTOCYTOMA MALIGNANT M9740/3

202.6# MASTOCYTOSIS M9741/3
5th digit: 202.6
0. Unspecified site, extranodal and solid organ sites
1. Lymph nodes of head, face, neck
2. Lymph nodes intrathoracic
3. Lymph nodes abdominal
4. Lymph nodes axilla and upper limb
5. Lymph nodes inguinal region and lower limb
6. Lymph nodes intrapelvic
7. Spleen
8. Lymph nodes multiple sites

757.33 MASTOCYTOSIS SYNDROME

611.71 MASTODYNIA

MASTOID

383.1 Caries
383.9 Disease
383.89 Disorders other
959.09 Injury
383.89 Perforation (antrum) cell
385.9 Process disease

MASTOIDECTOMY COMPLICATION

383.30 Unspecified
383.33 Chronic inflammation cavity
383.33 Granulations of postmastoidectomy cavity
383.31 Mucosal cyst
383.32 Recurrent cholesteatoma

MASTOIDITIS

383.9 Unspecified suppurative (hemorrhagic) (pneumoccocal) (streptococcal) (acute)
383.00 Acute
383.01 Acute with subperiostial abscess
383.02 Acute with other complications
383.1 Chronic
015.6# Tuberculous
5th digit: 015.6
0. Unspecified site, extranodal and solid organ sites
1. Lab not done
2. Lab pending
3. Microscopy positive (in sputum)
4. Culture positive - microscopy negative
5. Culture negative - microscopy positive
6. Culture and microscopy negative confirmed by other methods

307.9 MASTURBATION

0 MATERNAL DISORDERS SEE 'PREGNANCY COMPLICATIONS, MATERNAL CONDITIONS'

MATERNAL DISORDERS AFFECTING FETUS OR NEWBORN

In order to use the following codes, the medical record must specify that the maternal condition is a cause of morbidity or mortality in the fetus or newborn. The fact that the condition existed in the mother or complicated the pregnancy does not warrant the use of these codes on the newborn's record. Remember, codes 760-763 apply only to the infant and are never assigned to the mother's record. Conversely, never code the mother's condition with these fetal/newborn codes.

762.9 Unspecified abnormalities of chorion and amnion
761.9 Unspecified complications - due to current pregnancy
760.9 Unspecified conditions - unrelated to current pregnancy
762.6 Unspecified conditions of umbilical cord
763.9 Unspecified disorder - due to labor and delivery
761.4 Abdominal pregnancy
763.1 Abnormality bony
763.89 Abnormality soft tissues
761.8 Abortion spontaneous
762.1 Abruptio placentae
760.79 Adrenogenital iatrogenic syndrome affecting fetus or newborn
760.71 Alcohol transmitted via placenta or breast milk
762.1 Amniocentesis damage to placenta
762.8 Amnion adhesion to fetus
762.7 Amnionitis

MATERNAL DISORDERS AFFECTING FETUS OR NEWBORN (continued)

In order to use the following codes, the medical record must specify that the maternal condition is a cause of morbidity or mortality in the fetus or newborn. The fact that the condition existed in the mother or complicated the pregnancy does not warrant the use of these codes on the newborn's record. Remember, codes 760-763 apply only to the infant and are never assigned to the mother's record. Conversely, never code the mother's condition with these fetal/newborn codes.

763.5	Analgesics administered during labor and delivery
763.5	Anesthetics administered during labor and delivery
760.74	Antibiotics (anti-infectives) transmitted via placenta or breast milk
760.1	Bacteriuria
763.1	Bladder dilatation
762.1	Blood loss maternal
763.0	Breech delivery and extraction
761.7	Breech malpresentation before labor and delivery
760.8	Cervicitis
763.89	Cervix abnormality
761.0	Cervix incompetent
763.89	Cervix scar
763.1	Cervix scar obstructing labor
763.89	Cervix stenosis/stricture
763.1	Cervix stenosis/stricture obstructing labor
763.4	Cesarean delivery
763.89	Cesarean scar previous
762.1	Cesarean section damage (separation) (hemorrhage) to placenta
762.7	Chorioamnionitis
762.9	Chorion and amnion abnormality
762.8	Chorion and amnion abnormalities other specified
760.3	Circulatory disease maternal chronic
763.89	Cleidotomy fetal
760.75	Cocaine transmitted via placenta or breast milk
763.7	Contraction ring
760.75	Crack (cocaine) transmitted via placenta or breast milk
763.89	Cranioclasis, fetal
763.89	Craniotomy, fetal
763.89	Cystocele
763.1	Cystocele obstructing labor
761.6	Death (maternal)
763.89	Delayed birth or delivery NEC
763.89	Delayed birth or delivery second twin, triplet etc.
763.0	Delivery and extraction
763.6	Delivery rapid second stage
760.76	DES (diethylstilbestrol) transmitted via placenta or breast milk
763.89	Destructive operation or procedure on live fetus to facilitate delivery
775.0	Diabetes causing fetal hypoglycemia
760.76	Diethylstilbestrol (DES) transmitted via placenta or breast milk
763.5	Drug reaction maternal
761.4	Ectopic pregnancy
763.89	Endocervical OS stenosis/stricture
763.1	Endocervical OS stenosis/stricture obstructing labor
760.8	Endometritis
763.89	Exhaustion maternal
761.7	External version malpresentation before labor and delivery
763.89	Extraction fetal manual or with hook
762.3	Fetal blood loss due to placental transfusion [772.0]

MATERNAL DISORDERS AFFECTING FETUS OR NEWBORN (continued)

763.89	Forced birth
763.2	Forceps delivery
760.73	Hallucinogenic transmitted via placenta or breast milk
762.1	Hemorrhage complicating pregnancy, antepartum
763.89	Hemorrhage due to coagulation defect
760.8	Hepatitis maternal
761.3	Hydramnios acute (chronic)
760.0	Hypertensive disorders maternal
760.79	Immune sera transmitted via placenta or breast milk
763.89	Induction of labor (medical)
760.8	Infection genital tract other localized maternal
760.2	Infection maternal not manifested in fetus or newborn
760.1	Infection urinary tract
760.2	Influenza
763.89	Injury due to obstetrical trauma
760.5	Injury maternal
761.4	Intraperitoneal pregnancy
760.1	Kidney necrosis
760.8	Liver necrosis
761.7	Malpresentation/malposition before labor
763.1	Malpresentation/malposition during labor
761.6	Maternal death
760.79	Medicinal agents NEC transmitted via placenta or breast milk
762.7	Membranitis
763.89	Multiparity
761.5	Multiple pregnancy
763.5	Narcosis due to drug (correctly administered)
763.5	Narcotic reaction (intoxication) maternal during L&D
760.72	Narcotic transmitted via placenta or breast milk
760.70	Noxious substance unspecified transmitted via placenta or breast milk
760.79	Noxious substance other specified transmitted via placenta or breast milk
760.4	Nutritional deficiency disorders maternal
761.7	Oblique lie before labor and delivery
761.2	Oligohydramnios
763.5	Opiate reaction (intoxication) maternal during L&D
763.89	Os uteri stricture
763.1	Os uteri stricture obstructing labor
763.89	Ovarian cyst
763.1	Ovarian cyst obstructing labor
763.1	Pelvis bony
763.1	Pelvis contracted
763.89	Pelvis cyst
763.1	Pelvis cyst obstructing labor
763.89	Pelvis deformity
760.8	Pelvis inflammatory disease
763.89	Pelvis organs or soft tissue abnormality
763.89	Pelvis organs surgery previous
763.1	Pelvis Robert's
763.89	Pendulous abdomen
761.4	Peritoneal pregnancy
763.1	Persistent occipitoposterior position
762.1	Placenta damage
762.2	Placenta infarction
762.0	Placenta previa
762.3	Placenta transfusion syndromes
762.7	Placentitis
762.3	Polycythemia neonatorum placental transfusion [776.4]

M

MATERNAL DISORDERS AFFECTING FETUS OR NEWBORN (continued)

In order to use the following codes, the medical record must specify that the maternal condition is a cause of morbidity or mortality in the fetus or newborn. The fact that the condition existed in the mother or complicated the pregnancy does not warrant the use of these codes on the newborn's record. Remember, codes 760-763 apply only to the infant and are never assigned to the mother's record. Conversely, never code the mother's condition with these fetal/newborn codes.

761.3 Polyhydramnios
763.6 Precipitate delivery
760.0 Pre-eclampsia
761.1 Premature rupture of membranes
760.3 Respiratory disease maternal chronic
762.1 Rupture marginal sinus
760.8 Salpingitis
763.1 Shoulder dystocia
763.1 Shoulder presentation
763.1 Spondylolisthesis
763.1 Spondylolysis
760.6 Surgery maternal
762.1 Surgical induction with damage to placenta
760.70 Toxic substance NOS transmitted via placenta or breast milk
760.79 Toxic substance NEC transmitted via placenta or breast milk
763.5 Tranquilizer reaction (maternal)
761.7 Transverse lie before labor and delivery
763.1 Transverse lie-presentation during labor and delivery
761.5 Triplet pregnancy
761.4 Tubal pregnancy
761.5 Twin pregnancy
762.5 Umbilical cord entanglement (cord around neck, knot, torsion)
762.4 Umbilical cord prolapse (presentation)
762.6 Umbilical cord other and unspecified conditions
761.7 Unstable lie before labor and delivery
760.1 Urinary tract diseases maternal
763.89 Uterus abnormality
763.89 Uterus abscess (to abdominal wall)
763.89 Uterus adhesion
763.89 Uterus bicornis/double
763.89 Uterus body polyp (corpus) (mucous)
763.7 Uterus contractions abnormal
763.7 Uterus hypertonic/hypotonic
763.7 Uterus inertia-dysfunction
763.89 Uterus perforation with obstetrical trauma
763.1 Uterus prolapse
763.89 Uterus rupture
763.1 Uterus sacculation
763.89 Uterus shape abnormality
763.89 Uterus surgery previous
763.89 Uterus version
763.3 Vacuum extractor delivery
763.3 Vacuum rupture
763.89 Vagina abnormality
763.89 Vagina stenosis/stricture
763.1 Vagina stenosis/stricture obstructing labor
760.8 Vaginitis
763.89 Vulva abnormality

MATERNAL DISORDERS AFFECTING FETUS OR NEWBORN (continued)

762.8 Other specified abnormalities of chorion and amnion
761.8 Other specified complications - due to current pregnancy
760.8 Other specified conditions - unrelated to current pregnancy
762.6 Other specified conditions of umbilical cord
763.89 Other specified disorder - due to labor and delivery

315.1 MATHEMATICS DISORDER - DEVELOPMENTAL DELAY
100.0 MATHIEU'S DISEASE (LEPTOSPIRAL JAUNDICE)
732.3 MAUCLAIRE'S DISEASE
091.3 MAURIAC'S DISEASE (ERYTHEMA NODOSUM SYPHILITICUM)
081.0 MAXCY'S DISEASE

MAXILLA, MAXILLARY

524.09 Absence (congenital)
524.71 Alveolar hyperplasia
524.73 Alveolar hypoplasia
524.11 Asymmetry
473.0 Cloudy
524.07 Entire tuberosity
524.01 Hyperplasia
524.03 Hypoplasia
959.09 Injury
461.0 Sinus acute (abscess) (infection) (inflammation)
473.0 Sinus cloudy

288.2 MAY HEGGLIN SYNDROME
066.3 MAYARO FEVER (VIRAL)
610.8 MAZOPLASIA (MAMMARY)
277.85 MCAD (MEDIUM CHAIN ACYL COA DEHYDROGENASE DEFICIENCY)
271.0 MCARDLE'S (-SCHMID) (-PEARSON) DISEASE OR SYNDROME (GLYCOGENOSIS V)
756.59 MCCUNE-ALBRIGHT SYNDROME (OSTEITIS FIBROSA DISSEMINATA)
446.1 MCLS
648.9# MCLS MATERNAL CURRENT (CO-EXISTENT) IN PREGNANCY [446.1]

5th digit: 648.9
- **0. Episode of NOS or N/A**
- **1. Delivered**
- **2. Delivered with postpartum complication**
- **3. Antepartum complication**
- **4. Postpartum complication**

251.2 MCQUARRIE'S SYNDROME (IDIOPATHIC FAMILIAL HYPOGLYCEMIA)
V09.91 MDRO NOS (MULTIPLE DRUG RESISTANT ORGANISM)

MEASLES

055.9 NOS without complication
055.79 Complication other (rubeola mobilli)
055.8 Complication unspecified (rubeola mobilli)
055.0 Encephalitis (rubeola)
V01.79 Exposure
0 German see 'Rubella'
055.71 Keratitis (rubeola mobilli)
055.71 Keratoconjunctivitis (rubeola mobilli)
139.8 Late effect

M

MEASLES (continued)

647.6# Maternal complicating pregnancy **[055.#(#)]**
5th digit: 647.6
0. Episode of care unspecified or N/A
1. Delivered
2. Delivered with postpartum complication
3. Antepartum complication
4. Postpartum complication

4th or 4th and 5th digit: 055
0. Postmeasles encephalitis
1. Postmeasles pneumonia
2. Postmeasles otitis media
7#. Other specified complications
1. Measles keratoconjunctivitis
9. Other specified complication
8. Unspecified complication
9. Without mention of complication

055.2 Otitis media (rubeola)
055.1 Pneumonia (rubeola)
V73.2 Screening exam
V04.2 Vaccination measles alone
V06.4 Vaccination measles, mumps, rubella (MMR)

753.6 MEATUS URINARIUS ATRESIA (CONGENITAL)

751.0 MECKEL'S DIVERTICULUM CONGENITAL

MECONIUM

For code 770.12, use an additional code to identify any secondary pulmonary hypertension (416.8), if applicable.

770.11 Aspiration NOS
770.11 Aspiration below vocal cords
770.12 Aspiration below vocal cords with respiratory symptoms
770.12 Aspiration pneumonia/pneumonitis
770.12 Aspiration syndrome
770.12 Aspiration with respiratory symptoms
777.1 Ileus newborn
277.01 Ileus with cystic fibrosis
792.3 In liquor
656.8# In liquor fetal affecting management of mother
5th digit: 656.8
0. Episode of care unspecified or N/A
1. Delivered
3. Antepartum complication

770.11 Insufflation (inhalation)
770.12 Insufflation (inhalation) with respiratory symptoms
777.1 Obstruction newborn due to fecaliths
277.01 Obstruction newborn in mucoviscidosis
792.3 Passage
777.1 Passage delayed, newborn
763.84 Passage during delivery
777.6 Peritonitis
777.1 Plug syndrome
779.84 Staining

440.20 MEDIAL CALCIFICATION

440.20 MEDIAL CALCIFICATION WITH CHRONIC COMPLETE OR TOTAL OCCLLUSION [440.4]

MEDIAL COLLATERAL LIGAMENT

717.82 Disruption (old)
717.9 Relaxation
844.1 Tear (strain)(rupture) acute

726.31 MEDIAL EPICONDYLITIS

MEDIAL MENISCUS

717.3 Derangement (knee) unspecified (old)
717.1 Derangement (knee) anterior horn (old)
717.2 Derangement (knee) posterior horn (old)
717.3 Derangement (knee) other specified (old)
836.0 Tear bucket handle - acute
717.0 Tear bucket handle - old
836.0 Tear knee acute

MEDIAN

526.1 Anterior maxillary cyst
447.4 Arcuate ligament syndrome
600.90 Bar (prostate)
600.90 Bar (prostate) vesicle orifice

See 'LUTS' or 'Lower Urinary Tract Symptoms' for the additional code to identify the specific lower urinary tract symptoms.

600.91 Bar (prostate) vesicle orifice with urinary obstruction, retention or other lower urinary tract symptoms
600.91 Bar (prostate) with urinary obstruction, retention or other lower urinary tract symptoms
526.1 Palatal cyst

MEDIAN NERVE

526.1 Anterior maxillary cyst
447.4 Arcuate ligament syndrome
354.0 Carpal tunnel neuritis (neuralgia) (radiculitis)
354.1 Disorder NEC
354.0 Entrapment
955.1 Injury
354.1 Neuritis

0 MEDIASTINAL SEE 'MEDIASTINUM, MEDIASTINAL'

519.2 MEDIASTINITIS

MEDIASTINOPERICARDITIS

420.90 Acute
391.0 Acute rheumatic
393 Chronic rheumatic

MEDIASTINUM, MEDIASTINAL

785.6 Adenopathy
442.89 Artery (aneurysm) (A-V fistula) (cirsoid) (false) (varicose) (ruptured)
519.3 Disease NEC
519.3 Fibrosis syndrome
519.3 Hernia
862.29 Injury traumatic
862.39 Injury traumatic with open wound
519.3 Obstruction
519.3 Retraction
793.2 Shift (CXR)

MEDICAL

V68.09 Certificate issue
V70.0 Exam routine general
0 Exam see 'Exam'
V15.81 Treatment noncompliance history

M

MEDICAL CARE UNAVAILABLE

V63.9 Unspecified
V63.2 Awaiting care elsewhere
V60.4 Household member unable to render care
V63.1 In home
V63.0 No other facility
V63.8 Other specified reason
V63.0 Residence too remote

0 MEDICATION ERROR SEE 'POISONING'

Coumadin, Digoxin, chemotherapy drugs, and any other drug with a risk of severe adverse reactions are considered to be high risk medication. Code V67.51 is used to identify patients that have completed high risk medication therapy.

V58.83 MEDICATION HIGH RISK - DRUG MONITORING ENCOUNTER

V58.83 MEDICATION HIGH RISK - DRUG MONITORING ENCOUNTER WITH LONG TERM DRUG USE [V58.6#]

5th digit: V58.6
1. Anticoagulants
2. Antibiotics
3. Antiplatelets/antithrombotics
4. Anti-inflammatories non-steroidal (NSAID)
5. Steroids
6. Aspirin
7. Insulin
9. Other

V67.51 MEDICATION HIGH RISK FOLLOW UP - COMPLETED THERAPY

V58.6# MEDICATION HIGH RISK MANAGEMENT - CURRENT THERAPY (LONG TERM)

5th digit: V58.6
1. Anticoagulants
2. Antibiotics
3. Antiplatelets/antithrombotics
4. Anti-inflammatories non-steroidal (NSAID)
5. Steroids
6. Aspirin
7. Insulin
9. Other

V58.66 MEDICATION HIGH RISK MANAGEMENT - CURRENT THERAPY (LONG TERM) ASPIRIN

V58.67 MEDICATION HIGH RISK MANAGEMENT - CURRENT THERAPY (LONG TERM) INSULIN

V68.1 MEDICATION REPEAT PRESCRIPTION

760.79 MEDICINAL AGENTS NEC TRANSMITTED VIA PLACENTA OR BREAST MILK AFFECTING FETUS OR NEWBORN

045.9# MEDIN'S DISEASE (POLIOMYELITIS)

5th digit: 045.9
0. Unspecified
1. Type I
2. Type II
3. Type III

MEDITERRANEAN

282.49 Anemia
282.49 Disease with hemoglobinopathy
0 Fever see 'Brucella'
277.31 Fever familial
282.49 Syndrome
082.1 Tick fever

277.85 MEDIUM CHAIN ACYL COA DEHYDROGENASE DEFICIENCY (MCAD)

MEDULLARY

193 Carcinoma site NOS
0 Carcinoma site specified see 'Cancer', by site M8510/3
193 Carcinoma with amyloid stroma site NOS
0 Carcinoma with amyloid stroma site specified see 'Cancer', by site M8511/3
174.9 Carcinoma with lymphoid stroma site NOS
0 Carcinoma with lymphoid stroma site specified see 'Cancer', by site M8512/3
348.8 Center disease (idiopathic) (respiratory)
799.89 Failure
255.8 Hyperplasia (adrenal)
284.9 Hypoplasia NOS
344.89 Paralysis (tegmental)

MEDULLOBLASTOMA

191.6 Site NOS
0 Site specified see 'Cancer', by site M9470/3
191.6 Desmoplastic site NOS
0 Desmoplastic site specified see 'Cancer', by site M9471/3

MEDULLOEPITHELIOMA

199.1 Site NOS
0 Site specified see 'Cancer', by site M9501/3
199.1 Teratoid site NOS
0 Teratoid site specified see 'Cancer', by site M9502/3

191.6 MEDULLOMYOBLASTOMA SITE NOS
0 MEDULLOMYOBLASTOMA SITE SPECIFIED SEE 'CANCER', BY SITE M9472/3

756.83 MEEKEREN-EHLERS-DANLOS SYNDROME

MEGACOLON

564.7 NOS
751.3 Congenital
564.7 Functional
751.3 Hirschsprung's
556.5 Toxic

530.0 MEGAESOPHAGUS

MEGAKARYOCYTIC

287.30 Hypoplasia
238.79 Myelosclerosis uncertain behavior
207.2# Myelosis M9920/3

5th digit: 207.2
0. Without mention of remission
1. In remission

742.4 MEGALENCEPHALY CONGENITAL
751.5 MEGALOAPPENDIX CONGENITAL
751.5 MEGALODUODENUM CONGENITAL
750.7 MEGALOGASTRIA DUPLICATION CONGENITAL
753.22 MEGALOURETER CONGENITAL

MEIBOMIAN

373.2 Gland cyst
373.12 Gland cyst infected
373.12 Gland infection

757.0 MEIGE-MILROY DISEASE OR SYNDROME (CHRONIC HEREDITARY EDEMA)
333.82 MEIGE SYNDROME (BELPHAROSPASM-OROMANDIBULAR DYSTONIA)
296.90 MELANCHOLIA (PSYCHOSIS)
648.4# MELANCHOLIA MATERNAL CURRENT (CO-EXISTENT) IN PREGNANCY RECURRENT (PSYCHOSIS) **[296.3#]**
648.4# MELANCHOLIA MATERNAL CURRENT (CO-EXISTENT) IN PREGNANCY SINGLE EPISODE (PSYCHOSIS) **[296.2#]**

5th digit: 648.4
0. Episode of care unspecified or N/A
1. Delivered
2. Delivered with postpartum complication
3. Antepartum complication
4. Postpartum complication

5th digit: 296.2, 3
0. Unspecified
1. Mild
2. Moderate
3. Severe without mention of psychotic behavior
4. Severe specified as with psychotic behavior
5. In partial or unspecified remission
6. In full remission

791.9 MELANIN URINE ABNORMAL
172.# MELANOCARCINOMA M8720/3

4th digit: 172
0. Lip
1. Eyelid including canthus
2. Ear (auricle) auricular canal external (acoustic) meatus pinna
3. Unspecified parts of face external, cheek, chin, eyebrow, forehead, nose, temple
4. Scalp and neck
5. Trunk, axilla, breast, groin, perianal skin, perineum, umbilicus
6. Upper limb including shoulder
7. Lower limb including hip
8. Other specified skin sites, contiguous or overlapping, undetermined point of origin
9. Site unspecified

253.4 MELANOCYTE-STIMULATING HORMONE DEFICIENCY
253.1 MELANOCYTE-STIMULATING HORMONE OVERPRODUCTION
709.09 MELANODERMA
255.41 MELANODERMA ADDISON'S (PRIMARY ADRENAL INSUFFICIENCY)
521.05 MELANODONTIA INFANTILE
521.05 MELANODONTOCLASIA

MELANOMA BY CELL TYPE

172.# Melanoma M8720/3
172.# Amelanotic M8730/3
172.# Balloon cell M8722/3
172.# Epithelioid and spindle cell (mixed) M8775/3
172.# Epithelioid cell M8771/3
172.# In giant pigmented nevus M8761/3
172.# In Hutchinson's melanotic freckle M8742/3
172.# In junctional nevus (malignant) M8740/3
172.# In precancerous melanosis (malignant) M8741/3
0 Juvenile see 'Benign Neoplasm', skin, by site M8770/0
172.# Nodular M8721/3
172.# Spindle cell M8772/3

4th digit: 172
0. Lip
1. Eyelid including canthus
2. Ear (auricle) auricular canal external (acoustic) meatus pinna
3. Unspecified parts of face external, cheek, chin, eyebrow, forehead, nose, temple
4. Scalp and neck
5. Trunk, axilla, breast, groin, perianal skin, perineum, umbilicus
6. Upper limb including shoulder
7. Lower limb including hip
8. Other specified skin sites, contiguous or overlapping, undetermined point of origin
9. Site unspecified

190.0 Spindle cell type A site NOS M8773/3
190.0 Spindle cell type B site NOS M8774/3
172.# Superficial spreading M8743/3

4th digit: 172
0. Lip
1. Eyelid including canthus
2. Ear (auricle) auricular canal external (acoustic) meatus pinna
3. Unspecified parts of face external, cheek, chin, eyebrow, forehead, nose, temple
4. Scalp and neck
5. Trunk, axilla, breast, groin, perianal skin, perineum, umbilicus
6. Upper limb including shoulder
7. Lower limb including hip
8. Other specified skin sites, contiguous or overlapping, undetermined point of origin
9. Site unspecified

MELANOMA BY SITE

172.9 NOS
172.5 Abdominal wall
172.7 Ankle skin
154.3 Anus
154.2 Anus canal
172.5 Anus skin
172.6 Arm skin
172.2 Auricle canal
172.5 Axilla skin
172.5 Back skin
172.5 Breast skin
172.5 Buttock skin
172.3 Cheek (external) (skin)

M

MELANOMA BY SITE (continued)

172.5 Chest wall
172.3 Chin (skin)
172.2 Ear meatus external
172.2 Ear skin
172.2 External auditory canal skin
0 Eye see 'Cancer' eye
172.3 Eyebrow (skin)
172.1 Eyelid
172.1 Eyelid including canthus skin
172.3 Face skin
172.6 Finger skin
172.6 Fingernail NEC
172.5 Flank
172.7 Foot skin
172.6 Forearm skin
172.3 Forehead (skin)
187.1 Foreskin
184.4 Genitals female external
187.9 Genitals male
172.5 Groin
172.6 Hand skin
172.7 Heel skin
172.2 Helix
172.7 Hip skin
172.5 Intrascapular
172.3 Jaw
172.7 Knee skin
184.1 Labium majus
184.2 Labium minus
172.7 Leg skin
140.1 Lip lower vermilion border
140.0 Lip NOS vermilion border
140.0 Lip upper vermilion border
172.0 Lip skin
172.7 Lower limb skin
172.1 Meibomian gland
172.4 Neck (skin)
172.3 Nose (external) (skin)
172.8 Overlapping sites skin
187.4 Penis
172.5 Perianal skin
172.5 Perineum skin
172.2 Pinna (skin)
172.7 Popliteal area skin
187.1 Prepuce
172.5 Pubis
184.4 Pudendum
172.4 Scalp (skin)
187.7 Scrotum
172.3 Septum nasal
172.6 Shoulder skin
0 Site other than skin see 'Cancer', metastatic by site
172.9 Skin NOS
172.8 Skin other
172.5 Submammary fold
172.9 Superficial spreading site unspecified
172.3 Temple (skin)
172.7 Thigh skin
172.7 Toenail
172.7 Toe skin
172.5 Trunk skin
172.5 Umbilicus skin
172.6 Upper limb skin
184.0 Vaginal vault
184.4 Vulva

528.9 MELANOPLAKIA

MELANOSIS

255.41 Addisonian
017.6# Addisonian tuberculous
5th digit: 017.6
0. NOS
1. Lab not done
2. Lab pending
3. Microscopy positive (in sputum)
4. Culture positive - microscopy negative
5. Culture negative - microscopy positive
6. Culture and microscopy negative confirmed by other methods

255.41 Adrenal
569.89 Colon
372.55 Conjunctiva
743.49 Conjunctiva congenital
757.33 Corii degenerativa
371.12 Cornea
743.43 Cornea congenital
743.42 Cornea congenital interfering with vision
743.43 Cornea prenatal
743.42 Cornea prenatal interfering with vision
372.55 Eye
743.49 Eye congenital
709.09 Jute spinners'
757.33 Lenticularis progressiva
573.8 Liver
232.9 Precancerous site NOS
0 Precancerous site specified see 'Carcinoma In Situ' skin by site M8741/2
709.09 Riehl's
379.19 Sclera
743.47 Sclera congenital
255.41 Suprarenal
709.09 Tar
709.09 Toxic

229.9 MELANOTIC NEUROECTODERMAL TUMOR SITE NOS
0 MELANOTIC NEUROECTODERMAL TUMOR SITE SPECIFIED SEE 'BENIGN NEOPLASM', BY SITE M9363/0
791.9 MELANURIA
277.87 MELAS SYNDROME (MITOCHONDRIAL ENCEPHALOPATHY, LACTIC ACIDOSIS AND STROKE-LIKE EPISODES)
709.09 MELASMA
578.1 MELENA
777.3 MELENA DUE TO SWALLOWED MATERNAL BLOOD
772.4 MELENA PERINATAL
686.09 MELENEY'S GANGRENE OR ULCER (CHRONIC UNDERMINING)
025 MELIOIDOSIS
351.8 MELKERSSON'S (-ROSENTHAL) SYNDROME
762.7 MEMBRANITIS AFFECTING FETUS OR NEWBORN
0 MEMBRANITIS SEE 'AMNIONITIS'
464.4 MEMBRANOUS ANGINA
581.1 MEMBRANOUS GLOMERULAR DISEASE IDIOPATHIC

M

780.93 MEMORY DISTURBANCE (LOSS)
310.8 MEMORY DISTURBANCE MILD ORGANIC
256.39 MENARCHE DELAYED
259.1 MENARCHE PRECOCIOUS
258.0# MEN (MULTIPLE ENDOCRINE NEOPLASIA) SYNDROME
5th digit: 258.01-3
1. Type I
2. Type IIA
3. Type IIB
V18.11 MEN (MULTIPLE ENDOCRINE NEOPLASIA) SYNDROME FAMILY HISTORY
V84.81 MEN (MULTIPLE ENDOCRINE NEOPLASIA) SYNDROME SUSCEPTIBILITY GENETIC
270.2 MENDE'S SYNDROME (PTOSIS-EPICANTHUS)
668.0# MENDELSON'S SYNDROME DURING LABOR
5th digit: 668.0
0. Episode of care NOS or N/A
1. Delivered
2. Delivered with postpartum complication
3. Antepartum complication
4. Postpartum complication
997.3 MENDELSON'S SYNDROME RESULTING FROM A PROCEDURE
535.2 MENETRIER'S SYNDROME (HYPERTROPHIC GASTRITIS)

MENIERE'S DISEASE (SYNDROME)

386.00 Active NOS
386.02 Active cochlear
386.01 Active cochleovestibular
386.03 Active vestibular
386.04 In remission

349.2 MENINGEAL ADHESIONS (CEREBRAL) (SPINAL)
349.2 MENINGEAL CALCIFICATION (CEREBRAL)
0 MENINGEAL DISEASE SEE 'MENINGITIS'
088.81 MENINGIOENCEPHALITIS DUE TO LYME DISEASE [320.7]

MENINGIOMA

225.2 Site NOS
0 Site specified see 'Benign Neoplasm', by site M9530/0
225.2 Angiomatous site NOS
0 Angiomatous site specified see 'Benign Neoplasm', by site M9534/0
225.2 Fibrous site NOS
0 Fibrous site specified see 'Benign Neoplasm', By site M9532/0
225.2 Hemangioblastic site NOS
0 Hemangioblastic site specified see 'Benign Neoplasm', by site M9535/0
225.2 Hemangiopericytic site NOS
0 Hemangiopericytic site specified see 'Benign Neoplasm', by site M9536/0
192.1 Malignant site NOS
0 Malignant site specified see 'Cancer' by Site M9530/3
225.2 Meningotheliomatous site NOS
0 Meningotheliomatous site specified see 'Benign Neoplasm', by site M9531/0

MENINGIOMA (continued)

237.6 Papillary site NOS
0 Papillary site specified see 'Neoplasm Uncertain Behavior', by site M9538/1
225.2 Psammomatous site NOS
0 Psammomatous site specified see 'Benign Neoplasm', by site M9533/0
225.2 Transitional site NOS
0 Transitional site specified see 'Benign Neoplasm', by site M9537/0

237.6 MENINGIOMATOSIS SITE NOS
0 MENINGIOMATOSIS SITE SPECIFIED SEE 'NEOPLASM UNCERTAIN BEHAVIOR', BY SITE M9530/1
781.6 MENINGISM
781.6 MENINGISMUS (INFECTIONAL) (PNEUMOCOCCAL)
997.09 MENINGISMUS (INFECTIONAL) (PNEUMOCOCCAL) DUE TO SERUM OR VACCINE [321.8]

The code in the left margin always sequences first. The additional code in brackets to the right of the description is sequenced second. Underlining shows the code number that corresponds to the underlined description. Underlining never implies correct sequencing.

MENINGITIS

322.9 Unspecified
322.2 Unspecified cause chronic
047.9 Abacterial see also 'Meningitis', by specific virus
039.8 Actinomycotic [320.7]
049.1 Adenovirus
320.82 Aerobacter aerogenes
117.6 Allescheriosis [321.1]
320.81 Anaerobic (gram-negative)
066.9 Arbovirus NEC [321.2]
066.8 Arbovirus NEC other specified [321.2]
047.9 Aseptic
088.81 Aseptic due to lyme disease [320.7]
322.0 Aseptic noninfective
117.3 Aspergillosis [321.1]
320.89 Bacillus pyocyaneus
320.9 Bacterial
320.81 Bacteroides (fragilis) (oralis) (malaninogenicus)
111.3 Black piedra [321.1]
116.0 Blastomycotic [321.1]
198.4 Cancerous
112.83 Candidal
036.0 Cerebrospinal
V02.59 Cerebrospinal carrier (suspected of)
117.2 Chromoblastomycotic [321.1]
322.2 Chronic, cause unspecified
320.81 Clostridium (haemolyticum) (novyi) NEC
114.2 Coccidioidomycosis
047.0 Coxsackie virus
117.5 Cryptococcal [321.0]

M

MENINGITIS (continued)

117.8 Dematiacious fungi [321.1]
111.9 Dermatomycosis [321.1]
110.# Dermatophytosis [321.1]
4th digit: 110
0. Scalp and beard
1. Nail (unguium)
2. Hand (manuum)
3. Groin and perianal (cruris)
4. Foot (pedis)
5. Body (corporus)
6. Deep seated (granuloma trichophyticum)
8. Other specified site
9. Unspecified site

036.0 Diplococcal
036.0 Diplococcal gram negative
320.1 Diplococcal gram positive
997.09 Due to vaccination [321.8]
320.82 E. coli [041.4]
047.1 Echo virus
320.82 Enterobacter aerogenes
047.9 Enteroviral
047.8 Enteroviral specified type NEC
322.1 Eosinophilic
036.0 Epidemic
110.8 Epidermophyton [321.1]
320.81 Eubacterium
320.89 Eubacterium fibrinopurulent specified NEC
320.89 Fibrinopurulent NEC
320.82 Friedlander bacillus [041.3]
117.9 Fungal NEC [321.1]
320.81 Fusobacterium
098.82 Gonococcal
320.81 Gram-negative anaerobes [041.84]
320.82 Gram-negative bacteria NEC [041.85]
036.0 Gram-negative cocci
320.82 Gram-negative cocci specified NEC
320.9 Gram-negative cocci NEC
320.0 Hemophilus [041.5]
054.72 Herpes simplex
053.0 Herpes zoster
115.91 Histoplasma
115.01 Histoplasma capsulatum
115.11 Histoplasma duboisii
320.0 Influenzal
320.82 Klebsiella pneumoniae [041.3]
326 Late effect
100.81 Leptospiral (aseptic)
027.0 Listeriosis [320.7]
116.2 Lobomycotic [321.1]
088.81 Lyme disease [320.7]
049.0 Lymphocytic
049.0 Lymphocytic choriomeningitis virus
036.0 Meningococcal
047.1 Meningo - eruptive syndrome
110.8 Microsporum [321.1]
320.82 Mima polymorpha
047.9 Mollaret's
072.1 Mumps
117.9 Mycotic NOS [321.1]
117.4 Mycotic mycetomas [321.1]
110.1 Nail fungal disease [321.1]
036.0 Neisseria
321.8 Nonbacterial organisms classified elsewhere [100.81]
322.0 Nonpyogenic

MENINGITIS (continued)

116.1 Paracoccidioidomycotic [321.1]
320.81 Peptococcus
320.81 Peptostreptococcus
033.0 Pertussis [320.7]
117.8 Phaehyphomycotic [321.1]
111.0 Pityriasis versicolor [321.1]
320.1 Pneumococcal [041.2]
045.2# Poliovirus acute nonparalytic [321.2]
5th digit: 045.2
0. Poliovirus unspecified
1. Poliovirus type I
2. Poliovirus type II
3. Poliovirus type III

320.81 Proprionibacterium
320.82 Proteus morganii [041.6]
320.82 Pseudomonas [041.7]
320.89 Purulent specified organism NEC
320.89 Pyogenic specified organism NEC
117.0 Rhinosporidiosis [321.1]
003.21 Salmonella
135 Sarcoid [321.4]
320.9 Septic unspecified
320.89 Septic specified organism NEC
322.0 Serosa circumscipta NEC
320.82 Serratia (marcescens)
117.1 Sporotrichosis [321.1]
320.3 Staphylococcal [041.1#]
5th digit: 041.1
0. NOS
1. Aureus
9. Other staph

997.09 Sterile
320.2 Streptococcal [041.0#]
5th digit: 041.0
0. NOS
1. Group A
2. Group B
3. Group C
4. Group D (enterococcus)
5. Group G
9. Other strep

320.9 Suppurative NOS
320.89 Suppurative specified organism NEC
094.2 Syphilitic
091.81 Syphilitic acute secondary
090.42 Syphilitic congenital
094.2 Syphilitic meningovascular
111.2 Tinea blanca [321.1]
111.1 Tinea nigra [321.1]
111.0 Tinea versicolor [321.1]
117.5 Torula [321.0]
958.8 Traumatic late effect injury
320.81 Treponema (denticola) (macrodenticum)
110.8 Trichophyton [321.1]
086.# Trypanasomal [321.3]
4th digit: 086
0. American with heart involvement
1. American with involvement of organ other than heart
2. American NOS
3. Gambian
4. Rhodesian
5. African NOS
9. NOS

M

MENINGITIS (continued)

013.0# Tuberculosis
5th digit: 013.0
0. Unspecified
1. Lab not done
2. Lab pending
3. Microscopy positive (in sputum)
4. Culture positive - microscopy negative
5. Culture negative - microscopy positive
6. Culture and microscopy negative confirmed by other methods

002.0 Typhoid [320.7]
997.09 Vaccination complication [321.8]
320.81 Veillonella
320.82 Vibrio vulnificus
047.9 Viral unspecified
321.2 Viral not elsewhere classified
047.8 Viral other specified
033.0 Whooping cough [320.7]
322.0 With clear cerebrospinal fluid
117.7 Zygomatic (phycomosis) (mucormycosis) [321.1]
320.89 Other specified organism

047.1 MENINGO ERUPTIVE SYNDROME

MENINGOCELE

349.2 Acquired
742.0 Cerebral congenital
741.9# Spinal
741.0# With hydrocephalus
741.9# Without hydrocephalus
5th digit: 741.0, 9
0. Region NOS
1. Cervical
2. Dorsal
3. Lumbar

MENINGOCOCCAL

036.3 Adrenal syndrome
036.82 Arthritis
036.40 Carditis
V02.59 Carrier (suspected)
036.1 Encephalitis
036.42 Endocarditis
V01.84 Exposure
036.3 Hemorrhagic adrenalitis
036.0 Meningitis
036.2 Meningococcemia
036.43 Myocarditis
036.81 Optic neuritis
036.41 Pericarditis
036.2 Septicemia
036.3 Waterhouse Friderichsen syndrome
036.9 Infection
036.89 Infections other

036.2 MENINGOCOCCEMIA

MENINGOENCEPHALITIS

323.9 NOS
048 Acute NEC
039.8 Actinomycosis [320.7]
0 Bacterial, purulent, pyogenic, or septic see 'Meningitis'
116.0 Blastomycosis [323.41]
094.1 Chronic NEC
094.1 Diffuse NEC

MENINGOENCEPHALITIS (continued)

063.2 Diphasic
136.2 Due to free living ameba (Naegleria) [323.41]
088.81 Due to lyme disease [320.7]
036.0 Epidemic
136.2 Free living amebae
054.3 Herpes
048 Infectious (acute)
320.0 Influenzal
027.0 Listeria monocytogenes [320.7]
088.81 Lyme disease [320.7]
049.0 Lymphocytic (serous) (benign)
072.2 Mumps
136.2 Naegleria
123.9 Parasitic [323.41]
320.1 Pneumococcal
136.2 Primary amebic
056.01 Rubella
048 Serous
049.0 Serous lymphocytic
094.2 Specific
117.1 Sporotrichosis [321.1]
320.3 Staphylococcal
320.2 Streptococcal
094.2 Syphilitic
013.0# TB
5th digit: 013.0
0. NOS
1. Lab not done
2. Lab pending
3. Microscopy positive (in sputum)
4. Culture positive - microscopy negative
5. Culture negative - microscopy positive
6. Culture and microscopy negative confirmed by other methods

117.5 Torula [323.41]
989.9 Toxic NEC [323.71]
987.8 Toxic due to carbon tetrachloride [323.71]
961.3 Toxic due to hydroxyquinoline derivatives [323.71]
984.9 Toxic due to lead [323.71]
985.0 Toxic due to mercury [323.71]
985.8 Toxic due to thallium [323.71]
130.0 Toxoplasmosis (acquired)
771.2 Toxoplasmosis congenital (active) [323.41]
086.1 Trypanosomic [323.2]
048 Virus NEC
0 See also 'Encephalitis'

742.0 MENINGOENCEPHALOCELE CONGENITAL

348.39 MENINGOENCEPHALOPATHY (SEE ALSO MENINGOENCEPHALITIS)

0 MENINGOMYELITIS SEE 'MENINGOENCEPHALITIS'

0 MENINGOENCEPHALOMYELITIS SEE 'MENINGOENCEPHALITIS'

MENINGOMYELOCELE

741.0# With hydrocephalus
741.9# Without hydrocephalus
5th digit: 741.0, 9
0. Region NOS
1. Cervical
2. Dorsal
3. Lumbar

M

MENISCUS

0 Chondrocalcinosis see 'Chondrocalcinosis'
717.5 Discoid old
718.0# Disorder (derangement) (tear) (rupture) – old
5th digit: 718.0
0. Site unspecified
1. Shoulder region
2. Upper arm (elbow) (humerus)
3. Forearm (radius) (wrist) (ulna)
4. Hand (carpal) (metacarpal) (fingers)
5. Pelvic region and thigh (hip) (buttock) (femur)
7. Ankle and/or foot (metatarsals) (toes) (tarsals)
8. Other
9. Multiple

270.2 Disorder in ochronosis
717.5 Disorder knee (derangement) (tear) (rupture) - old (see also 'Meniscus', knee tear - old)
717.5 Knee congenital discoid
717.5 Knee cyst - semilunar cartilage
717.5 Knee derangement - semilunar cartilage
717.5 Knee derangement NEC - old

KNEE TEAR - ACUTE

836.2 Unspecified medial or lateral
836.1 Anterior horn lateral
836.0 Anterior horn medial
836.1 Bucket handle lateral
836.0 Bucket handle medial
836.1 Lateral NOS
836.0 Medial NOS
836.1 Posterior horn lateral
836.0 Posterior horn medial
836.1 Other specified lateral
836.0 Other specified medial

KNEE TEAR - OLD

717.5 Unspecified NEC
717.42 Anterior horn lateral
717.1 Anterior horn medial
717.41 Bucket handle lateral
717.0 Bucket handle medial
717.40 Lateral NOS
717.3 Medial NOS
717.43 Posterior horn lateral
717.2 Posterior horn medial
717.49 Other specified lateral
717.3 Other specified medial

759.89 MENKES' SYNDROME (GLUTAMIC ACID)
270.3 MENKES' SYNDROME-MAPLE SYRUP (URINE) DISEASE

MENOMETRORRHAGIA

626.2 NOS
627.0 Menopausal
626.3 Pubertal

MENOPAUSE, MENOPAUSAL

627.2 NOS
627.9 And postmenopausal disorder
627.8 And postmenopausal disorders other specified

MENOPAUSE, MENOPAUSAL (continued)

716.3# Arthritis
5th digit: 716.3
0. Site NOS
1. Shoulder region
2. Upper arm
3. Forearm
4. Hand
5. Pelvic region and thigh
6. Lower leg
7. Ankle and/or foot
8. Other
9. Multiple

627.4 Artificial
627.0 Bleeding
627.1 Bleeding post
627.2 Climacteric states
627.2 Crisis
296.3# Depression (melancholia) - recurrent
296.2# Depression (melancholia) - single episode
5th digit: 296.2-3
0. NOS
1. Mild
2. Moderate
3. Severe without mention of psychotic behavior
4. Severe with psychotic behavior
5. In partial or NOS remission
6. In full remission

627.4 Postartificial syndrome
V49.81 Postmenopausal status asymptomatic (natural) (age related)
256.31 Premature
256.2 Premature - postirradiation
256.2 Premature - postirradiation with artificial menopause [627.4]
256.2 Premature - postsurgical
256.2 Premature - postsurgical with artificial menopause [627.4]
627.4 States (artificial)
627.4 Surgical
627.2 Symptoms
627.2 Syndrome

MENORRHAGIA

626.2 NOS
626.2 Primary
627.0 Climacteric
627.0 Preclimacteric
627.0 Premenopausal
627.0 Menopausal
627.1 Postmenopausal
626.3 Pubertal

626.2 MENORRHEA
626.3 MENORRHEA PUBERTAL

MENSTRUATION, MENSTRUAL

626.0 Absence
625.3 Cramps
626.9 Disorder
306.52 Disorder psychogenic
626.8 Disorder other
625.4 Dysphoria

M

MENSTRUATION, MENSTRUAL (continued)

626.2 Excessive heavy periods
627.0 Excessive menopausal
626.3 Excessive onset of puberty
627.0 Excessive premenopausal
V25.3 Extraction
327.13 Hypersomnia
626.1 Infrequent
626.4 Irregular
625.4 Molimen
625.4 Migraine
625.3 Painful
625.4 PMDD (premenstrual dysphoric disorder)
625.4 PMS
626.8 Precocious
V25.3 Regulation
626.8 Retained
626.8 Suppression
625.4 Syndrome
626.8 Other specified disorder NEC

MENTAL DISORDER

291.9 Alcoholic induced NOS see also 'Psychosis Alcoholic'
291.89 Alcoholic induced other see also 'Psychosis Alcoholic'
V66.3 Convalescence
292.9 Drug induced NOS see also 'Psychosis Drug Induced
292.89 Drug induced other see also 'Psychosis Drug Induced
310.# Due to organic brain damage (nonpsychotic)
4th digit: 310
0. Frontal lobe syndrome
1. Organic personality syndrome
2. Postconcussion syndrome
8. Other specified nonpsychotic disorder NEC
9. Unspecified nonpsychotic disorder

V11.8 History

> ***648.4#: Use an additional code to identify the specific maternal mental disorder.***

648.4# Maternal current (co-existent) in pregnancy
5th digit: 648.4
0. Episode of care unspecified or N/A
1. Delivered
2. Delivered with postpartum complication
3. Antepartum complication
4. Postpartum complication

V23.89 Maternal previous affecting management of pregnancy
0 Neurotic see 'Neurosis, Neurotic'
300.9 Nonpsychotic unspecified
310.9 Nonpsychotic following organic brain damage
313.9 Of infancy, childhood or adolescence NOS
294.9 Persistent NOS in conditions classified elsewhere
294.8 Persistent other in conditions classified elsewhere
310.1 Presenile non psychotic
0 Psychotic see 'Psychosis'
V79.9 Screening (and developmental handicaps)
V79.8 Screening (and developmental handicaps) - other specified
293.9 Transient NOS in conditions classified elsewhere
293.89 Transient other in conditions classified elsewhere

MENTAL PROBLEM

V40.9 Unspecified
V40.2 Other specified

MENTAL RETARDATION

319 Unspecified
317 Mild IQ 50-70
318.0 Moderate IQ 35-49
318.1 Severe IQ 20-34
318.2 Profound
V18.4 Family history
V79.2 Screening

780.97 MENTAL STATUS ALTERED
780.93 MENTAL STATUS ALTERED-AMNESIA, MEMORY LOSS
304.0# MEPERIDINE DEPENDENCE
5th digit: 304.0
0. Unspecified
1. Continuous
2. Episodic
3. In remission

355.1 MERALGIA PARESTHETICA
758.89 MERFF SYNDROME
277.87 MERRF SYNDROME (MYOCLONUS WITH EPILEPSY AND WITH RAGGED RED FIBERS)
0 MERKEL CELL TUMOR SEE 'CANCER', BY SITE
330.0 MERZBACHER-PELIZAEUS DISEASE
305.3# MESCALINE ABUSE (NONDEPENDENT)
304.5# MESCALINE ADDICTION (DEPENDENT)
5th digit: 304.5, 305.3
0. Unspecified
1. Continuous
2. Episodic
3. In remission

344.89 MESENCEPHALIC PARALYSIS NEC
710.9 MESENCHYMAL DISEASE

MESENCHYMOMA

238.9 Site NOS
0 Site Specified see 'Neoplasm Uncertain Behavior', by site M8990/1
215.# Benign M8990/0
4th digit: 215
0. Head, face, neck
2. Upper limb including shoulder
3. Lower limb including hip
4. Thorax
5. Abdomen (wall), gastric, gastrointestinal, intestine, stomach
6. Pelvis, buttock, groin, inguinal region, perineum
7. Trunk NOS, back NOS, flank NOS
8. Other specified sites
9. Site unspecified

199.1 Malignant site NOS
0 Malignant site specified see 'Cancer', by site M8990/3

567.82 MESENTERITIS RETRACTILE (SCLEROSING)

M

Injury of a blood vessel can be a laceration, A-V fistula, aneurysm, or hematoma. Use the injury code found by anatomical site (the name of the blood vessel).

MESENTERY, MESENTERIC

027.2 Adenitis by pasteurella multocida
557.1 Arteritis
442.84 Artery (superior) aneurysm or A-V fistula (cirsoid) (false) (varicose)
557.1 Artery arteriosclerosis
557.0 Artery embolism
557.0 Artery infarction
557.0 Artery infarction (embolic) (thrombotic)
902.20 Artery injury - branch unspecified
902.27 Artery injury - inferior
908.4 Artery injury - late effect
902.25 Artery injury - superior
902.26 Artery injury - superior primary branches
902.29 Artery injury - other artery
557.0 Artery insufficiency acute
557.1 Artery insufficiency chronic
902.20 Artery laceration NOS traumatic (rupture) (hematoma) (avulsion) (aneurysm)
902.27 Artery laceration inferior traumatic (rupture) (hematoma) (avulsion) (aneurysm) (embolism) (thrombosis)
902.25 Artery laceration superior (rupture) (hematoma) (avulsion) (aneurysm) (embolism) (thrombosis) traumatic
557.0 Artery occlusion (with gangrene)
557.1 Artery superior syndrome
863.89 Injury (traumatic)
863.99 Injury (traumatic) with open wound
567.82 Panniculitis
751.4 Universal congenital
557.1 Vascular insufficiency syndrome (with gangrene)
902.39 Vein injury
902.32 Vein injury - inferior
902.31 Vein injury - superior

996.59 MESH EXTRUSION (REINFORCING)
524.23 MESIO-OCCLUSION
746.87 MESOCARDIA
199.1 MESODERMAL MIXED TUMOR SITE NOS
0 MESODERMAL MIXED TUMOR SITE SPECIFIED SEE 'CANCER', BY SITE M8951/3

MESONEPHRIC

752.89 Duct agenesis (congenital)
752.89 Duct persistence
238.9 Tumor site NOS
0 Tumor site specified see 'Neoplasm Uncertain Behavior', by site M9110/1

MESONEPHROMA

229.9 Benign site NOS
0 Benign site specified see 'Benign Neoplasm', by site M9110/0
199.1 Malignant site NOS
0 Malignant site specified see 'Cancer', by site M9110/3

867.6 MESOSALPINX INJURY TRAUMATIC
867.7 MESOSALPINX INJURY TRAUMATIC WITH OPEN WOUND

MESOTHELIOMA

229.9 Benign site NOS
0 Benign site specified see 'Benign Neoplasm', by site M9050/0
229.9 Biphasic type - benign site NOS
0 Biphasic type - benign site specified see 'Benign Neoplasm', by site M9050/0
199.1 Biphasic type - malignant site NOS
0 Biphasic type - malignant site specified see 'Cancer', by site M9053/3
229.9 Epithelioid - benign site NOS
0 Epithelioid - benign site specified see 'Benign Neoplasm', by site M9052/0
199.1 Epithelioid - malignant site NOS
0 Epithelioid - malignant site specified see 'Cancer', by site M9052/3
229.9 Fibrous - benign site NOS
0 Fibrous - benign site specified see 'Benign Neoplasm', by site M9051/0
199.1 Fibrous - malignant site NOS
0 Fibrous - malignant site specified see 'Cancer', by site M9051/3
199.1 Malignant site NOS
0 Malignant site specified see 'Cancer', by site M9050/3

0 METABOLIC SEE 'METABOLISM, METABOLIC'

METABOLISM, METABOLIC

276.2 Acidosis
V77.99 Disease screening
277.9 Disorder
669.0# Disorder complicating labor and delivery

5th digit: 669.0
- **0. Episode of care unspecified or N/A**
- **1. Delivered**
- **2. Delivered with postpartum complication**
- **3. Antepartum complication**
- **4. Postpartum complication**

277.85 Disorder fatty acid oxidation
639.4 Disorder following abortion, ectopic, molar pregnancy
V12.2 Disorder history
277.87 Disorder mitochondrial
0 Disorder see also specified disorder
277.89 Disorder other specified
775.9 Disturbances fetus and newborn
775.89 Disturbances neonatal other transitory
656.3# Fetal acidemia affecting management mother

5th digit: 656.3
- **0. Episode of care unspecified or N/A**
- **1. Delivered**
- **3. Antepartum complication**

783.9 Problem
V77.99 Screening for disease
V77.7 Screening for other inborn errors
783.9 Symptom other
277.7 Syndrome

755.28 METACARPALS AGENESIS
755.21 METACARPALS AGENESIS WITH ALL FINGERS COMPLETE

842.12 METACARPOPHALANGEAL SEPARATION (RUPTURE) (TEAR) (LACERATION)

842.12 METACARPOPHALANGEAL STRAIN (SPRAIN) (AVULSION)(HEMARTHROSIS)

121.5 METAGONIMIASIS

121.5 METAGONIMUS YOKOGAWAI INFECTION

709.00 METAL PIGMENTATION

502 METAL POLISHERS' DISEASE

360.24 METALLOSIS OTHER (GLOBE)

368.14 METAMORPHOPSIA

METAPLASIA

238.76 Agnogenic
530.85 Esophagus
537.89 Gastric mucosa
238.76 Megakaryocytic
289.89 Myelogenous
289.89 Myeloid
238.76 Myeloid with myelofibrosis
238.76 Myeloid with myelosclerosis

275.40 METASTATIC CALCIFICATION

METASTATIC CANCER M8010/6

199.1 Unspecified site
198.5 Coccyx
198.89 Coccygeal body
198.89 Hip
196.# Lymph node metastatic
4th digit: 196
0. Head, face, neck, cervical, supraclavicular, cervicofacial, scalene
1. Intrathoracic, intercostal, bronchopulmonary, mediastinal, tracheobronchial
2. Intrabdominal, mesenteric, retroperitoneal, intestinal
3. Axilla, upper limb, brachial, infraclavicular, pectoral, epitrochlear
5. Lower limb, inguinal, femoral, groin, popliteal, tibial
6. Intrapelvic, hypogastric, iliac, parametrial, obturator
8. Multiple sites
9. Lymph nodes NOS

197.# Respiratory and digestive
4th digit: 197
0. Lung, bronchus
1. Mediastinum
2. Pleura
3. Trachea or other respiratory organs
4. Small intestine, duodenum
5. Large intestine, rectum
6. Retroperitoneum and peritoneum
7. Liver, specified as secondary
8. Other digestive organs and spleen

METASTATIC CANCER M8010/6 (continued)

198.#(#) Other specified sites
4th or 4th and 5th digit: 198
0. Kidney
1. Other urinary organs
2. Skin and skin of breast or mastectomy site
3. Brain and spinal cord
4. Other parts of nervous system, meninges (cerebral) (spinal)
5. Bone and bone marrow
6. Ovary
7. Adrenal gland, suprarenal gland
8#. Other specified
81. Breast (soft) (connective) tissue, mastectomy site
82. Genital organs
89. Other

259.2 METASTATIC CARCINOID SYNDROME

726.70 METATARSALGIA

355.6 METATARSALGIA MORTON'S

755.38 METATARSALS AGENESIS (COMPLETE) (PARTIAL)

755.31 METATARSALS AGENESIS (COMPLETE) (PARTIAL) WITH COMPLETE ABSENCE OF DISTAL ELEMENTS

845.12 METATARSOPHALANGEAL SEPARATION (RUPTURE) (TEAR) (LACERATION)

845.12 METATARSOPHALANGEAL STRAIN (SPRAIN) (AVULSION)(HEMARTHROSIS)

764.60 METATARSUS ABDUCTUS VALGUS (CONGENITAL)

754.53 METATARSUS ABDUCTUS VARUS (CONGENITAL)

754.60 METATARSUS ADDUCTUS VALGUS (CONGENITAL)

754.53 METATARSUS ADDUCTUS VARUS (CONGENITAL)

754.52 METATARSUS PRIMUS VARUS CONGENITAL

754.53 METATARSUS VARUS (CONGENITAL)

173.# METATYPICAL CARCINOMA M8095/3
4th digit: 173
0. Skin of lip
1. Eyelid including canthus
2. Skin of ear, auricular canal external, external meatus pinna
3. Skin of unspecified parts of face external, chin, eyebrow, forehead, nose
4. Scalp and skin of neck
5. All skin trunk, axillary fold, perianal, abdominal wall, anus, back, breast (or mastectomy site), buttock
6. All skin upper limb, shoulder, arm, finger, forearm, hand
7. All skin lower limb, hip, ankle, foot, heel, knee, leg, thigh, toe, popiteal area
8. Other specified skin sites, contiguous, overlapping sites, undetermined point of origin
9. Site unspecified

M

304.0# METHADONE ADDICTION (DEPENDENT)
5th digit: 304.0
0. Unspecified
1. Continuous
2. Episodic
3. In remission

METHEMOGLOBINEMIA

289.7 Acquired
289.7 Acquired with sulfhemoglobinemia
289.7 Congenital
289.7 Hereditary
289.7 Toxic

V09.0 METHICILLIN RESISTANT STAPHYLOCOCCUS AUREUS (MRSA)
270.4 METHIONINEMIA
270.4 METHIONINE METABOLISM DISTURBANCES
270.4 METHYLENETETRAHYDROFOLATE REDUCTASE DEFICIENCY (MTHFR)
304.4# METHYLPHENIDATE DEPENDENCE
5th digit: 304.4
0. Unspecified
1. Continuous
2. Episodic
3. In remission

METRITIS (SEE ALSO 'ENDOMETRITIS')

615.9 NOS
615.0 Acute
615.1 Chronic

626.6 METRORRHAGIA
733.99 MEYENBURG-ALTHERR-UEHLINGER SYNDROME
759.89 MEYER-SCHWICKERATH AND WEYERS SYNDROME (DYSPLASIA OCULODENTODIGITALIS)

M

Acute myocardial infarction, 410.##, uses the following 5th digit subclassification.

0 "Episode of care unspecified": Use only when you have insufficient information to determine whether episode of care is initial or subsequent.

1 "Initial episode of care": Use to designate the acute phase of care, regardless of the location of treatment. This includes: 1) cases admitted to initial hospital 2) cases transferred for care or treatment or both 3) if transferred back to initial hospital during acute phase of care. Example: Acute MI admitted hospital 410.91, acute MI for heart catheter hospital 410.91, acute MI returned to hospital post, heart cath during acute phase of care 410.91, not during acute phase 410.92.

2 "Subsequent episode of care" Use to designate observation, treatment or evaluation of MI within 8 weeks of onset, but following the acute phase, or in the healing state where the episode of care may be for related or unrelated condition. Example: Patient admitted to hospital 4 weeks post acute MI for (PTCA) 410.92. Patient returned to hospital after (PTCA) angioplasty with stabilization of her MI. She has picked up virus infection in hospital. Diagnosis would be virus infection 079.99, acute MI, subsequent 410.92.

MI (MYOCARDIAL INFARCTION) ACUTE

STEMI (ST elevation)

410.9# Unspecified
410.0# Anterolateral
410.1# Anterior (wall)
410.1# Anterior other
410.1# Anteroapical
410.1# Anteroseptal
410.8# Atrium papillary or septum alone
410.5# Basolateral
410.4# Diaphragmatic
410.2# Inferolateral
410.3# Inferoposterior
410.4# Inferior wall
410.4# Inferior other
410.5# Lateral apical
410.5# Lateral other
410.6# Posterior (posterobasal)
410.3# Posteroinferior
410.5# Posterolateral

NSTEMI (non-ST elevation)

410.7# Non-Q wave
410.7# Nontransmural
410.7# Subendocardial
5th digit: 410.0-9
0. Episode unspecified
1. Initial episode
2. Subsequent episode

MI (MYOCARDIAL INFARCTION) ASSOCIATED DIAGNOSES

414.8 Chronic with symptoms > 8 weeks after infarction
412 Diagnosed on EKG
414.8 Diagnosed on EKG (old) presenting symptoms
V71.7 Evaluation, no MI found
412 History
411.1 Impending

MI (MYOCARDIAL INFARCTION) ASSOCIATED DIAGNOSES (continued)

When assigning a code for an intraoperative or postprocedural MI (Myocardial infarction), use an additional code for the acute MI to identify the specific site of of MI.

997.1 Intraoperative
0 Non-Q wave see, MI ('Myocardial Infarction) Acute', by site
412 Old
414.8 Old presenting symptoms
411.0 Post myocardial infarction syndrome
997.1 Postprocedural
0 Q wave see, 'MI (Myocardial Infarction) Acute', by site

757.39 MIBELLI'S DISEASE

MICE (JOINT)

718.1# NEC

5th digit: 718.1
0. Site NOS
1. Shoulder region
2. Upper arm (elbow) (humerus)
3. Forearm (radius) (wrist) (ulna)
4. Hand (carpal) (metacarpal) (fingers)
5. Pelvic region and thigh (hip) (buttock) (femur)
7. Ankle and/or foot (metatarsals) (toes) (tarsals)
8. Other specified sites
9. Multiple

717.6 Knee
724.9 Vertebral (facet)

282.49 MICHELI-RIETTE SYNDROME (THALASSEMIA MINOR)
721.5 MICHOTTE'S SYNDROME
742.1 MICRENCEPHALY CONGENITAL
362.14 MICROANEURYSMS RETINAL
795.39 MICROBIOLOGIC CULTURE NEC ABNORMAL
742.1 MICROCEPHALUS
744.82 MICROCHEILIA CONGENITAL
751.5 MICROCOLON CONGENITAL
743.41 MICROCORNEA
743.22 MICROCORNEA ASSOCIATED WITH BUPHTHALMOS
362.62 MICROCYSTOID DEGENERATION (RETINA)
758.33 MICRODELETION NEC
520.2 MICRODONTIA
282.49 MICRODREPANOCYTOSIS
362.33 MICROEMBOLISM RETINA SEE ALSO 'ATHEROEMBOLISM'
750.7 MICROGASTRIA DUPLICATION CONGENITAL
524.06 MICROGENIA
752.89 MICROGENITALIA (CONGENITAL)
191.9 MICROGLIOMA SITE NOS
0 MICROGLIOMA SITE SPECIFIED SEE 'CANCER', BY SITE M9710/3
750.16 MICROGLOSSIA CONGENITAL

MICROGNATHIA

524.00 Unspecified
756.0 Glossoptosis syndrome
524.04 Mandibular
524.74 Mandibular alveolar
524.03 Maxillary
524.73 Maxillary alveolar

742.2 MICROGYRIA CONGENITAL
516.2 MICROLITHIASIS PULMONARY ALVEOLAR
0 MICROORGANISMS RESISTANT TO DRUGS SEE 'DRUG RESISTANCE'
752.64 MICROPENIS CONGENITAL
743.36 MICROPHAKIA CONGENITAL

MICROPHTHALMOS

743.10 NOS (congenital)
743.11 Simple (congenital)
743.12 With other anomalies of eye and adnexa (congenital)

368.14 MICROPSIA
744.89 MICROSOMIA
110.9 MICROSPORIC TINEA
136.8 MICROSPORIDIA
111.1 MICROSPOROSIS NIGRA
110.# MICROSPORUM INFECTIONS

4th digit: 110
0. Scalp and beard
1. Nail (unguium)
2. Hand (manuum)
3. Groin and perianal (cruris)
4. Foot (pedis)
5. Body (corporus)
6. Deep seated (granuloma trichophyticum)
8. Other specified site
9. Unspecified site

744.84 MICROSTOMIA CONGENITAL
744.23 MICROTIA CONGENITAL
378.34 MICROTROPIA
0 MICROVASCULAR DISEASE – CODE TO CONDITION

MICTURITION

788.69 Disorder NEC
306.53 Disorder psychogenic
788.41 Frequency
788.43 Frequency nocturnal
788.1 Painful
306.53 Painful psychogenic

348.8 MIDBRAIN SYNDROME
344.89 MIDDLE ALTERNATING PARALYSIS

MIDDLE EAR

385.9 And mastoid disorder
385.89 And mastoid disorder other
959.09 Injury
382.2 Persistent mucosal disease (with posterior or superior marginal perforation of ear drum)

518.0 MIDDLE LOBE SYNDROME (LUNG) (RIGHT)
353.0 MIDDLE RADICULAR SYNDROME
524.29 MIDLINE DEVIATION
959.11 MIDTHORACIC REGION INJURY NOS

M

709.3 MIESCHER'S DISEASE OR SYNDROME-GRANULOMATOSIS DISCIFORMIS
701.2 MIESCHER'S SYNDROME-FAMILIAL ACANTHOSIS NIGRICANS
759.89 MIETEN'S SYNDROME

MIGRAINE

346.9# NOS
346.2# Abdominal
346.1# Atypical
346.2# Basilar
346.2# Bing Horton
346.0# Classic
346.2# Cluster
346.1# Common
346.8# Hemiplegic
346.2# Histamine
346.2# Lower half
625.4 Menstrual
346.8# Ophthalmoplegic
346.2# Retinal
346.0# Syndrome
346.2# Variant
346.0# With aura
346.0# With transient focal neurological phenomena
346.8# Other

5th digit: 346.0-2, 8
0. Without mention intractable migraine
1. With intractable migraine

V60.0 MIGRANT SOCIAL (HOMELESS PERSON)
770.7 MIKITY-WILSON SYNDROME (PULMONARY DYSMATURITY)
527.1 MIKULICZ'S DISEASE OR SYNDROME (DRYNESS OF MOUTH, DECREASED LACRIMATION)
783.42 MILESTONE DELAYED IN CHILDHOOD (LATE TALKER) (LATE WALKER)
705.1 MILIARIA RUBRA (TROPICALIS)
078.2 MILIARY FEVER
709.3 MILIA (UM) COLLOID
374.84 MILIA (UM) EYELID
706.2 MILIA (UM) SEBACEOUS SEE ALSO 'SEBACEOUS' CYST
275.42 MILK ALKALI SYNDROME (MILK DRINKERS')
690.11 MILK CRUST
423.1 MILK SPOTS PERICARDIUM
051.1 MILKERS' NODE
268.2 MILKMAN (-LOOSER) DISEASE OR SYNDROME (OSTEOMALACIA WITH PSEUDOFRACTURES)
344.89 MILLARD-GUBLER (MILLARD-GUBLER-FOVILLE) SYNDROME
758.33 MILLER-DIEKER SYNDROME
357.0 MILLER FISHER'S SYNDROME
268.2 MILLER'S DISEASE (OSTEOMALACIA)
335.29 MILL'S DISEASE
759.6 MILLES' SYNDROME (ENCEPHALOCUTANEOUS ANGIOMATOSIS)
757.0 MILROY'S DISEASE CONGENITAL (CHRONIC HEREDITARY EDEMA)
0 MIMA POLYMORPHA SEE 'BACTERIAL INFECTION' OR SPECIFIED CONDITION

985.0 MINAMATA DISEASE
500 MINERS' ASTHMA
727.2 MINER'S ELBOW
727.2 MINER'S KNEE

MINERAL

790.6 Abnormal blood level
269.3 Deficiency NEC
275.9 Metabolism disorder
275.8 Metabolism disorders other specified

255.41 MINERALOCORTICOID AND COMBINED GLUCOCORTICOID DEFICIENCY
255.42 MINERALOCORTICOID DEFICIENCY
282.0 MINKOWSKI CHAUFFARD SYNDROME
336.1 MINOR'S DISEASE
776.0 MINOT'S DISEASE (HEMORRHAGIC DISEASE NEWBORN)
379.42 MIOSIS PERSISTENT NOT DUE TO MIOTICS
576.2 MIRIZZI'S SYNDROME (HEPATIC DUCT STENOSIS)
0 MIRIZZI'S SYNDROME WITH CALCULUS, CHOLELITHIASIS OR STONES SEE 'CHOLEDOCHOLITHIASIS'
999.9 MISADVENTURE OF MEDICAL CARE
998.2 MISADVENTURE OF SURGERY (ACCIDENTAL PUNCTURE) OF ORGAN
0 MISCARRIAGE SEE 'ABORTION', SPONTANEOUS
365.83 MISDIRECTION AQUEOUS
313.1 MISERY OF CHILDHOOD AND ADOLESCENCE
632 MISSED ABORTION
632 MISSED ABORTION WITH COMPLICATION DURING TREATMENT [639.#]
639.# MISSED ABORTION WITH COMPLICATION FOLLOWING TREATMENT

4th digit: 639
0. Genital tract and pelvic infection
1. Delayed or excessive hemorrhage
2. Damage to pelvic organs and tissue
3. Renal failure
4. Metabolic disorders
5. Shock
6. Embolism
8. Other specified complication
9. Unspecified complication

656.4# MISSED DELIVERY (FETAL DEATH AFTER 22 WEEKS)

5th digit: 656.4
0. Episode of care NOS
1. Delivered with or without mention of antepartum condition
3. Antepartum condition

443.82 MITCHELL'S DISEASE (ERYTHROMELALGIA)
133.9 MITE INFESTATION
758.9 MITOCHONDRIAL CHROMOSOME ANOMALIES
277.87 MITOCHONDRIAL ENCEPHALOPATHY, LACTIC ACIDOSIS AND STROKE-LIKE EPISODES (MELAS SYNDROME)
277.87 MITOCHONDRIAL METABOLISM DISORDER
277.87 MITOCHONDRIAL NEUROGASTROINTESTINAL ENCEPHALOPATHY SYNDROME (MNGIE SYNDROME)

MITRAL (VALVE)

396.9 And aortic valve disease
396.8 And aortic valve disease multiple insufficiency and stenosis
746.89 Atresia
746.7 Atresia or hypoplasia of aortic orifice or valve, with hypoplasia of ascending aorta and defective development of left ventricle
785.2 Click (murmur) syndrome
394.9 Disease chronic
394.9 Failure
746.5 Fused congenital
0 Incompetence see 'Mitral Insufficiency'

INSUFFICIENCY

424.0 NOS
396.3 And aortic insufficiency (rheumatic)
396.2 And aortic stenosis (rheumatic)
421.0 Bacterial (acute) (chronic)
746.6 Congenital
394.1 Rheumatic
093.21 Syphilitic
396.3 With aortic valve disease

MITRAL (VALVE) (continued)

424.0 Prolapse disease or syndrome
0 Regurgitation see 'Mitral Insufficiency'

STENOSIS

394.0 NOS
396.1 And aortic insufficiency (rheumatic)
396.0 And aortic stenosis (rheumatic)
421.0 Bacterial (acute) (chronic)
746.5 Congenital
394.0 Rheumatic
093.21 Syphilitic
396.1 With aortic valve disease
394.2 With insufficiency (rheumatic)
421.0 With insufficiency bacterial (acute) (chronic)
093.21 With insufficiency syphilitic
394.2 With regurgitation
424.0 Other specified cause non rheumatic

625.2 MITTELSCHMERZ

0 MIXED FLORA SEE 'BACTERIAL INFECTION' OR SPECIFIED CONDITION

199.1 MIXED TUMOR MALIGNANT SITE NOS

0 MIXED TUMOR MALIGNANT SITE SPECIFIED SEE 'CANCER', BY SITE M8940/3

757.39 MLJET DISEASE (MAL DE MELEDA)

V06.4 MMR VACCINATION

277.87 MNGIE SYNDROME (MITROCHONDRIAL NEUROGASTROINTESTINAL ENCEPHALOPATHY SYNDROME)

426.13 MOBITZ (TYPE) I HEART BLOCK

426.12 MOBITZ (TYPE) II HEART BLOCK AV

346.8# MOBIUS' DISEASE OR SYNDROME (OPHTHALMOPLEGIC MIGRAINE)
5th digit: 346.8
0. Without mention intractable migraine
1. With intractable migraine

352.6 MOBIUS' SYNDROME (CONGENITAL OCULOFACIAL PARALYSIS)

267 MOELLER'S DISEASE (VITAMIN C DEFICIENCY)

529.4 MOELLER'S GLOSSITIS

759.89 MOHR'S SYNDROME (TYPES I AND II)

MOLAR PREGNANCY

631 NOS
631 NOS with complication during treatment **[639.#]**
639.# NOS with complication following treatment
4th digit: 639
0. Genital tract and pelvic infection
1. Delayed or excessive hemorrhage
2. Damage to pelvic organs and tissue
3. Renal failure
4. Metabolic disorders
5. Shock
6. Embolism
8. Other specified complication
9. Unspecified complication

631 Blighted ovum
631 Blighted ovum with complication during treatment **[639.#]**
639.# Blighted ovum with complication following treatment
4th digit: 639
0. Genital tract and pelvic infection
1. Delayed or excessive hemorrhage
2. Damage to pelvic organs and tissue
3. Renal failure
4. Metabolic disorders
5. Shock
6. Embolism
8. Other specified complication
9. Unspecified complication

631 Carneous mole
631 Carneous mole with complication during treatment **[639.#]**
639.# Carneous mole with complication following treatment
639.# Complication following molar pregnancy
4th digit: 639
0. Genital tract and pelvic infection
1. Delayed or excessive hemorrhage
2. Damage to pelvic organs and tissue
3. Renal failure
4. Metabolic disorders
5. Shock
6. Embolism
8. Other specified complication
9. Unspecified complication

631 Fleshy mole
631 Fleshy mole with complication during treatment **[639.#]**
639.# Fleshy mole with complication following treatment
630 Hydatidiform mole
236.1 Hydatidiform mole malignant
630 Hydatidiform mole with complication during treatment **[639.#]**
639.# Hydatidiform mole with complication following treatment
4th digit: 639
0. Genital tract and pelvic infection
1. Delayed or excessive hemorrhage
2. Damage to pelvic organs and tissue
3. Renal failure
4. Metabolic disorders
5. Shock
6. Embolism
8. Other specified complication
9. Unspecified complication

M

MOLAR PREGNANCY (continued)

631 Mole NOS
631 Mole NOS with complication during treatment [639.#]
639.# Mole NOS with complication following treatment
4th digit: 639
0. Genital tract and pelvic infection
1. Delayed or excessive hemorrhage
2. Damage to pelvic organs and tissue
3. Renal failure
4. Metabolic disorders
5. Shock
6. Embolism
8. Other specified complication
9. Unspecified complication

631 Stone mole
631 Stone mole with complication during treatment [639.#]
639.# Stone mole with complication following treatment
4th digit: 639
0. Genital tract and pelvic infection
1. Delayed or excessive hemorrhage
2. Damage to pelvic organs and tissue
3. Renal failure
4. Metabolic disorders
5. Shock
6. Embolism
8. Other specified complication
9. Unspecified complication

630 Trophoblastic disease NOS
630 Trophoblastic disease NOS with complication during treatment [639.#]
639.# Trophoblastic disease NOS with complication following treatment
4th digit: 639
0. Genital tract and pelvic infection
1. Delayed or excessive hemorrhage
2. Damage to pelvic organs and tissue
3. Renal failure
4. Metabolic disorders
5. Shock
6. Embolism
8. Other specified complication
9. Unspecified complicatioN

630 Vesicular mole
630 Vesicular mole with complication during treatment [639.#]
639.# Vesicular mole with complication following treatment
4th digit: 639
0. Genital tract and pelvic infection
1. Delayed or excessive hemorrhage
2. Damage to pelvic organs and tissue
3. Renal failure
4. Metabolic disorders
5. Shock
6. Embolism
8. Other specified complication
9. Unspecified complication

236.1 MOLE INVASIVE (PLACENTA)
0 MOLE PRODUCT OF CONCEPTION SEE 'MOLAR PREGNANCY'
0 MOLE SKIN BENIGN SEE 'BENIGN NEOPLASM', SKIN
0 MOLE SKIN MALIGNANT SEE 'MELANOMA BY SITE'
267 MOLLER'S DISEASE (INFANTILE SCURVY)
078.0 MOLLUSCUM CONTAGIOSUM

440.2# MONCKEBERG'S MEDIAL SCLEROSIS
440.2# MONCKEBERG'S MEDIAL SCLEROSIS WITH CHRONIC COMPLETE OR TOTAL OCCLUSION [440.4]
5th digit: 440.2
0. Unspecified
1. With intermittent claudication
2. With rest pain or rest pain and intermittent claudication
9. Other atherosclerosis extremities

> ***When coding atherosclerosis of the extremities use an additional code, if applicable to identify chronic complete or total occlusion of the artery of the extremities (440.4)***

440.24 MONCKEBERG'S MEDIAL SCLEROSIS WITH ISCHEMIC GANGRENE OR ISCHEMIC GANGRENE ULCERATION, OR ULCERATION AND INTERMITTENT CLAUDICATION, REST PAIN [707.#(#)]
440.23 MONCKEBERG'S MEDIAL SCLEROSIS WITH ULCERATION, OR ULCERATION AND INTERMITTENT CLAUDICATION, REST PAIN [707.#(#)]
4th or 4th and 5th digit: 707
1#. Lower limb except decubitus
10. Unspecified
11. Thigh
12. Calf
13. Ankle
14. Heel and midfoot
15. Other parts of foot, toes
19. Other
8. Chronic of other specified site
9. Chronic site NOS

440.3# MONCKEBERG'S MEDIAL SCLEROSIS BYPASS GRAFT
440.3# MONCKEBERG'S MEDIAL SCLEROSIS BYPASS GRAFT WITH CHRONIC COMPLETE OR TOTAL OCCLUSION [440.4]
5th digit: 440.3
0. Unspecified graft
1. Autologous vein bypass graft
2. Nonautologous biological bypass graft

744.05 MONDINI'S MALFORMATION (COCHLEA)
451.89 MONDOR'S DISEASE (THROMBOPHLEBITIS OF BREAST)
993.2 MONGE'S DISEASE
757.33 MONGOLIAN SPOT
758.0 MONGOLISM
757.4 MONILETHRIX CONGENITAL

MONILIASIS

771.7 Neonatal
112.1 Vulvovaginitis
0 See also 'Candidiasis'

057.8 MONKEYPOX
368.54 MONOCHROMATISM (CONE) (ROD)
075 MONOCYTIC ANGINA
V10.63 MONOCYTIC LEUKEMIA HISTORY
288.59 MONOCYTOPENIA
288.63 MONOCYTOSIS (SYMPTOMATIC)
378.34 MONOFIXATION SYNDROME

MONONEURITIS

355.9 NOS
378.54 Abducens (nerve)
352.4 Accessory nerve
388.5 Acoustic (8th nerve)
094.86 Acoustic syphilitic
353.0 Axillary nerve (nondiscogenic)
353.8 Costal region (nondiscogenic)
388.5 Eighth nerve
351.8 Facial nerve
352.1 Glossopharyngeal
274.89 Gouty [357.4]
355.79 Iliohypogastric
355.79 Ilioinguinal
355.8 Lower limb
355.79 Lower limb other
354.1 Median nerve
354.5 Multiplex
377.30 Ophthalmic
377.41 Optic (ischemic)
341.0 Optic in myelitis
377.30 Optic nerve
377.33 Optic nutritional
377.34 Optic toxic
355.5 Peritoneal
723.4 Radial (nerve)
094.85 Retrobulbar syphilitic
355.79 Saphenous
724.3 Sciatic (nerve)
351.8 Seventh nerve
723.4 Subscapular (nerve)
357.7 Toxic
350.8 Trigeminal
053.12 Trigeminal post herpetic
723.4 Ulnar (nerve)
354.9 Upper limb
354.8 Upper limb other
352.3 Vagus (nerve)
386.12 Vestibular
0 See also 'Neuropathy'

MONONUCLEOSIS

V01.79 Exposure
075 Infectious
075 Infectious with encephalitis [323.01]
075 Infectious with hepatitis [573.1]

MONOPLEGIA

344.5 NOS
306.0 Disorder psychogenic
344.3# Lower limb (old)
438.4# Lower limb (old) late effect of cerebrovascular disease
781.4 Transient
344.4# Upper limb (old)
438.3# Upper limb (old) late effect of cerebrovascular disease

5th digit: 344.3-4, 438.3-4
0. Unspecified side
1. Dominant side
2. Nondominant side

752.89 MONORCHISM CONGENITAL

MONSTER

740.0 Acephalic
759.4 Composite
759.4 Compound
759.4 Double
759.4 Twin
759.89 Specified type NEC
759.7 Single

813.03 MONTEGGIA'S FOREARM FRACTURE - CLOSED
813.13 MONTEGGIA'S FOREARM FRACTURE - OPEN
835.## MONTEGGIA'S HIP DISLOCATION

4th digit: 835
0. Closed
1. Open

5th digit: 835
0. Unspecified
1. Posterior
2. Obturator
3. Anterior

MOOD DISORDER

296.90 NOS
296.90 Episodic
296.99 Episodic other specified
296.99 Swings (psychosis)
0 See also 'Bipolar Disorder'
293.83 Transient in conditions classified elsewhere

345.5# MOORE'S SYNDROME

5th digit: 345.5
0. Without mention of intractable epilepsy
1. With intractable epilepsy

370.07 MOOREN'S ULCER (CORNEAL)
278.01 MORBID (SEVERE) OBESTIY
278.01 MORBID (SEVERE) OBESTIY WITH BODY MASS INDEX 25.0 AND ABOVE **[V85.#(#)]**

V85.#(#): These codes are for use in persons over 20 years old.

4th or 4th and 5th digit: V85
2#. 25-29
1. 25.0-25.9
2. 26.0-26.9
3. 27.0-27.9
4. 28.0-28.9
5. 29.0-29.9
3#. 30-39
0. 30.0-30.9
1. 31.0-31.9
2. 32.0-32.9
3. 33.0-33.9
4. 34.0-34.9
5. 35.0-35.9
6. 36.0-36.9
7. 37.0-37.9
8. 38.0-38.9
9. 39.0-39.9
4. 40 and over

799.9 MORBIDITY OR MORTALITY UNKNOWN CAUSE0
MORBILLI SEE 'MEASLES'
429.9 MORBUS CORDIS

295.9# MOREL-KRAEPELIN DISEASE (SEE ALSO 'SCHIZOPHRENIA')

5th digit: 295.9

0. NOS
1. Subchronic
2. Chronic
3. Subchronic with acute exacerbation
4. Chronic with acute
5. In remission

733.3 MOREL-MOORE SYNDROME (HYPEROSTOSIS FRONTALIS INTERNA)
733.3 MOREL-MORGAGNI SYNDROME (HYPEROSTOSIS FRONTALIS INTERNA)
426.9 MORGAGNI-ADAMS-STOKES SYNDROME (SYNCOPE WITH HEART BLOCK)
366.18 MORGAGNI CATARACT SENILE
733.3 MORGAGNI'S DISEASE (SYNDROME) (HYPEROSTOSIS FRONTALIS INTERNA)
607.3 MORNING PRIAPISM
643.0# MORNING SICKNESS

5th digit: 643.0

0. Episode of care unspecified or N/A
1. Delivered
3. Antepartum complication

317 MORON
701.0 MORPHEA
304.0# MORPHINE ADDICTION (DEPENDENT)

5th digit: 304.0

0. NOS
1. Continuous
2. Episodic
3. In remission

277.5 MORQUIO (-BRAILSFORD) (-ULLRICH) DISEASE OR SYNDROME (MUCOPOLYSACCHARIDOSIS IV)
259.5 MORRIS SYNDROME (TESTICULAR FEMINIZATION)
355.6 MORTON'S NEUROMA OR SYNDROME
336.0 MORVAN'S DISEASE
758.9 MOSAICISM, MOSAIC (CHROMOSOMAL)
758.5 MOSAICISM, MOSAIC AUTOSOMAL
758.81 MOSAICISM, MOSAIC SEX
446.6 MOSCHCOWITZ'S (-SINGER-SYMMERS) SYNDROME (THROMBOTIC THROMBOCYTOPENIC PURPURA)
0 MOSQUITO BITE SEE 'INSECT BITE NONVENOMOUS', BY SITE
V73.5 MOSQUITO BORNE DISEASE SCREENING EXAM

MOTION

0 Range (joint) limitation see 'Stiff, Stiffness', joint
994.6 Sickness - NOS
909.4 Sickness - late effect

315.4 MOTOR DEVELOPMENT DISORDER SPECIFIC
307.9 MOTOR DISORDER PSYCHOGENIC
335.20 MOTOR NEURON DISEASE (BULBAR) (MIXED TYPE)
335.29 MOTOR NEURON DISEASE OTHER
520.3 MOTTLED TEETH
732.5 MOUCHET'S DISEASE (JUVENILE OSTEOCHONDROSIS FOOT)

494.# MOUNIER-KUHN SYNDROME
519.19 MOUNIER-KUHN SYNDROME ACQUIRED
748.3 MOUNIER-KUHN SYNDROME CONGENITAL
494.# MOUNIER-KUHN SYNDROME WITH BRONCHIECTASIS

4th digit: 494

0. Without acute exacerbation
1. With acute exacerbation

993.2 MOUNTAIN SICKNESS
909.4 MOUNTAIN SICKNESS LATE EFFECT

MOUTH

528.3 Abscess
750.26 Anomalies other specified congenital
784.99 Breathing
524.59 Breathing malocclusion
528.2 Canker sore ulcer
528.00 Catarrh, catarrhal
528.3 Cellulitis
528.9 Denture sore
528.9 Disease (soft tissue)
528.9 Disease (soft tissue) other specified
523.8 Hyperplasia - gum
528.9 Hyperplasia - soft tissue NEC (inflammatory) (irritative) (mucosa)
529.8 Hyperplasia - tongue
528.00 Inflammation
959.09 Injury

MOVEMENT

781.0 Abnormal (dystonic) (involuntary)
655.7# Decrease fetal

5th digit: 655.7

0. Episode of care unspecified or N/A
1. Delivered
3. Antepartum complication

333.90 Disorder NEC
300.11 Disorder hysterical
333.90 Disorder medication induced NOS
780.58 Disorder sleep related unspecified
307.3 Disorder stereotypic (repetitive)
333.99 Disorder other
374.43 Paradoxical facial
327.51 Periodic limb disorder – sleep related
780.58 Sleep related unspecified
327.59 Sleep related other organic

437.5 MOYAMOYA DISEASE
V72.5 MRI
V09.0 MRSA (METHICILLIN RESISTANT STAPHYLOCOCCUS AUREUS)
340 MS
340 MS WITH DEMENTIA [294.1#]

5th digit: 294.1

0. Without behavioral disturbance or NOS
1. With behavioral disturbance

270.4 MTHFR (METHYLENETETRAHYDROFOLATE REDUCTASE DEFICIENCY)
066.3 MUCAMBO FEVER (VIRAL)
696.2 MUCHA'S (-HABERMAN) DISEASE OR SYNDROME (ACUTE PARAPSORIASIS VARIOLIFORMIS)
701.8 MUCINOSIS (CUTANEOUS) (PAPULAR)

199.1 MUCOCARCINOID TUMOR MALIGNANT SITE NOS
0 MUCOCARCINOID TUMOR MALIGNANT SITE SPECIFIED SEE 'CANCER', BY SITE M8243/3

MUCOCELE

543.9 Appendix
528.9 Buccal cavity
575.3 Gallbladder
375.43 Lacrimal
375.43 Orbit
527.6 Salivary gland
478.19 Sinus (nasal)
478.19 Sinus (nasal) accessory
478.19 Turbinate (middle) (nasal)
621.8 Uterus

446.1 MUCOCUTANEOUS LYMPH NODE SYNDROME (ACUTE) (FEBRILE) (INFANTILE) (MCLS)
564.9 MUCOENTERITIS

MUCOEPIDERMOID

199.1 Carcinoma site NOS
0 Carcinoma site specified see 'Cancer', by site M8430/3
238.9 Tumor site NOS
0 Tumor site specified see 'Neoplasm Uncertain Behavior', by site M8430/1

272.7 MUCOLIPIDOSIS (I) (II) (III) DISEASE
277.5 MUCOPOLYSACCHARIDE METABOLISM DISORDER
277.5 MUCOPOLYSACCHARIDOSIS
277.5 MUCOPOLYSACCHARIDOSIS CARDIOMYOPATHY [425.7]
277.5 MUCOPOLYSACCHARIDOSIS CEREBRAL DEGENERATION DISEASE OF CHILDHOOD [330.3]
117.7 MUCOR INFECTION

200.3# MUCOSA ASSOCIATED LYMPHOID TISSUE (MALT)
5th digit: 200.3
0. Unspecified site, extranodal and solid organ sites
1. Lymph nodes of head, face, neck
2. Lymph nodes intrathoracic
3. Lymph nodes abdominal
4. Lymph nodes axilla and upper limb
5. Lymph nodes inguinal region and lower limb
6. Lymph nodes intrapelvic
7. Spleen
8. Lymph nodes multiple sites

MUCOSITIS

528.00 NOS
528.3 Cellulitis and abscess of mouth
616.81 Cervix (ulcerative)
528.01 Due to antineoplastic therapy (ulcerative)
528.02 Due to other drugs (ulcerative)
538 Gastrointestinal (ulcerative)
0 Gingivitis see 'Gingivitis'
478.11 Nasal
288.09 Necroticans agranulocytica see also 'Agranulocytosis'
112.0 Oral thrush
695.1 Stevens-Johnson Syndrome
528.00 Ulcerative

MUCOSITIS (continued)

616.81 Vagina (ulcerative)
616.81 Vulva (ulcerative)
528.09 Other (ulcerative)

0 MUCOUS SEE 'MUCUS'
0 MUCOVISCIDOSIS SEE 'CYSTIC', FIBROSIS
792.1 MUCUS IN STOOL

For code 770.18, use an additional code to identify any secondary pulmonary hypertension (416.8), if applicable.

770.18 MUCUS ASPHYXIA OR SUFFOCATION NEWBORN
933.1 MUCUS PLUG (SEE ALSO 'ASPHYXIATION FOOD, MUCUS OR FOREIGN BODY INHALATION')
770.17 MUCUS PLUG ASPIRATION OF NEWBORN
519.19 MUCUS PLUG BRONCHIAL
519.19 MUCUS PLUG TRACHEOBRONCHIAL
770.18 MUCUS PLUG TRACHEOBRONCHIAL NEWBORN
079.81 MUERTO CANYON VIRUS
752.89 MULLERIAN DUCT CYST CONGENITAL
199.1 MULLERIAN MIXED TUMOR SITE NOS
0 MULLERIAN MIXED TUMOR SITE SPECIFIED SEE 'CANCER', BY SITE M8950/3
710.8 MULTIFOCAL FIBROSCLEROSIS (IDIOPATHIC) NEC
046.3 MULTIFOCAL LEUKOENCEPHALOPATHY

Elderly multigravida: Second or more pregnancy in a woman who will be 35 years of age or older at expected date of delivery.

659.6# MULTIGRAVIDA ELDERLY
5th digit: 659.6
0. Episode of care unspecified or N/A
1. Delivered
3. Antepartum complication

600.10 MULTINODULAR PROSTATE
600.11 MULTINODULAR PROSTATE WITH URINARY OBSTRUCTION (RETENTION)
763.89 MULTIPARITY AFFECTING FETUS OR NEWBORN
V61.5 MULTIPARITY CAUSING FAMILY CIRCUMSTANCE PROBLEM (REASON FOR ENCOUNTER)

659.4# MULTIPARITY GRAND
5th digit: 659.4
0. Episode of care unspecified or N/A
1. Delivered
3. Antepartum complication

V82.6 MULTIPHASIC SCREENING

MULTIPLE

919.0 Abrasions
919.1 Abrasions infected
260 Deficiency syndrome
V09.91 Drug resistant organism NOS (MDRO)
258.0# Endocrine neoplasia syndrome (MEN)
5th digit: 258.0
1. Type I
2. Type IIA
3. Type IIB
V18.11 Endocrine neoplasia syndrome (MEN) family history
V84.81 Endocrine neoplasia syndrome (MEN) susceptibility genetic

M

MULTIPLE (continued)

0	Gestation see 'Gestation', multiple
919.8	Injury other and unspecified superficial
919.9	Injury other and unspecified superficial infected
203.0#	Myeloma M9730/3
	5th digit: 203.0
	0. Without mention of remission
	1. In remission
301.51	Operation syndrome
300.14	Personality disorder
0	Pregnancy see 'Gestation', multiple
761.5	Pregnancy affecting fetus or newborn
340	Sclerosis
340	Sclerosis with dementia [**294.1#**]
	5th digit: 294.1
	0. Without behavioral disturbance or NOS
	1. With behavioral disturbance

MUMPS

072.9	Unspecified
072.2	Encephalitis
V01.79	Exposure
072.71	Hepatitis
072.1	Meningitis
072.2	Meningoencephalitis
072.0	Orchitis
072.3	Pancreatitis
072.9	Parotitis
072.72	Polyneuropathy
072.9	Uncomplicated
V04.6	Vaccination alone
072.8	With unspecified complication
072.79	With other specified complication

301.51	MUNCHAUSEN SYNDROME
728.11	MUNCHMEYER'S DISEASE OR SYNDROME (EXOSTOSIS LUXURIANS)
429.79	MURAL THROMBUS (ATRIAL) (VENTRICULAR) ACQUIRED FOLLOWING MYOCARDIAL INFARCTION <8 WEEKS [**410.##**]
	4th digit: 410
	0. Anterolateral
	1. Anterior (wall) anteroapical anteroseptal other anterior
	2. Inferolateral
	3. Inferoposterior
	4. Inferior other
	5. Lateral apical, basolateral, posterolateral, lateral other
	6. Posterior (posterobasal)
	7. Subendocardial
	8. Atrium papillary or septum alone
	9. Unspecified
	5th digit: 410
	0. Episode unspecified
	1. Initial episode
	2. Subsequent episode
429.79	MURAL THROMBUS (ATRIAL) (VENTRICULAR) ACQUIRED FOLLOWING MYOCARDIAL INFARCTION >8 WEEKS [414.8]
093.89	MURAL THROMBUS DUE TO SYPHILIS
412	MURAL THROMBUS HEALED OR OLD
0	MURCHISON-SANDERSON SYNDROME SEE 'HODGKIN'S DISEASE'
785.2	MURMUR HEART
283.2	MURRI'S DISEASE (INTERMITTENT HEMOGLOBINURIA)
062.4	MURRAY VALLEY ENCEPHALITIS

MUSCLE, MUSCULAR

756.81	Absence (pectoral) congenital
743.69	Absence eye (accessory) congenital
756.81	Absence with tendon absence congenital
756.82	Accessory congenital

ATROPHY

728.2	NOS (disuse)
335.21	Duchenne-Aran
728.2	Extremities
335.11	Familial spinal (juvenile)
728.2	General
335.0	Infantile spinal
356.1	Neuropathic
356.1	Peroneal
335.0	Progressive of infancy
335.21	Progressive pure
335.10	Spinal NOS
335.19	Spinal adult
335.0	Spinal infantile (progressive of infancy)
335.11	Spinal juvenile
335.19	Spinal other
095.6	Syphilitic

MUSCLE, MUSCULAR (continued)

728.10	Calcification and ossification
728.13	Calcification heterotopic postoperative
275.49	Calcium salt infiltrate
756.89	Contracture congenital
728.85	Contracture paralytic flaccid
958.6	Contracture posttraumatic
908.6	Contracture posttraumatic - late effect
728.85	Contracture NEC
729.82	Cramp (limb) (general)
994.1	Cramp due to immersion
300.11	Cramp hysterical
728.84	Diastasis
359.9	Disease
728.9	Disease inflammatory
728.9	Disorder
306.0	Disorder psychogenic
728.3	Disorder other specified
0	Division see 'Sprain', by site
0	Division with open wound see 'Laceration'

DYSTROPHY

359.1	NOS
359.0	Benign congenital myopathy
359.0	Congenital hereditary
359.1	Distal
359.1	Duchenne
359.1	Erb's
359.1	Fascioscapulohumeral
359.1	Gower's
359.1	Landouzy Dejerine
359.1	Limb girdle
359.21	Myotonic
359.22	Myotonic congenital
359.1	Ocular
359.1	Oculopharyngeal

MUSCLE, MUSCULAR (continued)

781.3 Incoordination
275.49 Infiltrate calcareous
728.83 Rupture nontraumatic
728.85 Spasm
728.87 Weakness (generalized)

955.4 MUSCULOCUTANEOUS NERVE INJURY

MUSCULOSKELETAL

729.89 Loss of function NEC
729.89 Symptoms in limbs other
781.99 Symptoms other
793.7 System abnormal (x-ray) (ultrasound) (thermography)
756.9 System anomaly (absence) congenital NEC
729.9 System disorder NEC
306.0 System disorder psychogenic

495.5 MUSHROOM WORKERS' LUNG

629.2# MUTILATION (CUTTING) GENITAL FEMALE STATUS
5th digit: 629.2
0. Unspecified
1. Type I (clitorectomy)
2. Type II (clitorectomy with excision of labia minora)
3. Type III (infibulation)
9. Type IV or other

MUTISM

309.83 Elective - adjustment reaction
300.11 Hysterical
313.23 Selective (elective) - emotional disturbance of childhood

V71.4 MVA EVALUATION NO APPARENT INJURY
424.0 MVP (MITRAL VALVE PROLAPSE)
751.3 MYA'S DISEASE (CONGENITAL DILATION COLON)
729.1 MYALGIA
710.5 MYALGIA EOSINOPHILIA SYNDROME
074.1 MYALGIA EPIDEMIC

MYASTHENIA

005.1 Botulani [358.1]
358.00 Gravis
358.00 Gravis pseudoparalytica
358.01 Gravis with (acute) exacerbation (crisis)
775.2 Gravis neonatal
244.# Hypothyroid [358.1]
4th digit: 244
0. Postsurgical
1. Postablative (irradiation)
2. Iodine ingestion
3. PAS, phenylbut, resorcinol
8. Secondary NEC
9. NOS

243 Hypothyroid congenital
358.1 Neoplastic
281.0 Pernicious anemia [358.1]
536.8 Stomach
306.4 Stomach psychogenic

MYASTHENIA (continued)

242.## Thyrotoxic [358.1]
4th digit: 242
0. Toxic diffuse goiter
1. Toxic uninodular goiter
2. Toxic multinodular goiter
3. Toxic nodular goiter unspecified
4. From ectopic thyroid nodule
8. Of other specified origin
9. Without goiter or other cause

5th digit: 242
0. Without storm
1. With storm

728.87 MYASTHENIC
117.4 MYCETOMAS MYCOTIC

MYCOBACTERIA

031.9 Atypical infection NOS
031.0 Avium infection pulmonary
031.2 Avium intracellulare complex infection disseminated (DMAC)
031.9 Diseases
031.1 Diseases cutaneous
031.0 Diseases pulmonary
031.8 Diseases other specified
031.0 Intracellulare (battey bacillus) infection
031.0 Kansasii infection
031.1 Marinum (M. Balnei) infection
031.1 Ulcerans infection

0 MYCOBACTERIUM LEPRAE INFECTION SEE 'LEPROSY'

0 MYCOPLASMA SEE 'BACTERIAL INFECTION' OR SPECIFIED CONDITION

MYCOSIS, MYCOTIC

117.9 Unspecified
111.9 Cutaneous NEC
202.1# Fungoides M9700/3
5th digit: 202.1
0. Unspecified site, extranodal and solid organ sites
1. Lymph nodes of head, face, neck
2. Lymph nodes intrathoracic
3. Lymph nodes abdominal
4. Lymph nodes axilla and upper limb
5. Lymph nodes inguinal region and lower limb
6. Lymph nodes intrapelvic
7. Spleen
8. Lymph nodes multiple sites

112.0 Mouth
117.4 Mycetomas
118 Opportunistic pathogenic to compromised hosts only
117.9 Pharynx
V75.4 Screening exam
111.9 Skin NEC
112.0 Stomatitis
117.9 Toenail
117.9 Tonsil
112.1 Vagina
117.9 Other

379.43 MYDRIASIS PERSISTENT NOT DUE TO MYDRIATICS
742.59 MYELATELIA CONGENITAL

M

136.9 MYELINOCLASIS PERIVASCULAR ACUTE (POSTINFECTIOUS) NEC [323.61]
323.51 MYELINOCLASIS PERIVASCULAR ACUTE (POSTINFECTIOUS) POSTIMMUNIZATION OR POSTVACCINAL
341.8 MYELINOSIS CENTRAL PONTINE

MYELITIS

323.9 NOS
341.20 Acute (transverse)
341.22 Acute (transverse) idiopathic
341.21 Acute (transverse) in conditions classified elsewhere
136.9 Due to infection classified elsewhere [323.42]
323.52 Due to vaccination (any)
323.02 Due to viral diseases classified elsewhere
054.74 Herpes simplex
053.14 Herpes zoster
341.22 Idiopathic transverse
323.2 In protozoal disease classified elsewhere
323.1 In rickettsial disease classified elsewhere
052.2 Postchickenpox
323.52 Postimmunization
136.9 Postinfectious [323.63]
323.52 Postvaccinal
052.2 Postvaricella
056.01 Rubella [323.02]
094.89 Syphilis [323.42]
989.9 Toxic [323.72]
323.82 Transverse NOS
341.22 Transverse idiopathic
013.6# Tuberculosis [323.72]

5th digit: 013.6
0. NOS
1. Lab not done
2. Lab pending
3. Microscopy positive (in sputum)
4. Culture positive - microscopy negative
5. Culture negative - microscopy positive
6. Culture and microscopy negative confirmed by other methods

756.89 MYELO-OSTEO-MUSCULODYSPLASIA HEREDITARIA

MYELOCELE

741.0# With hydrocephalus
741.9# Without hydrocephalus

5th digit: 741.0, 9
0. Region NOS
1. Cervical
2. Dorsal
3. Lumbar

MYELOCYSTOCELE

741.0# With hydrocephalus
741.9# Without hydrocephalus

5th digit: 741.0, 9
0. Region NOS
1. Cervical
2. Dorsal
3. Lumbar

742.59 MYELODYSPLASIA CONGENITAL
238.75 MYELODYSPLASTIC SYNDROME UNSPECIFIED
238.74 MYELODYSPLASTIC SYNDROME WITH 5Q DELETION
238.73 MYELODYSPLASTIC SYNDROME HIGH GRADE LESIONS
238.73 MYELODYSPLASTIC SYNDROME HIGH GRADE WITH 5Q DELETION
238.72 MYELODYSPLASTIC SYNDROME LOW GRADE LESIONS

289.83 MYELOFIBROSIS NOS
238.76 MYELOFIBROSIS IDIOPATHIC (CHRONIC)
238.79 MYELOFIBROSIS MEGAKARYOCYTIC
238.76 MYELOFIBROSIS PRIMARY
289.83 MYELOFIBROSIS SECONDARY
238.76 MYELOFIBROSIS WITH MYELOID METAPLASIA
289.89 MYELOID DYSPLASIA
V10.62 MYELOID LEUKEMIA HISTORY
289.89 MYELOID METAPLASIA
238.76 MYELOID METAPLASIA AGNOGENIC
238.76 MYELOID METAPLASIA MEGAKARYOCYTIC
288.09 MYELOKATHEXIS
214.9 MYELOLIPOMA SITE NOS
0 MYELOLIPOMA SITE SPECIFIED SEE 'BENIGN NEOPLASM', BY SITE M8870/0
203.0# MYELOMA M9730/3

5th digit: 203.0
0. Without mention of remission
1. In remission

238.6 MYELOMA SOLITARY UNCERTAIN BEHAVIOR M9731/1
203.0# MYELOMATOSIS M9730/3

5th digit: 203.0
0. Without mention of remission
1. In remission

338.0 MYELOPATHIC PAIN SYNDROME

If myelopathy is neoplastic, code the neoplasm first with the myelopathy second (336.3).

MYELOPATHY DISCOGENIC

722.70 Intervertebral NOS
722.71 Cervical
722.72 Dorsal thoracic
722.73 Lumbar

MYELOPATHY NONDISCOGENIC

336.9 Unspecified
336.8 Drug-induced
987.8 Due to carbon tetrachloride [323.72]
961.3 Due to hydroxyquinoline derivatives [323.72]
0 Due to infection see 'Encephalitis'
984.9 Due to lead [323.72]
985.0 Due to mercury [323.72]
0 Due to spondylosis see 'Spondylosis', by site with myelopathy
985.8 Due to thallium [323.72]
239.9 Neoplastic [336.3] see also 'Neoplasm', by site
281.0 Pernicious anemia [336.3]
336.8 Radiation-induced
336.1 Subacute necrotic
989.9 Toxic NEC [323.72]
323.82 Transverse see also 'Myelitis'
336.1 Vascular acute (embolism) (thrombosis) (infarction)
336.8 Other specified

M

284.2 MYELOPHTHISIS

MYELOPROLIFERATIVE

238.79 Disease or syndrome (chronic) site NOS M9960/1
0 Disease chronic site specified see 'Neoplasm Uncertain Behavior', by site M9960/1

MYELOSCLEROSIS

289.89 NOS
238.76 With myeloid metaplasia site NOS
0 With myeloid metaplasia site specified see 'Neoplasm Uncertain Behavior', by site M9961/1

207.0# MYELOSIS ERYTHREMIC (ACUTE)
5th digit: 207.0
0. Without mention of remission
1. With mention of remission

289.9 MYELOSUPPRESSION BONE MARROW DUE TO CHEMOTHERAPY

134.0 MYIASIS
600.20 MYOADENOMA PROSTATE

See 'LUTS' or 'Lower Urinary Tract Symptoms' for the additional code to identify the specific lower urinary tract symptoms.

600.21 MYOADENOMA PROSTATE WITH URINARY OBSTRUCTION, RETENTION OR OTHER LOWER URINARY TRACT SYMPTOMS

MYOCARDIAL

429.1 Atrophy
746.85 Bridge
861.01 Contusion
861.11 Contusion with open wound into thorax
277.39 Degeneration amyloid [425.7]
746.89 Degeneration congenital
429.1 Degeneration (fatty) (mural) (muscular) with arteriosclerosis [440.9]
779.89 Degeneration fetus or newborn
274.82 Degeneration gouty
402.#0 Degeneration hypertensive
4th digit: 402.#0
0. Malignant
1. Benign
9. Unspecified
402.#1 Degeneration hypertensive with heart failure **[428.#(#)]**
4th digit: 402.#1
0. Malignant
1. Benign
9. Unspecified

4th digit: 428
0. Congestive
1. Left
2#. Systolic
3#. Diastolic
4#. Combined systolic and diastolic
9. NOS

5th digit: 428.2-4
0. NOS
1. Acute
2. Chronic
3. Acute on chronic

MYOCARDIAL (continued)

0 Degeneration hypertensive with chronic kidney disease see 'Hypertensive', heart and chronic kidney disease with or without heart failure
093.82 Degeneration syphilitic
429.1 Degeneration with arteriosclerosis [440.9]
0 Degeneration see also 'Cardiomyopathy'
0 Disease see 'Cardiomyopathy'
V71.7 Evaluation no MI found
0 Failure see 'Heart Failure'
428.0 Insufficiency
429.4 Insufficiency due to cardiac prosthesis
997.1 Insufficiency post op immediate [428.0]
429.4 Insufficiency post op late
414.8 Ischemia (chronic)
411.89 Ischemia acute without MI
411.81 Ischemia acute without MI, with coronary (artery) occlusion
414.0# Ischemia chronic without MI, with coronary (artery) occlusion due to atherosclerosis
414.0# Ischemia chronic without MI, with coronary (artery) occlusion due to atherosclerosis with chronic complete or total occlusion [414.2]
5th digit: 414.0
0. Unspecified type of vessel, native or graft
1. Native coronary vessel
2. Autologous vein bypass graft
3. Nonautologous biological bypass graft
4. Autologous artery bypass graft (gastroepiploic) (internal mammary)
5. Unspecified type of bypass graft
6. Native vessel of transplanted heart
7. Bypass graft of transplanted heart

861.0# Laceration
861.1# Laceration with open wound into thorax
5th digit: 861.0-1
2. Without penetration of heart chambers
3. With penetration of heart chambers

0 Rupture (nontraumatic) see 'Myocardial Infarction Acute'
861.03 Rupture traumatic
861.13 Rupture traumatic with open wound into thorax

M

Acute myocardial infarction - 410.## - the following 5th digit subclassification is to be used with category 410.

0 - "Episode of care unspecified" - use only when you have insufficient information to determine whether episode of care is initial or subsequent.

1 - "Initial episode of care" - use to designate the acute phase of care, regardless of the location of treatment. This includes: 1) cases admitted to initial hospital 2) cases transferred for care or treatment or both 3) if transferred back to initial hospital during acute phase of care. Example: acute MI admitted hospital II - 410.91, acute MI for heart catheter hospital II - 410.91, acute MI returned to hospital I post, heart cath during acute phase of care - 410.91, not during acute phase - 410.92.

2 - "Subsequent episode of care" - use to designate observation, treatment or evaluation of MI within 8 weeks of onset, but following the acute phase, or in the healing state where the episode of care may be for related or unrelated condition. Example: patient admitted to hospital 4 weeks post acute MI for (PTCA) - 410.92. Patient returned to hospital I after (PTCA) angioplasty with stabilization of her MI. She has picked up virus infection in hospital II. Diagnosis would be virus infection 079.99, acute MI, subsequent 410.92.

MYOCARDIAL INFARCTION ACUTE

STEMI (ST elevation)

410.9# Unspecified
410.1# Anterior (wall) (contiguous with septum)
410.1# Anterior other (contiguous with septum)
410.1# Anteroapical (contiguous with septum)
410.0# Anterolateral
410.1# Anteroseptal (contiguous with septum)
410.8# Atrium papillary or septum alone
410.5# Basolateral
410.4# Diaphragmatic
410.4# Inferior (wall) (contiguous with septum)
410.2# Inferolateral
410.3# Inferoposterior
410.5# Lateral apical
410.5# Lateral high or posterior
410.6# Posterior true posterior (posterobasal)
410.5# Posterolateral

NSTEMI (non-ST elevation)

410.7# Non-Q wave
410.7# Nontransmural
410.7# Subendocardial

5th digit: 410.0-9
0. episode unspecified
1. Initial episode
2. Subsequent episode

MYOCARDIAL INFARCTION ASSOCIATED DIAGNOSES

414.8 Chronic with symptoms > 8 weeks after infarction
412 Diagnosed on EKG but presenting no symptoms
V71.7 Evaluation, no MI found
412 History
411.1 Impending

When assigning a code for an intraoperative or postprocedural MI (Myocardial infarction), use an additional code for the acute MI to identify the specific site of of MI.

997.1 Intraoperative

MYOCARDIAL INFARCTION ASSOCIATED DIAGNOSES (continued)

0 Non-Q wave see, 'Myocardial Infarction Acute', by site
412 Old
411.0 Post myocardial infarction syndrome
997.1 Postprocedural
0 Q wave see, 'Myocardial Infarction Acute', by site

If the diagnosis is not specified as acute on the record, the coder is required to select the chronic or NOS code. If the medical record indicates that the reason the patient sought care was due to an exacerbation of a chronic condition, consult the physician for further documentation.

MYOCARDITIS

429.0 Unspecified
422.90 Acute
422.92 Acute bacterial
422.91 Acute idiopathic
422.90 Acute interstitial
422.99 Acute other specified
429.0 Arteriosclerotic [440.9]
429.0 Chronic interstitial
425.4 Constrictive
422.91 Giant cell (acute) (subacute)
422.91 Granulomatous acute (isolated) (diffuse)
0 Hypertensive see 'Cardiomyopathy', hypertensive
422.91 Idiopathic granulomatous
422.92 Infective
487.8 Influenzal acute [422.0]
422.99 Malignant
036.43 Meningococcal
422.90 Nonrheumatic, active
422.90 Parenchymatous
422.92 Pneumococcal [041.2]
391.2 Rheumatic acute
398.0 Rheumatic chronic
422.92 Septic
422.92 Staphylococcal [041.1#]

5th digit: 041.1
0. NOS
1. Aureus
9. Other staph

391.2 Streptococcal [041.0#]

5th digit: 041.0
0. NOS
1. Group A
2. Group B
3. Group C
4. Group D (enterococcus)
5. Group G
9. Other strep

422.92 Suppurative
422.93 Toxic
422.91 Viral
074.23 Viral coxsackie
422.99 Other specified acute

MYOCARDITIS INFECTIOUS OR ASSOCIATED WITH OTHER DISEASES

074.23 Acute aseptic (of newborn)
422.99 Acute other
074.23 Aseptic newborn
074.23 Coxsackie
032.82 Diphtheria
422.91 Fiedler's

MYOCARDITIS INFECTIOUS OR ASSOCIATED WITH OTHER DISEASES (continued)

422.91 Giant cell acute
422.91 Granulomatous isolated (diffuse) acute
422.91 Idiopathic acute, subacute
093.82 Syphilis
130.3 Toxoplasmosis
017.9# Tuberculous acute [422.0]
5th digit: 017.9
0. Unspecified
1. Lab not done
2. Lab pending
3. Microscopy positive (in sputum)
4. Culture positive - microscopy negative
5. Culture negative - microscopy positive
6. Culture and microscopy negative confirmed by other methods

333.2 MYOCLONUS
333.2 MYOCLONUS FAMILIAL ESSENTIAL
277.87 MYOCLONUS WITH EPILEPSY AND WITH RAGGED RED FIBERS (MERRF SYNDROME)
421.9 MYOENDOCARDITIS (ACUTE) (SUBACUTE)
229.9 MYOEPITHELIOMA SITE NOS
0 MYOEPITHELIOMA SITE SPECIFIED SEE 'BENIGN NEOPLASM', BY SITE M8982/0
724.2 MYOFASCIAL PAIN LOWER BACK (MYOFASCIITIS)
729.1 MYOFASCIAL PAIN SYNDROME (MYOFASCITIS)
729.1 MYOFASCITIS (ACUTE)
724.2 MYOFASCITIS LOWER BACK
759.89 MYOFIBROMATOSIS INFANTILE

MYOFIBROSIS

728.2 NOS
726.2 Humeroscapular
726.2 Scapulohumeral

729.1 MYOFIBROSITIS
726.2 MYOFIBROSITIS SCAPULOHUMERAL
791.3 MYOGLOBINURIA (UNSPECIFIED)
351.8 MYOKYMIA FACIAL

MYOMA

215.# NOS M8895/0
4th digit: 215
0. Head, face, neck
2. Upper limb including shoulder
3. Lower limb including hip
4. Thorax
5. Abdomen (wall), gastric, gastrointestinal, intestine, stomach
6. Pelvis, buttock, groin, inguinal region, perineum
7. Trunk NOS, back NOS, flank NOS
8. Other specified sites
9. Site unspecified

218.9 Cervix unspecified
218.1 Cervix intramural
218.0 Cervix submucous
218.2 Cervix subserous

MYOMA (continued)

171.# Malignant M8811/3
4th digit: 171
0. Head, face, neck
2. Upper limb including shoulder
3. Lower limb including hip
4. Thorax
5. Abdomen (wall), gastric, gastrointestinal, intestine, stomach
6. Pelvis, buttock, groin, inguinal region, perineum
7. Trunk NOS, back NOS, flank NOS
8. Other specified sites
9. Site NOS

600.20 Prostate

See 'LUTS' or 'Lower Urinary Tract Symptoms' for the additional code to identify the specific lower urinary tract symptoms.

600.21 Prostate with urinary obstruction, retention or other lower urinary tract symptoms
218.9 Uterus unspecified
763.89 Uterus affecting fetus or newborn
763.1 Uterus causing obstructed labor affecting fetus or newborn
654.1# Uterus complicating pregnancy
660.2# Uterus complicating pregnancy causing obstructed labor [654.1#]
5th digit: 654.1
0. Episode of care NOS or N/A
1. Delivered
2. Delivered with postpartum complication
3. Antepartum complication
4. Postpartum complication

5th digit: 660.2
0. Episode of care NOS or N/A
1. Delivered
2. Delivered with postpartum complication
3. Antepartum complication

218.1 Uterus intramural
218.0 Uterus submucous
218.2 Uterus subserous

MYOMETRITIS (SEE ALSO 'ENDOMETRITIS')

615.9 NOS
615.0 Acute
615.1 Chronic
670.0# Maternal due to pregnancy
5th digit: 670.0
0. Unspecified
2. Delivered with postpartum complication
4. Postpartum complication

621.8 MYOMETRIUM ATROPHY
622.8 MYOMETRIUM ATROPHY CERVIX
040.0 MYONECROSIS, CLOSTRIDIAL

MYONEURAL

358.9 Disorders
358.8 Disorders other NEC
358.2 Disorders toxic

M

MYOPATHY

359.9 NOS
255.41 Addisonian [359.5]
277.39 Amyloid [359.6]
359.0 Benign congenital
359.0 Centronuclear
359.81 Critical illness
376.82 Extraocular muscles
252.01 Hyperparathyroidism [359.5]
253.2 Hypopituitary [359.5]
244.# Hypothyroid [359.5]
4th digit: 244
0. Postsurgical
1. Postablative (irradiation)
2. Iodine ingestion
3. PAS, phenylbut, resorcinol
8. Secondary NEC
9. NOS
359.89 Inflammatory
359.81 Intensive care
359.1 Limb-girdle
359.0 Myotubular
359.81 Necrotizing acute
359.1 Ocular (hereditary) (progressive)
446.0 Polyarteritis nodosa [359.6]
359.89 Primary
359.89 Progressive NEC
359.21 Proximal myotonic (PROMM)
359.81 Quadriplegic acute
714.0 Rheumatoid [359.6]
135 Sarcoid [359.6]
359.1 Scapulohumeral
710.1 Scleroderma [359.6]
242.## Thyrotoxic [359.5]
4th digit: 242
0. Toxic diffuse goiter
1. Toxic uninodular goiter
2. Toxic multinodular goiter
3. Toxic nodular goiter unspecified
4. From ectopic thyroid nodule
8. Of other specified origin
9. Without goiter or other cause
5th digit: 242
0. Without storm
1. With storm
359.4 Toxic
255.0 With Cushing's syndrome [359.5]
244.# With myxedema [359.5]
4th digit: 244
0. Postsurgical
1. Postablative (irradiation)
2. Iodine ingestion
3. PAS, phenylbut, resorcinol
8. Secondary NEC
9. NOS
359.89 Other

MYOPERICARDITIS

420.90 Acute
423.8 Chronic
391.0 Rheumatic acute
393 Rheumatic chronic

367.1 MYOPIA
360.21 MYOPIA MALIGNANT
360.21 MYOPIA PROGRESSIVE HIGH (DEGENERATIVE)

171.# MYOSARCOMA M8895/3
4th digit: 171
0. Head, face, neck
2. Upper limb including shoulder
3. Lower limb including hip
4. Thorax
5. Abdomen (wall), gastric, gastrointestinal, intestine, stomach
6. Pelvis, buttock, groin, inguinal region, perineum
7. Trunk NOS, back NOS, flank NOS
8. Other specified sites
9. Site NOS

MYOSITIS

729.1 NOS
040.0 Clostridial
074.1 Epidemic
728.0 Infective
728.81 Interstitial
729.1 Occupational
376.12 Orbital
728.19 Ossificans other
728.11 Ossificans progressive
728.12 Ossificans traumatic
729.1 Postural
728.0 Purulent
729.1 Rheumatoid
728.0 Suppurative
095.6 Syphilitic
729.1 Traumatic old
040.81 Tropical

MYOTONIA

728.85 NOS
359.21 Atrophica
359.22 Becker's Disease
359.22 Congenita (acetazolamide responsive) (dominant or recessive form)
359.22 Congenital chondrodystrophy
359.29 Disorder
359.24 Drug-induced
359.21 Dystrophica
359.29 Fluctuans
359.29 Levior
359.21 Muscular dystrophy
359.29 Paramyotonia congenital (of von Eulenburg)
359.29 Permanens
359.21 Proximal myopathy (PROMM)
359.23 Schwartz-Jampel Disease
359.21 Steinert's Disease
359.22 Thomsen's Disease
359.29 Other specified

359.0 MYOTUBULAR MYOPATHY

M

MYRINGITIS

384.00 Acute
384.09 Acute other specified
384.01 Bullosa hemorrhagic acute
384.1 Chronic
0 With otitis media see 'Otitis Media'

MYXEDEMA

244.9 NOS
244.# Adult
244.# Cerebellar ataxia [334.4]
244.# Cerebral degeneration [331.7]
243 Congenital
244.# Juvenile
293.0 Madness (acute) [**244.#**]
244.# Primary
4th digit: 244
0. Postsurgical
1. Postablative (irradiation)
2. Iodine ingestion
3. PAS, phenylbut, resorcinol
8. Secondary NEC
9. NOS

214.# MYXOLIPOMA M8852/0
4th digit: 214
0. Facial skin and subcutaneous tissue
1. Skin and subcutaneous tissue other
2. Intrathoracic organs
3. Intra-abdominal organs
4. Spermatic cord
8. Other specified sites
9. Unspecified site

MYXOMA

215.# NOS M8840/0
4th digit: 215
0. Head, face, neck
2. Upper limb including shoulder
3. Lower limb including hip
4. Thorax
5. Abdomen (wall), gastric, gastrointestinal, intestine, stomach
6. Pelvis, buttock, groin, inguinal region, perineum
7. Trunk NOS, back NOS, flank NOS
8. Other specified sites
9. Site unspecified

213.# Odontogenic M9320/0
4th digit: 213
0. Skull, face, upper jaw
1. Lower jaw

171.# MYXOSARCOMA M8840/3
4th digit: 171
0. Head, face, neck
2. Upper limb including shoulder
3. Lower limb including hip
4. Thorax
5. Abdomen (wall), gastric, gastrointestinal, intestine, stomach
6. Pelvis, buttock, groin, inguinal region, perineum
7. Trunk NOS, back NOS, flank NOS
8. Other specified sites
9. Site NOS

616.0 NABOTHIAN (GLAND) CYST OR FOLLICLE ECTROPION (NONOBSTETRICAL)
289.7 NADH [DPNH]-METHEMOGLOBIN-REDUCTASE DEFICIENCY CONGENITAL
287.1 NAEGELI'S DISEASE
136.2 NAEGLERIA MENINGOENCEPHALITIS
353.0 NAFFZIGER'S SYNDROME
756.0 NAGER-DE REYNIER SYNDROME (DYSOSTOSIS MANDIBULARIS)

NAIL

757.5 Absence congenital
703.8 Atrophy
757.5 Atrophy congenital
883.0 Avulsion finger or thumb
883.1 Avulsion finger or thumb complicated
893.0 Avulsion toe
893.1 Avulsion toe complicated
307.9 Biting
757.5 Clubnail congenital
757.5 Deformity - congenital (finger or toe)
703.8 Deformity - finger or toe
703.8 Deformity - spongiform
703.8 Discoloration
703.9 Disease unspecified
703.8 Disease other specified NEC
703.8 Hypertrophy
681.9 Infection
681.02 Infection finger (paronychia or onychia)
681.11 Infection toe (paronychia or onychia)
703.0 Ingrowing with infection
959.5 Injury finger
959.7 Injury toe
756.89 Patella (hereditary osteo-onychodysplasia)
703.8 Thickening

066.1 NAIROBI SHEEP DISEASE
691.0 NAPKIN DERMATITIS (RASH)
301.81 NARCISSISTIC PERSONALITY DISORDER

NARCOLEPSY

347.00 NOS
347.01 NOS with cataplexy

When using codes 347.10 and 347.11, code first the underlying condition.

347.10 In conditions elsewhere classified
347.11 In conditions elsewhere classified with cataplexy

786.09 NARCOSIS CO 2 (RESPIRATORY)
763.5 NARCOSIS DUE TO DRUG (CORRECTLY ADMINISTERED) AFFECTING FETUS OR NEWBORN
763.5 NARCOTIC REACTION (INTOXICATION) MATERNAL DURING L&D AFFECTING FETUS OR NEWBORN
760.72 NARCOTIC TRANSMITTED VIA PLACENTA OR BREAST MILK AFFECTING FETUS OR NEWBORN
748.0 NARES ATRESIA (CONGENITAL)
748.0 NARES STENOSIS CONGENITAL
277.87 NARP SYNDROME (NEUROPATHY, ATAXIA AND RETINITIS PIGMENTOSA SYNDROME)

0 NASAL SEE 'NOSE, NASAL'
0 NASOGASTRIC TUBE ENCOUNTER - CODE SPECIFIED CONDITION

NASOLACRIMAL DUCT

743.65 Anomaly or atresia congenital
375.56 Obstruction
743.65 Obstruction congenital
375.55 Obstruction neonatal
375.56 Stenosis acquired

526.1 NASOPALATINE CYST

NASOPHARYNGEAL

478.29 Abscess
748.8 Atresia
472.2 Atrophy
478.21 Cellulitis
478.26 Cyst
478.20 Disease
478.29 Disease other specified
478.25 Edema
959.09 Injury
478.29 Obstruction
478.29 Ulcer

NASOPHARYNGITIS

460 NOS
460 Acute (common cold)
460 Acute due to RSV (respiratory syncytial virus) [079.6]
460 Acute infective
472.2 Chronic
460 Infective
460 Subacute
034.0 Streptococcal
472.2 Suppurative (chronic)
472.2 Ulcerative chronic
472.1 With chronic pharyngitis

787.02 NAUSEA
787.01 NAUSEA WITH VOMITING
771.4 NAVEL CORD INFECTION PERINATAL
779.89 NAVEL DISEASE NEWBORN NEC
367.1 NEAR SIGHTEDNESS
780.2 NEAR-SYNCOPE
253.3 NEBECOURT'S SYNDROME
371.01 NEBULA CORNEA
743.43 NEBULA CORNEA CONGENITAL
743.42 NEBULA CORNEA CONGENITAL INTERFERING WITH VISION
126.1 NECATOR AMERICANUS INFECTION
126.9 NECATORIASIS

NECK

900.9 Blood vessel NOS injury
900.82 Blood vessel NEC injury - multiple
900.89 Blood vessel NEC injury - specified NEC
719.88 Calcification (cervical)
723.5 Contracture, see also 'Torticollis'
V48.1 Deficiency
738.2 Deformity acquired
744.9 Deformity congenital
744.89 Deformity congenital other specified

N

NECK (continued)

V48.7	Disfigurement
723.9	Disorder (neck region) (musculoskeletal)
959.09	Injury
925.2	Injury crush
910.8	Injury other and unspecified superficial
910.9	Injury other and unspecified superficial infected
723.1	Pain (nondiscogenic)
V48.9	Problem
V48.7	Problem disfigurement
V48.3	Problem mechanical and motor
V48.5	Problem sensory
V48.8	Problem other
0	See also 'Cervical'
847.0	Separation (rupture) (tear) (laceration)
723.5	Spasm
723.5	Stiff
847.0	Strain (sprain) (avulsion) (hemarthrosis)
784.2	Swelling, mass or lump
784.99	Symptom other
744.5	Webbing congenital

437.8	NECRENCEPHALUS
040.3	NECROBACILLOSIS
799.89	NECROBIOSIS
709.3	NECROBIOSIS LIPOIDICA
250.8#	NECROBIOSIS LIPOIDICA DIABETICORUM [709.3]

5th digit: 250.8

0. Type II, adult-onset, non-insulin dependent (even if requiring insulin), or unspecified; controlled

1. Type I, juvenile-onset or insulin-dependent; controlled

2. Type II, adult-onset, non-insulin dependent (even if requiring insulin); uncontrolled

3. Type I, juvenile-onset or insulin-dependent; uncontrolled

NECROSIS

785.4	NOS
567.82	Abdominal wall fat
255.8	Adrenal (capsule) (gland)
478.19	Antrum nasal sinus
441.9	Aortic (hyaline)
441.0#	Aortic dissecting cystic medial

5th digit: 441.0

0. Site NOS

1. Thoracic

2. Abdominal

3. Thoracoabdominal

441.5	Aortic ruptured
446.0	Arteritis
447.5	Artery

> ***731.3: Use an additional code to identify major osseous defect, if applicable.***

733.40	Aseptic - bone site NOS
733.42	Aseptic - femur head and neck
733.43	Aseptic - femur medial condyle
733.42	Aseptic - femur other
733.41	Aseptic - humerus (head)
733.45	Aseptic – jaw
733.44	Aseptic - talus
733.49	Aseptic - other bone site
0	Avascular see 'Necrosis', aseptic, by site

NECROSIS (continued)

596.8	Bladder (aseptic) (sphincter)
730.0#	Bone acute NOS

5th digit: 730.0

0. Site NOS

1. Shoulder region

2. Upper arm (elbow) (humerus)

3. Forearm (radius) (wrist) (ulna)

4. Hand (carpal) (metacarpal) (fingers)

5. Pelvic region and thigh (hip) (buttock) (femur)

6. Lower leg (fibula) (knee) (patella) (tibia)

7. Ankle and/or foot (metatarsals) (toes) (tarsal)

8. Other (head) (neck) (rib) (skull) (trunk)

9. Multiple

0	Bone aseptic see 'Necrosis', aseptic
730.1#	Bone due to osteomyelitis chronic (see also 'Osteomyelitis')

5th digit: 730.1

0. Site NOS

1. Shoulder region

2. Upper arm (elbow) (humerus)

3. Forearm (radius) (wrist) (ulna)

4. Hand (carpal) (metacarpal) (fingers)

5. Pelvic region and thigh (hip) (buttock) (femur)

6. Lower leg (fibula) (knee) (patella) (tibia)

7. Ankle and/or foot (metatarsals) (toes) (tarsal)

8. Other (head) (neck) (rib) (skull) (trunk)

9. Multiple

731.0	Bone due to Paget's disease
0	Bone due to tuberculosis see 'Tuberculosis', bone
0	Bone epiphyseal ischemic see 'Osteochondrosis'
478.19	Bone ethmoid (nose)
733.40	Bone ischemic
526.4	Bone jaw
733.45	Bone jaw aseptic
289.89	Bone marrow
437.8	Brain
611.3	Breast (aseptic) (fat) (segmental)
519.19	Bronchus
437.8	Central nervous system NEC
437.8	Cerebellar
437.8	Cerebral NOS
742.4	Cerebral congenital
437.8	Cerebrospinal
557.0	Colon
371.40	Cornea
521.09	Dental
0	Due to radiation/radium see 'Necrosis', by site
0	Due to swallowing corrosive substance see 'Burn', by site
983.9	Due to poisoning by phosphorus compounds
0	Due to tuberculosis see 'Tuberculosis'
385.24	Ear (ossicle)
0	Epiphyseal ischemic see 'Osteochondrosis'
530.89	Esophagus
478.19	Ethmoid (bone)
374.50	Eyelid

NECROSIS (continued)

272.8 Fatty (generalized)
567.82 Fatty abdominal wall
611.3 Fatty breast
569.89 Fatty intestine
567.82 Fatty mesentery
567.82 Fatty omentum
577.8 Fatty pancreas
567.82 Fatty peritoneum
709.3 Fatty skin (subcutaneous)
778.1 Fatty skin (subcutaneous) newborn
733.42 Femur (aseptic) (avascular)
733.42 Femur (aseptic) (avascular) - head
733.43 Femur (aseptic) (avascular) - medial condyle
733.42 Femur (aseptic) (avascular) - neck
575.0 Gallbladder (see also 'Cholecystitis' acute)
537.89 Gastric

> ***646.6#: Specify the maternal genital necrosis with an additional code.***

646.6# Genital organ or tract maternal complicating pregnancy
5th digit: 646.6
0. Episode of care unspecified or N/A
1. Delivered
2. Delivered with postpartum complication
3 Antepartum complication
4 Postpartum complication

478.79 Glottis
0 Heart (myocardial) (subendocardial) see 'Myocardial Infarction Acute'
570 Hepatic (see also 'Necrosis', liver)
733.42 Hip aseptic (avascular) (see also 'Necrosis', femur)
557.0 Intestine
785.4 Ischemic (see also 'Gangrene')
583.9 Kidney NOS (bilateral)
584.9 Kidney acute
583.6 Kidney cortical
584.6 Kidney cortical - acute
760.1 Kidney cortical - acute affecting fetus or newborn
646.2# Kidney cortical - acute complicating pregnancy [584.6]
5th digit: 646.2
0. Episode of care unspecified or N/A
1. Delivered
2. Delivered with postpartum complication
3. Antepartum complication
4. Postpartum complication

639.3 Kidney cortical - acute following abortion
639.3 Kidney cortical - acute following ectopic pregnancy
669.3# Kidney cortical - acute following labor and delivery
5th digit: 669.3
0. Episode of care unspecified or N/A
2. Delivered with postpartum complication
4. Postpartum complication

639.3 Kidney cortical - acute following molar pregnancy
0 Kidney cortical - acute with abortion see 'Abortion', by type, with renal failure
0 Kidney cortical - acute with ectopic pregnancy see 'Ectopic Pregnancy', by site with complication
0 Kidney cortical - acute with molar pregnancy see 'Molar Pregnancy', by type with complication

NECROSIS (continued)

590.80 Kidney medullary (see also 'Pyelonephritis')
584.7 Kidney medullary - acute renal failure
583.7 Kidney medullary - in glomerulonephritis NOS
584.5 Kidney tubular
760.1 Kidney tubular - affecting fetus or newborn
646.2# Kidney tubular - complicating pregnancy [584.5]
5th digit: 646.2
0. Episode of care unspecified or N/A
1. Delivered
2. Delivered with postpartum complication
3. Antepartum complication
4. Postpartum complication

997.5 Kidney tubular - due to a procedure
639.3 Kidney tubular - following abortion
639.3 Kidney tubular - following ectopic pregnancy
669.3# Kidney tubular - following labor and delivery
5th digit: 669.3
0. Episode of care unspecified or N/A
2. Delivered with postpartum complication
4. Postpartum complication

639.3 Kidney tubular - following molar pregnancy
958.5 Kidney tubular - traumatic
0 Kidney tubular - with abortion see 'Abortion', by type, with renal failure
0 Kidney tubular - with ectopic pregnancy see 'Ectopic Pregnancy', by site, with complication
0 Kidney tubular - with molar pregnancy see 'Molar Pregnancy', by type, with complication
478.79 Larynx
570 Liver (acute) (congenital) (diffuse) (massive) (subacute)
760.8 Liver afffecting fetus or newborn
646.7# Liver complicating pregnancy [570]
5th digit: 646.7
0. Episode of care unspecified or N/A
1. Delivered
3. Antepartum complication

639.8 Liver following abortion
639.8 Liver following ectopic pregnancy
639.8 Liver following molar pregnancy
674.8# Liver maternal due to pregnancy
5th digit: 674.8
0. Episode of care unspecified or N/A
2. Delivered with postpartum complication
4. Postpartum complication

639.8 Liver postabortal
573.3 Liver toxic (noninfectious)
0 Liver with abortion see 'Abortion', by type, with other specified complication
0 Liver with ectopic pregnancy see 'Ectopic Pregnancy', by site with complication
0 Liver with molar pregnancy see 'Molar Pregnancy', by type with complication
513.0 Lung
683 Lymphatic gland
611.3 Mammary gland
526.4 Mandible
383.1 Mastoid (chronic)
557.0 Mesentery
567.82 Mesentery fat
0 Mitral valve see 'Mitral Insufficiency'

N

NECROSIS (continued)

478.19 Nasal (septum)
478.19 Nasal sinus (antrum)
557.0 Omentum
567.82 Omentum fat
557.0 Omentum with mesenteric infarction
376.10 Orbit
385.24 Ossicles, ear (aseptic)
614.2 Ovary (see also 'Salpingo-oophoritis')
577.8 Pancreas (aseptic) (duct) (fat)
577.0 Pancreas acute (aseptic) (duct) (fat)
577.0 Pancreas infective (aseptic) (duct) (fat)
590.80 Papillary kidney (see also 'Pyelonephritis')
624.8 Perineum
557.0 Peritoneum
567.82 Peritoneum fat
557.0 Peritoneum with mesenteric infarction
462 Pharynx
288.09 Pharynx in granulocytopenia
253.2 Pituitary (gland) (postpartum) (sheehan)
656.7# Placenta affecting management of mother

5th digit: 656.7

0. Episode of care unspecified or N/A
1. Delivered
3. Antepartum complication

513.0 Pneumonia
513.0 Pulmonary
537.89 Pylorus
0 Radiation/radium (due to) see 'Necrosis', by site
0 Renal see 'Necrosis', kidney
379.19 Sclera
608.89 Scrotum
709.8 Skin or subcutaneous tissue
709.8 Skin or subcutaneous tissue due to burn see 'Burn', by site
785.4 Skin or subcutaneous tissue gangrenous
336.1 Spinal cord
730.18 Spine, spinal (column) acute
289.59 Spleen
537.89 Stomach
528.1 Stomatitis
709.3 Subcutaneous fat
778.1 Subcutaneous fat fetus or newborn
255.8 Suprarenal (capsule) (gland)
521.09 Tooth
522.1 Tooth pulp
608.89 Testes
254.8 Thymus (gland)
474.8 Tonsil
519.19 Trachea
0 Tuberculous see 'Tuberculosis'
584.5 Tubular (acute)
997.5 Tubular (acute) due to a procedure
762.6 Umbilical cord affecting fetus or newborn
623.8 Vagina

NECROSIS (continued)

730.18 Vertebra (acute) (lumbar)
015.0# Vertebral column due to tuberculosis [730.8#]

5th digit: 015.0

0. NOS
1. Lab not done
2. Lab pending
3. Microscopy positive (in sputum)
4. Culture positive - microscopy negative
5. Culture positive - microscopy positive
6. Culture and microscopy negative - confirmed by other methods

5th digit: 730.8

0. Site NOS
1. Shoulder region
2. Upper arm (elbow) (humerus)
3. Forearm (radius) (wrist) (ulna)
4. Hand (carpal) (metacarpal) (fingers)
5. Pelvic region and thigh (hip) (buttock) (femur)
6. Lower leg (fibula) (knee) (patella) (tibia)
7. Ankle and/or foot (metatarsals) (toes) (tarsal)
8. Other (head) (neck) (rib) (skull) (trunk)
9. Multiple

624.8 Vulva
0 X-ray see 'Necrosis', by site

288.09 NECROTICANS AGRANULOCYTICA MUCOSITIS SEE ALSO 'AGRANULOCYTOSIS'
777.5 NECROTIZING ENTEROCOLITIS IN FETUS OR NEWBORN
0 NECROTIZING FASCIITIS SEE 'FASCIITIS', NECROTIZING
584.7 NECROTIZING RENAL PAPILLITIS
446.4 NECROTIZING RESPIRATORY GRANULOMATOSIS
0 NEGLECT SEE 'ABUSE', ADULT OR CHILD
759.89 NEILL DINGWALL SYNDROME (MICROENCEPHALY AND DWARFISM)
359.0 NEMALINE BODY DISEASE
128.9 NEMATODE INFESTATION NEC CONJUNCTIVA
0 NEONATAL SEE SPECIFIED CONDITION
0 NEOPLASM BENIGN SEE 'BENIGN NEOPLASM', BY SITE
0 NEOPLASM IN SITU SEE 'CARCINOMA IN SITU', BY SITE
0 NEOPLASM MALIGNANT SEE 'CANCER', BY SITE
0 NEOPLASM METASTATIC SEE 'CANCER', BY SITE, METASTATIC.

Symptoms of a neoplasm such as pain or nausea should not replace the neoplasm code. Sequence the neoplasm first and the neoplasm or tumor related pain code second.

N

NEOPLASM UNCERTAIN BEHAVIOR - QUICK REFERENCE

235.# Digestive and respiratory

4th digit: 235

- **0. Salivary glands, major**
- **1. Lip, oral cavity, pharynx**
- **2. Stomach, intestines, rectum**
- **3. Liver, biliary passages, gallbladder**
- **4. Peritoneum, retroperitoneum**
- **5. Other and NOS digestive organs**
- **6. Larynx**
- **7. Trachea, bronchus, lung**
- **8. Pleura, thymus, lung**
- **9. Other and NOS respiratory organs**

236.#(#) Genitourinary

4th or 4th and 5th digit: 236

- **0. Uterus**
- **1. Placenta**
- **2. Ovary**
- **3. Other and NOS female genital organs**
- **4. Testes**
- **5. Prostate**
- **6. Other and NOS male genital organs**
- **7. Bladder**
- **9#. Other and NOS urinary organs**
  - **90. Urinary organ, unspecified**
  - **91. Kidney and ureter**
  - **99. Other specified**

237.#(#) Endocrine and nervous system

4th or 4th and 5th digit: 237

- **0. Pituitary and craniopharyngeal duct**
- **1. Pineal**
- **2. Adrenal, suprarenal**
- **3. Paraganglia (aortic, carotid, coccygeal, bodies), glomus jugulare**
- **4. Parathyroid, thyroid, other and NOS glands**
- **5. Brain and spinal cord**
- **6. Meninges**
- **7#. Neurofibromatosis**
  - **70. Not otherwise specified**
  - **71. Type 1**
  - **72. Type 2**
- **9. Cranial nerves, other and unspecified parts of the nervous system**

238.#(#) Other and unspecified sites

4th or 4th and 5th digit: 238

- **0. Bone and articular cartilage**
- **1. Connective and other soft tissue**
- **2. Skin**
- **3. Breast**
- **4. Polycythemia vera**
- **5. Histiocytic and mast cells**
- **6. Plasma cells**
- **7# Other lymphatic and hemopoietic tissues**
  - **1. Essential thrombocythemia**
  - **2. Low grade myelodysplastic syndrome lesions**
  - **3. High grade myelodysplastic syndrome lesions**
  - **4. Myelodysplastic syndrome with 5Q deletion**
  - **5. Myelodysplastic syndrome unspecified**
- **8. Eye, heart, other specified**
- **9. Site unspecified**

0 Benign see 'Benign Neoplasm', by site M8000/0

NEOPLASM UNCERTAIN BEHAVIOR - QUICK REFERENCE (continued)

203.8# Immunoproliferative

5th digit: 203.8

- **0. Without mention of remission**
- **1. In remission**

> ***Neoplasm uncertain behavior is coded when the ultimate behavior of the neoplasm cannot be determined as to whether it is benign or malignant by the pathologist.***

NEOPLASM UNCERTAIN BEHAVIOR

237.2	Adrenal gland
235.3	Ampulla of Vater
235.5	Anal canal
235.5	Anus NOS
238.2	Anus skin (margin) (perianal)
237.3	Aortic body
235.1	Aryepiglottic fold
235.6	Aryepiglottic fold laryngeal aspect
235.3	Bile ducts
235.3	Biliary passages
236.7	Bladder
238.0	Bone
237.5	Brain
238.2	Breast - skin
238.3	Breast - soft tissue
235.7	Bronchus
237.3	Carotid body
238.0	Cartilage NOS
238.0	Cartilage - articular
238.1	Cartilage - ear
238.1	Cartilage - eyelid
235.6	Cartilage - larynx
235.9	Cartilage - nose
237.5	Cerebellopontine angle
237.6	Cerebral meninges
236.0	Cervix stump
236.1	Chorioadenoma (Destruens)
237.3	Coccygeal body
238.8	Conjunctiva
238.1	Connective tissue
238.8	Cornea
237.9	Cranial nerve (central)
237.0	Craniopharyngeal duct
235.5	Digestive organs unspecified other
238.2	Ear external
238.1	Ear external cartilage
235.9	Ear internal
237.4	Endocrine
235.6	Epiglottis
235.5	Esophagus
238.8	Eye
238.1	Eyelid cartilage
238.1	Eyelid connective tissue
238.2	Eyelid skin
235.3	Gallbladder
238.1	Ganglia
236.3	Genital organs NEC - female
236.6	Genital organs NEC - male
235.1	Gingiva
237.3	Glomus jugular

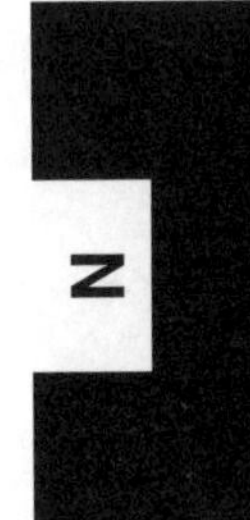

NEOPLASM UNCERTAIN BEHAVIOR (continued)

238.8 Heart
238.5 Histiocytic
235.1 Hypopharynx
235.2 Intestines
236.91 Kidney
235.6 Larynx
235.1 Lip
238.2 Lip skin
235.3 Liver
235.7 Lung
238.5 Mast cell
235.8 Mediastinum
237.6 Meninges
235.9 Middle ear
235.1 Mouth
235.1 Mouth gingiva
235.9 Nasal cavity
238.2 Nasal skin
235.1 Nasopharynx
238.1 Nerve - parasympathetic, peripheral, sympathetic
237.9 Nervous system other and unspecified (central)
237.7# Neurofibromatosis

5th digit: 237.7
0. NOS or multiple
1. Type I
2. Type II

235.1 Oral cavity
235.1 Oropharynx
236.2 Ovary
235.5 Pancreas
237.3 Paraganglia
237.4 Parathyroid
235.0 Parotid
238.8 Pericardium
235.4 Peritoneum
235.1 Pharynx
237.1 Pineal gland
237.0 Pituitary
236.1 Placenta
238.6 Plasma cell
235.8 Pleura
236.5 Prostate
235.2 Rectum
235.9 Respiratory organs other and NOS
235.4 Retroperitoneum
235.1 Salivary gland (minor)
235.0 Salivary glands major
235.9 Sinus (accessory)
238.2 Skin NOS
238.2 Skin anus
238.2 Skin breast
236.3 Skin genitalia - female
236.6 Skin genitalia - male
235.1 Skin lip (border) (vermilion)
238.1 Soft tissue site unspecified
237.5 Spinal cord
237.6 Spinal meninges
235.5 Spleen
235.2 Stomach

NEOPLASM UNCERTAIN BEHAVIOR (continued)

235.0 Sublingual gland
235.0 Submandibular gland
237.2 Suprarenal gland
238.1 Synovia
236.4 Testis
235.8 Thymus
237.4 Thyroid
235.1 Tongue
235.7 Trachea
235.7 Tracheobronchial
236.91 Ureter
236.90 Urinary organ unspecified
236.99 Urinary organ other
236.0 Uterus
236.3 Vaginal
236.2 Vesicovaginal
236.3 Vesicovaginal septum
235.6 Vocal cords (true) (false)
235.0 Wharton's duct
237.3 Zuckerkandl's organ
238.9 Other sites and tissues

NEOPLASM UNSPECIFIED NATURE - QUICK REFERENCE

239.# NOS

4th digit: 239
0. Digestive system, anal
1. Respiratory system
2. Bone, soft tissue, skin, (anal skin margin)
3. Breast
4. Bladder
5. Other genitourinary
6. Brain
7. Endocrine glands and other parts of nervous system
8. Other specified sites
9. Site unspecified

Neoplasm unspecified nature is coded when the behavior or the morphology is unspecified.

NEOPLASM UNSPECIFIED NATURE

239.9 Site unspecified
239.0 Anus
239.2 Anus margin skin perianal
239.4 Bladder
239.2 Bone
238.79 Bone marrow
239.6 Brain
239.7 Brain meninges
239.3 Breast
239.2 Breast skin
239.2 Cartilage NOS
239.1 Cartilage larynx
239.1 Cartilage nasal
239.9 Cells site unspecified
239.6 Cerebellopontine angle
239.8 Conjunctiva
239.2 Connective tissue
239.8 Cornea
239.7 Cranial nerves
239.0 Digestive system

N

NEOPLASM UNSPECIFIED NATURE (continued)

239.2 Ear external
239.8 Ear internal
239.7 Endocrine
239.2 Eyelid (skin of)
239.2 Ganglia
239.5 Genital
239.5 Genitourinary other specified
239.2 Great vessels
238.79 Hematopoietic tissue
239.1 Larynx
239.0 Lip vermilion border
238.79 Lymphatic tissues
239.7 Meninges
239.2 Nerves - peripheral/sympathic/parasympathic
239.7 Nerves - other specified
239.1 Nose
239.7 Optic nerve
239.8 Pericardium
239.1 Respiratory system
239.2 Skin NOS
239.5 Skin genital (female) (male)
239.2 Soft tissue
239.7 Spinal cord
239.0 Tongue
239.1 Tracheobronchial
239.5 Urinary tract
239.5 Vagina
239.5 Vesicovaginal septum
239.1 Vocal cords (true) (false)
239.5 Vulva
239.0 Wharton's duct
239.8 Other specified sites

334.4 NEOPLASTIC CEREBELLAR ATAXIA
117.4 NEOTESTUDINA ROSATII INFECTION
364.42 NEOVASCULARIZATION OF IRIS OR CILIARY BODY
V45.89 NEPHRECTOMY STATUS

NEPHRITIS

583.# NOS
4th digit: 583
0. Proliferative
1. Membranous
2. Membranoproliferative, hypocomplementemic persistent, lobular, mesangiocapillary, mixed membranous and proliferative
4. Rapidly progressive, necrotizing
6. With cortical necrosis
7. With medullary (papillary) necrosis
9. Unspecified lesion in kidney

580.# Acute
4th digit: 580
0. Proliferative or post streptococcal
4. Rapidly progressive necrotizing, extracapillary with epithelial crescents
9. Unspecified or hemorrhagic

NEPHRITIS (continued)

582.# Chronic
4th digit: 582
0. Proliferative
1. Membranous sclerosing, focal, segmental hyalinosis
2. Membranoproliferative, endothelial, hypocomplementemic persistent, lobular, mesangiocapillary, mixed membranous and proliferative
4. Rapidly progressive, necrotizing
9. Unspecified or hemorrhagic

581.# Nephrotic syndrome in glomerulonephritis
4th digit: 581
0. Proliferative
1. Membranous, epimembranous, idiopathic membranous, focal, sclerosing, segmental hyalinosis
2. Membranoproliferative, endothelial, hypocomplementemic persistent, lobular, mesangiocapillary, mixed membranous and proliferative
3. Minimal change, foot process disease, lipoid
9. Unspecified

NEPHRITIS DUE TO OTHER CAUSES

277.39 Amyloid NOS [583.81]
277.39 Amyloid chronic [582.81]
277.39 Amyloidosis [583.81]
277.39 Amyloidosis chronic [582.81]
583.89 Analgesic
0 Arteriolar (arteriosclerotic) see 'Hypertensive', chronic kidney disease
590.80 Ascending see also 'Pyelitis'
582.9 Atrophic
583.89 Basement membrane NEC
446.21 Basement membrane with pulmonary hemorrhage (Goodpasture's syndrome) [583.81]
592.0 Calculous, calculus
0 Cardiac, cardiovascular see 'Hypertensive', heart and chronic kidney disease
587 Cirrhotic
580.9 Croupous
250.4# Diabetic (nephropathy) [583.81]
250.4# Diabetic (nephropathy) with nephrotic syndrome [581.81]
5th digit: 250.4
0. Type II, adult-onset, non-insulin dependent (even if requiring insulin), or unspecified; controlled
1. Type I, juvenile-onset or insulin-dependent; controlled
2. Type II, adult-onset, non-insulin dependent (even if requiring insulin); uncontrolled
3. Type I, juvenile-onset or insulin-dependent; uncontrolled

032.89 Diphtheritic [580.81]
984.9 Due to lead
421.0 Endocarditis bacterial subacute (due to) [580.81]
585.6 End state (chronic) (terminal)
581.1 Epimembranous
583.89 Exudative NOS
580.89 Exudative acute
582.89 Exudative chronic
581.89 Exudative with nephrotic syndrome

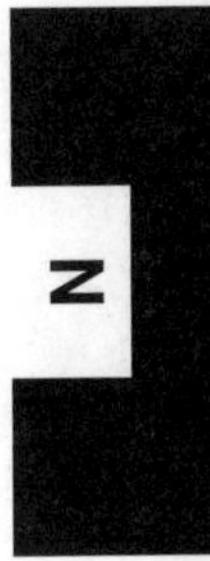

NEPHRITIS DUE TO OTHER CAUSES (continued)

098.19 Gonococcal infection (acute) [583.81]
098.39 Gonococcal infection chronic or lasting over two months [583.81]
274.10 Gouty
274.11 Gouty nephrolithiasis (uric acid stones) [582.81]
759.89 Hereditary
277.31 Hereditary amyloid
588.89 Hypercalcemic
0 Hypertensive (chronic) (interstitial) see 'Hypertensive', chronic kidney disease
588.89 Hypokalemic
583.9 IgA
583.89 Immune complex NEC
590.80 Infective see also 'Pyelonephritis'
583.89 Interstitial (diffuse) (focal) NOS
580.89 Interstitial (diffuse) (focal) acute
582.89 Interstitial (diffuse) (focal) chronic
581.89 Interstitial (diffuse) (focal) with nephrotic syndrome
984.9 Lead (toxic)
583.2 Lobular (hypocomplement) (mixed)
710.0 Lupus NOS [583.81]
710.0 Lupus acute [580.81]
710.0 Lupus chronic [582.81]
760.0 Maternal hypertension affecting fetus or newborn
760.1 Maternal renal disease affecting fetus or newborn
642.1# Maternal with hypertension complicating pregnancy

5th digit: 642.1
- **0. Episode of care unspecified or N/A**
- **1. Delivered**
- **2. Delivered with postpartum complication**
- **3. Antepartum complication**
- **4. Postpartum complication**

> ***646.2#: Specify the maternal nephritis with an additional code.***

646.2# Maternal without hypertension complicating pregnancy

5th digit: 646.2
- **0. Episode of care unspecified or N/A**
- **1. Delivered**
- **2. Delivered with postpartum complication**
- **3. Antepartum complication**
- **4. Postpartum complication**

072.79 Mumps (due to) [580.81]
581.89 Parenchymatous
753.12 Polycystic NOS
753.13 Polycystic adult type
753.13 Polycystic autosomal dominant
753.14 Polycystic autosomal childhood type (CPKD)
753.14 Polycystic autosomal infantile type
753.14 Polycystic autosomal recessive
588.89 Potassium depletion
588.89 Protein-losing
590.80 Purulent see also 'Pyelonephritis'
583.9 Renal necrosis
583.6 Renal necrosis cortical
583.7 Renal necrosis medullary (papillary)

NEPHRITIS DUE TO OTHER CAUSES (continued)

593.9 Salt losing
584.9 Saturnine
V81.5 Screening
590.80 Septic see also 'Pyelonephritis'
710.0 SLE (systemic lupus erythematosus) [583.81]
583.89 Specified pathology NEC
580.89 Specified pathology acute
582.89 Specified pathology chronic
581.89 Specified pathology with nephrotic syndrome
590.80 Staphylococcal see also 'Pyelonephritis'
039.8 Streptotrichosis [583.81]
581.9 Subacute
590.80 Suppurative
095.4 Syphilitic (late)
095.5 Syphilitic congenital [583.81]
091.69 Syphilitic early [583.81]
585.6 Terminal NEC (end-stage) (chronic)
584.5 Toxic see also 'Nephritis'
016.0# Tuberculosis [583.81]

5th digit: 016.0
- **0. NOS**
- **1. Lab not done**
- **2. Lab pending**
- **3. Microscopy positive (in sputum)**
- **4. Culture positive - microscopy negative**
- **5. Culture negative - microscopy positive**
- **6. Culture and microscopy negative confirmed by other methods**

002.0 Typhoid with nephrotic syndrome [581.81]
002.0 Typhoid fever acute [580.81]
580.9 War
588.89 Water-losing
581.9 With edema
581.89 With glomerulonephritis

NEPHROBLASTOMA

189.0 Site NOS
0 Site specified see 'Cancer', by site M8960/3
189.0 Epithelial site NOS
0 Epithelial site specified see 'Cancer', by site M8961/3
189.0 Mesenchymal site NOS
0 Mesenchymal site specified see 'Cancer', by site M8962/3

275.49 NEPHROCALCINOSIS

592.0 NEPHROLITHIASIS
274.11 NEPHROLITHIASIS URIC ACID

236.99 NEPHROMA MESOBLASTIC SITE NOS
0 NEPHROMA MESOBLASTIC SITE SPECIFIED SEE 'NEOPLASM UNCERTAIN BEHAVIOR' BY SITE M8960/1

753.16 NEPHRONOPTHISIS
0 NEPHROPATHY SEE ALSO 'NEPHRITIS'
593.0 NEPHROPTOSIS

N

NEPHROSCLEROSIS

587 NOS (senile)
274.10 Gouty
0 Hyperplastic see 'Hypertensive', chronic kidney disease
0 Hypertensive see 'Hypertensive', chronic kidney disease

NEPHROSIS

581.9 NOS
250.4# Diabetic [581.81]
5th digit: 250.4
0. Type II, adult-onset, non-insulin dependent (even if requiring insulin), or unspecified; controlled
1. Type I, juvenile-onset or insulin-dependent; controlled
2. Type II, adult-onset, non-insulin dependent (even if requiring insulin); uncontrolled
3. Type I, juvenile-onset or insulin-dependent; uncontrolled

759.89 Finnish type (congenital)
581.3 Lipoid
084.9 Malarial [581.81]
588.89 Osmotic (sucrose)
078.6 Syndrome with epidemic fever

When coding an infection of an ostomy, use an additional code to specify the organism. See 'Bacterial Infection'.

NEPHROSTOMY

V55.6 Care
V55.6 Catheter adjustment or repositioning
V55.6 Catheter removal or replacement
V55.6 Closure
996.39 Complication device mechanical
997.5 Complication stoma
997.5 Malfunction
V55.6 Removal or change
V44.6 Status
V55.6 Toilet stoma

NEPHROTIC SYNDROME

581.# NOS
4th digit: 581
0. Proliferative
1. Membranous (sclerosing) (hyalinosis)
2. Membranoproliferative (lobular) (hypocomplement)
3. Minimal change
9. Unspecified

277.39 Amyloid [581.81]
250.4# Diabetic [581.81]
5th digit: 250.4
0. Type II, adult-onset, non-insulin dependent (even if requiring insulin), or unspecified; controlled
1. Type I, juvenile-onset or insulin-dependent; controlled
2. Type II, adult-onset, non-insulin dependent (even if requiring insulin); uncontrolled
3. Type I, juvenile-onset or insulin-dependent; uncontrolled

NEPHROTIC SYNDROME (continued)

V13.03 History
710.0 Lupus (due to) [581.81]
084.9 Malarial [581.81]
446.0 Polyarteritis (due to) [581.81]
078.6 With epidemic hemorrhagic fever
581.89 With glomerulonephritis and nephritis (exudative) (interstitial) (diffuse)

NERVE

742.8 Absence (atrophy) congenital
742.8 Agenesis congenital
742.9 Anomaly
742.8 Anomaly NEC
355.9 Disorder NEC
355.79 Disorder - lower limb
354.8 Disorder - upper limb
0 Division see 'Nerve Injury', by site
996.2 Graft (peripheral) complication (mechanical)
996.63 Graft (peripheral) infection or inflammation
0 Injury see 'Nerve Injury'
0 Laceration see 'Nerve Injury', by specified site
0 Pinched see 'Neuropathy', entrapment
353.9 Root and plexus disorder (nondiscogenic)
353.8 Root and plexus disorders other (nondiscogenic)
794.10 Stimulation abnormal response

NERVE INJURY

957.9 Unspecified nerve
951.3 Abducens
951.6 Accessory
951.5 Acoustic
955.0 Axillary
953.4 Brachial plexus
767.6 Brachial plexus birth trauma
954.1 Celiac ganglion or plexus
953.0 Cervical root
954.0 Cervical sympathetic
951.# Cranial
4th digit: 951
0. Oculomotor (3rd)
1. Trochlear (4th)
2. Trigeminal (5th)
3. Abducens (6th)
4. Facial (7th)
5. Acoustic (8th)
6. Accessory (11th)
7. Hypoglossal (12th)
8. Other: glossopharyngeal (9th), olfactory (1st), pneumogastric (10th), vagus (10th)
9. Unspecified

950.0 Cranial optic (2nd nerve)
956.4 Cutaneous sensory, lower limb
955.5 Cutaneous sensory, upper limb
955.6 Digital
953.1 Dorsal root
951.5 Eighth cranial
951.6 Eleventh cranial
951.4 Facial
767.5 Facial birth trauma
956.1 Femoral
951.2 Fifth cranial
951.8 First cranial
951.1 Fourth cranial

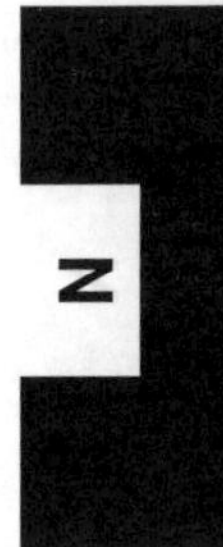

NERVE INJURY (continued)

951.8 Glossopharyngeal
957.0 Head and neck superficial
951.7 Hypoglossal
954.1 Inferior mesenteric plexus
907.9 Late effect - unspecified nerve
907.1 Late effect - cranial
907.3 Late effect - nerve root(s)
907.5 Late effect - pelvic girdle and lower limb peripheral
907.4 Late effect - shoulder girdle and upper limb peripheral
907.3 Late effect - spinal plexus
907.3 Late effect - trunk nerve
907.9 Late effect - other specified nerve
953.2 Lumbar root
953.5 Lumbosacral plexus
955.1 Median
954.1 Mesenteric plexus inferior
957.8 Multiple nerves NOS
953.8 Multiple nerve root sites
956.8 Multiple nerves of pelvic girdle and lower limb
955.8 Multiple nerves of shoulder girdle and upper limb
955.4 Musculocutaneous
951.8 Ninth cranial
951.0 Oculomotor
951.8 Olfactory
950.# Optic nerve and pathways

4th digit: 950
0. Optic nerve injury (2nd cranial nerve)
1. Optic chiasm
2. Optic pathways
3. Visual cortex
9. Unspecified

956.# Pelvic girdle and lower limb (peripheral nerves)

4th digit: 956
0. Sciatic
1. Femoral
2. Posterior tibial
3. Peroneal
4. Cutaneous sensory nerve, lower limb
5. Other specified
8. Multiple
9. Unspecified

956.3 Peroneal
951.8 Pneumogastric
956.2 Posterior tibial
955.3 Radial
953.# Roots and spinal plexus injury

4th digit: 953
0. Cervical root
1. Dorsal root
2. Lumbar root
3. Sacral root
4. Brachial plexus
5. Lumbosacral plexus
8. Multiple sites
9. Unspecified site

953.3 Sacral root
956.0 Sciatic
950.0 Second cranial
951.4 Seventh cranial

NERVE INJURY (continued)

955.# Shoulder girdle and upper limb (peripheral nerves)

4th digit: 955
0. Axillary
1. Median
2. Ulnar
3. Radial
4. Musculocutaneous
5. Cutaneous sensory nerve, upper limb
6. Digital
7. Other specified
8. Multiple
9. Unspecified

951.3 Sixth cranial
953.9 Spinal root
954.1 Splanchnic
954.1 Stellate ganglion
951.8 Tenth cranial
951.0 Third cranial
956.2 Tibial posterior
951.2 Trigeminal
951.1 Trochlear
954.9 Trunk - NOS
954.1 Trunk - celiac ganglion or plexus
954.0 Trunk - cervical sympathetic
954.1 Trunk - inferior mesenteric plexus
954.1 Trunk - splanchnic
954.1 Trunk - stellate ganglion
954.1 Trunk - other sympathetic
954.8 Trunk - other specified
951.7 Twelfth cranial
955.2 Ulnar
951.8 Vagus
951.8 Other specified cranial
956.5 Other specified pelvic girdle and lower limb
955.7 Other specified shoulder girdle and upper limb
954.8 Other specified trunk nerves
957.1 Other specified nerves

799.2 NERVES

NERVOUS SYSTEM

742.8 Absence (atrophy) congenital
742.9 Anomaly
V76.81 Cancer screening
349.1 Complication from surgically implanted device - nonmechanical
997.00 Complication postoperative immediate NOS
997.01 Complication postoperative immediate central nervous system (anoxic brain damage) (cerebral hypoxia)
997.02 Complication postoperative immediate CVA (stroke) (brain hemorrhage)
997.09 Complication postoperative immediate other specified
742.9 Deformity congenital
349.89 Degeneration
<u>277.39</u> Degeneration <u>amyloid</u> [357.4]
V53.09 Device (fitting and adjustment) (removal) (replacement)
996.63 Device, implant or graft (internal prosthetic) complication - infection or inflammation
996.2 Device, implant or graft complication - mechanical
996.75 Device, implant or graft (internal prosthetic) complication - other

NERVOUS SYSTEM (continued)

349.9 Disorder (central) NEC
337.9 Disorder - autonomic (peripheral)
352.9 Disorder - cranial
337.9 Disorder - parasympathetic
337.9 Disorder - sympathetic
337.9 Disorder - vegetative
V12.40 Disorder history NOS
V12.49 Disorder history other
349.89 Disorders other specifed NEC
781.99 Symptom other specified

799.2 NERVOUSNESS

757.1 NETHERTON'S SYNDROME (ICHTHYOSIFORM ERYTHRODERMA)

708.8 NETTLE RASH

757.33 NETTLESHIP'S DISEASE CONGENITAL (URTICARIA PIGMENTOSA)

694.4 NEUMANN'S DISEASE (PEMPHIGUS VEGETANS)

NEURALGIA

0 See also 'Neuritis'
729.2 Unspecified (acute) (rheumatic)
352.4 Accessory (nerve)
388.5 Acoustic (nerve)
355.8 Ankle
355.8 Anterior crural
787.99 Anus or rectum
723.4 Arm
388.5 Auditory (nerve)
353.0 Axilla
788.1 Bladder
723.4 Brachial
0 Brain see 'Neuralgia', cranial nerve
625.9 Broad ligament
0 Cerebral see 'Neuralgia' cranial nerve
346.2# Ciliary

5th digit: 346.2
0. Without mention intractable migraine
1. With intractable migraine

CRANIAL NERVE

352.9 NOS
352.0 First
377.49 Second
378.51 Third partial
378.52 Third total
378.53 Fourth
350.1 Fifth or trigeminal
378.54 Sixth
351.9 Seventh NEC
388.5 Eighth
352.2 Ninth
352.3 Tenth
352.4 Eleventh
352.5 Twelfth
352.6 Multiple

NEURALGIA (continued)

388.71 Ear
352.1 Ear middle
351.8 Facial
354.9 Finger
355.8 Flank
355.8 Foot
354.9 Forearm
350.1 Fothergill's
053.12 Fothergill's postherpetic
352.1 Glossopharyngeal (nerve)
355.8 Groin
354.9 Hand
355.8 Heel
346.2# Horton's

5th digit: 346.2
0. Without mention intractable migraine
1. With intractable migraine

053.11 Hunt's
352.5 Hypoglossal (nerve)
355.8 Iliac region
350.1 Infraorbital
355.8 Inguinal
353.8 Intercostal (nerve)
053.19 Intercostal (nerve) postherpetic
352.1 Jaw
788.0 Kidney
355.8 Knee
355.8 Loin
0 Malarial see 'Malaria'
385.89 Mastoid
352.1 Maxilla
354.1 Median thenar
355.6 Metatarsal
352.1 Middle ear
346.2# Migrainous

5th digit: 346.2
0. Without mention intractable migraine
1. With intractable migraine

355.6 Morton's
0 Nerve cranial see 'Neuralgia', cranial nerve
0 Nerve other specified see nerve by specific name, disorder
352.0 Nose
723.8 Occipital
352.0 Olfactory (nerve)
377.30 Ophthalmic
053.19 Ophthalmic postherpetic
377.30 Optic (nerve)
607.9 Penis
355.8 Perineum
511.0 Pleura
053.19 Postherpetic NEC
053.11 Postherpetic geniculate ganglion
053.19 Postherpetic ophthalmic
053.12 Postherpetic trifacial
053.12 Postherpetic trigeminal
355.8 Pubic region
723.4 Radial (nerve)
787.99 Rectum

N

NEURALGIA (continued)

724.3	Sacroiliac joint
724.3	Sciatic (nerve)
608.9	Scrotum
608.9	Seminal vesicle
354.9	Shoulder
337.0	Sluder's
608.9	Spermatic cord
337.0	Sphenopalatine (ganglion)
723.4	Subscapular (nerve)
723.4	Suprascapular (nerve)
608.89	Testis
354.1	Thenar (median)
355.8	Thigh
352.5	Tongue
350.1	Trifacial
350.1	Trigeminal (nerve)
053.12	Trigeminal (nerve) postherpetic
388.71	Tympanic plexus
723.4	Ulnar (nerve)
352.3	Vagus (nerve)
354.9	Wrist
300.89	Writers'
333.84	Writers' organic

353.5	NEURALGIC AMYOTROPHY (NONDISCOGENIC)
300.5	NEURASTHENIA
780.79	NEURASTHENIA POSTFEBRILE
780.79	NEURASTHENIA POSTVIRAL

NEURILEMMOMA

225.1	Acoustic (nerve) benign
192.0	Acoustic (nerve) malignant M9560/3
215.#	Benign M9560/0
171.#	Malignant M9560/3

4th digit: 171, 215
0. Head, face, neck
2. Upper limb including shoulder
3. Lower limb including hip
4. Thorax
5. Abdomen (wall), gastric, gastrointestinal, intestine, stomach
6. Pelvis, buttock, groin, inguinal region, perineum
7. Trunk NOS, back NOS, flank NOS
8. Other specified sites
9. Site NOS

171.9	NEURILEMMOSARCOMA SITE NOS
0	NEURILEMMOSARCOMA SITE SPECIFIED SEE 'CANCER', BY SITE SOFT TISSUE M9560/3
238.1	NEURINOMATOSIS SITE NOS
0	NEURINOMATOSIS SITE SPECIFIED SEE 'NEOPLASM UNCERTAIN BEHAVIOR', BY SITE M9560/1

NEURITIS

0	See also 'Neuralgia'
729.2	NOS
378.54	Abducens nerve
352.4	Accessory nerve
388.5	Acoustic nerve
094.86	Acoustic syphilitic
357.5	Alcoholic
291.1	Alcoholic with psychosis (see also 'Psychosis Alcoholic')
277.39	Amyloid [357.4]
355.8	Anterior crural
723.4	Arm
355.2	Ascending
0	Associated with other disorders see 'Neuritis Associated With Other Disorders'
388.5	Auditory
353.0	Axillary nerve (nondiscogenic)
723.4	Brachial NEC
722.0	Brachial NEC due to disc displacement
723.4	Cervical
722.0	Cervical due to displacement, prolapse, protrusion or rupture of intervertebral disc
353.8	Chest wall
353.8	Costal region (nondiscogenic)
356.0	Dejerine-Sottas
722.2	Discogenic syndrome NOS
722.2	Due to displacement, prolapse, protrusion or rupture of intervertebral disc site NOS
388.5	Eighth nerve
352.4	Eleventh nerve
351.8	Facial nerve
767.5	Facial nerve newborn
355.2	Femoral nerve
350.1	Fifth nerve
352.0	First nerve
378.53	Fourth nerve
0	General see 'Polyneuropathy'
351.1	Geniculate ganglion
053.11	Geniculate ganglion due to herpes
352.1	Glossopharyngeal
722.2	HNP (due to) site NOS
722.0	HNP cervical
722.10	HNP lumbar
722.11	HNP thoracic
352.5	Hypoglossal (nerve)
355.79	Iliohypogastric
355.8	Ilioinguinal
357.0	Infectious (multiple)
353.8	Intercostal
356.9	Interstitial hypertrophic progressive NEC
355.8	Leg
355.9	Limb site unspecified
355.8	Limb lower, unspecified
355.79	Limb lower, other specified
354.9	Limb upper, unspecified
354.8	Limb upper, other specified
724.4	Lumbar or lumbosacral
722.10	Lumbar or lumbosacral due to displacement, prolapse, protrusion or rupture of intervertebral disc
356.9	Multiple (acute) (infective)
354.5	Multiplex
354.1	Median nerve
729.2	Nerve root
352.1	Ninth nerve

N

NEURITIS (continued)

378.52 Oculomotor
352.0 Olfactory nerve
377.30 Ophthalmic
053.19 Ophthalmic postherpetic
377.30 Optic
377.41 Optic ischemic
341.0 Optic in myelitis
036.81 Optic meningoccal
377.30 Optic nerve
377.33 Optic nutritional
377.34 Optic toxic
066.42 Optic with West Nile Fever (Virus)
355.8 Pelvic
0 Peripheral (nerve) see 'Peripheral Neuropathy'
355.3 Peroneal
352.3 Pneumogastric
355.3 Popliteal lateral
355.4 Popliteal median
052.7 Postchickenpox
053.19 Postherpetic
356.9 Progressive hypertrophic interstitial NEC
723.4 Radial (nerve)
377.32 Retrobulbar
094.85 Retrobulbar syphilitic
729.2 Rheumatic (chronic)
355.8 Sacral
355.79 Saphenous
724.3 Sciatic (nerve) (sciatica)
722.10 Sciatic (nerve) (sciatica) due to displacement, prolapse, protrusion or rupture of intervertebral disc
355.0 Sciatic mononeuritis
377.30 Second nerve
999.5 Serum
351.8 Seventh nerve
767.5 Seventh nerve newborn
378.54 Sixth nerve
355.9 Spinal (nerve)
0 Spinal root see 'Radiculitis'
723.4 Subscapular (nerve)
723.4 Suprascapular (nerve)
095.8 Syphilitic
352.3 Tenth nerve
354.1 Thenar
378.52 Third nerve
724.4 Thoracic or thoracolumbar
722.11 Thoracic or thoracolumbar due to displacement, prolapse, protrusion or rupture of intervertebral disc
357.7 Toxic
350.1 Trigeminal
378.53 Trochlear
352.5 Twelfth nerve
723.4 Ulnar (nerve)
352.3 Vagus (nerve)
386.12 Vestibular
0 Specified nerve NEC see specified nerve by site, disorder

NEURITIS ASSOCIATED WITH OTHER CONDITIONS

729.2 Unspecified
357.5 Alcoholic
291.1 Alcoholic with psychosis (see also 'Psychosis Alcoholic')
277.39 Amyloid (any site) [357.4]
265.0 Beriberi (due to) [357.4]
250.6# Diabetic [357.2]

5th digit: 250.6

0. Type II, adult-onset, non-insulin dependent (even if requiring insulin), or unspecified; controlled
1. Type I, juvenile-onset or insulin-dependent; controlled
2. Type II, adult-onset, non-insulin dependent (even if requiring insulin); uncontrolled
3. Type I, juvenile-onset or insulin-dependent; uncontrolled

032.89 Diphtheritic [357.4]
274.89 Gouty [357.4]

> ***646.4#: Specify the maternal peripheral neuritis with an additional code.***

646.4# Maternal (peripheral) in pregnancy

5th digit: 646.4

0. Episode of care unspecified or N/A
1. Delivered
2. Delivered with postpartum complication
3. Antepartum complication
4. Postpartum complication

265.0 Multiplex endemica [357.4]
053.19 Postherpetic
729.2 Rheumatic
053.12 Trifacial (postherpetic)

194.0 NEUROBLASTOMA SITE NOS
0 NEUROBLASTOMA SITE SPECIFIED SEE 'CANCER', BY SITE M9500/3

306.2 NEUROCIRCULATORY DISORDER PSYCHOGENIC
759.6 NEUROCUTANEOUS SYNDROME

229.9 NEUROCYTOMA SITE NOS
0 NEUROCYTOMA SITE SPECIFIED SEE 'BENIGN NEOPLASM', BY SITE M9506/0

691.8 NEURODERMATITIS
691.8 NEURODERMATITIS DIFFUSE OF BROCQ

199.1 NEUROEPITHELIOMA SITE NOS
0 NEUROEPITHELIOMA SITE SPECIFIED SEE 'CANCER', BY SITE M9503/3

Carcinomas and neoplasms should be coded by site first, not cell type. If a site is not specified, then code by cell type. Code the 'site NOS' only if no site is mentioned. When no site is given, the code reverts to the histological origin .

NEUROFIBROMA

215.# NOS M9540/0
215.# Melanotic M9541/0
215.# Plexiform M9550/0

4th digit: 215
0. Head, face, neck
2. Upper limb including shoulder
3. Lower limb including hip
4. Thorax
5. Abdomen (wall), gastric, gastrointestinal, intestine, stomach
6. Pelvis, buttock, groin, inguinal region, perineum
7. Trunk NOS, back NOS, flank NOS
8. Other specified sites
9. Site NOS

NEUROFIBROMATOSIS

237.70 NOS M9540/1
171.# Malignant M9540/3

4th digit: 171
0. Head, face, neck
2. Upper limb including shoulder
3. Lower limb including hip
4. Thorax
5. Abdomen (wall), gastric, gastrointestinal, intestine, stomach
6. Pelvis, buttock, groin, inguinal region, perineum
7. Trunk NOS, back NOS, flank NOS
8. Other specified sites
9. Site NOS

237.71 Type I (Von Recklinghausen's disease)
237.72 Type II (acoustic neurofibromatosis)

171.# NEUROFIBROSARCOMA M9540/3

4th digit: 171
0. Head, face, neck
2. Upper limb including shoulder
3. Lower limb including hip
4. Thorax
5. Abdomen (wall), gastric, gastrointestinal, intestine, stomach
6. Pelvis, buttock, groin, inguinal region, perineum
7. Trunk NOS, back NOS, flank NOS
8. Other specified sites
9. Site NOS

596.54 NEUROGENIC BLADDER NOS
344.61 NEUROGENIC BLADDER WITH CAUDA EQUINA SYNDROME
0 NEUROGENIC BLADDER WITH INCONTINENCE SEE 'BLADDER DISORDERS WITH INCONTINENCE'
564.81 NEUROGENIC BOWEL
253.6 NEUROHYPOPHYSIS DISORDER NEC
332.1 NEUROLEPTIC INDUCED ACUTE AKATHISIA
333.72 NEUROLEPTIC INDUCED ACUTE DSYTONIA
332.1 NEUROLEPTIC INDUCED PARKINSONISM
333.85 NEUROLEPTIC INDUCED TARDIVE DYSKINESIA
333.92 NEUROLEPTIC MALIGNANT SYNDROME
781.8 NEUROLOGIC NEGLECT SYNDROME
V80.0 NEUROLOGICAL CONDITIONS SCREENING
781.99 NEUROLOGICAL DISORDER (SYMPTOM) (ILL DEFINED)

A neuroma is a tumor or growth on a nerve, composed of nerve cells and fibers.

NEUROMA

215.9 Site NOS
0 Site specified see 'Benign Neoplasm', by site M9570/0
225.1 Acoustic (8th nerve)
997.61 Amputation stump
355.6 Digital
355.6 Morton's
225.1 Optic nerve
355.6 Plantar
355.8 Surgical - lower extremity (nonneoplastic)
354.9 Surgical - upper extremity (nonneoplastic)
355.8 Traumatic old - lower extremity (nonneoplastic)
354.9 Traumatic old - upper extremity (nonneoplastic)
0 Traumatic other see 'Nerve Injury', by site

358.9 NEUROMUSCULAR DISORDER - NEC
359.1 NEUROMUSCULAR DISORDER - HEREDITARY NEC
358.8 NEUROMUSCULAR DISORDER - SPECIFIED NEC
358.2 NEUROMUSCULAR DISORDER - TOXIC
V49.89 NEUROMUSCULOSKELETAL IMPAIRMENT
729.1 NEUROMYALGIA
341.0 NEUROMYELITIS OPTICA
216.# NEURONEVUS M8725/0

4th digit: 216
0. Lip (skin of)
1. Eyelid including canthus
2. Ear (external) (auricle) (pinna)
3. Face (cheek) (nose) (eyebrow) (temple)
4. Scalp, neck
5. Trunk, back except scrotum
6. Upper limb including shoulder
7. Lower limb including hip
8. Other specified sites
9. Skin unspecified

V53.02 NEUROPACEMAKER (BRAIN) (PERIPHERAL NERVE) (SPINAL CORD) FITTING AND ADJUSTMENT
V45.89 NEUROPACEMAKER STATUS

NEUROPATHY

355.9 NOS
357.5 Alcoholic
291.1 Alcoholic with psychosis (see also 'Psychosis Alcoholic')
354.9 Arm NEC
277.87 Ataxia and retinitis pigmentosa syndrome
353.0 Axillary nerve
353.0 Brachial plexus
353.2 Cervical plexus
357.89 Chronic progressive segmentally demyelinating
357.89 Chronic relapsing demyelinating
356.2 Congenital sensory
356.0 Dejerine - Sottas

NEUROPATHY (continued)

250.6# Diabetic NOS [357.2]
250.6# Diabetic peripheral autonomic [337.1]
250.6# Diabetic polyneuropathy [357.2]
5th digit: 250.6
0. Type II, adult-onset, non-insulin dependent (even if requiring insulin), or unspecified; controlled
1. Type I, juvenile-onset or insulin-dependent; controlled
2. Type II, adult-onset, non-insulin dependent (even if requiring insulin); uncontrolled
3. Type I, juvenile-onset or insulin-dependent; uncontrolled

032.#(#) Diphtheritic [357.4]
4th or 4th and 5th digit: 032
0. Faucial (throat)
1. Nasopharyngeal
2. Anterior nasal
3. Laryngeal
81. Conjunctival
82. Myocarditis
83. Peritonitis
84. Cystitis
85. Cutaneous
89. Other

355.9 Entrapment
355.79 Entrapment iliohypogastric nerve
355.79 Entrapment ilioinguinal nerve
355.1 Entrapment lateral cutaneous nerve of thigh
354.0 Entrapment median
355.79 Entrapment obturator
355.3 Entrapment peroneal
355.5 Entrapment posterior tibial
354.3 Entrapment radial nerve
355.79 Entrapment saphenous
355.0 Entrapment sciatic
354.2 Entrapment ulnar
351.9 Facial nerve
356.9 Hereditary unspecified
356.0 Hereditary peripheral
356.2 Hereditary sensory (radicular)
356.# Hypertrophic
4th digit: 356
0. Dejerine-Sottas
1. Charcot-Marie-tooth
3. Refsum
9. Interstitial
251.2 Hypoglycemia [357.4]
337.0 Idiopathic peripheral autonomic
357.89 Inflammatory other
354.8 Intercostal
357.7 Jamaican (ginger)
355.8 Leg NEC, lower extremity
353.1 Lumbar plexus
250.6# Lumbar plexus with diabetes [353.1]
5th digit: 250.6
0. Type II, adult-onset, non-insulin dependent (even if requiring insulin), or unspecified; controlled
1. Type I, juvenile-onset or insulin-dependent; controlled
2. Type II, adult-onset, non-insulin dependent (even if requiring insulin); uncontrolled
3. Type I, juvenile-onset or insulin-dependent; uncontrolled

NEUROPATHY (continued)

710.0 Lupus (polyneuropathy) [357.1]
354.1 Median
357.82 Motor acute
356.9 Multiple NOS
356.1 Muscular atrophy
357.3 Neoplastic
377.3# Optic
5th digit: 377.3
3. Nutritional
4. Toxic
9. Other

377.41 Optic ischemia
265.2 Pellagra [357.4]
0 Peripheral see 'Neuropathy Peripheral'
355.6 Plantar nerves
446.0 Polyarteritis nodosa (polyneuropathy) [357.1]
277.1 Porphyric [357.4]
356.9 Progressive hypertrophic interstitial
0 Radicular see 'Radiculitis'
714.0 Rheumatoid (polyneuropathy) [357.1]
250.6# Sacral plexus with diabetes [353.1]
5th digit: 250.6
0. Type II, adult-onset, non-insulin dependent (even if requiring insulin), or unspecified; controlled
1. Type I, juvenile-onset or insulin-dependent; controlled
2. Type II, adult-onset, non-insulin dependent (even if requiring insulin); uncontrolled
3. Type I, juvenile-onset or insulin-dependent; uncontrolled

135 Sarcoid [357.4]
355.9 Spinal nerve
357.7 Toxic agent
357.89 Toxic other
586 Uremia NOS [357.89]
585.# Uremic (renal failure) (chronic) [357.4]
4th digit: 585
1. Stage I
2. Stage II (mild)
3. Stage III (moderate)
4. Stage IV (severe)
5. Stage V
6. End stage
9. Unspecified stage

357.89 Other inflammatory
357.89 Other toxic
0 See also 'Neuritis'

NEUROPATHY PERIPHERAL

356.9 NOS
337.9 Autonomic unspecified
277.39 Autonomic amyloidosis [337.1]
274.89 Autonomic gout [337.1]
242.9# Autonomic hyperthyroidism [337.1]
5th digit: 242.9
0. Without storm
1. With storm

337.0 Autonomic idiopathic
357.6 Drug induced
356.0 Hereditary
356.2 Hereditary sensory

NEUROPATHY PERIPHERAL (continued)

356.9 Idiopathic
356.4 Idiopathic progressive
356.8 Idiopathic other specified
356.9 Nerve NOS
354.9 Nerve arm NEC
907.4 Nerve injury late effect (shoulder girdle)
355.8 Nerve leg, lower extremity
0 Nerve see 'Polyneuropathy'
354.9 Nerve upper extremity
794.19 Nervous system abnormal findings function study

> ***646.4#: Specify the maternal peripheral neuritis with an additional code.***

646.4# Neuritis maternal complicating pregnancy
5th digit: 646.4
0. Episode of care unspecified or N/A
1. Delivered
2. Delivered with postpartum complication
3. Antepartum complication
4. Postpartum complication

353.1 Sacral plexus
250.6# Sacral plexus with diabetes [353.1]
5th digit: 250.6
0. Type II, adult-onset, non-insulin dependent (even if requiring insulin), or unspecified; controlled
1. Type I, juvenile-onset or insulin-dependent; controlled
2. Type II, adult-onset, non-insulin dependent (even if requiring insulin); uncontrolled
3. Type I, juvenile-onset or insulin-dependent; uncontrolled

355.0 Sciatic nerve
0 Spinal nerve root see 'Radiculitis'
357.7 Toxic induced (arsenic, lead, organophosphates)
354.2 Ulnar nerve

0 NEUROPRAXIA SEE 'NERVE INJURY'
363.05 NEURORETINITIS

NEUROSIS, NEUROTIC

300.9 NOS
300.16 Accident
300.3 Anancastic, anankastic
300.00 Anxiety NOS
300.02 Anxiety generalized
300.01 Anxiety panic type
300.5 Asthenic
306.53 Bladder
306.2 Cardiac (reflex)
306.2 Cardiovascular
627.2 Climacteric NOS
306.4 Colon
300.16 Compensatory
300.3 Compulsive
300.11 Conversion
300.89 Cramp
306.3 Cutaneous
300.6 Depersonalization
300.4 Depressive (reaction) (type)
300.89 Disorder other NEC
306.6 Endocrine
300.89 Environmental

NEUROSIS, NEUROTIC (continued)

300.5 Fatigue
306.9 Functional
306.4 Gastric (gastrointestinal)
306.50 Genitourinary
306.2 Heart
V11.2 History
300.7 Hypochondriacal
300.10 Hysterical
300.11 Hysterical conversion type
300.15 Hysterical dissociative type
300.3 Impulsive
306.0 Incoordination
306.1 Incoordination larynx
306.1 Incoordination vocal cord
306.4 Intestine
306.1 Larynx
300.11 Larynx hysterical
306.1 Larynx sensory
627.2 Menopause natural
627.4 Menopause artificial
300.89 Mixed NEC
306.0 Musculoskeletal
300.3 Obsessional
300.3 Obsessional phobia
300.3 Obsessive compulsive
300.89 Occupational
306.7 Ocular
307.0 Oral
306.9 Organ
306.1 Pharynx
300.20 Phobic
309.81 Posttraumatic (acute) (situational)
300.89 Psychasthenic
300.16 Railroad
306.4 Rectum
306.1 Respiratory
306.4 Rumination
300.89 Senile
302.70 Sexual
302.71 Sexual with inhibited sexual desire
302.72 Sexual with inhibited sexual excitement
300.89 Situational
300.9 State
300.6 State with depersonalization episode
306.4 Stomach
306.2 Vasomotor
306.4 Visceral
300.16 War
300.89 Other specified type

NEUROSYPHILIS:

WITH DEMENTIA [294.1#]

094.9 NOS
094.3 Asymptomatic
090.40 Congenital
094.1 General paresis
090.40 Juvenile
094.1 Paretic
094.0 Tabetic
094.89 Other

WITH DEMENTIA [294.1#]
5th digit: 294.1
0. Without behavioral disturbance or NOS
1. With behavioral disturbance

524.21 NEUTRO-OCCLUSION

When coding neutropenia (288.0#), use an additional code for any associated mucositis. See' Mucositis', by site.

NEUTROPENIA

288.00 NOS
288.09 Chronic (hypoplastic)
288.01 Congenital (nontransient)
288.02 Cyclic
288.03 Drug induced
288.04 Due to infection
288.00 Fever [780.6]
288.01 Genetic
288.00 Idiopathic
288.09 Immune
288.01 Infantile
288.09 Malignant
288.02 Periodic
288.00 Pernicious
288.00 Primary
289.53 Splenic
289.53 Splenomegaly
288.09 Toxic
288.09 Other

NEUTROPENIA NEONATAL

776.7 Isoimmune
776.7 Maternal transfer
776.7 Transient

288.00 NEUTROPHIL ABSENCE

288.1 NEUTROPHIL, POLYMORPHONUCLEAR DISORDER (FUNCTIONAL)

NEVUS BENIGN

216.# NOS M8720/0
216.# Achromic M8730/0
216.# Amelanotic M8730/0
228.00 Angiomatous M9120/0
216.# Balloon cell M8722/0
216.# Blue M8780/0
216.# Blue cellular M8790/0
216.# Blue giant M8790/0
216.# Blue Jadassohn's M8780/0
228.00 Capillary M9131/0
228.00 Cavernous M9121/0
216.# Cellular M8720/0
216.# Compound M8760/0
224.3 Conjunctiva M8720/0
216.# Dermal M8750/0
216.# Dermal and epithelioid M8760/0
216.# Epithelioid and spindle cell M8770/0
216.# Giant pigmented nevus M8761/0

4th digit: 216
0. Lip (skin of)
1. Eyelid including canthus
2. Ear (external) (auricle) (pinna)
3. Face (cheek) (nose) (eyebrow) (temple)
4. Scalp neck
5. Trunk, back except scrotum
6. Upper limb including shoulder
7. Lower limb including hip
8. Other specified sites
9. Skin unspecified

NEVUS BENIGN (continued)

216.# Hairy M8720/0
216.# Halo M8723/0
228.00 Hemangiomatous M9120/0
216.# Intradermal M8750/0
216.# Intraepidermal M8740/0
216.# Involutional M8724/0
216.# Junctional M8740/0
216.# Juvenile M8770/0
228.1 Lymphatic M9170/0
216.# Melanotic M8720/0
216.# Nonpigmented M8730/0
216.# Nonvascular M8720/0
216.# Papillaris M8720/0
216.# Papillomatosus M8720/0
216.# Pilosus M8720/0
216.# Pigmented M8720/0
216.# Spindle cell and epithelioid M8770/0
216.# Syringocystadenomatous papilliferous M8406/0

4th digit: 216
0. Lip (skin of)
1. Eyelid including canthus
2. Ear (external) (auricle) (pinna)
3. Face (cheek) (nose) (eyebrow) (temple)
4. Scalp neck
5. Trunk, back except scrotum
6. Upper limb including shoulder
7. Lower limb including hip
8. Other specified sites
9. Skin unspecified

173.# NEVUS BLUE MALIGNANT OR OTHER M8780/3

4th digit: 173
0. Lip
1. Eyelid including canthus
2. Ear (auricle) auricular canal external (acoustic)
3. Unspecified parts of face, cheek external, chin, eyebrow, forehead, nose external, temple
4. Scalp and neck
5. Trunk, axilla, breast (or mastectomy site), buttock, groin, perianal skin, perineum, umbilicus
6. Upper limb including shoulder
7. Lower limb including hip
8. Other specified skin sites, contiguous or overlapping, undetermined point of origin
9. Site NOS

NEVUS - OTHER

702.8 Acanthotic
709.09 Anemic, anemicus
448.1 Araneus
709.09 Avasculosus
757.33 Comedonicus
757.32 Flammeus
759.89 Flammeus osteohypertrophic
238.2 Giant pigmented site NOS M8761/1
0 Junctional in malignant melanoma see 'Melanoma', by site M8740/3
224.0 Magnocellular site NOS M8726/0
759.5 Multiplex

N

NEVUS - OTHER (continued)

448.1 Non-neoplastic
648.9# Non-neoplastic maternal current (co-existent) in pregnancy [448.1]
5th digit: 648.9
0. Episode of NOS or N/A
1. Delivered
2. Delivered with postpartum complication
3. Antepartum complication
4. Postpartum complication

750.26 Oral mucosa, white sponge
757.33 Pigmented systematicus
757.32 Portwine congenital
757.32 Sanguineous
702.8 Sebaceous, senile
448.1 Senile
448.1 Spider
448.1 Stellar
757.32 Strawberry
757.33 Unius lateris
757.32 Unna's
757.32 Vascular
757.33 Verrucous

0 NEWBORN DELIVERY OUTCOME, SEE 'OUTCOME OF DELIVERY'

0 NEWBORN EVALUATION FOR SUSPECTED CONDITION NOT FOUND SEE 'OBSERVATION NEWBORN/INFANT SUSPECTED CONDITION (UNDIAGNOSED) (UNPROVEN) NOT FOUND'

077.8 NEWCASTLE CONJUNCTIVITIS
279.13 NEZELOF'S SYNDROME (PURE ALYMPHOCYTOSIS)
099.4# NGU (NONGONOCCAL URETHRITIS)
5th digit: 099.4
0. Unspecified
1. Chlamydia trachomatis
9. Other specified organism

265.2 NIACIN DEFICIENCY
099.1 NICOLAS (-DURAND) -FAVRE DISEASE (CLIMATIC BUBO)
265.2 NICOTINAMIDE DEFICIENCY
265.2 NICOTINIC ACID DEFICIENCY
0 NIDDM (NON INSULIN DEPENDENT DIABETES MELLITUS) SEE 'DIABETES'
272.7 NIEMANN PICK CEREBRAL DEGENERATION [330.2]
272.7 NIEMANN PICK DISEASE OR SYNDROME (LIPID HISTIOCYTOSIS)

NIGHT BLINDNESS

368.60 NOS
368.63 Abnormal dark adaptation curve
368.62 Acquired
368.61 Congenital
368.63 Due to delayed adaptation of cones or rods
264.5 Due to vitamin A deficiency
368.69 Other

729.82 NIGHT CRAMPS (LIMB)
780.8 NIGHT SWEATS
307.46 NIGHT TERRORS
307.47 NIGHTMARES

352.2 NINTH CRANIAL NERVE ATROPHY
352.2 NINTH CRANIAL NERVE DISORDER NEC
951.8 NINTH CRANIAL NERVE INJURY

NIPPLE

757.6 Absence congenital
757.6 Accessory congenital
675.8# And breast infection other specified maternal due to pregnancy
675.9# And breast infection maternal due to pregnancy
5th digit: 675.8, 9
0. Episode of care unspecified or N/A
1. Delivered
2. Delivered with postpartum complication
3. Antepartum complication
4. Postpartum complication

757.6 Anomaly
0 Cracked see 'Nipple', fissure
611.79 Discharge nonpuerperal
611.9 Disorder
611.2 Fissure
676.1# Fissure (lactating) due to pregnancy
5th digit: 676.1
0. Episode of care unspecified or N/A
1. Delivered
2. Delivered with postpartum complication
3. Antepartum complication
4. Postpartum complication

675.0# Inflammation due to pregnancy
5th digit: 675.0
0. Episode of care unspecified or N/A
1. Delivered
2. Delivered with postpartum complication
3. Antepartum complication
4. Postpartum complication

611.0 Inflammation nonpuerperal
757.6 Inversion (retraction) congenital
676.0# Inversion (retraction) due to pregnancy
5th digit: 676.0
0. Episode of care unspecified or N/A
1. Delivered
2. Delivered with postpartum complication
3. Antepartum complication
4. Postpartum complication

611.79 Inversion (retraction) nonpuerperal
757.6 Supernumerary congenital

437.5 NISHIMOTO (-TAKEUCHI) DISEASE
458.29 NITRITOID CRISIS - ADVERSE EFFECT (POSTOPERATIVE) (PROPERLY TAKEN)
961.1 NITRITOID CRISIS - POISONING (OVERDOSE) (IMPROPERLY TAKEN)
790.6 NITROGEN DERIVATIVES, BLOOD ABNORMAL FINDINGS
270.9 NITROGEN METABOLISM DISORDER
289.89 NITROSOHEMOGLOBINEMIA
104.0 NJOVERA
333.92 NMS (NEUROLEPTIC MALIGNANT SYNDROME)
799.9 NO DIAGNOSIS FOR CAUSE OF DEATH
0 NOCARDIOSIS SEE 'ACTINOMYCOSIS'

N

788.43 NOCTURIA
788.36 NOCTURNAL ENURESIS
788.43 NOCTURNAL FREQUENCY (MICTURITION)
427.60 NODAL PREMATURE CONTRACTION
371.46 NODULAR DEGENERATION CORNEA
728.79 NODULAR FASCIITIS
202.0# NODULAR LYMPHOMA M9690\3
5th digit: 202.0
0. Unspecified site, extranodal and solid organ sites
1. Lymph nodes of head, face, neck
2. Lymph nodes intrathoracic
3. Lymph nodes abdominal
4. Lymph nodes axilla and upper limb
5. Lymph nodes inguinal region and lower limb
6. Lymph nodes intrapelvic
7. Spleen
8. Lymph nodes multiple sites

NODULE, NODE

039.9 Actinomycotic (see also 'Actinomycosis')
0 Arthritic see 'Arthritis Osteoarthritis (Degnerative)'
782.2 Cutaneous
715.04 Haygarth's
715.04 Heberden's
102.7 Juxta-articular
095.7 Juxta-articular - syphilitic
102.7 Juxta-articular - yaws
478.79 Larynx
518.89 Lung, solitary
492.8 Lung, solitary emphysematous
051.1 Milkers'
421.0 Osler's
600.10 Prostate
600.11 Prostate with urinary obstruction (retention)
729.89 Rheumatic
0 Rheumatoid see 'Rheumatoid Arthritis'
0 Schmorl's see 'Schmorl's Nodes'
608.4 Scrotum (inflammatory)
478.5 Singers'
782.2 Skin
518.89 Solitary, lung
492.8 Solitary, lung emphysematous
782.2 Subcutaneous
241.0 Thyroid (gland) (nontoxic) (uninodular)
242.1# Thyroid (gland) (nontoxic) (uninodular) with hyperthyroidism
242.1# Thyroid (gland) (nontoxic) (uninodular) with thyrotoxicosis
242.1# Thyroid (gland) (uninodular) toxic
242.1# Thyroid (gland) (uninodular) toxic with hyperthyroidism
5th digit: 242.1
0. Without mention of thyrotoxic crisis or storm
1. With mention of thyrotoxic crisis or storm

0 Tuberculous see 'Tuberculosis', lymph nodes
478.5 Vocal cords

388.10 NOISE EFFECTS (INNER EAR)
388.12 NOISE INDUCED HEARING LOSS
V15.81 NONCOMPLIANCE WITH MEDICAL TREATMENT (HISTORY)

099.4# NONGONOCOCCAL URETHRITIS (NGU)
5th digit: 099.4
0. Unspecified
1. Chlamydia trachomatis
9. Other specified organism

998.83 NON-HEALING SURGICAL WOUND
234.9 NONINFILTRATING INTRACYSTIC CARCINOMA SITE NOS
0 NONINFILTRATING INTRACYSTIC CARCINOMA SITE SPECIFIED SEE 'CA IN SITU', BY SITE M8504/2
757.0 NONNE-MILROY-MEIGE DISEASE OR SYNDROME (CHRONIC HEREDITARY EDEMA)
300.16 NONSENSE SYNDROME
V72.85 NONSTRESS TEST (FOR PREGNANCY)
733.82 NONUNION FRACTURE
759.89 NOONAN'S SYNDROME
259.3 NOREPINEPHRINE ECTOPIC SECRETION
289.89 NORMOBLASTOSIS
743.8 NORRIE'S DISEASE (CONGENITAL PROGRESSIVE OCULOACOUSTICOCEREBRAL DEGENERATION)
116.0 NORTH AMERICAN BLASTOMYCOSIS
082.2 NORTH ASIAN TICK FEVER
008.63 NORWALK VIRUS ENTERITIS

NOSE, NASAL

738.0 Absence
748.1 Absence congenital
748.1 Accessory congenital
478.19 Adhesions
748.1 Anomalies other congenital
738.0 Atresia
748.0 Atresia congenital
754.0 Bent congenital
784.7 Bleed
738.0 Bones overdevelopment
478.19 Calculus
748.1 Cleft congenital
478.19 Congestion
795.39 Culture positive
738.0 Deformity
748.1 Deformity congenital
754.0 Deviation nasal septum congenital
478.19 Degeneration
478.19 Discharge
478.19 Disease
478.19 Disorder
478.19 Dry
478.19 Hyperactive
478.19 Hyperplasia (lymphoid) (polypoid)
478.19 Hypertrophy mucous membrane, alae or cartilage
478.19 Infection (inflammation)
959.09 Injury
910.8 Injury other and unspecified superficial
910.9 Injury other and unspecified superficial infected
478.19 Irritation
478.11 Mucositis (ulcerative)
748.1 Notching of tip congenital
478.19 Obstruction
375.56 Obstruction duct
375.55 Obstruction duct neonatal
478.19 Occlusion
748.0 Occlusion congenital

N

NOSE, NASAL (continued)

478.19 Pain
471.9 Polyp
212.0 Polyp adenomatous
478.19 Redness
470 Septum - deviated
754.0 Septum - deviated congenital
478.19 Septum - necrosis
478.19 Septum - perforation
748.1 Septum - perforation congenital
095.8 Septum - perforation syphiltic
478.19 Septum - spur
478.19 Septum - ulcer (abscess) (necrosis)
456.8 Septum - varices
456.8 Septum - varicose ulcer
478.19 Sinus cyst (mucocele) (rhinolith)
748.1 Sinus deformity congenital
0 Sinus obstruction see 'Sinusitis'
748.1 Sinus perforation congenital
478.19 Spur (septum)
726.91 Spur bone
754.0 Squashed congenital
478.19 Stuffy
478.19 Synechia
478.0 Turbinate hypertrophy

378.52 NOTHNAGEL'S OPHTHALMOPLEGIA-CEREBELLAR ATAXIA SYNDROME

443.89 NOTHNAGEL'S VASOMOTOR ACROPARESTHESIA SYNDROME

0 NOXIOUS SUBSTANCE TRANSMITTED VIA PLACENTA OR BREAST MILK AFFECTING FETUS OR NEWBORN SEE 'PREGNANCY COMPLICATIONS, MATERNAL DISORDERS AFFECTING FETUS OR NEWBORN' BY SPECIFIED SUBSTANCE

0 NSTEMI (NON-ST ELEVATION MYOCARDIAL INFARCTION) SEE 'MYOCARDIAL INFARCTION ACUTE', BY SITE

597.80 NSU (NONSPECIFIC URETHRITIS)

781.6 NUCHAL RIGIDITY

366.16 NUCLEAR SCLEROSIS SENILE CATARACT

352.6 NUCLEUS AMBIGUOUS-HYPOGLOSSAL SYNDROME

782.0 NUMBNESS

832.01 NURSEMAID'S ELBOW

831.0# NURSEMAID'S SHOULDER

5th digit: 831.0
0. NOS
1. Anterior dislocation
2. Posterior dislocation
3. Inferior dislocation
4. Acromioclavicular (joint)
9. Other

573.8 NUTMEG LIVER

783.9 NUTRITION PROBLEM

NUTRITIONAL DEFICIENCY

269.9 Unspecified
261 Atrophy
783.7 Deficiency with failure to thrive – adult
783.41 Deficiency with failure to thrive – child
269.8 Deficiency other
V77.99 Disease screening
269.9 Disorder
760.4 Disorders maternal affecting fetus or newborn
783.3 Feeding problems
779.3 Feeding problems in newborn
V12.1 History
261 Marasmus
648.9# Maternal current (co-existent) in pregnancy

5th digit: 648.9
0. Episode of care NOS or N/A
1. Delivered
2. Delivered with postpartum complication
3. Antepartum complication
4. Postpartum complication

281.2 Megaloblastic anemia (of infancy)

368.60 NYCTALOPIA

788.43 NYCTURIA

302.89 NYMPHOMANIA

NYSTAGMUS

379.50 NOS
386.11 Benign positional
386.2 Central positional
379.51 Congenital
379.53 Deprivation (visual deprivation)
379.55 Dissociated
379.52 Latent
379.54 Vestibular (disorder of vestibular system)
379.56 Other forms

N

066.3 O'NYONG NYONG FEVER (VIRAL)
0 OA (OSTEOARTHRITIS) SEE 'OSTEOARTHRITIS'
270.2 OASTHOUSE URINE DISEASE
162.9 OAT CELL CARCINOMA SITE NOS
0 OAT CELL CARCINOMA SITE SPECIFIED SEE 'CANCER', BY SITE M8042/3
756.0 OAV SYNDROME (OCULOAURICULOVERTEBRAL DYSPLASIA)

OBESITY

278.00 NOS
255.8 Adrenal

> ***V65.3 Use an additional code to identify body mass index (BMI), if known. See 'Body Mass Index'.***

V65.3 Dietary counseling and surveillance
253.8 Due to adiposogenital dystrophy
259.9 Due to endocrine disturbance
783.6 Due to excessive eating
259.9 Due to hormone disturbance
278.00 Due to hyperalimentation
259.9 Due to infantilism disturbance
259.9 Endocrine in origin

> ***649.1#: Use an additional code to identify the obesity.***

649.1# Maternal in pregnancy
5th digit: 649.1
0. Episode of care unspecified or N/A
1. Delivered
2. Delivered with postpartum complication
3. Antepartum complication
4. Postpartum complication

278.00 Metabolic

> ***For code 278.01, use an additional code to identify Body Mass Index if known. These codes can be found under 'Body Mass Index'.***

278.01 Morbid
783.6 Polyphagic (hyperalimentation) (overeating)
V77.8 Screening
278.01 Severe
0 See also 'Weight', gain

OBLIQUE LIE

652.3# NOS
660.0# NOS obstructing labor **[652.3#]**
761.7 Affecting fetus or newborn before L&D
652.6# With multiple gestation
660.0# With multiple gestation obstructing labor **[652.6#]**
5th digit: 652.3, 6, 660.0
0. Episode of care unspecified or N/A
1. Delivered
3. Antepartum complication

599.84 OBLITERATION URETHRA
447.1 OBLITERATIVE VASCULAR DISEASE
291.2 OBS ALCOHOLIC (SEE ALSO 'PSYCHOSIS ALCOHOLIC')
294.9 OBS (CHRONIC)

> ***V71 - V71.9 are always sequenced first. They describe the evaluation and observation for suspected injury or illness. Example: Evaluation of a patient in a motor vehicle accident with no apparent injury.***

OBSERVATION FOR SUSPECTED CONDITION (UNDIAGNOSED) (UNPROVEN) NOT FOUND

V71.9 Unspecified
V71.81 Abuse - NOS child or adult
V71.6 Abuse - battery child or adult
V71.81 Abuse - neglect child or adult
V71.5 Abuse - rape child or adult
V71.3 Accident at work
V71.4 Accident NEC
V71.89 Acute abdomen
V71.82 Anthrax exposure
V71.01 Antisocial behavior - adult
V71.02 Antisocial behavior - child or adolescent
V71.6 Assault with no need for medical treatment
V71.89 Benign neoplasm
V71.83 Biological agent other exposure
V71.1 Cancer
V71.7 Cardiovascular disease
V71.4 Concussion - accidental
V71.6 Concussion - inflicted
V71.3 Concussion - work related
V71.89 CVA (cerebrovascular accident)
V71.82 Exposure anthrax
V71.83 Exposure SARS (severe acute respiratory syndrome)
V71.83 Exposure severe acute respiratory syndrome (SARS)
V71.83 Exposure other biological agent
V71.89 Foreign body ingestion
V71.01 Gang activity - adult without manifest psychiatric disorder
V71.02 Gang activity - child or adolescent without manifest psychiatric disorder
V71.89 Hemorrhage (non traumatic) (post op)
V71.89 Infectious disease not requiring isolation
V71.89 Ingestion of deleterious agent
V71.09 Mental condition
V71.4 MVA (motor vehicle accident) with no apparent injury
V71.7 Myocardial infarction

NEWBORN (28 DAYS OR LESS)

V29.9 Unspecified
V29.8 Cardiovascular disease
V29.8 Congenital abnormality
V29.3 Genetic condition
V29.8 Ingestion foreign object
V29.0 Infectious disease
V29.8 Injury
V29.3 Metabolic condition
V29.8 Neoplasm
V29.1 Neurological disease
V29.8 Poisoning
V29.2 Respiratory condition
V29.8 Specified NEC

OBSERVATION FOR SUSPECTED CONDITION (UNDIAGNOSED) (UNPROVEN) NOT FOUND (continued)

V71.02 Psychiatric disorder - adolescent or child with antisocial behavior (gang activity)
V71.01 Psychiatric disorder - adult with antisocial behavior (gang activity)
V71.09 Psychiatric disorder other
V71.5 Rape (alleged)
V71.89 Rupture of membranes premature
V71.5 Seduction (alleged)
V71.89 Sepsis
V71.89 Stroke
V71.89 Suicide attempt (alleged)
V71.2 Tuberculosis
V71.4 Other accident
V71.6 Other inflicted injury
V71.89 Other specified suspected conditions

301.4 OBSESSIONAL PERSONALITY
300.3 OBSESSIVE COMPULSIVE NEUROSIS (DISORDER) (SYNDROME)
300.3 OBSESSIVE COMPULSIVE REACTION

648.##: Use an additional code to identify the specific maternal back disorder or nutritional defeciency.

OBSTETRICAL

648.7# Bone disorder maternal current (co-existent) (back pelvis lower limbs)
5th digit: 648.7
0. Episode of care unspecified or N/A
1. Delivered
2. Delivered with postpartum complication
3. Antepartum complication
4. Postpartum complication

V13.29 Disorder history (nongravid)
V13.29 History poor
V23.49 History poor affecting current pregnancy supervision
V13.21 History of pre-term labor
V23.41 History of pre-term labor affecting current pregnancy supervision
648.9# Nutritional deficiencies maternal current (co-existent)
669.4# Surgery or medical procedures complication, other
5th digit: 648.9, 669.4
0. Episode of care unspecified or N/A
1. Delivered
2. Delivered with postpartum complication
3. Antepartum complication
4. Postpartum complication

0 Trauma see 'Labor and Delivery Complications Trauma Obstetrical'

0 OBSTIPATION SEE 'CONSTIPATION'
0 OBSTRUCTION SEE ANATOMICAL SITE, OBSTRUCTION
593.89 OBSTRUCTIVE NEPHROPATHY
599.60 OBSTRUCTIVE UROPATHY NOS
599.69 OBSTRUCTIVE UROPATHY NEC

553.8 OBTURATOR HERNIA
355.79 OBTURATOR MONONEUROPATHY
355.79 OBTURATOR NERVE COMPRESSION (ENTRAPMENT)
355.79 OBTURATOR NERVE DISORDER (LESION)
959.09 OCCIPITAL INJURY
723.8 OCCIPITAL NEURALGIA
739.0 OCCIPITOCERVICAL REGION SEGMENTAL OR SOMATIC DYSFUNCTION
0 OCCLUSION ARTERIES EXTREMITIES SEE 'ARTERY, ARTERIAL', OCCLUSION
0 OCCLUSION ARTERY SPECIFIED, SEE SPECIFIED ARTERY EMBOLISM, (THROMBOSIS) (INFARCTION) (OCCLUSION)
0 OCCLUSION SEE ANATOMICAL SITE, OCCLUSION
792.1 OCCULT BLOOD IN STOOL
727.2 OCCUPATIONAL BURSITIS
300.89 OCCUPATIONAL DISORDER PSYCHOGENIC
V70.5 OCCUPATIONAL EXAM (HEALTH)
V62.2 OCCUPATIONAL PROBLEM
V57.21 OCCUPATIONAL THERAPY
270.2 OCHRONOSIS AMINO ACID METABOLISM AROMATIC DISTURBANCES
270.2 OCHRONOSIS ARTHRITIS [713.0]

OCULAR

0 See also 'Eye'
360.32 Fistula (causing hypotony) (postinflammatory) (post op) (posttraumatic)
365.04 Hypertension
871.1 Laceration with prolapse of intraocular tissue
871.0 Laceration without prolapse
996.69 Lens prosthesis complication - infection or inflammation
996.53 Lens prosthesis complication - mechanical
996.79 Lens prosthesis complication - other
378.87 Motion disturbance
306.7 Motion disturbance psychogenic
743.69 Muscle absence (congenital)
743.9 Muscle deformity (congenital)
378.60 Muscle deformity acquired
378.9 Muscle disease
359.1 Muscular dystrophy
378.71 Retraction syndrome
781.93 Torticollis

364.24 OCULOCUTANEOUS SYNDROME
378.87 OCULOGYRIC CRISIS
306.7 OCULOGYRIC CRISIS PSYCHOGENIC

OCULOMOTOR

344.89 Alternating paralysis
794.14 Function study abnormal
378.51 Nerve disorder (atrophy) (palsy) - partial
378.52 Nerve disorder (atrophy) (palsy) - total
951.0 Nerve injury
344.89 Nerve paralysis
378.81 Syndrome

359.1 OCULOPHARYNGEAL MUSCULAR DYSTROPHY

099.3 OCULOURETHROARTICULAR SYNDROME

099.3 OCULOURETHROARTICULAR SYNDROME WITH ARTHROPATHY [711.1#]

5th digit: 711.1

0. Site NOS
1. Shoulder region
2. Upper arm (elbow) (humerus)
3. Forearm (radius) (wrist) (ulna)
4. Hand (carpal) (metacarpal) (fingers)
5. Pelvic region and thigh (hip) (buttock) (femur)
6. Lower leg (fibula) (knee) (patella) (tibia)
7. Ankle and/or foot (metatarsals) (toes) (tarsals)
8. Other (head) (neck) (rib) (skull) (trunk) (vertebrae)
9. Multiple

099.3 OCULOURETHROARTICULAR SYNDROME WITH CONJUNCTIVITIS [372.33]

732.1 ODELBERG'S DISEASE (JUVENILE OSTEOCHONDROSIS)

213.# ODONTOAMELOBLASTOMA M9311/0

4th digit: 213

0. Skull, face, upper jaw
1. Lower jaw

521.05 ODONTOCLASIA

520.5 ODONTOGENESIS IMPERFECTA

ODONTOGENIC

526.0 Cyst
213.# Cyst calcifying M9301/0
238.0 Tumor M9270/1
213.# Tumor adenomatoid M9300/0
213.# Tumor benign M9270/0
213.# Tumor epithelial M9340/0
170.# Tumor malignant M9270/3
213.# Tumor squamous M9312/0

4th digit: 170, 213

0. Skull, face, upper jaw
1. Lower jaw

ODONTOMA

213.# Unspecified M9280/0
213.# Complex M9282/0
213.# Compound M9281/0

4th digit: 213

0. Skull, face, upper jaw
1. Lower jaw

521.09 ODONTONECROSIS

170.# ODONTOSARCOMA AMELOBLASTIC M9290/3

4th digit: 170

0. Skull, face, upper jaw
1. Lower jaw

787.20 ODYNOPHAGIA

127.7 OESOPHAGOSTOMUM APIOSTOMUM AND RELATED SPECIES INFECTION

134.0 OESTRUS OVIS INFESTATION

560.89 OGILVIE'S SYNDROME (SYMPATHICOTONIC COLON OBSTRUCTION)

0 OGILVIE'S SYNDROME SEE 'OBSTRUCTION', BOWEL

368.61 OGUCHI'S (RETINA) DISEASE

021.9 OHARA'S DISEASE (SEE ALSO 'TULAREMIA')

797 OLD AGE (CAUSE OF MORBIDITY AND MORTALITY)

726.33 OLECRANON BURSITIS

OLFACTORY

352.0 Nerve atrophy
352.0 Nerve disorders
951.8 Nerve injury
352.0 Nerve neuritis
160.0 Neurogenic tumor site NOS
0 Neurogenic tumor site specified see 'Cancer', by site M9520/3

285.9 OLIGOCYTHEMIA

191.9 OLIGODENDROBLASTOMA SITE NOS

0 OLIGODENDROBLASTOMA SITE SPECIFIED SEE 'CANCER', BY SITE M9460/3

OLIGODENDROGLIOMA

191.9 Site NOS
0 Site specified see 'Cancer', by site M9450/3
191.9 Anaplastic type site NOS
0 Anaplastic type site specified see 'Cancer', by site M9451/3

520.0 OLIGODONTIA

658.0# OLIGOHYDRAMNIOS

5th digit: 658.0

0. Episode of care unspecified or N/A
1. Delivered
3. Antepartum complication

761.2 OLIGOHYDRAMNIOS AFFECTING FETUS OR NEWBORN

658.1# OLIGOHYDRAMNIOS DUE TO PREMATURE RUPTURE OF MEMBRANES

5th digit: 658.1

0. Episode of care unspecified or N/A
1. Delivered
3. Antepartum complication

705.0 OLIGOHYDROSIS

626.1 OLIGOMENORRHEA

606.1 OLIGOSPERMIA

OLIGURIA

788.5 NOS
0 Cardiac see 'Heart Failure'
646.2# Complicating pregnancy

5th digit: 646.2

0. Episode of care NOS or N/A
1. Delivered
2. Delivered with postpartum complication
3. Antepartum complication
4. Postpartum complication

0 Complicating pregnancy with hypertension see 'Hypertension Complicating Pregnancy' eclampsia
997.5 Due to a procedure [788.5]
997.5 Postoperative [788.5]
639.3 Post pregnancy (abortive) (ectopic) (molar)
669.3# Pueperal postpartum

5th digit: 669.3

0. Episode of care NOS or N/A
2. Delivered with postpartum complication
4. Postpartum complication

O

333.0 OLIVOPONTOCEREBELLAR ATROPHY OR DEGENERATION
756.4 OLLIER'S DISEASE CONGENITAL (CHONDRODYSPLASIA)
771.4 OMPHALITIS NEWBORN
771.3 OMPHALITIS TETANUS
756.79 OMPHALOCELE
751.0 OMPHALOMESENTERIC DUCT PERSISTENT (CONGENITAL)
125.3 ONCHOCERCA VOLVULUS INFECTION
125.3 ONCHOCERCIASIS
125.3 ONCHOCERCIASIS EYELID [373.6]
125.3 ONCHOCERCOSIS
295.4# ONEIROPHRENIA

5th digit: 295.4

0. Unspecified
1. Subchronic
2. Chronic
3. Subchronic with acute exacerbation
4. Chronic with acute
5. In remission

703.8 ONYCHAUXIS
757.5 ONYCHAUXIS CONGENITAL

ONYCHIA

681.02 Finger
681.11 Toe
112.3 Candidal digit NOS [681.9]
112.3 Candidal finger [681.02]
112.3 Candidal toe [681.11]
110.1 Dermatophytic
110.1 Tinea digit NOS [681.9]
110.1 Tinea finger [681.02]
110.1 Tinea toe [681.11]

703.0 ONYCHOCRYPTOSIS
703.8 ONYCHOGRYPOSIS
703.8 ONYCHOLYSIS
110.1 ONYCHOMYCOSIS (FINGER) (TOE)
110.1 ONYCHOMYCOSIS BLASTOMYCOSIS
112.3 ONYCHOMYCOSIS CANDIDAL
V59.7# OOCYTE DONOR (EGG) (OVUM)

4th digit: V59.7

0. Unspecified
1. Under age 35, NOS or anonymous recipient
2. Under age 35, designated recipient
3. Age 35 and over, NOS or anonymous recipient
4. Age 35 and over, designated recipient

V45.89 OOPHORECTOMY STATUS

OOPHORITIS

614.2 NOS
614.0 Acute
614.1 Chronic
072.79 Mumps

OOPHORITIS (continued)

016.6# Tuberculous

5th digit: 016.6

0. Unspecified
1. Lab not done
2. Lab pending
3. Microscopy positive (in sputum)
4. Culture positive - microscopy negative
5. Culture negative - microscopy positive
6. Culture and microscopy negative confirmed by other methods

524.24 OPEN BITE ANTERIOR
524.25 OPEN BITE POSTERIOR
525.61 OPEN MARGIN ON TOOTH RESTORATION
525.61 OPEN RESTORATION MARGINS

When an open wound or laceration is accompanied by cellulitis, two codes are needed. Report a code for the complicated open wound or laceration and a code for the cellulitis. Sequencing depends on which diagnosis required the major work and effort.

OPEN WOUND

0 See also 'Laceration', by site
879.8 NOS
879.9 NOS complicated
879.2 Abdomen wall anterior
879.3 Abdomen wall anterior complicated
879.4 Abdomen wall lateral
879.5 Abdomen wall lateral complicated
873.62 Alveolar (gum)
873.72 Alveolar (gum) complicated
891.0 Ankle
891.1 Ankle complicated
891.2 Ankle with tendon involvement
879.6 Anus (sphincter)
879.7 Anus (sphincter) complicated
569.43 Anus nontraumatic nonpuerperal
884.0 Arm NOS
884.1 Arm NOS complicated
884.2 Arm NOS with tendon involvement
0 Arm lower see 'Open Wound', forearm
884.0 Arm multiple sites
884.1 Arm multiple sites complicated
884.0 Arm multiple sites of one upper limb
884.2 Arm multiple sites with tendon involvement
880.03 Arm upper
880.13 Arm upper complicated
880.23 Arm upper with tendon involvement
0 Artery see specific artery
872.02 Auditory canal
872.12 Auditory canal complicated
872.01 Auricle (pinna)
872.11 Auricle (pinna) complicated

O

OPEN WOUND (continued)

880.02 Axilla
880.12 Axilla complicated
880.22 Axilla with tendon involvement

880.09 Axilla with other sites of upper arm
880.19 Axilla with other sites of upper arm complicated
880.29 Axilla with other sites of upper arm with tendon involvement

876.0 Back
876.1 Back complicated

0 Blood vessel see 'Blood Vessel Injury', by site

879.0 Breast
879.1 Breast complicated

0 Brow see 'Open Wound', eyebrow

873.61 Buccal mucosa
873.71 Buccal mucosa complicated

877.0 Buttock
877.1 Buttock complicated

891.0 Calf
891.1 Calf complicated
891.2 Calf with tendon involvement

870.8 Canaliculus lacrimalis
870.2 Canaliculus lacrimalis with laceration of eyelid

870.8 Canthus, eye

873.41 Cheek external
873.51 Cheek external complicated

873.61 Cheek internal
873.71 Cheek internal complicated

875.0 Chest wall
875.1 Chest wall complicated

873.44 Chin
873.54 Chin complicated

363.63 Choroid

878.8 Clitoris
878.9 Clitoris complicated

872.64 Cochlea
872.74 Cochlea complicated

871.9 Conjunctiva (alone)
0 Cornea see 'Open Wound', eyeball

875.0 Costal region
875.1 Costal region complicated

0 Descemet's membrane see 'Open Wound', eyeball

872.8 Ear
872.9 Ear complicated

872.01 Ear auricle (pinna)
872.11 Ear auricle (pinna) complicated

872.02 Ear canal
872.12 Ear canal complicated

872.61 Ear drum
872.71 Ear drum complicated

872.00 Ear external NOS
872.10 Ear external NOS complicated

OPEN WOUND (continued)

872.62 Ear ossicles (incus) (malleus) (stapes)
872.72 Ear ossicles (incus) (malleus) (stapes) complicated

872.69 Ear other and multiple sites
872.79 Ear other and multiple sites complicated

881.01 Elbow
881.11 Elbow complicated
881.21 Elbow with tendon involvement

878.2 Epididymis
878.3 Epididymis complicated

879.2 Epigastric region
879.3 Epigastric region complicated

874.01 Epiglottis
874.11 Epiglottis complicated

874.4 Esophagus cervical
874.5 Esophagus cervical complicated

872.63 Eustachian tube
872.73 Eustachian tube complicated

871.4 Eye
870.9 Eye ocular adnexa
870.8 Eye ocular adnexa other specified
870.3 Eye orbit penetrating
0 Eye with foreign body see 'Foreign Body', eye

871.9 Eyeball NOS
871.7 Eyeball penetrating NOS
0 Eyeball with foreign body see 'Foreign Body', eye
871.2 Eyeball with partial loss of intraocular tissue
871.1 Eyeball with prolapse of intraocular tissue
871.0 Eyeball without prolapse of intraocular tissue

873.42 Eyebrow
873.52 Eyebrow complicated
870.0 Eyelid and periocular area
870.1 Eyelid full thickness
870.2 Eyelid involving lacrimal passages

873.40 Face
873.50 Face complicated

873.49 Face other and multiple sites
873.59 Face other and multiple sites complicated

883.0 Finger (nail)
883.1 Finger (nail) complicated
883.2 Finger (nail) with tendon involvement
879.4 Flank
879.5 Flank complicated

892.0 Foot
892.1 Foot complicated
892.2 Foot with tendon involvement

881.00 Forearm
881.10 Forearm complicated
881.20 Forearm with tendon involvement

873.42 Forehead
873.52 Forehead complicated

878.8 Genitalia
878.9 Genitalia complicated

873.62 Gingiva
873.72 Gingiva complicated

0 Globe see 'Open Wound', eyeball

O

OPEN WOUND (continued)

Open wound includes laceration, puncture wound, animal bites, foreign body, or avulsion.

879.4	Groin
879.5	Groin complicated
873.62	Gum
873.72	Gum complicated
882.0	Hand
882.1	Hand complicated
882.2	Hand with tendon involvement
873.8	Head
873.9	Head complicated
0	Heel see 'Open Wound', foot
890.0	Hip
890.1	Hip complicated
890.2	Hip with tendon involvement
878.6	Hymen
878.7	Hymen complicated
879.4	Hypochondrium
879.5	Hypochondrium complicated
879.2	Hypogastric region
879.3	Hypogastric region complicated
879.4	Iliac region
879.5	Iliac region complicated
879.4	Inguinal region
879.5	Inguinal region complicated
892.0	Instep
892.1	Instep complicated
892.2	Instep with tendon involvement
0	Internal organ see specific organ
876.0	Interscapular region
876.1	Interscapular region complicated
0	Iris see 'Open Wound', eyeball
873.44	Jaw
873.54	Jaw complicated
891.0	Knee
891.1	Knee complicated
891.2	Knee with tendon involvement
878.4	Labia
878.5	Labia complicated
870.8	Lacrimal apparatus, gland or sac
870.2	Lacrimal apparatus, gland or sac with laceration of eyelid
874.##	Larynx **4th digit: 874** **0. Unspecified** **1. Complicated** **5th digit: 874** **0. Larynx with trachea** **1. Larynx**
906.1	Late effect extremities
906.0	Late effect head, neck or trunk
905.8	Late effect with tendon involvement

OPEN WOUND (continued)

891.0	Leg NOS or lower
891.1	Leg NOS or lower complicated
891.2	Leg NOS or lower with tendon involvement
890.0	Leg upper
890.1	Leg upper complicated
890.2	Leg upper with tendon involvement
894.0	Limb lower NOS or multiple sites
894.1	Limb lower NOS or multiple sites complicated
894.2	Limb lower NOS or multiple sites with tendon involvement
884.0	Limb upper NOS or multiple sites
884.1	Limb upper NOS or multiple sites complicated
884.2	Limb upper NOS or multiple sites with tendon involvement
873.43	Lip
873.53	Lip complicated
876.0	Loin
876.1	Loin complicated
876.0	Lumbar region
876.1	Lumbar region complicated
873.41	Malar
873.51	Malar complicated
873.44	Mandible
873.54	Mandible complicated
873.49	Mastoid
873.59	Mastoid complicated
875.0	Midthoracic region
875.1	Midthoracic region complicated
873.60	Mouth
873.70	Mouth complicated

When an open wound or laceration is accompanied by cellulitis, two codes are needed. Report a code for the complicated open wound or laceration and a code for the cellulitis. Sequencing depends on which diagnosis required the major work and effort.

873.64	Mouth floor
873.74	Mouth floor complicated
873.69	Mouth other and multiple sites
873.79	Mouth other and multiple sites complicated
879.8	Multiple
879.9	Multiple complicated
894.0	Multiple lower limb
894.1	Multiple lower limb complicated
894.2	Multiple lower limb with tendon involvement
884.0	Multiple upper limb
884.1	Multiple upper limb complicated
884.2	Multiple upper limb with tendon involvement
0	Nail see 'Open Wound', finger, thumb or toe
0	Nasal see 'Open Wound', nose
873.22	Nasopharynx
873.32	Nasopharynx complicated
874.8	Neck
874.9	Neck complicated

O

OPEN WOUND (continued)

874.8 Neck nape
874.9 Neck nape complicated

874.8 Neck other and unspecified
874.9 Neck other and unspecified complicated

0 Nerve see 'Laceration', nerve by site

998.83 Non-healing surgical

873.20 Nose
873.30 Nose complicated

873.22 Nose cavity
873.32 Nose cavity complicated

873.29 Nose multiple sites
873.39 Nose multiple sites complicated

873.21 Nose septum
873.31 Nose septum complicated

873.23 Nose sinus
873.33 Nose sinus complicated

0 Occipital region see 'Open Wound', scalp

870.9 Ocular adnexa
870.8 Ocular adnexa other specified

870.8 Orbit
870.3 Orbit penetrating
870.4 Orbit penetrating with foreign body
870.9 Orbital region

0 Organ internal see specific organ

872.62 Ossicles ear
872.72 Ossicles ear complicated

873.65 Palate
873.75 Palate complicated

When an open wound or laceration is accompanied by cellulitis, two codes are needed. Report a code for the complicated open wound or laceration and a code for the cellulitis. Sequencing depends on which diagnosis required the major work and effort.

0 Palm see 'Open Wound', hand

874.2 Parathyroid gland
874.3 Parathyroid gland complicated

0 Parietal region see 'Open Wound', scalp

879.6 Pelvic region
879.7 Pelvic region complicated

878.0 Penis
878.1 Penis complicated

879.6 Perineum
879.7 Perineum complicated

870.8 Periocular area
870.0 Periocular area with laceration of skin

874.4 Pharynx
874.5 Pharynx complicated

872.01 Pinna
872.11 Pinna complicated

891.0 Popliteal
891.1 Popliteal complicated
891.2 Popliteal with tendon involvement

OPEN WOUND (continued)

0 Prepuce see 'Open Wound', penis

879.2 Pubic region
879.3 Pubic region complicated

878.8 Pudenda
878.9 Pudenda complicated

878.8 Rectovaginal septum
878.9 Rectovaginal septum complicated

877.0 Sacral region
877.1 Sacral region complicated

0 Sacroiliac region see 'Open Wound', sacral region

873.69 Salivary (ducts) (gland)
873.79 Salivary (ducts) (gland) complicated

873.0 Scalp
873.1 Scalp complicated

880.01 Scapular
880.11 Scapular complicated
880.21 Scapular with tendon involvement

871.9 Sclera

878.2 Scrotum
878.3 Scrotum complicated

891.0 Shin
891.1 Shin complicated
891.2 Shin with tendon involvement

880.00 Shoulder
880.10 Shoulder complicated
880.20 Shoulder with tendon involvement

880.09 Shoulder and arm multiple sites
880.19 Shoulder and arm multiple sites complicated
880.29 Shoulder and arm multiple sites with tendon involvement

879.8 Skin NOS
879.9 Skin NOS complicated

0 Spermatic cord (scrotal) see 'Open Wound', scrotum

0 Spinal cord see 'Spinal Cord', injury, by site

875.0 Sternal region
875.1 Sternal region complicated

0 Submaxillary region see 'Open Wound', jaw
0 Submental region see 'Open Wound', jaw

0 Subungual see 'Open Wound', finger, thumb or toe

874.8 Supraclavicular region
874.9 Supraclavicular region complicated

0 Supraorbital see 'Open Wound', forehead

873.49 Temple
873.59 Temple complicated

0 Temporal region see 'Open Wound', temple

0 Tendon see 'Laceration', tendon by site

878.2 Testis
878.3 Testis complicated

890.0 Thigh
890.1 Thigh complicated
890.2 Thigh with tendon involvement

O

OPEN WOUND (continued)

875.0 Thorax external
875.1 Thorax external complicated

874.8 Throat
874.9 Throat complicated

883.0 Thumb (nail)
883.1 Thumb (nail) complicated
883.2 Thumb (nail) with tendon involvement

874.2 Thyroid gland
874.3 Thyroid gland complicated

893.0 Toe (nail)
893.1 Toe (nail) complicated
893.2 Toe (nail) with tendon involvement

873.64 Tongue
873.74 Tongue complicated

873.64 Tongue and floor of mouth
873.74 Tongue and floor of mouth complicated

874.## Trachea
4th digit: 874
0. Unspecified
1. Complicated
5th digit: 874
0. Trachea with larynx
2. Trachea

879.6 Trunk
879.7 Trunk complicated

> ***When an open wound or laceration is accompanied by cellulitis, two codes are needed. Report a code for the complicated open wound or laceration and a code for the cellulitis. Sequencing depends on which diagnosis required the major work and effort.***

878.2 Tunica vaginalis
878.3 Tunica vaginalis complicated

872.61 Tympanic membrane
872.71 Tympanic membrane complicated

879.2 Umbilical region
879.3 Umbilical region complicated

873.69 Uvula
873.79 Uvula complicated

878.6 Vagina
878.7 Vagina complicated

871.2 Vitreous (humor)

878.4 Vulva
878.5 Vulva complicated

881.02 Wrist
881.12 Wrist complicated
881.22 Wrist with tendon involvement

523.40 OPERCULITIS (CHRONIC)
523.30 OPERCULITIS ACUTE
709.01 OPHIASIS
771.6 OPHTHALMIA NEONATORUM
098.40 OPHTHALMIA NEONATORUM GONOCOCCAL
360.14 OPHTHALMIA NODOSA
370.31 OPHTHALMIA PHLYCTENULAR
377.30 OPHTHALMIC NEURITIS

OPHTHALMOPLEGIA

378.9 NOS
378.52 Cerebellar ataxia syndrome
242.## Exophthalmic [376.22]
4th digit: 242
0. Diffuse
1. Uninodular
2. Multinodular
3. Nodular unspecified
4. Ectopic thyroid nodule
8. Other specified
9. NOS

5th digit: 242
0. Without mention of thyrotoxic crisis or storm
1. With mention of thyrotoxic crisis or storm

378.55 External
378.86 Internuclear
378.72 Progressive external
333.0 Progressive supranuclear
378.56 Total
367.52 Total or complete internal

763.5 OPIATE REACTION (INTOXICATION) MATERNAL DURING L&D AFFECTING FETUS OR NEWBORN
305.5# OPIOID ABUSE (NONDEPENDENT)
304.0# OPIOID ADDICTION (DEPENDENT)
304.7# OPIOID ADDICTION MIXED WITH ANY OTHER DRUG DEPENDENCE
5th digit: 304.0, 7, 305.5
0. NOS
1. Continuous
2. Episodic
3. In remission

524.00 OPISTHOGNATHISM
121.0 OPISTHORCHIASIS
289.51 OPITZ'S DISEASE (CONGESTIVE SPLENOMEGALY)

305.5# OPIUM ABUSE (NONDEPENDENT)
304.0# OPIUM ADDICTION (DEPENDENT)
304.7# OPIUM ADDICTION MIXED WITH ANY OTHER DRUG DEPENDENCE
5th digit: 304.0, 7, 305.5
0. Unspecified
1. Continuous
2. Episodic
3. In remission

358.8 OPPENHEIM'S DISEASE (MYONEURAL DISORDER)
250.8# OPPENHEIM-URBACH DISEASE OR SYNDROME (NECROBIOSIS LIPOIDICA DIABETICORUM) [709.3]
5th digit: 250.8
0. Type II, adult-onset, non-insulin dependent (even if requiring insulin), or unspecified; controlled
1. Type I, juvenile-onset or insulin-dependent; controlled
2. Type II, adult-onset, non-insulin dependent (even if requiring insulin); uncontrolled
3. Type I, juvenile-onset or insulin-dependent; uncontrolled

313.81 OPPOSITIONAL DEFIANT DISORDER (EMOTIONAL DISTURBANCES OF CHILDHOOD OR ADOLESCENCE)
379.59 OPSOCLONUS

OPTIC ATROPHY

377.10 NOS
377.16 Hereditary
377.15 Partial
377.12 Postinflammatory
377.11 Primary
094.84 Syphilitic
090.49 Syphilitic congenital
094.0 Syphilitic tabes dorsalis
377.13 With retinal dystrophies

OPTIC CHIASM

377.54 Disorders with inflammatory disorders
377.52 Disorders with neoplasms NEC
377.51 Disorders with pituitary neoplasms and disorders
377.53 Disorders with vascular disorders
950.1 Injury

OPTIC DISC

743.57 Anomalies specified congenital
377.14 Atrophy (cupping) glaucomatous
377.23 Coloboma
743.57 Coloboma congenital
377.22 Crater-like holes
377.15 Pallor (temporal)

OPTIC NERVE

377.9 And visual pathways disorder
377.10 Atrophy - NOS
377.14 Atrophy - glaucomatous
377.16 Atrophy - hereditary
377.15 Atrophy - partial
377.12 Atrophy - postinflammatory
377.11 Atrophy - primary
094.84 Atrophy - syphilitic
090.49 Atrophy - syphilitic congenital
094.0 Atrophy - syphilitic tabes dorsalis
377.13 Atrophy - with retinal dystrophies
377.49 Compression
377.49 Disorder - NEC
377.41 Disorder - ischemic
377.33 Disorder - nutritional
377.34 Disorder - toxic
377.42 Hemorrhage sheaths
377.43 Hypoplasia
950.0 Injury
950.9 Injury unspecified
950.9 Traumatic blindness

OPTIC NEURITIS

377.30 NOS
341.0 In myelitis
377.41 Ischemic
036.81 Meningococcal
377.33 Nutritional
377.32 Retrobulbar acute
094.85 Retrobulbar syphilitic
377.34 Toxic
377.39 Other

377.31 OPTIC PAPILLITIS
950.2 OPTIC PATHWAYS INJURY
377.63 OPTIC RADIATION DISORDER
377.63 OPTIC TRACTS DISORDER
379.57 OPTOKINETIC RESPONSE ABNORMAL

ORAL

528.3 Abscess
528.9 Disease (soft tissue)
528.9 Disease (soft tissue) other specified
528.79 Dyskeratosis
528.79 Epithelium
528.72 Epithelium residual ridge mucosa - excessive
528.71 Epithelium residual ridge mucosa - minimal
759.89 Facial - digital syndrome
528.3 Fistula
528.79 Hyperplasia - epithelial
523.8 Hyperplasia - gum
528.9 Hyperplasia - irritative
528.9 Hyperplasia - soft tissue NEC (inflammatory) (irritative) (mucosa)
529.8 Hyperplasia – tongue
528.79 Keratinization
528.72 Keratinization residual ridge mucosa - excessive
528.71 Keratinization residual ridge mucosa - minimal
528.79 Leukoedema

ORBIT, ORBITAL

743.66 Anomalies specified congenital
376.45 Atrophy
376.33 Congestion
376.40 Deformity
376.44 Deformity associated with craniofacial deformities
376.47 Deformity due to trauma or surgery
376.43 Deformity local due to bone disease
376.9 Disorder
376.89 Disorders other
376.46 Enlargement
376.42 Exostosis
376.41 Hypertelorism
996.69 Implant complication - infection or inflammation
996.59 Implant complication - mechanical
996.79 Implant complication - other
376.00 Inflammation acute
376.10 Inflammation chronic
376.13 Parasitic infestation
376.11 Pseudotumor (inflammatory)
870.3 Wound penetrating
870.4 Wound penetrating with foreign body
376.6 Wound penetrating with foreign body retained (old)

ORCHITIS

604.90 NOS
032.89 Diphtheritic [604.91]
125.9 Filarial [604.91]
098.13 Gonococcal acute
098.33 Gonococcal chronic
072.0 Mumps
095.8 Syphilitic [604.91]

O

ORCHITIS (continued)

016.5# Tuberculous
5th digit: 016.5
0. Unspecified
1. Lab not done
2. Lab pending
3. Microscopy positive (in sputum)
4. Culture positive - microscopy negative
5. Culture negative - microscopy positive
6. Culture and microscopy negative confirmed by other methods

604.0 With abscess
0 With abscess of known organism see 'Abscess', testis
604.99 Other

759.89 ORDIGITOFACIAL SYNDROME
051.2 ORF
744.05 ORGAN OF CORTI ANOMALY (CONGENITAL)
V45.79 ORGAN OR SITE NOS ABSENCE ACQUIRED
759.89 ORGAN OR SITE NOS ABSENCE CONGENITAL

ORGANIC

293.83 Affective syndrome NEC
292.84 Affective syndrome drug induced
293.83 Affective syndrome transient depressive type
293.84 Anxiety syndrome

BRAIN SYNDROME

310.9 NOS
294.9 Chronic
291.2 Chronic alcoholic (see also 'Psychosis Alcoholic')
294.8 Due to dialysis
293.9 Due to dialysis transient
265.2 Due to nicotine acid deficiency
310.2 Due to trauma (postconcussional)
294.8 Epileptic [345.##]
4th digit: 345
0. Generalized nonconvulsive
1. Generalized convulsive
4. Partial, with impairment of consciousness
5. Partial, without impairment of consciousness
6. Infantile spasms
7. Epilepsia partialis continua
8. Other forms
9. Unspecified, NOS
5th digit: 345
0. Without mention of intractable epilepsy
1. With intractable epilepsy

294.8 Epileptic grand mal status [345.3]
294.8 Epileptic petit mal status [345.2]
294.8 Other specified

DELUSIONAL SYNDROME

293.81 NOS
291.5 Alcohol induced (see also 'Psychosis Alcoholic')
292.11 Drug induced (see also 'Psychosis Drug Induced')
290.42 Due to or associated with arteriosclerosis [437.0]
290.12 Due to or associated with presenile brain disease
290.20 Due to or associated with senility

ORGANIC (continued)

DEPRESSIVE SYNDROME

293.83 NOS
292.84 Drug induced
290.43 Due to or associated with arteriosclerosis [437.0]
290.13 Due to or associated with presenile brain disease
290.21 Due to or associated with senility

ORGANIC (continued)

293.82 Hallucinosis syndrome
292.84 Hallucinosis syndrome drug induced
799.89 Insufficiency
310.1 Personality syndrome
292.89 Personality syndrome drug induced
293.9 Psychosis due to or associated with physical condition
293.81 Psychosis due to or associated with physical condition with delusions
293.82 Psychosis due to or associated with physical condition with hallucinations
310.1 Psychosyndrome of nonpsychotic severity
293.84 Psychotic transient state - anxiety type

302.73 ORGASM FEMALE PSYCHOSEXUAL DISORDER
302.74 ORGASM MALE PSYCHOSEXUAL DISORDER
121.1 ORIENTAL LIVER FLUKE DISEASE
121.2 ORIENTAL LUNG FLUKE DISEASE
085.1 ORIENTAL SORE
593.4 ORMOND'S DISEASE OR SYNDROME
270.6 ORNITHINE METABOLISM DISORDERS

ORNITHOSIS

073.9 NOS
073.7 Encephalitis [323.01]
073.0 Lobular pneumonitis
073.0 Pneumonia
073.8 With unspecified complication
073.7 With other specified complications

066.3 OROPOUCHE FEVER (VIRAL)
088.0 OROYA FEVER
V53.4 ORTHODONTIC DEVICES FITTING AND ADJUSTMENT
V58.5 ORTHODONTICS AFTERCARE

ORTHOPEDIC

V54.9 Aftercare
V54.2# Aftercare fracture pathological healing
V54.1# Aftercare fracture traumatic healing
5th digit: V54.1-2
0. Arm
1. Arm upper
2. Arm lower
3. Hip
4. Leg
5. Leg upper
6. Leg lower
7. Vertebrae
9. Other (pelvis) (wrist) (ankle) (hand/foot) (fingers/toes)

O

ORTHOPEDIC (continued)

V54.81 Aftercare joint replacement **[V43.6#]**
5th digit: V43.6
0. Site unspecified
1. Shoulder
2. Elbow
3. Wrist
4. Hip
5. Knee
6. Ankle
9. Other

V54.89 Aftercare other
996.67 Device (internal) complication - infection or inflammation (pin) (rod) (screw)
996.4# Device (internal) complication – mechanical **[V43.6#]**
5th digit: 996.4
0. Unspecified device, implant or graft
Internal fixation nail, rod or plate
1. Loosening prosthetic joint
Aseptic loosening
2. Dislocation prosthetic joint
Instability, subluxation
3. Implant failure prosthetic joint
Breakage, fracture
4. Periprosthetic fracture around prosthetic joint
5. Periprosthetic osteolysis
6. Articular bearing surface wear prosthetic joint
Breakage, fracture
7. Other mechanical complication of prosthetic joint
9. Other mechanical complication of other device implant or graft
Bone graft
Cartilage graft
External fixation with internal components
Muscle graft
Tendon graft
5th digit: V43.6
0. Site unspecified
1. Shoulder
2. Elbow
3. Wrist
4. Hip
5. Knee
6. Ankle
9. Other

996.78 Device (internal) complication - other
V53.7 Device fitting and adjustment (brace) (cast) (corset) (shoes)
V54.02 Growth rod adjustment/lengthening
V54.01 Growth rod removal
V54.09 Internal fixation device aftercare other
V54.01 Internal fixation device removal
V52.0 Prosthesis fitting (removal) - arm
V52.1 Prosthesis fitting (removal) - leg
V52.8 Prosthesis fitting (removal) - other

786.02 ORTHOPNEA
V57.4 ORTHOPTIC TRAINING
333.0 ORTHOSTATIC HYPOTENSIVE-DYSAUTONOMIC DYSKINETIC SYNDROME
V57.81 ORTHOTIC TRAINING
0 OS CALCIS SEE 'CALCANEUS'
732.4 OSGOOD SCHLATTER DISEASE (TIBIA TUBERCLE)

421.0 OSLER'S NODE
238.4 OSLER (-VAQUEZ) DISEASE (POLYCYTHEMIA VERA) M9950/1
448.0 OSLER-WEBER-RENDU SYNDROME (FAMILIAL HEMORRHAGIC TELANGIECTASIA)
731.3 OSSEOUS DEFECTS - MAJOR
744.03 OSSEOUS MEATUS (EAR) ABSENCE OR ATRESIA
724.8 OSSIFICATION POSTERIOR LONGITUDINAL LIGAMENT
723.7 OSSIFICATION POSTERIOR LONGITUDINAL LIGAMENT CERVICAL REGION

OSTEITIS (SEE ALSO 'OSTEOMYELITIS')

730.2# NOS
5th digit: 730.2
0. Site unspecified
1. Shoulder region
2. Upper arm (elbow) (humerus)
3. Forearm (radius) (wrist) (ulna)
4. Hand (carpal) (metacarpal) (fingers)
5. Pelvic region and thigh (hip) (buttock) (femur)
6. Lower leg (fibula) (knee) (patella) (tibia)
7. Ankle and/or foot (metatarsals) (toes) (tarsals)
8. Other (head) (neck) (rib) (skull) (trunk) (vertebrae)
9. Multiple

733.5 Condensans
731.1 Deformans neoplastic (malignant) **[170.#]**
4th digit: 170
0. Skull and face
1. Mandible
2. Vertebral column
3. Ribs, sternum, clavicle
4. Scapula, long bones of upper limb
5. Short bones of upper limb
6. Pelvic bones, sacrum, coccyx
7. Long bones of lower limb
8. Short bones of lower limb
9. Site unspecified

731.0 Deformans without mention of bone tumor
250.8# Diabetic [731.8]
5th digit: 250.8
0. Type II, adult-onset, non-insulin dependent (even if requiring insulin), or unspecified; controlled
1. Type I, juvenile-onset or insulin-dependent; controlled
2. Type II, adult-onset, non-insulin dependent (even if requiring insulin); uncontrolled
3. Type I, juvenile-onset or insulin-dependent; uncontrolled

102.6 Due to yaws
252.01 Fibrosa cystica (osteoplastica) [737.4#]
5th digit: 737.4
0. Curvature unspecified
1. Kyphosis
2. Lordosis
3. Scoliosis

756.59 Fibrosa disseminate

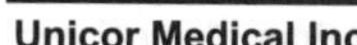

Osteoarthritis, often referred to as degenerative joint disease, is the most common type of arthritis. Classification is usually coded to localized (primary or secondary), or generalized.

OSTEOARTHRITIS

715.9# NOS
5th digit: 715.9
0. Site unspecified
1. Shoulder region
2. Upper arm (elbow) (humerus)
3. Forearm (radius) (wrist) (ulna)
4. Hand (carpal) (metacarpal) (fingers)
5. Pelvic region and thigh (hip) (buttock) (femur)
6. Lower leg (fibula) (knee) (patella) (tibia)
7. Ankle and/or foot (metatarsals) (toes)(tarsals)
8. Other (head) (neck) (rib) (skull) (trunk) (vertebrae)

715.0# Generalized
5th digit: 715.0
0. Site unspecified
4. Hand (carpal) (metacarpal) (fingers)
9. Multiple

715.3# Localized
715.1# Localized primary (by joint)
715.2# Localized secondary (by joint)
5th digit: 715.1-3
0. Site unspecified
1. Shoulder region
2. Upper arm (elbow) (humerus)
3. Forearm (radius) (wrist) (ulna)
4. Hand (carpal) (metacarpal) (fingers)
5. Pelvic region and thigh (hip) (buttock) (femur)
6. Lower leg (fibula) (knee) (patella) (tibia)
7. Ankle and/or foot (metatarsals) (toes)(tarsals)
8. Other (head) (neck) (rib) (skull) (trunk) (vertebrae)

715.8# Multiple sites (by joint) (not specified as generalized)
5th digit: 715.8
0. Site unspecified
9. Multiple

OSTEOARTHRITIS OF SPINE-WITH OSTEOPOROSIS [733.0#]

721.90 NOS
721.91 NOS with myelopathy (cord compression)
721.0 Cervical
721.1 Cervical with myelopathy (cord compression)
721.3 Lumbar
721.42 Lumbar with myelopathy (cord compression)
721.3 Lumbosacral
721.42 Lumbosacral with myelopathy (cord compression)
721.3 Sacral
721.42 Sacral with myelopathy (cord compression)
721.3 Sacrococcygeal
721.42 Sacrococcygeal with myelopathy (cord compression)
721.3 Sacroiliac
721.42 Sacroiliac with myelopathy (cord compression)
721.2 Thoracic
721.41 Thoracic with myelopathy (cord compression)
721.7 Traumatic
WITH OSTEOPOROSIS [733.0#]
5th digit: 733.0
0. Unspecified
1. Senile
2. Idiopathic
3. Disuse
9. Drug induced

0 OSTEOARTHROPATHY SEE 'OSTEOARTHRITIS'
731.2 OSTEOARTHROPATHY HYPERTROPHIC PULMONARY
0 OSTEOARTHROSIS SEE 'OSTEOARTHRITIS'
213.# OSTEOBLASTOMA M9200/0
4th digit: 213
0. Skull, face, upper jaw
1. Lower jaw
2. Spine
3. Rib, sternum, clavicle
4. Scapula, long bone of upper limb
5. Short bone of upper limb
6. Pelvis, sacrum, coccyx
7. Long bone of lower limb
8. Short bone of lower limb
9. Site unspecified

OSTEOCHONDRITIS

732.9 NOS
732.7 Dissecans
732.6 Juvenile

277.5 OSTEOCHONDRODYSTROPHY
213.# OSTEOCHONDROMA M9210/1
4th digit: 213
0. Skull, face, upper jaw
1. Lower jaw
2. Spine
3. Rib, sternum, clavicle
4. Scapula, long bone of upper limb
5. Short bone of upper limb
6. Pelvis, sacrum, coccyx
7. Long bone of lower limb
8. Short bone of lower limb
9. Site unspecified

238.0 OSTEOCHONDROMATOSIS SITE NOS
0 OSTEOCHONDROMATOSIS SITE SPECIFIED SEE 'NEOPLASM UNCERTAIN BEHAVIOR', BY SITE M9210/1
732.9 OSTEOCHONDROPATHY NOS

O

OSTEOCHONDROSIS

732.9 NOS
732.6 Site NOS juvenile
732.# Specified site (juvenile)

4th digit: 732
0. Spine
1. Hip and pelvis
3. Upper extremity
4. Lower extremity excluding foot
5. Foot
6. Other

737.0 Spine adolescent postural kyphosis
732.8 Spine adult
732.0 Spine juvenile
090.0 Syphilitic

757.39 OSTEODERMOPATHIC HYPEROSTOSIS SYNDROME

OSTEODYSTROPHY

588.0 Azotemic
756.50 Congenital
756.59 Congenital other
252.01 Parathyroid
588.0 Renal

252.01 OSTEOFIBROCYSTIC DISEASE
756.51 OSTEOGENESIS IMPERFECTA
213.# OSTEOID OSTEOMA M9191/0
213.# OSTEOMA M9180/0

4th digit: 213
0. Skull, face, upper jaw
1. Lower jaw
2. Spine
3. Rib, sternum, clavicle
4. Scapula, long bone of upper limb
5. Short bone of upper limb
6. Pelvis, sacrum, coccyx
7. Long bone of lower limb
8. Short bone of lower limb
9. Site unspecified

268.2 OSTEOMALACIA VITAMIN D DEFICIENCY
275.3 OSTEOMALACIA VITAMIN D RESISTANT

OSTEOMYELITIS

> ***731.3: Use an additional code to identify major osseous defect, if applicable.***

730.2# NOS
730.0# Acute
730.1# Chronic

5th digit: 730.0-2
0. Site unspecified
1. Shoulder region
2. Upper arm (elbow) (humerus)
3. Forearm (radius) (wrist) (ulna)
4. Hand (carpal) (metacarpal) (fingers)
5. Pelvic region and thigh (hip) (buttock) (femur)
6. Lower leg (fibula) (knee) (patella) (tibia)
7. Ankle and/or foot (metatarsals) (toes) (tarsals)
8. Other (head) (neck) (rib) (skull) (trunk) (vertebrae)
9. Multiple

OSTEOMYELITIS (continued)

250.8# Diabetic [731.8] **[730.0#]**

5th digit: 250.8
0. Type II, adult-onset, non-insulin dependent (even if requiring insulin), or unspecified; controlled
1. Type I, juvenile-onset or insulin-dependent; controlled
2. Type II, adult-onset, non-insulin dependent (even if requiring insulin); uncontrolled
3. Type I, juvenile-onset or insulin-dependent; uncontrolled

5th digit: 730.0
0. Site unspecified
1. Shoulder region
2. Upper arm (elbow) (humerus)
3. Forearm (radius) (wrist) (ulna)
4. Hand (carpal) (metacarpal) (fingers)
5. Pelvic region and thigh (hip) (buttock) (femur)
6. Lower leg (fibula) (knee) (patella) (tibia)
7. Ankle and/or foot (metatarsals) (toes) (tarsals)
8. Other (head) (neck) (rib) (skull) (trunk) (vertebrae)
9. Multiple

526.4 Jaw (acute) (chronic) (neonatal) (suppurative)
0 Old see 'Osteomyelitis', chronic
376.03 Orbital
383.20 Petrous
383.21 Petrous acute
383.22 Petrous chronic
003.24 Salmonella
0 Sclerosing of Garre see 'Osteomyelitis', chronic
095.5 Syphilitic

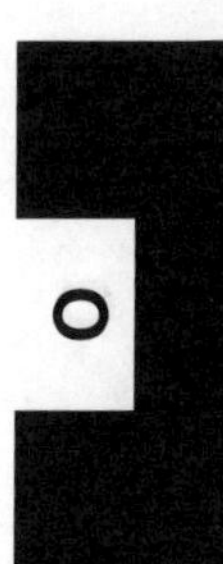

OSTEOMYELITIS (continued)

> *731.3: Use an additional code to identify major osseous defect, if applicable.*

015.## Tuberculous [730.8#]

4th digit: 015
- **0. Vertebral column**
- **1. Hip**
- **2. Knee**
- **5. Limb bones**
- **6. Mastoid**
- **7. Other specified bone**
- **8. Other specified joint**
- **9. Unspecified bones and joint**

5th digit: 015
- **0. Unspecified**
- **1. Lab not done**
- **2. Lab pending**
- **3. Microscopy positive (in sputum)**
- **4. Culture positive - microscopy negative**
- **5. Culture negative - microscopy positive**
- **6. Culture and microscopy negative confirmed by other methods**

5th digit: 730.8
- **0. Site unspecified**
- **1. Shoulder region**
- **2. Upper arm (elbow) (humerus)**
- **3. Forearm (radius) (wrist) (ulna)**
- **4. Hand (carpal) (metacarpal) (fingers)**
- **5. Pelvic region and thigh (hip) (buttock) (femur)**
- **6. Lower leg (fibula) (knee) (patella) (tibia)**
- **7. Ankle and/or foot (metatarsals) (toes) (tarsals)**
- **8. Other (head) (neck) (rib) (skull) (trunk) (vertebrae)**
- **9. Multiple**

002.0 Typhoid [730.8#]

5th digit: 730.8
- **0. Site unspecified**
- **1. Shoulder region**
- **2. Upper arm (elbow) (humerus)**
- **3. Forearm (radius) (wrist) (ulna)**
- **4. Hand (carpal) (metacarpal) (fingers)**
- **5. Pelvic region and thigh (hip) (buttock) (femur)**
- **6. Lower leg (fibula) (knee) (patella) (tibia)**
- **7. Ankle and/or foot (metatarsals) (toes) (tarsals)**
- **8. Other (head) (neck) (rib) (skull) (trunk) (vertebrae)**
- **9. Multiple**

289.89 OSTEOMYELOFIBROSIS
289.89 OSTEOMYELOSCLEROSIS

733.4# OSTEONECROSIS MEANING ASEPTIC NECROSIS

5th digit: 733.4
- **0. Site unspecified**
- **1. Head of humerus**
- **2. Head and neck of femur**
- **3. Medial femoral condyle**
- **4. Talus**
- **5. Jaw**
- **9. Other**

730.1# OSTEONECROSIS MEANING OSTEOMYELITIS

5th digit: 730.1
- **0. Site unspecified**
- **1. Shoulder region**
- **2. Upper arm (elbow) (humerus)**
- **3. Forearm (radius) (wrist) (ulna)**
- **4. Hand (carpal) (metacarpal) (fingers)**
- **5. Pelvic region and thigh (hip) (femur)**
- **6. Lower leg (fibula) (knee) (patella) (tibia)**
- **7. Ankle and/or foot (metatarsals) (toes) (tarsals)**
- **8. Other (head) (neck) (rib) (skull) (trunk) (vertebrae)**
- **9. Multiple**

045.## OSTEOPATHY DUE TO POLIOMYELITIS [730.7#]

4th digit: 045
- **0. Acute bulbar paralytic**
- **1. Acute with other paralysis**
- **2. Acute non paralytic**
- **9. Acute unspecified**

5th digit: 045
- **0. Poliovirus unspecified**
- **1. Poliovirus type I**
- **2. Poliovirus type II**
- **3. Poliovirus type III**

5th digit: 730.7
- **0. Site unspecified**
- **1 Shoulder region**
- **2. Upper arm (elbow) (humerus)**
- **3. Forearm (radius) (wrist) (ulna)**
- **4. Hand (carpal) (metacarpal) (fingers)**
- **5. Pelvic region and thigh (hip) (buttock) (femur)**
- **6. Lower leg (fibula) (knee) (patella) (tibia)**
- **7. Ankle and/or foot (metatarsals) (toes) (tarsals)**
- **8. Other (head) (neck) (rib) (skull) (trunk) (vertebrae)**
- **9. Multiple**

0 OSTEOPATHY SEE ALSO 'OSTEITIS'
733.90 OSTEOPENIA
756.52 OSTEOPETROSIS
0 OSTEOPHYTE SEE 'EXOSTOSIS'
756.53 OSTEOPOIKILOSIS

OSTEOPOROSIS

> *731.3: Use an additional code to identify major osseous defect, if applicable.*

733.00 NOS
733.03 Disuse
733.09 Drug induced
V17.81 Family history
733.02 Idiopathic

O

OSTEOPOROSIS (continued)

268.2 Osteomalacia syndrome
733.01 Postmenopausal
V82.81 Screening
V82.81 Screening with hormone therapy status (postmenopausal) [V07.4]
V82.81 Screening with postmenopausal (natural) status [V49.81]
733.01 Senile
733.00 Vertebra

526.89 OSTEORADIONECROSIS OF JAW

756.51 OSTEOPSATHYROSIS CONGENITAL

OSTEOSARCOMA

170.# NOS M9180/3
170.# Chondroblastic M9181/3
170.# Fibroblastic M9182/3
170.# In Paget's disease of bone M9184/3
170.# Juxtacortical M9190/3
170.# Telangiectatic M9183/3

4th digit: 170
0. Skull and face
1. Mandible
2. Vertebral column
3. Ribs, sternum, clavicle
4. Scapula, long bones of upper limb
5. Short bones of upper limb
6. Pelvic bones, sacrum, coccyx
7. Long bones of lower limb
8. Short bones of lower limb
9. Site NOS

756.52 OSTEOSCLEROSIS CONGENITAL

289.89 OSTEOSCLEROTIC ANEMIA

756.89 OSTERREICHER-TURNER (HEREDITARY OSTEO-ONYCHODYSPLASIA)

745.61 OSTIUM PRIMUM DEFECT CONGENITAL

745.5 OSTIUM SECUNDUM (PATENT) (PERSISTENT) CONGENITAL

> ***When coding an infection of an ostomy, use an additional code to specify the organism. See 'Bacterial Infection'***

OSTOMY

V55.9 Care (closure) (toilet) (attention) (removal or replacement)
V55.4 Care other digestive (closure) (toilet) (attention) (removal or replacement)
V55.6 Care other urinary (closure) (toilet) (attention) (removal or replacement)
V55.8 Care other specified site (closure) (toilet) (attention) (removal or replacement)
V44.9 Status unspecified ostomy
V44.4 Status other G.I. tract
V44.6 Status other urinary
V44.8 Status other ostomy
0 See also cecostomy, colostomy, cystostomy, enterostomy, esophagostomy, gastrostomy, ileostomy, jejunostomy, nephrostomy, tracheostomy, ureterostomy, urethrostomy

757.7 OSTOMYLOSIS ACROMEGLIOID

756.59 OSTRUM-FURST SYNDROME

V57.21 OT (OCCUPATIONAL THERAPY)

388.70 OTALGIA

388.11 OTIC BLAST INJURY

OTITIS

NOS

382.9 NOS (acute)
382.4 Purulent
381.4 Secretory (serous)
382.4 Suppurative
381.4 With effusion

CHRONIC

382.9 NOS
381.20 Mucoid, mucous
382.3 Purulent
381.3 Secretory
381.10 Serous
382.3 Suppurative
381.3 With effusion

OTITIS (continued)

136.8 Diffuse parasitic
0 Externa see 'Otitis Externa'
0 Insidiosa see 'Otosclerosis'
0 Interna see 'Labyrinthitis'
0 Media see 'Otitis Media'

OTITIS EXTERNA

380.10 NOS
380.22 Actinic
380.10 Acute
380.10 Acute infective
117.3 Aspergillosis [380.15]
112.82 Candida
380.22 Chemical
380.21 Cholesteatoma
380.23 Chronic
380.16 Chronic infective
380.22 Contact
111.3 Dermatomycotic (tinea) (ringworm) [380.15]
110.8 Dermatophytosis [380.15]
380.22 Eczematoid
035 Erysipelas [380.13]
680.0 Furuncular [380.13]
054.73 Herpes simplex
053.71 Herpes zoster
684 Impetigo [380.13]
380.14 Malignant
380.15 Mycotic
111.9 Otomycosis [380.15]
380.22 Reactive
690.10 Seborrheic dermatitis NOS [380.13]
690.11 Seborrheic dermatitis capitis [380.13]
690.12 Seborrheic dermatitis infantile [380.13]
690.18 Seborrheic dermatitis other [380.13]
380.12 Swimmer's ear
111.8 Tropical [380.15]
380.22 Other acute
380.23 Other chronic
380.16 Other chronic infective

O

Many carriers require verification of the presence of effusion (a dictated explanation by the physician) for any PE tubes placed for chronic nonsuppurative otitis media (381.3).

OTITIS MEDIA

382.9 NOS

ACUTE

382.9 NOS
381.00 NOS with effusion
0 Adhesive see 'Adhesion, Adhesive', otitis
381.04 Allergic
381.00 Exudative
487.8 Influenzal [382.02]
055.2 Measles (due to)
381.02 Mucoid
381.05 Mucoid allergic
381.03 Sanguinous
381.06 Sanguinous allergic
034.1 Scarlet fever (due to) [382.02]
381.01 Serous
381.04 Serous allergic
382.00 Suppurative
382.01 Suppurative with spontaneous rupture of ear drum

CHRONIC

382.9 NOS
381.3 Allergic
112.82 Candidal
381.20 Mucoid
381.29 Mucosanguinous
381.3 Nonsuppurative (allergic) (exudative) (transudative) (secretory) (mucoid) (catarrhal)
381.3 Nonsuppurative (allergic) (exudative) (transudative) (secretory) (mucoid) (catarrhal) with effusion
381.19 Serosanguinous
381.10 Serous simple
382.3 Suppurative
382.1 Suppurative tubotympanic with anterior perforation of ear drum
382.2 Suppurative with posterior or superior marginal perforation ear drum
017.4# Tuberculous chronic
5th digit: 017.4
0. Unspecified
1. Lab not done
2. Lab pending
3. Microscopy positive (in sputum)
4. Culture positive - microscopy negative
5. Culture negative - microscopy positive
6. Culture and microscopy negative confirmed by other methods

385.03 Tympanosclerosis (due to)

OTITIS MEDIA (continued)

993.0 Due to barotrauma
909.4 Due to barotrauma - late effect
381.4 Nonsuppurative (allergic) (exudative) (transudative) (secretory) (mucoid) (catarrhal)
381.4 Nonsuppurative with effusion (allergic) (exudative) (transudative) (secretory) (mucoid) (catarrhal)
055.2 Postmeasles
381.4 Serous (mucoid) (catarrhal)
382.4 Suppurative

386.8 OTOCONIA
388.71 OTOGENIC PAIN
386.19 OTOLITH SYNDROME
111.8 OTOMYCOSIS [380.15]
117.3 OTOMYCOSIS ASPERGILLUS [380.15]
112.82 OTOMYCOSIS CANDIDA
759.89 OTOPALATATODIGITAL SYNDROME
388.69 OTORRHAGIA
388.60 OTORRHEA
388.61 OTORRHEA CEREBROSPINAL FLUID

OTOSCLEROSIS

387.9 NOS
387.2 Cochlear
387.2 Otic capsule
387.0 Oval window
387.1 Oval window obliterative
387.2 Round window
387.8 Other

715.35 OTTO'S DISEASE

OUTCOME OF DELIVERY

V30.#(#) Single liveborn (code on infant's record)
V27.0 Single liveborn (code on mother's record)
V27.1 Single stillborn (code on mother's record)

V31.#(#) Twin mate, liveborn (code on infant's record)
V27.2 Twin mate, liveborn (code on mother's record)
V27.3 Twin mate, one liveborn one stillborn (code on mother's record)
V32.#(#) Twin mate, stillborn (code on infant's record)
V27.4 Twin mate, stillborn (code on mother's record)
V33.#(#) Twin, unspecified (code on infant's record)
V34.#(#) Other multiple, mates all liveborn (code on infant's record)
V27.5 Other multiple, mates all liveborn (code on mother's record)
V35.#(#) Other multiple, mates all stillborn (code on infant's record)
V27.7 Other multiple, mates all stillborn (code on mother's record)
V36.#(#) Other multiple, mates liveborn and stillborn (code on infant's record)
V27.6 Other multiple, mates liveborn and stillborn (code on mother's record)
V37.#(#) Other multiple, unspecified (code on infant's record)
V39.#(#) Unspecified (single or multiple) (code on infant's record)
V27.9 Unspecified (single or multiple) (code on mother's record)
4th or 4th and 5th digit: V30 - V39
0#. Born in hospital
0. Delivered without mention of cesarean section
1. Delivered by cesarean section
1. Born before admission to hospital
2. Born outside hospital and not hospitalized

353.0 OUTLET COMPRESSION SYNDROME (THORACIC)

O

653.3# OUTLET CONTRACTION PELVIS

660.1# OUTLET CONTRACTION PELVIS OBSTRUCTING LABOR **[653.3#]**

5th digit: 653.3, 660.1

0. Episode of care unspecified or N/A

1. Delivered

3. Antepartum condition or complication

OUT-TOEING (DUE TO)

754.62 Calcaneovalgus
755.63 Femoral retroversion
754.61 Flatfeet
755.69 Tibia torsion, external

282.1 OVALOCYTOSIS CONGENITAL

282.1 OVALOCYTOSIS HEREDITARY

0 OVARIAN SEE 'OVARY, OVARIAN'

OVARY, OVARIAN

V45.77 Absence acquired
752.0 Absence congenital
752.0 Accessory congenital
614.6 Adhesion
752.0 Adhesion congenital (to cecum, kidney, omentum)
620.4 And fallopian tube prolapse or hernia
902.81 Artery injury
908.4 Artery injury late effect
902.81 Artery laceration (rupture) (hematoma) (avulsion) (aneurysm) traumatic
908.4 Artery laceration late effect
620.3 Atrophy (senile)
620.8 Calcification
V76.46 Cancer screening
0 Cyst see 'Cyst', ovary
220 Cystadenoma
620.2 Cystoma simple
256.39 Deficiency
256.39 Deficiency with natural menopause [627.2]
620.9 Disease - NEC (noninflammatory)
620.2 Disease - cystic
256.4 Disease - polycystic
620.8 Disease - specified NEC
614.9 Disorder inflammatory - NOS
614.8 Disorder inflammatory - other
620.9 Disorder noninflammatory - NOS
620.8 Disorder noninflammatory - other
620.4 Displacement
752.0 Displacement - congenital
256.9 Dysfunction
256.2 Dysfunction postirradiation
256.2 Dysfunction postirradiation with artificial menopause [627.4]
256.8 Dysfunction other
758.6 Dysgenesis
752.0 Ectopic congenital
256.39 Failure
256.2 Failure iatrogenic (post irradiation) (postsurgical)
256.2 Failure iatrogenic (post irradiation) (postsurgical) with artificial menopause [627.4]
256.2 Failure postablative
256.2 Failure postablative with artificial menopause [627.4]
256.31 Failure premature
256.39 Failure primary
256.39 Failure with natural menopause [627.2]

OVARY, OVARIAN (continued)

256.1 Hyperfunction other
620.8 Hyperplasia
256.1 Hyperstimulation
256.39 Hypofunction
256.39 Hypofunction with natural menopause [627.2]
620.8 Infarction
908.2 Injury late effect
867.6 Injury traumatic
867.7 Injury traumatic with open wound into cavity
752.0 Malformation
256.1 Overstimulation
620.5 Pedicle torsion
633.20 Pregnancy
633.20 Pregnancy with complication during treatment **[639.#]**
639.# Pregnancy with complication following treatment
633.21 Pregnancy with intrauterine pregnancy
633.21 Pregnancy with intrauterine pregnancy with complication during treatment **[639.#]**
639.# Pregnancy with intrauterine pregnancy with complication following treatment

4th digit: 639

0. Genital tract and pelvic infection

1. Delayed or excessive hemorrhage

2. Damage to pelvic organs and tissue

3. Renal failure

4. Metabolic disorders

5. Shock

6. Embolism

8. Other specified complication

9. Unspecified complication

620.4 Prolapse (hernia)
620.8 Remnant syndrome
V50.42 Removal prophylactic
620.8 Rupture (nonpregnant)
620.8 Rupture with hemoperitoneum (non-traumatic) [568.81]
620.3 Senile involution
752.0 Streak congenital
620.5 Torsion
752.0 Torsion congenital
902.82 Vein injury
908.4 Vein injury late effect
902.82 Vein laceration (rupture) (hematoma) (avulsion)
908.4 Vein laceration late effect

596.51 OVERACTIVE BLADDER

314.01 OVERACTIVITY NOS (ADULT) (CHILD)

313.0 OVERANXIOUS DISORDER OF CHILDHOOD AND ADOLESCENCE

524.29 OVERBITE (DEEP) (EXCESSIVE) (HORIZONTAL) (VERTICAL)

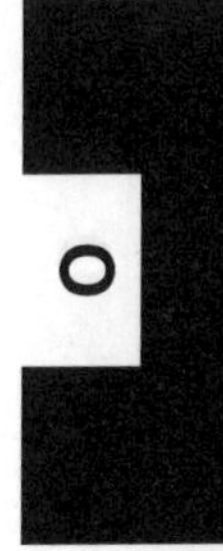

977.9 OVERDOSE DRUG UNSPECIFIED
0 OVERDOSE SEE APPENDIX B, DRUGS AND CHEMICALS

OVEREATING

783.6 NOS (unspecified cause)
307.51 Non-organic
278.00 With obesity
278.00 With obesity and body mass index above 25 [V85.#(#)]

V85.#(#): These codes are for use in persons over 20 years old.

4th or 4th and 5th digit: V85
2#. 25-29
1. 25.0-25.9
2. 26.0-26.9
3. 27.0-27.9
4. 28.0-28.9
5. 29.0-29.9
3#. 30-39
0. 30.0-30.9
1. 31.0-31.9
2. 32.0-32.9
3. 33.0-33.9
4. 34.0-34.9
5. 35.0-35.9
6. 36.0-36.9
7. 37.0-37.9
8. 38.0-38.9
9. 39.0-39.9
4. 40 and over

526.62 OVERFILL ENDODONTIC
788.38 OVERFLOW INCONTINENCE
525.62 OVERHANGING TOOTH RESTORATION
525.62 OVERHANGING UNREPAIRABLE DENTAL RESTORATIVE MATERIALS
524.29 OVERJET
524.26 OVERJET EXCESSIVE HORIZONTAL

OVERLOAD

276.6 Fluid
276.7 Potassium
276.0 Sodium

255.3 OVERPRODUCTION ACTH
255.0 OVERPRODUCTION CORTISOL
253.0 OVERPRODUCTION GROWTH HORMONE
242.8# OVERPRODUCTION TSH
5th digit: 242.8
0. Without thyrotoxic crisis or storm
1. With mention of throtoxic crisis or storm

747.21 OVERRIDING AORTA CONGENITAL
780.79 OVERSTRAINED
0 OVERUSE SYNDROME SEE 'BURSITIS', OCCUPATIONAL

278.02 OVERWEIGHT
278.02 OVERWEIGHT WITH BODY MASS INDEX 25.0 AND ABOVE [V85.#(#)]

V85.#(#): These codes are for use in persons over 20 years old.

4th or 4th and 5th digit: V85
2#. 25-29
1. 25.0-25.9
2. 26.0-26.9
3. 27.0-27.9
4. 28.0-28.9
5. 29.0-29.9
3#. 30-39
0. 30.0-30.9
1. 31.0-31.9
2. 32.0-32.9
3. 33.0-33.9
4. 34.0-34.9
5. 35.0-35.9
6. 36.0-36.9
7. 37.0-37.9
8. 38.0-38.9
9. 39.0-39.9
4. 40 and over

780.79 OVERWORK

OVIDUCT

752.19 Absence or atresia (congenital)
V45.77 Absence or atresia acquired
620.3 Atrophy (senile) acquired
619.2 Fistula external
628.2 Occlusion
752.19 Occlusion congenital

626.5 OVULATION BLEEDING
625.2 OVULATION PAIN
V59.7# OVUM DONOR (EGG) (OOCYTE)
4th digit: V59.7
0. Unspecified
1. Under age 35, NOS or anonymous recipient
2. Under age 35, designated recipient
3. Age 35 and over, NOS or anonymous recipient
4. Age 35 and over, designated recipient

286.3 OWREN'S (CONGENITAL) DISEASE OR SYNDROME
758.6 OX SYNDROME
271.8 OXALOSIS CARBOHYDRATE TRANSPORT DISORDERS
277.85 OXIDATION, FATTY ACID DISORDER
756.0 OXYCEPHALY
790.91 OXYGEN SATURATION ABNORMAL FINDING
V46.2 OXYGEN THERAPY (SUPPLEMENTAL) LONG TERM (DEPENDENCE)
127.4 OXYURIASIS
127.4 OXYURIS VERMICULARIS INFECTION
472.0 OZENA

O

756.59 PAAS' DISEASE

PACEMAKER (CARDIAC)

V53.31 Battery replacement
V53.39 Carotid sinus fitting and adjustment
996.61 Complication - infection or inflammation
996.01 Complication - mechanical (breakdown) (perforation) (displaced)
996.72 Complication - other
V53.31 Fitting and adjustment
V45.01 In situ status
996.01 Malfunction (breakdown) (perforation) (displaced)
V53.31 Reprogramming
V45.01 Status postsurgical (in situ)
429.4 Syndrome

427.61 PAC'S (PREMATURE ATRIAL CONTRACTIONS)
322.9 PACHYMENINGITIS
757.5 PACHYONYCHIA CONGENITAL
216.# PACINIAN TUMOR M9507/0

4th digit: 216
0. Lip (skin of)
1. Eyelid including canthus
2. Ear (external) (auricle) (pinna)
3. Face (cheek) (nose) (eyebrow) (temple)
4. Scalp, neck
5. Trunk, back except scrotum
6. Upper limb including shoulder
7. Lower limb including hip
8. Other specified sites
9. Skin unspecified

PAGET'S DISEASE

731.0 Bone (osteitis deformans)
0 Bone in osteosarcoma see 'Osteosarcoma' in Paget's disease of bone

> ***Use an additional code to identify estrogen receptor status. V86.0 Estrogen receptor positive status (ER+) or V86.1 Estrogen receptor negative status (ER-).***

174.# Breast infiltrating duct carcinoma M8541/3
174.# Breast soft/connective tissue M8540/3

4th digit: 174
0. Nipple and areola
1. Central portion
2. Upper inner quadrant
3. Lower inner quadrant
4. Upper outer quadrant
5. Lower outer quadrant
6. Axillary tail
8. Mastectomy site, inner lower midline outer upper ectopic sites, sites contiguous overlapping sites undetermined
9. Breast (female) site unspecified

199.1 Extra mammary (except Paget's disease of bone) site NOS
0 Extra mammary (except Paget's disease of bone) site specified see 'Cancer', by site M8542/3

453.8 PAGET-SCHROETTER SYNDROME (INTERMITTENT VENOUS CLAUDICATION)

> ***Pain codes usually sequence second, unless they are the reason for the encounter. Example: Encounter for a nerve block for acute postop pain following lumbar laminectomy with status fusion. 338.18 Pain postop acute and V45.4 Status lumbar fusion.***

PAIN

780.96 NOS
789.0# Abdominal (rebound tenderness)

5th digit: 789.0
0. Unspecified site
1. Upper right quadrant
2. Upper left quadrant
3. Lower right quadrant
4. Lower left quadrant
5. Periumbilic
6. Epigastric
7. Generalized
9. Other specified site (multiple)

338.1# Acute

5th digit: 338.1
1. Due to trauma
2. Post-thoracotomy
8. Other postoperative
9. Other

719.47 Ankle joint
569.42 Anus
729.5 Arch foot
729.5 Arm
729.5 Axillary
724.5 Back (postural)
724.2 Back low
788.9 Bladder
611.71 Breast
625.9 Broad ligament
338.3 Cancer associated (acute) (chronic)
337.0 Carotid artery
733.90 Cartilage NEC
723.3 Cervical - brachial (syndrome)
0 Chest see 'Chest Pain'
338.2# Chronic

5th digit: 338.2
1. Due to trauma
2. Post-thoracotomy
8. Other postoperative
9. Other

338.4 Chronic associated with psychosocial dysfunction
338.4 Chronic syndrome
724.79 Coccyx
786.52 Costochondral
786.52 Diaphragm
0 Due to device, implant, graft see 'Complications of an Internal Prosthetic Device, Implant or Graft – Other Specified'
338.3 Due to malignancy (primary or secondary) (acute) (chronic)
388.70 Ear
388.72 Ear referred
719.42 Elbow
789.06 Epigastric
729.5 Extremity (lower) (upper)
379.91 Eye
784.0 Face
350.2 Face atypical
351.8 Face neurogenic

P

PAIN (continued)

729.5 Finger
719.44 Finger joints
789.09 Flank
729.5 Foot
719.47 Foot joint
729.5 Forearm
780.96 Generalized
625.9 Genital female
608.9 Genital male
529.6 Glottic (tongue)
789.09 Groin
781.99 Growing
729.5 Hand
719.44 Hand joints
784.0 Head
719.45 Hip
526.9 Jaw
719.4# Joint

5th digit: 719.4

0. Site unspecified
1. Shoulder region
2. Upper arm (elbow) (humerus)
3. Forearm (radius) (wrist) (ulna)
4. Hand (carpal) (metacarpal) (fingers)
5. Pelvic region and thigh (hip) (buttock) (femur)
6. Lower leg (fibula) (knee) (patella) (tibia)
7. Ankle and/or foot (metatarsals) (toes) (tarsals)
8. Other
9. Multiple

788.0 Kidney
719.46 Knee
729.5 Leg
454.8 Leg due to varicose veins
729.5 Limb (lower) (upper)
0 Localized, unspecified type – code to pain by site
724.2 Lumbar
526.9 Maxilla
528.9 Mouth
729.1 Muscle
786.59 Muscle - intercostal
729.1 Musculoskeletal see also 'Pain', by site
729.1 Myofascial syndrome
478.19 Nasal
478.29 Nasopharynx
338.3 Neoplasm related (acute) (chronic)
723.1 Neck (nondiscogenic)
729.2 Nerve
729.1 Neuromuscular
478.19 Nose
379.91 Orbital
388.71 Otogenic
625.9 Ovary
719.45 Pelvic bone structures
625.9 Pelvic female (organic)
789.09 Pelvic male
607.9 Penis
789.05 Periumbilic
786.52 Pleuritic (chest)

PAIN (continued)

338.18 Postoperative
338.18 Postoperative acute
338.28 Postoperative chronic
338.12 Post-thoracotomy
338.12 Post-thoracotomy acute
338.22 Post-thoracotomy chronic
786.51 Precordial (chest)

In order to code psychogenic pain or pain exclusively attributed to psychological factors, code first the site of the physical pain and use an additional code (307.80) to identify the psychogenic pain.

307.80 Psychogenic site unspecified
306.3 Psychogenic skin
307.89 Psychogenic other
729.0 Rheumatic NEC
729.1 Rheumatic muscular
786.50 Rib
724.6 Sacroiliac
724.3 Sciatic
608.9 Scrotum
608.9 Seminal vesicle
719.41 Shoulder
478.19 Sinus
782.0 Skin
608.9 Spermatic cord
0 Spinal root see 'Radiculitis'
536.8 Stomach
338.4 Syndrome chronic
608.9 Testis
348.8 Thalamic
724.1 Thoracic spine (nonvertebral) (nondiscogenic)
724.4 Thoracic spine (nonvertebral) (nondiscogenic) with radicular and visceral pain
784.1 Throat
524.6# TMJ (temporomandibular joint)

5th digit: 524.6

0. Unspecified
1. Adhesions and ankylosis
2. Arthralgia
3. Articular disc disorder (reducing or non reducing)
4. Sounds on opening and/or closing the jaw
9. Other specified joint disorder

729.5 Toe
719.47 Toe joint
529.6 Tongue
525.9 Tooth
338.3 Tumor associated (acute) (chronic)
789.05 Umbilical
788.0 Ureter
788.0 Urinary organ (system)
625.9 Uterus
625.9 Vagina
454.8 Varicose veins
724.5 Vertebrogenic
625.9 Vulva
307.89 With psychological factors
719.43 Wrist

P

PAINFUL

162.3 Apicocostal vertebral syndrome M8010/3
726.19 Arc syndrome
786.52 Breathing
287.2 Bruising syndrome
625.0 Coitus female
608.89 Coitus male
302.76 Coitus psychogenic (female) (male)
0 Device, implant, graft see 'Complications of an Internal Prosthetic Device, Implant or Graft – Other Specified'
608.89 Ejaculation
302.79 Ejaculation psychogenic
607.3 Erection
266.2 Feet syndrome
0 Intercourse see 'Painful', coitus
625.2 Intermenstrual
625.3 Menstruation
306.52 Menstruation psychogenic
788.1 Micturition
378.55 Ophthalmoplegia
625.2 Ovulation
625.4 Premenstrual
786.52 Respiration
709.2 Scar
998.89 Sutures (wire)
788.1 Urination
998.89 Wire sutures

0 PAINT GUN INJURY SEE 'OPEN WOUND', BY SITE, COMPLICATED

PALATE

749.0# Cleft

5th digit: 749.0

0. NOS
1. Unilateral complete
2. Unilateral incomplete
3. Bilateral complete
4. Bilateral incomplete

749.2# Cleft with cleft lip

5th digit: 749.2

0. Palate with cleft lip unspecified
1. Palate unilateral complete
2. Palate unilateral incomplete
3. Palate bilateral complete
4. Palate bilateral incomplete
5. Palate other combinations

750.9 Deformity - congenital
526.89 Deformity - hard
528.9 Deformity - soft
528.9 Disease (soft) (hyperplasia)
528.9 Edema
0 Fissure see 'Palate', cleft
750.26 Flaccid congenital
526.89 Hypertrophy
528.9 Hypertrophy soft
959.09 Injury
524.89 Narrowing

719.3# PALINDROMIC RHEUMATISM

5th digit: 719.3

0. Site unspecified
1. Shoulder region
2. Upper arm (elbow) (humerus)
3. Forearm (radius) (wrist) (ulna)
4. Hand (carpal) (metacarpal) (fingers)
5. Pelvic region and thigh (hip) (buttock) (femur)
6. Lower leg (fibula) (knee) (patella) (tibia)
7. Ankle and/or foot (metatarsals) (toes) (tarsals)
8. Other
9. Multiple

362.63 PALISADE DEGENERATION RETINA

When using code V66.7, code the terminal illness first.

V66.7 PALLIATIVE CARE FOR END-OF-LIFE, HOSPICE OR TERMINAL CARE

782.61 PALLOR SKIN

PALMAR

903.4 Artery injury
908.3 Artery injury late effect
903.4 Artery laceration traumatic (rupture) (hematoma) (avulsion) (aneurysm)
908.3 Artery laceration late effect
726.4 Bursitis
757.2 Creases abnormal congenital
695.0 Erythema
728.6 Fascia contracture
693.0 Plantar erythrodysesthesia (PPE)

785.1 PALPITATIONS

PALSY

335.20 Atrophic diffuse
351.0 Bell's
993.3 Divers
351.0 Facial
767.5 Facial due to birth trauma
335.22 Progressive bulbar
335.23 Pseudobulbar
354.3 Radial nerve acute
356.8 Supranuclear NEC
333.0 Supranuclear progressive
354.2 Ulnar nerve tardy

201.9# PALTAUF-STERNBERG DISEASE

5th digit: 201.9

0. Unspecified site, extranodal and solid organ sites
1. Lymph nodes of head, face, neck
2. Lymph nodes intrathoracic
3. Lymph nodes abdominal
4. Lymph nodes axilla and upper limb
5. Lymph nodes inguinal region and lower limb
6. Lymph nodes intrapelvic
7. Spleen
8. Lymph nodes multiple sites

446.0 PANARTERITIS NODOSA
446.0 PANARTERITIS NODOSA POLYNEUROPATHY [357.1]
162.3 PANCOAST'S SYNDROME (CARCINOMA, PULMONARY APEX) M8010/3

P

556.6 PANCOLITIS

PANCREAS, PANCREATIC

577.0	Abscess
V45.79	Absence acquired (postoperative) (posttraumatic)
751.7	Absence congenital
751.7	Accessory congenital
751.7	Agenesis
751.7	Annular congenital
577.8	Atrophy
577.8	Calcification
577.2	Cyst or pseudocyst
577.9	Disease
577.2	Disease - cystic
751.7	Disease - cystic congenital
277.0#	Disease - cystic fibrosis

5th digit: 277.0
0. NOS
1. With meconium ileus
2. With pulmonary manifestations
3. With gastrointestinal manifestations
9. With other manifestations

251.9	Disorder of internal secretion (non-diabetic)
251.8	Disorder of internal secretion (non-diabetic) other
V59.8	Donor non-autogenous
577.8	Duct calculus
577.8	Duct obstruction
751.7	Ectopic
277.0#	Fibrocystic disease

5th digit: 277.0
0. NOS
1. With meconium ileus
2. With pulmonary manifestations
3. With gastrointestinal manifestations
9. With other manifestations

577.8	Fibrosis (atrophy) (calculus) (cirrhosis)
794.9	Function study abnormal
751.7	Heterotopia congenital
751.7	Hypoplasia congenital
863.8#	Injury
863.9#	Injury with open wound into cavity

5th digit: 863.8-9
1. Head
2. Body
3. Tail
4. Multiple and unspecified sites

908.1	Injury late effect
251.5	Islet alpha cells hyperplasia with gastrin excess
251.1	Islet beta cells hyperplasia
251.9	Islet cell hyperplasia
211.7	Islet cell tumor
577.8	Necrosis NOS (aseptic) (fat)
577.0	Necrosis acute or infective
577.8	Other specified diseases
442.84	Pancreaticoduodenal artery (aneurysm) (A-V fistula) (cirsoid) (false) (varicose)
794.9	Radioisotope study abnormal
794.9	Scan abnormal
579.4	Steatorrhea
996.86	Transplant rejection (failure)
V42.83	Transplant status

0 PANCREATIC SEE 'PANCREAS, PANCREATIC'

PANCREATITIS

577.0	NOS
577.0	Acute
577.0	Apoplectic
577.0	Calcereous
577.1	Chronic (infectious) (interstitial)
577.0	Gangrenous
577.0	Hemorrhagic
072.3	Mumps
577.1	Painless
577.0	Recurrent acute
577.1	Recurrent chronic
577.1	Relapsing
577.0	Subacute
577.0	Suppurative

577.8	PANCREATOLITHIASIS
284.1	PANCYTOPENIA (ACQUIRED)
284.09	PANCYTOPENIA CONGENITAL
284.09	PANCYTOPENIA WITH MALFORMATIONS
046.2	PANENCEPHALITIS SCLEROSING SUBACUTE
284.81	PANHEMATOPENIA
284.09	PANHEMATOPENIA CONGENITAL OR CONSTITUTIONAL
284.81	PANHEMOCYTOPENIA
284.09	PANHEMOCYTOPENIA CONGENITAL OR CONSTITUTIONAL
253.7	PANHYPOPITUITARISM IATROGENIC
253.2	PANHYPOPITUITARISM (POSTPARTUM) (SYNDROME)
300.01	PANIC ATTACK
0	PANIC ATTACK (TRANSIENT) DUE TO GROSS STRESS REACTION (ACUTE) SEE 'STRESS REACTION', ACUTE
300.01	PANIC DISORDER
300.21	PANIC DISORDER WITH AGORAPHOBIA
284.09	PANMYELOPATHY FAMILIAL CONSTITUTIONAL
284.2	PANMYELOPHTHISIS
284.81	PANMYELOPHTHISIS ACQUIRED (SECONDARY)
284.2	PANMYELOPHTHISIS CONGENITAL
238.79	PANMYELOSIS (ACUTE)
0	PANMYELOSIS ACUTE SITE SPECIFIED SEE 'NEOPLASM UNCERTAIN BEHAVIOR' BY SITE M9951/1
732.3	PANNER'S DISEASE (OSTEOCHONDROSIS)

PANNICULITIS

729.30	NOS
724.8	Back
729.31	Knee
567.82	Mesenteric
723.6	Neck
729.30	Nodular, nonsuppurative
724.8	Sacral
729.39	Other site

370.62	PANNUS (CORNEAL)
278.1	PANNUS ABDOMINAL (SYMPTOMATIC)
076.1	PANNUS TRACHOMATOUS
360.02	PANOPHTHALMITIS
461.8	PANSINUSITIS
360.12	PANUVEITIS

PAP SMEAR

795.02 ASC-H, cervix (atypical squamous cells cannot exclude high grade squamous intraepithelial lesion)
795.01 ASC-US, cervix (atypical squamous cells of undetermined significance)
795.00 Cervix abnormal NOS
795.00 Cervix abnormal glandular smear
795.09 Cervix and cervical HPV abnormal other
795.00 Cervix atypical endocervical or endometrial cell NOS
795.00 Cervix atypical glandular cells NOS
795.02 Cervix atypical squamous cells cannot exclude high grade squamous intraepithelial lesion (ASC-H)
795.01 Cervix atypical squamous cells of undetermined significance (ASC-US)
233.1 Cervix carcinoma in situ
795.09 Cervix dyskaryotic
622.10 Cervix dysplasia - NOS
622.11 Cervix dysplasia - mild
622.12 Cervix dysplasia - moderate
233.1 Cervix dysplasia - severe
795.05 Cervix high risk human papillomavirus (HPV) DNA test positive [079.4]
795.08 Cervix inadequate smear
795.09 Cervix low risk human papillomavirus (HPV) DNA test positive [079.4]
795.08 Cervix unsatisfactory smear
795.06 Cervix with cytologic evidence of carcinoma
622.11 CIN I
622.12 CIN II
233.1 CIN III
0 Follow up to previous treatment of a disorder without recurrence see 'Follow up Exam'
795.04 HGSIL cervix (high grade squamous intraepithelial lesion)
795.03 LGSIL cervix (low grade squamous intraepithelial lesion)
V72.31 Routine cervical and vaginal smears with GYN exam [V76.47]
V72.31 Routine cervical smear with GYN exam
V76.2 Routine cervix without GYN exam
V71.1 Suspected neoplasm (unproven) (undiagnosed)
V72.32 To confirm recent normal smear following initial abnormal smear
V76.47 Vaginal
V76.47 Vaginal following hysterectomy [V45.77]
V76.47 Vaginal following hysterectomy for nonmalignant condition [V45.77]
V67.01 Vaginal following hysterectomy for cancer **[V10.4#]** [V45.77]

5th digit: V10.4
- **0. Genital organ unspecified**
- **1. Cervix uteri**
- **2. Other part of uterus**
- **3. Ovary**
- **4. Genital organ other**

795.1 Other site abnormal

PAPILLARY CARCINOMA

199.1 Site NOS
0 Site specified see 'Cancer', by site M8050/3
234.9 In situ site NOS
0 In situ site specified see'Carcinoma In Situ'by Site M8050/2
183.0 Serous surface site NOS
0 Serous surface site specified see 'Cancer', by site M8461/3

PAPILLARY CARCINOMA (continued)

199.1 Squamous cell site NOS
0 Squamous cell site specified see 'Cancer', by site M8052/3
199.1 Transitional cell site NOS
0 Transitional cell site specified see 'Cancer', by site M8130/3

216.# PAPILLARY HYDROADENOMA M8405/0

4th digit: 216
- **0. Lip (skin of)**
- **1. Eyelid including canthus**
- **2. Ear external (auricle) (pinna)**
- **3. Face (cheek) (nose) (eyebrow) (temple)**
- **4. Scalp, neck**
- **5. Trunk, back except scrotum**
- **6. Upper limb including shoulder**
- **7. Lower limb including hip**
- **8. Other specified sites**
- **9. Skin unspecified**

PAPILLARY MUSCLE

429.81 Atrophy
429.81 Degeneration
429.81 Dysfunction (disorder)
429.81 Incompetence
429.81 Incoordination
410.8# Infarction acute

5th digit: 410.8
- **0. Episode unspecified**
- **1. Initial episode**
- **2. Subsequent episode**

429.6 Rupture
410.8# Rupture (dysfunction) (post infarction) acute, < 8 weeks

5th digit: 410.8
- **0. Episode unspecified**
- **1. Initial episode**
- **2. Subsequent episode**

429.79 Rupture (dysfunction) (post infarction) > 8 weeks [414.8]
429.81 Scarring
429.81 Syndrome
410.8# Syndrome with myocardial infarction

5th digit: 410.8
- **0. Episode unspecified**
- **1. Initial episode**
- **2. Subsequent episode**

216.# PAPILLARY SYRINGADENOMA M8406/0

4th digit: 216
- **0. Lip (skin of)**
- **1. Eyelid including canthus**
- **2. Ear external (auricle) (pinna)**
- **3. Face (cheek) (nose) (eyebrow) (temple)**
- **4. Scalp, neck**
- **5. Trunk, back except scrotum**
- **6. Upper limb including shoulder**
- **7. Lower limb including hip**
- **8. Other specified sites**
- **9. Skin unspecified**

PAPILLEDEMA

377.00 NOS
377.02 With decreased ocular pressure
377.01 With increased intracranial pressure
377.03 With retinal disorder

P

377.31	PAPILLITIS OPTIC

PAPILLOMA

229.9	Site NOS (except papilloma of urinary bladder)
0	Site specified see 'Benign Neoplasm', by site (except papilloma of urinary bladder) M8050/0
078.11	Acuminatum (male) (female)
217	Breast lactiferous duct (solitary) site NOS
0	Breast lactiferous duct (solitary) site specified see 'Benign Neoplasm', breast
225.0	Choroid plexus site NOS M9390/0
0	Choroid plexus site specified see 'Benign Neoplasm', by site
191.5	Choroid plexus malignant site NOS
0	Choroid plexus malignant site specified see 'Cancer', by site M9390/3
229.9	Intraductal site NOS
0	Intraductal site specified see 'Benign Neoplasm', by site M8503/0
229.9	Inverted site NOS
0	Inverted site specified see 'Benign Neoplasm', by site M8053/0
212.0	Schneiderian site NOS
0	Schneiderian site specified see 'Benign Neoplasm', by site M8121/0
220	Serous surface site NOS
0	Serous surface - benign site specified see 'Benign Neoplasm', by site M8461/0
236.2	Serous surface - borderline malignancy site NOS
0	Serous surface - borderline malignancy site specified see 'Neoplasm Uncertain Behavior', by site M8461/1
229.9	Squamous cell site NOS
0	Squamous cell site specified see 'Benign Neoplasm', by site M8052/0
229.9	Transitional cell site NOS
0	Transitional cell site specified see 'Benign Neoplasm', by site M8120/0
238.1	Transitional cell - inverted type site NOS
0	Transitional cell - inverted type site specified see 'Neoplasm Uncertain Behavior', by site M8121/1
238.9	Urothelial site NOS
0	Urothelial site specified see 'Neoplasm Uncertain Behavior', by site M8120/1
229.9	Verrucous site NOS
0	Verrucous site specified see 'Benign Neoplasm', by site M8051/0
0	Verrucous carcinoma site specified see 'Cancer', by site M8051/3
238.9	Villous site NOS
0	Villous site specified see 'Neoplasm Uncertain Behavior', by site M8261/1

PAPILLOMATOSIS

229.9	Site NOS
0	Site specified see 'Benign Neoplasm', by site M8060/0
229.9	Intraductal site NOS
0	Intraductal site specified see 'Benign Neoplasm', by site M8505/0
217	Subareolar duct site NOS
0	Subareolar duct site specified see 'Benign Neoplasm', by site M8506/0

079.4	PAPILLOMAVIRUS INFECTION
078.1#	PAPILLOMAVIRUS WART

5th digit: 078.1
- **0. Unspecified, condyloma NOS, verruca NOS, verruca vulgaris, warts (infectious)**
- **1. Condyloma acuminatum**
- **9. Other specified viral, genital NOS, verruca: plana, plantaris**

759.89	PAPILLON-LEAGE AND PSAUME (ORODIGITOFACIAL DYSOSTOSIS)
709.8	PAPULAR ERUPTION
747.42	PAPVR (PARTIAL ANOMALOUS PULMONARY VENOUS RETURN)
779.89	PAPYRACEOUS FETUS
772.0	PARABIOTIC (TRANSFUSION) SYNDROME-DONOR (TWIN)
776.4	PARABIOTIC (TRANSFUSION) SYNDROME-RECIPIENT (TWIN)
746.5	PARACHUTE DEFORMITY MITRAL VALVE CONGENITAL
116.1	PARACOCCIDIOIDOMYCOSIS PULMONARY
116.1	PARACOCCIDIOIDOMYCOSIS VISCERAL
374.43	PARADOXICAL FACIAL MOVEMENTS

PARAGANGLIOMA

237.3	Site NOS
0	Site specified see 'Neoplasm Uncertain Behavior', by site M8680/1
237.3	Extra adrenal site NOS
0	Extra adrenal site specified see 'Neoplasm Uncertain Behavior', by site M8693/1
194.6	Extra adrenal - malignant site NOS
0	Extra adrenal - malignant site specified see 'Cancer', by site M8693/3
194.6	Malignant site NOS
0	Malignant site specified see 'Cancer', by site M8680/3
237.3	Parasympathetic site NOS
0	Parasympathetic site specified see 'Neoplasm Uncertain Behavior', by site M8682/1
237.3	Sympathetic site NOS
0	Sympathetic site specified see 'Neoplasm Uncertain Behavior', by site M8681/1

781.1	PARAGEUSIA
121.2	PARAGONIMIASIS
121.2	PARAGONIMUS INFECTION
286.3	PARAHEMOPHILIA
079.89	PARAINFLUENZA VIRUS INFECTION
690.8	PARAKERATOSIS
696.2	PARAKERATOSIS VARIEGATA

PARALYSIS, PARALYTIC

344.9	Unspecified
355.9	Abdomen (muscles)
355.9	Abductor
352.4	Accessory nerve
344.9	Acquired (old) (cause other or unspecified)
332.0	Agitans (syndrome)
344.89	Alternating
355.8	Ankle
569.49	Anus (sphincter)

P

PARALYSIS, PARALYTIC (continued)

344.4# Arm (monoplegia)
5th digit: 344.4
0. Unspecified side
1. Dominant side
2. Nondominant side

344.2 Arms both (diplegia)
358.00 Asthenic bulbar
358.01 Asthenic bulbar with (acute) exacerbation (crisis)
333.71 Athetoid
355.9 Atrophy
344.89 Babinski-Nageotte's
355.9 Back (muscles)
344.89 Benedikt's
767.7 Birth injury
0 Bladder see 'Bladder Disorders', paralysis
767.6 Brachial plexus (birth trauma)
353.0 Brachial plexus (nondiscogenic)
437.8 Brain (cortical)
519.19 Bronchi
344.89 Brown-Sequard's
335.22 Bulbar (chronic) (progressive)
358.00 Bulbospinal
358.01 Bulbospinal with (acute) exacerbation (crisis)
428.9 Cardiac
0 Cerebral spastic infantile see 'Cerebral Palsy'
437.8 Cerebrocerebellar
337.0 Cervical sympathetic
344.89 Cestan-Chenais
378.81 Conjugate cortical (nuclear) (supranuclear)
378.83 Convergence
767.7 Cranial nerve due to birth trauma
344.89 Crossed leg
784.99 Deglutition
519.4 Diaphragm
564.89 Digestive organs NEC
344.2 Diplegia
781.4 Extremity transient
367.51 Eye intrinsic
378.51 Eye oblique
351.0 Facial nerve
767.5 Facial nerve due to birth trauma (congenital)
998.2 Facial nerve due to procedure
359.3 Familial periodic
354.9 Finger NEC
094.1 General (of the insane) (progressive)
353.4 Gluteal (nondiscogenic)
354.9 Hand
349.89 Hemifacial progressive
342.## Hemiplegia
4th digit: 342
0. Flaccid
1. Spastic
8. Other specified
9. Unspecified

5th digit: 342
0. Unspecified side
1. Dominant side
2. Nondominant side

359.3 Hyperkalemic periodic
359.3 Hypokalemic periodic
300.11 Hysterical (conversion)
560.1 Ileus
564.89 Intestinal
767.0 Intracranial (birth trauma)
364.89 Iris

PARALYSIS, PARALYTIC (continued)

344.89 Jackson's
478.30 Laryngeal nerve recurrent
478.30 Larynx
478.34 Larynx bilateral complete
478.33 Larynx bilateral partial
478.32 Larynx unilateral complete
478.31 Larynx unilateral partial
438.50 Late effect cerebrovascular disease - cauda equina syndrome [344.60]
438.50 Late effect cerebrovascular disease - cauda equina syndrome with neurogenic bladder [344.61]
438.2# Late effect cerebrovascular disease - hemiplegia or hemiparesis
438.53 Late effect cerebrovascular disease - locked in state [344.81]
438.4# Late effect cerebrovascular disease - monoplegia lower limb
438.3# Late effect cerebrovascular disease - monoplegia upper limb
5th digit: 438.2-4
0. Unspecified side
1. Dominant side
2. Nondominant side

438.5# Late effect cerebrovascular disease - other paralytic syndrome
5th digit: 438.5
0. Unspecified side
1. Dominant side
2. Nondominant side
3. Bilateral

438.53 Late effect cerebrovascular disease - quadriplegia [344.0#]
5th digit: 344.0
0. Unspecified
1. C1 - C4, complete
2. C1 - C4, incomplete
3. C5 - C7, complete
4. C5 - C7, incomplete
9. Other quadriplegia

984.9 Lead toxicity
781.4 Limb transient
344.81 Locked in state
344.1 Lower extremities (paraplegia)
344.3# Lower limb monoplegia (old)
5th digit: 344.3
0. Unspecified side
1. Dominant side
2. Nondominant side

354.1 Median nerve
344.89 Medullary (tegmental)
344.89 Mesencephalic
344.89 Mesencephalic tegmental
344.89 Millard-Gubler-Foville
344.5 Monoplegia unspecified
344.3# Monoplegia lower limb (old)
344.4# Monoplegia upper limb (old)
5th digit: 344.3-4
0. Unspecified side
1. Dominant side
2. Nondominant side

359.9 Muscle
344.89 Nuclear associated
378.9 Ocular NOS
352.6 Oculofacial (congenital)
344.89 Oculomotor alternating

P

PARALYSIS, PARALYTIC (continued)

359.3 Periodic
767.7 Peripheral nerve due to birth trauma
354.8 Phrenic nerve
767.7 Phrenic nerve due to birth trauma
344.89 Postepileptic (transitory)
359.3 Potassium sensitive periodic
094.1 Progressive (general)
335.23 Pseudobulbar
306.0 Psychogenic
379.49 Pupillary
355.8 Quadriceps
344.0# Quadriplegia

5th digit: 344.0
0. Unspecified
1. C1 - C4, complete
2. C1 - C4, incomplete
3. C5 - C7, complete
4. C5 - C7, incomplete
9. Other quadriplegia

354.3 Radial nerve
767.6 Radial nerve birth trauma
344.89 Respiratory center NEC
770.87 Respiratory fetus or newborn
359.3 Secondary periodic
344.9 Senile
355.9 Serratus (anterior)
354.9 Shoulder
327.43 Sleep related recurrent isolated
344.9 Spastic
344.89 Spinal cord late effect NEC
352.4 Sternomastoid
536.3 Stomach
352.3 Stomach nerve (nondiabetic)
354.8 Subscapularis
334.9 Superior nuclear NEC
344.89 Supranuclear
333.0 Supranuclear progressive
344.9 Syndrome NOS
344.89 Syndrome acquired specified NEC
094.89 Syphilitic
989.5 Tick
344.89 Todd's
529.8 Tongue
781.4 Transient extremity
781.4 Transient limb
352.4 Trapezius
354.9 Triceps
350.9 Trigeminal nerve
378.53 Trochlear nerve
354.2 Ulnar nerve
344.2 Upper extremities (diplegia)
344.4# Upper limb monoplegia (old)

5th digit: 344.4
0. Unspecified side
1. Dominant side
2. Nondominant side

352.3 Vagus nerve
0 Vesical see 'Bladder Disorders', paralysis
344.89 Weber's

PARAMETRITIS

614.3 Acute
614.4 Chronic or unspecified
639.0 Following ectopic molar or aborted pregnancy
016.7# Tuberculous

5th digit: 016.7
0. Unspecified
1. Lab not done
2. Lab pending
3. Microscopy positive (in sputum)
4. Culture positive - microscopy negative
5. Culture negative - microscopy positive
6. Culture and microscopy negative confirmed by other methods

614.4 PARAMETRIUM ABSCESS CHRONIC OR UNSPECIFIED
629.9 PARAMETRIUM DISEASE
780.93 PARAMNESIA
277.30 PARAMYLOIDOSIS
359.29 PARAMYOTONIA CONGENITA (OF VON EULENBURG)
0 PARANEOPLASTIC SYNDROME SEE SPECIFIC DISORDER

PARANOIA

297.1 NOS
291.5 Alcoholic
292.11 Drug induced
297.8 Querulans
293.81 Transient organic

PARANOID

297.9 Disorder
297.3 Disorder shared (induced)
301.0 Personality
297.9 Reaction
298.3 Reaction acute (psychotic)
295.3# Schizophrenic

5th digit: 295.3
0. Unspecified
1. Subchronic
2. Chronic
3. Subchronic with acute exacerbration
4. Chronic with acute
5. In remission

PARANOID STATES (DELUSIONAL DISORDERS)

297.9 NOS
291.5 Alcoholic
297.1 Delusional disorder
292.11 Induced by drugs
297.2 Involutional
297.1 Paranoid (chronic)
297.2 Paraphrenia
297.3 Shared psychotic disorder
297.0 Simple
297.8 Other specified

344.1 PARAPARESIS SEE ALSO PARAPLEGIA
784.3 PARAPHASIA
302.9 PARAPHILIA
605 PARAPHIMOSIS
297.2 PARAPHRENIA

P

344.1 PARAPLEGIA ACQUIRED (OLD) (CAUSE OTHER OR UNSPECIFIED)
343.0 PARAPLEGIA CONGENITAL
334.1 PARAPLEGIA HEREDITARY SPASTIC
438.53 PARAPLEGIA LATE EFFECT OF CEREBROVASCULAR DISEASE [344.1]
728.10 PARAPLEGIC CALCIFICATION (MASSIVE)
273.1 PARAPROTEINEMIA
696.2 PARAPSORIASIS
696.2 PARAPSORIASIS LICHENOIDES CHRONICA
057.8 PARASCARLATINA

PARASITIC DISEASE

136.9 NOS
123.9 Cerebral NEC
V01.89 Exposure
V12.00 History NOS
V18.8 History family
V12.09 History other specified
136.9 Infestation
129 Intestinal NOS
139.8 Late effect

647.8#: Use an additional code to identify the maternal parasitic disease.

647.8# Maternal current (co-existent) in pregnancy
5th digit: 647.8
0. Episode of care unspecified or N/A
1. Delivered
2. Delivered with postpartum complication
3. Antepartum complication
4. Postpartum complication

112.0 Mouth
V75.8 Screening exam parasitic infections other specified
134.9 Skin NEC
112.0 Tongue
136.8 Other specified

300.29 PARASITOPHOBIA

PARASOMNIA

307.47 Unspecified
291.82 Alcohol induced
327.41 Confusional arousals
292.85 Drug induced
307.47 Nonorganic
327.40 Organic NOS

327.44: Code first the underlying condition

327.44 Organic in conditions classified elsewhere
327.49 Organic other
327.43 Recurrent isolated sleep paralysis
327.42 REM sleep behavior disorder

752.69 PARASPADIAS CONGENITAL
351.8 PARASPASM FACIALIS
337.9 PARASYMPATHETIC NERVOUS SYSTEM DISORDER NEC

PARATHYROID

759.2 Gland absent (congenital)
252.8 Gland cyst
252.9 Gland disorder
252.8 Gland disorder specified NEC
252.8 Gland hemorrhage (infarct)
252.8 Hemorrhage
252.00 Hyperfunction
252.01 Hyperplasia (gland)
252.01 Hypertrophy
959.09 Injury (gland)
252.1 Tetany

252.1 PARATHYROIDITIS AUTOIMMUNE
077.0 PARATRACHOMA

PARATYPHOID FEVER

002.9 NOS
002.1 A
002.2 B
002.3 C

753.8 PARAURETHRAL DUCT ABSENCE
051.9 PARAVACCINIA
570 PARENCHYMATOUS LIVER DEGENERATION
V61.3 PARENT PROBLEM (AGED) (IN-LAW)
0 PARESIS SEE 'PARALYSIS'
782.0 PARESTHESIA SKIN
378.81 PARINAUD'S SYNDROME (PARALYSIS OF CONJUGATE UPWARD GAZE)
372.02 PARINAUD'S SYNDROME - OCULOGLANDULAR
759.6 PARKES WEBER AND DIMITRI SYNDROME (ENCEPHALOCUTANEOUS ANGIOMATOSIS)
0 PARKINSON'S (PARKINSONIAN) DISEASE OR SYNDROME SEE 'PARKINSONISM'

PARKINSONISM

332.0 NOS
331.82 Dementia [**294.1#**]
5th digit: 294.1
0. Without behavioral disturbance or NOS
1. With behavioral disturbance

332.1 Drug induced
332.0 Idiopathic
333.4 In Huntingdon's disease
332.0 In progressive supranuclear ophthalmogplegia
333.0 In Shy-Drager syndrome
332.1 Neuroleptic-induced
332.0 Primary
332.1 Secondary
094.82 Syphilitic
333.0 With orthostatic hypotension

523.9 PARODONTAL DISEASE
523.40 PARODONTITIS
681.02 PARONYCHIA FINGER
681.11 PARONYCHIA TOE
0 PARONYCHIA SEE ALSO 'ONYCHIA'
781.1 PAROSMIA

P

PAROTID

527.8 Duct atresia
750.23 Duct atresia congenital
527.8 Duct obstruction
750.21 Gland absence (congenital)
527.0 Gland atrophy
785.6 Gland swelling

PAROTITIS

527.2 NOS
527.2 Allergic
072.9 Epidemic
072.9 Infectious
072.9 Mumps
527.2 Surgical (postoperative) (not mumps)
527.2 Toxic

PAROXYSMAL

427.0 Atrial tachycardia
333.5 Choreoathetosis
780.39 Disorder (attack), mixed
427.2 Tachycardia
316 Tachycardia psychogenic [427.2]
427.1 Tachycardia ventricular

090.0 PARROT'S DISEASE (SYPHILITIC OSTEOCHONDRITIS)
0 PARROT FEVER SEE 'ORNITHOSIS'
242.0# PARRY'S DISEASE OR SYNDROME (EXOPHTHALMIC GOITER)
5th digit: 242.0
0. Without mention of thyrotoxic crisis or storm
1. With mention of thyrotoxic crisis or storm

349.89 PARRY-ROMBERG SYNDROME
242.0# PARSON'S DISEASE (EXOPHTHALMIC GOITER)
5th digit: 242.0
0. Without mention of thyrotoxic crisis or storm
1. With mention of thyrotoxic crisis or storm

353.5 PARSONAGE-ALDREN-TURNER SYNDROME
353.5 PARSONAGE-TURNER SYNDROME
363.21 PARS PLANITIS
353.5 PARSONAGE ALDREN TURNER SYNDROME (NONDISCOGENIC)
790.92 PARTIAL THROMBOPLASTIN TIME (PTT) ABNORMAL
553.1 PARUMBILICAL HERNIA
551.1 PARUMBILICAL HERNIA GANGRENOUS
552.1 PARUMBILICAL HERNIA INCARCERATED
079.83 PARVOVIRUS NOS (HUMAN) (B19)
301.84 PASSIVE AGGRESSIVE PERSONALITY
301.6 PASSIVE DEPENDENT PERSONALITY DISORDER
301.6 PASSIVE PERSONALITY
0 PASTEURELLA PESTIS SEE 'PLAGUE'
027.2 PASTEURELLA PSEUDOTUBERCULOSIS INFECTION
027.2 PASTEURELLA SEPTICA (CAT BITE) (DOG BITE)
0 PASTEURELLA TULAREMSIS SEE 'TULAREMIA'
027.2 PASTEURELLOSIS

427.0 PAT (PAROXYSMAL ATRIAL TACHYCARDIA)
316 PAT (PAROXYSMAL ATRIAL TACHYCARDIA) PSYCHOGENIC [427.0]
758.1 PATAU'S SYNDROME (TRISOMY D1)

PATELLA, PATELLAR

755.64 Absence congenital
755.64 Bipartite
717.7 Chondromalacia
719.66 Clunk syndrome
755.64 Rudimentary congenital
717.89 Slipping
844.8 Sprain
717.89 Sprain - old
726.64 Tedinitis
727.66 Tendon rupture nontraumatic
844.8 Tendon rupture traumatic
891.2 Tendon rupture traumatic with open wound

719.46 PATELLOFEMORAL STRESS SYNDROME
747.0 PATENT DUCTUS ARTERIOSUS
747.0 PATENT DUCTUS BOTALLI
745.5 PATENT FORAMEN BOTALLI
745.5 PATENT FORAMEN OVALE CONGENITAL
753.7 PATENT URACHUS CONGENITAL
V70.4 PATERNITY TESTING
280.8 PATERSON (-BROWN) (-KELLY) SYNDROME (SIDEROPENIC DYSPHAGIA)
301.7 PATHOLOGIC LIAR
301.9 PATHOLOGICAL PERSONALITY (DISORDER)
302.9 PATHOLOGICAL SEXUALITY
V72.6 PATHOLOGY
V64.2 PATIENT DECISION - PROCEDURE (SURGICAL) NOT CARRIED OUT
V62.6 PATIENT DECISION - PROCEDURE (SURGICAL) NOT CARRIED OUT FOR REASONS OF CONSCIENCE OR RELIGION
0 PATIENT SEE 'PERSON'
362.61 PAVING STONE DEGENERATION (RETINAL)
593.6 PAVY'S DISEASE
111.2 PAXTON'S DISEASE (WHITE PIEDRA)
569.89 PAYR'S SPLENIC FLEXURE SYNDROME
310.8 PBA (PSEUDOBULBAR AFFECT)
0 PCL (POSTERIOR CRUCIATE LIGAMENT) SEE 'POSTERIOR', CRUCIATE

PE TUBE (PRESSURE EQUALIZATION)

996.69 Complication - infection or inflammation
996.59 Complication - malfunction
996.79 Complication - other complication
V53.09 Removal
V53.09 Replacement

0 PEARL-WORKERS DISEASE SEE 'OSTEOMYELITIS', CHRONIC
447.8 PECTORAL GIRDLE SYNDROME
447.8 PECTORALIS MINOR SYNDROME

PECTUS

738.3 Carinatum acquired
754.82 Carinatum congenital
738.3 Excavatum acquired
754.81 Excavatum congenital
738.3 Recurvatum acquired
754.81 Recurvatum congenital

V65.11 PEDIATRIC PRE-BIRTH VISIT FOR EXPECTANT MOTHER

PEDICULOSIS

132.9 NOS
132.0 Capitis (head louse)
132.1 Corporis (body louse)
V01.89 Exposure
132.0 Eyelid [373.6]
132.3 Mixed infestation
132.2 Pubis (pubic louse)

302.2 PEDOPHILIA
302.2 PEDOPHILIC HOMOSEXUAL

PEG TUBE (PERCUTANEOUS ENDOSCOPIC GASTROSTOMY)

V55.1 Adjustment or repositioning
V55.1 Care
V55.1 Closure
536.40 Complication NOS
536.42 Complication mechanical
536.49 Complication other
V53.5 Device fitting and adjustment

When coding an infection of an ostomy, use an additional code to specify the organism. See 'Bacterial Infection'

536.41 Infection
536.41 Infection with cellulitis of abdomen [682.2]
536.41 Infection with septicemia [**038.#(#)**]

4th or 4th and 5th Digit Code for Organism: 038
.9 NOS
.3 Anaerobic
.3 Bacteroides
.3 Clostridium
.42 E. coli
.49 Enterobacter aerogenes
.40 Gram negative
.49 Gram negative other
.41 Hemophilus influenzae
.2 Pneumococcal
.49 Proteus
.43 Pseudomonas
.44 Serratia
.10 Staphylococcal NOS
.11 Staphylococcal aureus
.19 Staphylococcal other
.0 Streptococcal (anaerobic)
.49 Yersinia enterocolitica
.8 Other specified

536.42 Malfunction
V55.1 Removal
V55.1 Replacement
V44.1 Status
V55.1 Toilet stoma

0 PEL-EBSTEIN SEE 'HODGKIN'S DISEASE'
288.2 PELGER HUET SYNDROME (HEREDITARY HYPOSEGMENTATION)
287.0 PELIOSIS RHEUMATICA

330.0 PELIZAEUS MERZBACHER DISEASE
330.0 PELIZAEUS MERZBACHER DISEASE WITH DEMENTIA [**294.1#**]

5th digit: 294.1
0. Without behavioral disturbance or NOS
1. With behavioral disturbance

265.2 PELLAGRA (ALCOHOLIC)
270.0 PELLAGRA CEREBELLAR ATAXIA-RENAL AMINOACIDURIA SYNDROME
265.2 PELLAGRA POLYNEUROPATHY [357.4]
726.62 PELLEGRINI STIEDA SYNDROME (CALCIFICATION KNEE JOINT)
265.2 PELLAGROID SYNDROME
259.8 PELLIZZI'S SYNDROME (PINEAL)
0 PELVIC SEE 'PELVIS, PELVIC'

PELVIS, PELVIC

902.9 Blood vessel injury - NOS
902.87 Blood vessel injury - multiple
902.89 Blood vessel injury - specified NEC
763.1 Bony affecting fetus or newborn
653.0# Bony complicating pregnancy, L&D
660.1# Bony obstructing labor [**653.0#**]

5th digit: 653.0, 660.1
0. Episode of care unspecified or N/A
1. Delivered
3. Antepartum complication

614.4 Cellulitis female
614.3 Cellulitis female - acute
614.4 Cellulitis female - chronic
639.0 Cellulitis female - following abortion or ectopic/molar pregnancy
016.7# Celllulitis female - tuberculous

5th digit: 016.7
0. Unspecified
1. Lab not done
2. Lab pending
3. Microscopy positive (in sputum)
4. Culture positive - microscopy negative
5. Culture negative - microscopy positive
6. Culture and microscopy negative confirmed by other methods

567.21 Cellulitis male
625.5 Congestion (-fibrosis) syndrome
763.1 Contracted affecting fetus or newborn
653.1# Contracted - NOS complicating pregnancy childbirth or puerperium
660.1# Contracted - NOS obstructing labor [**653.1#**]
653.2# Contracted - inlet complicating pregnancy childbirth or puerperium
660.1# Contracted - inlet obstructing labor [**653.2#**]
653.8# Contracted - midplane (midpelvic) complicating pregnancy childbirth or puerperium
660.1# Contracted - midplane (midpelvic) obstructing labor [**653.8#**]
653.3# Contracted - outlet complicating pregnancy childbirth or puerperium
660.1# Contracted - outlet obstructing labor [**653.3#**]

5th digit: 653.1-3, 8, 660.1
0. Episode of care unspecified or N/A
1. Delivered
3. Antepartum complication

P

PELVIS, PELVIC (continued)

738.6 Deformity acquired
763.1 Deformity affecting fetus or newborn
755.60 Deformity congenital
629.9 Disease female NEC
614.9 Disease female inflammatory (PID) unspecified
614.8 Disease female inflammatory specified NEC
629.89 Disease female specified NEC
653.0# Disproportion in pregnancy (pelvic deformity unspecified)
660.1# Disproportion obstructing labor (bony pelvic deformity unspecified) **[653.0#]**
5th digit: 653.0, 660.1
0. Episode of care unspecified or N/A
1. Delivered
3. Antepartum complication

V72.31 Exam (annual) (periodic)
959.19 Floor injury
618.8# Floor relaxation
618.8# Floor relaxation with stress incontinence [625.6]
618.8# Floor relaxation with other urinary incontinence **[788.3#]**
5th digit: 618.8
1. Pubocervical tissue incompetence (weakening)
2. Rectovaginal tissue incompetence (weakening)
5th digit: 788.3
1. Urge incontinence
3. Mixed urge and stress
4. Without sensory awareness
5. Post-void dribbling
6. Nocturnal enuresis
7. Continuous leakage
8. Overflow incontinence
9. Other

654.4# Floor repair (previous) complicating pregnancy childbirth or pureperium
660.2# Floor repair (previous) obstructing labor **[654.4#]**
5th digit: 654.4
0. Episode of care unspecified or N/A
1. Delivered
2. Delivered with postpartum complication
3. Antepartum complication
4. Postpartum complication

5th digit: 660.2
0. Episode of care unspecified or N/A
1. Delivered
3. Antepartum complication

618.8# Incompetence
618.8# Incompetence with stress incontinence [625.6]
618.8# Incompetence with other urinary incontinence **[788.3#]**
5th digit: 618.8
1. Pubocervical tissue
2. Rectovaginal tissue
5th digit: 788.3
1. Urge incontinence
3. Mixed urge and stress
4. Without sensory awareness
5. Post-void dribbling
6. Nocturnal enuresis
7. Continuous leakage
8. Overflow incontinence
9. Other

PELVIS, PELVIC (continued)

614.9 Infection female NOS
614.9 Inflammatory disease female - NOS
614.3 Inflammatory disease female - acute
614.4 Inflammatory disease female - chronic
760.8 Inflammatory disease maternal - affecting fetus or newborn
670.0# Inflammatory disease maternal due to pregnancy NOS - major puerperal [614.9]
670.0# Inflammatory disease maternal due to pregnancy acute - major puerperal [614.3]
670.0# Inflammatory disease maternal due to pregnancy chronic - major puerperal [614.4]
5th digit: 670.0
0. Episode of care unspecified or N/A
2. Delivered with postpartum complication
4. Postpartum complication

639.0 Inflammatory disease maternal - following abortion or ectopic/molar pregnancy
0 Inflammatory disease maternal - in abortion see 'Abortion', by type with shock
646.6# Inflammatory disease maternal NOS - minor complicating pregnancy [614.9]
646.6# Inflammatory disease maternal acute - minor complicating pregnancy [614.3]
646.6# Inflammatory disease maternal chronic - minor complicating pregnancy [614.4]
5th digit: 646.6
0. Episode of care unspecified or N/A
1. Delivered
2. Delivered with postpartum complication
3. Antepartum complication
4. Postpartum complication

016.7# Inflammatory disease tuberculous
5th digit: 016.7
0. Unspecified
1. Lab not done
2. Lab pending
3. Microscopy positive (in sputum)
4. Culture positive - microscopy negative
5. Culture negative - microscopy positive
6. Culture and microscopy negative confirmed by other methods

614.8 Inflammatory disease - other specified
959.19 Injury
665.6# Joint and ligament damage obstetrical
5th digit: 665.6
0. Episode of care unspecified or N/A
1. Delivered
4. Postpartum complication

719.85 Joint calcification (pelvic region)
718.15 Joint loose body (pelvic region)
789.39 Mass

P

PELVIS, PELVIC (continued)

618.83 Muscle wasting
618.83 Muscle wasting with stress incontinence [625.6]
618.83 Muscle wasting with other urinary incontinence **[788.3#]**
5th digit: 788.3
1. Urge incontinence
3. Mixed urge and stress
4. Without sensory awareness
5. Post-void dribbling
6. Nocturnal enuresis
7. Continuous leakage
8. Overflow incontinence
9. Other

738.6 Obliquity
629.9 Organ disease female - NOS
629.89 Organ disease female - other specified NEC
867.8 Organ injury traumatic
867.9 Organ injury traumatic with open wound into cavity
908.2 Organ injury late effect
763.89 Organ or soft tissue abnormality affecting fetus or newborn
654.9# Organ or soft tissue abnormality complicating pregnancy
660.2# Organ or soft tissue abnormality obstructing labor **[654.9#]**
5th digit: 654.9
0. Episode of care unspecified or N/A
1. Delivered
2. Delivered with postpartum complication
3. Antepartum complication
4. Postpartum complication

5th digit: 660.2
0. Episode of care unspecified or N/A
1. Delivered
3. Antepartum complication

625.9 Pain female
789.09 Pain male
568.0 Peritoneal adhesions
560.81 Peritoneal adhesions with intestinal obstruction
614.6 Peritoneal adhesions - female
614.6 Peritoneal adhesions - female postoperative (postinfection)
614.7 Peritonitis chronic female
567.89 Peritonitis chronic male
016.7# Peritonitis female tuberculous
5th digit: 016.7
0. Unspecified
1. Lab not done
2. Lab pending
3. Microscopy positive (in sputum)
4. Culture positive - microscopy negative
5. Culture negative - microscopy positive
6. Culture and microscopy negative confirmed by other methods

639.0 Peritonitis following abortion or ectopic/molar pregnancy
567.21 Peritonitis male (acute)
739.5 Region segmental or somatic dysfunction

PELVIS, PELVIC (continued)

654.4# Rigid floor complicating pregnancy childbirth or pureperium
660.2# Rigid floor complicating pregnancy obstructing labor **[654.4#]**
5th digit: 654.4
0. Episode of care unspecified or N/A
1. Delivered
2. Delivered with postpartum complication
3. Antepartum complication
4. Postpartum complication

5th digit: 660.2
0. Episode of care unspecified or N/A
1. Delivered
3. Antepartum complication

848.5 Separation (rupture) (tear) (laceration)
665.6# Separation obstetrical
5th Digit for 665.6
0. Episode of care unspecified or N/A
1. Delivered
4. Postpartum complication

848.5 Strain (sprain) (avulsion) (hemarthrosis)
789.9 Symptom other
789.69 Tenderness
738.6 Tipping
763.1 Tipping affecting fetus or newborn
653.0# Tipping in pregnancy (bony pelvic deformity)
660.1# Tipping obstructing labor (bony pelvic deformity) **[653.0#]**
5th digit: 653.0, 660.1
0. Episode of care unspecified or N/A
1. Delivered
3. Antepartum complication

456.5 Varices

PEMPHIGOID

694.5 NOS
694.60 Benign mucous membrane
694.61 Benign mucous membrane with ocular involvement
694.5 Bullous
694.60 Cicatricial
694.61 Cicatricial with ocular involvement
694.2 Juvenile
694.60 Mucosynechial atrophic bullous dermatitis
694.61 Mucosynechial atrophic bullous dermatitis with ocular involvement

PEMPHIGUS

694.4 NOS
694.5 Benign
694.4 Brazilian
694.0 Circinatus
694.61 Conjunctiva
694.4 Erythematosus
694.4 Foliaceus
694.4 Frambesiodes
785.4 Gangrenous see also 'Gangrene'
694.4 Malignant
684 Neonatorum
694.61 Ocular
694.4 Papillaris
694.4 Seborrheic
694.4 South American
694.4 Vegetans
694.4 Vulgaris

243 PENDRED'S SYNDROME (FAMILIAL GOITER WITH DEAF-MUTISM)
701.9 PENDULOUS ABDOMEN
345.5# PENFIELD'S SYNDROME (SEE ALSO 'EPILEPSY')
5th digit: 345.5
0. Without mention of intractable epilepsy
1. With intractable epilepsy

V14.0 PENICILLIN ALLERGY (HISTORY)
V09.0 PENICILLIN RESISTANT INFECTION (SEE 'DRUG RESISTANCE')

0 PENILE SEE 'PENIS, PENILE'

PENIS, PENILE

V45.77 Absence acquired
752.69 Absence congenital
752.69 Accessory (congenital)
752.69 Agenesis (congenital)
752.69 Anomalies other
752.69 Atresia (congenital)
607.89 Atrophy
607.2 Boil (abscess) (carbuncle)
607.89 Calcification
607.2 Cellulitis
752.69 Cleft (congenital)
752.69 Closure imperfect (congenital)
752.65 Concealed (congenital)
752.69 Curvature (lateral) (congenital)
788.7 Discharge
607.9 Disorder
607.2 Disorder inflammatory
607.89 Disorder other specified
752.69 Double (congenital)
752.69 Elongation frenulum (congenital)
607.82 Embolism (hematoma) (hemorrhage) nontraumatic
607.83 Edema
607.89 Fibrosis
959.13 Fracture of corpus cavernosum
607.89 Gangrene noninfective
752.69 Glans division (congenital)
752.65 Hidden (congenital)
752.69 Hooded (congenital)
607.89 Hypertrophy
752.69 Hypoplasia congenital
607.1 Inflammation
607.81 Inflammation due to stricture
959.14 Injury other and NOS
911.8 Injury other and NOS superficial
911.9 Injury other and NOS superficial infected
607.0 Leukoplakia kraurosis
752.69 Malposition congenital
752.64 Micropenis (congenital)
607.81 Ossification
607.9 Pain
607.9 Pain psychogenic [307.80]
607.3 Painful erection
607.89 Phagedena
605 Phimosis
996.65 Prosthesis (implant) complication - infection or inflammation
996.39 Prosthesis (implant) complication - mechanical
996.76 Prosthesis (implant) complication - other
607.82 Thrombosis
607.89 Torsion
752.69 Torsion congenital

PENIS, PENILE (continued)

607.89 Ulcer (chronic)
607.82 Vascular disorders
752.69 Other specified anomaly congenital

758.81 PENTA X SYNDROME
282.2 PENTOSE PHOSPHATE PATHWAY DISORDER WITH ANEMIA
271.8 PENTOSURIA ESSENTIAL BENIGN
536.8 PEPTIC DISORDER ACID
536.9 PEPTIC DISORDER FUNCTIONAL - NEC
533.## PEPTIC ULCER (SYNDROME)
533.## PEPTIC ULCER DUE TO HELICOBACTER PYLORI INFECTION [041.86]
4th digit: 533
0. Acute with hemorrhage
1. Acute with perforation
2. Acute with hemorrhage and perforation
3. Acute
4. Chronic or unspecified with hemorrhage
5. Chronic or unspecified with perforation
6. Chronic or unspecified with hemorrhage and perforation
7. Chronic
9. Unspecified as acute or chronic
5th digit: 533
0. Without obstruction
1. Obstructed

V12.71 PEPTIC ULCER HISTORY
0 PEPTOCOCCUS SEE 'BACTERIAL INFECTION' OR SPECIFIED CONDITION
0 PEPTOSTREPTOCOCCUS SEE 'BACTERIAL INFECTION' OR SPECIFIED CONDITION
447.8 PERABDUCTION SYNDROME
0 PERCUTANEOUS TRANSLUMINAL CORONARY ANGIOPLASTY (PTCA) SEE 'PTCA'
V65.2 PEREGRINATING PATIENT

PERFORATION

473.0 Antrum (sinus)
540.0 Appendix
540.1 Appendix with peritoneal abscess
745.5 Atrial septum, multiple
384.22 Attic ear
384.81 Attic ear healed
576.3 Bile duct
575.4 Bile duct cystic
867.0 Bladder
639.2 Bladder following abortion, ectopic or molar pregnancy
596.6 Bladder nontraumatic (urinary)
665.5# Bladder obstetrical trauma
5th digit: 665.5
0. Episode of care unspecified or N/A
1. Delivered
4. Postpartum complication

867.0 Bladder traumatic
0 Bladder with abortion see 'Abortion', by type, with damage to pelvic organs or tissue
0 Bladder with ectopic pregnancy see 'Ectopic Pregnancy', by site with complication
0 Bladder with molar pregnancy see 'Molar Pregnancy', by type with complication

P

PERFORATION (continued)

569.83 Bowel
777.6 Bowel fetus or newborn
639.2 Bowel following abortion, ectopic or molar pregnancy
665.5# Bowel obstetrical trauma
5th digit: 665.5
0. Episode of care unspecified or N/A
1. Delivered
4. Postpartum complication

0 Bowel with abortion see 'Abortion', by type, with damage to pelvic organs or tissue
0 Bowel with ectopic pregnancy see 'Ectopic Pregnancy', by site with complication
0 Bowel with molar pregnancy see 'Molar Pregnancy', by type with complication
639.2 Broad ligament following abortion, ectopic or molar pregnancy
665.6# Broad ligament obstetrical trauma
5th digit: 665.6
0. Episode of care unspecified or N/A
1. Delivered
4. Postpartum complication

0 Broad ligament with abortion see 'Abortion', by type, with damage to pelvic organs or tissue
0 Broad ligament with ectopic pregnancy see 'Ectopic Pregnancy', by site with complication
0 Broad ligament with molar pregnancy see 'Molar Pregnancy', by type with complication
0 By device, implant or graft see 'Complication of a Device, Implant or Graft - Mechanical'
998.4 By foreign body left accidentally in operation wound
998.2 By instrument (any) during a procedure, accidental
540.0 Cecum
540.1 Cecum with peritoneal abscess
867.4 Cervix
639.2 Cervix following abortion, ectopic or molar pregnancy
665.3# Cervix obstetrical trauma
5th digit: 665.3
0. Episode of care unspecified or N/A
1. Delivered
4. Postpartum complication

0 Cervix with abortion see 'Abortion', by type, with damage to pelvic organs or tissue
0 Cervix with ectopic pregnancy see 'Ectopic Pregnancy', by site with complication
0 Cervix with molar pregnancy see 'Molar Pregnancy', by type with complication
569.83 Colon
576.3 Common duct (bile)
370.00 Cornea NOS
370.06 Cornea due to ulceration
575.4 Cystic duct
0 Diverticulum see anatomical site
0 Duodenum ulcer see 'Ulcer', duodenum with perforation
0 Ear drum see 'Perforation', tympanic membrane
0 Enteritis see 'Enteritis'
530.4 Esophagus
473.2 Ethmoid sinus
0 Eye traumatic see 'Eye', injuries
0 Foreign body - external site see 'Laceration', complicated
0 Foreign body - internal site, by ingested object see 'Foreign Body'
473.1 Frontal sinus

PERFORATION (continued)

575.4 Gallbladder
0 Gastric ulcer see 'Ulcer', gastric with perforation
0 Heart valve see 'Endocarditis'
569.83 Ileum
665.5# Ileum obstetrical trauma
5th digit: 665.5
0. Episode of care unspecified or N/A
1. Delivered
4. Postpartum complication

777.6 Ileum perinatal
0 Instrumental external see 'Laceration'
665.9# Instrumental pregnant uterus complicating delivery
5th digit: 665.9
0. Episode of care unspecified or N/A
1. Delivered
2. Delivered with postpartum complication
3. Antepartum complication
4. Postpartum complication

998.2 Instrumental surgical accidental
569.83 Intestine
665.5# Intestine obstetrical trauma
5th digit: 665.5
0. Episode of care unspecified or N/A
1. Delivered
4. Postpartum complication

777.6 Intestine perinatal
0 Intestine with abortion see 'Abortion', by type, with damage to pelvic organs or tissue
0 Intestine with ectopic pregnancy see 'Ectopic Pregnancy', by site with complication
0 Intestine with molar pregnancy see 'Molar Pregnancy', by type with complication
569.83 Intestine ulcerative NEC
569.83 Jejunum
665.5# Jejunum obstetrical trauma
5th digit: 665.5
0. Episode of care unspecified or N/A
1. Delivered
4. Postpartum complication

777.6 Jejunum perinatal
0 Jejunum ulcer see 'Ulcer', gastrojejunal with perforation
383.89 Mastoid (antrum) (cell)
473.0 Maxillary sinus
0 Membrana tympani see 'Perforation' tympanic membrane
478.19 Nasal septum
748.1 Nasal septum congenital
095.8 Nasal septum syphilitic
473.9 Nasal sinus NOS
748.1 Nasal sinus congenital
0 Organ internal traumatic see anatomical site
526.89 Palate hard
528.9 Palate soft
095.8 Palate syphilitic (hard) (soft)
526.89 Palatine vault
095.8 Palatine vault syphilitic
090.5 Palatine vault syphilitic congenital

PERFORATION (continued)

664.1# Pelvic floor obstetrical trauma
5th digit: 664.1
0. Episode of care unspecified or N/A
1. Delivered
4. Postpartum complication

0 Pelvic floor with abortion see 'Abortion', by type, with damage to pelvic organs or tissue
0 Pelvic floor with ectopic pregnancy see 'Ectopic Pregnancy', by site with complication
0 Pelvic floor with molar pregnancy see 'Molar Pregnancy', by type with complication
639.2 Pelvic organ following abortion, ectopic or molar pregnancy
665.5# Pelvic organ obstetrical trauma
5th digit: 665.5
0. Episode of care unspecified or N/A
1. Delivered
4. Postpartum complication

0 Pelvic organ with abortion see 'Abortion', by type, with damage to pelvic organs or tissue
0 Pelvic organ with ectopic pregnancy see 'Ectopic Pregnancy', by site with complication
0 Pelvic organ with molar pregnancy see 'Molar Pregnancy', by type with complication
879.6 Perineum
0 Periurethral tissue with abortion see 'Abortion', by type, with damage to pelvic organs or tissue
0 Periurethral tissue with ectopic pregnancy see 'Ectopic Pregnancy', by site with complication
0 Periurethral tissue with molar pregnancy see 'Molar Pregnancy', by type with complication
478.29 Pharynx
0 Pyloric ulcer see 'Ulcer', stomach with perforation
569.49 Rectum
526.61 Root canal space
569.83 Sigmoid
473.9 Sinus NOS
473.3 Sphenoidal sinus
0 Stomach due to ulcer see 'Ulcer', stomach with perforation
998.2 Surgical (accidental) (due to instrument)
384.20 Tympanic membrane (posttraumatic) (persistent) - NOS
384.22 Tympanic membrane (posttraumatic) (persistent) - attic
384.21 Tympanic membrane (posttraumatic) (persistent) - central
384.81 Tympanic membrane (posttraumatic) (persistent) - healed
384.24 Tympanic membrane (posttraumatic) (persistent) - multiple
384.22 Tympanic membrane (posttraumatic) (persistent) - pars flaccida
384.23 Tympanic membrane (posttraumatic) (persistent) - other marginal
0 Tympanic membrane (posttraumatic) (persistent) - with otitis media see 'Otitis Media'
384.25 Tympanic membrane (posttraumatic) (persistent) - total
872.61 Tympanic membrane - traumatic
872.71 Tympanic membrane - traumatic complicated
002.0 Typhoid, gastrointestinal

PERFORATION (continued)

0 Ulcer see 'Ulcer', by site with perforation
593.89 Ureter
639.2 Urethra following abortion, ectopic or molar pregnancy
665.5# Urethra obstetrical trauma
5th digit: 665.5
0. Episode of care unspecified or N/A
1. Delivered
4. Postpartum complication

867.0 Urethra traumatic
0 Urethra with abortion see 'Abortion', by type, with damage to pelvic organs or tissue
0 Urethra with ectopic pregnancy see 'Ectopic Pregnancy', by site with complication
0 Urethra with molar pregnancy see 'Molar Pregnancy', by type with complication
867.4 Uterus
996.32 Uterus by intrauterine contraceptive device
639.2 Uterus following abortion, ectopic or molar pregnancy
665.5# Uterus obstetrical trauma
5th digit: 665.5
0. Episode of care unspecified or N/A
1. Delivered
4. Postpartum complication

0 Uterus with abortion see 'Abortion', by type, with damage to pelvic organs or tissue
0 Uterus with ectopic pregnancy see 'Ectopic Pregnancy', by site with complication
0 Uterus with molar pregnancy see 'Molar Pregnancy', by type with complication
763.89 Uterus with obstetrical trauma affecting fetus or newborn
528.9 Uvula
095.8 Uvula syphilitic
665.4# Vagina complicating delivery NOS
665.4# Vagina complicating delivery with high vaginal wall or sulcus laceration
5th digit: 665.4
0. Episode of care unspecified or N/A
1. Delivered
4. Postpartum complication

664.## Vagina complicating delivery with perineal laceration
4th digit: 664
0. First degree
1. Second degree
2. Third degree
3. Fourth degree
4. Unspecified

5th digit: 664
0. Episode of care unspecified or N/A
1. Delivered
4. Postpartum complication

639.2 Vagina following abortion, ectopic or molar pregnancy
623.4 Vagina nonpuerperal, nontraumatic
623.4 Vagina old or postpartal
0 Vagina with abortion see 'Abortion', by type, with damage to pelvic organs or tissue
0 Vagina with ectopic pregnancy see 'Ectopic Pregnancy', by site with complication
0 Vagina with molar pregnancy see 'Molar Pregnancy', by type with complication
799.89 Viscus NEC
868.00 Viscus NEC traumatic
868.10 Viscus NEC traumatic with open wound into cavity

P

698.0 PERIANAL ITCH
522.9 PERIAPICAL TISSUES DISEASE NEC
446.0 PERIARTERITIS NODOSA
446.0 PERIARTERITIS NODOSA POLYNEUROPATHY [357.1]
726.2 PERIARTHRITIS SHOULDER
726.4 PERIARTHRITIS WRIST
0 PERICARDIAL SEE 'PERICARDIUM, PERICARDIAL'

PERICARDITIS

423.9 NOS
420.90 Acute
420.99 Acute bacterial
420.90 Acute infective
391.0 Acute rheumatic
392.0 Acute rheumatic with chorea
420.99 Acute septic
423.1 Adhesive
420.99 Bacterial (acute)
420.91 Benign (acute)
423.8 Cholesterol (chronic)
423.8 Chronic
393 Chronic rheumatic
423.2 Constrictive
098.83 Gonococcal
420.90 Hemorrhagic (acute)
420.91 Idiopathic (acute)
420.90 Infective (acute)
036.41 Meningococcal
420.90 Neoplastic (acute)
423.1 Obliterative

998.59: Postoperative pericarditis, use an additional code to identify the specific type of pericarditis.

998.59 Postoperative
420.99 Purulent (acute)
391.0 Rheumatic (acute)
392.0 Rheumatic (acute) with chorea
393 Rheumatic chronic (inactive) with chorea
420.99 Septic (acute)
420.90 Sicca (acute)
420.99 Suppurative (acute)
420.91 Viral acute

PERICARDITIS OTHER

039.8 Actinomycotic (acute) [420.0]
006.8 Amebic (acute) [420.0]
074.21 Coxsackie
411.0 Dressler's
115.93 Histoplasma
115.03 Histoplasma capsulatum
115.13 Histoplasma duboisii
039.8 Nocardia (due to) (acute) [420.0]
423.1 Obliterans obliterating (plastic)
420.99 Pneumococcal (acute) [041.2]

998.59: Postoperative pericarditis, use an additional code to identify the specific type of pericarditis.

998.59 Postoperative
420.99 Staphylococcal (acute) **[041.1#]**
5th digit: 041.1
0. NOS
1. Aureus
9. Other staph

PERICARDITIS OTHER (continued)

420.99 Streptococcal (acute) **[041.0#]**
5th digit: 041.0
0. NOS
1. Group A
2. Group B
3. Group C
4. Group D (enterococcus)
5. Group G
9. Other strep

093.81 Syphilis
017.9# TB [420.0]
5th digit: 017.9
0. Unspecified
1. Lab not done
2. Lab pending
3. Microscopy positive (in sputum)
4. Culture positive - microscopy negative
5. Culture negative - microscopy positive
6. Culture and microscopy negative confirmed by other methods

585.# Uremic (renal failure) (chronic) [420.0]
4th digit: 585
1. Stage I
2. Stage II (mild)
3. Stage III (moderate)
4. Stage IV (severe)
5. Stage V
6. End stage
9. Unspecified stage

PERICARDIUM, PERICARDIAL

746.89 Absence (congenital)
423.1 Adherent
423.1 Adhesion (nonrheumatic)
746.89 Anomaly (congenital)
423.8 Calcification
746.89 Defect congenital
423.9 Disease
0 Disease rheumatic see 'Rheumatic'
423.8 Disease specified type NEC
423.8 Diverticulum
746.89 Diverticulum congenital
423.9 Effusion
420.90 Effusion acute
391.0 Effusion acute rheumatic
393 Effusion chronic rhuematic
423.1 Fibrosis
423.8 Fistula
423.1 Milk spots
423.1 Soldiers' patches

523.40 PERICEMENTITIS NOS OR CHRONIC (SUPPURATIVE)
523.30 PERICEMENTITIS ACUTE
0 PERICHOLECYSTITIS SEE 'CHOLECYSITIS'

PERICHONDRITIS

380.00 Auricle
380.01 Auricle acute
380.02 Auricle chronic
478.71 Larynx
478.19 Nose
380.00 Pinna
380.01 Pinna acute
380.02 Pinna chronic

P

569.89 PERICOLITIS INTESTINE
523.40 PERICORONITIS NOS (CHRONIC)
523.30 PERICORONITIS ACUTE
375.32 PERIDACRYOCYSTITIS ACUTE
523.30 PERIDENTAL INFECTION
610.4 PERIDUCTAL MASTITIS
421.9 PERIENDOCARDITIS (ACUTE) (SUBACUTE)
704.8 PERIFOLLICULITIS
704.8 PERIFOLLICULITIS CAPITIS ABSCEDENS ET SUFFODIENS
704.8 PERIFOLLICULITIS SCALP
099.56 PERIHEPATITIS CHLAMYDIAL

PERIMETRITIS

615.9 NOS
615.0 Acute
615.1 Chronic
670.0# Maternal due to pregnancy
5th digit: 670.0
0. Unspecified
2. Delivered with postpartum complication
4. Postpartum complication

Further specify these perinatal diseases or disorders with an additional code(s) for the specific condition.

PERINATAL

779.9 Condition
779.89 Conditions other specified
777.9 Digestive system disorder
775.9 Endocrine and metabolic disorders
776.9 Hematological disorders
771.89 Infection other
778.9 Integumentary and temperature regulation disorders
0 Jaundice see 'Jaundice Neonatal'
V13.7 Problem history

0 PERINEAL SEE 'PERINEUM, PERINEAL'

PERINEOCELE

618.#(#) Female
618.#(#) Female with stress incontinence [625.6]
618.#(#) Female with other urinary incontinence **[788.3#]**
4th or 4th and 5th digit: 618
05. Without uterine prolapse
2. With incomplete uterine prolapse
3. With complete uterine prolapse
4. Uterine prolapse unspecified
5th digit: 788.3
1. Urge incontinence
3. Mixed urge and stress
4. Without sensory awareness
5. Post-void dribbling
6. Nocturnal enuresis
7. Continuous leakage
8. Overflow incontinence
9. Other

590.2 PERINEPHRIC ABSCESS

PERINEUM, PERINEAL

624.9 Disease female
616.9 Disease female - inflammatory
616.89 Disease female - inflammatory other specified NEC
624.8 Disease female - other specified NEC
682.2 Disease male - inflammatory
654.8# Fibrosis (rigid) complicating childbirth
660.2# Fibrosis obstructing labor **[654.8#]**
5th digit: 654.8
0. Episode of care unspecified or N/A
1. Delivered
2. Delivered with postpartum complication
3. Antepartum complication
4. Postpartum complication

5th digit: 660.2
0. Episode of care unspecified or N/A
1. Delivered
3. Antepartum complication

785.4 Gangrene
959.14 Injury
911.8 Injury other and NOS superficial
911.9 Injury other and NOS superficial infected
664.4# Laceration obstetrical
664.0# Laceration obstetrical - 1st degree
664.1# Laceration obstetrical - 2nd degree
664.2# Laceration obstetrical - 3rd degree
664.3# Laceration obstetrical - 4th degree
5th digit: 664.0-4
0. Episode of care unspecified or N/A
1. Delivered
4. Postpartum complication

879.6 Laceration traumatic
618.8# Prolapse female
618.8# Prolapse female with stress incontinence [625.6]
618.8# Prolapse female with other urinary incontinence **[788.3#]**
5th digit: 618.8
1. Pubocervical tissue incompetence (weakening)
2. Rectovaginal tissue incompetence (weakening)
3. Pelvic muscle wasting
4. Cervical stump
9. Other

5th digit: 788.3
1. Urge incontinence
3. Mixed urge and stress
4. Without sensory awareness
5. Post-void dribbling
6. Nocturnal enuresis
7. Continuous leakage
8. Overflow incontinence
9. Other

PERINEUM, PERINEAL (continued)

654.8# Surgery previous complicating pregnancy childbirth or pureperium

660.2# Surgery previous obstructing labor [654.8#]

5th digit: 654.8
0. Episode of care unspecified or N/A
1. Delivered
2. Delivered with postpartum complication
3. Antepartum complication
4. Postpartum complication

5th digit: 660.2
0. Episode of care unspecified or N/A
1. Delivered
3. Antepartum complication

664.9# Trauma - NOS during delivery
0 Trauma - laceration during delivery see 'Perineum, Perineal' laceration
664.8# Trauma - other specified during delivery

5th digit: 664.8-9
0. Episode of care unspecified or N/A
1. Delivered
4. Postpartum complication

380.02 PERIOCHONDRITIS AURICLE CHRONIC
380.02 PERIOCHONDRITIS PINNA CHRONIC
277.31 PERIODIC FAMILIAL (REIMANN'S) DISEASE NEC
359.3 PERIODIC (FAMILIAL) PARALYSIS
327.51 PERIODIC LIMB MOVEMENT DISORDER
277.31 PERIODIC SYNDROME
523.31 PERIODONTAL ABSCESS OR INFECTION
522.8 PERIODONTAL CYST
523.9 PERIODONTAL DISEASE NEC

648.9#: Use an additional code to identify the periodontal disease.

648.9# PERIODONTAL DISEASE MATERNAL CURRENT (CO-EXISTENT) IN PREGNANCY

5th digit: 648.9
0. Episode of care NOS or N/A
1. Delivered
2. Delivered with postpartum complication
3. Antepartum complication
4. Postpartum complication

523.8 PERIODONTAL DISEASE SPECIFIED NEC
523.8 PERIODONTAL OCCLUSION, TRAUMATIC

PERIODONTITIS

523.40 NOS
523.33 Acute
522.4 Acute apical (pulpal)
523.30 Agressive
523.32 Aggressive generalized
523.31 Aggressive localized
523.40 Chronic
522.6 Chronic apical
523.42 Generalized (chronic)
523.41 Localized (chronic)

523.5 PERIODONTOSIS
733.90 PERIOSTEAL DISORDER NOS

PERIOSTITIS

730.3# NOS

5th digit: 730.3
0. Site unspecified
1. Shoulder region
2. Upper arm (elbow) (humerus)
3. Forearm (radius) (wrist) (ulna)
4. Hand (carpal) (metacarpal) (fingers)
5. Pelvic region and thigh (hip) (buttock) (femur)
6. Lower leg (fibula) (knee) (patella) (tibia)
7. Ankle and/or foot (metatarsals) (toes) (tarsals)
8. Other (head) (neck) (rib) (skull) (trunk) (vertebrae)
9. Multiple

526.5 Alveolodental
102.6 Due to yaws
526.4 Jaw
376.02 Orbital
095.5 Syphilitic
091.61 Syphilitic secondary
0 With osteomyelitis see 'Osteomyelitis'

0 PERIOSTOSIS SEE 'PERIOSTITIS'

0 PERIPHERAL ARTERY OCCLUSION SEE 'ARTERY, ARTERIAL', OCCLUSION

V53.02 PERIPHERAL NERVE NEUROPACEMAKER (FITTING AND ADJUSTMENT) (REMOVAL) (REPLACEMENT)

PERIPHERAL NEUROPATHY

356.9 NOS
337.9 Autonomic unspecified
277.39 Autonomic amyloidosis [337.1]
274.89 Autonomic gout [337.1]
242.9# Autonomic hyperthyroidism [337.1]

5th digit: 242.9
0. Without storm
1. With storm

337.0 Autonomic idiopathic
357.6 Drug induced
356.0 Hereditary
356.2 Hereditary sensory
356.9 Idiopathic
356.4 Idiopathic progressive
356.8 Idiopathic other specified
356.9 Nerve NOS
354.9 Nerve arm NEC
907.4 Nerve injury late effect (shoulder girdle)
355.8 Nerve leg, lower extremity
0 Nerve see 'Polyneuropathy'
354.9 Nerve upper extremity
794.19 Nervous system abnormal findings function study
0 Spinal nerve root see 'Radiculitis'
357.7 Toxic induced, (arsenic, lead, organophosphates)

V42.82 PERIPHERAL STEM CELLS TRANSPLANT STATUS

P

You should not assume a cause and effect relationship between diabetes and peripheral vascular disease. Unless the physician states that the peripheral vascular disease is diabetic or due to diabetes, code the conditions separately or ask the physician to document the diagnosis clearly.

PERIPHERAL VASCULAR

747.6# Anomalies (congenital) (aberrant) (absence) (agenesis) (accessory) (aneurysm) (atresia) (deformity) (hypoplasia) (malposition)
5th digit: 747.6
0. Unspecified site
1. Gastrointestinal vessel
2. Renal vessel
3. Upper limb vessel
4. Lower limb vessel
9. Other specified site peripheral vascular

443.9 Disease NOS
250.7# Disease diabetic [443.81]
5th digit: 250.7
0. Type II, adult-onset, non-insulin dependent (even if requiring insulin), or unspecified; controlled
1. Type I, juvenile-onset or insulin-dependent; controlled
2. Type II, adult-onset, non-insulin dependent (even if requiring insulin); uncontrolled
3. Type I, juvenile-onset or insulin-dependent; uncontrolled

648.9#: Use an additional code to identify the peripheral vascular disease.

648.9# Disease maternal current (co-existent) in pregnancy
5th digit: 648.9
0. Episode of care NOS or N/A
1. Delivered
2. Delivered with postpartum complication
3. Antepartum complication
4. Postpartum complication

443.89 Disease specified type NEC

526.69 PERIRADICULAR PATHOLOGY ASSOCIATED WITH PREVIOUS ENDODONTIC TREATMENT
590.2 PERIRENAL ABSCESS
569.89 PERISIGMOIDITIS INTESTINE
289.59 PERISPLENITIS
787.4 PERISTALSIS REVERSE(D)
787.4 PERISTALSIS VISIBLE
0 PERITONEAL SEE 'PERITONEUM, PERITONEAL'

PERITONEUM, PERITONEAL

568.0 Adhesions
648.9# Adhesions complicating pregnancy, childbirth or puerperium
5th digit: 648.9
0. Episode of care NOS or N/A
1. Delivered
2. Delivered with postpartum complication
3. Antepartum complication
4. Postpartum complication

PERITONEUM, PERITONEAL (continued)

751.4 Adhesions congenital
614.6 Adhesions female
614.6 Adhesions female pelvic
614.6 Adhesions female postoperative (postinfection)
568.0 Adhesions male
614.6 Adhesions pelvic postoperative (postinfection)
568.0 Adhesions postoperative (postinfection)
568.89 Cyst
0 Dialysis see 'Dialysis' peritoneal
629.9 Disease pelvic female
629.89 Disease pelvic female - other specified
568.9 Disorder
629.9 Disorder pelvic female - NOS
629.89 Disorder pelvic female - other specified
568.82 Effusion (chronic) nonascites
V56.32 Equilibration test
792.9 Fluid abnormal
568.89 Granuloma
868.03 Injury
868.03 Injury - traumatic
868.13 Injury - traumatic with open wound into cavity
908.1 Injury - late effect
0 Pregnancy see 'Ectopic Pregnancy (Ruptured) (Unruptured)'
761.4 Pregnancy affecting fetus or newborn

When coding an infection, use an additional code, [041.#], to identify the organism. See 'Bacterial Infection'.

PERITONITIS

567.9 NOS
567.21 Acute
567.21 Acute generalized
567.29 Acute other suppurative
540.0 Appendicitis acute (with)
540.1 Appendicitis with peritoneal abscess
998.7 Aseptic - acute reaction to foreign substance accidentally left during a procedure
567.29 Bacterial
567.23 Bacterial spontaneous
277.31 Benign paroxysmal
567.81 Bile
998.7 Chemical - acute reaction to foreign substance accidentally left during a procedure
567.89 Chemical - talc
099.56 Chlamydial
567.89 Chronic proliferative
777.6 Congenital NEC
567.22 Diaphragmatic (subphrenic)
567.29 Diffuse NEC
032.83 Diphtheria
567.29 Disseminated NEC
567.29 Due to staphylococcal [041.1#]
5th digit: 041.1
0. NOS
1. Aureus
9. Other staph

567.29 Due to streptococcal [041.0#]
5th digit: 041.0
0. NOS
1. Group A
2. Group B
3. Group C
4. Group D (enterococcus)
5. Group G
9. Other strep

P

PERITONITIS (continued)

567.89 Due to talc
567.82 Fat necrosis
567.29 Fibrinopurulent (fibrinous) (fibropurulent)
098.86 Gonococcal
777.6 Meconium
567.89 Mesenteric saponification
0 Obstetrical see 'Peritonitis Obstetrical'
577.8 Pancreatic
614.5 Pelvic female (acute)
614.7 Pelvic female chronic
016.7# Pelvic female tuberculous
567.21 Pelvic male (acute)
016.5# Pelvic male tuberculous
016.9# Pelvic tuberculous NOS (female) (male)

5th digit: 016.5-9
0. Unspecified
1. Lab not done
2. Lab pending
3. Microscopy positive (in sputum)
4. Culture positive - microscopy negative
5. Culture negative - microscopy positive
6. Culture and microscopy negative confirmed by other methods

277.31 Periodic familial
567.29 Phlegmonous
567.1 Pneumococcal
998.7 Postoperative due to foreign substance accidentally left
998.59 Postoperative infective [567.21]
567.89 Proliferative (chronic)
567.29 Purulent (septic)
567.29 Subdiaphragmatic
567.29 Subphrenic
567.29 Suppurative
095.2 Syphilitic
090.0 Syphilitic congenital [567.0]
014.0# Tuberculous

5th digit: 014.0
0. NOS
1. Lab not pending
2. Lab pending
3. Microscopy positive (in sputum)
4. Culture positive - microscopy negative
5. Culture negative - microscopy positive
6. Culture and microscopy negative confirmed by other methods

567.89 Urine
567.21 With abscess
567.89 Other specified

PERITONITIS OBSTETRICAL

639.0 Following abortion
639.0 Following ectopic or molar pregnancy
638.0# In abortion failed/attempted
636.0# In abortion illegally induced
635.0# In abortion legally induced
634.0# In abortion spontaneous
635.0# In abortion therapeutic
637.0# In abortion unspecified

5th digit: 634.0, 635.0, 636.0, 637.0, 638.0
0. NOS
1. Incomplete
2. Complete

PERITONITIS OBSTETRICAL (continued)

670.0# Pelvic maternal due to pregnancy

5th digit: 670.0
0. Unspecified
2. Delivered with postpartum complication
4. Postpartum complication

475 PERITONSILLAR ABSCESS
475 PERITONSILLAR CELLULITIS

614.6 PERITUBAL ADHESIONS
614.6 PERITUBAL ADHESIONS POSTOPERATIVE (POSTINFECTION)

593.89 PERIURETERITIS
593.4 PERIURETHRAL FIBROSIS SYNDROME
639.2 PERIURETHRAL INJURY FOLLOWING ABORTION, ECTOPIC OR MOLAR PREGNANCY
362.18 PERIVASCULITIS RETINAL
779.7 PERIVENTRICULAR LEUKOMALACIA PERINATAL
686.8 PERLECHE
112.0 PERLECHE MONILIAL
266.0 PERLECHE RIBOFLAVIN DEFICIENCY

PERNICIOUS ANEMIA

281.0 NOS
281.0 Congenital
281.0 With combined subacute spinal cord degeneration [336.2]
281.0 With myelopathy (cord compression) [336.3]
281.0 With polyneuropathy [357.4]
281.0 With spinal degeneration [336.2]

991.5 PERNIOSIS ERYTHEMA
909.4 PERNIOSIS ERYTHEMA LATE EFFECT

PERONEAL

356.1 Muscular atrophy
355.3 Nerve disorder
956.3 Nerve injury
355.3 Neuritis (common)
726.79 Tendinitis
727.09 Tendons dislocating

277.86 PEROXISOMAL DISORDER
719.65 PERRIN-FERRATON DISEASE (SNAPPING HIP)
V62.4 PERSECUTION SOCIAL
751.5 PERSISTENT CLOACA CONGENITAL
747.83 PERSISTENT FETAL CIRCULATION SYNDROME
654.8# PERSISTENT HYMEN COMPLICATING CHILDBIRTH
660.2# PERSISTENT HYMEN COMPLICATING CHILDBIRTH OBSTRUCTING LABOR [**654.8#**]

5th digit: 654.8
0. Episode of care unspecified or N/A
1. Delivered
2. Delivered with postpartum complication
3. Antepartum complication
4. Postpartum complication

5th digit: 660.2
0. Episode of care unspecified or N/A
1. Delivered
3. Antepartum complication

757.4 PERSISTENT LANUGO CONGENITAL
752.89 PERSISTENT MESONEPHRIC DUCT (CONGENITAL)
763.1 PERSISTENT OCCIPITOPOSTERIOR POSITION AFFECTING FETUS OR NEWBORN
747.83 PERSISTENT PULMONARY HYPERTENSION CONGENITAL (FETAL)
745.0 PERSISTENT TRUNCUS ARTERIOSUS CONGENITAL HISTORY
752.89 PERSISTENT UROGENITALIS SINUS (CONGENITAL)
780.03 PERSISTENT VEGETATIVE STATE
743.51 PERSISTENT VITREOUS HYPERPLASIA CONGENITAL
752.89 PERSISTENT (CONGENITAL) WOLFFIAN DUCT
V60.3 PERSON LIVING ALONE
V60.6 PERSON LIVING IN RESIDENTIAL INSTITUTION
V60.4 PERSON UNABLE TO CARE FOR SELF
0 PERSONAL HISTORY SEE 'HISTORY'
310.1 PERSONALITY CHANGE DUE TO CONDITIONS CLASSIFIED ELSEWHERE

When coding a personality disorder, use an additional code for any associated neurosis, psychosis or physical condition.

PERSONALITY DISORDER

301.9 NOS
301.10 Affective
301.3 Aggressive
301.7 Amoral
301.4 Anancastic
301.7 Antisocial
301.7 Asocial
301.6 Asthenic
301.82 Avoidant
301.83 Borderline
301.4 Compulsive
301.13 Cycloid (cyclothymic)
301.6 Dependent
301.12 Depressive chronic
292.89 Drug induced [**304.##**]

4th digit: 304
0. Opioid
1. Sedative, hypnotic or anxiolytic
2. Cocaine
3. Cannabis
4. Amphetamine type
5. Hallucinogenic
6. Other specified
7. Mixed with opioid
8. Mixed
9. NOS

5th digit: 304
0. Unspecified
1. Continuous
2. Episodic
3. In remission

300.14 Dual
301.7 Dyssocial
301.89 Eccentric
301.59 Emotionally unstable
301.3 Epileptoid
301.3 Explosive

PERSONALITY DISORDER (continued)

301.0 Fanatic
301.50 Histrionic
301.11 Hyperthymic
301.11 Hypomanic chronic
301.50 Hysterical
301.89 Immature
301.6 Inadequate
301.21 Introverted
301.59 Labile
301.89 Masochistic
300.14 Multiple
301.51 Munchausen
301.81 Narcissistic
300.5 Neurasthenia
301.4 Obsessional
301.4 Obsessive - compulsive
301.0 Paranoid
301.6 Passive
301.84 Passive aggressive
301.6 Passive dependent
301.9 Pathological
301.9 Pattern disturbance
301.59 Psycho-infantile
301.9 Psychopathic
0 Psychotic see 'Psychosis'
301.20 Schizoid
301.21 Schizoid introverted
0 Schizophrenic see also 'Schizophrenia'
301.22 Schizotypal
301.59 Seductive
301.7 Sociopathic
301.9 Trait disturbance
301.4 Type A

732.1 PERTHES' DISEASE (CAPITAL FEMORAL OSTEOCHONDROSIS)

PERTUSSIS

033.0 Bordetella
033.1 Bordetella parapertussis
V01.89 Exposure
V74.8 Screening exam
V03.6 Vaccination (single)

PERVASIVE DEVELOPMENTAL DISORDER

299.9# NOS
299.0# Autistic
299.1# Childhood disintegrative
299.8# Other specified

5th digit: 299.0-9
0. Current or active state
1. Residual state

PES

726.61 Anserinus tendinitis
754.71 Cavus
754.69 Planovalgus (congenital)
736.79 Planovalgus acquired
754.61 Planus (congenital)
734 Planus (acquired) flat foot
736.79 Talipes deformity acquired NEC
754.50 Varus congenital
736.79 Other acquired NEC

020.8 PESTIS MINOR

P

782.7 PETECHIAE
772.6 PETECHIAE FETUS OR NEWBORN
743.44 PETERS' ANOMALY
710.3 PETGES-CLEJAT SYNDROME (POIKILODERMATOMYOSITIS)

345.0# PETIT MAL
5th digit: 345.0
0. Without mention of intractable epilepsy
1. With intractable epilepsy

345.2 PETIT MAL STATUS

0 PETIT'S DISEASE SEE 'HERNIA' LUMBAR
117.6 PETRIELLIDOSIS
383.20 PETROSITIS
383.21 PETROSITIS ACUTE
383.22 PETROSITIS CHRONIC
759.6 PEUTZ-JEGHERS SYNDROME
607.85 PEYRONIES DISEASE
075 PFEIFFER'S DISEASE (INFECTIOUS MONONUCLEOSIS)
755.55 PFEIFFER SYNDROME (ACROCEPHALOSYNDACTYLY)
117.8 PHAEHYPHOMYCOSIS INFECTION
785.4 PHAGEDENA

When coding arteriosclerosis of the extremities use an additional code, if applicable to identify chronic complete or total occlusion of the artery of the extremities (440.4)

440.24 PHAGEDENA ARTERIOSCLEROTIC ISCHEMIC GANGRENE (SENILE) WITH ULCER [707.#(#)]
4th or 4th and 5th digit: 707
1#. Lower limb except decubitus
10. Unspecified
11. Thigh
12. Calf
13. Ankle
14. Heel and midfoot
15. Other parts of foot, toes
19. Other
8. Chronic of other specified site
9. Chronic site NOS

440.3# PHAGEDENA DUE TO BYPASS GRAFT ARTERIOSCLEROSIS [785.4]
5th digit: 440.3
0. Unspecified graft
1. Autologous vein bypass graft
2. Nonautologous biological bypass graft

686.09 PHAGEDENA GEOMETRIC
099.8 PHAGEDENIC BUBO NEC

PHAKIA
996.69 Complication infection or inflammation
996.53 Complication mechanical
996.79 Complication other
996.53 Dislocated

0 PHALANGES SEE 'FINGER' OR 'THUMB' OR 'TOE'
353.6 PHANTOM LIMB (SYNDROME) (NONDISCOGENIC)
0 PHARYNGEAL SEE 'PHARYNX, PHARYNGEAL'

PHARYNGITIS
462 Acute
472.1 Atrophic
099.51 Chlamydial
472.1 Chronic
472.1 Chronic granular
074.0 Coxsackie virus
101 Fusospirochetal
462 Gangrenous (acute)
098.6 Gonococcal
054.79 Herpes simplex
472.1 Hypertrophic
462 Infective (acute)
487.1 Influenzal
074.8 Lymphonodular acute
075 Mononucleosis
462 Phlegmonous (acute)
462 Pneumococcal (acute)
034.0 Septic
462 Staphylococcal (acute)
034.0 Streptococcal
462 Suppurative (acute)
462 Ulcerative (acute)
074.0 Vesicular
462 Viral

077.2 PHARYNGOCONJUNCTIVAL FEVER
077.2 PHARYNGOCONJUNCTIVITIS VIRAL
530.6 PHARYNGOESOPHAGEAL DIVERTICULUM (ESOPHAGEAL)
465.8 PHARYNGOTRACHEITIS ACUTE
478.9 PHARYNGOTRACHEITIS CHRONIC

PHARYNX, PHARYNGEAL
478.29 Abscess
478.22 Abscess parapharyngeal
478.24 Abscess retropharyngeal
750.29 Anomaly other specified (congenital)
478.29 Atrophy
925.2 Crush injury
478.26 Cyst
478.20 Disease
478.29 Disease other NEC
750.27 Diverticulum congenital
478.25 Edema
478.29 Hyperplasia (lymphoid)
750.29 Imperforate congenital
959.09 Injury
478.29 Obstruction
474.00 Posterior lymphoid tissue infection
750.27 Pouch congenital
279.11 Pouch syndrome
478.29 Ulcer

305.9# PHENCYCLIDINE ABUSE
304.6# PHENCYCLIDINE ADDICTION (DEPENDENT)
5th digit: 304.6, 305.9
0. NOS
1. Continuous
2. Episodic
3. In remission

304.4# PHENMETRAZINE DEPENDENCE
5th digit: 304.4
0. Unspecified
1. Continuous
2. Episodic
3. In remission

P

995.21 PHENOMENON ARTHUS
270.1 PHENYLKETONURIA (PKU)
V77.3 PHENYLKETONURIA SCREENING (PKU)
270.1 PHENYLPYRUVIC OLIGOPHRENIA AMINO ACID DISORDER (METABOLIC)

PHEOCHROMOCYTOMA

227.0 Site NOS
0 Site specified see 'Benign Neoplasm', by site M8700/0
194.0 Malignant site NOS
0 Malignant site specified see 'Cancer', by site M8700/3
255.6 Syndrome

PHIALOPHORA INFECTION

117.8 Gougerotii
117.8 Jeanselmei
117.2 Verrucosa

605 PHIMOSIS
605 PHIMOSIS CONGENITAL
747.6# PHLEBECTASIA CONGENITAL PERIPHERAL VASCULAR
5th digit: 747.6
0. Peripheral vascular unspecified site
1. Gastrointestinal vessel
2. Renal vessel
3. Upper limb vessel
4. Lower limb vessel
9. Other specified site peripheral vascular

0 PHLEBECTASIA PERIPHERAL VASCULAR SEE 'VARICOSE VEINS' LOWER EXTREMITIES
0 PHLEBECTASIA OTHER SITES SEE 'VARICES' BY SPECIFIED SITE

PHLEBITIS

451.9 NOS
451.82 Antecubital vein
451.83 Arm deep
451.82 Arm superficial
451.84 Arm NEC
451.89 Axillary vein
451.82 Basilic vein
451.83 Brachial vein
451.82 Cephalic vein
997.2 During or resulting from a procedure
451.11 Femoral vein (deep) (superficial)
451.19 Femoropopliteal vein
999.2 Following infusion perfusion or transfusion
274.89 Gouty [451.9]
451.89 Hepatic vein
451.81 Iliac vein
451.11 Iliofemoral
326 Intracranial late effect
325 Intracranial sinus
451.89 Jugular vein
451.2 Leg
451.2 Lower extremities
451.19 Lower extremities deep vessels other specified

PHLEBITIS (continued)

648.9#: Use an additional code to identify the specific phlebitis.

648.9# Maternal current (co-existent) in pregnancy
671.9# Maternal due to pregnancy
5th digit: 648.9, 671.9
0. Episode of care unspecified or N/A
1. Delivered
2. Delivered with postpartum complication
3. Antepartum complication
4. Postpartum complication

451.19 Popliteal vein
572.1 Portal vein
997.2 Postoperative
451.83 Radial vein
362.18 Retinal
451.0 Saphenous vein (greater) (lesser)
451.89 Subclavian vein
451.19 Tibial vein
451.83 Ulnar vein
451.84 Upper extremities
451.83 Upper extremities deep vessels
451.82 Upper extremities superficial vessels

459.89 PHLEBOSCLEROSIS

PHLEBOTHROMBOSIS (DEEP-VEIN) COMPLICATING PREGNANCY OR THE PUERPERIUM

671.3# Maternal due to pregnancy antepartum
5th digit: 671.3
0. Episode of care NOS or N/A
1. Delivered
3. Antepartum complication

671.4# Maternal due to pregnancy postpartum
5th digit: 671.4
0. Unspecified
2. Delivered, wtih postpartum complication
4. Postpartum condition or complication

066.0 PHLEBOTOMUS FEVER
475 PHLEGMONOUS ANGINA
370.31 PHLYCTENULOSIS

PHOBIA

300.20 NOS
300.29 Acrophobia
300.22 Agoraphobia
300.21 Agoraphobia with panic attacks
300.29 Animal
300.29 Claustrophobia
300.29 Crowds
300.23 Eating in public
300.3 Obsessional (any)
300.21 Open spaces with panic attacks
300.29 Parasites
300.23 Public-speaking
300.23 Social
300.21 Streets with panic attacks
300.21 Travel with panic attacks
300.23 Washing in public
300.29 Other specific

610.1 PHOCAS' DISEASE

PHOCOMELIA

755.4 NOS
755.32 Lower limb
755.33 Lower limb complete
755.35 Lower limb distal
755.34 Lower limb proximal
755.22 Upper limb
755.23 Upper limb complete
755.25 Upper limb distal
755.24 Upper limb proximal

PHONOCARDIOGRAM

794.39 Abnormal
V71.7 For suspected disease
V72.81 Preoperative
V72.85 Routine

315.39 PHONOLOGICAL DISORDER (DEVELOPMENTAL SPEECH DISORDER)
275.3 PHOSPHATE ABNORMAL FINDINGS
588.0 PHOSPHATE LOSING TUBULAR DISORDERS
275.3 PHOSPHATE METABOLISM DISORDER
271.8 PHOSPHOENOLPYRUVATE CARBOXYKINASE DEFICIENCY
271.2 PHOSPHOFRUCTOKINASE DEFICIENCY
271.0 PHOSPHOGLUMOTASE DEFICIENCY
271.0 PHOSPHOHEXOSISOMERASE DEFICIENCY
271.8 PHOSPHOMANNOMUTASE DEFICIENCY
271.8 PHOSPHOMANNOSE ISOMERASE DEFICIENCY
271.8 PHOSPHOMANNOSYL MUTASE DEFICIENCY
275.3 PHOSPHORUS ABNORMAL FINDINGS
275.3 PHOSPHORUS METABOLISM DISORDER
692.72 PHOTOALLERGIC RESPONSE (ACUTE)
031.9 PHOTOCHROMOGENIC DISEASE (ACID-FAST BACILLI) – NONPULMONARY
031.0 PHOTOCHROMOGENIC DISEASE (ACID-FAST BACILLI) – PULMONARY
692.72 PHOTODERMATITIS SUN
692.82 PHOTODERMATITIS LIGHT OTHER
370.24 PHOTOKERATITIS
368.13 PHOTOPHOBIA
368.15 PHOTOPSIA
363.31 PHOTORETINITIS
363.31 PHOTORETINOPATHY
692.72 PHOTOSENSITIVITY SUNLIGHT
692.82 PHOTOSENSITIVITY LIGHT OTHER
692.72 PHOTOSENSITIZATION SUNLIGHT
692.82 PHOTOSENSITIZATION LIGHT OTHER
692.72 PHOTOTOXIC RESPONSE (ACUTE)
990 PHOTOTHERAPY COMPLICATION
530.89 PHRENIC AMPULLA
354.8 PHRENIC NERVE NEURITIS (DISORDER)
767.7 PHRENIC NERVE PARALYSIS NEWBORN (BIRTH TRAUMA)

017.3# PHTHISICAL CORNEA [371.05]

5th digit: 017.3
- **0. Unspecified**
- **1. Lab not done**
- **2. Lab pending**
- **3. Microscopy positive (in sputum)**
- **4. Culture positive - microscopy negative**
- **5. Culture negative - microscopy positive**
- **6. Culture and microscopy negative confirmed by other methods**

132.2 PHTHIRUS PUBIS (PUBIC LOUSE)
360.41 PHTHISIS BULBI
127.7 PHYSALOPTERIASIS INFECTION
306.9 PHYSICAL DISORDER PSYCHOGENIC
0 PHYSICAL EXAM SEE 'EXAM'
V57.1 PHYSICAL THERAPY THERAPEUTIC AND REMEDIAL EXERCISES (EXCEPT BREATHING)
935.2 PHYTOBEZOAR GASTRIC
936 PHYTOBEZOAR INTESTINE
102.1 PIANOMA SEE ALSO 'YAWS'
307.52 PICA
300.11 PICA HYSTERICAL

PICK'S DISEASE

331.11 NOS
331.11 NOS with dementia [**294.1#**]
331.11 Brain
331.11 Brain with dementia [**294.1#**]
331.11 Cerebral atrophy
331.11 Cerebral atrophy with dementia [**294.1#**]

5th digit: 294.1
- **0. Without behavioral disturbance or NOS**
- **1. With behavioral disturbance**

423.2 Heart (and liver) (syndrome)
272.7 Lipid histiocytosis
423.2 Pericardium (syndrome)

701.8 PICK-HERXHEIMER SYNDROME (DIFFUSE IDIOPATHIC CUTANEOUS ATROPHY)
278.8 PICKWICKIAN SYNDROME (CARDIOPULMONARY OBESITY)

PID (PELVIC INFLAMMATORY DISEASE)

614.9 NOS
614.3 Acute
614.4 Chronic
760.8 Maternal - affecting fetus or newborn
639.0 Maternal - following abortion or ectopic/molar pregnancy
0 Maternal - in abortion see 'Abortion', by type with shock
670.0# Maternal NOS - major puerperal [614.9]
670.0# Maternal acute - major puerperal [614.3]
670.0# Maternal chronic - major puerperal [614.4]

5th digit: 670.0
- **0. Episode of care unspecified or N/A**
- **2. Delivered with postpartum complication**
- **4. Postpartum complication**

P

PID (PELVIC INFLAMMATORY DISEASE) (continued)

646.6# Maternal NOS - minor complicating pregnancy [614.9]
646.6# Maternal acute - minor complicating pregnancy [614.3]
646.6# Maternal chronic - minor complicating pregnancy [614.4]
5th digit: 646.6
0. Episode of care unspecified or N/A
1. Delivered
2. Delivered with postpartum complication
3. Antepartum complication
4. Postpartum complication

016.9# Tuberculous unspecified (female) (male)
016.7# Tuberculous female
016.5# Tuberculous male
5th digit: 016.5, 7, 9
0. Unspecified
1. Lab not done
2. Lab pending
3. Microscopy positive (in sputum)
4. Culture positive - microscopy negative
5. Culture negative - microscopy positive
6. Culture and microscopy negative confirmed by other methods

614.8 Other specified

518.3 PIE SYNDROME (PULMONARY INFILTRATION WITH EOSINOPHILIA)
709.09 PIEBALDISM
111.3 PIEDRAIA HORTAI INFECTION
316 PIELINOSIS PSYCHOGENIC
731.2 PIERRE MARIE-BAMBERGER SYNDROME (HYPERTROPHIC PULMONARY OSTEOARTHROPATHY)
258.1 PIERRE MAURIAC'S SYNDROME (DIABETES-DWARFISM-OBESITY)
756.0 PIERRE ROBIN SYNDROME
732.1 PIERSON'S DISEASE (OSTEOCHONDROSIS)
754.82 PIGEON CHEST (BREAST) CONGENITAL
495.2 PIGEON FANCIERS' (BREEDERS') DISEASE
735.8 PIGEON TOE
364.53 PIGMENT DISPERSION SYNDROME, IRIS
333.0 PIGMENTARY PALLIDAL ATROPHY OR DEGENERATION BASAL GANGLIA

PIGMENTATION (ABNORMAL)

709.00 Anomaly NEC
0 Anomaly see 'Dyschromia'
709.09 Arsenical due to drug or correct substance properly administered
743.53 Choroid disorder, congenital
372.55 Conjunctiva
371.10 Cornea - NOS
371.11 Cornea - anterior
371.13 Cornea - posterior
371.12 Cornea - stromal
374.52 Eyelids acquired
757.33 Eyelids congenital
743.57 Optic papilla congenital
362.74 Retina acquired
743.53 Retina congenital

216.# PIGMENTED NEVUS M8720/0
4th digit: 216
0. Lip (skin of)
1. Eyelid including canthus
2. Ear external (auricle) (pinna)
3. Face (cheek) (nose) (eyebrow) (temple)
4. Scalp, neck
5. Trunk, back except scrotum
6. Upper limb including shoulder
7. Lower limb including hip
8. Other specified sites
9. Skin unspecified

757.4 PILI ANNULATI TORTI (CONGENITAL)
704.8 PILI INCARNATI
216.# PILOMATRIXOMA M8110/0
4th digit: 216
0. Lip (skin of)
1. Eyelid including canthus
2. Ear external (auricle) (pinna)
3. Face (cheek) (nose) (eyebrow) (temple)
4. Scalp, neck
5. Trunk, back except scrotum
6. Upper limb including shoulder
7. Lower limb including hip
8. Other specified sites
9. Skin unspecified

PILONIDAL

685.1 Cyst (sinus) (fistula)
685.0 Cyst with abscess
685.1 Fistula (sinus)
685.0 Fistula (sinus) with abscess

602.3 PIN I (PROSTATIC INTRAEPITHELIAL NEOPLASIA I)
602.3 PIN II (PROSTATIC INTRAEPITHELIAL NEOPLASIA II)
233.4 PIN III (PROSTATIC INTRAEPITHELIAL NEOPLASIA III)
V54.09 PIN AFTERCARE NEC (ORTHOPEDIC)
V54.01 PIN REMOVAL (ORTHOPEDIC)
0 PINCHED NERVE SEE 'NEUROPATHY', ENTRAPMENT
259.8 PINEAL CALCIFICATION
259.8 PINEAL GLAND DISEASE (DYSFUNCTION)
259.8 PINEAL SYNDROME
237.1 PINEALOMA SITE NOS
0 PINEALOMA SITE SPECIFIED SEE 'NEOPLASM UNCERTAIN BEHAVIOR', BY SITE M9360/1
194.8 PINEOBLASTOMA SITE NOS
0 PINEOBLASTOMA SITE SPECIFIED SEE 'CANCER', BY SITE M9362/3
237.1 PINEOCYTOMA SITE NOS
0 PINEOCYTOMA SITE SPECIFIED SEE 'NEOPLASM UNCERTAIN BEHAVIOR', BY SITE M9361/1
372.51 PINGUECULA
985.0 PINK DISEASE
492.8 PINK PUFFER SYNDROME
697.1 PINKUS' DISEASE (LICHEN NITIDUS)

PINNA

738.7 Acquired deformities (cauliflower ear)
380.32 Acquired deformities noninfections
274.81 Disorder gouty
380.30 Disorder noninfectious
380.39 Disorder noninfectious other specified
380.31 Hematoma of auricle
380.11 Infection acute

622.4 PINPOINT OS (UTERI) SEE ALSO 'CERVIX' STRICTURE

PINTA

103.9 NOS
103.0 Chancre (primary)
103.1 Erythematous plaques
103.1 Hyperkeratosis
103.1 Intermediate lesions
103.2 Late lesions
103.3 Mixed lesions
103.0 Papule (primary)
103.0 Primary lesions

103.0 PINTID OF PINTA

127.4 PINWORM INFECTION

270.7 PIPECOLIC ACIDEMIA

733.5 PIRIFORM SCLEROSIS OF ILIUM

355.0 PIRIFORMIS SYNDROME

066.8 PIRY FEVER

PITUITARY

253.2 Cachexia
253.9 Disease (gland)
253.7 Disorder iatrogenic
253.9 Disorder thalamic
253.4 Disorder thalamic - anterior NEC
253.7 Disorder thalamic - iatrogenic
253.7 Disorder thalamic - postablative
253.4 Disorders other (anterior)
253.3 Dwarfism
253.9 Dysfunction
259.3 Ectopic secretion (posterior)
253.8 Embolism
759.2 Gland absence (congenital)
253.4 Hormone deficiency anterior
253.1 Hyperfunction
253.2 Hypofunction
253.2 Insufficiency
253.7 Insufficiency iatrogenic
253.2 Necrosis postpartum
495.8 Snuff-takers' disease
253.0 Syndrome

PITYRIASIS

696.5 NOS
696.5 Alba (streptogenes)
690.11 Capitis
696.3 Circinata (et Maculata)
695.89 Hebra
696.2 Lichenoides et Varioliformis
696.8 Like disorder NEC
111.1 Nigra
696.3 Rosea
696.4 Rubra pilaris
690.18 Sicca
690.8 Simplex
111.0 Versicolor

066.3 PIXUNA FEVER (VIRAL)

270.1 PKU (PHENYLKETONURIA)

V77.3 PKU (PHENYLKETONURIA) SCREENING

Fetal or newborn codes (760-779), sometimes require an additional code to further specify the cause of the condition, the infecting organism, or complicating diagnoses. Whenever appropriate, describe the patient's medical situation as clearly and concisely as possible using multiple codes.

PLACENTA, PLACENTAL

656.9# Unspecified problem affecting management of mother
762.2 Abnormal - affecting fetus or newborn
762.1 Abnormal - affecting fetus or newborn with hemorrhage
656.7# Abnormal - affecting management of mother
5th digit: 656.7, 9
0. Episode of care unspecified or N/A
1. Delivered
3. Antepartum complication

794.9 Abnormal finding (radioisotope localization)
793.99 Abnormal finding (x-ray) (ultrasound) (thermography)
641.8# Abnormal - with hemorrhage affecting management of mother
641.2# Abruptio or ablatio
5th digit: 641.2, 8
0. Episode of care unspecified or N/A
1. Delivered
3. Antepartum complication

762.1 Abruptio or ablatio affecting fetus or newborn
0 Accreta see 'Placenta, Placental', retained
0 Adherent see 'Placenta, Placental', retained
0 Bipartita see 'Placenta, Placental', abnormal
762.1 Damaged due to amniocentesis, C-section, or surgical induction - affecting fetus or newborn
762.2 Disease affecting fetus or newborn
656.7# Disease affecting management of mother
5th digit: 656.7
0. Episode of care unspecified or N/A
1. Delivered
3. Antepartum complication

762.2 Dysfunction syndrome
794.9 Function study abnormal
762.2 Infarct affecting fetus or newborn
656.7# Infarct affecting management of mother
5th digit: 656.7
0. Episode of care unspecified or N/A
1. Delivered
3. Antepartum complication

762.2 Insufficiency affecting fetus or newborn
656.5# Insufficiency affecting management of mother
5th digit: 656.5
0. Episode of care unspecified or N/A
1. Delivered
3. Antepartum complication

762.2 Insufficiency syndrome
0 Low implantation see 'Placenta, Placental', previa
0 Low lying see 'Placenta, Placental', previa
762.1 Malformation affecting fetus or newborn
656.7# Malformation affecting management of mother
641.8# Malformation with hemorrhage affecting management of mother
5th digit: 641.8, 656.7
0. Episode of care unspecified or N/A
1. Delivered
3. Antepartum complication

P

PLACENTA, PLACENTAL (continued)

0 Malposition see 'Placenta, Placental', previa
658.4# Placentitis
5th digit: 658.4
0. Episode of care unspecified or N/A
1. Delivered
3. Antepartum complication

762.7 Placentitis affecting fetus or newborn
674.4# Polyp maternal due to pregnancy
5th digit: 674.4
0. Episode of care unspecified or N/A
2. Delivered with postpartum complication
4. Postpartum complication

0 Premature separation see 'Placenta, Placental', abruptio
762.0 Previa affecting fetus or newborn
641.0# Previa (during pregnancy) (before labor)
641.1# Previa with hemorrhage
5th digit: 641.0-1
0. Episode of care unspecified or N/A
1. Delivered
3. Antepartum complication

794.9 Radioisotope study abnormal
667.0# Retained
667.1# Retained fragments
666.0# Retained with postpartum hemorrhage
666.2# Retained with postpartum hemorrhage second stage
667.1# Retained products of conceptus
5th digit: 666.0, 2, 667.0-1
0. Episode of care unspecified or N/A
2. Delivered with postpartum complication
4. Postpartum complication

095.8 Syphilitic
762.3 Transfusion syndromes affecting fetus or newborn
762.3 Transfusion syndromes affecting fetus or newborn - with fetal blood loss [772.0]
762.3 Transfusion syndromes affecting fetus or newborn - with polycythemia neonatorum [776.4]
656.7# Varices
656.8# Other specified problems affecting management of mother
5th digit: 656.7-8
0. Episode of care unspecified or N/A
1. Delivered
3. Antepartum complication

658.4# PLACENTITIS
5th digit: 658.4
0. Episode of care unspecified or N/A
1. Delivered
3. Antepartum complication

762.7 PLACENTITIS AFFECTING FETUS OR NEWBORN
754.0 PLAGIOCEPHALY

PLAGUE

020.9 NOS
020.8 Abortive
020.8 Ambulatory
020.0 Bubonic
020.1 Cellulocutaneous
020.5 Pneumonia
020.3 Pneumonia primary
020.4 Pneumonia secondary

PLAGUE (continued)

V74.8 Screening exam
V03.3 Vaccination
020.8 Other specified types

736.79 PLANOVALGUS DEFORMITY (ACQUIRED)
754.69 PLANOVALGUS DEFORMITY CONGENITAL

PLANTAR

904.6 Artery injury (deep vessels)
908.3 Artery injury (deep vessels) - late effect
904.6 Blood vessel laceration deep vessels traumatic (rupture) (hematoma) (avulsion) (aneurysm)
908.3 Blood vessel laceration deep vessels late effect
728.71 Fascia contracture
728.71 Fasciitis (syndrome) (traumatic)
355.6 Nerve disorder
956.5 Nerve injury
907.5 Nerve injury - late effect
355.6 Nerve lesion
904.6 Vein injury (deep vessels)
908.3 Vein injury (deep vessels) - late effect
078.19 Warts

PLASMA CELL

610.4 Mastitis
203.0# Myeloma
5th digit: 203.0
0. Without mention of remission
1. In remission

0 Myeloma site specified see 'Cancer', by site M9730/3
229.9 Tumor benign site NOS
0 Tumor benign site specified see 'Benign Neoplasm', by site M9731/0
203.8# Tumor malignant site NOS
5th digit: 203.8
0. Without mention of remission
1. In remission

0 Tumor malignant site specified see 'Cancer', by site M7931/3
238.6 Tumor uncertain behavior unspecified

273.9 PLASMA PROTEIN METABOLIC DISORDER NOS
273.8 PLASMA PROTEIN METABOLIC DISORDER NEC
286.2 PLASMA THROMBOPLASTIN ANTECEDENT (PTA) DEFICIENCY
286.1 PLASMA THROMBOPLASTIN COMPONENT DEFICIENCY
203.1# PLASMACYTIC LEUKEMIA M9830/3
5th digit: 203.1
0. Without mention of remission
1. In remission

238.6 PLASMACYTOMA SITE NOS
0 PLASMACYTOMA SITE SPECIFIED SEE 'NEOPLASM UNCERTAIN BEHAVIOR', BY SITE M9731/1
0 PLASMACYTOMA BENIGN SITE SPECIFIED SEE 'BENIGN NEOPLASM', BY SITE M9731/0
203.8# PLASMACYTOMA MALIGNANT SITE NOS M9731/3
5th digit: 203.8
0. Without mention of remission
1. In remission

288.59 PLASMACYTOPENIA
288.64 PLASMACYTOSIS

P

V50.1 PLASTIC SURGERY (ELECTIVE) (FOR UNACCEPTABLE COSMETIC APPEARANCE)
V51 PLASTIC SURGERY REVISION OF OLD INJURY
V54.09 PLATE AFTERCARE NEC (ORTHOPEDIC)
V54.01 PLATE REMOVAL (ORTHOPEDIC)
287.1 PLATELET DEFECT
286.9 PLATELET STICKY SYNDROME
756.0 PLATYBASIA
756.19 PLATYSPONDYLIA SUPERNUMERARY VERTEBRA
199.1 PLEOMORPHIC CARCINOMA SITE NOS
0 PLEOMORPHIC CARCINOMA SITE SPECIFIED SEE 'CANCER', BY SITE M8022/3
782.62 PLETHORA
776.4 PLETHORA NEWBORN

PLEURA, PLEURAL

511.0 Adhesion
511.0 Calcification
786.52 Chest pain
511.0 Congestion
511.0 Disease (cavity) (see also 'Pleurisy')
V58.82 Drainage tube fitting
511.9 Effusion - unspecified
511.9 Effusion - fetus or newborn
197.2 Effusion - malignant
511.9 Effusion - pleurisy NOS
511.1 Effusion - pneumococcal [041.2]
997.3 Effusion - post op
511.1 Effusion - staphylococcal **[041.1#]**

5th digit: 041.1
0. Unspecified
1. Aureus
9. Other

511.1 Effusion - streptococcal **[041.0#]**

5th digit: 041.0
0. NOS
1. Group A
2. Group B
3. Group C
4. Group D (enterococcus)
5. Group G
9. Other strep

862.39 Effusion - traumatic with open wound
862.29 Effusion - traumatic without open wound
012.0# Effusion - tuberculous
010.1# Effusion - tuberculous primary progressive

5th digit: 010.1, 012.0
0. Unspecified
1. Lab not done
2. Lab pending
3. Microscopy positive (in sputum)
4. Culture positive - microscopy negative
5. Culture negative - microscopy positive
6. Culture and microscopy negative confirmed by other methods

511.0 Fibrin deposit
511.0 Fibrosis
792.9 Fluid abnormal
748.8 Folds anomaly congenital
786.7 Friction rub

PLEURA, PLEURAL (continued)

862.29 Injury
862.39 Injury with open wound
908.0 Injury late effect
748.8 Sacs and pericardial sacs abnormal communication
511.0 Thickening

PLEURISY

511.0 Unspecified
511.9 Unspecified with effusion
511.0 Acute
511.0 Acute (sterile) diaphragmatic
511.0 Acute (sterile) fibrinous
511.0 Acute (sterile) interlobular
511.0 Bacterial
511.1 Bacterial with effusion
511.8 Encysted
511.9 Exudative
511.8 Hemorrhagic
487.1 Influenzal
511.1 Pneumococcal with effusion [041.2]
511.9 Serous
511.1 Staphylococcal with effusion **[041.1#]**

5th digit: 041.1
0. NOS
1. Aureus
9. Other staph

511.1 Streptococcal with effusion **[041.0#]**

5th digit: 041.0
0. NOS
1. Group A
2. Group B
3. Group C
4. Group D (enterococcus)
5. Group G
9. Other strep

510.9 Suppurative (septic) (purulent) (fibrinopurulent)
012.0# Tuberculous
010.1# Tuberculous primary progressive

5th digit: 010.1, 012.0
0. Unspecified
1. Lab not done
2. Lab pending
3. Microscopy positive (in sputum)
4. Culture positive - microscopy negative
5. Culture negative - microscopy positive
6. Culture and microscopy negative confirmed by other methods

511.1 Other specified bacterial with effusion
511.8 Other specified with effusion

485 PLEUROBRONCHOPNEUMONIA
786.52 PLEURODYNIA
074.1 PLEURODYNIA EPIDEMIC
573.8 PLEUROHEPATITIS
420.90 PLEUROPERICARDITIS ACUTE
486 PLEUROPNEUMONIA
515 PLEUROPNEUMONIA CHRONIC
0 PLEUROPNEUMONIA LIKE ORGANISM (PPLO) SEE 'BACTERIAL INFECTION' OR SPECIFIED CONDITION

P

PLICA

727.83 Knee
132.0 Polonica
727.83 Syndrome
727.83 Synovium
474.8 Tonsil

335.24 PLS (PRIMARY LATERAL SCLEROSIS)
984.9 PLUMBISM
242.3# PLUMMER'S DISEASE (TOXIC NODULAR GOITER)
5th digit: 242.3
0. Without storm
1. With storm

280.8 PLUMMER-VINSON SYNDROME (SIDEROPENIC DYSPHAGIA)
260 PLURICARENTIAL (PLURIDEFICIENCY) OF INFANCY SYNDROME
258.8 PLURIGLANDULAR ATROPHY
258.8 PLURIGLANDULAR (COMPENSATORY) SYNDROME
625.4 PMDD (PREMENSTRUAL DYSPHORIC DISORDER)
625.4 PMS (PREMENSTRUAL SYNDROME)
786.09 PND (PAROXYSMAL NOCTURUAL DYSPNEA)
170.# PNET (PRIMITIVE NEUROECTODERMAL TUMOR)
4th digit: 170
0. Skull and face
1. Mandible
2. Vertebral column
3. Ribs, sternum, clavicle
4. Scapula, long bones of upper limb
5. Short bones of upper limb
6. Pelvic bones, sacrum, coccyx
7. Long bones of lower limb
8. Short bones of lower limb
9. Site NOS

958.0 PNEUMATHEMIA
908.6 PNEUMATHEMIA LATE EFFECT
348.8 PNEUMATOCELE INTRACRANIAL
518.89 PNEUMATOCELE LUNG
492.0 PNEUMATOCELE TENSION
599.84 PNEUMATURIA
348.8 PNEUMOCEPHALUS
0 PNEUMOCOCCAL ARTHRITIS SEE 'ARTHRITIS OTHER SPECIFIED' PYOGENIC
0 PNEUMOCOCCUS SEE 'BACTERIAL INFECTION' OR SPECIFIED CONDITION

PNEUMOCONIOSIS

505 NOS
503 Aluminum
501 Asbestos
495.1 Bagasse
503 Bauxite
503 Beryllium
500 Coal workers'
504 Cotton dust
506.9 Fumes vapors (from silo)
503 Graphite hard metal
503 Inorganic dust other
502 Mica talc
504 Organic dust NEC
502 Silica or silicates other due to

136.3 PNEUMOCYSTIS (CARINII) (JIROVECI)
136.3 PNEUMOCYSTOSIS (CARINII) (JIROVECI)
793.0 PNEUMOENCEPHALOGRAM ABNORMAL
352.3 PNEUMOGASTRIC NERVE ATROPHY
352.3 PNEUMOGASTRIC NERVE DISORDER
951.8 PNEUMOGASTRIC NERVE INJURY
511.8 PNEUMOHEMOTHORAX
860.4 PNEUMOHEMOTHORAX TRAUMATIC
860.5 PNEUMOHEMOTHORAX TRAUMATIC WITH OPEN WOUND
423.9 PNEUMOHYDROPERICARDIUM
518.1 PNEUMOMEDIASTINUM
770.2 PNEUMOMEDIASTINUM PERINATAL PERIOD
117.9 PNEUMOMYCOSIS

If the physician has not specified whether the organism causing the pneumonia is bacterial or viral, assign code 486, pneumonia unspecified. A more specific code may be assigned only if the medical record substantiates a more specific diagnosis.

PNEUMONIA

486 Unspecified
480.0 Adenoviral
518.3 Allergic
482.81 Anaerobic

When both aspiration pneumonia (507.0) and bacterial pneumonia (480-483) are documented on the same encounter, both conditions should be coded. Sequencing depends on the reason for encounter.

ASPIRATION

507.0 NOS

For codes 770.12, 770.14, 770.16, 770.18, 770.86, use an additional code to identify any secondary pulmonary hypertension (416.8), if applicable.

770.18 Fetal or newborn
770.16 Fetal or newborn due to blood
770.14 Fetal or newborn due to clear amniotic fluid
770.12 Fetal or newborn due to meconium
770.86 Fetal or newborn due to postnatal stomach contents
507.0 Food regurgitated
506.0 Fumes or vapors (chemical) (acute)
507.0 Gastric secretions
516.8 Lipoid endogenous
507.1 Lipoid exogenous

668.0#: When coding a maternal aspiration pneumonia/pneumonitis use an additional code to show the type of aspiration.

668.0# Obstetrical maternal (mother's record)
5th digit: 668.0
0. Episode of care NOS or N/A
1. Delivered
2. Delivered with postpartum complication
3. Antepartum complication
4. Postpartum complication

507.1 Oils or essences
997.3 Postoperative
507.0 Vomitus
507.8 Other solids or liquids

P

PNEUMONIA (continued)

482.9 Bacterial
482.89 Bacterial specified NEC
482.83 Bacterium anitratum
482.81 Bacteroides (melaninogenicus)
485 Brochopneumonia (confluent) (croupous) (diffuse) (disseminated) (lobar) (hemorrhagic) (terminal)
482.81 Butyrivibrio (fibriosolvens)
112.4 Candidiasis
466.19 Capillary
483.1 Chlamydial
482.81 Clostridium (haemolyticum) (novyi)
481 Community acquired
481 Diplococcal
483.0 Eaton's agent
482.82 Escherichia coli (E. coli)
482.81 Eubacterium
482.0 Friedlander's bacillus
482.81 Fusobacterium (nucleatum)
513.0 Gangrenous
482.81 Gram-negative anaerobic
482.83 Gram-negative bacteria NEC
482.83 Herellea
V12.61 History
0 Hypostatic – due to or specified as a specific type of pneumonia – code to the type of pneumonia
770.0 Infective acquired prenatally

In order to correctly code influenza with pneumonia (487.0), use an additional code from the pneumonia category to identify the type of pneumonia, if known. Ie., Influenza with e. coli pneumonia 487.0 and 482.82.

487.0 Influenza
516.8 Interstitial (desquamative) (lymphoid)
482.0 Klebsiella pneumoniae
482.84 Legionnaires'
481 Lobar
485 Lobular
038.8 Metastatic NEC [484.8]
483.8 Microorganism other specified
483.0 Mycoplasma pneumoniae
513.0 Necrotic
486 Obstructive (bronchogenic neoplasm)
480.2 Parainfluenza
514 Passive
482.81 Peptococcus
482.81 Peptostreptococcus
483.0 Pleuropneumonia-like organism (PPLO)
481 Pneumococcal
V03.82 Pneumococcal vaccination
997.3 Post op
483.0 PPLO
770.0 Prenatally acquired infective
486 Primary atypical
482.81 Propionibacterium
482.83 Proteus
482.1 Pseudomonas
480.1 Respiratory syncytial virus
997.3 Resulting from a procedure
480.3 SARS-associated coronavirus
485 Segmental
482.83 Serratia (marcescens)
480.3 Severe acute respiratory syndrome-associated coronavirus

PNEUMONIA (continued)

482.4# Staphylococcal
5th digit: 482.4
0. NOS
1. Aureus
9. Other staph

482.3# Streptococcal
482.3# Streptococcal betahemolytic
5th digit: 482.3
0. NOS
1. Group A
2. Group B
9. Other streptococcus

481 Streptococcus pneumoniae
V03.82 Streptococcus pneumoniae vaccination
958.8 Traumatic
908.6 Traumatic late effect
V03.82 Vaccination
052.1 Varicella
482.81 Veillonella
999.9 Ventilator associated
480.9 Viral
480.8 Viral NEC

In order to correctly code influenza with pneumonia (487.0), use an additional code from the pneumonia category to identify the type of pneumonia, if known. Ie., Influenza with e. coli pneumonia 487.0 and 482.82.

487.0 With influenza
482.89 Other specified bacteria
483.8 Other specified organism

The code in the left margin always sequences first. The additional code in brackets to the right of the description is sequenced second. Underlining shows the code number that corresponds to the underlined description. Underlining never implies correct sequencing.

PNEUMONIA - OTHER

039.1 Actinomycotic
022.1 Anthrax [484.5]
127.0 Ascaris [484.8]
117.3 Aspergilla [484.6]
482.89 Bacteria NEC [041.89]
112.4 Candidiasis lung
466.19 Capillary (bronchiolitis) (with bronchospasm or obstruction)
483.1 Chlamydial (pneumoniae) (trachomatis)
073.0 Chlamydial psittaci
078.5 CMV [484.1]
114.# Coccidioidomycosis
4th digit: 114
0. Acute (primary)
4. Chronic (secondary)
5. Unspecified

For codes 770.12, 770.18, use an additional code to identify any secondary pulmonary hypertension (416.8), if applicable.

770.18 Congenital aspiration see 'Pneumonia', aspiration fetal
078.5 Cytomegalic inclusion [484.1]
506.0 Due to fumes and vapors
518.3 Eosinophilic
117.9 Fungus [484.7]
513.0 Gangrenous

P

PNEUMONIA – OTHER (continued)

487.0 Grippal
083.0 Hiberno-vernal [484.8]
115.95 Histoplasmosis
115.05 Histoplasmosis capsulatum
115.15 Histoplasmosis duboisii
514 Hypostatic
136.9 Infectious diseases [484.8]
516.8 Interstitial (desquamative) (lymphoid)
0 Intrauterine see 'Pneumonia', aspiration fetal
516.8 Lipoid endogenous
507.1 Lipoid exogenous
770.12 Meconium aspiration
038.8 Metastatic due to blood bourne bacteria [484.8]
038.8 Metastatic due to septicemia [484.8]
117.9 Mycotic (other) (systemic) [484.7]
039.1 Nocardia
486 Organism unspecified
483.8 Organism other specified
073.0 Ornithosis
514 Passive
033.# Pertussis [484.3]

5th digit: 033

- **0. B. pertussis**
- **1. B. parapertussis**
- **8. B. bronchiseptica**
- **9. Unspecified organism**

136.3 Pneumocystis carinii
136.3 Pneumocystis jiroveci
055.1 Postmeasles
083.0 Q fever [484.8]
390 Rheumatic [517.1]
083.9 Rickettsia [484.8]
771.0 Rubella pneumonitis congenital
003.22 Salmonella
104.8 Spirochetal [484.8]
130.4 Toxoplasmosis
958.8 Traumatic
011.6# Tuberculous

5th digit: 011.6

- **0. Unspecified**
- **1. Lab not done**
- **2. Lab pending**
- **3. Microscopy positive (in sputum)**
- **4. Culture positive - microscopy negative**
- **5. Culture negative - microscopy positive**
- **6. Culture and microscopy negative confirmed by other methods**

021.2 Tularemia
483.1 Twar agent
002.# Typhoid [484.8]

4th digit: 002

- **0. Paratyphoid fever**
- **1. Paratyphoid fever A**
- **2. Paratyphoid fever B**
- **3. Paratyphoid fever C**
- **9. Paratyphoid fever unspecified**

052.1 Varicella
033.# Whooping cough [484.3]

5th digit: 033

- **0. B. pertussis**
- **1. B. parapertussis**
- **8. B. bronchiseptica**
- **9. Unspecified organism**

PNEUMONITIS

486 NOS
495.9 Allergic
495.8 Allergic other specified

ASPIRATION

507.0 NOS

> ***For codes 770.12, 770.14, 770.16, 770.18, 770.86, use an additional code to identify any secondary pulmonary hypertension (416.8), if applicable.***

770.18 Fetal or newborn
770.16 Fetal or newborn due to blood
770.14 Fetal or newborn due to clear amniotic fluid
770.12 Fetal or newborn due to meconium
770.86 Fetal or newborn due to postnatal stomach contents
507.0 Food regurgitated
506.0 Fumes or vapors (chemical) (acute)
507.0 Gastric secretions
516.8 Lipoid endogenous
507.1 Lipoid exogenous

> ***668.0#: When coding a maternal aspiration pneumonia/pneumonitis, use an additional code to show the type of aspiration.***

668.0# Obstetrical maternal (mother's record)

5th digit: 668.0

- **0. Episode of care NOS or N/A**
- **1. Delivered**
- **2. Delivered with postpartum complication**
- **3. Antepartum complication**
- **4. Postpartum complication**

507.1 Oils or essences
997.3 Postoperative
771.0 Rubella congenital
507.0 Vomitus
507.8 Other solids or liquids

PNEUMONITIS (continued)

506.0 Chemical (or fumes)
506.0 Crack (cocaine)
495.9 Hypersensitivity
515 Interstitial (chronic)
516.8 Interstitial lymphoid
770.12 Meconium fetus or newborn
508.0 Radiation
0 See also 'Pneumonia'
495.7 Ventilation

516.9 PNEUMONOPATHY ALVEOLAR AND PARIETOALVEOLAR
504 PNEUMONOPATHY - INHALATION OTHER DUST
527.8 PNEUMOPAROTID
420.90 PNEUMOPERICARDITIS ACUTE
770.2 PNEUMOPERICARDIUM PERINATAL PERIOD
568.89 PNEUMOPERITONEUM
770.2 PNEUMOPERITONEUM FETUS OR NEWBORN
420.99 PNEUMOPYOPERICARDIUM
503 PNEUMOSIDEROSIS (OCCUPATIONAL)

PNEUMOTHORAX

512.1 Accidental during a procedure
770.2 Congenital
512.1 Due to operative procedure
512.1 Iatrogenic
770.2 Perinatal period
512.1 Postoperative
512.8 Spontaneous
512.8 Spontaneous acute or chronic
512.1 Tension iatrogenic
512.1 Tension postoperative
512.0 Tension spontaneous
860.0 Tension traumatic
860.1 Tension traumatic with open wound into thorax
908.0 Tension traumatic late effect
860.0 Traumatic
860.4 Traumatic with hemothorax
860.1 Traumatic with open wound into thorax
908.0 Traumatic late effect
011.7# Tuberculous
5th digit: 011.7
0. Unspecified
1. Lab not done
2. Lab pending
3. Microscopy positive (in sputum)
4. Culture positive - microscopy negative
5. Culture negative - microscopy positive
6. Culture and microscopy negative confirmed by other methods

132.2 PHTHIRUS PUBIS
790.91 PO2 OXYGEN RATIO ABNORMAL
790.09 POIKILOCYTOSIS
790.09 POIKILOCYTOSIS ABNORMAL FINDINGS
709.09 POIKILODERMA
757.33 POIKILODERMA CONGENITAL
710.3 POIKILODERMATOMYOSITIS
744.29 POINTED EAR CONGENITAL
692.6 POISON IVY DERMATITIS
692.6 POISON OAK DERMATITIS
692.6 POISON SUMAC DERMATITIS
692.6 POISON VINE DERMATITIS

Poisoning - medicinal: Conditions caused by medicinal substances are classified as a poisoning when the substance involved is improperly taken. Code the poisoning from the section below first, then the manifestation, with an additional E-code to further classify the type of poisoning. (see appendix A, 'Poisoning').

POISONING - MEDICINAL

0 See also appendix B, drug and chemicals index
977.9 Unspecified drug or medicinal substances
965.#(#) Analgesics, antipyretics, and antirheumatics
4th or 4th and 5th digit: 965
0#. Opiates and related narcotics
00. Opium (alkaloids) unspecified
01. Heroin
02. Methadone
09. Other (codeine) (meperidine) (morphine)
1. Salicylates
4. Aromatic analgesics, NEC
5. Pyrazole derivatives
6#. Antirheumatics (antiphlogistics)
61. Propionic acid derivatives
69. Other antirheumatics
7. Other non-narcotic analgesics
8. Other specified analgesics and antipyretics
9. Unspecified analgesic and antipyretic

960.# Antibiotics
4th digit: 960
0. Penicillins
1. Antifungal antibiotics
2. Chloramphenicol group
3. Erythromycin and other macrolides
4. Tetracycline group
5. Cephalosporin group
6. Antimycobacterial group
7. Antineoplastic antibiotics
8. Other specified antibiotics
9. Unspecified antibiotics

961.# Other anti-infectives
4th digit: 961
0. Sulfonamides
1. Arsenical anti-infectives
2. Heavy metal anti-infectives
3. Quinoline and hydroxyquinoline derivatives
4. Antimalarials and drugs acting on other blood protozoa
5. Other antiprotozoal drugs
6. Anthelmintics
7. Antiviral drugs
8. Other antimycobacterial drugs
9. Other and unspecified anti-infectives

966.# Anticonvulsants and anti-Parkinsonism drugs
4th digit: 966
0. Oxazolidine derivatives
1. Hydantoin derivatives
2. Succinimides
3. Other and unspecified anticonvulsants
4. Anti-parkinsonism drugs

P

POISONING - MEDICINAL (continued)

971.# Autonomic nervous system drugs - (primarily affecting)
4th digit: 971
- **0. Parasympathomimetics (cholinergics)**
- **1. Parasympatholytics (anticholinergics and antimuscarinics) and spasmolytics**
- **2. Sympathomimetics (adrenergics)**
- **3. Sympatholytics (antiadrenergics)**
- **9. Unspecified drug primarily affecting autonomic nervous system**

964.# Blood constituent agents (primarily affecting)
4th digit: 964
- **0. Iron and its compounds**
- **1. Liver preparations and other antianemic agents**
- **2. Anticoagulants**
- **3. Vitamin K (phytonadione)**
- **4. Fibrinolysis-affecting drugs**
- **5. Anticoagulant antagonists and other coagulants**
- **6. Gamma globulin**
- **7. Natural blood and blood products**
- **8. Other specified agents affecting blood constituents**
- **9. Unspecified agents affecting blood constituents**

972.# Cardiovascular system drugs - (primarily affecting)
4th digit: 972
- **0. Cardiac rhythm regulators**
- **1. Cardiotonic glycosides and drugs of similar action**
- **2. Antilipemic and antiarteriosclerotic drugs**
- **3. Ganglion-blocking agents**
- **4. Coronary vasodilators**
- **5. Other vasodilators**
- **6. Other antihypertensive agents**
- **7. Antivaricose drugs, including sclerosing agents**
- **8. Capillary-active drugs**
- **9. Other and NOS agents primarily affecting the cardiovascular system**

973.# Gastrointestinal system drugs (primarily affecting)
4th digit: 973
- **0. Antacids and antigastric secretion drugs**
- **1. Irritant cathartics**
- **2. Emollient cathartics**
- **3. Other cathartics, including intestinal atonia drugs**
- **4. Digestants**
- **5. Antidiarrheal drugs**
- **6. Emetics**
- **8. Other specified agents**
- **9. Unspecified agent affecting the gastrointestinal system**

POISONING - MEDICINAL (continued)

962.# Hormones and synthetic substitutes
4th digit: 962
- **0. Adrenal cortical steroids**
- **1. Androgens and anabolic congeners**
- **2. Ovarian hormones and synthetic substitutes**
- **3. Insulins and antidiabetic agents**
- **4. Anterior pituitary hormones**
- **5. Posterior pituitary hormones**
- **6. Parathyroid and parathyroid derivatives**
- **7. Thyroid and thyroid derivatives**
- **8. Antithyroid agents**
- **9. Other and unspecified hormones and synthetic substitutes**

967.# Sedatives and hypnotics
4th digit: 967
- **0. Barbiturates**
- **1. Chloral hydrate group**
- **2. Paraldehyde**
- **3. Bromine compounds**
- **4. Methaqualone compounds**
- **5. Glutethimide group**
- **6. Mixed sedatives, NEC**
- **8. Other sedatives and hypnotics**
- **9. Unspecified sedative or hypnotic**

968.# Other depressants and anesthetics (central nervous system)
4th digit: 968
- **0. CNS muscle tone depressants**
- **1. Halothane**
- **2. Other gaseous anesthetics**
- **3. Intravenous anesthetics**
- **4. Other and unspecified general anesthetics**
- **5. Surface (topical) and infiltration anesthetics**
- **6. Peripheral nerve- and plexus-blocking anesthetics**
- **7. Spinal anesthetics**
- **9. Other and unspecified local anesthetics**

969.# Psychotropic agents
4th digit: 969
- **0. Antidepressants**
- **1. Phenothiazine-based tranquilizers**
- **2. Butyrophenone-based tranquilizers**
- **3. Other antipsychotics, neuroleptics, and major tranquilizers**
- **4. Benzodiazepine-based tranquilizers**
- **5. Other tranquilizers**
- **6. Psychodysleptics, (hallucinogens)**
- **7. Psychostimulants**
- **8. Other specified psychotropic agents**
- **9. Unspecified psychotropic agent**

POISONING - MEDICINAL (continued)

976.# Skin and mucous membrane, ophthalmological, otorhinolaryngological, and dental drugs - (primarily affecting)
4th digit: 976
0. Local anti-infectives and anti-inflammatory drugs
1. Antipruritics
2. Local astringents and local detergents
3. Emollients, demulcents, and protectants
4. Keratolytics, keratoplastics, other hair treatment drugs and preparations
5. Eye anti-infectives and other eye drugs
6. Anti-infectives and other drugs and preparations for ear, nose, and throat
7. Dental drugs topically applied
8. Other agents primarily affecting skin and mucous membrane
9. Unspecified agent primarily affecting skin and mucous membrane

975.# Smooth muscles, skeletal muscles, respiratory system drugs (primarily acting on)
4th digit: 975
0. Oxytocic agents
1. Smooth muscle relaxants
2. Skeletal muscle relaxants
3. Other and unspecified drugs acting on muscles
4. Antitussives
5. Expectorants
6. Anti-common cold drugs
7. Antiasthmatics
8. Other and unspecified respiratory drugs

970.# Stimulants (central nervous system)
4th digit: 970
0. Analeptics
1. Opiate antagonists
8. Other specified CNS stimulants
9. Unspecified CNS stimulants

963.# Systemic agents (primarily)
4th digit: 963
0. Antiallergic and antiemetic drugs
1. Antineoplastic and immunosuppressive drugs
2. Acidifying agents
3. Alkalizing agents
4. Enzymes NEC
5. Vitamins NEC (A) (D)
8. Other specified systemic agents
9. Unspecified systemic agents

978.# Vaccines bacterial
4th digit: 978
0. BCG
1. Typhoid and paratyphoid
2. Cholera
3. Plague
4. Tetanus
5. Diphtheria
6. Pertussis vaccine combinations with a pertussis component
8. Other and unspecified bacterial vaccine
9. Mixed bacterial vaccines except combinations with pertussis component

POISONING - MEDICINAL (continued)

979.# Other vaccines and biological substances
4th digit: 979
0. Smallpox vaccine
1. Rabies vaccine
2. Typhus vaccine
3. Yellow fever vaccine
4. Measles vaccine
5. Poliomyelitis vaccine
6. Other and unspecified viral and rickettsial vaccines
7. Mixed viral-rickettsial and bacterial vaccines, except combinations with a pertussis component
9. Other and unspecified vaccines and biological substances

974.# Water, mineral, and uric acid metabolism drugs
4th digit: 974
0. Mercurial diuretics
1. Purine derivative diuretics
2. Carbonic acid anhydrase inhibitors
3. Saluretics
4. Other diuretics
5. Electrolytic, caloric, and water-balance agents
6. Other mineral salts, NEC
7. Uric acid metabolism drugs

977.# Other drugs and medicinal substances
4th digit: 977
0. Dietetics
1. Lipotropics
2. Antidotes and chelating agents, NEC
3. Alcohol deterrents
4. Pharmaceutical excipients
8. Other specified drugs and medicinals
9. Unspecified drug or medicinal substance

989.9 Unspecified substance chiefly nonmedicinal as to source

POISONING - NONMEDICINAL

982.8 Acetone (solvent)
989.7 Aflatoxin and other mycotoxin (food contaminants)
980.9 Alcohol
980.2 Alcohol isopropyl (rubbing)
980.8 Alcohol other specified
989.2 Aldrin
985.4 Antimony and its compounds
985.1 Arsenic and its compounds
989.81 Asbestos
982.0 Benzene and homologues (solvent)
981 Benzine
988.2 Berries and other plants
985.3 Beryllium and its compounds
985.8 Brass fumes
987.5 Bromobenzyl cyanide
987.0 Butane
985.5 Cadmium and its compounds
989.3 Carbamate
989.3 Carbaryl
983.0 Carbolic acid or phenol
982.2 Carbon bisulfide (solvent)
982.2 Carbon disulfide (solvent)
986 Carbon monoxide from any source
982.1 Carbon tetrachloride (solvent)
983.9 Caustic
989.2 Chlordane
989.9 Chlorinated hydrocarbon
987.6 Chlorine gas

P

POISONING - NONMEDICINAL (continued)

987.5	Chloroacetophenone
985.6	Chromium
985.8	Copper salts
983.0	Cresol
989.2	DDT
989.6	Detergents
987.4	Dichloromonofluoromethane
989.3	Dichlorvos
989.2	Dieldrin
980.2	Dimethyl carbinol
796.0	Drugs (heavy metals) abnormal
981	Ether petroleum

> ***980.0 Ethyl alcohol:** Use an additional code to identify associated drunkenness. See 'Drunkenness.'*

980.0	Ethyl alcohol
987.5	Ethyliodoacetate
988.0	Fish and shellfish
987.4	Freon
980.3	Fusel oil
987.9	Gas fume or vapor
981	Gasoline
987.1	Hydrocarbon gas other
983.1	Hydrochloric acid (liquid)
987.7	Hydrocyanic acid gas (fumes) (vapors)
989.4	Insecticide mixtures
985.8	Iron compounds
980.2	Isopropanol
981	Kerosene
909.1	Late effect nonmedical substances
989.82	Latex
984.1	Lead (tetraethyl)
984.1	Lead acetate
984.9	Lead compound
984.8	Lead compounds other
984.0	Lead dioxide
984.0	Lead salts
983.2	Lye
989.3	Malathion
985.2	Manganese and its compounds
985.0	Mercury and its compounds
985.9	Metal
980.1	Methanol
988.1	Mushrooms
981	Naptha petroleum
985.8	Nickel compounds
983.1	Nitric acid
987.2	Nitrogen dioxide
982.4	Nitroglycol (solvent)
987.2	Nitrous fumes
988.8	Noxious substances eaten as food other specified
989.3	Organophosphate and carbamate
981	Paraffin wax
989.3	Parathion
989.4	Pesticides NEC other
981	Petroleum (spirit)
989.3	Phorate
989.3	Phosdrin
987.8	Phosgene
987.8	Polyester fumes
989.0	Potassium cyanide
983.2	Potassium hydroxide
987.0	Propane

POISONING - NONMEDICINAL (continued)

> ***989.83 Silicone:** For silicone used in medical devices, implants and grafts see 'Complication Of A Device, Implant Or Graft.'*

989.83	Silicone
989.6	Soaps and detergents
989.0	Sodium cyanide
983.2	Sodium hydroxide
982.8	Solvent (nonpetroleum based) other
989.1	Strychnine and salts
987.3	Sulfur dioxide
983.1	Sulfuric acid
987.5	Tear gas
982.3	Tetrachloroethylene (solvent)
989.84	Tobacco
982.3	Trichloroethylene (solvent)
989.5	Venom
989.89	Other substances chiefly nonmedicinal as to source

0	POISONING SEE ALSO APPENDIX B, DRUG AND CHEMICALS INDEX
0	POLIO SEE 'POLIOMYELITIS'
045.0#	POLIOENCEPHALITIS BULBAR ACUTE, PARALYTIC
045.0#	POLIOENCEPHALOMYELITIS BULBAR ACUTE ANTERIOR, PARALYTIC

5th digit: 045.0
0. Unspecified
1. Type I
2. Type II
3. Type III

POLIOMYELITIS

045.9#	Acute unspecified
045.2#	Acute anterior nonparalytic
045.1#	Acute atrophic
045.2#	Acute epidemic nonparalytic
045.1#	Acute epidemic paralytic
045.1#	Acute infantile paralytic
138	Acute late effects
045.2#	Acute nonparalytic
045.1#	Acute paralytic
045.1#	Acute spinal paralytic
045.0#	Bulbar acute anterior paralytic
045.0#	Bulbar acute anterior polioencephalomyelitis paralytic
045.0#	Bulbar acute infantile paralytic
045.0#	Bulbar acute paralytic
045.0#	Bulbar acute polioencephalitis paralytic
045.1#	Other paralysis acute

5th digit: 045.0-2, 9
0. Unspecified
1. Type I
2. Type II
3. Type III

V01.2	Exposure
V12.02	History
V73.0	Screening exam
V04.0	Vaccination

704.3	POLIOSIS
704.3	POLIOSIS CIRCUMSCRIPTA ACQUIRED
V62.4	POLITICAL DISCRIMINATION CAUSING ENCOUNTER
788.41	POLLAKIURIA

P

705.83 POLLITZER'S DISEASE (HIDRADENITIS SUPPURATIVA)
729.9 POLYALGIA

POLYARTERITIS

446.0 Nodosa
446.0 Nodosa myopathy [359.6]
446.0 Nodosa with dementia **[294.1#]**
5th digit: 294.1
0. Without behavioral disturbance or NOS
1. With behavioral disturbance

446.0 Nodosa with polyneuropathy [357.1]
648.9# Maternal current (co-existent) in pregnancy [446.0]
5th digit: 648.9
0. Episode of care NOS or N/A
1. Delivered
2. Delivered with postpartum complication
3. Antepartum complication
4. Postpartum complication

POLYARTHRITIS

716.5# NOS
5th digit: 716.5
0. Site NOS
1. Shoulder region
2. Upper arm (elbow) (humerus)
3. Forearm (radius) (wrist) (ulna)
4. Hand (carpal) (metacarpal) (fingers)
5. Pelvic region (hip) (buttock) (femur)
6. Lower leg (fibula) (knee) (patella) (tibia)
7. Ankle and/or foot (metatarsals) (toes) (tarsals)
8. Other (head) (neck) (rib) (skull) (trunk) (vertebrae)
9. Multiple

714.0 Atrophic
714.9 Inflammatory
714.89 Inflammatory NEC
714.31 Juvenile acute
714.30 Juvenile chronic

260 POLYCARENTIAL OF INFANCY SYNDROME
733.99 POLYCHONDRITIS RELAPSING

POLYCYSTIC DISEASE

759.89 NOS (congenital)
753.12 Kidney (congenital)
753.13 Kidney (congenital) - adult type (APKD)
753.13 Kidney (congenital) - autosomal dominant
753.14 Kidney (congenital) - autosomal recessive
753.14 Kidney (congenital) - childhood type (infantile) (CPKD)
V18.61 Kidney family history
751.62 Liver congenital
518.89 Lung (pulmonary)
748.4 Lung (pulmonary) - congenital
256.4 Ovaries
759.0 Spleen

POLYCYTHEMIA

289.0 NOS
289.0 Acquired
289.0 Benign
289.6 Benign familial
776.4 Due to donor twin transfusion
289.0 Due to fall in plasma volume

POLYCYTHEMIA (continued)

289.0 Due to high altitude
776.4 Due to maternal twin transfusion
289.0 Emotional
289.6 Erythrocytosis benign familial
289.0 Erythropoietin
289.0 Erythropoeitin induced
289.6 Familial
289.0 Hemoglobin
289.0 High oxygen affinity
289.0 Hypoxemic
238.4 Primary
776.4 Neonatorum
762.3 Neonatorum placental transfusion [776.4]
289.0 Nephrogenous
289.0 Relative
776.4 Secondary
289.0 Secondary acquired
289.0 Spurious
289.0 Stress
238.4 Vera site NOS
0 Vera site specified see 'Neoplasm Uncertain Behavior', by site M9950/1

POLYDACTYLY

755.00 Digits
755.01 Fingers
755.02 Toes

783.5 POLYDIPSIA
199.1 POLYEMBRYOMA SITE NOS
0 POLYEMBRYOMA SITE SPECIFIED SEE 'CANCER', BY SITE M9072/3
258.9 POLYGLANDULAR DYSFUNCTION (ENDOCRINE)
258.8 POLYGLANDULAR DYSFUNCTION OR SYNDROME OTHER SPECIFIED (ENDOCRINE)
199.1 POLYGONAL CELL CARCINOMA SITE NOS
0 POLYGONAL CELL CARCINOMA SITE SPECIFIED SEE 'CANCER', BY SITE M8034/3
657.0# POLYHYDRAMNIOS
5th digit: 657.0
0. Episode of care unspecified or N/A
1. Delivered
3. Antepartum complication

761.3 POLYHYDRAMNIOS AFFECTING FETUS OR NEWBORN
626.2 POLYMENORRHEA
692.72 POLYMORPHOUS LIGHT ERUPTION (ACUTE)
725 POLYMYALGIA RHEUMATICA

POLYMYOSITIS

710.4 NOS
728.19 Ossificans
710.3 Skin involvement

POLYNEURITIS

357.0 Acute infective
291.1 Alcoholic psychosis
291.5 Alcoholic psychosis with delusions
291.3 Alcoholic psychosis with hallucinations
352.6 Cranialis
357.81 Demyelinating chronic inflammatory
357.0 Guillain-Barre syndrome
357.0 Postinfectious
0 See also 'Polyneuropathy'

P

POLYNEUROPATHY

357.9	NOS
357.5	Alcoholic
277.39	Amyloid [357.4]
265.0	Beriberi [357.4]
357.82	Critical illness
266.2	Deficiency of B-complex [357.4]
266.9	Deficiency of vitamin B [357.4]
266.1	Deficiency of vitamin B6 [357.4]
269.2	Deficiency of vitamin [357.4]
357.81	Demyelinating chronic inflammatory
250.6#	Diabetic [357.2]

5th digit: 250.6
- **0. Type II, adult-onset, non-insulin dependent (even if requiring insulin), or unspecified; controlled**
- **1. Type I, juvenile-onset or insulin-dependent; controlled**
- **2. Type II, adult-onset, non-insulin dependent (even if requiring insulin); uncontrolled**
- **3. Type I, juvenile-onset or insulin-dependent; uncontrolled**

032.#(#)	Diphtheritic [357.4]

4th or 4th and 5th digit:032
- **.0 Faucial (throat)**
- **.1 Nasopharyngeal**
- **.2 Anterior nasal**
- **.3 Laryngeal**
- **.81 Conjunctival**
- **.82 Myocarditis**
- **.83 Peritonitis**
- **.84 Cystitis**
- **.85 Cutaneous**
- **.89 Other**

357.6	Due to drugs
710.0	Due to lupus erythematous [357.1]
356.0	Hereditary
356.3	Hereditary ataxic
251.2	Hypolycemia [357.4]
356.9	Idiopathic
356.4	Idiopathic progressive
269.2	In avitaminosis [357.4]
269.1	In avitaminosis specified NEC [357.4]
710.9	In collagen vascular disease [357.1]
199.1	Malignant (neoplastic) [357.3]
072.72	Mumps
265.2	Pellagra [357.4]
446.0	Polyarteritis nodosa [357.1]
277.1	Porphyria [357.4]
053.13	Postherpetic
724.4	Radicular thoracic NEC
714.0	Rheumatoid arthritis [357.1]
353.1	Sacral plexus
250.6#	Sacral plexus with diabetes [353.1]

5th digit: 250.6
- **0. Type II, adult-onset, non-insulin dependent (even if requiring insulin), or unspecified; controlled**
- **1. Type I, juvenile-onset or insulin-dependent; controlled**
- **2. Type II, adult-onset, non-insulin dependent (even if requiring insulin); uncontrolled**
- **3. Type I, juvenile-onset or insulin-dependent; uncontrolled**

135	Sarcoidosis [357.4]

P

POLYNEUROPATHY (continued)

355.0	Sciatic
356.2	Sensory (hereditary)
356.8	Specified NOS
355.9	Spinal nerve NEC
729.2	Spinal nerve root
0	Spinal nerve root see 'Radiculitis'
357.7	Toxic agents
350.8	Trigeminal sensory
354.2	Ulnar nerve
354.9	Upper extremity NEC
586	Uremia NOS [357.4]
266.2	Vitamin B12 [357.4]
281.0	Vitamin B12 with anemia (pernicious) [357.4]
368.15	POLYOPIA REFRACTIVE
752.89	POLYORCHISM CONGENITAL
756.54	POLYOSTOTIC FIBROUS DYSPLASIA BONE
744.1	POLYOTIA CONGENITAL

Polyps of sites not listed below should be coded to disease of the specified anatomical site.

POLYP

471.8	Accessory sinus
212.0	Accessory sinus adenomatous
199.1	Adenocarcinoma site NOS
0	Adenocarcinoma site specified see 'Cancer', by site M8210/3
471.0	Adenoid
212.0	Adenoid adenomatous
0	Adenomatous unspecified see 'Benign Neoplasm', by site M8210/0
211.4	Anal (canal) adenomatous
569.0	Anal (canal) nonadenomatous
471.8	Antrum
212.0	Antrum adenomatous
211.3	Appendix
624.6	Bartholin's gland
620.8	Broad ligament or fallopian tube (nonpregnant)
211.3	Cecum
622.7	Cervix
219.0	Cervix adenomatous
622.7	Cervix mucous
0	Cervix (maternal) see cervix abnormality maternal
471.0	Choanal
212.0	Choanal adenomatous
575.6	Cholesterol
624.6	Clitoris
211.3	Colon adenomatous M/8210/0
569.89	Colon nonadenomatous
211.4	Colon rectosigmoid junction adenomatous
621.0	Corpus uteri
575.6	Cystic duct
522.0	Dental pulp
211.2	Duodenum nonadenomatous
385.30	Ear (middle)
621.0	Endometrium
471.8	Ethmoid sinus
212.0	Ethmoid sinus adenomatous
620.8	Fallopian tube
624.8	Female genital organs NEC
471.8	Frontal sinus
212.0	Frontal sinus adenomatous
575.6	Gallbladder
624.8	Genital organs (female) NEC

POLYP (continued)

523.8 Gingival
523.8 Gum
211.3 Ileocecal valve
211.2 Ileum
211.2 Intestine small
569.9 Intestine small nonadenomatous
211.2 Jejunum
624.6 Labia and vulva
478.4 Larynx
212.1 Larynx adenomatous
471.8 Maxillary sinus
212.0 Maxillary sinus adenomatous
229.9 Multiple adenomatous site NOS
0 Multiple adenomatous site specified see 'Benign Neoplasm', by site M8221/0
621.0 Myometrium
212.0 Nares adenomatous
471.9 Nares anterior
471.0 Nares posterior
471.9 Nasal (mucous)
212.0 Nasal (mucous) adenomatous
471.0 Nasal cavity
212.0 Nasal cavity adenomatous
471.9 Nasal septum
212.0 Nasal septum adenomatous
471.0 Nasal choanal
212.0 Nasal choanal adenomatous
471.0 Nasopharyngeal
212.0 Nasopharyngeal adenomatous
0 Neoplastic see 'Benign Neoplasm', by site M/8210/0
620.8 Oviduct
620.8 Paratubal
478.29 Pharynx
750.29 Pharynx congenital
674.4# Placental maternal due to pregnancy

5t digit: 674.4
0. Unspecified
2. Delivered with postpartum complication
4. Postpartum complication

600.20 Prostate

> ***See 'LUTS' or 'Lower Urinary Tract Symptoms' for the additional code to identify the specific lower urinary tract symptoms.***

600.21 Prostate with urinary obstruction, retention or other lower urinary tract symptoms
624.6 Pudendal
569.0 Rectal
211.4 Rectosigmoid (adenomatous)
0 Rectosigmoid malignant see 'Cancer', rectosigmoid
569.0 Rectal nonadenomatous
471.8 Sinus NOS
471.8 Sphenoidal sinus
212.0 Sphenoidal sinus adenomatous
211.1 Stomach M8210/0
471.8 Turbinate (mucous membrane)
212.0 Turbinate (mucous membrane) adenomatous
593.89 Ureter
599.3 Urethra
621.0 Uterine
620.8 Uterine ligament
620.8 Uterine tube
763.89 Uterus body (corpus) (mucous) affecting fetus or newborn

POLYP (continued)

654.1# Uterus body (corpus) (mucous) in pregnancy
660.2# Uterus body (corpus) (mucous) obstructing labor **[654.1#]**

5th digit: 654.1
0. Episode of care unspecified or N/A
1. Delivered
2. Delivered with postpartum complication
3. Antepartum complication

5th digit: 660.2
0. Episode of care unspecified or N/A
1. Delivered
3. Antepartum complication

623.7 Vagina
478.4 Vocal cord
212.1 Vocal cord adenomatous
624.6 Vulva

783.6 POLYPHAGIA ORGANIC
471.1 POLYPOID SINUS DEGENERATION
357.0 POLYRADICULITIS (ACUTE)
066.42 POLYRADICULITIS DUE TO WEST NILE FEVER (VIRUS)
278.00 POLYSARCIA WITH BODY MASS INDEX 25 OR ABOVE **[V85.0#(#)]**

4th or 4th and 5th digit: V85
2#. 25-29
1. 25.0-25.9
2. 26.0-26.9
3. 27.0-27.9
4. 28.0-28.9
5. 29.0-29.9
3#. 30-39
0. 30.0-30.9
1. 31.0-31.9
2. 32.0-32.9
3. 33.0-33.9
4. 34.0-34.9
5. 35.0-35.9
6. 36.0-36.9
7. 37.0-37.9
8. 38.0-38.9
9. 39.0-39.9
4. 40 and over

277.31 POLYSEROSITIS PERIODIC FAMILIAL (RECURRENT)
277.31 POLYSEROSITIS PAROXYSMAL FAMILIAL
759.0 POLYSPLENIA SYNDROME
704.1 POLYTRICHIA
788.42 POLYURIA
271.0 POMPE'S DISEASE (GLYCOGENOSIS II)
705.81 POMPHOLYX
015.9# PONCET'S DISEASE (TUBERCULOUS RHEUMATISM) (SEE ALSO 'TUBERCULOSIS')

5th digit: 015.9
0. Unspecified
1. Lab not done
2. Lab pending
3. Microscopy positive (in sputum)
4. Culture positive - microscopy negative
5. Culture negative - microscopy positive
6. Culture and microscopy negative confirmed by other methods

P

433.8# PONTINE ARTERY OCCLUSION OR SYNDROME

433.8# PONTINE ARTERY THROMBOSIS (EMBOLISM) (DEFORMANS)
5th digit: 433.8
0. Without cerebral infarction
1. With cerebral infarction

431 PONTINE HEMORRHAGE (CEREBRAL)

674.0# PONTINE HEMORRHAGE MATERNAL DUE TO PREGNANCY
5th digit: 674.0
0. Episode of care unspecified or N/A
1. Delivered
2. Delivered with postpartum complication
3. Antepartum complication
4. Postpartum complication

Injury of a blood vessel can be a laceration, A-V fistula, aneurysm, or hematoma. Use the injury code found by anatomical site (the name of the blood vessel).

POPLITEAL

442.3 Artery aneurysm

440.2# Artery arteriosclerosis

440.2# Artery arteriosclerosis with chronic complete or total occlusion [440.4]
5th digit: 440.2
0. Unspecified
1. With intermittent claudication
2. With rest pain or rest pain and intermittent claudication
9. Other atherosclerosis extremities

When coding arteriosclerosis of the extremities use an additional code, if applicable to identify chronic complete or total occlusion of the artery of the extremities (440.4)

440.24 Artery arteriosclerosis with ischemic gangrene or ischemic gangrene and ulceration, or ulceration and intermittent claudication, rest pain **[707.1#]**

440.23 Artery arteriosclerosis with ulceration, or ulceration and intermittent claudication, rest pain **[707.1#]**
5th digit: 707.1
0. Unspecified
1. Thigh
2. Calf
3. Ankle
4. Heel and midfoot
5. Other parts of foot, toes
9. Other

440.3# Artery bypass graft arteriosclerosis

440.3# Artery bypass graft arteriosclerosis with chronic complete or total occlusion [440.4]
5th digit: 440.3
0. Unspecified graft
1. Autologous vein bypass graft
2. Nonautologous biological bypass graft

444.22 Artery embolism (thrombosis) (occlusion) (infarction)

447.8 Artery entrapment (syndrome)

904.41 Artery injury

908.3 Artery injury late effect

443.9 Artery spasm

904.42 Vein injury

908.3 Vein injury late effect

POPLITEAL (continued)

904.40 Vessel injury vessel unspecified

908.3 Vessel injury late effect

756.89 Web syndrome

POPLITEAL NERVE

355.3 Disorder lateral

355.4 Disorder medial

355.3 Neuritis lateral

355.4 Neuritis medial

348.0 PORENCEPHALY

742.4 PORENCEPHALY CONGENITAL

123.0 PORK TAPEWORM (ADULT) (INFECTION)

757.39 POROKERATOSIS

692.75 POROKERATOSIS DISSEMINATED SUPERFICIAL ACTINIC (DSAP)

277.1 PORPHYRIA

277.1 PORPHYRIA POLYNEUROPATHY [357.4]

277.1 PORPHYRIN METABOLISM DISORDER

277.1 PORPHYRINURIA

PORTAL

571.5 Cirrhosis

571.5 Cirrhosis with esophageal varices **[456.2#]**

572.3 Hypertension

572.3 Hypertension with esophageal varices **[456.2#]**
5th digit: 456.2
0. With bleeding
1. Without bleeding

452 Obstruction

572.2 Systemic encephalopathy

572.1 Thrombophlebitis

747.49 Vein absence (atresia)

452 Vein embolism

902.33 Vein injury

908.4 Vein injury late effect

452 Vein obstruction

572.1 Vein phlebitis

572.1 Vein thrombophlebitis

452 Vein thrombosis

093.89 Vein thrombosis due to syphilis

572.1 Vein thrombosis infectional or septic

757.32 PORTWINE STAIN CONGENITAL

114.9 POSADAS-WERNICKE DISEASE

V46.8 POSSUM DEPENDENCE

627.4 POSTARTIFICIAL MENOPAUSE SYNDROME

429.4 POSTCARDIAC INJURY SYNDROME – POSTCARDIOTOMY

411.0 POSTCARDIAC INJURY SYNDROME – POSTMYOCARDIAL INFARCTION

429.4 POSTCARDIOTOMY SYNDROME

576.0 POSTCHOLECYSTECTOMY SYNDROME

626.7 POSTCOITAL BLEEDING

429.4 POSTCOMMISSUROTOMY SYNDROME

310.2 POSTCONCUSSION SYNDROME (POSTCONTUSIONAL SYNDROME) (MENTAL DISORDER)

310.8 POSTENCEPHALITIS SYNDROME (MENTAL DISORDER)

372.64 POSTENUCLEATION CONTRACTION EYE SOCKET

POSTERIOR

723.2 Cervical sympathetic syndrome
433.8# Communicating artery obstruction (thrombosis)
5th digit: 433.8
0. Without cerebral infarction
1. With cerebral infarction

844.2 Cruciate ligament sprain, strain acute
717.84 Cruciate ligament sprain, strain old
348.4 Fossa compression syndrome
436 Inferior cerebellar artery syndrome
524.29 Lingual occlusion mandibular teeth
348.39 Reversible Encephalopathy Syndrome (PRES)
743.54 Segment congenital folds and cysts
904.53 Tibial artery injury
908.3 Tibial artery injury late effect
355.5 Tibial nerve compression
956.2 Tibial nerve injury
907.5 Tibial nerve injury late effect
904.54 TIbial vein injury
908.3 Tibial vein injury late effect

564.2 POSTGASTRECTOMY SYNDROME (DUMPING) (POSTGASTRIC SURGERY)

780.79 POSTHEPATITIS SYNDROME

053.11 POSTHERPETIC (NEURALGIA) GENICULATE GANGLION (SYNDROME)

053.19 POSTHERPETIC (NEURALGIA) INTERCOSTAL (ZOSTER) OPHTHALMICA (SYNDROME)

053.12 POSTHERPETIC TRIGEMINAL NEURALGIA

411.0 POSTINFARCTION SYNDROME

780.79 POSTINFLUENZA (ASTHENIA) SYNDROME

990 POSTIRRADIATION SYNDROME

Postlaminectomy syndrome is the continuous progression of scar tissue formation at the laminectomy site. This condition is marked by constant pain due to the scar tissue and is a basically untreatable condition. Assign a code from this section when the physician states that the pain is due to scar tissue.

POSTLAMINECTOMY SYNDROME

722.80 NOS
722.81 Cervical
722.83 Lumbar
722.82 Thoracic

310.0 POSTLEUKOTOMY SYNDROME (STATE)

310.0 POSTLOBOTOMY SYNDROME

457.0 POSTMASTECTOMY LYMPHEDEMA SYNDROME

POSTMATURE PREGNANCY

766.21 Affecting fetus or newborn >40 completed weeks to 42 completed weeks
766.22 Affecting fetus or newborn >42 completed weeks
645.1# Post-term (> 40 completed weeks to 42 completed weeks gestation)
645.2# Prolonged (> 42 completed weeks gestation)
5th digit: 645.1-2
0. Episode of care unspecified or N/A
1. Delivered
3. Antepartum complication

766.21 Syndrome (of newborn) >40 completed weeks to 42 completed weeks
766.22 Syndrome (of newborn) >42 completed weeks

POSTMENOPAUSAL

627.1 Bleeding
627.4 Bleeding - artificial menopause
627.9 Disorder unspecified
627.8 Disorder other specified NEC
V07.4 Hormone replacement therapy (prophylactic)
V49.81 Status asymptomatic (age-related) (natural)

411.0 POSTMYOCARDIAL INFARCTION SYNDROME

784.91 POSTNASAL DRIP

0 POSTNASAL DRIP DUE ALLERGIC RHINITIS SEE 'RHINITIS', ALLERGIC

460 POSTNASAL DRIP DUE TO COMMON COLD

530.81 POSTNASAL DRIP DUE TO GASTROESOPHAGEAL REFLUX

0 POSTNASAL DRIP DUE TO NASOPHARYNGITIS SEE 'NASOPHARYNGITIS'

0 POSTNASAL DRIP DUE TO OTHER KNOWN CONDITION – CODE TO CONDITION

0 POSTNASAL DRIP DUE TO SINUSITIS SEE 'SINUSITIS'

579.2 POSTOPERATIVE BLIND LOOP SYNDROME

998.9 POSTOPERATIVE COMPLICATION OR SYNDROME NOS (SEE ALSO 'COMPLICATION')

998.89 POSTOPERATIVE COMPLICATION SPECIFIED NEC (SEE ALSO 'COMPLICATION')

338.18 POSTOPERATIVE PAIN ACUTE

338.28 POSTOPERATIVE PAIN CHRONIC

0 POSTOPERATIVE STATUS SEE 'STATUS'

POSTPARTUM

648.2# Anemia
674.5# Cardiomyopathy
5th digit: 648.2, 674.5
0. Episode of care unspecified or N/A
1. Delivered
2. Delivered with postpartum complication
3. Antepartum complication
4. Postpartum complication

V24.0 Care immediately after delivery (routine)
V24.1 Care lactating mother
V24.2 Care routine follow-up
648.4# Blues
648.4# Depression - NOS [311]
648.4# Depression - psychotic - recurrent **[296.3#]**
648.4# Depression - psychotic - single episode **[296.2#]**
253.2 Panhypopituitary syndrome
668.8# Spinal headache
5th digit: 648.4, 668.8
0. Episode of care NOS
1. Delivered with or without mention of antepartum condition
2. Delivered with mention of postpartum complication
3. Antepartum condition
4. Postpartum complication

5th digit: 296.2-3
0. Unspecified
1. Mild
2. Moderate
3. Severe without mention of psychotic behavior
4. Severe specified as with psychotic behavior
5. In partial or unspecified remission

P

999.8 POSTPERFUSION SYNDROME (REACTION) (SHOCK)
996.85 POSTPERFUSION BONE MARROW SYNDROME NEC
429.4 POSTPERICARDIOTOMY SYNDROME

POSTPHLEBITIS SYNDROME

459.10 NOS
459.10 Asymptomatic
648.9# Maternal current (co-existent) in pregnancy **[459.1#]**

5th digit: 648.9
0. Episode of care NOS or N/A
1. Delivered
2. Delivered with postpartum complication
3. Antepartum complication
4. Postpartum complication

5th digit: 459.1
0. NOS
1. With ulcer
2. With inflammation
3. With ulcer and inflammation
4. With other complication

459.12 With inflammation
459.12 With stasis dermatitis
459.13 With stasis dermatitis with ulcer
459.11 With ulcer
459.13 With ulcer and inflammation
459.19 With other complication

138 POST POLIO SYNDROME
138 POSTPOLIOMYELITIS SYNDROME
V58.49 POSTSURGICAL AFTERCARE NEC
244.0 POSTSURGICAL HYPOTHYROIDISM
V45.89 POSTSURGICAL STATUS NEC
766.21 POST TERM INFANT >40 COMPLETED WEEKS TO 42 COMPLETED WEEKS
766.22 POST TERM INFANT >42 COMPLETED WEEKS
645.1# POST-TERM PREGNANCY (OVER 40 COMPLETED WEEKS TO 42 COMPLETED WEEKS GESTATION)

5th digit: 645.1
0. Episode of care unspecified or N/A
1. Delivered
3. Antepartum complication

338.12 POST-THORACOTOMY PAIN ACUTE
338.22 POST-THORACOTOMY PAIN CHRONIC
998.11 POST TONSILLECTOMY HEMORRHAGE
287.4 POSTTRANSFUSION PURPURA
310.2 POSTTRAUMATIC BRAIN SYNDROME NONPSYCHOTIC
309.81 POSTTRAUMATIC STRESS DISORDER (PTSD) (ACUTE) (BRIEF)
309.81 POSTTRAUMATIC STRESS SYNDROME (PTSS) (ACUTE) (BRIEF)
337.2# POSTTRAUMATIC SYMPATHETIC DYSTROPHY

5th digit: 337.2
0. Unspecified
1. Upper limb
2. Lower limb
9. Other specified site

958.3 POSTTRAUMATIC WOUND INFECTION
908.6 POSTTRAUMATIC WOUND INFECTION LATE EFFECT

781.92 POSTURE ABNORMAL
564.2 POSTVAGOTOMY SYNDROME
429.4 POSTVALVULOTOMY SYNDROME
780.79 POSTVIRAL SYNDROME (ASTHENIA) (MALAISE OR FATIGUE)
514 POTAIN'S DISEASE (PULMONARY EDEMA)
536.1 POTAIN'S SYNDROME (GASTRECTASIS WITH DYSPEPSIA)

POTASSIUM

276.8 Deficiency (hypokalemia)
269.3 Deficiency nutritional
276.7 Elevated, excess (hyperkalemia)
276.7 Intoxication syndrome

POTT'S DISEASE (TUBERCULOSIS OF THE SPINE)

015.0# NOS [730.88]
015.0# Osteomyelitis [730.88]
015.0# Paraplegia [730.88]
015.0# Spinal curvature [737.43]
015.0# Spondylitis [720.81]

5th digit: 015.0
0. Unspecified
1. Lab not done
2. Lab pending
3. Microscopy positive (in sputum)
4. Culture positive - microscopy negative
5. Culture negative - microscopy positive
6. Culture and microscopy negative confirmed by other methods

When coding atherosclerosis of the extremities use an additional code, if applicable to identify chronic complete or total occlusion of the artery of the extremities (440.4)

440.24 POTT'S ISCHEMIC GANGRENE AND ULCERATION **[707.#(#)]**

4th or 4th and 5th digit: 707
1#. Lower limb except decubitus
10. Unspecified
11. Thigh
12. Calf
13. Ankle
14. Heel and midfoot
15. Other parts of foot, toes
19. Other
8. Chronic of other specified site
9. Chronic site NOS

753.0 POTTER'S DISEASE OR SYNDROME
754.0 POTTER'S FACIES
714.2 POULET'S DISEASE
V60.2 POVERTY
063.8 POWASSAN ENCEPHALITIS
795.5 PPD (PURIFIED PROTEIN DERIVATIVE) POSITIVE (WITHOUT ACTIVE TB)
693.0 PPE (PALMAR PLANTAR ERYTHRODYSESTHESIA)
0 PPLO (PLEUROPNEUMONIA LIKE ORGANISMS) SEE 'BACTERIAL INFECTION' OR SPECIFIED CONDITION
V03.82 PPV (PNEUMOCOCCAL POLYSACCHARIDE VACCINE) VACCINATION

759.81 PRADER (-LABHART) -WILLI (-FANCONI) SYNDROME
744.1 PREAURICULAR APPENDAGE CONGENITAL
744.47 PREAURICULAR CYST CONGENITAL
744.46 PREAURICULAR SINUS OR FISTULA CONGENITAL
0 PRECANCEROUS MELANOSIS SEE 'CARCINOMA IN SITU' SKIN BY SITE M8741/2
433.9# PRECEREBRAL ARTERY EMBOLISM, THROMBOSIS, OBSTRUCTION OR OCCLUSION
433.3# PRECEREBRAL ARTERY EMBOLISM, THROMBOSIS, OBSTRUCTION OR OCCLUSION MULTIPLE AND BILATERAL
433.8# PRECEREBRAL ARTERY EMBOLISM, THROMBOSIS, OBSTRUCTION OR OCCLUSION OTHER SPECIFIED

5th digit: 433.3, 8-9
0. Without cerebral infarction
1. With cerebral infarction

763.6 PRECIPITATE DELIVERY AFFECTING FETUS OR NEWBORN
661.3# PRECIPITATE LABOR

5th digit: 661.3
0. Episode of care unspecified or N/A
1. Delivered
3. Antepartum complication

259.1 PRECOCIOUS ADRENARCHE NEC

PRECOCIOUS PUBERTY

259.1 NOS
255.2 Cortical hyperfunction (adrenal)
256.1 Ovarian hyperfunction
256.0 Ovarian hyperfunction estrogen (hyperestrogenism)
259.8 Pineal tumor
257.0 Testicular hyperfunction

786.51 PRECORDIAL CHEST PAIN
786.51 PRECORDIAL CHEST PAIN PSYCHOGENIC [307.80]
785.3 PRECORDIAL FRICTION
790.29 PREDIABETES
775.89 PREDIABETES COMPLICATING FETUS OR NEWBORN

Use an additional code, if applicable, for associated insulin use (V58.67), when using code 648.8#.

648.8# PREDIABETES IN PREGNANCY

5th digit: 648.8
0. Episode of care unspecified or N/A
1. Delivered
2. Delivered with postpartum complication
3. Antepartum complication
4. Postpartum complication

PRE-ECLAMPSIA

642.4# NOS
760.0 Affecting fetus or newborn
642.4# Mild
642.7# Or eclampsia with pre-existing hypertension
642.5# Severe

5th digit: 642.4-5, 7
0. Episode of care unspecified or N/A
1. Delivered
2. Delivered with postpartum complication
3. Antepartum complication
4. Postpartum complication

V70.5 PREEMPLOYMENT EXAM (HEALTH)
365.00 PREGLAUCOMA

PREGNANCY

0 Abdominal see 'Ectopic Pregnancy'
0 Complications see also 'Labor and Delivery Complications' (for complications of L&D)
0 Complications see also 'Pregnancy Complications'
646.9# Complication unspecified

5th digit: 646.9
0. Episode of care unspecified or N/A
1. Delivered
3. Antepartum complication

761.9 Complication unspecified affecting fetus or newborn

646.8#: Specify the maternal complication with an additional code.

646.8# Complication other specified

5th digit: 646.8
0. Episode of care unspecified or N/A
1. Delivered
2. Delivered with postpartum complication
3. Antepartum complication
4. Postpartum complication

761.8 Complication other specified affecting fetus or newborn
0 Cornual see 'Ectopic Pregnancy'
0 Ectopic see 'Ectopic Pregnancy'
V72.41 Exam or test - negative result
V72.42 Exam or test - positive result
V72.40 Exam or test - possible, unconfirmed pregnancy
300.11 False
V61.6 Illegitimate causing family problems
V22.2 Incidental finding
677 Late effect
645.1# Late - post-term (> 40 completed weeks to 42 completed weeks gestation)
645.2# Late - prolonged (> 42 completed weeks gestation)
0 Ovarian see 'Ectopic Pregnancy'
645.1# Post-term (> 40 completed weeks to 42 completed weeks gestation)
645.2# Prolonged (> 42 completed weeks gestation)

5th digit: 645.1-2
0. Episode of care unspecified or N/A
1. Delivered
3. Antepartum complication

779.6 Termination causing fetal death
V72.41 Test - negative result
V72.42 Test - positive result
V72.40 Test - unconfirmed
0 Tubal see 'Ectopic Pregnancy'
V61.7 Unwanted

PREGNANCY COMPLICATIONS
ABNORMALITIES OF PELVIC ORGANS OR TISSUE: COMPLICATING PREGNANCY, (CHILDBIRTH) (PUERPERIUM)

654.4# Bladder dilatation
660.2# Bladder dilatation obstructing labor **[654.4#]**
654.5# Cervical incompetence
660.2# Cervical incompetence obstructing labor **[654.5#]**
654.6# Cervical polyp
660.2# Cervical polyp obstructing labor **[654.6#]**
654.6# Cervical stenosis
660.2# Cervical stenosis obstructing labor **[654.6#]**
654.6# Cervix abnormality
660.2# Cervix abnormality obstructing labor **[654.6#]**
654.6# Cervix cicatrix
660.2# Cervix cicatrix obstructing labor **[654.6#]**
654.6# Cervix rigid
660.2# Cervix rigid obstructing labor **[654.6#]**
654.6# Cervix tumor
660.2# Cervix tumor obstructing labor **[654.6#]**
654.2# Cesarean section (previous)
660.2# Cesarean section (previous) obstructing labor **[654.2#]**
654.4# Cystocele
660.2# Cystocele obstructing labor **[654.4#]**
654.4# Kidney ectopic
660.2# Kidney ectopic obstructing labor **[654.4#]**
654.6# Locked twins
660.5# Locked twins obstructing labor **[654.6#]**
654.9# Other and unspecified abnormality
660.2# Other and unspecified abnormality obstructing labor **[654.9#]**
654.4# Pendulous abdomen
660.2# Pendulous abdomen obstructing labor **[654.4#]**
654.8# Perineal fibrosis
660.2# Perineal fibrosis obstructing labor **[654.8#]**
654.8# Perineum rigid
660.2# Perineum rigid obstructing labor **[654.8#]**

5th digit: 654.4-6, 8-9
- **0. Episode of care unspecified or N/A**
- **1. Delivered**
- **2. Delivered with postpartum complication**
- **3. Antepartum complication**
- **4. Postpartum complication**

5th digit: 660.2, 654.2
- **0. Episode of care unspecified or N/A**
- **1. Delivered**
- **3. Antepartum complication**

PREGNANCY COMPLICATIONS
ABNORMALITIES OF PELVIC ORGANS OR TISSUE: COMPLICATING PREGNANCY, (CHILDBIRTH) (PUERPERIUM) (continued)

654.8# Persistent hymen
660.2# Persistent hymen obstructing labor **[654.8#]**
654.2# Previous C section
660.2# Previous C section obstructing labor **[654.2#]**
654.4# Rectocele
660.2# Rectocele obstructing labor **[654.4#]**
654.7# Septate vagina
660.2# Septate vagina obstructing labor **[654.7#]**
654.5# Shirodkar suture
660.2# Shirodkar suture obstructing labor **[654.5#]**
654.0# Uterine abnormality congenital
660.2# Uterine abnormality congenital obstructing labor **[654.0#]**
654.0# Uterine bicornis
660.2# Uterine bicornis obstructing labor **[654.0#]**
654.1# Uterine fibroid
660.2# Uterine fibroid obstructing labor **[654.1#]**
654.4# Uterine sacculation
660.2# Uterine sacculation obstructing labor **[654.4#]**
654.4# Uterus prolapse
660.2# Uterus prolapse obstructing labor **[654.4#]**
654.3# Uterus retroverted (incarcerated)
660.2# Uterus retroverted (incarcerated) obstructing labor **[654.3#]**
654.7# Vagina abnormality
660.2# Vagina abnormality obstructing labor **[654.7#]**
654.7# Vaginal prolapse
660.2# Vaginal prolapse obstructing labor **[654.7#]**
654.7# Vaginal stenosis
660.2# Vaginal stenosis obstructing labor **[654.7#]**
654.7# Vaginal tumor
660.2# Vaginal tumor obstructing labor **[654.7#]**
654.8# Vulva abnormality
660.2# Vulva abnormality obstructing labor **[654.8#]**
654.8# Vulva tumor
660.2# Vulva tumor obstructing labor **[654.8#]**
671.1# Vulva varicose veins
660.2# Vulva varicose veins obstructing labor **[671.1#]**

5th digit: 654.0-1, 3-5, 7-8, 671.1
- **0. Episode of care unspecified or N/A**
- **1. Delivered**
- **2. Delivered with postpartum complication**
- **3. Antepartum complication**
- **4. Postpartum complication**

5th digit: 660.2, 654.2
- **0. Episode of care unspecified or N/A**
- **1. Delivered**
- **3. Antepartum complication**

P

PREGNANCY COMPLICATIONS
DELIVERY PROBLEMS:
MALPRESENTATION/MALPOSITION

652.2# Breech delivery
660.0# Breech delivery obstructing labor [652.2#]
652.1# Breech or malpresentation converted to cephalic
660.0# Breech or malpresentation converted to cephalic obstructing labor [652.1#]
652.2# Breech presentation without version
660.0# Breech presentation obstructing labor [652.2#]
652.6# Breech presentation with multiple gestation
660.0# Breech presentation with multiple gestation obstructing labor [652.6#]
652.4# Brow presentation
660.0# Brow presentation obstructing labor [652.4#]
652.2# Buttocks presentation
660.0# Buttocks presentation obstructing labor [652.2#]
652.1# Cephalic version
660.0# Cephalic version obstructing labor [652.1#]
652.4# Chin presentation
660.0# Chin presentation obstructing labor [652.4#]
652.2# Complete breech presentation
660.0# Complete breech presentation obstructing labor [652.2#]
652.8# Compound presentation
660.0# Compound presentation obstructing labor [652.8#]
652.6# Compound presentation with multiple gestation
660.0# Compound presentation with multiple gestation obstructing labor [652.6#]
652.4# Extended head presentation
660.0# Extended head presentation obstructing labor [652.4#]
652.4# Face presentation
660.0# Face presentation obstructing labor [652.4#]
652.8# Face to pubes presentation
660.0# Face to pubes presentation obstructing labor [652.8#]
652.8# Footling presentation
660.0# Footling presentation obstructing labor [652.8#]
652.2# Frank breech presentation
660.0# Frank breech presentation obstructing labor [652.2#]
652.5# High head at term
652.8# Incomplete breech presentation
660.0# Incomplete breech presentation obstructing labor [652.8#]
652.6# Locked twins
660.0# Locked twins obstructing labor [652.6#]
652.9# Malpresentation NOS
660.0# Malpresentation NOS obstructing labor [652.9#]
652.3# Oblique lie
660.0# Oblique lie obstructing labor [652.3#]
652.7# Prolapse arm
660.0# Prolapse arm obstructing labor [652.7#]
652.8# Prolapse foot
660.0# Prolapse foot obstructing labor [652.8#]
652.8# Prolapse leg
660.0# Prolapse leg obstructing labor [652.8#]
660.3# Transverse arrest and persistent occipitoposterior position
652.3# Transverse lie
660.0# Transverse lie obstructing labor [652.3#]

5th digit: 652.0-9, 660.0, 3
0. Episode of care unspecified or N/A
1. Delivered
3. Antepartum complication

PREGNANCY COMPLICATIONS
DELIVERY PROBLEMS:
MALPRESENTATION/MALPOSITION (continued)

652.0# Unstable lie
660.0# Unstable lie obstructing labor [652.0#]

5th digit: 652.0, 660.0
0. Episode of care unspecified or N/A
1. Delivered
3. Antepartum complication

PREGNANCY COMPLICATIONS
DISPROPORTION

653.4# Cephalopelvic disproportion
660.1# Cephalopelvic disproportion obstructing labor [653.4#]
653.9# Disproportion NOS
660.1# Disproportion NOS obstructing labor [653.9#]
653.7# Conjoined twins
660.1# Conjoined twins obstructing labor [653.7#]
653.7# Fetal ascites
660.1# Fetal ascites obstructing labor [653.7#]
653.7# Fetal hydrops
660.1# Fetal hydrops obstructing labor [653.7#]
656.6# Fetal "large for dates" affecting management of mother
653.5# Fetal "large for dates" causing disproportion
660.1# Fetal "large for dates" (exceptionally large) obstructing labor [653.5#]
653.7# Fetal myelomeningocele
660.1# Fetal myelomeningocele obstructing labor [653.7#]
653.7# Fetal sacral teratoma
660.1# Fetal sacral teratoma obstructing labor [653.7#]
653.7# Fetal tumor
660.1# Fetal tumor obstructing labor [653.7#]
653.4# Fetopelvic disproportion
660.1# Fetopelvic disproportion obstructing labor [653.4#]
653.7# Fetus abnormality (other)
660.1# Fetus abnormality (other) obstructing labor [653.7#]
655.0# Fetus hydrocephalic (known/suspected) affecting management of mother
653.6# Fetus hydrocephalic causing disproportion
660.1# Fetus hydrocephalic obstructing labor [653.6#]
653.2# Inlet contraction (pelvis)
660.1# Inlet contraction (pelvis) obstructing labor [653.2#]
653.3# Outlet contraction pelvis
660.1# Outlet contraction pelvis obstructing labor [653.3#]
653.0# Pelvic deformity NOS
660.1# Pelvic deformity NOS obstructing labor [653.0#]
653.1# Pelvis contracted
660.1# Pelvis contracted obstructing labor [653.1#]
653.8# Shoulder dystocia, causing disproportion
660.1# Shoulder dystocia, causing disproportion obstructing labor [653.8#]
660.4# Shoulder girdle dystocia obstructing labor
653.8# Other disproportion
660.1# Other disproportion obstructing labor [653.8#]

5th digit: 653.0-9, 655.0, 656.6, 660.1, 660.4
0. Episode of care unspecified or N/A
1. Delivered
3. Antepartum complication

P

PREGNANCY COMPLICATIONS
LABOR PROBLEMS

669.9# Complication NOS
5th digit: 669.9
0. Episode of care unspecified or N/A
1. Delivered
2. Delivered with postpartum complication
3. Antepartum complication
4. Postpartum complication

659.3# Bacteremia during labor
660.6# Failed trial
5th digit: 659.3, 660.6
0. Episode of care unspecified or N/A
1. Delivered
3. Antepartum complication

644.1# False > 37 weeks
644.0# False> 22 and < 37 weeks
5th digit: 644.0-1
0. Episode of care unspecified or N/A
3. Antepartum complication

When coding other obstructed labor (660.8#), use an additional code to identify the specific condition.

660.8# Obstructed by other causes
661.3# Precipitate
5th digit: 661.3, 660.8
0. Episode of care unspecified or N/A
1. Delivered
3. Antepartum complication

644.2# Premature with onset of delivery < 37 weeks
5th digit: 644.2
0. Episode of care unspecified or N/A
1. Delivered

644.0# Premature without delivery > 22 and < 37 weeks
5th digit: 644.0
0. Episode of care unspecified or N/A
3. Antepartum complication

662.1# Prolonged
662.0# Prolonged first stage
662.2# Prolonged second stage
659.2# Pyrexia or fever during labor
5th digit: 659.2, 662.0-2
0. Episode of care unspecified or N/A
1. Delivered
3. Antepartum complication

669.1# Shock during labor and delivery
5th digit: 669.1
0. Episode of care unspecified or N/A
1. Delivered
2. Delivered with postpartum complication
3. Antepartum complication
4. Postpartum complication

644.1# Threatened > 37 weeks
644.0# Threatened > 22 and < 37 weeks
5th digit: 644.0-1
0. Episode of care unspecified or N/A
3. Antepartum complication

PREGNANCY COMPLICATIONS
LABOR PROBLEMS (continued)

663.0# Umbilical cord prolapse
665.0# Uterus rupture before onset of labor
5th digit: 665.0, 663.0
0. Episode of care unspecified or N/A
1. Delivered
3. Antepartum complication

665.1# Uterus rupture unspecified
665.1# Uterus rupture during labor
5th digit: 665.1
0. Episode of care unspecified or N/A
1. Delivered

669.8# Complication other
5th digit: 669.8
0. Episode of care unspecified or N/A
1. Delivered
2. Delivered with postpartum complication
3. Antepartum complication
4. Postpartum complication

PREGNANCY COMPLICATIONS
MATERNAL CONDITIONS

When coding a maternal condition using a code listed below in the categories of 646.##, 647.## or 648.##, use an additional code to identify the specific condition.

646.9# Unspecified

Elderly multigravida: Second or more pregnancy in a woman who will be 35 years of age or older at expected date of delivery.

659.6# Age advanced - elderly multigravida

Elderly primigravida: First pregnancy in a woman who will be 35 years of age or older at expected date of delivery.

659.5# Age advanced - elderly primigravida

Young maternal age: Pregnancy in female who is less than 16 years old at expected date of delivery.

659.8# Age young maternal complicating labor and delivery
5th digit: 646.9, 659.5-6, 8
0. Episode of care unspecified or N/A
1. Delivered
3. Antepartum complication

647.6# AIDS current (co-existent) [042]
648.2# Anemia current (co-existent)
648.9# Appendditis
647.8# Bacteremia current (co-existent)
646.5# Bacteriuria asymptomatic
649.2# Bariatric surgery for obesity status
646.8# Biliary problems
654.4# Bladder dilatation
648.7# Bone and joint disorder back pelvis and lower limbs current (co-existent)
5th digit: 646.5, 8, 647.6, 8, 648.2, 7, 9, 649.2, 654.4
0. Episode of care NOS or N/A
1. Delivered
2. Delivered with postpartum complication
3. Antepartum complication
4. Postpartum complication

P

PREGNANCY COMPLICATIONS

MATERNAL CONDITIONS (continued)

674.5# Cardiomyopathy peripartum/postpartum
648.6# Cardiovascular disease other specified current (co-existent)
648.5# Cardiovascular disorder congenital current (co-existent)
641.3# Coagulation defect causing antepartum hemorrhage

> ***649.3#: Use an additional code to identify the specific coagulation defect.***

649.3# Coagulation defect not associated with antepartum hemorrhage
648.0# Diabetes current (co-existent)
648.8# Diabetes gestational
669.0# Distress (L&D)

5th digit: 647.5 648.0, 6, 8, 669.0, 674.5
- **0. Episode of care NOS or N/A**
- **1. Delivered**
- **2. Delivered with postpartum complication**
- **3. Antepartum complication**
- **4. Postpartum complication**

648.3# Drug dependence current (co-existent)
0 Eclampsia see 'Eclampsia'
646.1# Edema without mention of hypertension

5th digit: 646.1, 648.3
- **0. Episode of care NOS or N/A**
- **1. Delivered**
- **2. Delivered with postpartum complication**
- **3. Antepartum complication**
- **4. Postpartum complication**

670.0# Endometritis

5th digit: 670
- **0. Episode of care NOS or N/A**
- **2. Delivered with postpartum complication**
- **4. Postpartum complication**

> ***649.4#: Use an additional code to identify the specific type of epilepsy.***

649.4# Epilepsy
649.2# Gastric banding or bypass surgery for obesity status
648.9# Genital mutilation status

> ***Use an additional code, if applicable, for associated insulin use (V58.67), when using code 648.8#.***

648.8# Glucose test abnormal (fasting) (non fasting) (tolerance test)
647.1# Gonorrhea current (co-existent)

5th digit: 646.1, 647.1, 648.3, 8-9, 649.2, 4
- **0. Episode of care NOS or N/A**
- **1. Delivered**
- **2. Delivered with postpartum complication**
- **3. Antepartum complication**
- **4. Postpartum complication**

PREGNANCY COMPLICATIONS

MATERNAL CONDITIONS (continued)

641.9# Hemorrhage antepartum NOS
640.9# Hemorrhage antepartum < 22 weeks
641.3# Hemorrhage antepartum associated with coagulation defects
641.8# Hemorrhage antepartum other

5th digit: 640.9, 641.3, 8-9
- **0. Episode of care NOS or N/A**
- **1. Delivered**
- **3. Antepartum complication**

648.9# Hemorrhoids current (co-existent)
671.8# Hemorrhoids due to pregnancy

5th digit: 648.9, 671.8
- **0. Episode of care unspecified or N/A**
- **1. Delivered**
- **2. Delivered with postpartum complication**
- **3. Antepartum complication**
- **4. Postpartum complication**

646.7# Hepatitis

5th digit: 646.7
- **0. Episode of care unspecified or N/A**
- **1. Delivered**
- **3. Antepartum complication**

647.6# Hepatitis viral current (co-existent)
647.6# HIV asymptomatic current (co-existent) [V08]
647.6# HIV symptomatic current (co-existent) [042]
0 Hypertension see 'Hypertension Complicating Pregnancy'
648.0# Hypoglycemic reaction diabetic (dietary) current (co-existent) [251.2]
648.8# Hypoglycemic reaction gestational diabetes (dietary) [251.2]
669.2# Hypotension syndrome

5th digit: 647.6, 648.0, 8, 669.2
- **0. Episode of care unspecified or N/A**
- **1. Delivered**
- **2. Delivered with postpartum complication**
- **3. Antepartum complication**
- **4. Postpartum complication**

> ***When coding a maternal condition using a code listed below in the categories of 646.##, 647.## or 648.##, use an additional code to identify the specific condition.***

646.6# Infection genitourinary
647.9# Infection or infestation condition or diseases - NOS current (co-existent)
647.8# Infection or infestation condition or diseases - other specified current (co-existent)

5th digit: 646.6, 647.8-9
- **0. Episode of care unspecified or N/A**
- **1. Delivered**
- **2. Delivered with postpartum complication**
- **3. Antepartum complication**
- **4. Postpartum complication**

P

PREGNANCY COMPLICATIONS MATERNAL CONDITIONS (continued)

670.0# Infection major puerperal, endometritis due to pregnancy
670.0# Infection major puerperal, pelvic cellulitis due to pregnancy
670.0# Infection major puerperal, pelvic sepsis due to pregnancy
670.0# Infection major puerperal, peritonitis due to pregnancy
670.0# Infection major puerperal, pyemia due to pregnancy
670.0# Infection major puerperal, salpingitis due to pregnancy
5th digit: 670.0
0. Episode of care unspecified or N/A
2. Delivered with postpartum complication
4. Postpartum complication

647.6# Infection viral current (co-existent)
648.9# Injury-trauma non-obstetrical current (co-existent)
5th digit: 647.6, 648.9
0. Episode of care unspecified or N/A
1. Delivered
2. Delivered with postpartum complication
3. Antepartum complication
4. Postpartum complication

646.7# Liver disorder
5th digit: 646.7
0. Episode of care unspecified or N/A
1. Delivered
3. Antepartum complication

648.9# Lymphatic disorder current (co-existent)
646.1# Maternal obesity syndrome
648.4# Mental disorder current (co-existent)
5th digit: 646.1, 648.4, 9
0. Episode of care unspecified or N/A
1. Delivered
2. Delivered with postpartum complication
3. Antepartum complication
4. Postpartum complication

Elderly multigravida: Second or more pregnancy in a woman who will be 35 years of age or older at expected date of delivery.

659.6# Multigravida elderly
5th digit: 659.6
0. Episode of care unspecified or N/A
1. Delivered
3. Antepartum complication

646.4# Neuritis peripheral
648.9# Nutritional deficiencies current (co-existent)
649.1# Obesity metabolic [278.00]
649.1# Obesity morbid [278.01]
649.2# Obesity surgery status
647.9# Parasitic diseases - NOS current (co-existent)
647.8# Parasitic diseases - other specified current (co-existent)
648.9# Pelvic peritoneal adhesions
648.9# Periodontal disease
648.9# Phlebitis (any type) current (co-existent)
5th digit: 646.1, 4, 647.8, 9, 648.9
0. Episode of care NOS or N/A
1. Delivered
2. Delivered with postpartum complication
3. Antepartum complication
4. Postpartum complication

671.3# Phlebitis deep (vein) due to pregnancy
5th digit: 671.3
0. Episode of care NOS or N/A
1. Delivered
3. Antepartum complication

671.9# Phlebitis due to pregnancy
671.2# Phlebitis superficial (vein) due to pregnancy
671.5# Phlebitis other due to pregnancy
648.9# Phlebothrombosis current (co-existent)
5th digit: 648.9, 671.2, 5, 9
0. Episode of care unspecified or N/A
1. Delivered
2. Delivered with postpartum complication
3. Antepartum complication
4. Postpartum complication

671.3# Phlebothrombosis deep-vein antepartum due to pregnancy
5th digit: 671.3
0. Episode of care NOS or N/A
1. Delivered
3. Antepartum complication

671.4# Phlebothrombosis deep-vein postpartum due to pregnancy
674.8# Postpartum complication - other specified
674.9# Postpartum complication - unspecified
5th digit: 671.4, 674.8-9
0. Unspecified
2. Delivered, with postpartum complication
4. Postpartum condition or complication

When coding a maternal condition using a code listed below in the categories of 646.##, 647.## or 648.##, use an additional code to identify the specific condition.

642.4# Pre-eclampsia (NOS) (mild)
642.5# Pre-eclampsia severe
642.7# Pre-eclampsia with pre-existing hypertension
5th digit: 642.4-5, 7
0. Episode of care unspecified or N/A
1. Delivered
2. Delivered with postpartum complication
3. Antepartum complication
4. Postpartum complication

Elderly primigravida: First pregnancy in a woman who will be 35 years of age or older at expected date of delivery.

659.5# Primigravida elderly
5th digit: 659.5
0. Episode of care unspecified or N/A
1. Delivered
3. Antepartum complication

646.8# Pruritus (PUPP)
5th digit: 646.8
0. Episode of care unspecified or N/A
1. Delivered
2. Delivered with postpartum complication
3. Antepartum complication
4. Postpartum complication

PREGNANCY COMPLICATIONS
MATERNAL CONDITIONS (continued)

659.2# Pyrexia or fever during labor
5th digit: 659.2
0. Episode of care unspecified or N/A
1. Delivered
3. Antepartum complication

646.2# Renal disease without mention of hypertension
647.5# Rubella current (co-existent)
649.0# Smoking complicating pregnancy
5th digit: 646.2, 647.5, 649.0
0. Episode of care unspecified or N/A
1. Delivered
2. Delivered with postpartum complication
3. Antepartum complication
4. Postpartum complication

649.5# Spotting complicating pregnancy
5th digit: 649.5
0. Episode of care unspecified or N/A
1. Delivered
3. Antepartum complication

> ***When coding a maternal condition using a code listed below in the categories of 646.##, 647.## or 648.##, use an additional code to identify the specific condition.***

647.0# Syphilis current (co-existent)
649.0# Tobacco use disorder complicating pregnancy
648.9# Thrombosis (any type) current (co-existent)
671.3# Thrombosis deep (vein) due to pregnancy
671.9# Thrombosis due to pregnancy
671.2# Thrombosis superficial (vein) due to pregnancy
671.5# Thrombosis other due to pregnancy
648.1# Thyroid dysfunction current (co-existent)
647.3# Tuberculosis current (co-existent)
646.2# Uremia
646.8# Uterine irritability complicating pregnancy
649.6# Uterine size - date discrepancy complicating pregnancy
648.9# Varicose veins any site current (co-existent)
671.0# Varicose veins due to pregnancy
671.1# Varicose veins vulva and perineum due to pregnancy
648.9# Vascular disorder current (co-existent)
647.6# Viral disease current (co-existent)
646.1# Weight gain excessive
648.9# Other current (co-existent) condition (disease)
646.8# Other specified complication arising during pregnancy
647.8# Other specified infectious and parasitic disease current (co-existent)
647.2# Other specified venereal disease current (co-existent)
647.6# Other specified viral disease current (co-existent)
5th digit: 646.1, 2, 8, 647.0, 2, 3, 6, 8, 648.1, 9, 649.0, 6, 671.0, 2, 3, 5, 9
0. Episode of care unspecified or N/A
1. Delivered
2. Delivered with postpartum complication
3. Antepartum complication
4. Postpartum complication

PREGNANCY COMPLICATIONS
MATERNAL DISORDERS AFFECTING FETUS OR NEWBORN

> ***In order to use the following codes, the medical record must specify that the maternal condition is a cause of morbidity or mortality in the fetus or newborn. The fact that the condition existed in the mother or complicated the pregnancy does not warrant the use of these codes on the newborn's record. Remember, codes 760-763 apply only to the infant and are never assigned to the mother's record. Conversely, never code the mother's condition with these fetal/newborn codes.***

762.9 Unspecified abnormalities of chorion and amnion
761.9 Unspecified complications - due to current pregnancy
760.9 Unspecified conditions - unrelated to current pregnancy
762.6 Unspecified conditions of umbilical cord
763.9 Unspecified disorder - due to labor and delivery
761.4 Abdominal pregnancy
763.1 Abnormality bony
763.89 Abnormality soft tissues
761.8 Abortion spontaneous
762.1 Abruptio placentae
760.79 Adrenogenital iatrogenic syndrome affecting fetus or newborn
760.71 Alcohol transmitted via placenta or breast milk
762.1 Amniocentesis damage to placenta
762.8 Amnion adhesion to fetus
762.7 Amnionitis
763.5 Analgesics administered during labor and delivery
763.5 Anesthetics administered during labor and delivery
760.74 Antibiotics (anti-infectives) transmitted via placenta or breast milk
760.1 Bacteriuria
763.1 Bladder dilatation
762.1 Blood loss maternal
763.0 Breech delivery and extraction
761.7 Breech malpresentation before labor and delivery
760.8 Cervicitis
763.89 Cervix abnormality
761.0 Cervix incompetent
763.89 Cervix scar
763.1 Cervix scar obstructing labor
763.89 Cervix stenosis/stricture
763.1 Cervix stenosis/stricture obstructing labor
763.4 Cesarean delivery
763.89 Cesarean scar previous
762.1 Cesarean section damage (separation) (hemorrhage) to placenta
762.7 Chorioamnionitis
762.9 Chorion and amnion abnormality
762.8 Chorion and amnion abnormalities other specified
760.3 Circulatory disease maternal chronic
763.89 Cleidotomy fetal
760.75 Cocaine transmitted via placenta or breast milk
763.7 Contraction ring
760.75 Crack (cocaine) transmitted via placenta or breast milk
763.89 Cranioclasis, fetal
763.89 Craniotomy, fetal
763.89 Cystocele
763.1 Cystocele obstructing labor
761.6 Death (maternal)
763.89 Delayed birth or delivery NEC
763.89 Delayed birth or delivery second twin, triplet etc.
763.0 Delivery and extraction
763.6 Delivery rapid second stage

P

PREGNANCY COMPLICATIONS MATERNAL DISORDERS AFFECTING FETUS OR NEWBORN (continued)

In order to use the following codes, the medical record must specify that the maternal condition is a cause of morbidity or mortality in the fetus or newborn. The fact that the condition existed in the mother or complicated the pregnancy does not warrant the use of these codes on the newborn's record. Remember, codes 760-763 apply only to the infant and are never assigned to the mother's record. Conversely, never code the mother's condition with these fetal/newborn codes.

760.76	DES (diethylstilbestrol) transmitted via placenta or breast milk
763.89	Destructive operation or procedure on live fetus to facilitate delivery
775.0	Diabetes causing fetal hypoglycemia
760.76	Diethylstilbestrol (DES) transmitted via placenta or breast milk
763.5	Drug reaction maternal
760.70	Drugs transmitted via placenta or breast milk
761.4	Ectopic pregnancy
763.89	Endocervical os stenosis/stricture
763.1	Endocervical os stenosis/stricture obstructing labor
760.8	Endometritis
763.89	Exhaustion maternal
761.7	External version malpresentation before labor and delivery
763.89	Extraction fetal manual or with hook
762.3	Fetal blood loss due to placental transfusion [772.0]
763.89	Forced birth
763.2	Forceps delivery
760.73	Hallucinogenic transmitted via placenta or breast milk
762.1	Hemorrhage complicating pregnancy, antepartum
763.89	Hemorrhage due to coagulation defect
760.8	Hepatitis maternal
761.3	Hydramnios acute (chronic)
760.0	Hypertensive disorders maternal
760.79	Immune sera transmitted via placenta or breast milk
763.89	Induction of labor (medical)
760.8	Infection genital tract other localized maternal
760.2	Infection maternal not manifested in fetus or newborn
760.1	Infection urinary tract
760.2	Influenza
763.89	Injury due to obstetrical trauma
760.5	Injury maternal
761.4	Intraperitoneal pregnancy
760.1	Kidney necrosis
760.8	Liver necrosis
761.7	Malpresentation/malposition before labor
763.1	Malpresentation/malposition during labor
761.6	Maternal death
760.79	Medicinal agents NEC transmitted via placenta or breast milk
762.7	Membranitis
763.89	Multiparity
761.5	Multiple pregnancy
763.5	Narcosis due to drug (correctly administered)
763.5	Narcotic reaction (intoxication) maternal during L&D
760.72	Narcotic transmitted via placenta or breast milk
760.70	Noxious substance unspecified transmitted via placenta or breast milk
760.79	Noxious substance other specified transmitted via placenta or breast milk
760.4	Nutritional deficiency disorders maternal
761.7	Oblique lie before labor and delivery
761.2	Oligohydramnios
763.5	Opiate reaction (intoxication) maternal during L&D
763.89	Os uteri stricture
763.1	Os uteri stricture obstructing labor
763.89	Ovarian cyst
763.1	Ovarian cyst obstructing labor
763.1	Pelvis bony
763.1	Pelvis contracted
763.89	Pelvis cyst
763.1	Pelvis cyst obstructing labor
763.89	Pelvis deformity
760.8	Pelvis inflammatory disease
763.89	Pelvis organs or soft tissue abnormality
763.89	Pelvis organs surgery previous
763.1	Pelvis Robert's
763.89	Pendulous abdomen
761.4	Peritoneal pregnancy
763.1	Persistent occipitoposterior position
762.1	Placenta damage
762.2	Placenta infarction
762.0	Placenta previa
762.3	Placenta transfusion syndromes
762.7	Placentitis
762.3	Polycythemia neonatorum placental transfusion [776.4]
761.3	Polyhydramnios
766.22	Postmaturity (>42 completed weeks)
766.21	Post-term (>40 completed weeks to 42 completed weeks)
763.6	Precipitate delivery
760.0	Pre-eclampsia
761.1	Premature rupture of membranes
760.3	Respiratory disease maternal chronic
762.1	Rupture marginal sinus
760.8	Salpingitis
763.1	Shoulder dystocia
763.1	Shoulder presentation
763.1	Spondylolisthesis
763.1	Spondylolysis
760.6	Surgery maternal
762.1	Surgical induction with damage to placenta
760.70	Toxic substance NOS transmitted via placenta or breast milk
760.79	Toxic substance NEC transmitted via placenta or breast milk
763.5	Tranquilizer reaction (maternal)
761.7	Transverse lie before labor and delivery
763.1	Transverse lie-presentation during labor and delivery
761.5	Triplet pregnancy
761.4	Tubal pregnancy
761.5	Twin pregnancy
762.5	Umbilical cord entanglement (cord around neck, knot, torsion)
762.4	Umbilical cord prolapse (presentation)
762.6	Umbilical cord other and unspecified conditions
761.7	Unstable lie before labor and delivery
760.1	Urinary tract diseases maternal
763.89	Uterus abnormality
763.89	Uterus abscess (to abdominal wall)
763.89	Uterus adhesion
763.89	Uterus bicornis/double
763.89	Uterus body polyp (corpus) (mucous)

P

PREGNANCY COMPLICATIONS
MATERNAL DISORDERS AFFECTING FETUS OR NEWBORN (continued)

763.7 Uterus contractions abnormal
763.7 Uterus hypertonic/hypotonic
763.7 Uterus inertia-dysfunction
763.89 Uterus perforation with obstetrical trauma
763.1 Uterus prolapse
763.89 Uterus rupture
763.1 Uterus sacculation
763.89 Uterus shape abnormality
763.89 Uterus surgery previous
763.89 Uterus version
763.3 Vacuum extractor delivery
763.3 Vacuum rupture
763.89 Vagina abnormality
763.89 Vagina stenosis/stricture
763.1 Vagina stenosis/stricture obstructing labor
760.8 Vaginitis
763.89 Vulva abnormality
762.8 Other specified abnormalities of chorion and amnion
761.8 Other specified complications - due to current pregnancy
760.8 Other specified conditions - unrelated to current pregnancy
762.6 Other specified conditions of umbilical cord
763.89 Other specified disorder - due to labor and delivery

PREGNANCY SUPERVISION

V22.0 Normal - first
V22.1 Normal - other than first
V23.9 High risk
V23.2 High risk - abortion history
V23.49 High risk - difficult delivery history

> ***Elderly multigravida:** second or more pregnancy in a woman who will be 35 years of age or older at expected date of delivery.*

V23.82 High risk - elderly multigravida

> ***Elderly primigravida:** first pregnancy in a woman who will be 35 years of age or older at expected date of delivery.*

V23.81 High risk - elderly primigravida
V23.49 High risk - forceps delivery history
V23.3 High risk - grand multiparity
V23.49 High risk - hemmorhage antepartum history
V23.49 High risk - hemmorhage postpartum history
V23.1 High risk - hydatidiform mole history
V23.0 High risk - infertility history
V23.89 High risk - mental disorder history
V23.49 High risk - molar pregnancy history
V23.5 High risk - neonatal death history
V23.49 High risk - poor obstetrical history
V23.7 High risk - prenatal care poor or none
V23.41 High risk - pre-term delivery history
V23.41 High risk - pre-term labor history
V23.5 High risk - stillbirth history
V23.1 High risk - trophoblastic disease history
V23.1 High risk - vesicular mole history

PREGNANCY SUPERVISION (continued)

> ***Young multigravida:** Second or more pregnancy in a female who is less than 16 years old at expected date of delivery.*

V23.84 High risk - young multigravida

> ***Young primigravida:** First pregnancy in a female who is less than 16 years old at expected date of delivery.*

V23.83 High risk - young primigravida
V23.89 High risk - other specified

V22.2 PREGNANT STATE (INCIDENTAL FINDING)
411.1 PREINFARCTION ANGINA
411.1 PREINFARCTION SYNDROME
733.09 PREISER'S DISEASE (OSTEOPOROSIS)
238.75 PRELEUKEMIC SYNDROME
754.32 PRELUXATION OF HIP
524.04 PREMAXILLAR RETRUSION (DEVELOPMENTAL)

PREMATURE

427.61 Atrial contractions
427.60 Beats
756.0 Closure cranial sutures
644.2# Delivery <37 weeks
5th digit: 644.2
0. Episode of care unspecified or N/A
1. Delivered

302.75 Ejaculation (psychosexual)
704.3 Grey hair
0 Infant see 'Premature Infant'
427.60 Junctional contractions
644.0# Labor false >22 and <37 weeks
644.1# Labor false >37 weeks
644.0# Labor threatened >22 and <37 weeks
644.1# Labor threatened >37 weeks
5th digit: 644.0-1
0. Episode of care unspecified or N/A
3. Antepartum complication

644.2# Labor with delivery <37 weeks
5th digit: 644.2
0. Episode of care unspecified or N/A
1. Delivered

256.31 Menopause
256.31 Menopause with natural menopause [627.2]
761.1 Rupture of membranes - affecting fetus
V71.89 Rupture of membranes - evaluation, not found
658.1# Rupture of membranes obstetrical
5th digit: 658.1
0. Episode of care unspecified or N/A
1. Delivered
3. Antepartum complication

259.8 Senility syndrome
427.69 Ventricular contractions

P

> *765.##: Use an additional code if necessary, to further specify the condition of the premature infant.*

PREMATURE INFANT

765.10 Weight unspecified weeks gestation [765.2#]
765.14 1000-1249 grams weeks gestation [765.2#]
765.15 1250-1499 grams weeks gestation [765.2#]
765.16 1500-1749 grams weeks gestation [765.2#]
765.17 1750-1999 grams weeks gestation [765.2#]
765.18 2000-2499 grams weeks gestation [765.2#]
765.19 2500 grams and over weeks gestation [765.2#]

5th digit: 765.2
0. Unspecified
1. Less than 24 completed
2. 24 completed
3. 25 - 26 completed
4. 27 - 28 completed
5. 29 - 30 completed
6. 31 - 32 completed
7. 33 - 34 completed
8. 35 - 36 completed
9. 37 or more completed

PREMATURE INFANT EXTREME

765.00 Weight unspecified weeks gestation [765.2#]
765.01 Less than 500 grams weeks gestation [765.2#]
765.02 500-749 grams weeks gestation [765.2#]
765.03 750-999 grams weeks gestation [765.2#]

5th digit: 765.2
0. Unspecified
1. Less than 24 completed
2. 24 completed
3. 25 - 26 completed
4. 27 - 28 completed
5. 29 - 30 completed
6. 31 - 32 completed
7. 33 - 34 completed
8. 35 - 36 completed
9. 37 or more completed

627.0 PREMENOPAUSAL MENORRHAGIA
625.4 PREMENSTRUAL (TENSION) SYNDROME
625.4 PREMENSTRUAL DYSPHORIC DISORDER
625.4 PREMENSTRUAL TENSION

PRENATAL

V23.7 Care poor (insufficient) or none
V22.0 Care normal first
V22.1 Care normal other than first
520.6 Teeth

> *V72.#, Preoperative Examination identifies the type of exam done rather than the type of surgery to be performed. The preoperative examination codes should be listed first followed by the code for the condition necessitating the surgery.*

PREOPERATIVE (PRE-PROCEDURAL) EXAMINATION

V72.84 Unspecified or general
V72.81 Cardiovascular
V72.82 Respiratory
V72.83 Other specified

726.65 PREPATELLAR BURSITIS
959.14 PREPUCE INJURY
362.56 PRERETINAL FIBROSIS

388.01 PRESBYACUSIS
605 PREPUCE ADHERENT
348.39 PRES (POSTERIOR REVERSIBLE ENCEPHALOPATHY SYNDROME)
530.89 PRESBYESOPHAGUS
310.1 PRESBYOPHRENIA
367.4 PRESBYOPIA
V70.5 PRESCHOOL CHILDREN HEALTH EXAM
V68.1 PRESCRIPTION REPEAT ISSUE MEDS
0 PRESENTATION (ABNORMAL) SEE 'MALPOSITION/MALPRESENTATION'
756.11 PRESPONDYLOLISTHESIS (LUMBOSACRAL) CONGENITAL
786.59 PRESSURE CHEST

PRESSURE EQUALIZATION (PE) TUBE

996.69 Complication - infection or inflammation
996.59 Complication - malfunction
996.79 Complication - other
V53.09 Removal
V53.09 Replacement

781.99 PRESSURE INTRACRANIAL INCREASED
365.00 PRESSURE INTRAOCULAR INCREASED (GLAUCOMA SUSPECT)
780.2 PRESYNCOPE
100.89 PRETIBIAL FEVER
536.9 PRE ULCER SYNDROME
607.3 PRIAPISM
782.0 PRICKLING SENSATION SKIN
770.4 PRIMARY ATELECTASIS
334.2 PRIMARY CEREBELLAR DEGENERATION
335.24 PRIMARY LATERAL SCLEROSIS
661.0# PRIMARY UTERINE INERTIA

> *Elderly primigravida: First pregnancy in a woman who will be 35 years of age or older at expected date of delivery.*

659.5# PRIMIGRAVIDA ELDERLY

5th digit: 659.5, 661.0
0. Episode of care unspecified or N/A
1. Delivered
3. Antepartum complication

436 PRIND (PROLONGED REVERSIBLE ISCHEMIC NEUROLOGIC DEFICIT)
V12.54 PRIND (PROLONGED REVERSIBLE ISCHEMIC NEUROLOGICAL DEFICIT) HISTORY
759.5 PRINGLE'S DISEASE (TUBEROUS SCLEROSIS)
413.1 PRINZMETAL'S ANGINA
786.52 PRINZMETAL-MASSUMI ANTERIOR CHEST WALL SYNDROME
V70.5 PRISONER HEALTH EXAM
286.3 PROACCELERIN DEFICIENCY

PROBLEM WITH

V49.9 Condition influencing health status NOS

HEAD

V48.9 NOS
V48.0 Deficiency
V48.6 Disfigurement
V48.2 Mechanical and motor

PROBLEM WITH (continued)

HEAD (continued)

V48.4 Sensory
V48.8 Other

INTERNAL ORGANS

V47.9 NOS
V47.2 Cardiovascular (respiratory) exercise intolerance at rest
V47.0 Deficiency
V47.3 Digestive
V47.5 Genital
V47.1 Mechanical and motor
V47.4 Urinary NEC

LIFESTYLE

V69.9 NOS
V69.1 Diet and eating habits inappropriate
V69.3 Gambling and betting
V69.5 Insomnia of childhood
V69.0 Physical exercise (lack of)
V69.8 Self-damaging behavior
V69.2 Sexual behavior high risk
V69.4 Sleep, lack of
V69.8 Other

LIMB

V49.9 NOS
V49.0 Deficiency
V49.4 Disfigurement
V49.1 Mechanical
V49.2 Motor
V49.3 Sensory
V49.5 Other

MENTAL/BEHAVIORAL

V40.9 Behavioral
V40.3 Behavioral other specified
V40.1 Communication
V40.0 Learning
V40.9 Mental
V40.2 Mental other specified
V40.1 Speech

NECK

V48.9 NOS
V48.1 Deficiency
V48.7 Disfigurement
V48.3 Mechanical and motor
V48.5 Sensory
V48.8 Other

SOCIAL

V62.3 Academic
V62.4 Acculturation
V61.29 Adopted child
V61.3 Aged parents or in-laws
V61.49 Care of sick or handicapped family member
V61.29 Concerning adopted or foster child other
V62.3 Educational circumstances
V61.41 Family alcoholism
V61.9 Family circumstance unspecified
V61.8 Family members NEC
V61.29 Foster child
V61.6 Illegitimacy to family
V62.89 Intellectual function borderline

PROBLEM WITH (continued)

SOCIAL (continued)

V62.81 Interpersonal NEC
V62.5 Legal
V62.89 Life circumstance
V62.4 Maladjustment
V61.10 Marital
V61.5 Multiparity in family
V62.2 Occupational other circumstances or maladjustment
V61.20 Parent-child relationship
V61.10 Partner
V62.89 Phase of life
V62.9 Psychosocial
V62.81 Relational
V61.10 Relationship marital
V61.20 Relationship parent-child
V61.10 Relationship partner
V61.8 Relationship sibling
V62.6 Religious regarding medical care
V62.89 Religious other than medical care
V61.8 Sibling relational
V62.89 Spiritual
V62.0 Unemployment (as cause of)
V61.7 Unwanted pregnancy in family
V62.1 Work environment (adverse effects)

SPECIAL SENSES AND FUNCTION

V41.9 NOS
V41.3 Ear other specified
V41.1 Eye other specified
V41.2 Hearing
V41.6 Mastication
V41.7 Sexual function
V41.0 Sight
V41.5 Smell
V41.6 Swallowing
V41.5 Taste
V41.4 Voice (with production)
V41.8 Other specified

TRUNK

V48.9 NOS
V48.1 Deficiency
V48.7 Disfigurement
V48.3 Mechanical and motor
V48.5 Sensory
V48.8 Other

PROBLEM WITH (continued)

V49.89 Other specified condition influencing health status

PROCEDURE (SURGICAL) NOT DONE

V64.3 NEC
V64.43 Arthroscopic converted to open procedure
V64.1 Due to contraindication
V64.41 Laparoscopic converted to open procedure
V64.2 Patient decision
V64.6 Patient decision for reasons of conscience or religion
V64.42 Thoracoscopic converted to open procedure
V64.3 Other reasons NEC

569.1 PROCIDENTIA ANUS RECTUM (SPHINCTER)
537.89 PROCIDENTIA STOMACH
286.3 PROCONVERTIN DEFICIENCY CONGENITAL

V26.41 PROCREATIVE COUNSELING USING NATURAL FAMILY PLANNING
V26.49 PROCREATIVE COUNSELING NEC
V26.81 PROCREATIVE MANAGEMENT ENCOUNTER FOR ASSISTED REPRODUCTIVE FERTILITY PROCEDURE CYCLE
V26.89 PROCREATIVE MANAGEMENT SPECIFIED NEC

PROCTALGIA

569.42 NOS
564.6 Fugax
564.6 Spasmodic
564.6 Spasmodic psychogenic [307.80]

569.49 PROCTITIS
555.1 PROCTITIS GRANULOMATOUS
556.2 PROCTITIS ULCERATIVE (CHRONIC)

PROCTOCELE

618.#(#) Female
618.#(#) Female with stress incontinence [625.6]
618.#(#) Female with other urinary incontinence **[788.3#]**

4th or 4th and 5th digit: 618
04. Without uterine prolapse
2. With incomplete uterine prolapse
3. With complete uterine prolapse
4. Uterine prolapse unspecified

5th digit: 788.3
1. Urge incontinence
3. Mixed urge and stress
4. Without sensory awareness
5. Post-void dribbling
6. Nocturnal enuresis
7. Continuous leakage
8. Overflow incontinence
9. Other

556.2 PROCTOCOLITIS IDIOPATHIC
556.3 PROCTOSIGMOIDITIS ULCERATIVE
729.9 PROFICHET'S SYNDROME
259.8 PROGERIA (SYNDROME)
524.10 PROGNATHISM

PROGRESSIVE

335.22 Bulbar palsy
046.3 Multifocal leukoencephalopathy
335.21 Muscular atrophy
335.0 Muscular atrophy of infancy
333.2 Myoclonic epilepsy
333.0 Pallidal degeneration
709.09 Pigmentary dermatosis
288.1 Septic granulomatosis
333.0 Supranuclear ophthalmoplegia
333.0 Supranuclear palsy

PROLACTIN

253.4 Deficiency
253.1 Excess

PROLAPSE

569.1 Anal
756.71 Bladder congenital (mucosa) (female) (male)
0 Bladder female see 'Cystocele', female
596.8 Bladder male
569.69 Cecostomy

PROLAPSE (continued)

618.84 Cervical stump
618.84 Cervical stump with stress incontinence [625.6]
618.84 Cervical stump with other urinary incontinence **[788.3#]**

5th digit: 788.3
1. Urge incontinence
3. Mixed urge and stress
4. Without sensory awareness
5. Post-void dribbling
6. Nocturnal enuresis
7. Continuous leakage
8. Overflow incontinence
9. Other

569.69 Colostomy
372.73 Conjunctiva
537.89 Duodenal
569.69 Enterostomy
996.59 Eye implant (orbital)
537.89 Gastric (mucosa)
618.9 Genital female
618.9 Genital female with stress incontinence [625.6]
618.9 Genital female with other urinary incontinence **[788.3#]**

5th digit: 788.3
1. Urge incontinence
3. Mixed urge and stress
4. Without sensory awareness
5. Post-void dribbling
6. Nocturnal enuresis
7. Continuous leakage
8. Overflow incontinence
9. Other

618.8# Genital female other specified
618.8# Genital female other specified with stress incontinence [625.6]
618.8# Genital female other specified with other urinary incontinence **[788.3#]**

5th digit: 618.8
1. Pubocervical tissue incompetence (weakening)
2. Rectovaginal tissue incompetence (weakening)
3. Pelvic muscle wasting
4. Cervical stump prolapse
9. Other

5th digit: 788.3
1. Urge incontinence
3. Mixed urge and stress
4. Without sensory awareness
5. Post-void dribbling
6. Nocturnal enuresis
7. Continuous leakage
8. Overflow incontinence
9. Other

360.81 Globe
569.69 Ileostomy
569.89 Intestine
364.89 Iris
871.1 Iris traumatic (acute)
569.69 Jejunostomy
996.53 Lens implant (ocular)
424.0 Mitral valve
620.4 Ovary and fallopian tube

P

PROLAPSE (continued)

618.8# Pelvic floor female
618.8# Pelvic floor female with stress incontinence [625.6]
618.8# Pelvic floor female with other urinary incontinence [788.3#]
618.8# Perineum female
618.8# Perineum female with stress incontinence [625.6]
618.8# Perineum female with other urinary incontinence [788.3#]

5th digit: 618.8
1. Pubocervical tissue incompetence (weakening)
2. Rectovaginal tissue incompetence (weakening)
3. Pelvic muscle wasting
4. Cervical stump prolapse
9. Other

5th digit: 788.3
1. Urge incontinence
3. Mixed urge and stress
4. Without sensory awareness
5. Post-void dribbling
6. Nocturnal enuresis
7. Continuous leakage
8. Overflow incontinence
9. Other

569.1 Rectal
593.89 Ureter
599.5 Urethra
618.1 Uterus
618.4 Uterus and vagina
618.3 Uterus and vagina complete
618.2 Uterus and vagina incomplete
618.1 Uterus first degree
618.1 Uterus second degree
618.1 Uterus third degree
618.0# Vaginal (without uterine prolapse)
618.0# Vaginal (without uterine prolapse) with stress incontinence [625.6]
618.0# Vaginal (without uterine prolapse) with other urinary incontinence [788.3#]

5th digit: 618.0
0. Unspecified
1. Cystocele, midline
2. Cystocele, lateral (paravaginal)
3. Urethrocele
4. Rectocele (proctocele)
5. Perineocele
9. Other

5th digit: 788.3
1. Urge incontinence
3. Mixed urge and stress
4. Without sensory awareness
5. Post-void dribbling
6. Nocturnal enuresis
7. Continuous leakage
8. Overflow incontinence
9. Other

618.5 Vaginal after hysterectomy

PROLAPSE COMPLICATING PREGNANCY

652.7# Arm
660.0# Arm obstructing labor **[652.7#]**
652.6# Arm with multiple gestation
660.0# Arm with multiple gestation obstructing labor **[652.6#]**
762.4 Cord affecting fetus or newborn
652.8# Foot
660.0# Foot obstructing labor **[652.8#]**
652.8# Leg
660.0# Leg obstructing labor **[652.8#]**
663.0# Umbilical cord

5th digit: 652.6-8, 660.0, 663.0
0. Episode of care unspecified or N/A
1. Delivered
3. Antepartum complication

654.4# Uterus complicating pregnancy
660.2# Uterus obstructing labor **[654.4#]**
654.4# Vaginal (puerperal)
660.2# Vaginal (puerperal) obstructing labor **[654.4#]**

5th digit: 654.4
0. Episode of care unspecified or N/A
1. Delivered
2. Delivered with postpartum complication
3. Antepartum complication
4. Postpartum complication

5th digit: 660.2
0. Episode of care unspecified or N/A
1. Delivered
3. Antepartum complication

728.79 PROLIFERATIVE FIBROMATOSIS (SARCOMATOUS)
270.8 PROLINE METABOLISM DISORDERS
270.8 PROLINEMIA
270.8 PROLINURIA
766.21 PROLONGED GESTATION SYNDROME OVER 40 COMPLETED WEEKS TO 42 COMPLETED WEEKS
766.22 PROLONGED GESTATION SYNDROME OVER 42 COMPLETED WEEKS
645.2# PROLONGED PREGNANCY (> 42 COMPLETED WEEKS GESTATION)

5th digit: 645.2
0. Episode of care unspecified or N/A
1. Delivered
3. Antepartum complication

794.31 PROLONGED QT INTERVAL
426.82 PROLONGED QT INTERVAL SYNDROME
434.91 PROLONGED REVERSIBLE ISCHEMIC NEUROLOGICAL DEFICIT (PRIND)
V12.54 PROLONGED REVERSIBLE ISCHEMIC NEUROLOGICAL DEFICIT (PRIND) HISTORY
359.21 PROMM (PROXIMAL MYOTONIC MYOTONIA)
736.79 PRONATION ANKLE (FOOT)
755.67 PRONATION ANKLE FOOT CONGENITAL

PROPHYLACTIC

V07.39 Antibiotic administration
V07.2 Antivenin administration
V50.41 Breast removal
V50.41 Breast removal due to family history cancer breast [V16.3]

P

PROPHYLACTIC (continued)

V07.39 Chemotherapeutic agent administration NEC
V58.11 Chemotherapeutic agent maintenance following disease
V07.39 Drug administration
V07.31 Fluoride administration
V07.2 Gamma globulin administration
V07.4 Hormone replacement therapy (postmenopausal)
0 Immunization see 'Vaccination'
V07.0 Isolation
V07.9 Measure NOS
V07.8 Measure other specified
V07.39 Medication administration
V50.49 Organ removal other specified
V50.42 Ovary removal
V50.42 Ovary removal due to family history of ovarian cancer [V16.41]
V07.2 Rhogam administration
V07.2 Tetanus antitoxin administration
V07.8 Toxoxifen administration due to family history cancer breast [V16.3]
0 Vaccination or inoculation see 'Vaccination'

0 PROPIONIBACTERIUM SEE 'BACTERIAL INFECTION' OR SPECIFIED CONDITION
376.30 PROPTOSIS OCULAR
V62.5 PROSECUTION PROBLEM (REASON FOR ENCOUNTER)
079.81 PROSPECT HILL VIRUS

PROSTATE

601.2 Abscess
V45.77 Absence acquired
752.89 Absence congenital

See 'LUTS' or 'Lower Urinary Tract Symptoms' for the additional code to identify the specific lower urinary tract symptoms.

600.20 Adenofibromatous hypertrophy
600.21 Adenofibromatous hypertrophy with urinary obstruction, retention or other lower urinary tract symptoms
600.20 Adenomyoma
600.21 Adenomyoma with urinary obstruction, retention or other lower urinary tract symptoms
752.89 Anomaly
752.89 Aplasia congenital
602.2 Atrophy
600.20 Benign adenoma
600.21 Benign adenoma with obstruction, retention or other lower urinary tract symptoms
600.00 Benign hypertrophy
752.89 Benign hypertrophy congenital
600.01 Benign hypertrophy with obstruction, retention or other lower urinary tract symptoms
222.2 Benign neoplasm
222.2 Benign neoplasm with incontinence [788.3#]
602.0 Calculus
V76.44 Cancer screening
602.1 Congestion or hemorrhage
602.9 Disorder
602.8 Disorder specified type NEC
602.3 Dysplasia
600.00 Enlargement, simple (smooth) (soft)
600.01 Enlargement, simple (smooth) (soft) with obstruction, retention or other lower urinary tract symptoms

PROSTATE (continued)

600.20 Fibroadenoma, fibroma
600.21 Fibroadenoma, fibroma with obstruction, retention or other lower urinary tract symptoms
600.10 Hard, firm
600.11 Hard, firm with obstruction, retention or other lower urinary tract symptoms
600.90 Hyperplasia unspecified
600.91 Hyperplasia unspecified with obstruction, retention or other lower urinary tract symptoms
600.20 Hyperplasia benign
600.21 Hyperplasia benign with obstruction, retention or other lower urinary tract symptoms
600.90 Hypertrophy (NOS) (asymptomatic) (early) (recurrent)
600.91 Hypertrophy (NOS) (asymptomatic) (early) (recurrent) with obstruction, retention or other lower urinary tract symptoms
600.20 Hypertrophy adenofibromatous
600.21 Hypertrophy adenofibromatous with obstruction, retention or other lower urinary tract symptoms
602.8 Infarction
867.6 Injury
600.00 Hypertrophy benign
600.01 Hypertrophy benign with urinary obstruction, retention or other lower urinary tract symptoms
867.7 Injury with open wound into cavity
908.2 Injury late effect
602.3 Intraepithelial neoplasia I
602.3 Intraepithelial neoplasia II
233.4 Intraepithelial neoplasia III
600.90 Median bar
600.91 Median bar with urinary obstruction, retention or other lower urinary tract symptoms
600.10 Multinodular
600.11 Multinodular with urinary obstruction, retention or other lower urinary tract symptoms
600.20 Myoma
600.21 Myoma with urinary obstruction, retention or other lower urinary tract symptoms
600.10 Nodule (nodular)
600.11 Nodule (nodular) with urinary obstruction, retention or other lower urinary tract symptoms
600.90 Obstruction NOS
600.91 Obstruction NOS with urinary obstruction, retention or other lower urinary tract symptoms
600.20 Polyp
600.21 Polyp with urinary obstruction, retention or other lower urinary tract symptoms
790.93 PSA (prostatic specific antigen) elevated
V76.44 PSA (prostatic specific antigen) screening
790.93 Specific antigen (PSA) elevated
602.8 Stricture
016.5# Tuberculosis [608.81]

5th digit: 016.5
0. Unspecified
1. Lab not done
2. Lab pending
3. Microscopy positive (in sputum)
4. Culture positive - microscopy negative
5. Culture negative - microscopy positive
6. Culture and microscopy negative confirmed by other methods

596.0 Valve obstruction (prostatic) (urinary)
602.8 Other specified disorder NEC

P

See 'LUTS' or 'Lower Urinary Tract Symptoms' for the additional code to identify the specific lower urinary tract symptoms.

600.91 PROSTATISM WITH URINARY OBSTRUCTION, RETENTION OR OTHER LOWER URINARY TRACT SYMPTOMS

PROSTATITIS

601.9 NOS
601.0 Acute
039.8 Actinomycotic [601.4]
116.0 Blastomycotic [601.4]
601.8 Cavitary
099.54 Chlamydial
601.1 Chronic
601.8 Diverticular
600.90 Fibrous
600.91 Fibrous with urinary obstruction, retention or other lower urinary tract symptoms
098.12 Gonococcal acute
098.32 Gonococcal chronic
601.8 Granulomatous
600.00 Hypertrophic
600.01 Hypertrophic with urinary obstruction, retention or lower urinary tract symptoms
112.2 Monilial
095.8 Syphilitic [601.4]
131.03 Trichomonal

601.3 PROSTATOCYSTITIS

PROSTHESIS (FITTING AND ADJUSTMENT) (REMOVAL)

V52.9 NOS
V52.0 Arm
V52.4 Breast
V52.3 Dentures
V52.2 Eye
V52.1 Leg
V52.8 Other specified

PROSTHESIS (STATUS)

V43.5 Bladder
V43.82 Breast
V45.83 Breast removal
0 Complication see 'Complication'
V43.0 Eye globe
V43.1 Eye lens
V43.22 Heart artificial fully implantable
V43.21 Heart assist device
V43.3 Heart valve
V43.4 Heart vessel
V45.85 Insulin pump
V43.89 Intestine
V43.60 Joint
V54.81 Joint aftercare [V43.6#]

5th digit: V43.6
0. Site unspecified
1. Shoulder
2. Elbow
3. Wrist
4. Hip
5. Knee
6. Ankle
9. Other

PROSTHESIS (STATUS) (continued)

V43.66 Joint ankle
V43.62 Joint elbow
V43.69 Joint finger
V43.64 Joint hip
V43.65 Joint knee
V43.61 Joint shoulder
V43.63 Joint wrist
V43.69 Joint other
V43.89 Kidney
V43.81 Larynx
V43.7 Limb
V43.89 Liver
V43.89 Lung
V43.89 Organ other
V43.89 Pancreas
V43.83 Skin artificial
V43.89 Tissue other
V43.89 Other organ or tissue

V70.5 PROSTITUTES HEALTH EXAM

PROSTRATION

780.79 NOS
992.5 Heat
992.4 Heat - salt depletion
992.4 Heat - salt and water depletion
992.3 Heat - water depletion
300.5 Nervous
779.89 Newborn
797 Senile

368.51 PROTAN DEFECT
368.51 PROTANOMALY
368.51 PROTANOPIA
0 PROTECTION (AGAINST) (FROM) – SEE PROPHYLACTIC

PROTEIN

790.95 C reactive elevated (CRP)
289.81 C resistant
289.81 C deficiency
273.8 Plasma metabolism abnormality specified NEC
273.9 Plasma metabolism disorder
289.81 S deficiency
790.99 Serum abnormal findings NEC
273.8 Transport abnormality

790.99 PROTEINEMIA
272.8 PROTEINOSIS LIPID

PROTEINURIA

791.0 NOS
791.0 Bence-Jones
646.2# Maternal (gestational) complicating pregnancy without mention of hypertension

5th digit: 646.2
0. Episode of care unspecified or N/A
1. Delivered
2. Delivered with postpartum complication
3. Antepartum complication
4. Postpartum complication

593.6 Orthostatic
593.6 Postural benign

P

0 PROTEUS MIRABILIS MORGANII SEE 'BACTERIAL INFECTION' OR SPECIFIED CONDITION
757.39 PROTEUS SYNDROME (DERMAL HYPOPLASIA)
0 PROTEUS VULGARIS SEE 'BACTERIAL INFECTION' OR SPECIFIED CONDITION

PROTHROMBIN

286.3 Deficiency congenital
286.7 Deficiency due to liver disease
289.81 Gene mutation
286.7 Time increased due to liver disease
790.92 Time (prolonged)

790.92 PROTIME ABNORMAL
286.7 PROTIME TIME INCREASED DUE TO LIVER DISEASE
277.1 PROTOCOPROPORPHYRIA
277.1 PROTOPORPHYRIA
136.8 PROTOZOAL DISEASE OTHER SPECIFIED NEC
007.9 PROTOZOAL INTESTINAL DISEASE
007.8 PROTOZOAL INTESTINAL DISEASES OTHER SPECIFIED
701.5 PROUD FLESH
359.21 PROXIMAL MYOTONIC MYOTONIA (PROMM)
756.71 PRUNE BELLY SYNDROME

PRURIGO

698.2 NOS
691.8 Asthma syndrome
691.8 Besnier's (infantile eczema)
691.8 Eczematodes allergicum
692.72 Estivalis
698.2 Hebra's
692.72 Hutchinson's
698.2 Mitis
698.3 Nodularis
698.2 Prurigo
698.2 Simplex

PRURITUS

698.9 NOS
698.0 Ani
698.9 Ear
379.99 Eye
698.1 Genital organs
698.8 Hiemalis

646.8#: Specify the maternal pruritus with an additional code.

646.8# Maternal complicating pregnancy
5th digit: 646.8
0. Episode of care unspecified or N/A
1. Delivered
2. Delivered with postpartum complication
3. Antepartum complication
4. Postpartum complication

306.3 Psychogenic
698.1 Scrotum
306.3 Scrotum psychogenic
698.8 Senilis
698.8 Uremic
698.1 Vulva

790.93 PSA (PROSTATIC SPECIFIC ANTIGEN) ELEVATED ABNORMAL FINDINGS
V76.44 PSA (PROSTATIC SPECIFIC ANTIGEN) SCREENING
0 PSEUDOANEURYSM SEE 'ANEURYSM'
733.82 PSEUDARTHROSIS
V45.4 PSEUDARTHROSIS FOLLOWING FUSION (STATUS)
272.7 PSEUDO-HURLER'S (MUCOLIPIDOSIS III)
799.89 PSEUDOATAXIA
310.8 PSEUDOBULBAR AFFECT (PBA)
335.23 PSEUDOBULBAR PALSY
727.89 PSEUDOBURSA
701.8 PSEUDOCANTHOSIS NIGRICANS
354.0 PSEUDOCARPAL TUNNEL SYNDROME (SUBLIMIS)
289.89 PSEUDOCHOLINESTERASE DEFICIENCY (INSUFFICIENCY)
705.89 PSEUDOCHROMIDROSIS
051.1 PSEUDOCOWPOX
732.1 PSEUDOCOXALGIA
300.11 PSEUDOCYESIS
577.2 PSEUDOCYST PANCREAS
361.19 PSEUDOCYST RETINA
518.89 PSEUDOEMPHYSEMA
265.1 PSEUDOENCEPHALITIS SUPERIOR (ACUTE) HEMORRHAGIC
268.2 PSEUDOFRACTURE (IDIOPATHIC) (MULTIPLE) (SPONTANEOUS)(SYMMETRICAL)
025 PSEUDOGLANDERS
360.44 PSEUDOGLIOMA
0 PSEUDOGOUT SEE 'CHONDROCALCINOSIS'
780.1 PSEUDOHALLUCINATION
782.0 PSEUDOHEMIANESTHESIA

PSEUDOHEMOPHILIA

287.8 Hereditary capillary fragility
287.8 Type A
286.4 Type B
287.8 Vascular

PSEUDOHERMAPHRODITISM

255.2 Adrenal female
752.7 Congenital
255.2 Female (adrenocortical)
257.9 Male with gonadal disorder
259.5 Male with testicular feminization
256.4 Stein leventhal (polycystic ovary)
255.2 Virilism-hirsutism syndrome

348.2 PSEUDOHYDROCEPHALUS
275.49 PSEUDOHYPOPARATHYROIDISM
285.8 PSEUDOLEUKEMIA INFANTILE
101 PSEUDOMEMBRANOUS ANGINA
008.45 PSEUDOMEMBRANOUS COLITIS
777.5 PSEUDOMEMBRANOUS ENTEROCOLITIS IN NEWBORN
349.2 PSEUDOMENINGOCELE, ACQUIRED (SPINAL)
997.01 PSEUDOMENINGOCELE, ACQUIRED (SPINAL) POSTPROCEDURAL
626.8 PSEUDOMENSTRUATION

PSEUDOMONAS

008.42 Gastroenteritis
041.7 Infection
024 Infection mallei
025 Infection pseudomallei
038.43 Infection with septicemia

197.6 PSEUDOMYXOMA PERITONEI SITE NOS
0 PSEUDOMYXOMA PERITONEI SITE SPECIFIED SEE 'CANCER', BY SITE M8480/6
377.24 PSEUDONEURITIS (OPTIC NERVE) (PAPILLA)
564.89 PSEUDOOBSTRUCTION INTESTINE (CHRONIC) (IDIOPATHIC) (INTERMITTENT SECONDARY) (PRIMARY)
560.89 PSEUDOOBSTRUCTION INTESTINE ACUTE
377.24 PSEUDOPAPILLEDEMA
358.00 PSEUDOPARALYTICA SYNDROME
358.01 PSEUDOPARALYTICA SYNDROME WITH (ACUTE) EXACERBATION (CRISIS)
704.09 PSEUDOPELADE
V43.1 PSEUDOPHAKIA
556.4 PSEUDOPOLYPOSIS COLON
348.0 PSEUDOPORENCEPHALY
275.49 PSEUDOPSEUDOHYPOPARATHYROIDISM
372.52 PSEUDOPTERYGIUM
374.34 PSEUDOPTOSIS
362.65 PSEUDORETINITIS PIGMENTOSA
057.8 PSEUDORUBELLA

PSEUDOSARCOMATOUS

199.1 Carcinoma site NOS
0 Carcinoma site specified see 'Cancer', by site M8033/3
728.79 Fibromatosis (proliferative) (subcutaneous)

057.8 PSEUDOSCARLATINA
046.1 PSEUDOSCLEROSIS (JAKOB'S) (SPASTIC) BRAIN
046.1 PSEUDOSCLEROSIS SPASTIC (JAKOB'S) (SPASTIC) BRAIN WITH DEMENTIA [**294.1#**]

5th digit: 294.1
0. Without behavioral disturbance or NOS
1. With behavioral disturbance

780.39 PSEUDOSEIZURE
300.11 PSEUDOSEIZURE PSYCHOGENIC
799.89 PSEUDOTABES
780.39 PSEUDOTETANUS (SEE ALSO 'CONVULSIONS')
348.2 PSEUDOTUMOR CEREBRI
376.11 PSEUDOTUMOR ORBIT (INFLAMMATORY)
759.89 PSEUDO-TURNER'S SYNDROME
305.3# PSILOCYBIN ABUSE (NONDEPENDENT)
304.5# PSILOCYBIN ADDICTION (DEPENDENT)

5th digit: 304.5, 305.3
0. Unspecified
1. Continuous
2. Episodic
3. In remission

073.9 PSITTACOSIS
726.5 PSOAS TENDINITIS

PSORIASIS

696.1 NOS
696.0 Arthritic
696.0 Arthropathic
528.6 Buccal
696.1 Flexural
696.1 Follicular
528.6 Mouth
691.0 Napkin eruption
696.1 Pustulosa continua
316 Psychogenic [696.1]
696.1 Vulgaris
696.8 Other specified

136.4 PSOROSPERMIASIS
427.0 PSVT (PAROXYSMAL SUPRAVENTRICULAR TACHYCARDIA)
300.89 PSYCHASTHENIA
300.89 PSYCHASTHENIC NEUROSIS
V70.1 PSYCHIATRIC EXAM GENERAL REQUESTED BY AUTHORITY
V70.2 PSYCHIATRIC EXAM GENERAL OTHER AND UNSPECIFIED

PSYCHOGENIC

316 Cause of (or associated with) other organic disease
300.9 Disorder (neurotic) NEC

In order to code psychogenic pain or pain exclusively attributed to psychological factors, code first the site of the physical pain and use an additional code (307.80) to identify the psychogenic pain.

307.80 Pain disorder related to psychological factor unspecified site
307.89 Pain disorder related to psychological factor other
307.80 Pain site unspecified
316 Pielinosis
306.7 Special sense organs disorder
0 See specified condition psychogenic

301.59 PSYCHOINFANTILE PERSONALITY
V15.4# PSYCHOLOGICAL TRAUMA HISTORY

5th digit: V15.4
1. Physical abuse, rape
2. Emotional abuse, neglect
9. Other

300.11 PSYCHOMOTOR DISORDER NEC - HYSTERICAL
307.9 PSYCHOMOTOR DISORDER NEC - PSYCHOGENIC
300.9 PSYCHONEUROSIS
301.89 PSYCHONEUROTIC PERSONALITY DISORDER

PSYCHO-ORGANIC SYNDROME

293.9 NOS
293.0 Acute
293.84 Anxiety type
293.83 Depressive type
293.82 Hallucinatory type
310.1 Nonpsychotic severity
310.8 Nonpsychotic severity, specified focal (partial)
293.81 Paranoid type
293.1 Subacute
293.89 Other specified

P

301.9 PSYCHOPATHIC PERSONALITY DISORDER

306.9 PSYCHOPHYSIOLOGIC DISORDER

PSYCHOSEXUAL DYSFUNCTION

302.70 NOS
302.76 Dyspareunia psychogenic
302.72 Female arousal disorder
302.73 Female orgasmic disorder
302.72 Frigidity
302.71 Hypoactive sexual desire disorder
302.6 Identity disorder NOS
302.85 Identity disorder adolescent
302.85 Identity disorder adult
302.6 Identity disorder childhood
302.72 Impotence
302.72 Male erectile disorder
302.74 Male orgasmic disorder
302.75 Premature ejaculation
302.79 Sexual aversion disorder
306.51 Vaginismus
302.72 With inhibited sexual excitement
302.79 Other specified

PSYCHOSIS

298.9 NOS
296.90 Affective see also 'Mood Disorder'
295.4# Confusional type

5th digit: 295.4

0. NOS
1. Subchronic
2. Chronic
3. Subchronic with acute exacerbation
4. Chronic with acute
5. In remission

298.9 Disorder NOS
298.8 Disorder brief
296.90 Melancholic

Psychosis alcoholic, 291.#(#), requires two codes. Code the psychosis first with an additional code for the dependence/non dependence. See 'Alcohol Abuse', (dependent) (non dependent).

PSYCHOSIS ALCOHOLIC

291.9 NOS
291.0 Acute with delirium
291.3 Acute with hallucination
291.1 Amnestic persisting disorder
291.0 Delirium (tremens)
291.5 Delusions
291.2 Dementia persisting
291.3 Hallucinosis
291.4 Intoxication pathologic (idiosyncratic)
291.5 Jealousy
291.1 Korsakoff's
291.2 Organic brain syndrome
291.5 Paranoid
291.1 Polyneuritic
291.5 Polyneuritic with delusions
291.3 Polyneuritic with hallucinations
291.1 With amnestic persisting disorder
291.89 With anxiety disorder
291.89 With mood disorder or disturbance
291.82 With sleep disorder or disturbance
291.0 Withdrawal delirium
291.3 Withdrawal hallucinosis
291.81 Withdrawal syndrome

PSYCHOSIS ARTERIOSCLEROTIC

290.40 NOS [437.0]
290.41 Acute [437.0]
290.42 Paranoid or delusional [437.0]
290.40 Uncomplicated [437.0]
290.41 With confusional state [437.0]
290.41 With delirium [437.0]
290.42 With delusion [437.0]
290.43 With depressed mood [437.0]
290.43 With depression [437.0]

PSYCHOSIS CHILDHOOD

299.9# NOS
299.8# Atypical
299.0# Autistic
299.8# Borderline
299.1# Disintegrative
299.0# Infantile
299.8# Other specified

5th digit: 299.0-9

0. Current or active state
1. Residual state

PSYCHOSIS DRUG INDUCED

292.9 NOS
292.11 Delusional
292.12 Hallucinatory
292.2 Pathological drug intoxication (brief)
292.83 With amnestic persisting disorder
292.89 With anxiety
292.81 With delerium
292.11 With delusions
292.82 With dementia persisting
292.12 With hallucination
292.84 With mood disorder
292.85 With sleep disorder or disturbance
292.0 Withdrawl
292.89 Other

PSYCHOSIS NON ORGANIC (STRESS INDUCED)

298.9 NOS
298.9 Atypical
298.8 Brief reactive
297.1 Delusional disorder
298.0 Depressive type
298.9 Disorder NOS
298.8 Disorder brief
298.1 Excitative type
298.1 Hysterical (acute)
298.8 Hysterical brief reactive
298.8 Incipient
298.8 Involutional
298.9 Nonorganic
297.9 Paranoid
298.3 Paranoid acute psychogenic
297.1 Paranoid chronic
298.4 Paranoid psychogenic chronic
298.3 Paranoid psychogenic protracted
298.8 Psychogenic
298.8 Reactive brief hysterical
298.2 Reactive confusion
298.0 Reactive depressive
298.4 Reactive paranoid, protracted

P

PSYCHOSIS ORGANIC

294.9 NOS
291.2 Alcoholic
293.9 Infective
294.8 Mixed paranoid and affective states
293.9 Posttraumatic

PSYCHOSIS ORGANIC TRANSIENT

293.9 NOS
293.84 Anxiety type
293.0 Associated with endocrine, metabolic, or cerebrovascular disorder acute
293.1 Associated with endocrine or metabolic disorder subacute
293.9 Associated with physical condition
293.81 Associated with physical condition with delusions
293.82 Associated with physical condition with hallucinations
293.0 Delirium due to conditions classified elsewhere
293.1 Delirium subacute
293.81 Delusional syndrome
293.83 Depressive type
293.82 Hallucinosis syndrome
293.0 Infective acute
293.1 Infective subacute
293.0 Organic reaction acute
293.1 Organic reaction subacute
293.81 Paranoid type
293.0 Posttraumatic acute
293.1 Posttraumatic subacute
293.89 Other specified type

PSYCHOSIS ORGANIC - OTHER

330.1 Cerebral lipidoses with dementia **[294.1#]**
294.8 Epileptic **[345.##]**
345.3 Epileptic grand mal status with dementia **[294.1#]**
294.8 Epileptic petit mal status [345.2]
345.2 Epileptic petit mal status with dementia **[294.1#]**
345.## Epileptic with dementia **[294.1#]**

4th digit: 345
- **0. Generalized nonconvulsive**
- **1. Generalized convulsive**
- **4. Partial, with impairment of consciousness**
- **5. Partial, without impairment of consciousness**
- **6. Infantile spasms**
- **7. Epilepsia partialis continua**
- **8. Other forms**
- **9. Unspecified, NOS**

5th digit: 345
- **0. Without mention of intractable epilepsy**
- **1. With intractable epilepsy**

5th digit: 294.1
- **0. Without behavioral disturbance or NOS**
- **1. With behavioral disturbance**

275.1 Hepatolenticular degeneration with dementia **[294.1#]**
333.4 Huntington's chorea with dementia **[294.1#]**
046.1 Jakob Creutzfeldt disease (syndrome) (new variant) (presenile) with dementia **[294.1#]**
0 Manic depressive see 'Manic Depressive Psychosis'

5th digit: 294.1
- **0. Without behavioral disturbance or NOS**
- **1. With behavioral disturbance**

PSYCHOSIS ORGANIC - OTHER (continued)

340 Multiple sclerosis with dementia **[294.1#]**
294.9 Organic brain syndrome chronic
446.0 Polyarteritis nodosa with dementia **[294.1#]**
094.1 Syphilitic with dementia **[294.1#]**

5th digit: 294.1
- **0. Without behavioral disturbance or NOS**
- **1. With behavioral disturbance**

> *290.#(#) psychosis: Code first any associated neurological condition.*

PSYCHOSIS PRESENILE

290.10 Uncomplicated
290.12 Paranoid
295.7# Schizoaffective disorder

5th digit: 295.7
- **0. Unspecified**
- **1. Subchronic**
- **2. Chronic**
- **3. Subchronic with acute exacerbation**
- **4. Chronic with acute**
- **5. In remission**

290.11 With delirium
290.12 With delusions
290.13 With depressive features

PSYCHOSIS SENILE

290.20 NOS
290.20 Delusional
290.20 Paranoid
290.8 Presbyophrenic
094.1 Syphilitic with dementia **[294.1#]**

5th digit: 294.1
- **0. Without behavioral disturbance or NOS**
- **1. With behavioral disturbance**

290.3 With delerium
290.21 With depression

> *Specify the maternal psychosis with an additional code. See 'Psychosis'.*

PSYCHOSIS WITH PREGNANCY

648.4# NOS
648.4# Major depressive - recurrent **[296.3#]**
648.4# Major depressive - single episode **[296.2#]**

5th digit: 648.4
- **0. Episode of care unspecified or N/A**
- **1. Delivered**
- **2. Delivered with postpartum complication**
- **3. Antepartum complication**
- **4. Postpartum complication**

5th digit: 296.2-3
- **0. Unspecified**
- **1. Mild**
- **2. Moderate**
- **3. Severe without mention of psychotic behavior**
- **4. Severe specified as with psychotic behavior**
- **5. In partial or unspecified remission**

306.9 PSYCHOSOMATIC DISORDER
306.9 PSYCHOSOMATIC REACTION
V67.3 PSYCHOTHERAPY AND OTHER TREATMENT FOLLOW UP EXAM
V66.3 PSYCHOTHERAPY CONVALESCENCE
V57.1 PT (PHYSICAL THERAPY)
790.92 PT (PROTHROMBIN TIME) PROLONGED
286.7 PT (PROTHROMBIN TIME) PROLONGED DUE TO LIVER DISEASE
286.2 PTA (PLASMA THROMBOPLASTIN ANTECEDENT) DEFICIENCY
286.1 PTC (PLASMA THROMBOPLASTIN COMPONENT) DEFICIENCY

PTCA (PERCUTANEOUS TRANSLUIMINAL CORONARY ANGIOPLASTY)

998.2 Accidental puncture or laceration during a procedure
996.61 Complication - infection
996.09 Complication - mechanical
996.72 Complication - other
410.## MI acute during procedure

4th digit: 410
0. Anterior lateral
1. Anterior
2. Inferior lateral
3. Inferior posterior
4. Inferior other
5. Lateral
6. Posterior
7. Subendocardial
8. Other site
9. Site NOS

5th digit: 410
0. Episode of care
1. Initial episode of care
2. Subsequent episode of care

V45.82 Status

PTERYGIUM

372.40 NOS
372.43 Central
744.5 Colli congenital
372.44 Double
372.42 Peripheral progressive
372.41 Peripheral stationary
372.52 Pseudopterygium
372.45 Recurrent

758.6 PTERYGOLYMPHANGIECTASIA SYNDROME
0 PTHIRUS SEE 'PEDICULOSIS'

PTOSIS

611.8 Breast
270.2 Epicanthus syndrome
569.89 Intestine

PTOSIS OF THE EYE

374.30 NOS
743.61 Congenital
374.33 Mechanical
374.32 Myogenic
374.31 Paralytic
374.34 Pseudoptosis

309.81 PTSD (POSTTRAUMATIC STRESS DISORDER) (ACUTE) (BRIEF)
309.81 PTSS (POSTTRAUMATIC STRESS SYNDROME) (ACUTE) (BRIEF)
790.92 PTT (PARTIAL THROMBOPLASTIN TIME) PROLONGED
286.7 PTT (PARTIAL THROMBOPLASTIN TIME) PROLONGED DUE TO LIVER DISEASE
848.8 PUBALGIA

PUBERTY

259.9 Abnormal
626.3 Bleeding
259.0 Delayed
259.1 Precocious - NOS
255.2 Precocious - cortical hyperfunction (adrenal)
256.1 Precocious - ovarian hyperfunction
256.0 Precocious - ovarian hyperfunction estrogen (hyperestrogenism)
259.8 Precocious - pineal tumor
257.0 Precocious - testicular hyperfunction
259.1 Premature - NOS
255.2 Premature - cortical hyperfunction (adrenal)
259.8 Premature - pineal tumor
253.1 Premature - pituitary (anterior) hyperfunction
V21.1 State

665.6# PUBIC BONE SEPARATION (OBSTETRICAL)

5th digit: 665.6
0. Episode of care unspecified or N/A
1. Delivered
4. Postpartum complication

132.2 PUBIC LICE
959.19 PUBIC REGION INJURY NOS/NEC
739.5 PUBIC REGION SEGMENTAL OR SOMATIC DYSFUNCTION
848.5 PUBIC SYMPHYSIS SEPARATION
959.14 PUDENDA INJURY
553.8 PUDENDAL HERNIA
099.2 PUDENDAL ULCER
528.5 PUENTE'S (SIMPLE GLANDULAR CHEILITIS)
672.0# PUERPERAL FEVER
670.0# PUERPERAL FEVER SEPTIC

4th digit: 670.0, 672.0
0. Unspecified
2. Delivered with postpartum complication
4. Postpartum complication

PULMONARY

235.7 Adenomatous tumor site NOS
0 Adenomatous tumor site specified see 'Neoplasm Uncertain Behavior', by site M8250/1
516.2 Alveolar microlithiasis
516.0 Alveolar proteinosis
416.0 Arteriosclerosis syndrome
747.3 Artery - absence congenital
747.3 Artery - agenesis congenital
417.1 Artery - aneurysm
747.3 Artery - anomaly congenital
417.8 Artery - arteritis
747.3 Artery - atresia congenital
747.3 Artery - coarctation congenital
417.9 Artery - disease
417.8 Artery - endarteritis
747.3 Artery - hypoplasia congenital

PULMONARY (continued)

415.19 Artery - infarction
415.11 Artery - infarction iatrogenic
415.11 Artery - infarction postoperative
901.41 Artery - injury
908.4 Artery - injury late effect
901.41 Artery - laceration (rupture) (hematoma) (avulsion)
908.4 Artery - laceration late effect
417.8 Artery - rupture
417.8 Artery - stenosis (stricture) acquired
747.3 Artery - stenosis congenital
417.8 Artery - stricture
668.0# Aspiration following anesthesia or other sedation in L&D
5th digit: 668.0
0. Episode of care unspecified or N/A
1. Delivered
2. Delivered with postpartum complication
3. Antepartum complication
4. Postpartum complication

417.9 Blood vessel - circulation disease
901.40 Blood vessel - injury
908.4 Blood vessel - injury or laceration late effect
901.40 Blood vessel - laceration (rupture) (hematoma) (avulsion) (aneurysm) traumatic
417.8 Blood vessel - rupture
518.0 Collapse
770.5 Collapse perinatal
514 Congestion
861.21 Contusion
861.31 Contusion with open wound into thorax
908.0 Contusion late effect
417.9 Disease circulation
416.9 Disease heart
416.0 Disease hypertensive vascular (cardiovascular)
277.39 Disease in amyloidosis [517.8]
496 Disease obstructive chronic (see also 'COPD')
491.21 Disease obstructive chronic with exacerbation NEC (acute)
491.2# Disease obstructive chronic with bronchitis (chronic)
5th digit: 491.2
0. NOS
1. With (acute) exacerbation
2. With acute bronchitis

424.3 Disease valve
508.0 Disorder due to radiation acute
508.1 Disorder due to radiation chronic
508.8 Disorder due to other external agents
508.9 Disorder due to unspecified external agents
0 Edema see 'Pulmonary Edema'
415.19 Embolism NOS
V12.51 Embolism history
415.11 Embolism iatrogenic
0 Embolism obsterical see 'Embolism Complicating Pregnancy'
415.11 Embolism postoperative

PULMONARY (continued)

415.12 Embolism septic
038.#(#) Embolism septic with septicemia [415.12]
4th or 4th and 5th digit code for organism: 038
.9 NOS
.3 Anaerobic
.3 Bacteroides
.3 Clostridium
.42 E. coli
.49 Enterobacter aerogenes
.40 Gram negative
.49 Gram negative other
.41 Hemophilus influenzae
.2 Pneumococcal
.49 Proteus
.43 Pseudomonas
.44 Serratia
.10 Staphylococcal NOS
.11 Staphylococcal aureus
.19 Staphylococcal other
.0 Streptococcal (anaerobic)
.49 Yersinia enterocolitica
.8 Other specified

415.19 Embolism other specified
417.8 Endarteritis
515 Fibrosis - chronic or unspecified
506.4 Fibrosis - due to fumes and vapors
508.1 Fibrosis - due to radiation
508.0 Fibrosis - due to radiation acute
508.1 Fibrosis - due to radiation chronic
508.8 Fibrosis - due to other external agents
508.9 Fibrosis - due to unspecified external agents
516.3 Fibrosis - idiopathic (interstitial) (diffuse)
770.7 Fibrosis - interstitial of prematurity
710.1 Fibrosis - sclerosis due to scleroderma [517.2]
770.89 Function abnormality of newborn
V71.89 Function studies to evaluate respiratory disease or insufficiency
794.2 Function study abnormal
416.8 Heart disease chronic other
770.3 Hemorrhage perinatal
747.83 Hypertension persistent congenital
416.0 Hypertension primary chronic
416.0 Hypertension primary chronic idiopathic
747.83 Hypertension primary of newborn
416.8 Hypertension secondary chronic
731.2 Hypertrophic osteoarthropathy
769 Hypoperfusion syndrome (idiopathic)
770.4 Immaturity
424.3 Incompetence
415.19 Infarction
415.11 Infarction iatrogenic
415.11 Infarction postoperative

P

PULMONARY (continued)

415.12 Infarction septic
038.#(#) Infarction septic with septicemia [415.12]

4th or 4th and 5th digit code for organism:
038
- **.9 NOS**
- **.3 Anaerobic**
- **.3 Bacteroides**
- **.3 Clostridium**
- **.42 E. coli**
- **.49 Enterobacter aerogenes**
- **.40 Gram negative**
- **.49 Gram negative other**
- **.41 Hemophilus influenzae**
- **.2 Pneumococcal**
- **.49 Proteus**
- **.43 Pseudomonas**
- **.44 Serratia**
- **.10 Staphylococcal NOS**
- **.11 Staphylococcal aureus**
- **.19 Staphylococcal other**
- **.0 Streptococcal (anaerobic)**
- **.49 Yersinia enterocolitica**
- **.8 Other specified**

518.3 Infiltrate
793.1 Infiltrate x-ray finding
861.20 Injury NOS
861.30 Injury NOS with open wound into thorax
908.0 Injury NOS late effect
518.82 Insufficiency acute
770.89 Insufficiency newborn
0 Insufficiency valve see 'Pulmonary', valve insufficiency
861.22 Laceration
861.32 Laceration with open wound into thorax
908.0 Laceration late effect
518.89 Nodule
731.2 Osteoarthropathy hypertrophic
V81.4 Perfusion screening
424.3 Regurgitation see also 'Pulmonary' valve insufficiency
446.21 Renal (hemorrhagic) syndrome
415.19 Thrombosis NOS
415.11 Thrombosis postoperative (iatrogenic)
415.12 Thrombosis septic
038.#(#) Thrombosis septic with septicemia [415.12]

4th or 4th and 5th digit code for organism:
038
- **.9 NOS**
- **.3 Anaerobic**
- **.3 Bacteroides**
- **.3 Clostridium**
- **.42 E. coli**
- **.49 Enterobacter aerogenes**
- **.40 Gram negative**
- **.49 Gram negative other**
- **.41 Hemophilus influenzae**
- **.2 Pneumococcal**
- **.49 Proteus**
- **.43 Pseudomonas**
- **.44 Serratia**
- **.10 Staphylococcal NOS**
- **.11 Staphylococcal aureus**
- **.19 Staphylococcal other**
- **.0 Streptococcal (anaerobic)**
- **.49 Yersinia enterocolitica**
- **.8 Other specified**

415.19 Thrombosis other specified

PULMONARY (continued)

746.01 Valve - absence (congenital)
746.00 Valve - anomaly (congenital)
746.01 Valve - atresia (congenital)

Pulmonic incompetence and pulmonic regurgitation are synonyms for pulmonic insufficiency.

424.3 Valve insufficiency
421.0 Valve insufficiency - bacterial (acute) (chronic)
746.09 Valve insufficiency - congenital
397.1 Valve insufficiency - rheumatic
093.24 Valve insufficiency - syphilitic
424.3 Valve obstruction (see also 'Endocarditis', pulmonary)
424.3 Valve stenosis
421.0 Valve stenosis - bacterial (acute) (chronic)
746.02 Valve stenosis - congenital
746.83 Valve stenosis - congenital infundibular
746.83 Valve stenosis - congenital subpulmonary
397.1 Valve stenosis - rheumatic
093.24 Valve stenosis - syphilitic
424.3 Valve stenosis - with insufficiency
421.0 Valve stenosis - with insufficiency bacterial (acute) (chronic)
397.1 Valve stenosis - with insufficiency rheumatic
093.24 Valve stenosis - with insufficiency syphilitic
747.49 Vein - absence or atresia (congenital)
747.42 Vein - anomalous return (connection) (partial)
747.40 Vein - anomaly congenital
901.42 Vein - avulsion (aneurysm) traumatic
415.19 Vein - infarction
415.11 Vein - infarction iatrogenic
415.11 Vein - infarction postoperative
901.42 Vein - injury
901.42 Vein - laceration (rupture) (hematoma)
908.4 Vein - late effect of avulsion, injury or laceration
747.49 Vein - obstruction
747.42 Vein - return partial anomalous connection (return)
747.41 Vein - return total anomalous connection (return)
417.8 Vein - stricture
747.49 Vein - transposition
770.89 Ventilation abnormality of newborn

PULMONARY EDEMA

514 NOS
518.4 Acute
507.0 Acute aspiration
428.1 Acute cardiogenic
506.1 Acute chemical or fumes
518.4 Acute due to pneumonia
518.4 Acute postoperative
428.0 Acute with CHF (right heart failure)
402.91 Acute with hypertensive heart failure **[428.#(#)]**
402.11 Acute with hypertensive heart failure benign **[428.#(#)]**
402.01 Acute with hypertensive heart failure malignant **[428.#(#)]**

4th digit: 428
- **0. Congestive**
- **1. Left**
- **2#. Systolic**
- **3#. Diastolic**
- **4#. Combined systolic and diastolic**
- **9. NOS**

5th digit: 428.2-4
- **0. NOS**
- **1. Acute**
- **2. Chronic**
- **3. Acute on chronic**

P

PULMONARY EDEMA (continued)

428.1 Acute with left heart failure
518.5 Adult respiratory distress syndrome associated with shock
507.0 Associated with aspiration pneumonia [518.82]
514 Associated with hypostatic pneumonia
518.82 Associated with other conditions
518.81 Associated with respiratory failure - acute in other conditions
518.84 Associated with respiratory failure - acute and chronic in other conditions
518.83 Associated with respiratory failure - chronic in other conditions
514 Chronic
506.4 Chronic due to chemical fumes/vapor
518.4 Due to ARDS [518.82]
518.4 Due to ARDS drug overdose
518.5 Due to ARDS post op with shock
518.5 Due to ARDS traumatic [518.4]
993.2 Due to high altitude
994.1 Due to near drowning
508.1 Due to radiation chronic
508.0 Due to radiation pneumonitis
518.4 Due to renal failure [585.#]

4th digit: 585
1. Stage I
2. Stage II (mild)
3. Stage III (moderate)
4. Stage IV (severe)
5. Stage V
6. End stage
9. Unspecified stage

518.5 Due to shock lung
518.5 Due to shock traumatic
508.8 Due to other external agents
508.9 Due to unspecified external agents
518.5 Following trauma and surgery
518.4 Postoperative acute
518.4 Postoperative acute due to fluid overload [276.6]
391.8 Rheumatic acute
398.91 Rheumatic chronic
392.0 Rheumatic with chorea
428.1 With heart disease or failure, left
428.#(#) With heart disease or failure

4th digit: 428
0. Congestive
1. Left
2#. Systolic
3#. Diastolic
4#. Combined systolic and diastolic
9. NOS

5th digit: 428.2-4
0. NOS
1. Acute
2. Chronic
3. Acute on chronic

522.9 PULP (DENTAL) DISEASE NOS
0 PULP (DENTAL) SEE ALSO 'TOOTH PULP AND PERIAPICAL DISORDERS'
522.1 PULP GANGRENE
522.0 PULPITIS (TOOTH)
785.0 PULSE RAPID
779.82 PULSE RAPID NEONATAL
427.89 PULSE SLOW
785.9 PULSE WEAK
446.7 PULSELESS DISEASE OR SYNDROME
375.52 PUNCTA LACRIMALIA OCCLUSION
0 PUNCTURE WOUND SEE 'OPEN WOUND'

PUPIL

743.46 Atresia congenital
364.75 Deformed
379.43 Dilatation
379.40 Dysfunction
379.49 Dysfunction hippus
379.46 Dysfunction tonic
364.75 Ectopic
364.76 Fixed
364.75 Rupture sphincter

PUPILLARY

364.74 Membrane
743.46 Membrane persistent
364.74 Occlusion
379.49 Paralysis
379.46 Reaction (myotonic) (tonic)
364.74 Seclusion

646.8# PUPP (PRURITIC URTICARIAL PAPULES AND PLAQUES OF PREGNANCY) COMPLICATING PREGNANCY

5th digit: 646.8
0. Episode of care unspecified or N/A
1. Delivered
2. Delivered with postpartum complication
3. Antepartum complication
4. Postpartum complication

277.2 PURINE AMINO ACID DISORDER (METABOLISM) NEC

PURPURA

287.2 NOS
287.0 Abdominal
287.0 Allergic
287.0 Anaphylactoid
709.1 Annularis telangiectodes
287.2 Autoerythrocyte sensitization
287.0 Autoimmune
287.0 Bacterial
273.2 Cryoglobulinemic
287.2 Devil's pinches
287.1 Due to qualitative platelet defects
286.6 Fibrinolytic
286.6 Fulminans
287.39 Hemorrhagic
287.0 Henoch's
287.0 Henoch Schonlein
273.0 Hypergammaglobulinemic
287.31 Idiopathic
287.31 Immune
287.2 Nonthrombocytopenic
287.0 Nonthrombocytopenic hemorrhagic
287.0 Nonthrombocytopenic idiopathic
709.09 Pigmentaria
287.4 Posttransfusion
287.2 Red cell membrane sensitivity
287.0 Rheumatica
287.2 Senile
287.2 Simplex
287.1 Thrombasthenia
287.1 Thrombocytasthenia

P

PURPURA (continued)

287.1 Thrombocytopathy

666.3# Thrombocytopenic (puerperium) (postpartum)
5th digit: 666.3
0. Unspecified
2. Delivered with postpartum complication
4. Postpartum complication

287.30 Thrombocytopenic (essential) (primary)

287.33 Thrombocytopenic congenital

287.31 Thrombocytopenic hereditary (idiopathic) (immune)

446.6 Thrombocytopenic thrombotic

287.1 Thrombopathy

287.0 Toxic

050.0 Variolosa

287.0 Vascular

287.0 Visceral symptoms

792.1 PUS IN STOOL

791.9 PUS IN URINE

022.0 PUSTULE MALIGNANT

686.9 PUSTULE SKIN/SUBCUTANEOUS (NONMALIGNANT)

696.1 PUSTULOSA CONTINUA

281.0 PUTNAM'S DISEASE OR SYNDROME (SUBACUTE COMBINED SCLEROSIS WITH PERNICIOUS ANEMIA) [336.2]

427.69 PVC'S

593.89 PYELECTASIA

0 PYELITIS SEE 'PYELONEPHRITIS'

593.89 PYELOCALIECTASIS

PYELONEPHRITIS

590.80 NOS

590.10 Acute

590.11 Acute with renal medullary necrosis

112.2 Candidal

590.00 Chronic

590.01 Chronic with renal medullary necrosis

590.01 Chronic with renal medullary necrosis with vesicoureteral reflux [593.7#]
5th digit: 593.7
0. Unspecified
1. With reflux nephropathy, unilateral
2. With reflux nephropathy, bilateral
3. With reflux nephropathy, unspecified

590.00 Chronic with vesicoureteral reflux [593.7#]
5th digit: 593.7
0. Unspecified
1. With reflux nephropathy, unilateral
2. With reflux nephropathy, bilateral
3. With reflux nephropathy, unspecified

> ***646.6#: Specify the maternal pyelonephritis with an additional code.***

646.6# Maternal complicating pregnancy
5th digit: 646.6
0. Episode of care NOS or N/A
1. Delivered
2. Delivered with postpartum complication
3. Antepartum complication
4. Postpartum complication

PYELONEPHRITIS (continued)

016.0# Tuberculous [590.81]
5th digit: 016.0
0. NOS
1. Lab not done
2. Lab pending
3. Microscopy positive (in sputum)
4. Culture positive - microscopy negative
5. Culture negative - microscopy positive
6. Culture and microscopy negative confirmed by other methods

590.3 PYELOURETERITIS CYSTICA

PYEMIA

771.81 Newborn

0 Obstructive see 'Sepsis'

572.1 Portal (vein)

> ***999.39 Other infection - Use an additional code to identify the specified infection such as septicemia, (038.#(#)).***

999.39 Postvaccinal

0 See 'Sepsis'

759.4 PYGOPAGUS

345.0# PYKNO EPILEPSY PYKNOLEPSY (IDIOPATHIC)
5th digit: 345.0
0. Without mention of intractable epilepsy
1. With intractable epilepsy

756.89 PYLE (-COHN) DISEASE (CRANIOMETAPHYSEAL DYSPLASIA)

572.1 PYLEPHLEBITIS SUPPURATIVE

572.1 PYLETHROMBOPHLEBITIS

PYLORIC

537.0 Constriction

537.0 Obstruction or occlusion

537.0 Stenosis hypertrophic

537.0 Stenosis hypertrophic noninfantile

537.0 Stricture

PYLORIC STENOSIS CONGENITAL OR INFANTILE

750.5 Constriction

750.5 Hypertrophy

750.5 Spasm

750.5 Stenosis

750.5 Stenosis hypertrophic

750.5 Stricture

537.89 PYLORODUODENAL SYNDROME

537.81 PYLOROSPASM

750.5 PYLOROSPASM CONGENITAL

686.0# PYODERMA, PYODERMATITIS
5th digit: 686.0
0. Unpecified
1. Gangrenous
9. Other

686.1 PYOGENIC GRANULOMA
528.9 PYOGENIC GRANULOMA OF ORAL MUCOSA
615.9 PYOMETRA UTERUS - NOS
615.0 PYOMETRA UTERUS - ACUTE
615.1 PYOMETRA UTERUS - CHRONIC
420.99 PYOPERICARDITIS
510.9 PYOPNEUMOTHORAX
567.29 PYOPNEUMOTHORAX SUBDIAPHRAGMATIC OR SUBPHRENIC
523.40 PYORRHEA (ALVEOLAR) (ALVEOLARIS)
614.2 PYOSALPINX
510.9 PYOTHORAX
333.90 PYRAMIDAL TRACT DISEASE
332.0 PYRAMIDOPALLIDONIGRAL SYNDROME
117.4 PYRENOCHAETA ROMEROI INFECTION
780.6 PYREXIA
659.2# PYREXIA MATERNAL DURING LABOR
5th digit: 659.2
0. Episode of care unspecified or N/A
1. Delivered
3. Antepartum complication
778.4 PYREXIA NEWBORN ENVIRONMENTALLY INDUCED
672.0# PYREXIA PUERPERAL
670.0# PYREXIA PUERPERAL SEPTIC
4th digit: 670.0, 672.0
0. Unspecified
2. Delivered with postpartum complication
4. Postpartum complication
0 PYREXIA SEE ALSO 'FEVER'
266.1 PYRIDOXINE DEFICIENCY (PYRIDOXAL, PYRIDOXAMINE)
355.0 PYRIFORMIS SYNDROME
277.2 PYRIMIDINE AMINO ACID DISORDER (METABOLISM) NEC
312.33 PYROMANIA
787.1 PYROSIS
277.1 PYRROLOPORPHYRIA
271.8 PYRUVATE CARBOXYLASE (DEHYDROGENASE) DEFICIENCY
791.9 PYURIA (BACTERIAL)

083.0 Q FEVER
426.82 Q-T INTERVAL PROLONGATION SYNDROME
368.46 QUADRANT ANOPSIA

QUADRICEPS

890.2 Tendon laceration
891.2 Tendon laceration knee
727.65 Tendon rupture
843.8 Tendon rupture traumatic - hip and thigh
844.8 Tendon rupture traumatic - knee and leg

0 QUADRIPARESIS SEE 'QUADRIPLEGIA'
728.87 QUADRIPARESIS MEANING MUSCLE WEAKNESS

QUADRIPLEGIA

344.0# Acquired (long standing) any cause
5th digit: 344.0
0. Unspecified
1. C1 - C4, complete
2. C1 - C4, incomplete
3. C5 - C7, complete
4. C5 - C7, incomplete
9. Other quadriplegia

434.1# Cerebral embolic (current)
5th digit: 434.1
0. Without cerebral infarction
1. With cerebral infarction

437.8 Cerebral injury
767.0 Cerebral injury birth trauma (newborn)
434.0# Cerebral thrombotic
5th digit: 434.0
0. Without cerebral infarction
1. With cerebral infarction

438.53 Late effect of cerebrovascular disease **[344.0#]**
5th digit: 344.0
0. Unspecified
1. C1 - C4, complete
2. C1 - C4, incomplete
3. C5 - C7, complete
4. C5 - C7, incomplete
9. Other quadriplegia

344.81 Locked in state
344.0# Spinal acquired (long standing)
5th digit: 344.0
0. Unspecified
1. C1 - C4, complete
2. C1 - C4, incomplete
3. C5 - C7, complete
4. C5 - C7, incomplete
9. Other quadriplegia

767.4 Spinal injury birth trauma (newborn)
0 Spinal injury current see 'Spinal Cord', injury

651.2# QUADRUPLET GESTATION
651.7# QUADRUPLET GESTATION FOLLOWING (ELECTIVE) FETAL REDUCTION
651.5# QUADRUPLET WITH ONE OR MORE LOSSES
5th digit: 651.2, 5, 7
0. Episode of care NOS or N/A
1. Delivered
3. Antepartum complication

301.3 QUARRELSOMENESS
082.3 QUEENSLAND TICK TYPHUS

727.04 QUERVAIN'S TENDON SHEATH
245.1 QUERVAIN'S THYROID (SUBACUTE GRANULOMATOUS THYROIDITIS)
233.5 QUEYRAT'S ERYTHROPLASIA SITE NOS
0 QUEYRAT'S ERYTHROPLASIA SITE SPECIFIED SEE 'CA IN SITU', BY SITE M8080/2
0 QUINCKE'S SEE 'ANGIONEUROTIC EDEMA'
704.09 QUINQUAUD DISEASE (ACNE DECALVANS)
083.1 QUINTAN FEVER

651.8# QUINTUPLET GESTATION
651.7# QUINTUPLET GESTATION FOLLOWING (ELECTIVE) FETAL REDUCTION
5th digit: 651.7, 8
0. Episode of care NOS or N/A
1. Delivered
3. Antepartum complication

0 RA (RHEUMATOID ARTHRITIS) SEE 'ARTHRITIS RHEUMATOID'
0 RABBIT FEVER SEE 'TULAREMIA'

RABIES

071 NOS
V01.5 Exposure
V04.5 Vaccination

RACHISCHISIS

741.0# With hydrocephalus
741.9# Without hydrocephalus
5th digit: 741.0, 9
0. Region NOS
1. Cervical
2. Dorsal
3. Lumbar

0 RADIAL SEE 'RADIUS, RADIAL'

RADIATION

0 Burn see 'Burn', by site
595.82 Cystitis
692.82 Dermatitis (see also 'Dermatitis')
558.1 Enterocolitis
V82.5 Exposure screening
508.1 Fibrosis pulmonary
909.2 Late effect
990 Sickness
990 Therapy complication

RADICULAR SYNDROME

729.2 NOS
724.4 Lower limbs
723.4 Upper limbs
767.4 Upper limbs newborn

RADICULITIS

729.2 NOS
723.4 Accessory nerve
724.4 Anterior crural
723.4 Brachial (nondiscogenic)

RADICULITIS (continued)

723.4 Cervical (nondiscogenic)
724.4 Leg
724.4 Lumbar
724.4 Thoracic

357.0 RADICULOMYELITIS (ACUTE)
0 RADICULOPATHY SEE 'RADICULITIS'
990 RADIOACTIVE FALLOUT
909.2 RADIOACTIVE FALLOUT LATE EFFECT
0 RADIOACTIVE IODINE THERAPY CODE THE UNDERLYING DISEASE
V82.5 RADIOACTIVE SUBSTANCE INGESTION SCREENING

RADIOCARPAL

0 Joint dislocation, see 'Dislocation', wrist
842.02 Separation (rupture) (tear) (laceration)
842.02 Strain (sprain) (avulsion) (hemarthrosis)

692.82 RADIODERMATITIS

RADIOHUMERAL

841.2 Separation (rupture) (tear) (laceration)
841.2 Strain (sprain) (avulsion) (hemarthrosis)

V15.08 RADIOGRAPHIC DYE ALLERGY HISTORY
794.19 RADIOISOTOPE SCAN ABNORMAL

RADIOLOGICAL EXAM

793.#(#) Abnormal findings (nonspecific)
4th or 4th <u>and</u> 5th digit: 793
0. Skull and head
1. Lung field
2. Other intrathoracic
3. Biliary tract
4. Gastrointestinal tract
5. Genitourinary organs
6. Abdominal area including retroperitoneum
7. Musculoskeletal system
8#.Breast
80. Unspecified
81. Mammographic microcalcification
89. Other abnormal findings (calcification) (calculus)
9#. Other
91. Inconclusive due to excess body fat
99. Other abnormal findings (placenta) (skin) (subcutaneous)

> *When using code 793.91, Image test inconclusive due to excess body fat, use additional code to identify body mass index (BMI) which can be found at 'Body Mass Index'.*

V72.5 Exam NEC
V71.2 Exam for TB

> *If enounter is for radiotherapy sequence the radiotherapy first, with an additional code for the cancer.*

RADIOTHERAPY

V58.0 Admission
990 Complication
V66.1 Convalescence
V67.1 Follow up exam
V58.0 Encounter
V58.0 Maintenance
V58.0 Session
0 Session for radioactive implant code the cancer by site
0 Session for radioactive iodine therapy code the underlying disease

755.53 RADIOULNAR SYNOSTOSIS

RADIUS, RADIAL

755.26 Agenesis (congenital)
755.21 Agenesis (congenital) - with absence complete distal elements
755.26 Agenesis - with absence incomplete distal elements
755.25 And ulna absence congenital
442.0 Artery aneurysm (ruptured) (cirsoid) (varix) (false)
440.2# Artery arteriosclerosis (degeneration)
440.2# Artery arteriosclerosis (degeneration) with <u>chronic complete</u> or <u>total occlusion</u> <u>[440.4]</u>
5th digit: 440.2
0. Unspecified
1. With intermittent claudication
2. With rest pain or rest pain and intermittent claudication
9. Other atherosclerosis extremities

> *When coding arteriosclerosis of the extremities use an additional code, if applicable to identify chronic complete or total occlusion of the artery of the extremities (440.4)*

440.24 Artery arteriosclerosis (degeneration) with ischemic gangrene or ischemic gangrene and <u>ulceration</u>, intermittent claudication, rest pain <u>[707.8]</u>
440.23 Artery arteriosclerosis (degeneration) with <u>ulceration</u>, intermittent claudication, rest pain <u>[707.8]</u>
440.3# Artery bypass graft arteriosclerosis
440.3# Artery bypass graft arteriosclerosis with <u>chronic complete</u> or <u>total occlusion</u> <u>[440.4]</u>
5th digit: 440.3
0. Unspecified graft
1. Autologous vein bypass graft
2. Nonautologous biological bypass graft
444.21 Artery embolism (thrombosis) (occlusion) (infarction)
903.2 Artery injury
908.3 Artery injury late effect
903.2 Blood vessels injury
908.3 Blood vessels injury late effect
903.2 Blood vessels laceration (rupture) (hematoma)
908.3 Blood vessels laceration late effect
736.00 Deformity
755.50 Deformity congenital
354.3 Nerve disorder (palsy) (lesion)
955.3 Nerve injury
907.4 Nerve injury late effect
723.4 Nerve neuritis

Q-R

RADIUS, RADIAL (continued)

354.3 Nerve palsy acute
354.3 Nerve paralysis
767.6 Nerve paralysis birth trauma
727.04 Styloid tenosynovitis
903.2 Vein injury
908.3 Vein injury late effect
451.83 Vein phlebitis

446.7 RAEDER-HARBITZ PULSELESS DISEASE OR SYNDROME

022.1 RAG SORTER'S DISEASE

786.7 RALES

334.2 RAMSAY HUNT'S DYSSYNERGIA CEREBELLARIS MYOCLONICA SYNDROME

053.11 RAMSAY HUNT'S HERPETIC GENICULATE GANGLIONITIS SYNDROME

0 RAMUS SEE ALSO 'MANDIBLE, MANDIBULAR'

0 RANGE OF MOTION (JOINT) LIMITATION SEE 'STIFF, STIFFNESS', JOINT'

527.6 RANULA

750.26 RANULA CONGENITAL

V71.5 RAPE EXAM FOR ALLEGED RAPE

0 RAPE IN AN ABUSIVE RELATIONSHIP SEE 'ABUSE', CHILD OR 'ABUSE', ADULT

V21.0 RAPID GROWTH IN CHILDHOOD

327.35 RAPID TIME ZONE CHANGE SYNDROME

078.89 RASH ECHO 9 VIRUS

782.1 RASH NONSPECIFIC

026.9 RAT BITE FEVER

026.0 RAT BITE FEVER DUE TO SPIRILLUM MINOR (S. MINUS)

026.1 RAT BITE FEVER DUE TO STREPTOBACILLUS MONILIFORMIS

989.5 RATTLESNAKE BITE

995.0 RATTLESNAKE BITE WITH ANAPHYLAXIS [989.5]

433.8# RAYMOND (-CESTAN) SYNDROME

5th digit: 433.8
- **0. Without cerebral infarction**
- **1. With cerebral infarction**

443.0 RAYNAUD'S SYNDROME/PHENOMENON (PAROXYSMAL DIGITAL CYANOSIS)

648.9# RAYNAUD'S SYNDROME/PHENOMENOM (PAROXYSMAL DIGITAL CYANOSIS) MATERNAL CURRENT (CO-EXISTENT) IN PREGNANCY [443.0]

5th digit: 648.9
- **0. Episode of care NOS or N/A**
- **1. Delivered**
- **2. Delivered with postpartum complication**
- **3. Antepartum complication**
- **4. Postpartum complication**

443.0 RAYNAUD'S SYNDROME (PAROXYSMAL DIGITAL CYANOSIS) WITH GANGRENE [785.4]

426.4 RBBB (RIGHT BUNDLE BRANCH BLOCK)

769 RDS NEWBORN (RESPIRATORY DISTRESS SYNDROME)

493.90 REACTIVE AIRWAY DISEASE (SEE ALSO 'ASTHMA')

313.89 REACTIVE ATTACHMENT DISORDER OF INFANCY OR EARLY CHILDHOOD

300.4 REACTIVE DEPRESSION

READING DISORDER

315.00 NOS
315.01 Alexia
315.02 Developmental dyslexia
315.09 Spelling
315.09 Other specified

789.6# REBOUND TENDERNESS

5th digit: 789.6
- **0. Unspecified site**
- **1. Upper right quadrant**
- **2. Upper left quadrant**
- **3. Lower right quadrant**
- **4. Lower left quadrant**
- **5. Periumbilic**
- **6. Epigastric**
- **7. Generalized**
- **9. Other specified site (multiple)**

524.06 RECESSION CHIN

0 RECKLINGHAUSEN'S DISEASE SEE 'VON RECKLINGHAUSEN'S'

610.1 RECLUS' DISEASE (CYSTIC)

081.1 RECRUDESCENT TYPHUS

0 RECTAL SEE 'RECTUM, RECTAL'

RECTOCELE

618.#(#) Female
618.#(#) Female with stress incontinence [625.6]
618.#(#) Female with other urinary incontinence **[788.3#]**

4th or 4th and 5th digit: 618
- **04. Without uterine prolapse**
- **2. With incomplete uterine prolapse**
- **3. With complete uterine prolapse**
- **4. Uterine prolapse unspecified**

5th digit: 788.3
- **1. Urge incontinence**
- **3. Mixed urge and stress**
- **4. Without sensory awareness**
- **5. Post-void dribbling**
- **6. Nocturnal enuresis**
- **7. Continuous leakage**
- **8. Overflow incontinence**
- **9. Other**

654.4# Complicating pregnancy
660.2# Obstructing labor **[654.4#]**

5th digit: 654.4
- **0. Episode of care NOS or N/A**
- **1. Delivered**
- **2. Delivered with postpartum complication**
- **3. Antepartum complication**
- **4. Postpartum complication**

5th digit: 660.2
- **0. Episode of care NOS or N/A**
- **1. Delivered**
- **3. Antepartum complication**

0 Gravid see 'Uterus, Uterine Disorders Complicating Pregnancy', abnormality in shape or position

569.49 Male

RECTOSIGMOID (JUNCTION)

562.10 Diverticula
751.5 Diverticula congenital
569.89 Lesion
560.9 Obstruction (see also 'Intestine, Intestinal' obstruction)
211.4 Polyp (adenomatous)
0 Polyp malignant see 'Cancer', rectosigmoid

569.89 RECTOSIGMOIDITIS
556.3 RECTOSIGMOIDITIS ULCERATIVE (CHRONIC)
752.49 RECTOVAGINAL FISTULA CONGENITAL
959.14 RECTOVAGINAL SEPTUM INJURY NOS/NEC

RECTUM, RECTAL

V45.79 Absence acquired
751.2 Absence congenital
751.2 Atresia congenital
569.3 Bleeding
564.89 Contracture (sphincter)
306.4 Contracture psychogenic
569.49 Crypt
569.49 Disease NEC
306.4 Disorder psychogenic
562.10 Diverticula
569.49 Ectropion
565.1 Fistula
569.49 Granuloma (rupture) (papillary hypertrophy)
751.2 Imperforate congenital
569.49 Infection
569.49 Inflammation
863.45 Injury
863.55 Injury - with open wound
908.1 Injury - late effect
863.46 Injury - multiple sites
863.56 Injury - multiple sites with open wound
863.49 Injury - other
863.59 Injury - other with open wound into cavity
564.89 Irritabilty
569.49 Lesion
787.99 Mass
787.99 Neuralgia
569.49 Obstruction
569.42 Pain
211.4 Polyp adenomatous
569.0 Polyp nonadenomatous
569.1 Prolapse (sphincter)
569.49 Rupture
455.9 Skin tags (hemorrhoidal)
787.99 Sphincter impairment
564.89 Stasis
569.2 Stricture/stenosis
751.2 Stricture - congenital
947.3 Stricture - due to chemical burn
569.2 Stricture - due to radiation burn
098.7 Stricture - gonococcal
099.1 Stricture - inflammatory
095.8 Stricture - syphilitic
787.99 Swelling
455.9 Tag (hemorrhoidal)
787.99 Tenesmus
564.89 Tightness
569.41 Ulcer

087.9 RECURRENT FEVER (RELAPSING)
352.3 RECURRENT LARYNGEAL NERVE DISORDER

RED BLOOD CELL

284.9 Absence (idiopathic)
284.01 Absence congenital (hereditary)
790.09 Count abnormal
790.09 Morphology abnormal
790.09 Sickling abnormal
790.09 Volume abnormal

133.8 RED BUG BITE
284.81 RED CELL ABSENCE OR APLASIA ACQUIRED (ADULT) (SECONDARY) (WITH THYMOMA)
284.01 RED CELL APLASIA CONGENITAL (HEREDITARY) (OF INFANTS) (PRIMARY) (PURE)
V68.81 REFERRAL OF PATIENT WITHOUT EXAMINATION OR TREATMENT
796.1 REFLEX ABNORMAL (DISORDER)
337.2# REFLEX SYMPATHETIC DYSTROPHY

5th digit: 337.2
0. Unspecified
1. Upper limb
2. Lower limb
9. Other specified site

REFLUX

530.81 Esophageal acid
530.11 Esophagitis
530.81 Gastroesophageal

REFRACTIVE

367.81 Change transient
368.15 Diplopia
367.9 Disorder (see also specific disorder)
367.89 Disorder drug induced or toxic
367.89 Disorder other specified
368.15 Polypia

356.3 REFSUM'S DISEASE OR SYNDROME (HEREDOPATHIA ATACTICA POLYNEURITIFORMIS)
<u>356.3</u> <u>REFSUM'S</u> RETINAL DYSTROPHY [362.72]
V70.5 REFUGEES HEALTH EXAM
V15.81 REFUSAL OF TREATMENT AGAINST MEDICAL ADVICE
V62.6 REFUSAL OF TREATMENT RELIGION BASED
V64.2 REFUSAL OF TREATMENT (SURGERY) (PROCEDURE) PATIENT'S DECISION

REGIONAL ENTERITIS

555.9 NOS
555.1 Large intestine
555.0 Small intestine
555.2 Small intestine with large intestine

520.4 REGIONAL ODONTODYSPLASIA
787.03 REGURGITATION
779.3 REGURGITATION OF FOOD NEONATAL
307.53 REGURGITATION PSYCHOGENIC ORIGIN OF FOOD WITH RESWALLOWING

When a code from V57.#, rehabilitation, is assigned as the principal diagnosis, a secondary code (s) should be assigned to identify and explain the condition(s) requiring the rehabilitation services.

V57.4 Orthoptic training following healing traumatic hip fracture V54.13.

REHABILITATION

V57.9 NOS
V57.0 Breathing exercises
V57.89 Cardiac
V57.81 Gait or orthotic training
V57.89 Multiple types
V57.21 Occupational therapy
V57.4 Orthoptic training
V57.1 Physical therapy
V57.9 Procedure
V57.89 Procedure other (multiple)
V57.3 Speech therapy
V57.22 Vocational therapy
V57.89 Other

536.8 REICHMANN'S DISEASE OR SYNDROME (GASTROSUCCORRHEA)
245.3 REIDEL'S THYROIDITIS
259.5 REIFENSTEIN'S SYNDROME (HEREDITARY FAMILIAL HYPOGONADISM, MALE)
337.9 REILLY'S PHENOMENON OR SYNDROME
277.31 REIMANN'S (PERIODIC) DISEASE

REITER'S

099.3 Disease or syndrome
099.3 Disease or syndrome with arthropathy **[711.1#]**
5th digit: 711.1
0. Site NOS
1. Shoulder region
2. Upper arm (elbow) (humerus)
3. Forearm (radius) (wrist) (ulna)
4. Hand (carpal) (metacarpal) (fingers)
5. Pelvic region and thigh (hip) (buttock) (femur)
6. Lower leg (fibula) (knee) (patella) (tibia)
7. Ankle and/or foot (metatarsals) (toes) (tarsals)
8. Other (head) (neck) (rib) (skull) (trunk) (vertebrae)
9. Multiple

099.3 Disease or syndrome with conjunctivitis [372.33]
655.4# Disease maternal (with known/suspected damage to fetus)
5th digit: 655.4
0. Episode of care NOS or N/A
1. Delivered
3. Antepartum complication

647.2# Disease maternal current (co-existent) in pregnancy
5th digit: 647.2
0. Episode of care NOS or N/A
1. Delivered
2. Delivered with postpartum complication
3. Antepartum complication
4. Postpartum complication

RELAPSING FEVER

087.9 NOS
087.0 Louse borne
087.1 Tick borne

313.3 RELATIONSHIP PROBLEM (EMOTIONAL DISTURBANCE OF CHILDHOOD OR ADOLESCENCE)

0 RELATIONSHIP PROBLEM WITH CONDUCT DISORDER SEE 'CONDUCT DISORDER'

RELAXATION

728.4 Back ligaments
596.59 Bladder
0 Bladder with incontinence see 'Bladder Disorders With Incontinence'
530.89 Cardioesophageal
519.4 Diaphragmatic
734 Foot (arch)
724.6 Lumbosacral (joint)
618.8# Pelvis (pelvic floor)
618.8# Pelvis (pelvic floor) with stress incontinence [625.6]
618.8# Pelvis (pelvic floor) with other urinary incontinence **[788.3#]**
618.8# Perineum
618.8# Perineum with stress incontinence [625.6]
618.8# Perineum with other urinary incontinence **[788.3#]**
5th digit: 618.8
1. Pubocervical tissue incompetence (weakening)
2. Rectovaginal tissue incompetence (weakening)
3. Pelvic muscle wasting
9. Other

5th digit: 788.3
1. Urge incontinence
3. Mixed urge and stress
4. Without sensory awareness
5. Post-void dribbling
6. Nocturnal enuresis
7. Continuous leakage
8. Overflow incontinence
9. Other

724.6 Sacroiliac (joint)
599.84 Urethra
618.8# Uterus (vagina)
618.8# Uterus (vagina) with stress incontinence [625.6]
618.8# Uterus (vagina) with other urinary incontinence **[788.3#]**
5th digit: 618.8
1. Pubocervical tissue incompetence (weakening)
2. Rectovaginal tissue incompetence (weakening)
3. Pelvic muscle wasting
9. Other

5th digit: 788.3
1. Urge incontinence
3. Mixed urge and stress
4. Without sensory awareness
5. Post-void dribbling
6. Nocturnal enuresis
7. Continuous leakage
8. Overflow incontinence
9. Other

596.59 Vesical
0 Vesical with incontinence see 'Bladder Disorders With Incontinence'

V62.4 RELIGIOUS DISCRIMINATION CAUSING ENCOUNTER
V62.6 RELIGIOUS PROBLEM REGARDING MEDICAL CARE
V62.89 RELIGIOUS PROBLEM OTHER THAN MEDICAL CARE
327.42 REM SLEEP BEHAVIOR DISORDER

RENAL

590.2 Abscess
753.0 Agenesis (congenital)
593.7# Agenesis (congenital) with vesicoureteral reflux [753.0]
5th digit: 593.7
0. Unspecified
1. With reflux nephropathy, unilateral
2. With reflux nephropathy, bilateral
3. With reflux nephropathy, unspecified

747.62 Anomaly peripheral vascular (aberrant) (absence) (agenesis) (accessory) (aneurysm) (atresia) (deformity) (hypoplasia) (malposition)

ARTERY

747.62 Absence NEC (agenesis) (congenital)
747.62 Anomaly (multiple) (aberrant) (accessory) (congenital)
442.1 Aneurysm (A-V fistula) (cirsoid) (false) (varicose) (ruptured)
747.62 Aneurysm congenital
440.1 Arteriosclerosis (degeneration) (deformans) (arteritis)
747.62 Deformity NEC (congenital)
443.23 Dissection
593.81 Embolism
593.81 Hemorrhage
447.3 Hyperplasia
747.62 Hypoplasia (congenital)
593.81 Infarction (hemorrhage)
902.41 Injury
908.4 Injury late effect
593.81 Ischemia
908.4 Laceration late effect
902.41 Laceration traumatic (rupture) (hematoma) (avulsion) (aneurysm)
747.62 Malposition (congenital)
593.81 Occlusion
440.1 Stenosis
440.1 Stricture
593.81 Thrombosis

RENAL (continued)

587 Atrophy
583.89 Basement membrane disease NEC
593.89 Calcification
592.0 Calculus
274.11 Calculus - uric acid
189.0 Cell carcinoma site NOS
0 Cell carcinoma site specified see 'Cancer', by site M8312/3
587 Cirrhosis
788.0 Colic
866.01 Contusion
908.1 Contusion late effect
866.11 Contusion with open wound into cavity
593.81 Crisis
593.2 Cyst
591 Cyst - calyceal or pyelogenic
753.10 Cyst congenital
753.19 Cyst congenital - multicystic

RENAL (continued)

753.11 Cyst congenital - single or solitary
V45.1 Dialysis status

DISEASE

593.9 NOS
593.9 Acute
277.39 Amyloidosis [583.81]
585.# Chronic
4th digit: 585
1. Stage I
2. Stage II (mild)
3. Stage III (moderate)
4. Stage IV (severe)
5. Stage V
6. End stage
9. Unspecified stage

753.10 Cystic congenital
250.4# Diabetic [583.81]
5th digit: 250.4
0. Type II, adult-onset, non-insulin dependent (even if requiring insulin), or unspecified; controlled
1. Type I, juvenile-onset or insulin-dependent; controlled
2. Type II, adult-onset, non-insulin dependent (even if requiring insulin); uncontrolled
3. Type I, juvenile-onset or insulin-dependent; uncontrolled

585.6 End stage
593.9 Functional
098.19 Gonococcal [583.81]
274.10 Gouty
0 Hypertensive see 'Hypertensive'
710.0 Lupus (systemic lupus) erythematosus (due to) [583.81]
760.1 Maternal affecting fetus or newborn

646.2#: Specify the maternal renal disease with an additional code.

646.2# Maternal complicating pregnancy
5th digit: 646.2
0. Episode of care NOS or N/A
1. Delivered
2. Delivered with postpartum complication
3. Antepartum complication
4. Postpartum complication

0 Maternal hypertensive see 'Eclampsia' or 'Pre-eclampsia'
588.0 Phosphate-losing (tubular)
753.12 Polycystic (congenital)
753.13 Polycystic (congenital) - adult type (APKD)
753.13 Polycystic (congenital) - autosomal dominant
753.14 Polycystic (congenital) - autosomal recessive
753.14 Polycystic (congenital) - childhood type (infantile) (CPKD)
0 See also 'Nephritis'
095.4 Syphilitic

RENAL (continued)

DISEASE (continued)

016.0# Tuberculous [583.81]
5th digit: 016.0
0. NOS
1. Lab not done
2. Lab pending
3. Microscopy positive (in sputum)
4. Culture positive - microscopy negative
5. Culture negative - microscopy positive
6. Culture and microscopy negative confirmed by other methods

584.5 Tubular
581.9 With edema

RENAL (continued)

588.9 Disorder due to impaired function
588.89 Disorder other specified
593.89 Diverticulum
588.0 Dwarfism
753.15 Dysplasia
593.7# Dysplasia with vesicoureteral reflux [753.15]
5th digit: 593.7
0. Unspecified
1. With reflux nephropathy, unilateral
2. With reflux nephropathy, bilateral
3. With reflux nephropathy unspecified

FAILURE

586 NOS
584.# Acute
4th digit: 584
5. With acute tubular necrosis
6. With cortical necrosis
7. With medullary (papillary) necrosis
8. With other specified pathological lesion in kidney
9. Renal failure unspecified

669.3# Acute following L&D
5th digit: 669.3
0. Episode of care NOS or N/A
2. Delivered with postpartum complication
4. Postpartum complication

584.# Acute with hypertension [**401.#**]
4th digit: 584
5. With acute tubular necrosis
6. With cortical necrosis
7. With medullary necrosis
8. With other specified pathological lesion in kidney
9. Renal failure unspecified
4th digit: 401
0. Malignant, accelerated
1. Benign
9. NOS

RENAL (continued)

FAILURE (continued)

584.# Acute non-hypertensive with hypertensive renal (kidney) disease [**403.##**]
4th digit: 584
5. With acute tubular necrosis
6. With cortical necrosis
7. With medullary necrosis
8. With other specified pathological lesion in kidney
9. Renal failure unspecified

4th digit: 403
0. Malignant
1. Benign
9. Unspecified

5th digit: 403
0. Without chronic kidney disease
1. With chronic kidney disease

585.9 Chronic
585.9 Chronic with neuropathy [357.4]
585.9 Chronic with pericarditis [420.0]
585.9 Chronic with polyneuropathy [357.4]
958.5 Crush injury (due to)
908.6 Crush injury late effect (due to)
997.5 Due to procedure chronic [585.9]
997.5 Due to procedure acute [**584.#**]
4th digit: 584
5. With acute tubular necrosis
6. With cortical necrosis
7. With medullary necrosis
8. With other specified pathological lesion in kidney
9. Renal failure unspecified

0 Hypertensive associated with abortion see 'Abortion'
0 Hypertensive see 'Hypertensive
584.7 Necrotizing renal papillitis
639.3 Post pregnancy (abortive) (ectopic) (molar)
997.5 Post op
997.5 Post op NOS [586]
997.5 Post op acute [**584.#**]
4th digit: 584
5. With acute tubular necrosis
6. With cortical necrosis
7. With medullary necrosis
8. With other specified pathological lesion in kidney
9. Renal failure unspecified

997.5 Post op chronic [585.9]
639.3 Shutdown post pregnancy (abortive) (ectopic) (molar)
958.5 Traumatic
908.6 Traumatic late effect
0 With SIRS see 'SIRS', with renal failure

RENAL (continued)

593.81 Embolism
753.19 Fibrocystic disease
587 Fibrosis
588.9 Function impaired disorder NOS
588.89 Function impaired disorder other specified
794.4 Function test abnormal

RENAL (continued)

250.4# Glomerulohyalinosis - diabetic syndrome [583.81]
5th digit: 250.4
0. Type II, adult-onset, non-insulin dependent (even if requiring insulin), or unspecified; controlled
1. Type I, juvenile-onset or insulin-dependent; controlled
2. Type II, adult-onset, non-insulin dependent (even if requiring insulin); uncontrolled
3. Type I, juvenile-onset or insulin-dependent; uncontrolled

593.81 Hemorrhage
753.0 Hypoplasia
588.0 Infantilism
593.81 Infarction
866.## Injury
4th digit: 866
0. Closed
1. With open wound into cavity
5th digit: 866
0. Injury NOS
1. Contusion/hematoma
2. Laceration
3. Rupture

908.1 Injury late effect
593.9 Insufficiency acute
585.9 Insufficiency chronic
866.02 Laceration
908.1 Laceration late effect
866.12 Laceration with open wound into cavity
592.0 Lithiasis
593.9 Mass
593.89 Obstruction
588.0 Osteodystrophy
788.0 Pain
593.89 Polyp
588.0 Rickets
587 Sclerosis
0 Sclerosis hypertensive see 'Hypertensive', renal disease
593.81 Thrombosis
588.89 Transport disorder NEC
270.0 Transport amino acid disorder NEC (metabolic)
588.89 Tubular acidosis (Lightwood's)

VEIN (VESSEL)

747.62 Absence NEC (agenesis) (congenital)
747.62 Anomaly (multiple) (congenital) (aberrant) (accessory)
747.62 Aneurysm (congenital)
747.62 Deformity NEC (congenital)
747.62 Hypoplasia (congenital)
747.62 Malposition (congenital)
902.42 Vein injury
908.4 Vein injury late effect
908.4 Vein laceration late effect
902.42 Vein laceration traumatic (rupture) (hematoma) (avulsion) (aneurysm)
453.3 Vein thrombosis (embolism)

RENAL (continued)

VEIN (VESSEL) (continued)

902.40 Vessel injury - NOS
908.4 Vessel injury - late effect
902.49 Vessel injury - other NEC
908.4 Vessel NOS laceration late effect
902.40 Vessel NOS laceration traumatic (rupture) (hematoma) (avulsion) (aneurysm)

RENAL (continued)

0 See also 'Kidney'

790.99 RENIN ELEVATED

753.0 RENOFACIAL SYNDROME (CONGENITAL BILIARY FIBROANGIOMATOSIS)

253.8 RENON-DELILLE SYNDROME

RENOVASCULAR DISEASE

0 Due to hypertension (arteriosclerotic) see 'Hypertensive', chronic kidney disease
405.91 With secondary hypertension - unspecified
405.11 With secondary hypertension - benign
405.01 With secondary hypertension - malignant

727.2 REPETITIVE USE SYNDROME BURSITIS

REPLACEMENT STATUS

V43.5 Bladder (artificial) (prosthesis)
V43.4 Blood vessel (artificial) (prosthesis)
V43.82 Breast (artificial) (prosthesis)
V43.0 Eye globe (artificial) (prosthesis)
V43.21 Heart assist device
V43.22 Heart fully implantable (artificial) (prosthesis)
V43.3 Heart valve (artificial) (prosthesis)
V43.89 Intestine (artificial) (prosthesis)
V43.60 Joint
V54.81 Joint aftercare [V43.6#]
5th digit: V43.6
0. Site unspecified
1. Shoulder
2. Elbow
3. Wrist
4. Hip
5. Knee
6. Ankle
9. Other

V43.66 Joint ankle
V43.62 Joint elbow
V43.69 Joint finger
V43.64 Joint hip
V43.65 Joint knee
V43.61 Joint shoulder
V43.63 Joint wrist
V43.69 Joint other
V43.89 Kidney (artificial) (prosthesis)
V43.81 Larynx (artificial) (prosthesis)
V43.1 Lens (artificial) (prothesis)
V43.7 Limb (artificial) (prosthesis)
V43.89 Liver (artificial) (prosthesis)
V43.89 Lung (artificial) (prosthesis)
V43.89 Organ other (artificial) (prosthesis)
V43.89 Pancreas (artificial) (prosthesis)
V43.83 Skin artificial
V43.89 Tissue other (artificial) (prosthesis)
V43.89 Other organ or tissue (artificial) (prosthesis)

0 RESISTANCE TO DRUGS BY MICROORGANISMS SEE 'DRUG RESISTANCE'

RESPIRATION, RESPIRATORY

786.00 Abnormality
748.9 Anomaly (system) unspecified congenital
748.8 Anomaly (system) other specified congenital
799.1 Arrest
799.1 Arrest cause uncertain
770.87 Arrest fetus
770.87 Arrest newborn

DISORDER

519.9 Unspecified
770.9 Unspecified fetus and newborn
465.9 Acute (upper) NEC
519.9 Chronic
770.7 Chronic arising in perinatal period
760.3 Chronic maternal affecting fetus or newborn
508.9 Due to aspiration of liquids or solids
506.9 Due to fumes and vapors
506.3 Due to fumes and vapors - acute/subacute
506.4 Due to fumes and vapors - chronic
508.0 Due to radiation acute
508.1 Due to radiation chronic
508.8 Due to other external agents
508.9 Due to unspecified external agents
0 Failure see 'Respiratory', failure
V12.60 History NOS
V12.69 History other
306.1 Psychogenic
V81.3 Screening (for chronic bronchitis and emphysema)
V81.4 Screening (for other respiratory diseases)
519.8 Specified NEC

DISTRESS

786.09 NOS
518.82 Acute
518.82 Acute NEC
770.89 Newborn
770.89 Perinatal period
518.5 Syndrome adult (following shock, surgery or trauma)
518.82 Syndrome adult (following shock, surgery or trauma) specified NEC
769 Syndrome newborn
770.6 Syndrome newborn type II

FAILURE

518.81 NOS
518.81 Acute
518.84 Acute and chronic (acute on chronic)
518.83 Chronic
518.5 Due to trauma/surgery/shock
770.84 Newborn
770.84 Perinatal

INFECTION, UPPER

465.9 Acute
487.1 Acute influenzal
465.0 Acute laryngopharyngitis
465.8 Acute multiple sites
034.0 Acute streptococcal
519.8 Chronic

RESPIRATION, RESPIRATORY (continued)

INSUFFICIENCY

786.09 NOS
518.82 Acute
770.89 Newborn
518.82 NEC

RESPIRATION, RESPIRATORY (continued)

786.09 Kussmaul (air hunger)
786.09 Narcosis CO 2 (carbon dioxide)
519.8 Obstruction (airway) NEC
496 Obstruction (chronic) COPD
934.9 Obstruction due to foreign body
748.8 Obstruction upper congenital
748.9 Organ absence congenital
786.52 Painful
344.89 Paralysis (system)
786.09 Periodic
327.22 Periodic high altitude
786.06 Rapid
079.82 Severe acute syndrome-associated coronavirus (SARS)
786.9 Symptoms (system)
079.6 Syncytial virus
466.11 Syncytial virus bronchiolitis
<u>460</u> Syncytial virus <u>common cold-like</u> [079.6]
<u>460</u> Syncytial virus <u>nasopharyngitis acute</u> [079.6]
480.1 Syncytial virus pneumonia (bronchopneumonia)
<u>466.0</u> Syncytial virus <u>tracheobronchitis</u> [079.6]
V04.82 Syncytial virus vaccination
519.9 System disorder NOS
519.8 System disorder NEC
306.1 System disorder psychogenic
478.9 Tract upper atrophy

V46.1# RESPIRATOR DEPENDENCE
5th digit: V46.1
1. Status
2. Encounter during power failure
3. Encounter for weaning from
4. Mechanical complication

0 RESPIRATORY SEE 'RESPIRATION, RESPIRATORY'

333.94 RESTLESS LEGS (SYNDROME) (RLS)
799.2 RESTLESSNESS
V60.1 RESTRICTION OF SPACE (INADEQUATE HOUSING)
518.89 RESTRICTIVE LUNG DISEASE
667.0# RETAINED PLACENTA
666.0# RETAINED PLACENTA WITH POSTPARTUM HEMORRHAGE
666.2# RETAINED PLACENTA WITH POSTPARTUM HEMORRHAGE SECOND STAGE
667.1# RETAINED PRODUCTS OF CONCEPTUS
5th digit: 666.0, 2, 667.0-1
0. NOS
2. Delivered with postpartum complication
4. Postpartum complication

0 RETARDATION DEVELOPMENTAL LANGUAGE OR LEARNING SKILLS - SEE 'DEVELOPMENTAL DISORDER'

0 RETARDATION FETAL GROWTH SEE 'FETAL - INFANT'S RECORD', GROWTH RETARDATION

RETARDATION MENTAL

319 Unspecified
V18.4 Family history
317 Mild IQ 50-70
318.0 Moderate IQ 35-49
318.2 Profound
V79.2 Screening
318.1 Severe IQ 20-34

783.43 RETARDATION PHYSICAL (GROWTH) CHILD

276.2 RETENTION CARBON DIOXIDE

788.2# RETENTION URINE

997.5 <u>RETENTION URINE</u> POSTOPERATIVE [788.2#]

5th digit: 788.2
0. Unspecified
1. Incomplete bladder emptying
9. Other specified retention

362.64 RETICULAR DEGENERATION SENILE

701.8 RETICULATA ATROPHIC

790.99 RETICULOCYTOSIS

0 RETICULOENDOTHELIAL CYTOMYCOSIS SEE 'HISTOPLASMOSIS'

289.9 RETICULOENDOTHELIAL HYPERPLASIA (CELL)

289.89 RETICULOENDOTHELIAL SYSTEM DEGENERATION

202.5# RETICULOENDOTHELIOSIS INFANTILE ACUTE M9722/3

202.3# RETICULOENDOTHELIOSIS MALIGNANT M9720/3

277.89 RETICULOHISTIOCYTOMA (GIANT CELL)

200.8# RETICULOLYMPHOSARCOMA (DIFFUSE) M9613/3

5th digit: 200.8, 202.3, 5
0. Unspecified site, extranodal and solid organ sites
1. Lymph nodes of head, face, neck
2. Lymph nodes intrathoracic
3. Lymph nodes abdominal
4. Lymph nodes axilla and upper limb
5. Lymph nodes inguinal region and lower limb
6. Lymph nodes intrapelvic
7. Spleen
8. Lymph nodes multiple sites

RETICULOSARCOMA

200.0# NOS M9640/3

5th digit: 200.0, 202.0
0. Unspecified site, extranodal and solid organ sites
1. Lymph nodes of head, face, neck
2. Lymph nodes intrathoracic
3. Lymph nodes abdominal
4. Lymph nodes axilla and upper limb
5. Lymph nodes inguinal region and lower limb
6. Lymph nodes intrapelvic
7. Spleen
8. Lymph nodes multiple sites

V10.71 History (not in remission)

RETICULOSARCOMA (continued)

200.0# Nodular M9642/3
200.0# Pleomorphic cell type M9641/3

5th digit: 200.0
0. Unspecified site, extranodal and solid organ sites
1. Lymph nodes of head, face, neck
2. Lymph nodes intrathoracic
3. Lymph nodes abdominal
4. Lymph nodes axilla and upper limb
5. Lymph nodes inguinal region and lower limb
6. Lymph nodes intrapelvic
7. Spleen
8. Lymph nodes multiple sites

288.4 RETICULOSIS FAMILIAL HEMOPHAGOCYTIC

202.3# RETICULOSIS MALIGNANT M9720/3

202.5# RETICULOSIS OF INFANCY ACUTE M9722/3

5th digit: 202.3, 5
0. Unspecified site, extranodal and solid organ sites
1. Lymph nodes of head, face, neck
2. Lymph nodes intrathoracic
3. Lymph nodes abdominal
4. Lymph nodes axilla and upper limb
5. Lymph nodes inguinal region and lower limb
6. Lymph nodes intrapelvic
7. Spleen
8. Lymph nodes multiple sites

RETINA, RETINAL

0 Ablatio see 'Retina, Retinal', detachment
794.11 Abnormal function studies
362.17 Aneurysm
743.58 Aneurysm congenital

ARTERITIS/VARICES

362.18 Arteritis
362.18 Endarteritis
362.14 Microaneurysms
362.16 Neovascularization
362.18 Perivasculitis
362.18 Phlebitis
362.15 Telangiectasia
362.17 Varices
362.18 Vasculitis

ARTERY OCCLUSION (OBSTRUCTION)

362.30 NOS
362.32 Branch
362.31 Central
362.33 Partial
362.34 Transient
362.32 Tributary

RETINA, RETINAL (continued)

362.30 Artery spasm
0 Atrophy see 'Retina, Retinal', degeneration
0 Atrophy hereditary see 'Retina, Retinal', dystrophy
361.30 Break NOS
743.56 Changes other congenital
362.89 Congestion
368.34 Correspondence abnormal with binocular vision disorder
362.83 Cotton wool spots

RETINA, RETINAL (continued)

361.19 Cyst
361.13 Cyst primary
361.14 Cyst secondary

DEFECT

361.30 Without detachment
361.32 Horseshoe tear without detachment
361.33 Multiple without detachment
361.31 Round hole without detachment
0 With detachment see 'Retina, Retinal', detachment

DEGENERATION

0 Hereditary see 'Retina, Retinal', dystrophy hereditary
362.63 Lattice (palisade)
362.62 Microcystoid
362.61 Paving stone
362.60 Peripheral
362.65 Secondary pigmentary
362.66 Secondary vitreoretinal
362.64 Senile (reticular)
0 With retinal defect see 'Retina, Retinal', detachment

DETACHMENT

361.9 NOS
361.06 Old delimited
361.06 Old partial
361.07 Old total or subtotal
361.00 Partial retinal defect
361.03 Partial with giant tear
361.01 Partial with single defect
361.02 Partial with multiple defects
362.43 Pigment epithelium hemorrhagic
362.42 Pigment epithelium serous
361.04 Recent with retinal dialysis
361.05 Recent total or subtotal
361.2 Serous
362.41 Serous with central serous retinopathy
361.81 Traction
361.81 Traction with vitreoretinal organization
361.2 Without retinal defect
361.89 Other form

RETINA, RETINAL (continued)

361.04 Dialysis (juvenile) (with detachment)
362.9 Disorder
362.89 Disorder specified NEC

DYSTROPHY

272.5 Bassen Kornzweig [362.72]
330.1 Cerebroretinal [362.71]
362.70 Hereditary
362.74 Hereditary - albipunctate
362.77 Hereditary - drusen
362.76 Hereditary - fundus flavimaculatus
362.77 Hereditary - hyaline
362.74 Hereditary - pigmentary
362.76 Hereditary - primarily involving retinal pigment epithelium
362.77 Hereditary - primarily of Bruch's membrane
362.75 Hereditary - progressive cone (-rod)
362.77 Hereditary - pseudoinflammatory foveal
362.75 Hereditary - Stargardt's disease
362.76 Hereditary - vitelliform
362.73 Hereditary - vitreoretinal

RETINA, RETINAL (continued)

DYSTROPHY (continued)

356.3 Refsum's disease [362.72]
272.7 Systemic lipidoses (due to) [362.71]

RETINA, RETINAL (continued)

362.83 Edema cystoid (localized) (macular) (peripheral)
362.53 Edema (localized) (macular) (peripheral)
362.82 Exudates and deposits
228.03 Hemangioma
362.81 Hemorrhage (periretinal) (deep) (subretinal)
362.84 Infarction
921.3 Injury contusion
362.84 Ischemia
362.13 Light reflex increased
362.14 Microaneurysms
362.33 Microembolisms
362.16 Neovascularization
362.85 Nerve fiber bundle defects
361.32 Operculum
361.01 Operculum with detachment
362.42 Pigment epithelium detachment exudative
362.43 Pigment epithelium detachment hemorrhagic
362.42 Pigment epithelium detachment serous
361.19 Pseudocyst
361.30 Rupture
0 Rupture with detachment see 'Retina, Retinal', detachment
363.30 Scar
363.35 Scar disseminated
363.33 Scar of posterior pole
363.34 Scar peripheral
363.31 Scar solar
362.17 Sclerosis (senile) (vascular)
362.40 Separation layer unspecified
362.13 Silver wire arteries

TEAR

361.30 NOS
361.00 NOS with detachment
361.03 Giant
361.32 Horseshoe
361.33 Multiple
361.02 Multiple with detachment
361.06 Old partial
361.07 Old total
361.31 Round hole without detachment
361.05 Total
361.07 Total old
0 With detachment see 'Retina, Retinal', detachment

RETINA, RETINAL (continued)

362.89 Tessellated fundus (tigroid)
362.30 Vascular occlusion
362.13 Vascular sheathing
362.37 Vein engorgement

VEIN OCCLUSION (OBSTRUCTION)

362.30 NOS
362.36 Branch
362.35 Central (total)
362.35 Central (total) causing glaucoma [365.63]
362.37 Incipient
362.37 Partial
362.36 Tributary

Q-R

RETINA, RETINAL (continued)

362.17 Vessel tortuous acquired
743.58 Vessel tortuous congenital

RETINITIS

363.20 NOS
585.9 Albuminurica [363.10]
363.10 Disseminated
363.14 Disseminated metastatic
363.00 Focal
363.05 Focal juxtapapillary (and retinochoroiditis)
363.06 Focal macular or paramacular (and retinochoroiditis)
363.07 Focal other posterior pole (and retinochoroiditis)
363.08 Focal peripheral pole (and retinochoroiditis)
115.92 Histoplasma
115.02 Histoplasma capsulatum
115.12 Histoplasma duboisii
362.74 Pigmentosa hereditary
362.29 Proliferans
585.9 Renal [363.13]
0 See also 'Chorioretinitis'
094.84 Syphilitic

RETINOBLASTOMA

190.5 Site NOS
0 Site specified see 'Cancer', by site M9510/3
190.5 Differentiated type site NOS
0 Differentiated type site specified see 'Cancer', by site M9511/3
190.5 Familial Syndrome
190.5 Undifferentiated type site NOS
0 Undifferentiated type site specified see 'Cancer', by site M9512/3

0 RETINOCHORIORETINITIS SEE 'RETINITIS'

RETINOCHOROIDITIS

363.10 Disseminated NOS
363.15 Disseminated epitheliopathy (pigmentary)
130.2 Due to acquired toxoplasmosis
363.00 Focal
094.83 Syphilitic

RETINOPATHY

440.8 Arteriosclerotic [362.13]
362.10 Background
362.41 Central serous
250.5# Diabetic [**362.0#**]
250.5# Diabetic with edema [**362.0#**] [362.07]

5th digit: 250.5

0. Type II, adult-onset, non-insulin dependent (even if requiring insulin), or unspecified; controlled
1. Type I, juvenile-onset or insulin-dependent; controlled
2. Type II, adult-onset, non-insulin dependent (even if requiring insulin); uncontrolled
3. Type I, juvenile-onset or insulin-dependent; uncontrolled

4th digit: 362.0

1. Background or NOS
2. Proliferative
3. Nonproliferative NOS
4. Nonproliferative mild
5. Nonproliferative moderate
6. Nonproliferative severe

RETINOPATHY (continued)

362.12 Exudative
362.11 Hypertensive
362.14 Microaneurysms
362.21 Of prematurity
362.17 Other intraretinal microvascular abnormalities
362.29 Proliferative (other) (nondiabetic)
282.60 Proliferative due to sickle cell anemia [362.29]
363.31 Solar
362.13 Vascular (changes)

RETINOSCHISIS

361.10 NOS
361.12 Bullous
361.11 Flat
362.73 Juvenile hereditary

752.52 RETRACTILE TESTIS (CONGENITAL)
378.71 RETRACTION SYNDROME (DUANE'S)
094.85 RETROBULBAR NEURITIS SYPHILITIC
753.4 RETROCAVAL URETER CONGENITAL
524.10 RETROGNATHISM
362.21 RETROLENTAL FIBROPLASIA

RETROPERITONEAL

567.38 Abscess
568.89 Cyst
593.4 Fibrosis idiopathic (syndrome)
568.81 Hemoperitoneum nontraumatic
553.8 Hernia
560.81 Hernia due to adhesion with obstruction
551.8 Hernia gangrenous
552.8 Hernia incarcerated
868.04 Herniation traumatic
908.1 Herniation traumatic late effect
868.14 Herniation traumatic with open wound into cavity
567.39 Infection other
868.04 Injury
868.14 Injury with open wound into cavity
908.1 Injury late effect
789.39 Mass
789.09 Pain
789.69 Tenderness

567.39 RETROPERITONITIS
621.6 RETROVERTED UTERUS
654.3# RETROVERTED UTERUS (INCARCERATED) COMPLICATING CHILDBIRTH

5th digit: 654.3

0. Episode of care NOS or N/A
1. Delivered
2. Delivered with postpartum complication
3. Antepartum complication
4. Postpartum complication

V08 RETROVIRAL SEROCONVERSION SYNDROME (ACUTE)

AIDS, ARC and symptomatic HIV infections all code to 042. This code should be sequenced as the principal diagnosis with an additional code for any manifestation. Exception: If the encounter is for an unrelated condition such as a trauma, sequence the trauma as the principal diagnosis, followed by the 042 with additional codes for the manifestations.

RETROVIRUS

079.50 Unspecified
042 HIV 1 (human immunodeficiency virus, type 1)
079.53 HIV 2 (human immunodeficiency virus, type 2)
079.51 HTLV 1 (human T-cell lymphotrophic virus type 1)
079.52 HTLV 2 (human T-cell lymphotrophic virus type 2)
042 HTLV 3 (human T-cell lymphotrophic virus type 3)
042 LAV (lymphadenopathy-associated virus)
079.59 Other specified retrovirus

524.04 RETRUSION PREMAXILLA (DEVELOPMENTAL)
330.8 RETT'S SYNDROME
434.91 REVERSIBLE ISCHEMIC NEUROLOGICAL DEFICIT (RIND)
V12.54 REVERSIBLE ISCHEMIC NEUROLOGICAL DEFICIT (RIND) HISTORY
331.81 REYE'S SYNDROME
331.81 REYE'S SYNDROME WITH DEMENTIA [**294.1#**]
5th digit: 294.1
0. Without behavioral disturbance or NOS
1. With behavioral disturbance

253.2 REYE-SHEEHAN SYNDROME (POSTPARTUM PITUITARY NECROSIS)

RH INCOMPATIBILITY

773.0 Causing hemolytic disease (fetus) (newborn)
773.0 Fetus or newborn
999.7 Infusion or transfusion reaction
656.1# Maternal affecting management of mother
5th digit: 656.1
0. Episode of care NOS or N/A
1. Delivered
3. Antepartum complication

728.88 RHABDOMYOLYSIS (IDIOPATHIC)

RHABDOMYOMA

215.# NOS M8900/0
215.# Adult M8904/0
215.# Fetal M8903/0
4th digit: 215
0. Head, face, neck
2. Upper limb including shoulder
3. Lower limb including hip
4. Thorax
5. Abdomen (wall), gastric, gastrointestinal, intestine, stomach
6. Pelvis, buttock, groin, inguinal region, perineum
7. Trunk NOS, back NOS, flank NOS
8. Other specified sites
9. Site NOS

RHABDOMYOSARCOMA

171.# NOS M8900/0
171.# Alveolar M8920/3
171.# Embryonal M8910/3
171.# Mixed type M8902/3
171.# Pleomorphic M8901/3
4th digit: 171
0. Head, face, neck
2. Upper limb including shoulder
3. Lower limb including hip
4. Thorax
5. Abdomen (wall), gastric, gastrointestinal, intestine, stomach
6. Pelvis, buttock, groin, inguinal region, perineum
7. Trunk NOS, back NOS, flank NOS
8. Other specified sites
9. Site NOS

0 RHEGMATOGENOUS RETINAL DETACHMENT SEE 'RETINAL DETACHMENT'

RHEUMATIC

396.9 Aortic and mitral valve disease NOS
395.1 Aortic insufficiency
396.3 Aortic insufficiency and mitral insufficiency
395.0 Aortic stenosis
395.2 Aortic stenosis with insufficiency
396.2 Aortic stenosis and mitral insufficiency
396.0 Aortic stenosis and mitral stenosis
395.9 Aortic valve disease chronic
V82.2 Disorder screening
0 Heart failure see 'Heart Failure'
396.8 Other aortic stenosis and/or insufficiency with mitral stenosis and/or insufficiency
394.1 Mitral insufficiency
396.3 Mitral insufficiency and aortic insufficiency
394.0 Mitral stenosis
396.1 Mitral stenosis and aortic insufficiency
394.2 Mitral stenosis with insufficiency
394.9 Mitral valve disease other and unspecified
729.1 Myositis
397.0 Tricuspid disease
397.0 Tricuspid insufficiency
397.0 Tricuspid stenosis
396.8 Other mitral stenosis and/or insufficiency with aortic stenosis and/or insufficiency

RHEUMATIC ACUTE

390 Arthritis
391.9 Carditis
392.9 Chorea
392.0 Chorea with heart involvement
391.8 Disease active with other or multiple types of heart involvement
391.1 Endocarditis
390 Fever (without mention of heart involvement)
391.9 Heart disease
391.8 Heart disease other (with other or multiple)
0 Heart failure see 'Heart Failure'
391.2 Myocarditis
391.8 Pancarditis
391.0 Pericarditis

RHEUMATIC CHRONIC

398.90 Carditis
397.9 Endocarditis
398.90 Heart disease
398.99 Heart disease other
0 Heart failure see 'Heart Failure'
393 Mediastinopericarditis
398.0 Myocarditis
393 Myopericarditis
393 Pericarditis
397.1 Pulmonic insufficiency (regurgitation)
397.1 Pulmonic stenosis
V82.2 Screening

729.0 RHEUMATISM

RHEUMATOID

714.2 Carditis
714.81 Lung
714.0 Myopathy [359.6]

RHEUMATOID ARTHRITIS

714.0 Adult
714.30 Juvenile chronic or unspecified
714.33 Juvenile monoarticular
714.32 Juvenile pauciarticular
714.31 Juvenile polyarticular acute
V82.1 Screening
720.0 Spine
714.2 With visceral or systemic involvement

RHINITIS

472.0 NOS
460 Acute
460 Acute infective
477.9 Allergic
477.2 Allergic due to animal (cat) (dog) dander and hair
477.8 Allergic due to dust mites
477.1 Allergic due to food
477.0 Allergic due to pollen
477.8 Allergic due to other allergen
493.9# Allergic with asthma
493.0# Allergic with asthma with stated cause

5th digit: 493.0, 9
0. NOS
1. With status asthmaticus
2. With (acute) exacerbation

472.0 Atrophic
472.0 Chronic
472.0 Chronic atrophic
472.0 Chronic granulomatous
472.0 Hypertrophic
472.0 Obstructive
472.0 Ulcerative
477.9 Vasomotor

478.19 RHINOLITH SINUS (NASAL)

478.19 RHINOMEGALY

RHINOPHARYNGITIS

460 Acute
472.2 Chronic
102.5 Mutilans (destructive ulcerating)

695.3 RHINOPHYMA

RHINORRHEA

478.19 NOS
349.81 Cerebrospinal fluid
0 See 'Rhinitis'

040.1 RHINOSCLEROMA
117.0 RHINOSPORIDIOSIS
117.0 RHINOSPORIDIUM SEEBERI INFECTION
079.3 RHINOVIRUS (INFECTION) (INFECTING AGENT)
277.86 RHIZOMELIC CHONDRODYSPLASIA PUNCTATA
117.7 RHIZOPUS INFECTION
238.72 RHOADS AND BOMFORD ANEMIA (REFRACTORY)
086.4 RHODESIAN SLEEPING SICKNESS
V07.2 RHOGAM ADMINISTRATION (PROPHYLACTIC)
701.8 RHYTIDOSIS FAVALIS
701.8 RHYTIDS

RIB

748.3 Absence
756.3 Absence congenital
756.3 Accessory
756.3 Cage malposition congenital
739.8 Cage segmental or somatic dysfunction
719.88 Calcification
738.3 Deformity acquired
756.3 Extra
756.3 Fusion congenital
848.3 Separation (rupture) (tear) (laceration)
733.99 Slipped
848.3 Strain (sprain) (avulsion) (hemarthrosis)
756.3 Supernumerary congenital
353.0 Syndrome cervical

266.0 RIBOFLAVIN DEFICIENCY

RICE BODIES (OLD)

718.1# NOS

5th digit: 718.1
0. Site NOS
1. Shoulder region
2. Upper arm (elbow) (humerus)
3. Forearm (radius) (wrist) (ulna)
4. Hand (carpal) (metacarpal) (fingers)
5. Pelvic region and thigh (hip) (buttock) (femur)
7. Ankle and/or foot (metatarsals) (toes) (tarsals)
8. Other specified sites
9. Multiple

717.6 Knee (joint)
724.9 Vertebral facet

RICKETS

268.0 Active
268.0 Acute
268.0 Adolescent
268.0 Adult
579.0 Celiac (disease)
268.0 Chest wall
268.0 Congenital
268.0 Current
756.4 Fetal
267 Hemorrhagic
270.0 Hypophosphatemic with nephrotic-glycosuric dwarfism
268.0 Infantile
268.0 Intestinal

RICKETS (continued)

588.0 Kidney
268.1 Late effect
588.0 Renal
267 Scurvy
275.3 Vitamin D-resistant

RICKETTSIAL, RICKETTSIOSIS

083.9 Disease NOS
083.8 Disease other specified type
083.2 Pox
083.0 Q fever
V75.0 Screening exam

TICK-BORNE

082.9 NOS
082.1 Boutonneuse fever
082.40 Ehrlichiosis NOS
082.41 Ehrlichiosis Chaffeensis (E. Chaffeensis)
082.49 Ehrlichiosis other
082.2 North asian fever
082.3 Queensland fever
082.0 Spotted fever
082.8 Other specified

RICKETTSIAL, RICKETTSIOSIS (continued)

083.1 Trench fever
083.2 Vesicular

368.16 RIDDOCH'S SYNDROME (VISUAL DISORIENTATION)
733.99 RIDER'S BONE CALCIFICATION
744.29 RIDGE EAR CONGENITAL
428.1 RIDLEY'S SYNDROME
245.3 RIEDEL'S DISEASE (LIGNEOUS THYROIDITIS)
751.69 RIEDEL'S LOBE LIVER
743.44 RIEGER'S ANOMALY OR SYNDROME (MESODERMAL DYSGENESIS, ANTERIOR OCULAR SEGMENT)
709.09 RIEHL'S MELANOSIS
282.49 RIETTI-GREPPI-MICHELI SYNDROME (THALASSEMIA MINOR)
066.3 RIFT VALLEY FEVER (VIRAL)
529.0 RIGA (-FEDE) DISEASE (CACHECTIC APHTHAE)
523.40 RIGGS' DISEASE (COMPOUND PERIODONTITIS)
426.4 RIGHT BUNDLE BRANCH BLOCK
428.0 RIGHT HEART FAILURE (SECONDARY TO LEFT HEART FAILURE)
518.0 RIGHT MIDDLE LOBE SYNDROME
428.0 RIGHT VENTRICULAR FAILURE
429.3 RIGHT VENTRICULAR HYPERTROPHY
0 RIGHT VENTRICULAR OBSTRUCTION SYNDROME SEE 'HEART FAILURE'

789.4# RIGIDITY ABDOMEN

5th digit: 789.4
- **0. Unspecified site**
- **1. Upper right quadrant**
- **2. Upper left quadrant**
- **3. Lower right quadrant**
- **4. Lower left quadrant**
- **5. Periumbilic**
- **6. Epigastric**
- **7. Generalized**
- **9. Other specified site (multiple)**

780.99 RIGORS
742.8 RILEY-DAY SYNDROME (FAMILIAL DYSAUTONOMIA)
434.91 RIND (REVERSIBLE ISCHEMIC NEUROLOGICAL DEFICIT)
V12.54 RIND (REVERSIBLE ISCHEMIC NEUROLOGICAL DEFICIT) HISTORY

661.4# RING CONTRACTION COMPLICATING DELIVERY

5th digit: 661.4
- **0. Episode of care NOS or N/A**
- **1. Delivered**
- **3. Antepartum complication**

110.9 RINGWORM
0 RINGWORM SEE 'TINEA'
695.1 RITTER LYELL SYNDROME (SSSS)
695.81 RITTER'S DISEASE
039.3 RIVALTA'S DISEASE (CERVICOFACIAL ACTINOMYCOSIS)
333.94 RLS (RESTLESS LEG SYNDROME)
755.69 ROBERT'S PELVIS
763.1 ROBERT'S PELVIS AFFECTING FETUS
653.0# ROBERT'S PELVIS WITH DISPROPORTION
660.1# ROBERT'S PELVIS WITH DISPROPORTION CAUSING OBSTRUCTION [653.0#]

5th digit: 653.0, 660.1
- **0. Episode of care NOS or N/A**
- **1. Delivered**
- **3. Antepartum complication**

756.0 ROBIN'S SYNDROME
125.3 ROBLES' DISEASE (ONCHOCERCIASIS) [360.13]
0 ROCHALIMEA SEE 'RICKETSIOSIS
082.0 ROCKY MOUNTAIN SPOTTED FEVER
370.07 RODENT ULCER CORNEA
0 RODENT ULCER SKIN SEE 'CANCER', SKIN
745.4 ROGER'S DISEASE (CONGENITAL INTERVENTRICULAR SEPTAL DEFECT)
570 ROKITANSKY'S DISEASE (SEE ALSO 'NECROSIS', LIVER)
752.49 ROKITANSKY-KUSTER-HAUSER SYNDROME (CONGENITAL ABSENCE, VAGINA)
426.82 ROMANO-WARD SYNDROME (PROLONGED Q-T INTERVAL)
720.1 ROMANUS LESION
349.89 ROMBERG'S DISEASE OR SYNDROME

ROSACEA

695.3 NOS
695.3 Acne
695.3 Conjunctivitis [372.31]
695.3 Keratitis [370.49]

516.0 ROSEN-CASTLEMAN-LIEBOW SYNDROME (PULMONARY PROTEINOSIS)
286.2 ROSENTHAL'S DISEASE (FACTOR XI DEFICIENCY)
057.8 ROSEOLA
058.10 ROSEOLA INFANTUM
058.11 ROSEOLA INFANTUM DUE TO HUMAN HERPESVIRUS 6
058.12 ROSEOLA INFANTUM DUE TO HUMAN HERPESVIRUS 7
066.3 ROSS RIVER FEVER (VIRAL)

536.8 ROSSBACH'S DISEASE (HYPERCHLORHYDRIA)
306.4 ROSSBACH'S DISEASE (HYPERCHLORHYDRIA) - PSYCHOGENIC

ROTATOR CUFF

727.61 Capsule rupture nontraumatic
840.4 Capsule rupture traumatic
726.10 Disorder unspecified
726.19 Disorder other specified
726.19 Impingement
727.61 Rupture complete nontraumatic
840.4 Rupture traumatic
840.4 Separation (rupture) (tear) (laceration)
840.4 Sprain
840.4 Strain (sprain) (avulsion) (hemarthrosis)
726.10 Syndrome NOS
726.10 Tear degenerative
727.61 Tear nontraumatic
840.4 Tear traumatic

008.61 ROTAVIRUS ENTERITIS
355.1 ROTH (-BERNHARDT) DISEASE OR SYNDROME
757.33 ROTHMUND'S SYNDROME (CONGENITAL POIKILODERMA)
277.4 ROTOR'S SYNDROME (IDIOPATHIC HYPERBILIRUBINEMIA)
752.89 ROUND LIGAMENT ABSENCE (AGENSIS) (APLASIA) (CONGENITAL)
752.89 ROUND LIGAMENT ANOMALY (CONGENITAL)
867.6 ROUND LIGAMENT INJURY TRAUMATIC
867.7 ROUND LIGAMENT INJURY TRAUMATIC WITH OPEN WOUND
629.89 ROUND LIGAMENT SHORT
646.8# ROUND LIGAMENT SYNDROME COMPLICATING PREGNANCY [625.9]
5th digit: 646.8
0. Episode of care NOS or N/A
1. Delivered
2. Delivered with postpartum complication
3. Antepartum complication
4. Postpartum complication
127.0 ROUNDWORM INFECTION
334.3 ROUSSY-LEVY SYNDROME
757.39 ROY (-JUTRAS) SYNDROME (ACROPACHYDERMA)

RSV (RESPIRATORY SYNCYTIAL VIRUS)

079.6 NOS
466.11 Bronchiolitis
460 Common cold-like [079.6]
460 Nasopharyngitis acute [079.6]
480.1 Pneumonia (bronchopneumonia)
466.0 Tracheobronchitis [079.6]
V04.82 Vaccination

751.2 RS WADE SYNDROME

RUBELLA

056.9 NOS
056.71 Arthritis
771.0 Congenital or perinatal
056.01 Encephalitis
V01.4 Exposure
760.2 Maternal affecting fetus
056.01 Menigoencephalitis

RUBELLA (continued)

056.00 Neurological complication NOS (rubeola mobilli)
056.09 Neurological complication other specified
V73.3 Screening exam
771.0 Syndrome (congenital)
V04.3 Vaccination alone
056.8 With complication NOS
056.79 With complication other specified

RUBELLA COMPLICATING PREGNANCY

760.2 Maternal affecting fetus
771.0 Maternal affecting fetus with infant rubella pneumonitis congenital
655.3# Maternal affecting management of pregnancy, suspected damage to fetus
5th digit: 655.3
0. Episode of care NOS or N/A
1. Delivered
3. Antepartum complication

647.5#: Use an additional code to identify the maternal rubella.

647.5# Maternal current (coexistent)
5th digit: 647.5
0. Episode of care NOS or N/A
1. Delivered
2. Delivered with postpartum complication
3. Antepartum complication
4. Postpartum complication

0 RUBEOLA SEE 'MEASLES'
364.42 RUBEOSIS IRIDIS
759.89 RUBINSTEIN-TAYBI'S SYNDROME (BRACHYDACTYLIA, SHORT STATURE AND MENTAL RETARDATION)
759.89 RUD'S SYNDROME (MENTAL DEFICIENCY, EPILEPSY AND INFANTILISM)
755.22 RUDIMENTARY ARM
272.7 RUITER-POMPEN (-WYERS) SYNDROME (ANGIOKERATOMA CORPORIS DIFFUSUM)

RUMINATION

307.53 Disorder
300.3 Neurotic
300.3 Obsessional
307.53 Psychogenic

281.0 RUNEBERG'S DISEASE (PROGRESSIVE PERNICIOUS ANEMIA)
766.22 RUNGE'S SYNDROME (POSTMATURITY) (OVER 42 COMPLETED WEEKS)
726.69 RUNNER'S KNEE
784.99 RUNNY NOSE

RUPTURE

799.89 Abdominal visera NEC
845.09 Achilles tendon (traumatic)
727.67 Achilles tendon nontraumatic
441.5 Aorta NOS
441.1 Aorta ascending
441.5 Aorta descending
093.0 Aorta syphilitic
441.1 Aortic arch
424.1 Aortic valve
447.2 Artery
0 Artery traumatic see specific artery, injury

RUPTURE (continued)

840.8	Biceps long head (traumatic)
727.62	Biceps long head nontraumatic
576.3	Bile duct
867.0	Bladder (traumatic)
867.1	Bladder (traumatic) with open wound
596.6	Bladder nontraumatic
459.0	Blood vessel
996.54	Breast prosthesis
429.5	Chordae tendineae
363.63	Choroid
0	Collateral ligaments see 'Sprain'
0	Coronary artery thrombotic see 'MI Acute'
575.4	Cystic duct
872.61	Ear drum (traumatic)
872.71	Ear drum (traumatic) complicated
384.20	Ear drum (post trauma/post infective)
862.22	Esophagus (traumatic)
862.32	Esophagus (traumatic) with open wound into cavity
871.1	Eye with exposure of intraocular tissue
871.2	Eye with partial loss of intraocular tissue
620.8	Fallopian tube hydatid of Morgagni congenital
575.4	Gallbladder
537.89	Gastric or duodenal
422.90	Heart due to infection
0	Heart see 'Myocardial Infarction', acute
0	Heart traumatic see 'Myocardial', rupture (traumatic)
623.8	Hymen
0	Internal organ traumatic see specific organ, injury
0	Joint see 'Sprain'
866.03	Kidney (traumatic)
866.13	Kidney (traumatic) with open wound into cavity
767.8	Kidney birth trauma
593.89	Kidney nontraumatic
0	Ligaments of joint nontraumatic see 'Articular Cartilage Derangement'
0	Ligaments of joint traumatic see 'Sprain'
864.04	Liver (traumatic)
864.14	Liver (traumatic) with open wound into cavity
573.8	Liver nontraumatic
762.1	Marginal sinus affecting fetus or newborn
761.1	Membranes premature affecting fetus (see also 'Rupture Obstetrical', membranes)
0	Meniscus (knee), see 'Meniscus', knee tear, acute or old
424.0	Mitral valve
728.83	Muscle nontraumatic
0	Muscle NEC traumatic see 'Sprain', by site
0	Muscle traumatic with open wound see 'Laceration', by site
840.4	Musculotendinous cuff (nontraumatic) (shoulder)

RUPTURE (continued)

0	Myocardium (nontraumatic) see 'Myocardial Infarction Acute'
861.03	Myocardium traumatic
861.13	Myocardium traumatic with open wound into thorax
998.32	Operative wound
998.32	Operative wound external
998.31	Operative wound internal
620.8	Ovary or fallopian tube (nonpregnant)
620.8	Ovary with hemoperitoneum (non traumatic) [568.81]
620.8	Oviduct
577.8	Pancreas
429.6	Papillary muscle
844.8	Patellar tendon (traumatic)
624.8	Perineum
424.3	Pulmonary valve
417.8	Pulmonary vessel
844.8	Quadriceps (traumatic)
843.8	Quadriceps tendon - hip and thigh (traumatic)
844.8	Quadriceps tendon - knee and leg (traumatic)
569.49	Rectal sphincter
840.4	Rotator cuff (capsule) (traumatic)
727.61	Rotator cuff (capsule) complete nontraumatic
747.29	Sinus of valsalva congenital
767.4	Spine or spinal cord birth trauma
289.59	Spleen (spontaneous) (posttraumatic)
767.8	Spleen birth trauma
084.9	Spleen malarial
865.04	Spleen traumatic
865.14	Spleen traumatic with open wound into cavity
767.8	Stomach birth trauma
727.50	Synovium NOS
727.59	Synovium other specified
0	Tendon nontraumatic see 'Tendon', rupture
0	Tendon traumatic see 'Sprain'
457.8	Thoracic duct
474.8	Tonsil
424.2	Tricuspid valve
599.84	Urethra
0	Uterus obstetrical see 'Rupture Obstetrical'
0	Vein traumatic see specific vein, injury
0	Ventricle see 'MI Acute'
799.89	Viscus
998.32	Wound operative
998.32	Wound operative external
998.31	Wound operative internal

RUPTURE OBSTETRICAL

665.5# Bladder traumatic
5th digit: 665.5
0. Episode of care unspecified or N/A
1. Delivered
4. Postpartum condition or complication

674.1# C - section (uterine) (internal) (external)
674.2# Episiotomy
5th digit: 674.1-2
0. Episode of care NOS or N/A
2. Delivered with mention of postpartum complication
4. Postpartum condition or complication

658.3# Membranes artificial with delayed delivery
V71.89 Membranes evaluation, not found
658.1# Membranes premature
658.2# Membranes spontaneous with delayed delivery
5th digit: 658.1-3
0. Episode of care NOS or N/A
1. Delivered
3. Antepartum complication

674.2# Perineal
5th digit: 674.2
0. Episode of care NOS or N/A
2. Delivered with mention of postpartum complication
4. Postpartum condition or complication

RUPTURE OBSTETRICAL (continued)

665.5# Urethra traumatic
5th digit: 665.5
0. Episode of care unspecified or N/A
1. Delivered
4. Postpartum condition or complication

665.1# Uterus NOS
665.1# Uterus during labor
5th digit: 665.1
0. Episode of care NOS or N/A
1. Delivered

665.0# Uterus before onset of labor
5th digit: 665.0
0. Episode of care NOS or N/A
1. Delivered
3. Antepartum complication

759.89 RUSSELL (-SILVER) SYNDROME (CONGENITAL HEMIHYPERTROPHY AND SHORT STATURE)
063.0 RUSSIAN SPRING SUMMER (TAIGA) ENCEPHALITIS
0 RUST'S DISEASE SEE 'TUBERCULOSIS', SPONDYLOPATHY
203.0# RUSTITSKII'S MULTIPLE MYELOMA M9730/3
5th digit: 203.0
0. Without mention of remission
1. In remission

751.3 RUYSCH'S DISEASE CONGENITAL
426.0 RYTAND-LIPSITCH SYNDROME (COMPLETE ATRIOVENTRICULAR BLOCK)

379.57 SACCADIC EYE MOVEMENTS DEFICIENCY
330.1 SACH'S (-TAY) DISEASE
270.7 SACCHAROPINURIA
756.15 SACRALIZATION-SCOLIOSIS-SCIATICA SYNDROME
0 SACRAL SEE 'SACRUM, SACRAL'
739.4 SACROCOCCYGEAL REGION SEGMENTAL OR SOMATIC DYSFUNCTION

SACROILIAC

755.69 Deformity congenital
755.69 Fusion congenital
724.6 Joint disorder NEC (nonvertebral) (nondiscogenic)
724.6 Joint slipping
959.19 Ligament injury NEC
846.1 Ligament separation (rupture) (tear) (laceration)
846.1 Ligament strain (sprain) (avulsion) (hemarthrosis)
739.4 Region segmental or somatic dysfunction
846.9 Region separation (rupture) (tear) (laceration) unspecified site
846.8 Region separation (rupture) (tear) (laceration) other specified sites
846.9 Region strain (sprain) (avulsion) (hemarthrosis) unspecified site
846.8 Region strain (sprain) (avulsion) (hemarthrosis) other specified sites
724.6 Syndrome

720.2 SACROILIITIS
846.2 SACROSPINATUS SEPARATION (RUPTURE) (TEAR) (LACERATION)
846.2 SACROSPINATUS STRAIN (SPRAIN) (AVULSION) (HEMARTHROSIS)
846.3 SACROTUBEROUS SEPARATION (RUPTURE) (TEAR) (LACERATION)
846.3 SACROTUBEROUS STRAIN (SPRAIN) (AVULSION) (HEMARTHROSIS)

SACRUM, SACRAL

756.13 Absence congenital
724.6 Ankylosis (nonvertebral) (nondiscogenic)
724.6 Disorder
959.19 Injury NEC
724.6 Instability (nonvertebral) (nondiscogenic)
953.3 Nerve root injury
739.4 Region segmental or somatic dysfunction
847.3 Separation (rupture) (tear) (laceration)
847.3 Strain (sprain) (avulsion) (hemarthrosis)

309.1 SAD (SEASONAL AFFECTIVE DISORDER)
302.84 SADISM SEXUAL
370.04 SAEMISCH'S ULCER
379.46 SAENGER'S SYNDROME
0 SAH (SUBARACHNOID HEMORRHAGE) SEE 'SUBARACHNOID', HEMORRHAGE
692.74 SAILORS' SKIN
117.7 SAKSENAEA INFECTION
345.6# SALAAM ATTACKS

5th digit: 345.6
0. Without mention of intractable epilepsy
1. With intractable epilepsy

781.0 SALAAM TIC
792.4 SALIVA ABNORMAL

SALIVARY DUCT

527.8 Atresia
750.23 Atresia congenital
527.0 Atrophy
527.9 Disease NEC
750.23 Imperforate congenital
078.5 Inclusion disease
034.0 Inclusion streptococcal
959.09 Injury
527.8 Obstruction
527.5 Obstruction with calculus
527.8 Stenosis
527.8 Stricture
078.5 Virus disease

SALIVARY GLAND

527.3 Abscess
750.21 Absence congenital
750.22 Accessory congenital
527.8 Atresia
750.23 Atresia congenital
527.0 Atrophy
527.9 Disease NEC
527.7 Disturbance salivary secretion
527.4 Fistula
750.24 Fistula congenital
527.1 Hyperplasia
527.1 Hypertrophy
078.5 Inclusion disease
034.0 Inclusion streptococcal
959.09 Injury
527.8 Lymphoepithelial lesion benign
527.6 Mucocele
078.5 Virus disease

527.5 SALIVARY SYSTEM CALCULUS
527.7 SALIVATION ABNORMAL (EXCESSIVE) (HYPOSECRETION)

SALMONELLA

003.23 Arthritis
V02.3 Carrier
003.0 Gastroenteritis
003.9 Infection
003.20 Infection localized
003.29 Infections localized other
003.8 Infections other specified
771.89 Intra-amniotic newborn (fetus) [003.9]
771.89 Intra-amniotic perinatal [003.9]
003.21 Meningitis
003.24 Osteomyelitis
003.22 Pneumonia
003.1 Sepsis

SALPINGITIS

614.2 NOS
614.0 Acute
614.0 Acute and oophoritis
760.8 Affecting fetus or newborn
614.1 Chronic
614.1 Chronic and oophoritis
614.1 Follicularis
639.0 Following abortion or ectopic/molar pregnancy
098.17 Gonococcal acute
098.37 Gonococcal chronic
614.1 Isthmica nodosa

S

S

SALPINGITIS (continued)

670.0# Maternal due to pregnancy
5th digit: 670.0
0. NOS
2. Delivered with postpartum complication
4. Postpartum complication

016.6# Tuberculous
5th digit: 016.6
0. NOS
1. Lab not done
2. Lab pending
3. Microscopy positive (in sputum)
4. Culture positive - microscopy negative
5. Culture negative - microscopy positive
6. Culture and microscopy negative confirmed by other methods

SALPINGO-OOPHORITIS

614.2 NOS
614.0 Acute
614.1 Chronic

620.4 SALPINGOCELE
992.8 SALT DEPLETION SYNDROME DUE TO HEAT
992.4 SALT DEPLETION SYNDROME DUE TO HEAT CAUSING HEAT EXHAUSTION OR PROSTRATION
593.9 SALT LOSING (DEPLETION) SYNDROME
0 SALTER (HARRIS) INJURY (SLIPPED EPIPHYSEAL GROWTH PLATE), SEE 'FRACTURE', BY SITE, CLOSED
371.46 SALZMANN'S NODULAR DYSTROPHY
114.# SAN JOAQUIN VALLEY FEVER
4th digit: 114
0. Acute (primary)
4. Chronic (secondary)
5. Unspecified
134.1 SAND FLEA INFESTATION
297.1 SANDER'S DISEASE (DELUSIONAL DISORDER)
066.0 SANDFLY FEVER
330.1 SANDHOFF'S DISEASE
126.9 SANDWORM DISEASE
277.5 SANFILIPPO'S SYNDROME
334.2 SANGER BROWN CEREBELLA DEGENERATION
082.0 SAO PAULO FEVER

SAPHENOUS

904.7 Artery injury
908.3 Artery injury late effect
355.79 Mononeuropathy
355.79 Nerve compression (entrapment)
355.79 Nerve disorder (lesion) (neuritis)
904.3 Vein (greater) (lesser) injury
908.3 Vein (greater) (lesser) injury late effect
904.3 Vein (greater) (lesser) laceration
908.3 Vein (greater) (lesser) laceration late effect
451.0 Vein phlebitis

477.0 SAR (SEASONAL ALLERGIC RHINITIS)
136.5 SARCOCYSTIS LINDEMANNI INFECTION

SARCOID, SARCOIDOSIS

135 Any site or unspecified
135 Lung involvement [517.8]

SARCOID, SARCOIDOSIS (continued)

135 Meningitis [321.4]
135 Myopathy [359.6]
135 Polyneuropathy [357.4]
V82.89 Screening exam
V82.89 Test

SARCOMA

171.9 Site NOS
0 Site specified see 'Cancer', connective tissue, by site M8800/3
171.# Alveolar soft part M9581/3
4th digit: 171
0. Head, face, neck
2. Upper limb including shoulder
3. Lower limb including hip
4. Thorax
5. Abdomen (wall), gastric, gastrointestinal, intestine, stomach
6. Pelvis, buttock, groin, inguinal region, perineum
7. Trunk NOS, back NOS, flank NOS
8. Other specified sites
9. Site NOS

191.6 Cerebellar site NOS
0 Cerebellar site specified see 'Cancer', by site M9480/3
171.# Clear cell of tendons and aponeuroses M9044/3
171.# Embryonal M8991/3
4th digit: 171
0. Head, face, neck
2. Upper limb including shoulder
3. Lower limb including hip
4. Thorax
5. Abdomen (wall), gastric, gastrointestinal, intestine, stomach
6. Pelvis, buttock, groin, inguinal region, perineum
7. Trunk NOS, back NOS, flank NOS
8. Other specified sites
9. Site NOS

182.1 Endometrial isthmus M8930/3
182.0 Endometrial stroma uterine body, NOS M8930/3
171.# Epithelioid cell M8804/3
4th digit: 171
0. Head, face, neck
2. Upper limb including shoulder
3. Lower limb including hip
4. Thorax
5. Abdomen (wall), gastric, gastrointestinal, intestine, stomach
6. Pelvis, buttock, groin, inguinal region, perineum
7. Trunk NOS, back NOS, flank NOS
8. Other specified sites
9. Site NOS

170.# Ewing's M9260/3
4th digit: 170
0. Skull and face
1. Mandible
2. Vertebral column
3. Ribs, sternum, clavicle
4. Scapula, long bones of upper limb
5. Short bones of upper limb
6. Pelvic bones, sacrum, coccyx
7. Long bones of lower limb
8. Short bones of lower limb
9. Site NOS

SARCOMA (continued)

171.# Giant cell (except of bone)
4th digit: 171
0. Head, face, neck
2. Upper limb including shoulder
3. Lower limb including hip
4. Thorax
5. Abdomen (wall), gastric, gastrointestinal, intestine, stomach
6. Pelvis, buttock, groin, inguinal region, perineum
7. Trunk NOS, back NOS, flank NOS
8. Other specified sites
9. Site NOS

202.9# Follicular dendritic cell M8800/3
202.9# Interdigitating dendritic cell M8800/3
5th digit: 202.9
0. Unspecified site, extranodal and solid organ sites
1. Lymph nodes of head, face, neck
2. Lymph nodes intrathoracic
3. Lymph nodes abdominal
4. Lymph nodes axilla and upper limb
5. Lymph nodes inguinal region and lower limb
6. Lymph nodes intrapelvic
7. Spleen
8. Lymph nodes multiple sites

0 Internal organs see 'Cancer', by specified site

176.# Kaposi's M9140/3
4th digit: 176
0. Skin
1. Soft tissue
2. Soft palate
3. Gastrointestinal
4. Lung
5. Lymph nodes
8. Other specified sites (external genitalia) (scrotum) (vulva)
9. Site unspecified

155.0 Kupffer cell site NOS
202.9# Langerhans cell M8800/3
5th digit: 202.9
0. Unspecified site, extranodal and solid organ sites
1. Lymph nodes of head, face, neck
2. Lymph nodes intrathoracic
3. Lymph nodes abdominal
4. Lymph nodes axilla and upper limb
5. Lymph nodes inguinal region and lower limb
6. Lymph nodes intrapelvic
7. Spleen
8. Lymph nodes multiple sites

0 Mast cell see 'Cancer', by site M9740/3
191.9 Monstrocellular site NOS
0 Monstrocellular site specified see 'Cancer', by site M9481/3
205.3# Myeloid M9930/3
5th digit: 205.3
0. Without mention of remission
1. In remission

0 Osteogenic see 'Cancer', bone by site

SARCOMA (continued)

200.0# Reticulum cell NOS M9640/3
200.0# Reticulum cell pleomorphic cell type M9641/3
5th digit: 200.0
0. Unspecified site, extranodal and solid organ sites
1. Lymph nodes of head, face, neck
2. Lymph nodes intrathoracic
3. Lymph nodes abdominal
4. Lymph nodes axilla and upper limb
5. Lymph nodes inguinal region and lower limb
6. Lymph nodes intrapelvic
7. Spleen
8. Lymph nodes multiple sites

171.# Small cell M8803/3
171.# Spindle cell M8801/3
171.# Synovial M9040/3
171.# Synovial biphasic type M9043/3
171.# Synovial epithelioid cell type M9042/3
171.# Synovial spindle cell M9041/3
4th digit: 171
0. Head, face, neck
2. Upper limb including shoulder
3. Lower limb including hip
4. Thorax
5. Abdomen (wall), gastric, gastrointestinal, intestine, stomach
6. Pelvis, buttock, groin, inguinal region, perineum
7. Trunk NOS, back NOS, flank NOS
8. Other specified sites
9. Site NOS

SARCOMATOSIS

171.# NOS M8800/9
4th digit: 171
0. Head, face, neck
2. Upper limb including shoulder
3. Lower limb including hip
4. Thorax
5. Abdomen (wall), gastric, gastrointestinal, intestine, stomach
6. Pelvis, buttock, groin, inguinal region, perineum
7. Trunk NOS, back NOS, flank NOS
8. Other specified sites
9. Site NOS

192.1 Meningeal site NOS
0 Meningeal site specified see 'Cancer', by site M9539/3

133.0 SARCOPTES SCABIEI INFESTATION
133.0 SARCOPTIC ITCH SCABIES
270.8 SARCOSINEMIA
136.5 SARCOSPORIDIOSIS
079.82 SARS-ASSOCIATED CORONAVIRUS (SEVERE ACUTE RESPIRATORY SYNDROME)
V01.82 SARS-ASSOCIATED CORONAVIRUS (SEVERE ACUTE RESPIRATORY SYNDROME) EXPOSURE
480.3 SARS-ASSOCIATED CORONAVIRUS (SEVERE ACUTE RESPIRATORY SYNDROME) PNEUMONIA
780.94 SATIETY EARLY
354.3 SATURDAY NIGHT SYNDROME
302.89 SATYRIASIS

695.89 SAVILL'S DISEASE (EPIDEMIC EXFOLIATIVE DERMATITIS)
421.0 SBE (SUBACUTE BACTERIAL ENDOCARDITIS)
133.0 SCABIES (NORWEGIAN)
277.85 SCAD (SHORT CHAIN ACYL COA DEHYDROGENASE DEFICIENCY)
253.0 SCAGLIETTI-DAGNINI SYNDROME (ACROMEGALIC MACROSPONDYLITIS)
0 SCALD INJURY SEE 'BURN', BY SITE
695.1 SCALDED SKIN SYNDROME STAPHYLOCOCCAL (SSSS)
353.0 SCALENUS ANTICUS SYNDROME (NONDISCOGENIC)

S

SCALP INJURY

959.09 NOS
767.19 Birth trauma due to forceps
767.11 Birth trauma epicranial subaponeurotic hemorrhage (massive) (subgaleal)
767.19 Birth trauma other
910.8 Other and unspecified superficial
910.9 Other and unspecified superficial infected

767.8 SCALPEL WOUND (BIRTH TRAUMA)

SCAPULAR

755.59 Absence congenital
755.52 Elevation congenital
959.2 Injury unspecified (scapular region)
912.8 Region injury other and unspecified superficial
912.9 Region injury other and unspecified superficial infected

354.8 SCAPULOCOSTAL SYNDROME

SCAPULOHUMERAL

726.2 Fibrositis
726.2 Impingement
726.2 Myofibrosis
359.1 Myopathy

359.1 SCAPULOPERONEAL SYNDROME
723.4 SCAPULOVERTEBRAL SYNDROME

SCAR

709.2 NOS
654.6# Cervix complicating pregnancy
660.2# Cervix obstructing labor [654.6#]

5th digit: 654.6
0. Episode of care NOS or N/A
1. Delivered
2. Delivered with postpartum complication
3. Antepartum complication
4. Postpartum complication

5th digit: 660.2
0. Episode of care NOS or N/A
1. Delivered
3. Antepartum complication

SCAR (continued)

763.1 Cervix obstructing labor affecting fetus or newborn
654.2# Cesarean previous
660.2# Cesarean previous obstructing labor [654.2#]

5th digit: 654.2
0. Episode of care NOS or N/A
1. Delivered
2. Delivered with postpartum complication
3. Antepartum complication
4. Postpartum complication

5th digit: 660.2
0. Episode of care NOS or N/A
1. Delivered
3. Antepartum complication

763.89 Cesarean previous complicating pregnancy affecting fetus or newborn
701.4 Cheloid
363.3# Chorioretinal

5th digit: 363.3
0. NOS
2. Macular
3. Posterior pole NEC
4. Peripheral
5. Disseminated

0 Choroid see 'Scar', chorioretinal
423.9 Compression pericardial
757.39 Congenital NOS
372.64 Conjunctiva (post enucleation)
371.00 Cornea
264.6 Cornea due to vitamin A deficiency
264.6 Cornea xerophthalmic
709.2 Disfiguring
537.3 Duodenal (bulb) (cap)
571.9 Hepatic postnecrotic
701.4 Keloid
624.4 Labia
571.9 Liver postnecrotic
518.89 Lung (base)
363.32 Macula
363.35 Macula disseminated
363.34 Macula peripheral
728.89 Muscle
412 Myocardium post MI
709.2 Painful
429.81 Papillary muscle
423.9 Pericardial compression
363.33 Posterior pole retina
571.9 Postnecrotic hepatic
571.9 Postnecrotic liver
V15.4# Psychological history

5th digit: V15.4
1. Physical abuse, rape
2. Emotional abuse, neglect
9. Other

363.30 Retina
363.35 Retina disseminated
363.32 Retina other macular
363.33 Retina other posterior pole
363.34 Retina peripheral
363.31 Retina solar
0 Revision using plastic surgery (of old injury) - code 'Scar', by site

SCAR (continued)

709.2 Skin (adherent) (atrophic) (fibrosis)
709.2 Skin causing disfigurement
701.4 Skin keloid
478.9 Trachea
621.8 Uterine NEC
654.9# Uterine complicating pregnancy and childbirth
5th digit: 654.9
0. Episode of care NOS or N/A
1. Delivered
2. Delivered with postpartum complication
3. Antepartum complication
4. Postpartum complication

763.89 Uterine complicating pregnancy affecting fetus or newborn
0 Uterine from previous cesarean delivery see 'Scar', cesarean previous
623.4 Vagina
624.4 Vulva (old)

134.1 SCARABIASIS
034.1 SCARLATINAL ANGINA
695.0 SCARLATINIFORM ERYTHEMA
034.1 SCARLET FEVER
034.1 SCARLET FEVER OTITIS MEDIA [382.02]
V17.41 SCD (SUDDEN CARDIAC DEATH) FAMILY HISTORY
709.09 SCHAMBERG'S DISEASE (PROGRESSIVE PIGMENTARY DERMATOSIS)
530.3 SCHATZKI'S RING
750.3 SCHATZKI'S RING CONGENITAL
135 SCHAUMANN'S SYNDROME (SARCOIDOSIS)
277.5 SCHEIE'S SYNDROME (MUCOPOLYSACCHARIDOSIS IS)
117.1 SCHENCK'S DISEASE (SPOROTRICHOSIS)
732.0 SCHEUERMANN'S DISEASE (OSTEOCHONDROSIS)
755.59 SCHEUTHAUER-MARIE-SAINTON SYNDROME (CLEIDOCRANIALIS DYSOSTOSIS)
V74.3 SCHICK SCREENING EXAM
341.1 SCHILDER'S DISEASE
610.1 SCHIMMELBUSCH'S DISEASE (HYPERPLASIA)
759.6 SCHIRMER'S SYNDROME (ENCEPHALOCUTANEOUS ANGIOMATOSIS)
756.79 SCHISTOCELIA

SCHISTOSOMA, SCHISTOSOMIASIS

120.9 Infection
120.2 Asiatic
120.0 Bladder
120.8 Bovis infection
120.3 Cercariae infection
120.8 Chestermani
120.1 Colon
120.3 Cutaneous
120.3 Dermatitis
120.2 Eastern
120.0 Genitourinary tract
120.0 Haematobium
120.8 Intercalatum
120.1 Intestinal
120.2 Japonicum
120.2 Katayama
120.2 Lung
120.1 Mansoni

SCHISTOSOMA, SCHISTOSOMIASIS (continued)

120.8 Mattheii
120.2 Oriental
120.2 Pulmonary
V75.5 Screening exam
120.8 Spindale infection
120.0 Vesical
120.8 Other specified

742.4 SCHIZENCEPHALY
0 SCHIZO-AFFECTIVE DISORDER SEE 'SCHIZOPHRENIA'
313.22 SCHIZOID DISORDER CHILDHOOD / ADOLESCENCE
301.20 SCHIZOID PERSONALITY DISORDER
301.21 SCHIZOID PERSONALITY DISORDER - INTROVERTED
301.22 SCHIZOID PERSONALITY DISORDER - SCHIZOTYPAL
0 SCHIZOMYCETOMA (ACTINOMYCOTIC) SEE 'ACTINOMYCOSIS'

SCHIZOPHRENIA

295.9# NOS
295.8# Atypical
295.2# Catalepsy
295.2# Catatonic
295.8# Cenesthopathic
299.90 Childhood type NOS, active state
299.91 Childhood type NOS, residual state
295.6# Chronic undifferentiated
295.7# Cyclic NOS
295.4# Cyclic acute
295.1# Disorganized type
295.2# Flexibilitas cerea
295.1# Hebephrenic
V11.0 History
295.5# Latent (borderline) (incipient) (prepsychotic)
5th digit: 295.1-2, 4-9
0. NOS
1. Subchronic
2. Chronic
3. Subchronic with acute exacerbation
4. Chronic with acute
5. In remission

Specify the maternal schizophrenia with an additional code. See 'Schizophrenia'.

648.4# Maternal current (co-existent) in pregnancy
5th digit: 648.4
0. Episode of care NOS or N/A
1. Delivered
2. Delivered with postpartum complication
3. Antepartum complication
4. Postpartum complication

295.9# Mixed
295.7# Mixed with affective psychosis
5th digit: 295.3, 5-7, 9
0. NOS
1. Subchronic
2. Chronic
3. Subchronic with acute exacerbation
4. Chronic with acute
5. In remission

SCHIZOPHRENIA (continued)

295.3# Paranoid
295.3# Paraphrenic
295.5# Prodromal
295.5# Pseudoneurotic
295.5# Pseudopsychopathic
295.9# Reaction
295.6# Residual type
295.6# Restzustand
295.7# Schizoaffective disorder
301.20 Schizoid personality
295.9# Schizophrenic reaction acute
295.8# Schizophrenic undifferentiated acute
295.4# Schizophreniform attack
295.9# Schizophreniform psychosis acute
295.7# Schizophreniform psychosis,affective type
295.4# Schizophreniform psychosis, confusional type
295.0# Simple
299.90 Syndrome of childhood, active state
299.91 Syndrome of childhood, residual state
295.8# Undifferentiated acute
295.9# Undifferentiated type

5th digit: 295.0, 4, 7-9
0. NOS
1. Subchronic
2. Chronic
3. Subchronic with acute exacerbation
4. Chronic with acute
5. In remission

301.22 SCHIZOTYPAL PERSONALITY DISORDER
732.4 SCHLATTER-OSGOOD DISEASE
732.4 SCHLATTER'S TIBIA (TUBERCLE)
567.29 SCHLOFFER'S TUMOR SEE ALSO PERITONITIS
352.6 SCHMIDT'S SYNDROME (SPHALLO-PHARYNGO-LARYNGEAL HEMIPLEGIA)
258.1 SCHMIDT'S SYNDROME (THYROID-ADRENOCORTICAL INSUFFICIENCY)
352.6 SCHMIDT'S SYNDROME (VAGOACCESSORY)

SCHMORL'S NODES

722.30 NOS
722.32 Lumbar
722.31 Thoracic
722.39 Other

047.9 SCHNEIDER'S SYNDROME
160.0 SCHNEIDERIAN CARCINOMA SITE NOS
0 SCHNEIDERIAN CARCINOMA SITE SPECIFIED SEE 'CANCER', BY SITE M8121/3
273.1 SCHNITZLER SYNDROME
567.29 SCHOFFER'S TUMOR SEE ALSO PERITONITIS
259.2 SCHOLTE'S SYNDROME (MALIGNANT CARCINOID)
330.0 SCHOLZ'S (-BIELSCHOWSKY-HENNEBERG) DISEASE OR SYNDROME
287.0 SCHONLEIN (-HENOCH) DISEASE (PURPURA RHEUMATICA)
V70.5 SCHOOL EXAM (HEALTH)
002.9 SCHOTTMULLER'S DISEASE (SEE ALSO 'PARATYPHOID FEVER')
255.3 SCHROEDER'S SYNDROME (ENDOCRINE-HYPERTENSIVE)
277.89 SCHULLER-CHRISTIAN DISEASE OR SYNDROME (CHRONIC HISTIOCYTOSIS X)
288.09 SCHULTZ'S DISEASE OR SYNDROME (AGRANULOCYTOSIS)
V74.8 SCHULTZ CHARLTON SCREENING EXAM
288.02 SCHWACHMAN'S SYNDROME
333.6 SCHWALBE ZIEHEN OPPENHEIM DISEASE
0 SCHWANNOMA BENIGN SEE 'BENIGN NEOPLASM', BY SITE M9560/0
0 SCHWANNOMA MALIGNANT SEE 'CANCER', BY SITE M9560/3
359.23 SCHWARTZ (-JAMEL) SYNDROME
253.6 SCHWARTZ-BARTTER SYNDROME (INAPPROPRIATE SECRETION OF ANTIDIURETIC HORMONE)
701.3 SCHWENINGER-BUZZI DISEASE (MACULAR ATROPHY)

SCIATIC

0 Hernia see 'Hernia', sciatic
355.0 Nerve disorder
355.0 Nerve entrapment
956.0 Nerve injury
355.0 Nerve lesion
724.3 Nerve neuralgia (sciatica unspecified)
724.3 Nerve neuritis
355.0 Neuropathy

SCIATICA

722.10 Discogenic
722.73 Discogenic with myelopathy
355.0 Due to specified lesion
724.3 Nonvertebral (nondiscogenic)
724.3 Wallet

794.19 SCIATIPHOTOGRAPHY ABNORMAL
747.49 SCIMITAR SYNDROME (ANOMALOUS VENOUS DRAINAGE, RIGHT LUNG TO INFERIOR VENA CAVA)
368.12 SCINTILLATING SCOTOMA
199.1 SCIRRHOUS ADENOCARCINOMA SITE NOS
0 SCIRRHOUS ADENOCARCINOMA SITE SPECIFIED SEE 'CANCER', BY SITE M8141/3

SCLERA, SCLERAL

379.09 Abscess
743.47 Anomalies specified congenital
743.47 Blue (congenital)
379.16 Calcification
379.16 Disorders degenerative other
379.19 Disorders other
379.11 Ectasia
379.11 Staphyloma
379.14 Staphyloma - anterior localized
379.13 Staphyloma - equatorial
379.12 Staphyloma - posticum
379.15 Staphyloma - ring

778.1 SCLEREMA NEONATORUM

SCLERITIS

379.00 NOS
379.02 And episcleritis nodular
379.01 And episcleritis periodica fugax
379.03 Anterior
379.06 Brawny
379.05 Corneal involvement
379.01 Periodica fugax
379.07 Posterior
095.0 Syphilitic

256.4 SCLEROCYSTIC OVARY SYNDROME

701.0 SCLERODACTYLIA

SCLERODERMA

710.1 NOS
701.0 Circumscribed
701.0 Circumscribed or localized
710.1 Myopathy [359.6]
710.1 With lung involvement [517.2]

379.04 SCLEROMALACIA PERFORANS

379.05 SCLEROPERIKERATITIS

193 SCLEROSING CARCINOMA (NONENCAPSULATED) SITE NOS

0 SCLEROSING CARCINOMA (NONENCAPSULATED) SITE SPECIFIED SEE 'CANCER', BY SITE M8350/3

SCLEROSIS

255.8 Adrenal (gland)
331.0 Alzheimer's
331.0 Alzheimer's with dementia [**294.1#**]
5th digit: 294.1
0. Without behavioral disturbance or NOS
1. With behavioral disturbance

335.20 Amyotrophic (lateral)
424.1 Annularis fibrosi aortic
424.0 Annularis fibrosi mitral
440.0 Aorta, aortic
424.1 Aortic valve see also 'Endocarditis Aortic'
340 Ascending multiple
341.1 Balo's (concentric)
733.99 Bone (localized) NEC
0 Brain see 'Brain', sclerosis
340 Bulbar progressive
426.50 Bundle of HIS NOS
426.3 Bundle of HIS left
426.4 Bundle of HIS right
404.90 Cardiorenal
429.2 Cardiovascular
404.90 Cardiovascular renal
330.0 Centrolobar familial
340 Cerebrospinal (disseminated) (multiple)
437.0 Cerebrovascular
363.40 Choroid
363.56 Choroid diffuse
341.1 Concentric balos
370.54 Cornea
0 Coronary see 'Arteriosclerosis, Arteriosclerotic', coronary
624.8 Corpus cavernosum female
607.89 Corpus cavernosum male
424.1 Dewitzky's aortic
424.0 Dewitzky's mitral
341.1 Diffuse NEC
0 Disease heart see 'Arteriosclerosis, Arteriosclerotic', coronary
340 Disseminated
340 Dorsal
621.8 Endometrium
333.90 Extrapyramidal
366.16 Eye nuclear (senile)

SCLEROSIS (continued)

334.0 Friedreich's (spinal cord)
608.89 Funicular (spermatic cord)
535.4# Gastritis
5th digit: 535.4
0. Without hemorrhage
1. With hemorrhage

457.8 Gland (lymphatic)
571.9 Hepatic
334.2 Hereditary cerebellar
334.0 Hereditary spinal
730.1# Idiopathic cortical (Garre's)
5th digit: 730.1
0. Site NOS
1. Shoulder region
2. Upper arm (elbow) (humerus)
3. Forearm (radius) (wrist) (ulna)
4. Hand (carpal) (metacarpal) (fingers)
5. Pelvic region and thigh (hip) (buttock) (femur)
6. Lower leg (fibula) (knee) (patella) (tibia)
7. Ankle and/or foot (metatarsals) (toes)
8. Other (head) (neck) (rib) (skull) (vertebrae)
9. Multiple

733.5 Ilium piriform
340 Insular
251.8 Insular pancreas
251.8 Islands of langerhans
478.79 Larynx
571.9 Liver
515 Lung NOS
383.1 Mastoid
440.20 Monckeberg's (medial) see also 'Arteriosclerosis, Arteriosclerotic', extremities
340 Multiple (brain stem) (cerebral) (generalized) (spinal cord)
366.16 Nuclear (senile) eye
620.8 Ovary
577.8 Pancreas
607.89 Penis
440.20 Peripheral arteries NEC
440.20 Peripheral arteries NEC with chronic complete or total occlusion [440.4]
733.5 Piriform of ilium
340 Plaques
258.8 Pluriglandular
258.8 Polyglandular
094.0 Posterior (spinal cord) (syphilitic)
607.89 Prepuce
335.24 Primary lateral
710.1 Progressive systemic
710.1 Progressive systemic with lung involvement [517.2]
710.1 Progressive systemic with myopathy [359.6]
515 Pulmonary
416.0 Pulmonary artery
424.3 Pulmonary valve
587 Renal
362.17 Retina (senile) (vascular)
395.9 Rheumatic aortic valve
394.9 Rheumatic mitral valve
341.1 Schilder's

S

SCLEROSIS (continued)

SPINAL

336.8 NOS (cord) (general) (progressive) (transverse)
357.0 Ascending
340 Disseminated
334.0 Hereditary (Friedreich's) (mixed)
335.24 Lateral
340 Multiple
094.0 Posterior (syphilitic)

SCLEROSIS (continued)

537.89 Stomach
425.3 Subendocardial congenital
710.1 Systemic progressive
710.1 Systemic progressive with lung involvement [517.2]
759.5 Tuberous (brain)
385.00 Tympanic membrane see also 'Tympanosclerosis'
459.89 Vein

379.07 SCLEROTENONITIS

SCOLIOSIS

737.30 NOS
737.30 And kyphoscoliosis idiopathic
737.43 Associated with other conditions
356.1 Charcot Marie tooth [737.43]
737.33 Due to radiation
737.31 Infantile idiopathic (resolving)
277.5 Mucopolysaccharidosis [737.43]
237.7# Neurofibromatosis [737.43]

5th digit: 237.7
0. Unspecified
1. Type I
2. Type II

252.01 Osteitis fibrosa cystica [737.43]
733.0# Osteoporosis [737.43]

5th digit: 733.0
0. Unspecified
1. Senile
2. Idiopathic
3. Disuse
9. Other

045.## Poliomyelitis acute [737.43]

4th digit: 045
0. Acute bulbar paralytic
1. Acute with other paralysis
2. Acute non paralytic
9. Acute unspecified

5th digit: 045
0. NOS
1. Type I
2. Type II
3. Type III

138 Poliomyelitis late effect [737.43]
754.2 Postural congenital
737.32 Progressive infantile idiopathic
737.34 Thoracogenic
237.7# Von Recklinghausen's disease [737.43]

5th digit: 237.7
0. NOS or multiple
1. Type I
2. Type II

737.39 Other

SCOTOMA

368.44 NOS
368.43 Arcuate
368.43 Bjerrum
368.42 Blind spot area
368.41 Central
368.41 Centrocecal
368.42 Paracecal
368.41 Paracentral
368.12 Scintillating
368.43 Seidel

784.99 SCRATCHY THROAT

SCREENING

V82.9 Unspecified condition
V79.1 Alcoholism
V28.1 Alpha fetoprotein levels in amniotic fluid
V78.0 Anemia
V78.1 Anemia deficiency unspecified
V82.89 Anomaly, congenital
V28.9 Antenatal - NOS
V28.1 Antenatal - alphafetoprotein level by amniocentesis
V28.2 Antenatal - amniocentesis
V28.0 Antenatal - chromosomal anomaly by amniocentesis
V28.9 Antenatal – of mother
V28.8 Antenatal - other specified
V73.5 Arthropod borne viral
V81.4 Asthma
V74.5 Bacterial and spirochetal
V74.8 Bacterial spirochetal diseases other specified
V81.5 Bacteriuria asymptomatic
V28.2 Based on amniocentesis other
V78.9 Blood disorders
V78.8 Blood disorders other specified
V78.9 Blood forming organs disorder
V78.8 Blood forming organs disorder other specified
V81.3 Bronchitis (chronic)
V74.8 Brucellosis
V76.9 Cancer NOS
V76.3 Cancer bladder
V76.89 Cancer blood
V76.10 Cancer breast unspecified
V76.11 Cancer breast mammogram for high risk patient
V76.12 Cancer breast mammogram NEC
V76.19 Cancer breast specified type NEC
V76.2 Cancer cervix
V76.51 Cancer colon
V76.51 Cancer colorectal
V76.89 Cancer hematopoietic system
V76.50 Cancer intestinal - unspecified
V76.51 Cancer intestinal - colon
V76.52 Cancer intestinal - small
V76.89 Cancer lymph (glands)
V76.81 Cancer nervous system
V76.42 Cancer oral cavity
V76.46 Cancer ovary
V76.44 Cancer prostate
V76.41 Cancer rectal
V76.0 Cancer respiratory organs
V76.43 Cancer skin
V76.45 Cancer testis
V76.47 Cancer vagina
V76.49 Cancer other sites
V81.2 Cardiovascular conditions
V80.2 Cataract
V75.3 Chagas' disease

SCREENING (continued)

V82.5 Chemical poisoning and other contamination
V73.98 Chlamydia
V73.88 Chlamydia other specified
V74.0 Cholera
V77.91 Cholesterol
V28.0 Chromosomal anomalies by amniocentesis
V82.4 Chromosomal anomalies maternal postnatal
V82.89 Congenital anomaly
V82.3 Congenital hip dislocation
V74.4 Conjunctivitis (bacterial)
V77.6 Cystic fibrosis
V73.5 Dengue fever
V79.0 Depression
V79.9 Developmental handicaps
V79.3 Developmental handicaps in early childhood
V79.8 Developmental handicaps other
V77.1 Diabetes mellitus
V74.3 Diphtheria
V70.3 Drug administrative
V70.4 Drug medicolegal
V80.3 Ear diseases
V81.3 Emphysema
V73.5 Encephalitis viral (mosquito borne) (tick borne)
V77.99 Endocrine disorder
V80.2 Eye anomaly congenital
V80.2 Eye conditions other
V28.4 Fetal growth retardation using ultrasonics
V75.6 Filariasis
V77.4 Galactosemia
V81.6 Genitourinary conditions other and unspecified
V80.1 Glaucoma
V77.5 Gout
V82.5 Heavy metal poisoning
V75.7 Helminthiasis intestinal
V76.89 Hematopoietic malignancy
V78.3 Hemoglobinopathies other
V73.5 Hemorrhagic fever
V73.89 HIV
V76.89 Hodgkin's disease
V73.81 HPV (human papillomavirus)
V73.81 Human papillomavirus (HPV)
V77.91 Hypercholesterolemia
V77.91 Hyperlipidemia
V81.1 Hypertension
V77.99 Immunity disorders
V75.9 Infectious disease
V78.0 Iron deficiency anemia
V81.0 Ischemic heart disease
V28.5 Isoimmunization antenatal
V75.2 Leishmaniasis
V74.2 Leprosy
V74.8 Leptospirosis
V76.89 Leukemia
V77.91 Lipoid disorders
V76.89 Lymphoma
V80.2 Macular senile lesions
V75.1 Malaria
V28.3 Malformation using ultrasonics antenatal
V77.2 Malnutrition
V76.11 Mammogram for high risk patient
V76.12 Mammogram NEC
V73.2 Measles
V79.9 Mental disorders
V79.8 Mental disorders other
V79.2 Mental retardation

SCREENING (continued)

V77.99 Metabolic disorders
V77.7 Metabolism (other inborn errors)
V77.6 Mucoviscidosis
V82.6 Multiphasic
V75.4 Mycotic infections
V76.89 Neoplasms other (benign) (tumors)
V80.0 Neurological conditions
V77.99 Nutritional disorders
V77.8 Obesity
V82.81 Osteoporosis
V82.81 Osteoporosis with hormone therapy status (postmenopausal) [V07.4]
V82.81 Osteoporosis with postmenopausal (natural) status [V49.81]
V75.8 Parasitic infections other
V77.3 Phenylketonuria
V74.8 Plague
V82.5 Poisoning from contaminated water supply
V73.0 Poliomyelitis
V82.5 Radiation exposure
V82.5 Radioactive substance ingestion
V81.4 Respiratory conditions
V82.2 Rheumatic disorders
V82.1 Rheumatoid arthritis
V75.0 Rickettsial diseases
V73.3 Rubella
V75.5 Schistosomiasis
V74.5 Sexually transmitted disease NOS (bacterial and spirochetal)
V78.2 Sickle cell disease or trait
V82.0 Skin conditions
V75.3 Sleeping sickness
V73.1 Smallpox
V28.6 Streptococcus B antenatal
V74.5 Syphilis
V74.8 Tetanus
V77.0 Thyroid disorders
V73.6 Trachoma
V74.1 Tuberculosis
V74.5 Venereal disease
V73.99 Viral disease unspecified
V73.89 Viral disease other specified
V82.5 Water supply contamination
V74.8 Whooping cough
V74.6 Yaws
V73.4 Yellow fever
V82.89 Other specified conditions

V54.09 SCREW AFTERCARE NEC (ORTHOPEDIC)
V54.01 SCREW REMOVAL (ORTHOPEDIC)
017.2# SCROFULA
017.0# SCROFULODERMA

5th digit: 017.0, 2
0. NOS
1. Lab not done
2. Lab pending
3. Microscopy positive (in sputum)
4. Culture positive - microscopy negative
5. Culture negative - microscopy positive
6. Culture and microscopy negative confirmed by other methods

S

S

SCROTUM, SCROTAL

608.4 Abscess (cellulitis) (boil) (carbuncle)
752.89 Absence (agenesis) congenital
752.9 Anomaly congenital NOS
752.89 Anomaly congenital NEC
608.89 Atrophy (fibrosis) (hypertrophy) (ulcer)
752.89 Bifid
608.4 Cellulitis
608.9 Disorder NOS
608.83 Hemorrhage (thrombosis) (hematoma) nontraumatic
959.14 Injury NEC
878.2 Injury traumatic
878.3 Injury traumatic with open wound
911.8 Injury other and unspecified superficial
911.9 Injury other and unspecified superficial infected
608.89 Necrosis
608.4 Nodule inflammatory
752.81 Transposition
456.4 Varices

081.2 SCRUB TYPHUS
267 SCURVY (VITAMIN C DEFICIENCY)
272.7 SEA-BLUE HISTIOCYTE SYNDROME
275.49 SEABRIGHT-BANTAM SYNDROME (PSEUDOHYPOPARATHYROIDISM)
994.6 SEASICKNESS
909.4 SEASICKNESS LATE EFFECT
989.5 SEA SNAKE BITE
<u>995.0</u> SEA SNAKE BITE WITH <u>ANAPHYLAXIS</u> [989.5]
309.1 SEASONAL AFFECTIVE DISORDER (SAD)
477.0 SEASONAL ALLERGIC RHINITIS

SEBACEOUS

706.2 Cyst
610.8 Cyst breast
374.84 Cyst eyelid
629.89 Cyst genital organs NEC - female
608.89 Cyst genital organs NEC - male
706.2 Cyst scrotum
706.9 Gland disease NEC
706.8 Gland disease other specified

SEBORRHEA, SEBORRHEIC

706.3 NOS
690.11 Capitis
695.4 Congestiva
706.3 Corporis
690.10 Dermatitis NOS
690.12 Dermatitis infantile
690.18 Dermatitis other
690.18 Eczema
690.12 Eczema infantile
702.1# Keratosis
5th digit: 702.1
1. Inflamed
9. Other

705.89 Nigricans
690.18 Sicca
702.1# Wart
5th digit: 702.1
1. Inflamed
9. Other

759.89 SECKEL'S SYNDROME

377.10 SECOND CRANIAL NERVE ATROPHY
377.49 SECOND CRANIAL NERVE DISORDER OTHER NEC
426.13 SECOND DEGREE HEART BLOCK AV OTHER
664.1# SECOND DEGREE LACERATION (PERINEAL)
5th digit: 664.1
0. Episode of care NOS or N/A
1. Delivered
4. Postpartum complication

362.65 SECONDARY PIGMENTARY RETINAL DEGENERATION
661.1# SECONDARY UTERINE INERTIA
5th digit: 661.1
0. Episode of care NOS or N/A
1. Delivered
3. Antepartum complication

362.66 SECONDARY VITREORETINAL DEGENERATION
782.3 SECRETAN'S DISEASE OR SYNDROME (POSTTRAUMATIC EDEMA)
710.2 SECRETOINHIBITOR SYNDROME (KERATOCONJUNCTIVITIS SICCA)

668.##: Use an additional code to further specify the complication of anesthesia or other sedation.

SEDATION COMPLICATING L&D

668.9# NOS
668.1# Cardiac
668.2# Central nervous system
668.0# Pulmonary
668.8# Other specified
5th digit: 668.0-9
0. Episode of care NOS or N/A
1. Delivered
2. Delivered with postpartum complication
3. Antepartum complication
4. Postpartum complication

305.4# SEDATIVE ABUSE NONDEPENDENT
304.1# SEDATIVE ADDICTION NEC (DEPENDENT)
5th digit: 304.1, 305.4
0. NOS
1. Continuous
2. Episodic
3. In remission

790.1 SED RATE ELEVATED
790.1 SEDIMENTATION RATE ELEVATED
301.59 SEDUCTIVE PERSONALITY DISORDER
757.1 SEELIGMANN'S SYNDROME (ICHTHYOSIS CONGENITA)
0 SEGMENTAL DYSFUNCTION SEE 'SOMATIC DYSFUNCTION'

SEIZURE

780.39 NOS
780.39 Convulsive
780.39 Disorder
438.89 Due to stroke
0 Epileptic see 'Seizure Epileptic'
780.39 Epileptiform, epileptoid
780.31 Febrile NOS (simple)
780.32 Febrile complex (atypical) (complicated)
345.3 Febrile with status epilepticus
780.39 Infantile

SEIZURE (continued)

779.0 Newborn
345.9# Recurrent
5th digit: 345.0-9
0. Without mention of intractable epilepsy
1. With intractable epilepsy
780.39 Repetitive
780.39 Unknown etiology

SEIZURE EPILEPTIC

345.9# NOS
345.7# Epilepsia partialis continua
345.5# Focal (motor)
345.1# Generalized grand mal convulsive
345.0# Generalized petit mal nonconvulsive
345.3 Grand mal status
345.6# Infantile spasms
345.4# Partial with impairment of consciousness
345.5# Partial without impairment of consciousness
345.2 Petit mal status
345.8# Other
5th digit: 345.0-9
0. Without mention of intractable epilepsy
1. With intractable epilepsy

V69.8 SELF-DAMAGING BEHAVIOR PROBLEM

300.9 SELF-MUTILATION

792.2 SEMEN ABNORMAL

608.82 SEMEN BLOODY

780.09 SEMICOMA

780.09 SEMICONSCIOUSNESS

SEMILUNAR CARTILAGE

717.89 Calcification
717.5 Derangement (knee) old
717.5 Disease cystic
836.2 Tear (knee) acute

SEMINAL VESICLE

608.0 Abscess (cellulitis)
V45.77 Absence acquired
752.89 Absence congenital
752.89 Agenesis congenital
752.89 Anomaly (duct) (tract)
752.89 Atresia congenital
608.89 Atrophy (fibrosis) (hypertrophy) (ulcer)
608.9 Disorder
608.83 Hemorrhage (thrombosis) (hematoma) nontraumatic
867.6 Injury (traumatic)
867.7 Injury with open wound into cavity
908.2 Injury late effect

SEMINAL VESICULITIS

608.0 NOS
098.14 Gonococcal acute
098.34 Gonococcal chronic

257.2 SEMIFEROUS TUBULE FAILURE (ADULT)

SEMINOMA

186.9 Site NOS
0 Site specified see 'Cancer', by site M9061/3
186.9 Anaplastic type site NOS
0 Anaplastic type site specified see 'Cancer', by site M9062/3
186.9 Spermatocytic site NOS
0 Spermatocytic site specified see 'Cancer', by site M9063/3

694.4 SENEAR-USHER DISEASE OR SYNDROME (PEMPHIGUS ERYTHEMATOSUS)

797 SENESCENCE CAUSE OF MORBIDITY AND MORTALITY

SENILE

797 Asthenia cause of morbidity and mortality
797 Atrophy
701.8 Atrophy skin
701.3 Atrophy skin degenerative
371.41 Corneal changes
797 Debility cause of morbidity and mortality
331.2 Degeneration of brain
331.2 Degeneration of brain with dementia [294.1#]
5th digit: 294.1
0. Without behavioral disturbance or NOS
1. With behavioral disturbance
701.3 Degenerative atrophy
694.5 Dermatitis herpetiformis
709.3 Dermatosis
797 Exhaustion cause of morbidity and mortality
362.52 Macular degeneration disciform
362.64 Reticular degeneration
702.0 Wart

SENILE PSYCHOSIS (DEMENTIA)

290.9 NOS
290.0 Uncomplicated
290.20 Delusional
290.3 With delirium
290.20 With delusion
290.21 With depressive features
290.8 Other

702.0 SENILIS KERATOSIS

259.8 SENILISM SYNDROME

310.1 SENILITY NONPSYCHOTIC

797 SENILITY WITHOUT PSYCHOSIS CAUSE OF MORBIDITY AND MORTALITY

Use additional code to identify the altered sensation.

438.6 SENSATION DISTURBANCE LATE EFFECT OF CVA

782.0 SENSATION DISTURBANCE SKIN

521.89 SENSITIVE DENTINE

297.8 SENSITIVER BEZIEHUNGSWAHN

313.21 SENSITIVITY REACTION OF CHILDHOOD AND ADOLESCENCE

289.89 SENSITIVITY SUXAMETHONIUM

SENSORY

780.39 And motor attack
781.8 Extinction

Code first hearing and/or visual impairment.

V49.85 Impairment dual blindness with deafness (combined visual impairment)
781.8 Neglect
V48.4 Problem - head
V48.5 Problem - neck
V48.5 Problem - trunk

079.81 SEOUL VIRUS

0 SEPARATION SEE 'DISLOCATION'

309.21 SEPARATION ANXIETY

When coding sepsis, the underlying cause of the systemic infection (038.#(#)) or trauma should be reported first. The SIRS code (995.##) sequences next. The initial localized infection, if known, would be reported after the SIRS code. In a case where an unspecified sepsis is documented, code first 038.9 unspecified organism, followed by the SIRS code. When coding sepsis in a fetus, newborn or pregnancy it is not necessary to assign the 995.## codes.

SEPSIS

038.#(#) NOS [995.91]
4th or 4th and 5th digit code for organism: 038
.9 NOS
.3 Anaerobic
.3 Bacteroides
.3 Clostridium
.42 E. coli
.49 Enterobacter aerogenes
.40 Gram negative
.49 Gram negative other
.41 Hemophilus influenzae
.2 Pneumococcal
.49 Proteus
.43 Pseudomonas
.44 Serratia
.10 Staphylococcal NOS
.11 Staphylococcal aureus
.19 Staphylococcal other
.0 Streptococcal (anaerobic)
.49 Yersinia enterocolitica
.8 Other specified

771.81 Fetus intrauterine
639.0 Following abortion/ectopic/molar pregnancy

999.39 Other infection - Use an additional code to identify the specified infection such as septicemia, (038.#(#)).

999.39 Following infusion injection transfusion or vaccination
771.81 Naval newborn
771.81 Newborn (fetus) - gonococcal [098.89]
771.81 Newborn (fetus) - herpetic [054.5]
771.81 Newborn (fetus) - salmonella [003.1]
771.81 Newborn (fetus) - viral NOS [079.99]
771.81 Newborn (fetus) - other
999.39 Post transfusion
998.59 Postoperative

SEPSIS (continued)

0 Severe see 'SIRS', due to infectious process, with organ dysfunction
0 Severe with multiple organ dysfunction see 'SIRS', due to infectious process with multiple organ dysfunction
771.81 Umbilical newborn
038.#(#) Urinary meaning sepsis [995.91]
4th or 4th and 5th digit code for organism: 038
.9 NOS
.3 Anaerobic
.3 Bacteroides
.3 Clostridium
.42 E. coli
.49 Enterobacter aerogenes
.40 Gram negative
.49 Gram negative other
.41 Hemophilus influenzae
.2 Pneumococcal
.49 Proteus
.43 Pseudomonas
.44 Serratia
.10 Staphylococcal NOS
.11 Staphylococcal aureus
.19 Staphylococcal other
.0 Streptococcal (anaerobic)
.49 Yersinia enterocolitica
.8 Other specified

599.0 Urinary meaning urinary tract infection
079.99 Viral
0 With acute organ dysfunction see 'SIRS', due to infectious process with specified acute organ dysfunction
0 With shock see 'SIRS', due to infectious process with shock

SEPSIS COMPLICATING LABOR, PREGNANCY, PUERPERIUM

771.81 Fetus or newborn - gonococcal [098.89]
771.81 Fetus or newborn - herpetic [054.5]
771.81 Fetus or newborn - salmonella [003.1]
771.81 Fetus or newborn - viral NOS [079.99]
771.81 Fetus or newborn - other
639.0 Following abortion/ectopic/molar pregnancy
647.8# Maternal current (coexistent) (major infection)
5th digit: 647.8
0. Episode of care NOS or N/A
1. Delivered
2. Delivered with postpartum complication
3. Antepartum complication
4. Postpartum complication

670.0# Maternal due to pregnancy postpartum (puerperal) (major infection)
5th digit: 670.0
0. NOS
2. Delivered with postpartum complication
4. Postpartum complication

659.3# Maternal during labor
5th digit: 659.3
0. Episode of care NOS or N/A
1. Delivered
3. Antepartum complication

639.0 Post abortion or ectopic/molar pregnancy

0 SEPTAL SEE 'SEPTUM, SEPTAL'

654.7# SEPTATE VAGINA COMPLICATING CHILDBIRTH AND PREGNANCY

660.2# SEPTATE VAGINA OBSTRUCTING LABOR **[654.7#]**

5th digit: 654.7
0. Episode of care NOS or N/A
1. Delivered
2. Delivered with postpartum complication
3. Antepartum complication
4. Postpartum complication

5th digit: 660.2
0. Episode of care NOS or N/A
1. Delivered
3. Antepartum complication

034.0 SEPTIC ANGINA

999.8 SEPTIC SHOCK DUE TO TRANSFUSION

034.0 SEPTIC SORE THROAT

SEPTICEMIA

038.9 NOS
038.49 Aerobacter aerogenes
038.3 Anaerobic
038.0 Anaerobic streptococcal
022.3 Anthrax
038.42 Bacillus coli
038.3 Bacteroides
569.61 Cecostomy **[038.#(#)]**
038.3 Clostridium
569.61 Colostomy **[038.#(#)]**
038.9 Cryptogenic
038.42 E coli
038.49 Enterobacter aerogenes
569.61 Enterostomy **[038.#(#)]**
027.1 Erysipelothrix insidiosa (E. Rhusiopathiae)
038.42 Escherichia coli
771.81 Fetus intrauterine
639.0 Following abortion/ectopic/molar pregnancy

999.39 Other infection - Use an additional code to identify the specified infection such as septicemia, (038.#(#)).

999.39 Following infusion, injection, transfusion or vaccination
038.49 Friedlander's (bacillus)
038.9 Gangrenous
536.41 Gastrostomy **[038.#(#)]**
098.89 Gonococcal
038.40 Gram negative
038.3 Gram negative anaerobic
038.49 Gram negative other
038.41 Hemophilus influenzae
054.5 Herpes simplex

SEPTICEMIA (continued)

569.61 Ileostomy **[038.#(#)]**
569.61 Jejunostomy **[038.#(#)]**

4th or 4th and 5th digit code for organism: 038
.9 NOS
.3 Anaerobic
.3 Bacteroides
.3 Clostridium
.42 E. coli
.49 Enterobacter aerogenes
.40 Gram negative
.49 Gram negative other
.41 Hemophilus influenzae
.2 Pneumococcal
.49 Proteus
.43 Pseudomonas
.44 Serratia
.10 Staphylococcal NOS
.11 Staphylococcal aureus
.19 Staphylococcal other
.0 Streptococcal (anaerobic)
.49 Yersinia enterocolitica
.8 Other specified

027.0 Listeria monocytogenes
036.2 Meningococcal
038.9 Nadir
771.81 Navel newborn
771.81 Newborn
771.81 Newborn (fetus) - gonococcal [098.89]
771.81 Newborn (fetus) - herpetic [054.5]
771.81 Newborn (fetus) - salmonella [003.1]
771.81 Newborn (fetus) - viral NOS [079.99]
771.81 Newborn (fetus) - other
020.2 Plague
038.2 Pneumococcal

999.39 Other infection - Use an additional code to identify the specified infection such as septicemia, (038.#(#).).

999.39 Post transfusion
998.59 Postoperative **[038.#(#)]**
038.49 Proteus vulgaris
038.43 Pseudomonas
003.1 Salmonella
038.44 Serratia
004.9 Shigella
038.8 Specified oganism NEC
038.1# Staphylococcal

5th digit: 038.1
0. NOS
1. Aureus
9. Other staph

038.0 Streptococcal
038.2 Streptococcus pneumoniae
003.1 Suipestifer

S

SEPTICEMIA (continued)

519.01 Tracheostomy [038.#(#)]
4th or 4th and 5th digit code for organism: 038
.9 NOS
.3 Anaerobic
.3 Bacteroides
.3 Clostridium
.42 E. coli
.49 Enterobacter aerogenes
.40 Gram negative
.49 Gram negative other
.41 Hemophilus influenzae
.2 Pneumococcal
.49 Proteus
.43 Pseudomonas
.44 Serratia
.10 Staphylococcal NOS
.11 Staphylococcal aureus
.19 Staphylococcal other
.0 Streptococcal (anaerobic)
.49 Yersinia enterocolitica
.8 Other specified

771.81 Umbilical newborn
038.9 Urinary meaning sepsis
599.0 Urinary meaning urinary tract infection
079.99 Viral
038.49 Yersinia enterocolitica
038.8 Other specified

SEPTICEMIA COMPLICATING LABOR, PREGNANCY, PUERPERIUM

771.81 Fetus or newborn - gonococcal [098.89]
771.81 Fetus or newborn - herpetic [054.5]
771.81 Fetus or newborn - salmonella [003.1]
771.81 Fetus or newborn - viral NOS [079.99]
771.81 Fetus or newborn - other
639.0 Following ectopic/molar or aborted pregnancy
647.8# Maternal current (coexistent) (major infection)
5th digit: 647.8
0. Episode of care NOS or N/A
1. Delivered
2. Delivered with postpartum complication
3. Antepartum complication
4. Postpartum complication

670.0# Maternal due to pregnancy postpartum (puerperal) (major infection)
5th digit: 670.0
0. NOS
2. Delivered with postpartum complication
4. Postpartum complication

659.3# Maternal during labor
5th digit: 659.3
0. Episode of care NOS or N/A
1. Delivered
3. Antepartum complication

639.0 Post abortion or ectopic/molar pregnancy

SEPTUM, SEPTAL

745.69 Absence (congenital) - atrial
745.7 Absence (congenital) - atrial and ventricular
745.0 Absence (congenital) - between aorta and pulmonary artery
745.3 Absence (congenital) - ventricular
429.71 Defect heart – acquired
429.71 Defect heart - acquired post MI acute (< 8 weeks) [410.##]
4th digit: 410
0. Anterolateral
1. Anterior (wall) anteroapical anteroseptal other anterior
2. Inferolateral
3. Inferoposterior
4. Inferior other
5. Lateral apical, basolateral, posterolateral, lateral other
6. Posterior (posterobasal)
7. Subendocardial
8. Atrium papillary or septum alone
9. Unspecified

5th digit: 410
0. Episode unspecified
1. Initial episode
2. Subsequent episode

429.71 Defect heart - acquired following myocardial infarction (>8 weeks) [414.8]
745.9 Defect heart - NOS congenital
745.8 Defect heart - closure congenital
745.4 Defect heart - interventricular congenital
745.8 Defect heart - other congenital
470 Nasal deviated
754.0 Nasal deviated congenital
0 Nasal see also 'Nose, Nasal', septum

0 SEQUESTRUM (OF BONE) SEE 'OSTEOMYELITIS'
495.8 SEQUOIOSIS OR RED CEDAR ASTHMA
0 SERRATIA (MARCESCENS) SEE 'BACTERIAL INFECTION' OR SPECIFIED CONDITION
270.7 SERINE METABOLISM DISTURBANCES
795.6 SEROLOGY FOR SYPHILIS FALSE POSITIVE
0 SEROLOGY FOR SYPHILIS POSITIVE FOLLOW-UP OF LATENT SYPHILIS SEE 'SYPHILIS LATENT'
998.13 SEROMA COMPLICATING A PROCEDURE
998.51 SEROMA POSTOPERATIVE INFECTED
333.99 SEROTONIN SYNDROME
362.42 SEROUS DETACHMENT RETINAL PIGMENT EPITHELIUM
348.2 SEROUS MENINGITIS SYNDROME
370.04 SERPIGINOUS ULCER
041.85 SERRATIA (MARCESCENS) INFECTION OR ORGANISM
038.44 SERRATIA SEPTICEMIA

SERTOLI

186.9 Cell carcinoma site NOS
0 Cell carcinoma site specified see 'Cancer', by site M8640/3
606.0 Cell syndrome (germinal aplasia)

SERTOLI (continued)

220 Leydig cell tumor female site NOS
0 Leydig cell tumor female site specified see 'Benign Neoplasm', by site M8631/0
222.0 Leydig cell tumor male site NOS
0 Leydig cell tumor male site specified see 'Benign Neoplasm', by site M8631/0

SERUM

999.5 Allergy
V14.7 Allergy history
790.99 Blood NEC abnormal
999.5 Disease NEC
790.5 Enzymes NEC abnormal
070.3# Hepatitis
070.2# Hepatitis with coma
5th digit: 070.2-3
0. Acute or unspecified
1. Acute or unspecified with delta
2. Chronic
3. Chronic with delta

999.5 Intoxication
790.99 Protein abnormal
790.99 Protein (total) abnormal
790.99 Protein NEC abnormal
999.5 Protein sickness
999.5 Rash, urticaria
999.5 Reaction
999.4 Shock anaphylactic
999.5 Sickness

733.99 SESAMOIDITIS
V61.10 SEVEN YEAR ITCH
351.8 SEVENTH NERVE ATROPHY
351.9 SEVENTH NERVE DISORDER UNSPECIFIED
767.5 SEVENTH NERVE DISORDER BIRTH TRAUMA
951.4 SEVENTH NERVE INJURY
351.8 SEVENTH NERVE NEURITIS
351.0 SEVENTH NERVE PARALYSIS
997.09 SEVENTH NERVE PARALYSIS POSTOPERATIVE
732.5 SEVER'S DISEASE (OSTEOCHONDROSIS CALCANEUM)
079.82 SEVERE ACUTE RESPIRATORY SYNDROME-ASSOCIATED CORONAVIRUS (SARS)
V01.82 SEVERE ACUTE RESPIRATORY SYNDROME-ASSOCIATED CORONAVIRUS (SARS) EXPOSURE
480.3 SEVERE ACUTE RESPIRATORY SYNDROME-ASSOCIATED CORONAVIRUS (SARS) PNEUMONIA
758.81 SEX CHROMOSOME ANOMALIES OTHER CONDITIONS DUE TO SEX CHROMOSOME
758.81 SEX CHROMOSOME MOSAICISM (SYNDROME)
238.9 SEX CORD STROMAL TUMOR SITE NOS
0 SEX CORD STROMAL TUMOR SITE SPECIFIED SEE 'NEOPLASM UNCERTAIN BEHAVIOR', BY SITE M8590/1
302.5# SEX REASSIGNMENT SURGERY STATUS
5th digit: 302.5
0. With unspecified sexual history
1. With asexual history
2. With homosexual history
3. With heterosexual history

651.8# SEXTUPLET GESTATION
651.7# SEXTUPLET GESTATION FOLLOWING (ELECTIVE) FETAL REDUCTION
5th digit: 651.7, 8
0. Episode of care NOS or N/A
1. Delivered
3. Antepartum complication

SEXUAL

302.72 Arousal disorder psychosexual
302.79 Aversion disorder
V69.2 Behavior high risk
V65.49 Counseling NEC
302.71 Desire decreased psychosexual disorder
259.0 Development delay NEC
302.9 Deviation unspecified
302.89 Deviation other specified
V62.4 Discrimination causing encounter
302.9 Disorder NOS (psychosexual)
302.70 Dysfunction NOS
0 Dysfunction psychological see 'Psychosexual Dysfunction'
V41.7 Function problem
302.9 Pathological sexuality
302.0 Orientation conflict disorder
302.0 Orientation ego-dystonic
259.1 Precocity (idiopathic) (cryptogenic)
255.2 Precocity male with adrenal hyperplasia
0 See also 'Psychosexual Dysfunction'
V65.45 Transmitted disease counseling
V74.5 Transmitted disease screening (bacterial) (spirochetal)
0 See also Venereal Disease

202.2# SEZARY'S DISEASE OR SYNDROME (RETICULOSIS) M9701/3
5th digit: 202.2
0. Unspecified site, extranodal and solid organ sites
1. Lymph nodes of head face neck
2. Lymph nodes intrathoracic
3. Lymph nodes abdominal
4. Lymph nodes axilla and upper limb
5. Lymph nodes inguinal region and lower limb
6. Lymph nodes intrapelvic
7. Spleen
8. Lymph nodes multiple sites

790.4 SGOT ABNORMAL
790.4 SGPT ABNORMAL
995.55 SHAKEN INFANT SYNDROME
503 SHAVER'S DISEASE OR SYNDROME (BAUXITE PNEUMOCONIOSIS)
253.2 SHEEHAN'S SYNDROME (POSTPARTUM PITUITARY NECROSIS)
520.5 SHELL TEETH
V74.3 SHICK TEST

SHIGELLA

004.9 Infection NOS
004.2 Boydii - group C
V02.3 Carrier
004.0 Dysenteriae - group A (Schmitz) (Shiga)
004.1 Flexneri - group B
004.3 Sonnei - group D
004.8 Other specified infections

S

081.2 SHIMAMUSHI DISEASE (SCRUB TYPHUS)

> ***Shin splints are painful inflammation of muscles, tendons and periosteum of the lower legs. Both types; anteriolateral and posteromedial are classified to code 844.9 (sprain leg NOS).***

844.9 SHIN SPLINTS
053.9 SHINGLES
077.1 SHIPYARD DISEASE
654.5# SHIRODKAR SUTURE COMPLICATING PREGNANCY
660.2# SHIRODKAR SUTURE OBSTRUCTING LABOR [654.5#]

5th digit: 654.5
- **0. Episode of care NOS or N/A**
- **1. Delivered**
- **2. Delivered with postpartum complication**
- **3. Antepartum complication**
- **4. Postpartum complication**

5th digit: 660.2
- **0. Episode of care NOS or N/A**
- **1. Delivered**
- **3. Antepartum complication**

SHOCK

785.50 NOS
995.0 Allergic NOS
995.0 Anaphylactic
999.4 Anaphylactic due to serum
909.9 Anaphylactic late effect
779.89 Birth fetus or newborn
785.51 Cardiogenic
250.8# Diabetic hypoglycemic

5th digit: 250.8
- **0. Type II, adult-onset, non-insulin dependent (even if requiring insulin), or unspecified; controlled**
- **1. Type I, juvenile-onset or insulin-dependent; controlled**
- **2. Type II, adult-onset, non-insulin dependent (even if requiring insulin); uncontrolled**
- **3. Type I, juvenile-onset or insulin-dependent; uncontrolled**

995.4 Due to anesthesia
909.9 Due to anesthesia late effect
995.0 Due to drug, medicine correctly administered
909.9 Due to drug, medicine correctly administered late effect
977.9 Due to drug, medicine incorrectly administered (overdose)
909.0 Due to drug, medicine incorrectly administered (overdose) late effect
995.6# Due to nonpoisonous food

5th digit: 995.6
- **0. Unspecified food**
- **1. Peanuts**
- **2. Crustaceans**
- **3. Fruits and vegetables**
- **4. Tree nuts and seeds**
- **5. Fish**
- **6. Food additives**
- **7. Milk products**
- **8. Eggs**
- **9. Other specified food**

SHOCK (continued)

909.9 Due to food late effect
995.0 Due to nonmedical substance correctly administered
909.9 Due to nonmedical substance correctly administered late effect
994.8 Electric
909.4 Electric late effect
0 Electric with burns see 'Burn'

> ***When coding septic, endotoxic, or gram negative infectious shock, report first the underlying systemic infection (038.#(#)) or trauma. The SIRS code (995.92) would sequence next, followed by 785.52 shock. Codes for the initial localized infection such as pneumonia and any associated organ dysfunction should also be assigned.***

038.#(#) Endotoxic infectious 995.92 [785.52]
779.89 Fetus birth
639.5 Following abortion/ectopic/molar pregnancy
038.#(#) Gram negative 995.92 [785.52]
785.59 Hypovolemic (nontraumatic)
584.5 Kidney syndrome
958.5 Kidney syndrome following crush injury
518.5 Lung traumatic or postsurgical (syndrome)
998.89 Misadventure therapeutic
909.3 Misadventure therapeutic late effect
308.9 Neurogenic syndrome
779.89 Newborn birth
669.1# Obstetric (L&D)

5th digit: 669.1
- **0. Episode of care NOS or N/A**
- **1. Delivered**
- **2. Delivered with postpartum complication**
- **3. Antepartum complication**
- **4. Postpartum complication**

998.0 Postoperative endotoxic during or resulting from surgery
998.0 Postoperative hypovolemic during or resulting from surgery
998.0 Postoperative septic during or resulting from surgery
909.3 Postoperative late effect
308.9 Psychic syndrome
038.#(#) Septic (severe) infectious 995.92 [785.52]

4th or 4th and 5th digit code for organism: 038
- **.9 NOS**
- **.3 Anaerobic**
- **.3 Bacteroides**
- **.3 Clostridium**
- **.42 E. coli**
- **.49 Enterobacter aerogenes**
- **.40 Gram negative**
- **.49 Gram negative other**
- **.41 Hemophilus influenzae**
- **.2 Pneumococcal**
- **.49 Proteus**
- **.43 Pseudomonas**
- **.44 Serratia**
- **.10 Staphylococcal NOS**
- **.11 Staphylococcal aureus**
- **.19 Staphylococcal other**
- **.0 Streptococcal (anaerobic)**
- **.49 Yersinia enterocolitica**
- **.8 Other specified**

SHOCK (continued)

999.8 Septic due to transfusion
909.3 Septic due to transfusion late effect
958.4 Syndrome (traumatic)

When coding an infection, use an additional code, [041.#(#)], to identify the organism. See 'Bacterial Infection'.

040.82 Toxic syndrome
958.4 Traumatic
908.6 Traumatic late effect
785.59 Other

287.0 SHONLEIN'S PURPURIC DEMATOGRAPHICA
579.3 SHORT BOWEL SYNDROME
277.85 SHORT CHAIN ACYL COA DEHYDROGENASE DEFICIENCY (SCAD)
426.81 SHORT P-R INTERVAL SYNDROME
756.89 SHORT STATURE HOMEOBOX GENE (SHOX) DEFICIENCY WITH DYSCHONDROSTEOSIS
783.43 SHORT STATURE HOMEOBOX GENE (SHOX) DEFICIENCY WITH SHORT STATURE (IDIOPATHIC)
758.6 SHORT STATURE HOMEOBOX GENE (SHOX) DEFICIENCY WITH TURNER'S SYNDROME
783.43 SHORT STATURE IN CHILDHOOD
786.05 SHORTNESS OF BREATH

SHOULDER

V49.67 Amputation status
337.9 Arm syndrome see also 'Neuropathy Peripheral', autonomic
0 Blade see 'Scapular'
736.89 Deformity (acquired) NEC
718.31 Dislocation, recurrent

763.1 Dystocia affecting fetus or newborn
652.8# Dystocia complicating pregnancy
660.0# Dystocia obstructing labor **[652.8#]**
660.4# Dystocia (shoulder girdle) obstructing labor
5th digit: 652.8, 660.0, 4
0. Episode of care NOS or N/A
1. Delivered
3. Antepartum complication

726.2 Fibrositis
726.0 Frozen
755.59 Girdle absence congenital
723.4 Girdle syndrome
337.9 Hand syndrome see also 'Neuropathy Peripheral', autonomic
726.2 Impingement syndrome
959.2 Injury
912.8 Injury other and unspecified superficial
912.9 Injury other and unspecified superficial infected

0 Joint see also 'Joint'
719.81 Joint (region) calcification
718.81 Joint instability
718.91 Joint ligament relaxation
0 Joint ligament tear see 'Sprain'
718.11 Joint (region) loose body
V54.81 Joint replacement aftercare [V43.61]
V43.61 Joint replacement status

726.19 Ligament or muscle instability
726.2 Periarthritis
763.1 Presentation affecting fetus or newborn

SHOULDER (continued)

0 Rotator cuff see 'Rotator Cuff'

840.9 Separation (rupture) (tear) (laceration) site unspecified
840.8 Separation (rupture) (tear) (laceration) other specified sites

840.7 SLAP lesion
840.9 Strain (sprain) (avulsion) (hemarthrosis) site unspecified
840.8 Strain (sprain) (avulsion) (hemarthrosis) other specified sites

726.19 Other specified disorder

333.93 SHUDDERING ATTACKS (BENIGN)
288.02 SHWACHMAN'S SYNDROME
333.0 SHY-DRAGER SYNDROME (ORTHOSTATIC HYPOTENSION WITH MULTISYSTEM DEGENERATION)
313.21 SHYNESS DISORDER OF CHILDHOOD
527.2 SIALOADENITIS
527.5 SIALOLITHIASIS
527.7 SIALORRHEA
527.8 SIALOSIS
065.4 SIBERIAN HEMORRHAGIC FEVER
082.2 SIBERIAN TICK TYPHUS
313.3 SIBLING JEALOUSY
V61.8 SIBLING RELATIONAL PROBLEM
352.6 SICARD'S SYNDROME
710.2 SICCA SYNDROME (KERATOCONJUNCTIVITIS)
799.9 SICK
276.1 SICK CELL SYNDROME
759.89 SICK CILIA SYNDROME
V61.49 SICK PERSON PROBLEM (IN FAMILY) (IN HOUSEHOLD)
427.81 SICK SINUS SYNDROME

When coding Sickle cell disease with crisis; it is necessary to report an additional code to indicate the manifestation of the crisis.

SICKLE CELL

282.60 NOS
282.62 NOS with crisis
282.60 Anemia NOS
282.60 Anemia NOS with retinopathy [362.29]
282.62 Crisis NOS
282.60 Disease NOS
282.62 Disease NOS with crisis
282.68 Disease other
282.69 Disease other with acute chest syndrome [517.3]
282.69 Disease other with crisis or vaso-occlusive pain
282.69 Disease other with splenic sequestration [289.52]
282.60 Elliptocytosis
282.63 Hb-C disease
282.64 Hb-C disease with acute chest syndrome [517.3]
282.64 Hb-C disease with crisis or vaso-occlusive pain
282.64 Hb-C disease with splenic sequestration [289.52]
282.68 Hb-D
282.69 Hb-D with acute chest syndrome [517.3]
282.69 Hb-D with crisis or vaso-occlusive pain
282.69 Hb-D with splenic sequestration [289.52]

SICKLE CELL (continued)

282.68	Hb-E
282.69	Hb-E with acute chest syndrome [517.3]
282.69	Hb-E with crisis or vaso-occlusive pain
282.69	Hb-E with splenic sequestration [289.52]
282.61	Hb-S disease
282.61	Hb-SS NOS
282.62	Hb-SS with acute chest syndrome [517.3]
282.62	Hb-SS with crisis or vaso-occlusive pain
282.62	Hb-SS with splenic sequestration [289.52]
282.63	Hb-S/Hb-C
282.64	Hb-S/Hb-C with acute chest syndrome [517.3]
282.64	Hb-S/Hb-C with crisis or vaso-occlusive pain
282.64	Hb-S/Hb-C with splenic sequestration [289.52]
282.68	Hb-S/Hb-D
282.69	Hb-S/Hb-D with acute chest syndrome [517.3]
282.69	Hb-S/Hb-D with crisis or vaso-occlusive pain
282.69	Hb-S/Hb-D with splenic sequestration [289.52]
282.68	Hb-S/Hb-E
282.69	Hb-S/Hb-E with acute chest syndrome [517.3]
282.69	Hb-S/Hb-E with crisis or vaso-occlusive pain
282.69	Hb-S/Hb-E with splenic sequestration [289.52]
V78.2	Screening for disease or trait
282.60	Spherocytosis
282.41	Thalassemia NOS
282.42	Thalassemia with acute chest syndrome [517.3]
282.42	Thalassemia with crisis or vaso-occlusive pain
282.42	Thalassemia with splenic sequestration [289.52]
282.5	Trait
282.49	Trait with thalassemia

If a manifestation of an adverse effect is known, it should be coded as the principal diagnosis.

790.09	SICKLING OF RED BLOOD CELLS
995.20	SIDE EFFECT NOS TO DRUG (CORRECTLY ADMINISTERED SUBSTANCE)
909.9	SIDE EFFECT NOS TO DRUG (CORRECTLY ADMINISTERED SUBSTANCE) LATE EFFECT
280.8	SIDEROPENIC DYSPHAGIA OR SYNDROME
360.23	SIDEROSIS GLOBE
503	SIDEROSIS OCCUPATIONAL
798.0	SIDS (SUDDEN INFANT DEATH SYNDROME)
0	SIDS (SUDDEN INFANT DEATH SYNDROME) NEAR MISS - CODE INDIVIDUAL SYMPTOM(S)
277.31	SIEGAL-CATTAN-MAMOU DISEASE (PERIODIC)
757.31	SIEMENS' ECTODERMAL DYSPLASIA SYNDROME
757.39	SIEMENS' KERATOSIS FOLLICULARIS SPINULOSA (DECALVANS) SYNDROME
V41.0	SIGHT PROBLEM

SIGMOID

569.89	Colon lesion
562.10	Diverticula
751.5	Diverticula congenital
569.89	Hypertrophy
560.9	Obstruction (see also 'Intestine, Intestinal', obstruction)

SIGMOIDITIS

558.9	NOS, noninfective
558.3	Allergic
558.3	Allergic due to ingested foods [V15.0#]

5th digit: V15.0
1. Peanuts
2. Milk products
3. Eggs
4. Seafood
5. Other foods

SIGNET RING CELL

199.1	Carcinoma site NOS
0	Carcinoma site specified see 'Cancer', by site M8490/3
199.1	Carcinoma metastatic site NOS
0	Carcinoma metastatic site specified see 'Cancer', by site, metastatic M8490/6
756.50	SILFVERSKIOLD'S SYNDROME (OSTEOCHONDRODYSTROPHY, EXTREMITIES)
502	SILICOSIS OCCUPATIONAL
506.9	SILO FILLERS' DISEASE
759.89	SILVER'S SYNDROME (CONGENITAL HEMIHYPERTROPHY AND SHORT STATURE)
282.49	SILVESTRONI-BIANCO SYNDROME (THALASSEMIA MINIMA)
054.3	SIMIAN B DISEASE
253.2	SIMMOND'S DISEASE (PITUITARY CACHEXIA)
272.6	SIMONS' DISEASE (PROGRESSIVE LIPODYSTROPHY)
462	SIMPLE ANGINA – THROAT
079.81	SIN NOMBRE VIRUS
732.4	SINDING-LARSEN DISEASE (JUVENILE OSTEOPATHIA PATELLAE)
478.5	SINGER'S NODES
279.8	SINGLE COMPLEMENT (C1-C9) DISORDER
786.8	SINGULTUS
427.81	SINOATRIAL NODE DYSFUNCTION

SINUS

426.6	Arrest

BRADYCARDIA

427.89	NOS
427.81	Chronic
427.81	Persistent
427.81	Severe

SINUS (continued)

478.19	Disease specified NEC
0	Infection nasal see 'Sinusitis'
478.19	Nasal congestion
471.1	Nasal degeneration polypoid
959.09	Nasal injury
473.9	Nasal obstruction
744.46	Preauricular congenital
686.9	Skin infected
707.9	Skin non-infected (see also 'Ulcer, Ulceration Skin')
427.89	Tachycardia
427.81	Tachycardia - bradycardia syndrome
726.79	Tarsi syndrome
752.89	Urogenitalis persistence
0	See also 'Fistula'

SINUSITIS

473.9 NOS
461.9 Acute
461.2 Acute ethmoidal
461.1 Acute frontal
461.0 Acute maxillary
461.3 Acute sphenoidal
461.8 Acute other or pansinusitis
0 Allergic see 'Hay Fever'
759.3 Bronchiectasis-situs inversus syndrome
473.9 Chronic
473.2 Chronic ethmoidal
473.1 Chronic frontal
473.0 Chronic maxillary
473.3 Chronic sphenoidal
473.8 Chronic other
473.8 Chronic other or pansinusitis
478.19 Influenzal
461.8 Pansinusitis acute
473.8 Pansinusitis chronic
471.1 Woakes' ethmoiditis

258.02 SIPPLE'S SYNDROME (MEDULLARY THYROID CARCINOMA-PHEOCHROMOCYTOMA) (MUTIPLE ENDOCRINE NEOPLASIA, TYPE IIA)

992.0 SIRIASIS

909.4 SIRIASIS LATE EFFECT

085.0 SIRKARI'S DISEASE

When coding SIRS, report first the underlying systemic infection (038.#(#)) or trauma code. The SIRS code (995.92, 995.94) should follow the infection/trauma code(s). Code next any known specific localized infection such as pneumonia. Specific organ dysfunction codes sequence next.

SIRS (SYSTEMIC INFLAMMATORY RESPONSE SYNDROME)

038.#(#) NOS 995.90
038.#(#) Due to infectious process 995.91
038.#(#) Due to infectious process with acute organ dysfunction [995.92]
038.#(#) Due to infectious process with disseminated intravascular coagulopathy (DIC) [995.92] [286.6]
038.#(#) Due to infectious process with encephalopathy [995.92] [348.31]
038.#(#) Due to infectious process with hepatic failure [995.92] [570]
995.92 Due to infectious process with multiple organ dysfunction (MOD)
038.#(#) Due to infectious process with myopathy critical illness [995.92] [359.81]
038.#(#) Due to infectious process with polyneuropathy critical illness [995.92] [357.82]
038.#(#) Due to infectious process with renal failure acute [995.92] [**584.#**]

4th digit: 584
5. With lesion of tubular necrosis
6. With lesion of renal cortical necrosis
7. With lesion of renal medullary necrosis
8. With other specified pathological lesion in kidney
9. Acute

SIRS (SYSTEMIC INFLAMMATORY RESPONSE SYNDROME) (continued)

038.#(#) Due to infectious process with respiratory failure acute [995.92] [518.81]
038.#(#) Due to infectious process with septic shock [995.92] [785.52]

4th or 4th and 5th digit code for organism: 038
.9 NOS
.3 Anaerobic
.3 Bacteroides
.3 Clostridium
.42 E. coli
.49 Enterobacter aerogenes
.40 Gram negative
.49 Gram negative other
.41 Hemophilus influenzae
.2 Pneumococcal
.49 Proteus
.43 Pseudomonas
.44 Serratia
.10 Staphylococcal NOS
.11 Staphylococcal aureus
.19 Staphylococcal other
.0 Streptococcal (anaerobic)
.49 Yersinia enterocolitica
.8 Other specified

995.93 Due to non infectious process
995.94 Due to non infectious process with acute organ dysfunction
577.0 Due to non infectious process with acute pancreatitis with acute organ dysfunction [995.94]
577.0 Due to non infectious process with acute pancreatitis without acute organ dysfunction [995.93]
995.94 Due to non infectious process with disseminated intravascular coagulopathy [286.6]
995.94 Due to non infectious process with encephalopathy [348.31]
995.94 Due to non infectious process with hepatic failure [570]
995.94 Due to non infectious process with myopathy critical illness [359.81]
995.94 Due to non infectious process with polyneuropathy critical illness [357.82]
995.94 Due to non infectious process with renal failure acute [**584.#**]

4th digit: 584
5. With lesion of tubular necrosis
6. With lesion of renal cortical necrosis
7. With lesion of renal medullary necrosis
8. With other specified pathological lesion in kidney
9. Acute

995.94 Due to non infectious process with respiratory failure acute [518.81]

0 SITUATIONAL ADJUSTMENT REACTION SEE 'ADJUSTMENT REACTION

308.3 SITUATIONAL REACTION ACUTE DUE TO STRESS

SITUS INVERSUS

759.3 Abdominalis
759.3 Sinusitis and bronchiectasis
759.3 Thoracis

S

058.10 SIXTH DISEASE (EXANTHEMA SUBITUM) NOS
058.11 SIXTH DISEASE (EXANTHEMA SUBITUM) DUE TO HUMAN HERPESVIRUS 6
058.12 SIXTH DISEASE (EXANTHEMA SUBITUM) DUE TO HUMAN HERPESVIRUS 7
378.54 SIXTH NERVE ATROPHY
951.3 SIXTH NERVE CRANIAL INJURY
378.54 SIXTH NERVE DISORDER (PALSY)
649.6# SIZE - DATE UTERUS DISCREPANCY COMPLICATING PREGNANCY

5th digit: 649.6
0. Episode of care NOS or N/A
1. Delivered
2. Delivered with postpartum complication
3. Antepartum complication
4. Postpartum complication

SJOGREN'S

710.2 Disease
710.2 (-Gougerot) syndrome (keratoconjunctivitis sicca)
757.1 Larsson syndrome (ichthyosis congenital)

597.89 SKENE'S ADENITIS
131.02 SKENE'S ADENITIS TRICHOMONAL
989.5 SKEVAS-ZERFUS DISEASE
378.87 SKEW DEVIATION CONJUGATE GAZE

SKIN

757.39 Absence (congenital)
793.99 Abnormal (x-ray) (ultrasound) (thermography)
782.3 Anasarca
782.0 Anesthesia
757.39 Aplasia (congenital)
706.2 Atheroma
701.8 Atrophy (senile)
701.3 Atrophy degenerative
782.62 Blushing
782.0 Burning or prickling sensation
709.3 Calcifications subcutaneous
709.3 Calcinosis circumscripta
709.3 Calcinosis cutis
V76.43 Cancer screening
782.4 Cholemia
709.2 Cicatrix
V82.0 Conditions screening
782.5 Cyanosis
770.83 Cyanosis fetus or newborn
706.2 Cyst
692.79 Damage solar NOS
692.72 Damage solar acute
692.74 Damage solar chronic
709.3 Degeneration
277.39 Degeneration amyloid
709.3 Deposits
0 Dermatitis see 'Dermatitis'
709.3 Dermatosis senile
709.9 Disorder
709.3 Disorder - degenerative
778.9 Disorder - fetus or newborn
778.8 Disorder - fetus or newborn other NEC
306.3 Disorder - psychogenic (allergic) (eczematous) (pruritic)
709.1 Disorder - vascular
709.8 Disorder - other NEC
V59.1 Donor non-autogenous

SKIN (continued)

782.3 Dropsy
772.6 Ecchymoses newborn
782.7 Ecchymoses spontaneous
782.3 Edema localized
778.5 Edema newborn
782.1 Eruption nonspecific
782.1 Exanthem
709.2 Fibrosis
709.8 Fissure
686.9 Fissure streptococcal
782.62 Flushing
709.4 Foreign body granuloma
996.55 Graft artificial failure or rejection (dislodgement) (displacement) (non-adherence) (poor incorporation) (shearing)
996.55 Graft decellularized allodermis failure or rejection (dislodgement) (displacement) (non-adherence) (poor incorporation) (shearing)
996.52 Graft failure or rejection
996.69 Graft infection (inflammation)
V13.3 History of skin disease
782.0 Hyperesthesia
782.0 Hypoesthesia
782.4 Icterus
782.8 Induration
686.9 Infection NOS
686.8 Infection other
134.9 Infestation
0 Jaundice see 'Jaundice'
709.9 Lesion
709.8 Lesion other specified
782.2 Lump superficial
782.2 Mass superficial
782.2 Nodule subcutaneous
782.0 Numbness
782.61 Pallor
709.8 Papule
134.9 Parasites
782.0 Paresthesia
782.7 Petechiae
757.33 Pigmentary anomaly
782.0 Prickling
782.1 Rash
782.0 Sensation disturbance

Use additional code to identify the altered sensation.

438.6 Sensation disturbance late effect of CVA
686.9 Sinus infected
707.9 Sinus non-infected (see also 'Ulcer, Ulceration Skin')
782.2 Subcutaneous nodules
686.00 Suppuration diffuse
782.2 Swelling superficial
701.9 Tag
757.39 Tag accessory congenital
V82.89 Test Kveim
795.79 Test positive
795.5 Test positive tuberculin (without active TB)
V82.89 Test sarcoidosis
782.8 Texture changes
782.8 Thickening
782.0 Tingling
V42.3 Transplant (status)
V43.83 Transplant artificial (status)
707.9 Ulcer unspecified (see also 'Ulcer, Ulceration Skin')

SKIN (continued)

709.1 Vascular lesion
701.8 Wrinkling
782.9 Other symptoms

SKULL

756.0 Bones absence
738.19 Deformity (acquired)
756.0 Deformity congenital
754.0 Depressions congenital
756.0 Imperfect fusion congenital
793.0 X-ray abnormal

840.7 SLAP LESION (SUPERIOR GLENOID LABRUM)

286.5 SLE (SYSTEMIC LUPUS ERYTHEMATOSUS) INHIBITOR

0 SLE (SYSTEMIC LUPUS ERYTHEMATOSUS) SEE 'LUPUS', ERYTHEMATOSUS .

SLEEP DISORDER / DISTURBANCE

780.50 Unspecified cause
291.82 Alcohol induced
780.57 Apnea NEC
770.81 Apnea newborn
770.82 Apnea newborn obstructive
770.81 Apnea newborn sleep
770.82 Apnea newborn other
780.53 Apnea with hypersomnia
780.51 Apnea with hyposomnia
780.51 Apnea with insomnia
780.57 Apnea with sleep disturbance NEC
327.41 Arousal confusional
307.46 Arousal disorder
780.56 Arousal dysfunction
307.40 Child
0 Circadian rhythm disruption see 'Circadian Rhythm Sleep Disorder'
V69.4 Deprivation
780.55 Disruption of 24-hour sleep-wake cycle unspecified
0 Disruption of 24-hour sleep-wake cycle circadian rhythm see 'Circadian Rhythm Sleep Disorder'
780.55 Disruption of 24-hour sleep-wake cycle, phase shift, unspecified
292.85 Drug induced
307.47 Drunkenness (sleep)
780.56 Dysfunction sleep stages
0 Hypersomnia see 'Hypersomnia'
0 Hyposomnia see 'Hyposomnia'
780.52 Insomnia (see also 'Insomnia')
307.48 Intrusion repetitive, atypical polysomnographic features
307.48 Intrusion repetitive environmental disturbances
307.48 Intrusion repetitive REM-sleep
307.45 Jet lag syndrome
V69.4 Lack of
780.58 Movement disorder unspecified
347.00 Narcolepsy
347.01 Narcolepsy with cataplexy

> *When using codes 347.10 and 347.11, code first the underlying condition.*

347.10 Narcolepsy in conditions elsewhere classified
347.11 Narcolepsy in conditions elsewhere classified with cataplexy
307.46 Night terrors
307.47 Nightmares
307.40 Nonorganic
327.8 Organic other

SLEEP DISORDER / DISTURBANCE (continued)

0 Parasomnia see 'Parasomnia'
0 Paroxysmal see 'Sleep Disorder/Disturbance', narcolepsy
327.51 Periodic limb movement
524.59 Postures causing malocclusion
307.40 Psychogenic
307.41 Psychogenic, initiation or maintenance
307.42 Psychogenic, initiation or maintenance - persistent
307.41 Psychogenic, initiation or maintenance - transient
327.53 Related bruxism
327.52 Related leg cramps
780.58 Related movement disorder unspecified
327.42 REM-sleep disorder
307.48 REM-sleep interruptions, repeated
307.47 REM-sleep type dysfunction
327.39 Rhythm inversion
307.49 Short sleeper
780.56 Sleep stages dysfunction
327.39 Sleep-wake rhythm inversion undetermined cause
327.39 Sleep-wake rhythm irregular undetermined cause
307.46 Sleep walking
300.13 Sleep walking hysterical
307.42 Sleeplessness persistent associated with anxiety, depression, or psychosis
307.41 Sleeplessness transient due to emotional conflict/ reaction
307.46 Somnambulism
307.46 Terror disorder
307.45 Time-zone change rapid
307.44 Wakefulness disorder persistent associated with depression
307.43 Wakefulness disorder transient due to emotional conflict/reaction
327.36 Work-sleep schedule shift
307.49 Other disturbance nonorganic NEC
780.59 Other disturbance/disruption
780.57 Other disturbance/disruption with sleep apnea

347.00 SLEEPING DISEASE
347.01 SLEEPING DISEASE WITH CATAPLEXY

> *When using codes 347.10 and 347.11, code first the underlying condition.*

347.10 SLEEPING DISEASE IN CONDITIONS ELSEWHERE CLASSIFIED

347.11 SLEEPING DISEASE IN CONDITIONS ELSEWHERE CLASSIFIED WITH CATAPLEXY

086.# SLEEPING SICKNESS (SEE ALSO 'TRYPANOSOMIASIS')

4th digit: 086

0. American with heart involvement
1. American with involvement of organ other than heart
2. American NOS
3. Gambian
4. Rhodesian
5. African NOS
9. NOS

V75.3 SLEEPING SICKNESS SCREENING EXAM

0 SLEEPLESSNESS SEE 'INSOMNIA'

0 SLIPPED CAPITAL FEMORAL EPIPHYSIS SEE 'EPIPHYSIS, EPIPHYSEAL', SLIPPED

255.3 SLOCUMB'S SYNDROME

779.3 SLOW FEEDING NEONATAL
046.9 SLOW VIRUS INFECTION CNS
788.62 SLOWING OF URINARY STREAM
337.0 SLUDER'S SYNDROME
784.5 SLURRED SPEECH

SMALL CELL CARCINOMA

199.1 Site NOS
0 Site specified see 'Cancer', by site M8041/3
199.1 Fusiform cell type site NOS
0 Fusiform cell type site specified see 'Cancer', by site M8043/3

656.5# SMALL FOR DATES AFFECTING MANAGEMENT OF MOTHER
5th digit: 656.5
0. Episode of care NOS or N/A
1. Delivered
3. Antepartum complication

0 SMALL FOR DATES PERINATAL SEE 'LIGHT FOR DATES'
115.0 SMALL FORM HISTOPLASMOSIS

SMALL INTESTINE

751.1 Absence congenital
562.00 Diverticulum
751.5 Diverticulum congenital
863.3# Injury with open wound into cavity
863.2# Injury without mention of open wound into cavity
5th digit: 863.2-3
0. Unspecified site
1. Duodenum
9. Other
908.1 Injury late effect
751.1 Obstruction congenital
560.81 Obstruction due to adhesions
560.81 Obstruction due to adhesions postoperative (postinfection)
751.1 Stenosis congenital
751.1 Stricture congenital

SMALLPOX

050.9 NOS
050.1 Alastrim
V01.3 Exposure
050.0 Hemorrhagic (pustular)
050.0 Malignant
050.2 Modified
V73.1 Screening exam
V04.1 Vaccination
050.0 Variola major
050.1 Variola minor

008.64 SMALL ROUND VIRUS NOS ENTERITIS (SRV'S)
443.9 SMALL VESSEL DISEASE
781.1 SMELL AND TASTE DISTURBANCES OF SENSATION
438.6 <u>SMELL</u> <u>DISTURBANCES</u> LATE EFFECT OF CVA <u>[781.1]</u>
V41.5 SMELL PROBLEM
759.89 SMITH-LEMLI-OPITZ SYNDROME (CEREBROHEPATORENAL SYNDROME)
758.33 SMITH-MAGENIS SYNDROME
270.2 SMITH-STRANG DISEASE (OASTHOUSE URINE)

987.9 SMOKE INHALATION
491.0 SMOKERS' COUGH
305.1 SMOKERS' SYNDROME (TOBACCO ABUSE, NONDEPENDENT)
V65.49 SMOKING CESSATION COUNSELING
649.0# SMOKING COMPLICATING PREGNANCY
5th digit: 649.0
0. Episode of care unspecified or N/A
1. Delivered
2. Delivered with postpartum complication
3. Antepartum complication
4. Postpartum complication

305.1 SMOKING CURRENT (TOBACCO DEPENDENT)
V15.82 SMOKING HISTORY
989.5 SNAKE BITE VENOMOUS
<u>995.0</u> SNAKE BITE VENOMOUS WITH <u>ANAPHYLAXIS</u> [989.5]
0 SNAKE BITE NONVENOMOUS, SEE 'OPEN WOUND', BY SITE
0 SNAPPING JOINT SEE 'JOINT', SNAPPING
694.1 SNEDDON WILKINSON DISEASE OR SYNDROME (SUBCORNEAL PUSTULAR DERMATOSIS)
784.99 SNEEZING
478.19 SNEEZING INTRACTABLE
786.09 SNORING
370.24 SNOW BLINDNESS
495.8 SNUFF TAKERS' DISEASE
786.05 SOB (SHORTNESS OF BREATH)
313.22 SOCIAL DISORDER OF CHILDHOOD AND ADOLESCENCE
V62.4 SOCIAL ISOLATION/ PERSECUTION
V62.4 SOCIAL MALADJUSTMENT (REASON FOR ENCOUNTER)
301.7 SOCIOPATHIC PERSONALITY

SODIUM

790.6 Abnormal
276.1 Deficiency abnormal findings
276.1 Deficiency hyponatremia
276.1 Deficiency nutritional
276.0 Excess abnormal findings
276.0 Excess hypernatremia
276.9 Metabolism disorder
276.0 Overload

026.0 SODOKU
366.51 SOEMMERING'S RING
729.9 SOFT TISSUE DISORDER OTHER AND UNSPECIFIED
524.81 SOFT TISSUE IMPINGEMENT - ANTERIOR
524.82 SOFT TISSUE IMPINGEMENT - POSTERIOR

SOLAR

0 Dermatitis see 'Dermatitis Solar'
692.74 Elastosis
702.0 Keratosis
363.31 Retinopathy
692.79 Skin damage NOS
692.72 Skin damage NOS acute
692.74 Skin damage NOS chronic
692.71 Sunburn due to solar radiation NOS (first degree)
692.76 Sunburn due to solar radiation second degree
692.77 Sunburn due to solar radiation third degree
692.82 Sunburn due to tanning bed

193 SOLID CARCINOMA SITE NOS
0 SOLID CARCINOMA SITE SPECIFIED SEE 'CANCER', BY SITE M8230/3
238.6 SOLITARY MYELOMA UNCERTAIN BEHAVIOR SITE NOS M9731/1
733.21 SOLITARY CYST BONE
593.2 SOLITARY CYST KIDNEY
312.1# SOLITARY STEALING
5th digit: 312.1
0. NOS
1. Mild
2. Moderate
3. Severe

SOMATIC DYSFUNCTION

739.9 Abdominal area and other
739.1 Cervical region
739.0 Head region
739.5 Hip
739.6 Lower extremities
739.3 Lumbar region
739.0 Occipitocervical region
739.5 Pelvic region
739.5 Pubic region
739.8 Rib cage
739.4 Sacral region
739.2 Thoracic region
739.7 Upper extremities

300.81 SOMATIZATION DISORDER
306.9 SOMATIZATION REACTION
300.81 SOMATOFORM DISORDER
300.82 SOMATOFORM DISORDER ATYPICAL (UNDIFFERENTIATED)
300.81 SOMATOFORM DISORDER SEVERE
300.89 SOMATOFORM DISORDER OTHER
307.46 SOMNAMBULISM
780.09 SOMNOLENCE
004.3 SONNEI DYSENTERY - GROUP D SHIGELLA
0 SORE THROAT SEE 'PHARYNGITIS'
253.0 SOTO'S SYNDROME (CEREBRAL GIGANTISM)
425.2 SOUTH AFRICAN CARDIOMYOPATHY SYNDROME
133.8 SOUTH AFRICAN CREEPING DISEASE
116.1 SOUTH AMERICAN BLASTOMYCOSIS
784.2 SPACE-OCCUPYING LESION INTRACRANIAL
V60.1 SPACE RESTRICTION (INADEQUATE HOUSING)
754.89 SPADE LIKE HAND CONGENITAL
123.5 SPARGANOSIS
123.5 SPARGANUM MANSONI PROLIFERUM INFECTION

SPASM

781.0 NOS
367.53 Accommodation
564.6 Anal
306.4 Anal psychogenic

Artery

443.9 NOS
435.0 Basilar
435.8 Carotid

SPASM (continued)

Artery (continued)

435.9 Cerebral NOS
435.8 Cerebral NEC
362.30 Ophthalmic
443.9 Peripheral
362.30 Retinal
435.1 Vertebral
435.3 Vertobasilar
443.9 NEC

SPASM (continued)

724.8 Back
724.8 Back muscle
306.0 Back psychogenic
596.8 Bladder (sphincter)
564.9 Bowel
306.4 Bowel psychogenic
519.11 Bronchus
781.7 Carpopedal
564.9 Cecum
306.4 Cecum psychogenic
661.4# Cervix complicating labor
5th digit: 661.4
0. Episode of care unspecified or N/A
1. Delivered
3. Antepartum complication

367.53 Ciliary body (of accommodation)
564.1 Colon
306.4 Colon psychogenic
378.82 Conjugate
378.84 Convergence
786.8 Diaphragm
306.1 Diaphragm psychogenic
564.89 Duodenal bulb
564.89 Duodenum
530.5 Esophageal
306.4 Esophageal psychogenic
351.8 Facial (nerve)
728.85 Facial muscle
536.8 Gastrointestinal (tract)
306.4 Gastrointestinal (tract) psychogenic
478.75 Glottis
300.11 Glottis hysterical
306.1 Glottis psychogenic
0 Habit see 'Tic'
378.51 Internal oblique
564.9 Intestinal
306.4 Intestinal psychogenic
478.75 Laryngeal
300.11 Laryngeal hysterical
306.1 Laryngeal psychogenic
333.81 Levator palberae superioris
724.6 Lumbosacral
728.85 Muscle
724.8 Muscle back
306.0 Muscle psychogenic
723.5 Neck
378.87 Oculogyric
362.30 Ophthalmic artery
478.29 Pharynx (reflex)
300.11 Pharynx (reflex) hysterical
306.1 Pharynx (reflex) psychogenic
306.0 Psychogenic

S

SPASM (continued)

537.81 Pylorus
537.0 Pylorus adult hypertrophic
750.5 Pylorus congenital/infantile
306.4 Pylorus psychogenic
564.6 Rectum (sphincter)
306.4 Rectum (sphincter) psychogenic
724.6 Sacroiliac
564.9 Sigmoid
306.4 Sigmoid psychogenic
576.5 Sphincter of oddi
385.89 Stapedius
536.8 Stomach
306.4 Stomach neurotic
529.8 Tongue
593.89 Ureter
599.84 Urethra (sphincter)
625.8 Uterus
661.4# Uterus (abnormal) complicating labor
5th digit: 661.4
0. Episode of care unspecified or N/A
1. Delivered
2. Delivered with postpartum complication
3. Antepartum complication
4. Postpartum complication

625.1 Vaginal
306.51 Vaginal psychogenic
443.9 Vascular NEC
459.89 Vein NEC
596.8 Vesical (internal) (external) (sphincter)

378.82 SPASMODIC UPWARD MOVEMENT, EYE(S) SYNDROME

307.20 SPASMODIC WINKING SYNDROME

307.3 SPASMUS NUTANS

564.9 SPASTIC COLON (COLITIS)

316 SPASTIC COLON (COLITIS) PSYCHOGENIC [564.9]

781.2 SPASTIC GAIT

V53.1 SPECTACLES FITTING AND ADJUSTMENT

SPEECH

Use an additional code to indentify the type of hearing loss. See 'HEARING LOSS'

315.34 Developmental delay due to hearing loss
784.5 Disorder NEC
315.39 Disorder developmental - articulation
315.31 Disorder developmental - expressive
315.32 Disorder developmental - mixed receptive-expressive
315.39 Disorder developmental - other
438.1# Disorder late effect of cerebrovascular disease
5th digit: 438.1
0. Unspecified
1. Aphasia
2. Dysphasia
9. Other

784.5 Impediment
307.9 Impediment psychogenic
V40.1 Problem
784.5 Slurred
V57.3 Therapy

315.09 SPELLING DIFFICULTY SPECIFIC (DELAY IN DEVELOPMENT)

780.39 SPELLS

078.82 SPENCER'S DISEASE (EPIDEMIC VOMITING)

426.9 SPENS' SYNDROME (SYNCOPE WITH HEART BLOCK)

SPERM

792.2 Abnormal
606.0 Azoospermia
608.82 Bloody
V26.22 Count following sterilization reversal
V26.21 Count for fertility evaluation
V25.8 Count post vasectomy
V59.8 Donor
606.1 Oligospermia

SPERMATIC CORD

608.4 Abscess (boil) (carbuncle) (cellulitis)
752.89 Absence (congenital)
752.9 Anomaly (congenital) NOS
752.89 Anomaly (congenital) NEC
608.89 Atrophy (fibrosis) (hypertrophy) (ulcer)
608.83 Hematoma (hemorrhage) nontraumatic
0 Hydrocele see 'Hydrocele', spermatic cord
867.6 Injury traumatic
867.7 Injury traumatic with open wound
608.85 Stricture
608.83 Thrombosis
608.22 Torsion (intravaginal)
608.21 Torsion extravaginal

608.1 SPERMATOCELE

752.89 SPERMATOCELE CONGENITAL

SPERMATOGENIC

606.0 Arrest complete
606.1 Arrest incomplete
606.0 Azoospermia
606.1 Oligospermia

0 SPERMATOZOA SEE 'SPERM'

461.3 SPHENOIDAL SINUS (ABSCESS) (INFECTION) (INFLAMMATION) ACUTE

282.0 SPHEROCYTIC ANEMIA CONGENITAL HEMOLYTIC

282.0 SPHEROCYTOSIS (FAMILIAL)

282.0 SPHEROCYTOSIS HEREDITARY

199.1 SPHEROIDAL CELL CARCINOMA SITE NOS

0 SPHEROIDAL CELL CARCINOMA SITE SPECIFIED SEE 'CANCER', BY SITE M8035/3

759.89 SPHEROPHAKIA-BRACHYMORPHIA SYNDROME CONGENITAL

743.36 SPHEROPHAKIA CONGENITAL

787.6 SPHINCTER ANI INCONTINENCE

576.5 SPHINCTER OF ODDI SPASM

576.2 SPHINCTER OF ODDI STENOSIS

564.89 SPHINCTERAL (DIGESTIVE) ACHALASIA

272.7 SPHINGOLIPIDOSIS CEREBRAL DEGENERATION [330.2]

448.1 SPIDER ANGIOMA

V15.06 SPIDER BITE ALLERGY HISTORY

0 SPIDER BITE NONVENOMOUS SEE 'INSECT BITE NONVENOMOUS'

330.1 SPIELMEYER (-VOGT) (-STOCK) DISEASE

SPINA BIFIDA

741.0# Cerebral degeneration (hydrocephalic) [331.7]
5th digit: 741.0
0. Region NOS
1. Cervical region
2. Dorsal (thoracic) region
3. Lumbar region

655.0# Fetalis with myelomeningocele affecting pregnancy management
5th digit: 655.0
0. Episode of care NOS or N/A
1. Delivered
3. Antepartum complication

756.17 Occulta
741.0# With hydrocephalus
741.9# Without hydrocephalus
5th digit: 741.0, 9
0. Region NOS
1. Cervical region
2. Dorsal (thoracic) region
3. Lumbar region

SPINAL

442.89 Artery (aneurysm) (A-V fistula) (cirsoid) (false) (varicose) (ruptured)
747.82 Artery anomaly (aberrant) (absence) (accessory) (agenesis) (atresia)
721.1 Artery anterior - compression syndrome
433.8# Artery anterior - obstruction or occlusion
433.8# Artery anterior - syndrome
433.8# Artery anterior - thrombosis (embolism) (deformans)
5th digit: 433.8
0. Without cerebral infarction
1. With cerebral infarction

336.8 Atrophy (cord)
733.99 Atrophy column
0 Atrophy muscular see 'Spinal', muscular atrophy
738.5 Deformity NOS
724.9 Disorder NEC (nonvertebral) (nondiscogenic)
336.1 Embolism (thrombosis) (occlusion) (infarction)
720.1 Enthesopathy
792.0 Fluid abnormal
997.09 Fluid leakage at lumbar puncture site
724.9 Joint disorder (nonvertebral) (nondiscogenic)
724.8 Ligament hypertrophy
720.1 Ligamentous or mucscular attachments disorder - peripheral
742.59 Meninges anomaly congenital

Spinal cord injury can be hematomyelia, paralysis, paraplegia, quadriplegia, or spinal concussion.

MUSCULAR ATROPHY

335.10 NOS
335.19 Adult
335.11 Familial
335.11 Juvenile
335.19 Other

SPINAL (continued)

355.9 Nerve disorder
724.9 Nerve root compression NEC (nonvertebral) (nondiscogenic)
907.3 Nerve root(s) spinal plexus(es) and other nerves of trunk (injury) late effect

SPINAL (continued)

997.09 Puncture lumbar fluid leakage
349.0 Puncture reaction (headache)

STENOSIS (NONVERTEBRAL) (NONDISCOGENIC)

724.00 NOS
723.0 Cervical
0 Discogenic see 'Herniated Disc (HNP)'
0 Due to spondylosis see 'Spondylosis'
724.01 Thoracic (dorsal)
724.02 Lumbar
724.09 Other

SPINAL (continued)

747.82 Vein anomaly (aberrant) (absence) (accessory) (agenesis)
747.82 Vessel anomaly other

SPINAL CORD

742.59 Absence congenital
742.9 Anomaly
336.8 Atrophy (acute)
733.99 Atrophy column
335.10 Atrophy muscular - NOS
335.19 Atrophy muscular - adult
335.11 Atrophy muscular - familial
335.11 Atrophy muscular - juvenile
335.19 Atrophy muscular - other
336.9 Compression
742.9 Deformity (congenital)
336.8 Deformity acquired
336.8 Degeneration (familial) (fatty) (hereditary)
277.39 Degeneration due to amyloidosis [336.3]
266.2 Degeneration due to B12 deficiency [336.2]
281.1 Degeneration due to B12 deficiency anemia [336.2]
281.0 Degeneration due to pernicious anemia [336.2]
742.51 Diastematomyelia congenital
336.9 Disease NOS
0 Disease combined system see 'Spinal Cord', degeneration
742.9 Disease congenital
0 Division see 'Spinal Cord', injury, by site
742.53 Hydromyelia congenital
742.53 Hydrorhachis congenital
742.59 Hypoplasia congenital

A spinal cord injury can be hematomyelia, paralysis, paraplegia, quadriplegia or spinal concussion

INJURY

952.9 Site unspecified
806.8 Site unspecified with fracture closed
806.9 Site unspecified with fracture open
767.4 Birth trauma
952.4 Cauda equina
806.6# Cauda equina with fracture closed
806.7# Cauda equina with fracture open
5th digit: 806.6-7
0. Unspecified injury
1. Complete cauda equina injury
2. Other cauda equina injury
9. Other spinal cord injury

SPINAL CORD (continued)

INJURY (continued)

952.0# Cervical
806.0# Cervical with fracture closed
806.1# Cervical with fracture open
5th digit: 806.0-1, 952.0
0. C1-C4 with cord injury NOS
1. C1-C4 with complete cord lesion
2. C1-C4 with anterior cord syndrome
3. C1-C4 with central cord lesion
4. C1-C4 with incomplete cord lesion NOS or posterior cord syndrome
5. C5-C7 with cord injury NOS
6. C5-C7 complete lesion of cord
7. C5-C7 with anterior cord syndrome
8. C5-C7 with central cord syndrome
9. C5-C7 with incomplete cord lesion NOS or posterior cord syndrome

952.1# Dorsal
806.2# Dorsal with fracture closed
806.3# Dorsal with fracture open
5th digit: 806.2-3, 952.1
0. T1-T6 with cord injury NOS
1. T1-T6 with complete lesion of cord
2. T1-T6 with anterior cord syndrome
3. T1-T6 with central cord syndrome
4. T1-T6 with incomplete cord lesion NOS or posterior cord syndrome
5. T7-T12 with cord injury NOS
6. T7-T12 with complete lesion of cord
7. T7-T12 with anterior cord syndrome
8. T7-T12 with central cord syndrome
9. T7-T12 with spinal cord lesion NOS or posterior cord syndrome

331.3 Fluid malabsorption syndrome (acquired) (hydrocephalus communicating)
331.3 Fluid malabsorption syndrome (acquired) (hydrocephalus communicating) with dementia **[294.1#]**
5th digit: 294.1
0. Without behavioral disturbance or NOS
1. With behavioral disturbance

907.2 Late effect
952.2 Lumbar
806.4 Lumbar with fracture closed
806.5 Lumbar with fracture open
952.8 Multiple sites
952.3 Sacral
806.6# Sacrum/coccyx closed
806.7# Sacrum/coccyx open
5th digit: 806.6-7
0. Unspecified injury
1. Complete cauda equina injury
2. Other cauda equina injury
9. Other spinal cord injury

0 Syndrome see 'Spinal Cord', injury, by site
0 Thoracic see 'Spinal Cord', injury, dorsal

SPINAL CORD (continued)

V53.02 Neuropacemaker fitting and adjustment
742.59 Tethered spinal cord syndrome
0 Tuberculosis see 'Tuberculosis', central nervous system, other specified

199.1 SPINDLE CELL CARCINOMA SITE NOS
0 SPINDLE CELL CARCINOMA SITE SPECIFIED SEE 'CANCER' By SITE M8032/3

SPINE

756.13 Absence congenital
756.10 Anomaly congenital
738.5 Deformity unspecified acquired
756.15 Fusion congenital
767.4 Injury birth trauma
721.8 Other allied disorders

SPINE CURVATURE ABNORMALITY

737.9 Curvature unspecified
754.2 Curvature congenital
356.1 Charcot Marie tooth **[737.4#]**
5th digit: 737.4
0. Curvature unspecified
1. Kyphosis
2. Lordosis
3. Scoliosis

737.9 Hunchback
277.5 Mucopolysaccharidosis **[737.4#]**
237.7# Neurofibromatosis **[737.4#]**
5th digit: 237.7
0. NOS or multiple
1. Type I
2. Type II
5th digit: 737.4
0. Curvature unspecified
1. Kyphosis
2. Lordosis
3. Scoliosis

731.0 Osteitis deformans **[737.4#]**
252.01 Osteitis fibrosa cystica **[737.4#]**
733.0# Osteoporosis **[737.4#]**
5th digit: 733.0
0. Unspecified
1. Senile
2. Idiopathic
3. Disuse
9. Other
5th digit: 737.4
0. Curvature unspecified
1. Kyphosis
2. Lordosis
3. Scoliosis

045.9# Poliomyelitis **[737.4#]**
5th digit: 045.9
0. Unspecified
1. Type I
2. Type II
3. Type III
5th digit: 737.4
0. Curvature unspecified
1. Kyphosis
2. Lordosis
3. Scoliosis

237.7# Von Recklinghausen's disease **[737.4#]**
5th digit: 237.7
0. NOS or multiple
1. Type I
2. Type II
5th digit: 737.4
0. Curvature unspecified
1. Kyphosis
2. Lordosis
3. Scoliosis

737.8 Other specified

334.9 SPINOCEREBELLAR DISEASE
334.8 SPINOCEREBELLAR DISEASE OTHER
216.# SPIRADENOMA (ECCRINE) M8403/0
4th digit: 216
0. Lip (skin of)
1. Eyelid including canthus
2. Ear (external) (auricle) (pinna)
3. Face (cheek) (nose) (eyebrow) (temple)
4. Scalp, neck
5. Trunk, back except scrotum
6. Upper limb including shoulder
7. Lower limb including hip
8. Other specified sites
9. Skin NOS

026.0 SPIRILLARY FEVER
104.9 SPIROCHETAL INFECTION
104.8 SPIROCHETAL INFECTIONS OTHER SPECIFIED NONSYPHILITIC NONRELAPSING FEVER
123.5 SPIROMETRA LARVAE INFECTION
954.1 SPLANCHNIC NERVES INJURY

SPLEEN, SPLENIC

759.0 Aberrant
V45.79 Absence acquired
759.0 Absence congenital
759.0 Accessory congenital
277.39 Amyloid disease
442.83 Artery (aneurysm) (A-V fistula) (cirsoid) (false) (varicose) (ruptured)
902.23 Artery injury
908.4 Artery injury late effect
902.23 Artery laceration (rupture) (hematoma) (avulsion) (aneurysm) traumatic
908.4 Artery laceration late effect
289.59 Atrophy
289.59 Calcification
865.02 Capsule tear traumatic
865.12 Capsule tear traumatic with open wound into cavity
289.51 Congestion
865.01 Contusion
865.11 Contusion with open wound into cavity
277.39 Degeneration amyloid lardaceous
289.50 Disease (organic) (postinfectional)
289.59 Disease (organic) (postinfectional) specified NEC
120.0 Disease with bilharzial splenic
759.0 Ectopic congenital
789.2 Enlargement
289.59 Fibrosis
569.89 Flexure syndrome
794.9 Function study abnormal
865.01 Hematoma traumatic
865.11 Hematoma traumatic with open wound into cavity
289.4 Hypersplenism (syndrome)
289.59 Infarction
865.0# Injury (traumatic)
865.1# Injury (traumatic) with open wound into cavity
5th digit: 865.0-1
0. Unspecified injury
1. Hematoma without rupture of capsule
2. Capsular tears, without major disruption of parenchyma
3. Laceration extending into parenchyma
4. Massive parenchymal disruption
9. Other
908.1 Injury late effect

SPLEEN, SPLENIC (continued)

865.03 Laceration
865.13 Laceration with open wound into cavity
289.59 Lien migrans
759.0 Lobulation congenital
289.53 Neutropenia syndrome
759.0 Polycystic congenital
794.9 Radioisotope study abnormal
767.8 Rupture - birth trauma
289.59 Rupture - nontraumatic
865.04 Rupture - traumatic
865.14 Rupture - traumatic with open wound into cavity
277.39 Sago
794.9 Scan abnormal
289.52 Sequestration syndrome
282.64 Sequestration syndrome due to sickle cell/Hb-C disease with crisis or vaso-occlusive pain [289.52]
282.62 Sequestration syndrome due to sickle cell/Hb-SS disease with crisis or vaso-occlusive pain [289.52]
282.69 Sequestration syndrome due to sickle cell disease other specified with crisis or vaso-occlusive pain [289.52]
282.42 Sequestration syndrome due to sickle cell thalassemia [289.52]
289.51 Splenomegaly chronic congestive
902.34 Vein injury
908.4 Vein injury late effect
908.4 Vein laceration late effect
902.34 Vein laceration (rupture) (hematoma) (avulsion) (aneurysm) traumatic
289.59 Wandering

289.59 SPLENITIS

SPLENOMEGALY

789.2 Unspecified
289.51 Chronic congestive
759.0 Congenital
289.53 Neutropenic
789.2 Unknown etiology

SPLINT

V54.89 Aftercare
V54.89 Change
V54.89 Removal

0 SPLINTER SEE 'FOREIGN BODY', BY SITE, SUPERFICIAL

788.61 SPLITTING OF URINARY STREAM

SPONDYLITIS

0 See also 'Spondylosis'
720.9 NOS
720.0 Ankylopoietica
720.0 Ankylosing (chronic)
720.9 Atrophic (ligamentous)
721.90 Chronic (traumatic)
721.90 Deformans (chronic)
098.53 Gonococcal
274.0 Gouty
721.90 Hypertrophic
720.9 Infectious NEC
720.0 Juvenile (adolescent)
721.7 Kummell's
720.0 Marie Strumpell (ankylosing)
720.9 Muscularis
721.6 Ossificans ligamentosa

S

SPONDYLITIS (continued)

721.90 Osteoarthritica
721.7 Posttraumatic
720.0 Proliferative
720.0 Rhizomelica
720.0 Rheumatoid
720.2 Sacroiliac NEC
721.90 Senescent
721.90 Senile
721.90 Static
721.90 Traumatic (chronic)
015.0# Tuberculosis [720.81]
5th digit: 015.0
0. NOS
1. Lab not done
2. Lab pending
3. Microscopy positive (in sputum)
4. Culture positive - microscopy negative
5. Culture negative - microscopy positive
6. Culture and microscopy negative confirmed by other methods
002.0 Typhosa [720.81]

721.1 SPONDYLOGENIC COMPRESSION OF CERVICAL SPINAL CORD

721.91 SPONDYLOGENIC COMPRESSION OF SPINAL CORD

SPONDYLOLISTHESIS

738.4 Acquired
763.1 Affecting fetus or newborn
756.12 Congenital
738.4 Degenerative
653.3# Maternal with fetopelvic disproportion
660.1# Maternal with fetopelvic disproportion obstructing labor [653.3#]
5th digit: 653.3, 660.1
0. Episode of care NOS or N/A
1. Delivered
3. Antepartum complication
738.4 Traumatic

SPONDYLOLYSIS

738.4 Acquired
763.1 Affecting fetus or newborn
756.19 Cervical congenital
756.11 Congenital
756.11 Lumbosacral congenital
653.3# Maternal with fetopelvic disproportion
660.1# Maternal with fetopelvic disproportion obstructing labor [653.3#]
5th digit: 653.3, 660.1
0. Episode of care NOS or N/A
1. Delivered
3. Antepartum complication

SPONDYLOPATHIES

720.9 Inflammatory NOS
720.89 Inflammatory other

SPONDYLOPATHIES (continued)

015.0# Tuberculous [720.81]
5th digit: 015.0
0. NOS
1. Lab not done
2. Lab pending
3. Microscopy positive (in sputum)
4. Culture positive - microscopy negative
5. Culture negative - microscopy positive
6. Culture and microscopy negative confirmed by other methods

SPONDYLOSIS: WITH OSTEOPOROSIS [733.0#]

721.0 Cervical
721.1 Cervical with myelopathy (cord compression)
721.3 Lumbar
721.42 Lumbar with myelopathy (cord compression)
721.3 Lumbosacral
721.42 Lumbosacral with myelopathy (cord compression)

648.7#: Specify the maternal spondylosis with an additional code.

648.7# Maternal current (co-existing) in pregnancy
5th digit: 648.7
0. Episode of care NOS or N/A
1. Delivered
2. Delivered with postpartum complication
3. Antepartum complication
4. Postpartum complication

653.3# Maternal with disproportion
660.1# Maternal with disproportion obstructing labor [653.3#]
5th digit: 653.3, 660.1
0. Episode of care NOS or N/A
1. Delivered
3. Antepartum complication

721.3 Sacral
721.42 Sacral with myelopathy (cord compression)
721.3 Sacrococcygeal
721.42 Sacrococcygeal with myelopathy (cord compression)
721.3 Sacroiliac
721.42 Sacroiliac with myelopathy (cord compression)
721.90 Spine
721.91 Spine with myelopathy (cord compression)
721.2 Thoracic
721.41 Thoracic with myelopathy (cord compression)
721.7 Traumatic
With Osteoporosis [733.0#]
5th digit: 733.0
0. Unspecified
1. Senile
2. Idiopathic
3. Disuse
9. Drug induced

989.5 SPONGE DIVERS' DISEASE

SPONGIOBLASTOMA

191.9 Site NOS
0 Site specified see 'Cancer', by site M9422/3
191.9 Polare site NOS
0 Polare site specified see 'Cancer', by site M9423/3
191.9 Primitive polar site NOS
0 Primitive polar site specified see 'Cancer', by site

0 SPONGIOCYTOMA SEE 'CANCER', BY SITE
199.1 SPONGIONEUROBLASTOMA SITE NOS
0 SPONGIONEUROBLASTOMA SITE SPECIFIED SEE 'CANCER', BY SITE M9504/3
0 SPONTANEOUS FRACTURE SEE 'FRACTURE PATHOLOGICAL'
117.1 SPOROTHRIX (SPOROTRICHUM) SCHENCKII INFECTION

SPOROTRICHOSIS

117.1 Bone
117.1 Cutaneous
117.1 Disseminated
117.1 Lymphocutaneous
117.1 Pulmonary

649.5# SPOTTING COMPLICATING PREGNANCY

5th digit: 649.5

0. Episode of care unspecified or N/A
1. Delivered
3. Antepartum complication

Medically, a sprain occurs when excessive force causes injury to a ligament, and a strain occurs when excessive force causes injury to a muscle or tendon. In ICD-9, sprain is the term used to cover all sprains, strains, avulsions, hemarthroses, tears and ruptures. In Easy Coder you'll find that codes for all of the above conditions are listed by site under the heading, sprain.

SPRAIN

848.9 NOS
848.8 Abdominal muscles
845.09 Achilles tendon
840.0 Acromioclavicular (joint) (ligament)
843.8 Adductor thigh (magnus)
845.00 Ankle - NOS
845.02 Ankle - calcaneofibular (ligament)
845.01 Ankle - deltoid (ligament)
845.01 Ankle - internal collateral (ligament)
845.03 Ankle - tibiofibular (ligament) distal
845.09 Ankle - other specified
845.00 Ankle and foot
844.2 Anterior cruciate ligament
717.83 Anterior cruciate ligament old
840.9 Arm
840.9 Arm (upper) and shoulder unspecified
840.8 Arm (upper) and shoulder other specified
840.4 Arm rotator cuff
845.00 Astragalus
847.0 Atlanto-axial (joints)
847.0 Atlanto-occipital (joints)
847.0 Atlas
847.0 Axis
847.9 Back - NOS
847.0 Back - cervical
847.4 Back - coccyx
846.9 Back - low
847.2 Back - lumbar (spine)
846.0 Back - lumbosacral
724.6 Back - lumbosacral chronic (joint) (ligament) (old)
846.9 Back - sacroiliac (region)
724.6 Back - sacroiliac chronic (old)
846.1 Back - sacroiliac ligament
846.8 Back - sacroiliac region other specified sites

SPRAIN (continued)

846.2 Back - sacrospinatus (ligament)
846.3 Back - sacrotuberous (ligament)
847.3 Back - sacrum
847.1 Back - thoracic
840.8 Biceps arm (brachii)
843.8 Biceps leg (femoris)
848.40 Breast bone
843.8 Buttock
845.02 Calcaneofibular (ligament)
844.8 Calf
717.85 Capsular ligament old (knee)
842.01 Carpal (joint)
842.11 Carpometacarpal (joint)
847.0 Cervical spine acute
848.3 Chest wall
848.3 Chondrocostal
848.42 Chondrocostal involving sternum
848.42 Chondrosternal (joint)
840.9 Clavicle
847.4 Coccyx
840.9 Collar bone
844.0 Collateral ligaments - lateral (knee)
844.1 Collateral ligaments - medial (knee)
717.89 Collateral ligaments old - NOS (knee)
717.81 Collateral ligaments old - lateral (knee)
717.82 Collateral ligaments old - medial (knee)
840.8 Coracoacromial
840.1 Coracoclavicular (ligament)
840.2 Coracohumeral (ligament)
840.9 Coracoid (process)
844.8 Coronary knee
848.3 Costal cartilage
848.42 Costal cartilage involving sternum
848.3 Costochondral
848.2 Cricoarytenoid (joint) (ligament)
848.2 Cricothyroid (joint) (ligament)
844.2 Cruciate ligament - acute
717.83 Cruciate ligament - anterior old
717.84 Cruciate ligament - posterior old
717.89 Cruciate ligament - old
845.01 Deltoid ankle (ligament)
840.8 Deltoid shoulder
847.1 Dorsal spine
848.8 Ear cartilage
841.9 Elbow
841.0 Elbow radial collateral ligament
841.2 Elbow radiohumeral
841.1 Elbow ulnar collateral ligament
841.3 Elbow ulnohumeral
841.8 Elbow other specified sites
844.9 Femur distal
843.9 Femur proximal
845.00 Fibula distal
844.9 Fibula proximal
842.13 Finger
842.13 Finger interphalangeal
845.10 Foot - NOS
845.13 Foot - interphalangeal (joint) toe
845.12 Foot - metatarsophalangeal (joint)
845.11 Foot - tarsometatarsal (joint) (ligament)
845.19 Foot - other
845.00 Foot and ankle
841.9 Forearm
841.8 Forearm other specified sites
844.8 Gastrocnemius

S

S

SPRAIN (continued)

840.8	Glenoid (shoulder)
840.7	Glenoid (shoulder) SLAP lesion
843.8	Gluteus maximus
848.8	Groin
843.8	Hamstring
842.10	Hand
842.11	Hand carpometacarpal
842.13	Hand interphalangeal (joint)
842.12	Hand metacarpophalangeal
842.19	Hand midcarpal
842.19	Hand other joint
843.9	Hip - NOS
843.0	Hip - iliofemoral (ligament)
843.1	Hip - ischiocapsular (ligament)
843.8	Hip - ligamentum teres femoris
843.8	Hip - other specified sites
841.9	Humerus distal
840.9	Humerus proximal
843.0	Iliofemoral (ligament)
840.3	Infraspinatus (muscle) (tendon)
848.8	Inguinal
843.9	Innominate acetabulum
848.5	Innominate pubic junction
846.1	Innominate sacral junction
842.13	Interphalangeal (joint) hand
843.1	Ischiocapsular (ligament)
848.1	Jaw (cartilage) (meniscus)
524.69	Jaw (cartilage) (meniscus) - old

KNEE ACUTE (CURRENT INJURY)

844.9	Unspecified
844.2	Cruciate ligament
844.0	Lateral collateral ligament
844.1	Medial collateral ligament
844.8	Patellar ligament
844.3	Tibiofibular ligament (joint), Superior

KNEE OLD

717.89	Unspecified
717.81	Collateral ligament lateral
717.82	Collateral ligament medial
717.83	Cruciate ligament anterior
717.84	Cruciate ligament posterior
717.89	Patellar ligament
717.85	Other ligaments

SPRAIN (continued)

905.7	Late effect
905.8	Late effect with tendon injury
844.0	Lateral collateral ligament knee
717.81	Lateral collateral ligament knee - old
844.9	Leg
843.8	Ligamentum teres femoris
846.9	Low back
847.2	Lumbar
846.0	Lumbosacral (joint) (ligament)
724.6	Lumbosacral (joint) (ligament) - old
848.1	Mandible
524.69	Mandible - old
848.1	Maxilla
844.1	Medial collateral ligament knee
717.82	Medial collateral ligament knee - old
0	Meniscus see 'Meniscus', knee tear
842.10	Metacarpal
842.12	Metacarpal distal
842.11	Metacarpal proximal

SPRAIN (continued)

842.12	Metacarpophalangeal (joint)
845.10	Metatarsal
845.12	Metatarsophalangeal (joint)
842.19	Midcarpal (joint)
845.19	Midtarsal (joint)
847.0	Neck
848.0	Nose septal cartilage
847.0	Occiput from atlas
843.8	Orbicular hip
844.8	Patellar
717.89	Patellar - old
848.8	Pectorals
848.5	Pelvis
0	Phalanx see 'Sprain', finger or 'Sprain', toe
844.2	Posterior cruciate ligament
717.84	Posterior cruciate ligament old
843.8	Quadriceps
841.0	Radial collateral ligament
842.02	Radiocarpal (joint) (ligament)
841.2	Radiohumeral (joint)
841.9	Radioulnar
842.09	Radioulnar joint distal
842.00	Radius distal
841.9	Radius proximal
842.09	Radius and ulna distal
841.9	Radius and ulna proximal
841.0	Radius collateral (ligament)
848.8	Rectus abdominis
848.3	Rib
848.42	Rib with sternal involvement
840.4	Rotator cuff (capsule)
843.8	Round ligament femur
847.3	Sacrococcygeal (ligament)
846.1	Sacroiliac ligament
724.6	Sacroiliac ligament - old (chronic)
846.9	Sacroiliac region
846.8	Sacroiliac region other specified sites
846.2	Sacrospinatus (ligament)
846.2	Sacrospinous
846.3	Sacrotuberous (ligament)
847.3	Sacrum
845.00	Scaphoid ankle
840.9	Scapula
844.8	Semilunar cartilage knee
717.5	Semilunar cartilage knee - old
840.9	Shoulder
840.9	Shoulder and upper arm
840.9	Shoulder blade
840.8	Shoulder and upper arm other specified sites
847.9	Spine
848.41	Sternoclavicular (joint) (ligament)
848.40	Sternum NOS
848.49	Sternum other specified
840.7	Subglenoid SLAP lesion
840.5	Subscapularis (muscle)
840.6	Supraspinatus (muscle) (tendon)
848.1	Symphysis jaw (mandible)
524.69	Symphysis jaw (mandible) - old
848.5	Symphysis pubis
845.09	Talofibular
845.10	Tarsal
845.11	Tarsometatarsal (joint) (ligament)
848.1	Temporomandibular
524.69	Temporomandibular - old

SPRAIN (continued)

843.8 Teres ligamentum femoris
840.8 Teres major or minor
843.9 Thigh NOS
843.9 Thigh and hip
844.9 Thigh distal
843.9 Thigh proximal
847.1 Thoracic spine
848.8 Thorax
842.13 Thumb
842.13 Thumb interphalangeal
848.2 Thyroid region cartilage
845.00 Tibia distal
844.9 Tibia proximal
845.03 Tibiofibular distal
844.3 Tibiofibular ligament (joint), superior
717.85 Tibiofibular ligament (old)
845.13 Toe
845.13 Toe interphalangeal (joint)
848.8 Trachea
840.8 Trapezoid
842.01 Triangular fibrocartilage complex
719.83 Triangular fibrocartilage complex - old
840.8 Triceps
842.00 Ulnar distal
841.9 Ulnar proximal
841.1 Ulnar collateral ligament
841.3 Ulnohumeral (joint)
842.00 Wrist
842.01 Wrist carpal
842.02 Wrist radiocarpal (joint) (ligament)
842.09 Wrist other
848.49 Xiphoid cartilage
848.8 Other specified sites

755.52 SPRENGEL'S DEFORMITY

0 SPROM SEE 'PREMATURE', RUPTURE OF MEMBRANES OBSTETRICAL

SPRUE

579.1 Unspecified
579.0 Nontropical
579.1 Tropical

SPUR

726.91 NOS
726.73 Calcaneus
726.30 Elbow
726.73 Foot
726.4 Hand
726.73 Heel
726.5 Hip
726.5 Iliac crest
726.60 Knee
478.19 Nose
726.33 Olecranon
726.69 Prepatellar or subpatellar
478.19 Septal
726.4 Wrist
726.8 Other specified site

756.51 SPURWAY'S SYNDROME (BRITTLE BONES AND BLUE SCLERA)

786.4 SPUTUM ABNORMAL (COLOR) (EXCESS) (ODOR)

795.39 SPUTUM CULTURE POSITIVE

> ***Carcinomas and neoplasms should be coded by site first. If a site is not specified then code by cell type. Do not try to code by cell type first. Whenever possible, Easy Coder also provides the site menus for your convenience.***

SQUAMOUS CELL CARCINOMA

199.1 Site NOS
0 Site specified See 'CANCER', by site M8070/3
180.9 Adenoid site NOS
0 Adenoid site specified see 'Cancer', by site M8075/3
234.9 In situ site NOS
0 In situ site specified see 'Carcinoma In Situ', by site M8070/2
233.1 In situ with questionable stromal invasion site NOS
0 In situ with questionable stromal invasion specified site see 'Carcinoma In Situ', by site M8076/2
0 Intraepidermal bowen's type see 'Cancer' skin by site M8076/2
180.9 Keratinizing type site NOS
0 Keratinizing type site specified see 'Cancer', by site M8071/3
180.9 Large cell (nonkeratinizing type) site NOS
0 Large cell (nonkeratinizing type) site specified see 'Cancer', by site M8072/3
199.1 Metastatic site NOS
0 Metastatic site specified see 'Cancer', by site, metastatic M8070/6
180.9 Micro invasive site NOS
0 Micro invasive site specified see 'Cancer', by site M8076/3
199.1 Papillary site NOS
0 Papillary site specified see 'Cancer', by site M8052/3
180.9 Small cell (nonkeratinizing type) site NOS
0 Small cell (nonkeratinizing type) site specified see 'Cancer', by site M8073/3
180.9 Spindle cell type site NOS
0 Spindle cell type site specified see 'Cancer', by site M8074/3

754.0 SQUASHED OR BENT NOSE CONGENITAL

008.64 SRV ENTERITIS (SMALL ROUND VIRUS) NOS

427.81 SSS - SICK SINUS SYNDROME

695.1 SSSS - SCALDED SKIN SYNDROME

0 ST ELEVATION MYOCARDIAL INFARCTION SEE 'MYOCARDIAL INFARCTION ACUTE', BY SITE

062.3 ST. LOUIS ENCEPHALITIS

0 STAB WOUND SEE 'OPEN WOUND', BY SITE

0 STAB WOUND WITH INJURY TO INTERNAL ORGAN SEE SPECIFIED ORGAN/ANATOMICAL SITE, INJURY

592.0 STAGHORN CALCULUS KIDNEY

371.11 STAHLI'S LINES

307.0 STAMMERING

025 STANTON'S DISEASE (MELIOIDOSIS)

385.22 STAPES FIXED

S

STAPHYLOCOCCAL

462 Angina, throat
0 Arthritis see 'Arthritis Other Specified', pyogenic
V02.59 Carrier
008.41 Gastroenteritis
041.1# Infection or organism
482.4# Pneumonia
695.1 Scalded skin syndrome
038.1# Septicemia
5th digit: 038.1, 041.1, 482.4
0. NOS
1. Aureus
9. Other staph

038.1# STAPHYLOCOCCEMIA
5th digit: 038.1
0. Unspecified
1. Aureus
9. Other

686.00 STAPHYLODERMA (SKIN)
371.73 STAPHYLOMA CORNEAL

STAPHYLOMA SCLERA

379.11 NOS
379.13 Equatorial
379.14 Localized (anterior)
379.12 Posticum
379.15 Ring

362.75 STARGARDT'S DISEASE

759.89 STARTLE DISEASE

994.2 STARVATION
909.4 STARVATION LATE EFFECT

STASIS

0 Cardiac see 'Heart Failure'
459.81 Dermatitis (venous)
459.81 Dermatitis (venous) <u>ulcerated</u> **[707.#(#)]**
4th or 4th and 5th digit: 707
1#. Lower limb except decubitus
10. Unspecified
11. Thigh
12. Calf
13. Ankle
14. Heel and midfoot
15. Other parts of foot, toes
19. Other
8. Chronic of other specified site
9. Chronic site NOS

454.1 Dermatitis varicose
459.12 Dermatitis varicose due to postphlebitic syndrome
459.13 Dermatitis varicose due to postphlebitic syndrome with ulcer
454.8 Dermatitis varicose with edema
454.8 Dermatitis varicose with pain
454.8 Dermatitis varicose with swelling
454.2 Dermatitis varicose with ulcer
0 Edema see 'Hypertension', venous

STASIS (continued)

459.81 <u>Ulcer</u> **[707.#(#)]**
4th or 4th and 5th digit: 707
1#. Lower limb except decubitus
0. Unspecified
1. Thigh
2. Calf
3. Ankle
4. Heel and midfoot
5. Other parts of foot, toes
9. Other
8. Chronic of other specified site
9. Chronic site NOS

454.0 Ulcer varicose - NOS site
454.0 Ulcer varicose - lower extremity
454.2 Ulcer varicose - lower extremity infected

783.9 STATURE LARGE
783.43 STATURE SHORT

STATUS

V45.7# Absence organ (acquired) (postsurgical)
5th digit: V45.7
1. Breast
2. Intestine (large) (small)
3. Kidney
4. Other parts of urinary tract (bladder)
5. Stomach
6. Lung
7. Genital organs
8. Eye
9. Other organ

V49.7# Amputation lower limb
5th digit: V49.7
0. Unspecified level
1. Great toe
2. Other toe(s)
3. Foot
4. Ankle
5. Below knee
6. Above knee
7. Hip

V49.6# Amputation upper limb
5th digit: V49.6
0. Unspecified level
1. Thumb
2. Other finger(s)
3. Hand
4. Wrist
5. Below elbow
6. Above elbow
7. Shoulder

V45.3 Anastomosis intestinal bypass
V45.82 Angioplasty (PTCA)
V43.66 Ankle prosthesis
V54.81 Ankle prosthesis <u>aftercare</u> <u>[V43.66]</u>
V45.81 Aortocoronary bypass
V45.81 Aortocoronary shunt
V45.1 Arteriovenous shunt for dialysis renal
V43.4 Artery device
V45.4 Arthrodesis
V44.9 Artificial opening unspecified
V44.8 Artificial opening other specified
V46.0 Aspirator
V45.86 Bariatric surgery
V49.84 Bed confinement

STATUS (continued)

V43.5 Bladder device
V42.89 Blood vessel transplant
V42.81 Bone marrow transplant
V42.4 Bone tissue transplant
V43.82 Breast implant
V45.83 Breast implant removal
V45.81 Bypass coronary
V45.02 Cardiac defibrillator in situ
V45.00 Cardiac device in situ
V45.09 Cardiac device other specified in situ
V45.01 Cardiac pacemaker in situ
V45.09 Carotid sinus stimulator in situ
0 Carrier or suspected carrier of infectious disease see 'Carrier'
V45.61 Cataract extraction
V45.61 Cataract extraction with artificial lens status [V43.1]
V45.2 Cerebrospinal fluid drainage device
V45.2 Cerebrospinal fluid shunt
V45.4 Cervical fusion
V66.2 Chemotherapy
V58.69 Chemotherapy current
0 Clitorectomy see 'Mutilation Genital Female Status'
V44.3 Colostomy
V45.59 Contraceptive device NEC
V45.51 Contraceptive device intrauterine
V45.52 Contraceptive device subdermal
V45.69 Corneal surgery
V42.5 Corneal transplant
V45.82 Coronary angioplasty (PTCA)
V45.81 Coronary bypass
V45.89 Coronary stent/shunt
V44.50 Cystostomy - NOS
V44.52 Cystostomy - appendico-vesicostomy
V44.51 Cystostomy - cutaneous-vesicostomy
V44.59 Cystostomy - other
V45.84 Dental crowns (fillings)
V45.84 Dental restoration
V49.82 Dental sealant
V45.1 Dialysis (hemo) (peritoneal)
0 Donor see 'Donor'
V43.62 Elbow prosthesis
V54.81 Elbow prosthesis aftercare [V43.62]
345.3 Epilepticus
V44.4 Enterostomy
V86.1 Estrogen receptor negative (ER-)
V86.0 Estrogen receptor positive (ER+)
V43.0 Eye globe replacement
V45.69 Eye surgery and adnexa
0 Female Mutilation see 'Mutilation Genital Female Status'
V45.69 Filtering bleb eye (postglaucoma)
V43.69 Finger joint prosthesis
V54.81 Finger joint prosthesis aftercare [V43.69]
V45.86 Gastric banding
V45.86 Gastric bypass surgery for obesity
V44.1 Gastrostomy
V83.81 Genetic carrier cystic fibrosis
V83.89 Genetic carrier other defect
629.2# Genital mutilation (cutting) status female

5th digit: 629.2

0. Unspecified
1. Type I (clitorectomy)
2. Type II (clitorectomy with excision of labia minora)
3. Type III (infibulation)
9. Type IV or other

STATUS (continued)

V44.3 Hartmann's pouch intestine
V43.22 Heart artificial fully implantable
V43.21 Heart assist device
V43.3 Heart valve prosthesis
V45.1 Hemodialysis
V43.64 Hip prosthesis
V54.81 Hip prosthesis aftercare [V43.64]
V08 HIV infection (asymptomatic)
V45.89 Hysterectomy
V44.2 Ileostomy
0 Infection with drug-resistant organism see 'Drug Resistance'
V45.85 Insulin pump
V45.3 Intestinal bypass or anastomosis
V43.89 Intestine device
V42.84 Intestine transplant
V45.51 Intrauterine contraceptive device
V45.51 IUD (intrauterine device)
V44.4 Jejunostomy
V45.4 Joint fusion
V43.60 Joint prosthesis unspecified
V54.81 Joint prosthesis unspecified aftercare [V43.60]
V43.69 Joint prosthesis other specified
V54.81 Joint prosthesis other specified aftercare [V43.69]
V43.89 Kidney device
V43.65 Knee joint prosthesis
V54.81 Knee joint prosthesis aftercare [V43.65]
V43.81 Larynx device
V45.61 Lens intraocular following cataract extraction [V43.1]
V43.7 Limb prosthesis
V43.89 Liver device
V45.89 Lobectomy
V21.3# Low birth weight

5th digit: V21.3

0. Unspecified
1. Less than 500 grams
2. 500-999 grams
3. 1000-1499 grams
4. 1500-1999 grams
5. 2000-2500 grams

V45.4 Lumbar fusion
V43.89 Lung device
333.79 Marmoratus
V45.89 Nephrectomy
V44.6 Nephrostomy
V45.89 Neuropacemaker
V45.86 Obesity surgery
V45.89 Oophorectomy
V42.89 Organ specified site NEC transplant
V43.89 Organ tissue - other replacement (mechanical) (artificial) (prosthesis)
V44.9 Ostomy NOS
V44.4 Ostomy GI tract (other specified)
V44.8 Ostomy other
V45.89 Other surgery
V46.2 Oxygen therapy (supplemental) long term use
V45.89 Pacemaker brain
V45.01 Pacemaker cardiac (in situ)
V45.89 Pacemaker specified site NEC
V43.89 Pancreas device
V42.83 Pancreas transplant
V45.82 Percutaneous transluminal coronary angioplasty
V42.82 Peripheral stem cells transplant
V45.1 Peritoneal dialysis
310.2 Postcommotio cerebri
V49.81 Postmenopausal (natural) asymptomatic, age related

S

STATUS (continued)

V24.2 Postpartum NEC
V45.89 Postprocedural NEC
V45.89 Postsurgical NEC
V22.2 Pregnant state (incidental)
V45.82 PTCA (percutaneous transluminal coronary angioplasty)
V45.1 Renal dialysis
V43.60 Replacement - joint NOS
V54.81 Replacement - joint NOS aftercare [V43.60]
V43.66 Replacement - ankle joint
V54.81 Replacement - ankle joint aftercare [V43.66]
V43.62 Replacement - elbow joint
V54.81 Replacement - elbow joint aftercare [V43.62]
V43.69 Replacement - finger joint
V54.81 Replacement - finger joint aftercare [V43.69]
V43.64 Replacement - hip joint
V54.81 Replacement - hip joint aftercare [V43.64]
V43.65 Replacement - knee joint
V54.81 Replacement - knee joint aftercare [V43.65]
V43.61 Replacement - shoulder joint
V54.81 Replacement - shoulder joint aftercare [V43.61]
V43.63 Replacement - wrist joint
V54.81 Replacement - wrist joint aftercare [V43.63]
V43.69 Replacement - other joint
V54.81 Replacement - other joint aftercare [V43.69]
V46.1# Respirator
5th digit: V46.1
1. Status
2. Encounter during power failure
3. Encounter for weaning from
4. Mechanical complication

302.5# Sex reassignment surgery
5th digit: 302.5
0. With unspecified sexual history
1. With asexual history
2. With homosexual history
3. With heterosexual history

V43.61 Shoulder prosthesis
V54.81 Shoulder prosthesis aftercare [V43.61]
V43.83 Skin artificial replacement
V42.82 Stem cells peripheral transplant
V45.52 Subdermal contraceptive implant
V45.89 Surgery other
V45.4 Thoracic fusion
V42.89 Tissue specified type NEC transplant
V43.89 Tissue replacement NEC
V44.0 Tracheostomy
V42.#(#) Transplant organ
4th or 4th and 5th digit: V42
0. Kidney
1. Heart
2. Heart valve
3. Skin
4. Bone
5. Cornea
6. Lung
7. Liver
8#. Other specified
81. Bone marrow
82. Peripheral stem cells
83. Pancreas
84. Intestine
89. Other specified
9. Unspecified

STATUS (continued)

V49.83 Transplant organ - waiting
V43.83 Transplant skin artificial
V26.51 Tubal ligation
V44.6 Ureterostomy
V44.6 Urethrostomy
V44.6 Urinary tract artificial opening other
V44.7 Vagina artificial
V45.89 Vascular shunt NEC
V26.52 Vasectomy
V43.4 Vein device
V46.1# Ventilator
5th digit: V46.1
1. Status
2. Encounter during power failure
3. Encounter for weaning from
4. Mechanical complication

V45.2 Ventricular device cerebral (communicating) for drainage
V42.89 Vessel blood transplant
V43.63 Wrist prosthesis
V54.81 Wrist prosthesis aftercare [V43.63]

V65.45 STD (SEXUALLY TRANSMITTED DISEASE) COUNSELING
996.73 STEAL SYNDROME, ARTERIOVENOUS
435.2 STEAL SYNDROME, SUBCLAVIAN
312.1# STEALING SOLITARY
5th digit: 312.1
0. NOS
1. Mild
2. Moderate
3. Severe

987.9 STEAM INHALATION
706.2 STEATOCYSTOMA MULTIPLEX

STEATORRHEA

579.8 Chronic
579.0 Idiopathic
579.4 Pancreatic
579.1 Tropical

333.0 STEELE-RICHARDSON (-OLSZEWSKI) SYNDROME
256.4 STEIN (-LEVENTHAL) SYNDROME (POLYCYSTIC OVARY)
359.21 STEINERT'S DISEASE
337.9 STEINBROCKER'S SYNDROME (SEE ALSO 'NEUROPATHY PERIPHERAL', AUTONOMIC)
V54.89 STEINMANN PIN CHANGE, CHECKING, OR REMOVAL
121.6 STELLANTCHASMUS FALCATUS INFECTION
954.1 STELLATE GANGLION INJURY
V59.02 STEM CELL DONOR NON-AUTOGENOUS
V42.82 STEM CELLS PERIPHERAL TRANSPLANT STATUS
0 STEMI (ST ELEVATION MYOCARDIAL INFARCTION) SEE 'MYOCARDIAL INFARCTION ACUTE', BY SITE

STENOSIS

0 See also 'Stricture'
799.89 NOS
576.2 Ampulla of vater
751.61 Ampulla of vater congenital
0 Ampulla of vater with calculus see 'Choledocholithiasis'

STENOSIS (continued)

569.2 Anus
751.2 Anus congenital (infantile)
747.10 Aorta - arch congenital
440.0 Aorta - arteriosclerotic
747.22 Aorta - ascending congenital
440.0 Aorta - calcified

AORTIC VALVE

424.1 NOS
396.0 Atypical
421.0 Bacterial acute
421.0 Bacterial chronic
746.3 Congenital
746.7 Congenital in hypoplastic left heart
746.81 Congenital subaortic
747.22 Congenital supravalvular
425.1 Hypertrophic subaortic - idiopathic
395.0 Rheumatic
395.2 Rheumatic with insufficiency
093.22 Syphilitic
424.1 With insufficiency
421.0 With insufficiency bacterial (acute) (chronic)
093.22 With insufficiency syphilitic
396.2 With mitral insufficiency
396.2 With mitral insufficiency rheumatic
093.22 With mitral insufficiency syphilitic
396.0 With mitral stenosis
396.0 With mitral stenosis rheumatic
093.22 With mitral stenosis syphilitic
396.8 With other valve multiple involvement, stenosis/insufficiency

STENOSIS (continued)

331.4 Aqueduct of sylvius
331.4 Aqueduct of sylvius with dementia [**294.1#**]
5th digit: 294.1
0. Without behavioral disturbance or NOS
1. With behavioral disturbance

742.3 Aqueduct of sylvius congenital
0 Aqueduct of sylvius congenital with spina bifida see 'Spina Bifida'
447.1 Artery NEC
380.50 Auditory canal acquired
433.0# Basilar artery
433.3# Basilar artery bilateral or multiple
5th digit: 433.0, 3
0. Without cerebral infarction
1. With cerebral infarction

576.2 Bile duct
751.61 Bile duct congenital
751.61 Bile duct congenital with jaundice [774.5]
0 Bile duct with calculus see 'Choledocholithiasis'
596.0 Bladder neck
753.6 Bladder neck congenital
0 Bladder neck with incontinence see 'Bladder Disorders With Incontinence'
560.9 Bowel NOS
751.2 Bowel congenital large
751.1 Bowel congenital small
0 Bowel see also 'Intestine, Intestinal', obstruction
348.8 Brain
519.19 Bronchus
748.3 Bronchus congenital
095.8 Bronchus syphilitic

STENOSIS (continued)

537.89 Cardia (stomach)
750.7 Cardia (stomach) congenital
429.2 Cardiovascular
433.1# Carotid artery
433.3# Carotid artery bilateral or multiple
5th digit: 433.1, 3
0. Without cerebral infarction
1. With cerebral infarction

560.9 Cecum NOS
751.2 Cecum congenital
0 Cecum see also 'Intestine, Intestinal', obstruction
447.4 Celiac artery
437.0 Cerebral artery NOS
434.1# Cerebral artery due to embolism
434.0# Cerebral artery due to thrombus
5th digit: 434.0, 1
0. Without cerebral infarction
1. With cerebral infarction

622.4 Cervix
654.6# Cervix - complicating pregnancy
5th digit: 654.6
0. Episode of care unspecified or N/A
1. Delivered
2. Delivered with postpartum complication
3. Antepartum complication
4. Postpartum complication

763.89 Cervix - complicating pregnancy affecting fetus or newborn
660.2# Cervix - complicating pregnancy obstructing labor [**654.6#**]
5th digit: 654.6
0. Episode of care unspecified or N/A
1. Delivered
2. Delivered with postpartum complication
3. Antepartum complication
4. Postpartum complication
5th digit: 660.2
0. Episode of care unspecified or N/A
1. Delivered
3. Antepartum complication

752.49 Cervix - congenital
763.1 Cervix - obstructing labor affecting fetus or newborn
560.9 Colon
751.2 Colon congenital
0 Colon see also 'Intestine, Intestinal', obstruction
569.62 Colostomy
576.2 Common bile duct
751.61 Common bile duct congenital
751.61 Common bile duct congenital with jaundice [774.5]
0 Common bile duct with calculus see 'Choledocholithiasis'
0 Coronary see 'Arteriosclerosis, Arteriosclerotic', coronary
575.2 Cystic duct
751.61 Cystic duct congenital
751.61 Cystic duct congenital with jaundice [774.5]
0 Cystic duct with calculus see 'Cholelithiasis'
0 Due to any device, implant or graft see 'Complication Of An Internal Prosthetic Device, Implant or Graft - (embolus) (fibrosis) (hemorrhage) (pain) (stenosis) (thrombus)'
537.3 Duodenum
751.1 Duodenum congenital

S

STENOSIS (continued)

380.50	Ear canal (external) - acquired NOS
380.53	Ear canal (external) - postinflammation
380.52	Ear canal (external) - postsurgical
380.51	Ear canal (external) - posttraumatic
380.89	Ear canal (external) - other acquired
608.89	Ejaculatory duct
622.4	Endocervical os
752.49	Endocervical os congenital
654.6#	Endocervical os complicating pregnancy
660.2#	Endocervical os obstructing labor [654.6#]
	5th digit: 654.6
	0. Episode of care unspecified or N/A
	1. Delivered
	2. Delivered with postpartum complication
	3. Antepartum complication
	4. Postpartum complication
	5th digit: 660.2
	0. Episode of care unspecified or N/A
	1. Delivered
	3. Antepartum complication
763.89	Endocervical os complicating pregnancy affecting fetus or newborn
763.1	Endocervical os obstructing labor affecting fetus or newborn
569.62	Enterostomy
530.87	Esophagostomy
530.3	Esophagus
750.3	Esophagus - congenital
095.8	Esophagus - syphilitic
090.5	Esophagus - syphilitic congenital
0	Eustachian tube see 'Eustachian', obstruction
628.2	Fallopian tube
098.17	Fallopian tube gonococcal acute
098.37	Fallopian tube gonococcal chronic
0	Fallopian tube tuberculous see 'Tuberculosis', oophoritis
575.2	Gallbladder
751.69	Gallbladder congenital
751.69	Gallbladder congenital with jaundice [774.5]
0	Gallbladder with calculus see 'Cholelithiasis'
536.42	Gastrostomy
478.74	Glottis
424.90	Heart or cardiac valve NOS
746.89	Heart or cardiac valve NOS congenital
576.2	Hepatic duct
751.61	Hepatic duct congenital
751.61	Hepatic duct congenital with jaundice [774.5]
0	Hepatic duct with calculus see 'Choledocholithiasis'
537.6	Hourglass, of stomach
623.3	Hymen
425.1	Hypertrophic subaortic
569.62	Ileostomy
746.83	Infundibulum cardiac
560.9	Intestine NOS
751.2	Intestine congenital large
751.1	Intestine congenital small
0	Intestine see also 'Intestine, Intestinal', obstruction
569.62	Jejunostomy
375.53	Lacrimal canaliculi
743.65	Lacrimal canaliculi congenital
375.56	Lacrimal duct
743.65	Lacrimal duct congenital
375.52	Lacrimal punctum
743.65	Lacrimal punctum congenital

STENOSIS (continued)

375.54	Lacrimal sac
743.65	Lacrimal sac congenital
375.56	Lacrimonasal duct
743.65	Lacrimonasal duct congenital
375.55	Lacrimonasal duct neonatal
478.74	Larynx
748.3	Larynx congenital
095.8	Larynx syphilitic
090.5	Larynx syphilitic congenital
518.89	Lung
380.50	Meatus osseous acquired
598.9	Meatus urinarius
753.6	Meatus urinarius congenital

MITRAL VALVE

394.0	NOS
396.1	And aortic insufficiency
396.1	And aortic insufficiency rheumatic
396.0	And aortic stenosis
396.0	And aortic stenosis rheumatic
421.0	Bacterial (acute) (chronic)
746.5	Congenital
394.0	Rheumatic
093.21	Syphilitic
394.2	With insufficiency
421.0	With insufficiency bacterial (acute) (chronic)
394.2	With insufficiency rheumatic
093.21	With insufficiency syphilitic
394.2	With regurgitation
424.0	Specified cause non rheumatic

STENOSIS (continued)

429.1	Myocardial NOS
425.1	Myocardial hypertrophic subaortic (idiopathic)
478.19	Nares
748.0	Nares congenital
375.56	Nasal duct
743.65	Nasal duct congenital
375.55	Nasal duct neonatal
743.65	Nasolacrimal congenital
375.56	Nasolacrimal duct
375.55	Nasolacrimal neonatal
095.8	Nasopharynx syphilitic
478.19	Nose
748.0	Nose congenital
478.19	Nostril
748.0	Nostril congenital
380.50	Osseous meatus acquired
628.2	Oviduct
098.17	Oviduct gonococcal acute
098.37	Oviduct gonococcal chronic
0	Oviduct tuberculous see 'Tuberculosis', oophoritis
576.2	Papilla of vater
751.61	Papilla of Vater congenital
0	Papilla of Vater with calculus see 'Choledocholithiasis'
593.3	Pelviureteric junction
433.9#	Precerebral artery unspecified
433.3#	Precerebral artery multiple or bilateral
433.8#	Precerebral artery other specified
	5th digit: 433.3, 8-9
	0. Without cerebral infarction
	1. With cerebral infarction

STENOSIS (continued)

417.8 Pulmonary artery
747.3 Pulmonary artery congenital
745.2 Pulmonary artery congenital in tetralogy of fallot
745.2 Pulmonary artery congenital with ventricular septal defect, dextraposition of aorta and hypertrophy of right ventricle
746.83 Pulmonary infundibular congenital
746.83 Pulmonary subvalvular congenital

PULMONARY VALVE

424.3 NOS
421.0 Bacterial (acute) (chronic)
746.02 Congenital
397.1 Rheumatic
093.24 Syphilitic
424.3 With insufficiency
421.0 With insufficiency bacterial (acute) (chronic)
397.1 With insufficiency rheumatic
093.24 With insufficiency syphilitic

STENOSIS (continued)

417.8 Pulmonary vein or vessel
747.49 Pulmonary vein congenital
537.0 Pylorus
750.5 Pylorus congenital or infantile
569.2 Rectum and anus
751.2 Rectum congenital
569.2 Rectum due to irradiation
095.8 Rectum syphilitic
440.1 Renal artery
527.8 Salivary duct
576.2 Sphincter of Oddi
751.61 Sphincter of Oddi congenital
751.61 Sphincter of Oddi congenital with jaundice [774.5]
0 Sphincter of Oddi with calculus see 'Choledocholithiasis'
724.00 Spinal - unspecified region
723.0 Spinal - cervical
724.02 Spinal - lumbar or lumbosacral
724.9 Spinal - nerve (root) NEC
724.01 Spinal - thoracic or thoracolumbar
724.09 Spinal - other specified region NEC
537.89 Stomach
750.7 Stomach congenital
537.6 Stomach, hourglass
746.81 Subaortic
425.1 Subaortic hypertrophic (idiopathic)
433.8# Subclavian artery

5th digit: 433.8
0. Without cerebral infarction
1. With cerebral infarction

478.74 Subglottic
747.22 Supra (valvular)-aortic
095.8 Syphilitic NEC
519.19 Trachea
748.3 Trachea congenital
095.8 Trachea syphilitic
0 Trachea tuberculous see 'Tuberculosis', respiratory other specified
519.02 Tracheostomy

TRICUSPID VALVE

424.2 NOS
746.1 And atresia congenital
421.0 Bacterial
746.1 Congenital

STENOSIS (continued)

TRICUSPID VALVE (continued)

397.0 Rheumatic
093.23 Syphilitic
421.0 With insufficiency bacterial (acute) (chronic)
093.23 With insufficiency syphilitic

STENOSIS (continued)

628.2 Tubal
098.17 Tubal gonococcal acute
098.37 Tubal gonococcal chronic
0 Tubal tuberculous see 'Tuberculosis', oophoritis
593.3 Ureter
753.29 Ureter congenital
593.3 Ureter postoperative
593.3 Ureteropelvic junction
753.21 Ureteropelvic junction congenital
593.3 Ureterovesical orifice
753.22 Ureterovesical orifice congenital
598.9 Urethra
753.6 Urethra - congenital
753.6 Urethra - valve congenital
0 Urethra - with incontinence congenital see 'Urethra, Urethral Disorders With Incontinence'
598.9 Urinary meatus
753.6 Urinary meatus congenital
621.5 Uterus
623.2 Vagina
752.49 Vagina congenital
654.7# Vagina complicating pregnancy

5th digit: 654.7
0. Episode of care unspecified or N/A
1. Delivered
2. Delivered with postpartum complication
3. Antepartum complication
4. Postpartum complication

763.89 Vagina complicating pregnancy affecting fetus or newborn
660.2# Vagina complicating pregnancy and obstructing labor [654.7#]

5th digit: 654.7
0. Episode of care unspecified or N/A
1. Delivered
2. Delivered with postpartum complication
3. Antepartum complication
4. Postpartum complication

5th digit: 660.2
0. Episode of care unspecified or N/A
1. Delivered
3. Antepartum complication

763.1 Vagina obstructing labor affecting fetus or newborn
0 Valve heart or cardiac see by specific valve
753.6 Valve urethra congenital
752.89 Vas deferens congenital
996.1 Vascular graft or shunt-mechanical complication
996.74 Vascular graft or shunt-embolism, occlusion or thrombus
459.2 Vein
459.2 Vena cava
747.49 Vena cava congenital
996.2 Ventricular shunt - mechanical complication

S

S

STENOSIS (continued)

433.2#	Vertebral artery
433.3#	Vertebral artery bilateral or multiple
	5th digit: 433.2-3
	0. Without cerebral infarction
	1. With cerebral infarction
596.0	Vesicourethral orifice
753.6	Vesicourethral orifice congenital
624.8	Vulva

527.8	STENSEN'S DUCT OBSTRUCTION
996.61	STENT CARDIAC COMPLICATION - INFECTION
996.09	STENT CARDIAC COMPLICATION - MECHANICAL
996.72	STENT CARDIAC COMPLICATION – OTHER
560.39	STERCOLITH NOS (SEE ALSO FECALITH)
543.9	STERCOLITH APPENDIX
368.33	STEREOPSIS DEFECT WITH VISUAL FUSION
307.3	STEREOTYPIES
0	STERILITY SEE 'INFERTILITY'
V25.2	STERILIZATION
V26.22	STERILIZATION REVERSAL AFTER CARE
V26.51	STERILIZATION STATUS - TUBAL LIGATION
V26.52	STERILIZATION STATUS – VASECTOMY
0	STERNBERG'S DISEASE SEE 'HODGKIN'S DISEASE'
739.8	STERNOCHONDRAL REGION SEGMENTAL OR SOMATIC DYSFUNCTION

STERNOCLAVICULAR

739.7	Region segmental or somatic dysfunction
848.41	Separation (rupture) (tear) (laceration)
848.41	Strain (sprain) (avulsion) (hemarthrosis)
754.1	STERNOCLEIDOMASTOID CONTRACTURE CONGENITAL
754.1	STERNOCLEIDOMASTOID MUSCLE DEFORMITY CONGENITAL
754.1	STERNOMASTOID TORTICOLLIS CONGENITAL
754.1	STERNOMASTOID TUMOR CONGENITAL

STERNUM, STERNAL

756.3	Absence congenital
756.3	Bifidum congenital
756.3	Fissure congenital
959.11	Injury NEC
786.9	Retraction during respiration
848.40	Separation (rupture) (tear) (laceration)
848.40	Strain (sprain) (avulsion) (hemarthrosis)
784.99	STERNUTATION
255.41	STEROID EFFECTS (ADVERSE) (IATROGENIC) WITHDRAWAL TO CORRECT SUBSTANCE PROPERLY ADMINISTRATED
255.2	STEROID METABOLISM DISORDER
V58.83	STEROIDAL DRUG MONITORING ENCOUNTER
V58.83	STEROIDAL DRUG MONITORING ENCOUNTER WITH <u>LONG TERM USE</u> [V58.65]
V67.51	STEROIDAL FOLLOW UP EXAM - COMPLETED THERAPY
V58.65	STEROIDAL FOLLOW UP EXAM - CURRENT THERAPY
695.1	STEVENS JOHNSON SYNDROME (ERYTHEMA MULTIFORME EXUDATIVUM)
733.3	STEWART-MOREL SYNDROME (HYPEROSTOSIS FRONTALIS INTERNA)
057.0	STICKER'S DISEASE (ERYTHEMA INFECTIOSUM)
759.89	STICKLER SYNDROME
286.9	STICKY PLATELET SYNDROME
726.62	STIEDA'S DISEASE (CALCIFICATION KNEE JOINT)

STIFF, STIFFNESS

759.89	Baby syndrome
724.8	Back NOS
719.5#	Joint NEC
	5th digit: 719.5
	0. Site NOS
	1. Shoulder region
	2. Upper arm (elbow) (humerus)
	3. Forearm (radius) (wrist) (ulna)
	4. Hand (carpal) (metacarpal) (fingers)
	5. Pelvic region and thigh (hip) (buttock) (femur)
	6. Lower leg (fibula) (knee) (patella) (tibia)
	7. Ankle and/or foot (metatarsals) (toes) (tarsals)
	8. Other
	9. Multiple
724.6	Lumbosacral
333.91	Man syndrome
524.52	Mandible
723.5	Neck
724.6	Sacroiliac
724.9	Spine
714.30	STILL'S DISEASE (JUVENILE RHEUMATOID ARTHRITIS)
714.1	STILL-FELTY DISEASE OR SYNDROME (JUVENILE RHEUMATOID ARTHRITIS WITH SPLENOMEGALY AND LEUKOPENIA)
779.9	STILLBIRTH NEC
V23.5	STILLBIRTH HISTORY AFFECTING PREGNANCY SUPERVISION
656.4#	STILLBORN (FETAL DEATH) AFFECTING MANAGEMENT OF MOTHER
	5th digit: 656.4
	0. Episode of care NOS or N/A
	1. Delivered
	3. Antepartum complication
780.79	STILLER'S DISEASE (ASTHENIA)
378.71	STILLING-TURK-DUANE SYNDROME (OCULAR RETRACTION SYNDROME)

STING VENOMOUS

0	See also 'Bite Venomous'
989.5	Agua mala
<u>995.0</u>	Agua mala with <u>anaphylaxis</u> [989.5]
989.5	Ant bite
<u>995.0</u>	Ant bite with <u>anaphylaxis</u> [989.5]
989.5	Arthropod NEC
<u>995.0</u>	Arthropod NEC with <u>anaphylaxis</u> [989.5]
989.5	Bee
<u>995.0</u>	Bee with <u>anaphylaxis</u> [989.5]
989.5	Caterpillar
<u>995.0</u>	Caterpillar with <u>anaphylaxis</u> [989.5]
989.5	Centipede
<u>995.0</u>	Centipede with <u>anaphylaxis</u> [989.5]
989.5	Coral
<u>995.0</u>	Coral with <u>anaphylaxis</u> [989.5]
989.5	Fire ant
<u>995.0</u>	Fire ant with <u>anaphylaxis</u> [989.5]

STING VENOMOUS (continued)

989.5 Hornet
995.0 Hornet with anaphylaxis [989.5]
989.5 Insect poisonous
995.0 Insect poisonous with anaphylaxis [989.5]
989.5 Jellyfish
995.0 Jellyfish with anaphylaxis [989.5]
989.5 Krait
995.0 Krait with anaphylaxis [989.5]
909.1 Late effect
909.9 Late effect with anaphylaxis
989.5 Marine animals or plants
995.0 Marine animals or plants with anaphylaxis [989.5]
989.5 Marine plant
995.0 Marine plant with anaphylaxis [989.5]
989.5 Millipede (tropical)
995.0 Millipede (tropical) with anaphylaxis [989.5]
989.5 Nematocyst
995.0 Nematocyst with anaphylaxis [989.5]
989.5 Scorpion
995.0 Scorpion with anaphylaxis [989.5]
989.5 Sea anemone
995.0 Sea anemone with anaphylaxis [989.5]
989.5 Sea cucumber
995.0 Sea cucumber with anaphylaxis [989.5]
989.5 Sea urchin
995.0 Sea urchin with anaphylaxis [989.5]
989.5 Snake
995.0 Snake with anaphylaxis [989.5]
989.5 Wasp
995.0 Wasp with anaphylaxis [989.5]

STITCH

998.59 Abscess postoperative
998.32 Burst
674.1# Burst C section (uterine) (internal) (external)
674.2# Burst episiotomy
998.32 Burst external
998.31 Burst internal
674.2# Burst perineal obstetrical
674.1# Burst uterine obstetrical
5th digit: 674.1-2
0. Episode of care NOS or N/A
2. Delivered with mention of postpartum complication
4. Postpartum condition or complication

998.89 Granuloma postoperative - external
998.89 Granuloma postoperative - internal
998.4 Inadvertently left in wound
998.89 Pain (wire)
V58.32 Removal

098.86 STOJANO'S (SUBCOSTAL) SYNDROME

242.0# STOKES' DISEASE (EXOPHTHALMIC GOITER)
5th digit: 242.0
0. Without mention of thyrotoxic crisis or storm
1. With mention of thyrotoxic crisis or storm

426.9 STOKES-ADAMS SYNDROME (SYNCOPE WITH HEART BLOCK)

289.7 STOKVIS' DISEASE OR SYNDROME (ENTEROGENOUS CYANOSIS)

STOMACH

V45.75 Absence (acquired) (partial) (postoperative)
750.7 Absence (acquired) (partial) (postoperative) - congenital
564.2 Absence (acquired) (partial) (postoperative) - with postgastric surgery syndrome
536.8 Ache
536.3 Atony
537.89 Atrophy
536.8 Contraction
750.7 Contraction congenital
306.4 Contraction psychogenic
789.06 Cramp
277.39 Degeneration lardaceous
536.1 Dilatation acute
536.1 Distention acute
537.9 Disorder
536.9 Disorder functional
306.4 Disorder functional psychogenic
750.7 Displacement congenital
537.1 Diverticulum
750.7 Diverticulum congenital
750.7 Duplication congenital
536.8 Engorgement
793.4 Filling defect
536.3 Gastroparesis
750.7 Hourglass anomaly congenital
863.0 Injury
908.1 Injury late effect
863.1 Injury with open wound
277.39 Lardaceous
537.89 Obstruction
536.1 Obstruction acute
750.7 Obstruction congenital
536.8 Spasm
750.7 Transposition congenital

STOMATITIS

528.00 NOS
101 Acute necrotizing (ulcerative)
528.2 Aphthous
528.00 Catarrhal
528.3 Cellulitis and abscess of mouth
528.9 Denture
032.0 Diphtheritic
078.4 Epizootic
528.00 Follicular
528.1 Gangrenous
0 Gingivitis see 'Gingivitis'
054.2 Herpes (simplex)
528.2 Herpetiformis
528.00 Malignant
528.00 Membranous acute
112.0 Oral thrush
528.00 Septic
101 Spirochetal
695.1 Stevens-Johnson Syndrome
528.00 Supprative (acute)
528.00 Ulcerative
528.00 Vesicular
101 Vincent's
528.09 Other

282.8 STOMATOCYTOSIS

0 STONE COMMON DUCT SEE 'CHOLEDOCHOLITHIASIS'

0 STONE SEE 'CALCULUS'

S

428.1 STONE HEART SYNDROME

502 STONEMASONS' DISEASE

STOOL

787.7 Abnormal
792.1 Abnormal content
578.1 Blood
792.1 Blood occult
787.7 Bulky
792.1 Color abnormal
792.1 Culture positive
792.1 Fat elevated abnormal
792.1 Melenotic
772.4 Melenotic of newborn due to fetal G.I. hemorrhage
777.3 Melenotic of newborn due to swallowed maternal blood
792.1 Mucus elevated abnormal
792.1 Pus elevated abnormal

368.01 STRABISMIC AMBLYOPIA

STRABISMUS MECHANICAL

378.60 NOS
378.63 Associated with other conditions
378.61 Brown's tendon syndrome
378.62 From other musculofacial disorders

STRABISMUS OTHER ETIOLOGY OR UNSPECIFIED

378.9 NOS
378.71 Duane's syndrome
378.72 Due to other neuromuscular disorders
378.72 Due to progressive external ophthalmoplegia
378.73 In other neuromuscular disorders
0 See also 'Esotropia' or 'Exotropia'

STRABISMUS PARALYTIC

378.50 NOS
378.55 External (ophthalmoplegia)
378.53 Fourth nerve palsy
378.54 Sixth nerve palsy
378.51 Third nerve palsy partial
378.52 Third nerve palsy total
378.56 Total paralysis (ophthalmoplegia)

756.19 STRAIGHT-BACK SYNDROME

Medically, a sprain occurs when excessive force causes injury to a ligament. A strain occurs when excessive force causes injury to a muscle or tendon. In ICD-9, sprain is the term used to cover all sprains, strains, avulsions, hemarthroses, tears and ruptures. In Easy Coder you'll find that codes for all of the above conditions are listed by site under the heading, sprain.

STRAIN

847.9 Back - NOS
847.0 Back - cervical
846.9 Back - low
847.2 Back - lumbar (spine)
846.0 Back - lumbosacral
724.6 Back - lumbosacral (joint) (ligament) chronic (old)
846.9 Back - sacroiliac (region)
724.6 Back - sacroiliac chronic (old)
846.1 Back - sacroiliac ligament
846.8 Back - sacroiliac region other specified sites
846.2 Back - sacrospinatus (ligament)
846.3 Back - sacrotuberous (ligament)
368.13 Eye NEC
0 Late effect see 'Late Effect', sprain

STRAIN (continued)

V62.89 Physical NEC
V62.89 Psychological NEC
0 See also 'Sprain'

788.65 STRAINING ON URINATION
994.7 STRANGULATION
909.4 STRANGULATION LATE EFFECT
788.1 STRANGURY
757.32 STRAWBERRY NEVUS CONGENITAL
026.1 STREPTOBACILLARY FEVER

STREPTOCOCCAL

034.0 Angina
0 Arthritis see 'Arthritis Other Specified', pyogenic
V02.51 B carrier
V28.6 B screening antenatal
V02.51 Carrier group B
V02.52 Carrier other
V01.89 Exposure
041.0# Infection or organism
771.89 Intra-amniotic newborn (fetus) **[041.0#]**
771.89 Intra-amniotic perinatal **[041.0#]**

5th digit: 041.0
0. NOS
1. Group A
2. Group B
3. Group C
4. Group D (Enterococcus)
5. Group G
9. Other strep

034.0 Laryngitis
034.0 Pharyngitis
482.3# Pneumonia

5th digit: 482.3
0. NOS
1. Group A
2. Group B
9. Other streptococcus

V03.82 Pneumoniae vaccination
V06.6 Pneumoniae and influenza vaccination
038.0 Septicemia
034.0 Sore throat
034.0 Tonsillitis

686.00 STREPTODERMA (SKIN)
0 STREPTOMYCES SEE 'ACTINOMYCOSIS'
308.3 STRESS DISORDER ACUTE
309.81 STRESS DISORDER POSTTRAUMATIC NOS

Stress fractures result from a crack in the bone caused by overexertion placed on a bone structure of the limb or metatarsal bone or from the pull of muscle on bone. These fractures are also called march fractures. (stress fracture metatarsal 733.94).

733.9# STRESS FRACTURE

5th digit: 733.9
3. Tibia or fibula
4. Metatarsals
5. Other bone

625.6 STRESS INCONTINENCE FEMALE
788.32 STRESS INCONTINENCE MALE

STRESS REACTION

308.9 Acute unspecified
308.2 Acute agitation
308.0 Acute anxiety
308.3 Acute disorder
308.0 Acute emotional crisis
308.1 Acute fugues
308.4 Acute mixed disorder
308.9 Acute reaction
308.3 Acute situational disturbances
308.2 Acute stupor
308.1 Acute with disturbances of consciousness
308.0 Acute with panic anxiety
308.3 Acute other
0 Chronic see also 'Adjustment Reaction'
308.0 Depressed
309.81 Posttraumatic NOS (acute) (brief)
308.2 Psychomotor

STRESS - REASON FOR ENCOUNTER

V62.89 Borderline intellectual functioning
V62.3 Educational
V62.81 Interpersonal
V62.5 Legal
V62.89 Life circumstance
V62.82 Loss of loved one
V62.2 Occupational
V62.89 Physical NEC
V62.89 Psychological NEC
V62.81 Relational problems NOS
V62.89 Religious problem
V62.4 Social maladjustment
V62.89 Spiritual problem
V62.84 Suicide ideation
V62.0 Unemployment (due to)
V62.1 Work

701.3 STRETCH MARK
701.3 STRIAE ATROPHICAE
701.3 STRIAE DISTENSAE
333.0 STRIATONIGRAL ATROPHY OR DEGENERATION BASAL GANGLIA
333.90 STRIATOPALLIDAL SYSTEM DISEASE
333.89 STRIATOPALLIDAL SYSTEM DISEASE SPECIFIED NEC

STRICTURE

0 See also 'Stenosis'
799.89 NOS
576.2 Ampulla of vater
0 Ampulla of vater with calculus see 'Choledocholithiasis'
569.2 Anus
751.2 Anus congenital or infantile
747.22 Aorta (ascending)
747.10 Aorta arch
440.0 Aorta arteriosclerotic or calcified
424.1 Aortic valve
746.3 Aortic valve congenital
331.4 Aqueduct of sylvius
331.4 Aqueduct of sylvius with dementia [294.1#]
5th digit: 294.1
0. Without behavioral disturbance or NOS
1. With behavioral disturbance

742.3 Aqueduct of sylvius congenital
0 Aqueduct of sylvius congenital with spina bifida see 'Spina Bifida'

STRICTURE (continued)

447.1 Artery NEC
747.6# Artery peripheral vascular congenital
5th digit: 747.6
0. Peripheral vascular unspecified site
1. Gastrointestinal vessel
2. Renal vessel
3. Upper limb vessel
4. Lower limb vessel
9. Other specified site peripheral vascular

380.50 Auditory canal
744.02 Auditory canal congenital
433.0# Basilar artery
433.3# Basilar artery bilateral or multiple
5th digit: 433.0, 3
0. Without cerebral infarction
1. With cerebral infarction

576.2 Bile duct
751.61 Bile duct congenital
751.61 Bile duct congenital with jaundice [774.5]
0 Bile duct with calculus see 'Choledocholithiasis'
596.8 Bladder
753.6 Bladder congenital
596.0 Bladder neck
753.6 Bladder neck congenital
0 Bladder neck with incontinence see 'Bladder Disorders With Incontinence'
560.9 Bowel NOS
751.2 Bowel congenital large
751.1 Bowel congenital small
0 Bowel see also 'Intestine, Intestinal', obstruction
348.8 Brain
519.19 Bronchus
095.8 Bronchus syphilitic
537.89 Cardia (stomach)
750.7 Cardia (stomach) congenital
429.2 Cardiovascular
433.1# Carotid artery
433.3# Carotid artery bilateral or multiple
5th digit: 433.1, 3
0. Without cerebral infarction
1. With cerebral infarction

560.9 Cecum NOS
751.2 Cecum congenital
0 Cecum see also 'Intestine, Intestinal', obstruction
447.4 Celiac artery
437.0 Cerebral artery NOS
747.81 Cerebral artery congenital
434.1# Cerebral artery due to embolism
434.0# Cerebral artery due to thrombus
5th digit: 434.0, 1
0. Without cerebral infarction
1. With cerebral infarction

S

STRICTURE (continued)

622.4 Cervix
654.6# Cervix - complicating pregnancy
763.89 Cervix - complicating pregnancy affecting fetus or newborn
<u>660.2#</u> Cervix – complicating pregnancy <u>obstructing</u> <u>labor</u> [654.6#]

5th digit: 654.6
- **0. Episode of care unspecified or N/A**
- **1. Delivered**
- **2. Delivered with postpartum complication**
- **3. Antepartum complication**
- **4. Postpartum complication**

5th digit: 660.2
- **0. Episode of care unspecified or N/A**
- **1. Delivered**
- **3. Antepartum complication**

752.49 Cervix - congenital
763.1 Cervix - obstructing labor affecting fetus or newborn
560.9 Colon
751.2 Colon congenital
0 Colon see also 'Intestine, Intestinal', obstruction
569.62 Colostomy
576.2 Common bile duct
751.61 Common bile duct congenital
751.61 Common bile duct congenital with <u>jaundice</u> <u>[774.5]</u>
0 Common bile duct with calculus see 'Choledocholithiasis'
746.85 Coronary artery congenital
0 Coronary see 'Arteriosclerosis, Arteriosclerotic', coronary
575.2 Cystic duct
751.61 Cystic duct congenital
751.61 Cystic duct congenital with <u>jaundice</u> <u>[774.5]</u>
0 Cystic duct with calculus see 'Cholelithiasis'
0 Due to any device, implant or graft see 'Complication Of An Internal Prosthetic Device, Implant Or Graft - (Embolus) (Fibrosis) (Hemorrhage) (Pain) (Stenosis) (Thrombus)'
997.5 Cystostomy
751.8 Digestive organs NEC, congenital
537.3 Duodenum
751.1 Duodenum congenital
380.50 Ear canal
744.02 Ear canal - congenital
380.53 Ear canal - postinflammation
380.52 Ear canal - postsurgical
380.51 Ear canal - posttraumatic
608.85 Ejaculatory duct
622.4 Endocervical os
752.49 Endocervical os congenital
654.6# Endocervical os complicating pregnancy
<u>660.2#</u> Endocervical os <u>obstructing</u> <u>labor</u> [654.6#]

5th digit: 654.6
- **0. Episode of care unspecified or N/A**
- **1. Delivered**
- **2. Delivered with postpartum complication**
- **3. Antepartum complication**
- **4. Postpartum complication**

5th digit: 660.2
- **0. Episode of care unspecified or N/A**
- **1. Delivered**
- **3. Antepartum complication**

STRICTURE (continued)

763.89 Endocervical os complicating pregnancy affecting fetus or newborn
763.1 Endocervical os obstructing labor affecting fetus or newborn
569.62 Enterostomy
530.87 Esophagostomy
530.3 Esophagus
750.3 Esophagus - congenital
095.8 Esophagus - syphilitic
090.5 Esophagus - syphilitic congenital
0 Eustachian tube see 'Eustachian', obstruction
0 Eustachian tube congenital see 'Eustachian', anomaly
628.2 Fallopian tube
098.17 Fallopian tube - gonococcal acute
098.37 Fallopian tube - gonococcal chronic
0 Fallopian tube - tuberculous see 'Tuberculosis', oophoritis
575.2 Gallbladder
751.69 Gallbladder congenital
751.69 Gallbladder congenital with <u>jaundice</u> <u>[774.5]</u>
0 Gallbladder with calculus see 'Cholelithiasis'
536.42 Gastrostomy
478.74 Glottis
746.89 Heart valve NOS congenital
576.2 Hepatic duct
751.61 Hepatic duct - congenital
751.61 Hepatic duct - congenital with <u>jaundice</u> <u>[774.5]</u>
0 Hepatic duct - with calculus see 'Choledocholithiasis'
537.6 Hourglass, of stomach
623.3 Hymen
425.1 Hypertrophic subaortic
478.29 Hypopharynx
569.62 Ileostomy
746.83 Infundibulum cardiac
560.9 Intestine - NOS
751.2 Intestine - congenital large
751.1 Intestine - congenital small
557.1 Intestine - ischemic
0 Intestine - see also 'Intestine, Intestinal', obstruction
569.62 Jejunostomy
375.53 Lacrimal canaliculi
743.65 Lacrimal canaliculi congenital
375.56 Lacrimal duct
743.65 Lacrimal duct congenital
375.52 Lacrimal punctum
743.65 Lacrimal punctum congenital
375.54 Lacrimal sac
743.65 Lacrimal sac congenital
375.56 Lacrimonasal duct
743.65 Lacrimonasal duct congenital
375.55 Lacrimonasal duct neonatal
478.79 Larynx
748.3 Larynx congenital
095.8 Larynx syphilitic
090.5 Larynx syphilitic congenital
518.89 Lung
380.50 Meatus ear
744.02 Meatus ear - congenital
380.53 Meatus ear - postinflammation
380.52 Meatus ear - postsurgical
380.51 Meatus ear - posttraumatic
380.50 Meatus osseous
744.03 Meatus osseous congenital
598.9 Meatus urinarius
753.6 Meatus urinarius congenital

STRICTURE (continued)

394.0 Mitral valve NOS
746.5 Mitral valve congenital
424.0 Mitral valve specified cause except rheumatic
093.21 Mitral valve syphilitic
429.1 Myocardial NOS
425.1 Myocardial hypertrophic subaortic (idiopathic)
478.19 Nares
748.0 Nares congenital
375.56 Nasal duct
743.65 Nasal duct congenital
375.55 Nasal duct neonatal
375.56 Nasolacrimal duct
743.65 Nasolacrimal congenital
375.55 Nasolacrimal neonatal
478.29 Nasopharynx
095.8 Nasopharynx syphilitic
997.5 Nephrostomy
478.19 Nose, nostril
748.0 Nose, nostril congenital
622.4 Os uteri
752.49 Os uteri congenital
654.6# Os uteri complicating pregnancy
660.2# Os uteri obstructing labor [**654.6#**]

5th digit: 654.6
- **0. Episode of care unspecified or N/A**
- **1. Delivered**
- **2. Delivered with postpartum complication**
- **3. Antepartum complication**
- **4. Postpartum complication**

5th digit: 660.2
- **0. Episode of care unspecified or N/A**
- **1. Delivered**
- **3. Antepartum complication**

763.89 Os uteri complicating pregnancy affecting fetus or newborn
763.1 Os uteri obstructing labor affecting fetus or newborn
380.50 Osseous meatus
744.03 Osseous meatus congenital
628.2 Oviduct
098.17 Oviduct gonococcal acute
098.37 Oviduct gonococcal chronic
0 Oviduct tuberculous see 'Tuberculosis', oophoritis
576.2 Papilla of vater
0 Papilla of vater with calculus see 'Choledocholithiasis'
593.3 Pelviureteric junction
478.29 Pharynx
433.9# Precerebral artery unspecified
433.3# Precerebral artery multiple or bilateral
433.8# Precerebral artery other specified

5th digit: 433.3, 8-9
- **0. Without cerebral infarction**
- **1. With cerebral infarction**

602.8 Prostate
417.8 Pulmonary artery
747.3 Pulmonary artery congenital
746.83 Pulmonary infundibular congenital
746.83 Pulmonary subvalvular congenital
424.3 Pulmonary valve
746.02 Pulmonary valve congenital
417.8 Pulmonary vein or vessel
747.49 Pulmonary vein congenital
537.0 Pylorus
750.5 Pylorus congenital or infantile
569.89 Rectosigmoid

STRICTURE (continued)

569.2 Rectum
751.2 Rectum - congenital
947.3 Rectum - due to chemical burn
569.2 Rectum - due to irradiation
099.1 Rectum - due to lymphogranuloma venereum
098.7 Rectum - gonococcal
099.1 Rectum - inflammatory
095.8 Rectum - syphilitic
0 Rectum - tuberculous see 'Tuberculosis', rectum
440.1 Renal artery
747.62 Renal artery congenital
743.58 Retinal artery congenital
527.8 Salivary duct
608.85 Spermatic cord
576.2 Sphincter of oddi
751.61 Sphincter of oddi congenital
751.61 Sphincter of oddi congenital with jaundice [774.5]
0 Sphincter of oddi with calculus see 'Choledocholithiasis'
747.82 Spinal artery congenital
537.89 Stomach
750.7 Stomach congenital
537.6 Stomach, hourglass
746.81 Subaortic congenital
425.1 Subaortic hypertrophic acquired (idiopathic)
478.74 Subglottic
747.22 Supra (valvular)-aortic
095.8 Syphilitic NEC
727.81 Tendon (sheath)
519.19 Trachea
748.3 Trachea congenital
095.8 Trachea syphilitic
0 Trachea tuberculous see 'Tuberculosis', respiratory other specified
519.02 Tracheostomy
0 Tricuspid see 'Tricuspid', stenosis
628.2 Tubal
098.17 Tubal gonococcal acute
098.37 Tubal gonococcal chronic
0 Tubal tuberculous see 'Tuberculosis', oophoritis
608.85 Tunica vaginalis
747.5 Umbilical artery congenital
593.3 Ureter
753.29 Ureter congenital
593.3 Ureter postoperative
593.3 Ureteropelvic junction
753.21 Ureteropelvic junction congenital
997.5 Ureterostomy
593.3 Ureterovesical orifice
753.22 Ureterovesical orifice congenital
598.9 Urethra NOS
753.6 Urethra congenital (meatus or bladder neck)
098.2 Urethra gonococcal or gonorrheal [598.01]
598.00 Urethra infection NOS (due to)
598.1 Urethra late effect of injury
615.9 Urethra myometritis (due to) [598.01]
598.2 Urethra postcatheterization
598.1 Urethra postobstetric
598.2 Urethra postoperative
598.1 Urethra posttraumatic
614.2 Urethra salpingo-oophoritis NOS (due to) [598.01]
614.0 Urethra salpingo-oophoritis acute (due to) [598.01]
614.1 Urethra salpingo-oophoritis chronic (due to) [598.01]
120.9 Urethra schistosomal [598.01]
095.8 Urethra syphilitic [598.01]

S

S

STRICTURE (continued)

598.8 Urethra specified cause NEC
753.6 Urethra valvular congenital
0 Urethra with incontinence see 'Urethra, Urethral Disorders With Incontinence'
598.9 Urinary meatus
753.6 Urinary meatus congenital
621.5 Uterus
623.2 Vagina
654.7# Vagina complicating pregnancy
5th digit: 654.7
0. Episode of care NOS or N/A
1. Delivered
2. Delivered with postpartum complication
3. Antepartum complication
4. Postpartum complication
763.89 Vagina complicating pregnancy affecting fetus or newborn
660.2# Vagina complicating pregnancy obstructing labor [654.7#]
5th digit: 654.7
0. Episode of care NOS or N/A
1. Delivered
2. Delivered with postpartum complication
3. Antepartum complication
4. Postpartum complication
5th digit: 660.2
0. Episode of care NOS or N/A
1. Delivered
3. Antepartum complication

752.49 Vagina congenital
763.1 Vagina obstructing labor affecting fetus or newborn
424.90 Valve heart or cardiac NOS (see also 'Stenosis', by valve)
746.89 Valve heart or cardiac NOS congenital
746.3 Valve aortic congenital
746.5 Valve mitral congenital
746.02 Valve pulmonary congenital
746.1 Valve tricuspid congenital
753.6 Valve urethra congenital
608.85 Vas deferens
752.89 Vas deferens congenital
996.1 Vascular graft or shunt-mechanical complication
996.74 Vascular graft or shunt-embolism, occlusion or thrombus
459.2 Vein
459.2 Vena cava
747.49 Vena cava congenital
996.2 Ventricular shunt-mechanical complication
433.2# Vertebral artery
433.3# Vertebral artery bilateral or multiple
5th digit: 433.2-3
0. Without cerebral infarction
1. With cerebral infarction

596.0 Vesicourethral orifice
753.6 Vesicourethral orifice congenital
624.8 Vulva

786.1 STRIDOR
748.3 STRIDOR LARYNGEAL CONGENITAL

Remember, CVA, stroke and cerebral infarction with occlusion NOS are all indexed to code 434.91. Do not use code 436.

When using the 434.91 code, remember to code also any residual effects due to the stroke.

STROKE

434.91 NOS
434.91 Acute
434.11 Embolic
0 Hemorrhagic see 'Hemorrhage', brain
V17.1 History family
997.02 Iatrogenic
435.9 Impending (transient ischemic attack)
434.91 In evolution
434.91 Ischemic
434.91 Lacunar infarct
0 Late effect see 'Late Effect', cerebrovascular disease
435.9 Little syndrome
0 Old with residual see 'Late Effect', cerebrovascular disease
V12.54 Old without residual
997.02 Postoperative
434.01 Thrombotic

127.2 STRONGYLOIDES STERCORALIS INFECTION
127.2 STRONGYLOIDIASIS
127.6 STRONGYLOIDIASIS TRICHOSTRONGYLIASIS
779.89 STROPHULUS
793.99 STRUCTURE ABNORMAL-BODY (ECHOGRAM) (THERMOGRAM) (ULTRASOUND) (X-RAY)
245.3 STRUMA FIBROSA
245.2 STRUMA LYMPHOMATOSA

241.9 STRUMA NODOSA (SIMPLEX)
242.3# STRUMA NODOSA TOXIC OR WITH HYPERTHYROIDISM
5th digit: 242.3
0. Without storm
1. With storm

STRUMA OVARII

220 Site NOS
0 Site specified see 'Benign Neoplasm', by site M9090/0
183.0 Malignant site NOS
0 Malignant site specified see 'Cancer', by site M9090/3

720.0 STRUMPELL-MARIE DISEASE (ANKYLOSING SPONDYLITIS)
286.3 STUART-PROWER DISEASE (CONGENITAL FACTOR X DEFICIENCY)
V70.5 STUDENT EXAM (HEALTH)
478.19 STUFFY NOSE
780.09 STUPOR
308.2 STUPOR, ACUTE REACTION TO STRESS
298.8 STUPOR PSYCHOGENIC

759.6 STURGE -KALISCHER-WEBER SYNDROME (ENCEPHALOTRIGEMINAL ANGIOMATOSIS)
759.6 STURGE -WEBER (-DIMITRI) SYNDROME (ENCEPHALOCUTANEOUS ANGIOMATOSIS)
307.0 STUTTERING
100.89 STUTTGART DISEASE
373.11 STYE

SUBACUTE

336.1 Necrotic myelopathy
330.8 Necrotizing encephalopathy or encephalomyelopathy
046.2 Sclerosing panencephalitis
046.1 Spongiform encephalopathy

746.81 SUBAORTIC STENOSIS CONGENITAL

SUBARACHNOID

851.8# Contusion (with hemorrhage)
851.9# Contusion with open intracranial wound (with hemorrhage)
430 Hematoma (nontraumatic)
852.0# Hematoma (hemorrhage) traumatic
852.1# Hematoma (hemorrhage) traumatic with open intracranial wound

5th digit: 851.8-9, 852.0-1
0. Level of consciousness (LOC) NOS
1. No LOC
2. LOC < 1 hr
3. LOC 1 - 24 hrs
4. LOC > 24 hrs with return to prior level
5. LOC > 24 hrs without return to prior level: or death before regaining consciousness, regardless of duration of LOC
6. LOC duration NOS
9. With concussion NOS

430 Hemorrhage (rupture berry aneurysm)
772.2 Hemorrhage fetus or newborn
674.0# Hemorrhage maternal due to pregnancy

5th digit: 674.0
0. Episode of care NOS or N/A
1. Delivered
2. Delivered with postpartum complication
3. Antepartum complication
4. Postpartum complication

094.87 Hemorrhage syphilitic
852.0# Hemorrhage traumatic
852.1# Hemorrhage traumatic with open intracranial wound
851.8# Laceration (with hemorrhage)
851.9# Laceration (with hemorrhage) with open intracranial wound

5th digit: 851.8-9, 852.0-1
0. Level of consciousness (LOC) NOS
1. No LOC
2. LOC < 1 hr
3. LOC 1 - 24 hrs
4. LOC > 24 hrs with return to prior level
5. LOC > 24 hrs without return to prior level: or death before regaining consciousness, regardless of duration of LOC
6. LOC duration NOS
9. With concussion NOS

SUBCLAVIAN

442.82 Artery (aneurysm) (A-V fistula) (cirsoid) (false) (varicose) (ruptured)
444.21 Artery embolism (thrombosis) (occlusion)
901.1 Artery injury
908.4 Artery injury late effect
908.4 Artery laceration late effect
901.1 Artery laceration (rupture) (hematoma) (avulsion) (aneurysm) traumatic
446.7 Carotid obstruction syndrome (chronic)
996.62 Line complication - infection or inflammation
996.1 Line complication - mechanical
996.74 Line complication - other
435.2 Steal syndrome (insufficiency)
453.8 Vein embolism (thrombosis) (occlusion)
901.3 Vein injury
908.4 Vein injury late effect
908.4 Vein laceration late effect
901.3 Vein laceration (rupture) (hematoma) (avulsion) (aneurysm) traumatic
451.89 Vein phlebitis (thrombophlebitis)

372.73 SUBCONJUNCTIVAL EDEMA
372.72 SUBCONJUNCTIVAL HEMORRHAGE
447.8 SUBCORACOID-PECTORALIS MINOR SYNDROME
694.1 SUBCORNEAL PUSTULAR DERMATOSIS
431 SUBCORTICAL HEMORRHAGE (CEREBRAL)
098.86 SUBCOSTAL SYNDROME
354.8 SUBCOSTAL NERVE COMPRESSION SYNDROME

SUBCUTANEOUS

793.99 Abnormal finding tissue (x-ray) (ultrasound) (thermography)
701.9 Atrophy
709.3 Calcification
998.81 Emphysema post op
909.3 Emphysema post op late effect
958.7 Emphysema traumatic
908.6 Emphysema traumatic late effect
782.2 Mass
782.2 Nodules
V13.3 Tissue disease history

V25.43 SUBDERMAL CONTRACEPTIVE DEVICE - CHECKING, REINSERTION OR REMOVAL
V45.52 SUBDERMAL CONTRACEPTIVE DEVICE - IN SITU
V25.5 SUBDERMAL CONTRACEPTIVE DEVICE – INSERTION

530.6 SUBDIAPHRAGMATIC DIVERTICULUM (ESOPHAGEAL)

S

SUBDURAL

851.8# Contusion (with hemorrhage)
851.9# Contusion with open intracranial wound (with hemorrhage)
432.1 Hematoma (hemorrhage)
852.2# Hematoma (hemorrhage) traumatic
852.3# Hematoma (hemorrhage) traumatic with open intracranial wound
5th digit: 851.8-9, 852.2-3
0. Level of consciousne (LOC) NOS
1. No LOC
2. LOC < 1 hr
3. LOC 1 - 24 hrs
4. LOC > 24 hrs with return to prior level
5. LOC > 24 hrs without return to prior level: or death before regaining consciousness, regardless of duration of LOC
6. LOC duration NOS
9. With concussion NOS

767.0 Hemorrhage fetus or newborn birth trauma (intrapartum hypoxia/anoxia)
674.0# Hemorrhage maternal due to pregnancy
5th digit: 674.0
0. Episode of care NOS or N/A
1. Delivered
2. Delivered with postpartum complication
3. Antepartum complication
4. Postpartum complication

852.2# Hemorrhage traumatic
852.3# Hemorrhage traumatic with open intracranial wound
851.8# Laceration (with hemorrhage)
851.9# Laceration with open intracranial wound (with hemorrhage)
5th digit: 851.8-9, 852.2-3
0. Level of consciousness (LOC) NOS
1. No LOC
2. LOC < 1 hr
3. LOC 1 - 24 hrs
4. LOC > 24 hrs with return to prior level
5. LOC > 24 hrs without return to prior level: or death before regaining consciousness, regardless of duration of LOC
6. LOC duration NOS
9. With concussion NOS

410.7# SUBENDOCARDIAL INFARCTION
5th digit: 410.7
0. Episode unspecified
1. Initial episode
2. Subsequent episode

411.89 SUBENDOCARDIAL ISCHEMIA
495.3 SUBEROSIS
0 SUBGLOTTIC SEE 'SUBGLOTTIS, SUBGLOTTIC'

SUBGLOTTIS, SUBGLOTTIC

478.6 Edema
228.09 Hemangioma
748.2 Webbing of larynx congenital

286.0 SUBHEMOPHILIA
621.1 SUBINVOLUTION UTERUS
674.8# SUBINVOLUTION UTERUS MATERNAL DUE TO PREGNANCY
5th digit: 674.8
0. Episode of care NOS or N/A
2. Delivered with postpartum complication
4. Postpartum complication

SUBLINGUAL

527.8 Duct atresia
750.23 Duct atresia congenital
527.0 Gland atrophy
456.3 Varices

SUBLUXATION (SEE ALSO DISLOCATION)

839.0# Cervical spine (vertebra)
5th digit: 839.0
0. Cervical vertebra unspecified
1. First cervical vertebra
2. Second cervical vertebra
3. Third cervical vertebra
4. Fourth cervical vertebra
5. Fifth cervical vertebra
6. Sixth cervical vertebra
7. Seventh cervical vertebra
8. Multiple cervical vertebra

839.41 Coccyx
832.0# Elbow
5th digit: 832.0
0. Unspecified
1. Anterior
2. Posterior
3. Medial
4. Lateral
9. Other

754.33 Hip bilateral congenital
754.32 Hip unilateral congenital
754.35 Hip with dislocation other hip congenital
836.5# Knee
5th digit: 836.5
0. Unspecified
1. Anterior
2. Posterior
3. Medial
4. Lateral end
9. Other or rotatory

718.26 Knee pathological
718.36 Knee recurrent old
379.32 Lens nonsurgical
839.20 Lumbar vertebra
836.3 Patella
718.36 Patella recurrent old
839.69 Pelvic
839.42 Sacroiliac (joint)
839.42 Sacrum
839.21 Thoracic vertebra

527.2 SUBMANDIBULAR GLAND INFECTION

SUBMAXILLARY

527.8 Duct or gland atresia
750.23 Duct or gland atresia congenital
750.21 Gland absence (congenital)
527.0 Gland (duct) atrophy
527.8 Gland (duct) dilatation
527.8 Gland (duct) obstruction
527.5 Gland (duct) obstruction with calculus
959.09 Region injury

994.1 SUBMERSION
909.4 SUBMERSION LATE EFFECT

566 SUBMUCOSAL ABSCESS RECTUM
528.8 SUBMUCOSAL FIBROSIS ORAL INCLUDING TONGUE

726.69 SUBPATELLAR BURSITIS
267 SUBPERIOSTEAL HEMATOMA SYNDROME
751.4 SUBPHRENIC INTERPOSITION SYNDROME

362.81 SUBRETINAL HEMORRHAGE
362.16 SUBRETINAL NEOVASCULARIZATION

723.4 SUBSCAPULAR NEURITIS
840.5 SUBSCAPULARIS SEPARATION (RUPTURE) (TEAR) (LACERATION)
840.5 SUBSCAPULARIS STRAIN (SPRAIN) (AVULSION) (HEMARTHROSIS)

> ***Substance abuse is the term used to describe the practice of using drugs or alcohol to excess without having reached a stage of physical dependence. Substance dependence is addiction. Dependence involves loss of control and judgment to use in moderate amounts.***

SUBSTANCE ABUSE

303.0# Alcohol (dependent) acute drunkenness
303.9# Alcohol (dependent) chronic
305.0# Alcohol (nondependent)

5th digit: 303.0, 9, 305.0
- **0. NOS**
- **1. Continuous**
- **2. Episodic**
- **3. In remission**

V65.42 Counseling
304.## Drug dependent – addiction

4th digit: 304
- **0. Opioid**
- **1. Sedative, hypnotic or anxiolytic**
- **2. Cocaine**
- **3. Cannabis**
- **4. Amphetamine type**
- **5. Hallucinogenic**
- **6. Other specified**
- **7. Mixed with opioid**
- **8. Mixed**
- **9. NOS**

5th digit: 304
- **0. NOS**
- **1. Continuous**
- **2. Episodic**
- **3. In remission**

SUBSTANCE ABUSE (continued)

305.## Drug nondependent - abuse

4th digit: 305
- **0. Alcohol**
- **2. Cannabis**
- **3. Hallucinogen**
- **4. Sedative, hypnotic or anxiolytic**
- **5. Opioid**
- **6. Cocaine**
- **7. Amphetamine type**
- **8. Antidepressant type**
- **9. Mixed or other specified**

5th digit: 305
- **0. NOS**
- **1. Continuous**
- **2. Episodic**
- **3. In remission**

305.1 Tobacco dependent

300.11 SUBSTITUTION DISORDER
923.3 SUBUNGUAL HEMATOMA FINGERNAIL (THUMB NAIL)
924.3 SUBUNGUAL HEMATOMA TOENAIL
796.1 SUCKING REFLEX POOR (NEWBORN)
271.3 SUCROSE ISOMALTOSE INTOLERANCE OR MALABSORPTION
705.1 SUDAMINA
V17.41 SUDDEN CARDIAC DEATH (SCD) FAMILY HISTORY
674.9# SUDDEN DEATH (PUERPERAL) MATERNAL DUE TO PREGNANCY

5th digit: 674.9
- **0. NOS**
- **2. Delivered with postpartum complication**
- **4. Postpartum complication**

798.0 SUDDEN INFANT DEATH SYNDROME (SIDS)
0 SUDDEN INFANT DEATH SYNDROME (SIDS) NEAR MISS - CODE INDIVIDUAL SYMPTOM(S)
798.2 SUDDEN UNEXPLAINED DEATH (SUDS)
368.11 SUDDEN VISUAL LOSS
733.7 SUDECK (-LERICHE) ATROPHY OR SYNDROME
798.2 SUDS

SUFFOCATION

994.7 Bedclothes
994.7 Cave-in
994.7 Constriction
909.4 Late effect
994.7 Mechanical
994.7 Plastic bag
994.7 Pressure
994.7 Strangulation
0 See also 'Asphyxiation Food, Mucus, or Foreign Body Inhalation'

SUICIDE

300.9 Attempt
V62.84 Ideation
V71.89 Observation for alleged attempt
300.9 Risk
300.9 Tendencies

V14.2 SULFA ALLERGY (HISTORY)
289.7 SULFHEMOGLOBINEMIA
270.0 SULFITE OXIDASE DEFICIENCY

V14.2 SULFONAMIDE ALLERGY (HISTORY)
V09.6 SULFONAMIDES RESISTANT INFECTION (SEE 'DRUG RESISTANCE')
692.72 SUMMER ACNE
692.72 SUMMER PRURIGO
992.0 SUN STROKE
909.4 SUN STROKE LATE EFFECT
692.7# SUNBURN

5th digit: 692.7
- **1. NOS (first degree)**
- **6. Second degree**
- **7. Third degree**

692.82 SUNBURN TANNING BED
360.24 SUNFLOWER CATARACT [366.34]
651.9# SUPERFECUNDATION GESTATION
651.7# SUPERFECUNDATION GESTATION FOLLOWING (ELECTIVE) FETAL REDUCTION

5th digit: 651.7, 9
- **0. Episode of care NOS or N/A**
- **1. Delivered**
- **3. Antepartum complication**

651.9# SUPERFETATION GESTATION
651.7# SUPERFETATION GESTATION FOLLOWING (ELECTIVE) FETAL REDUCTION

5th digit: 651.7, 9
- **0. Episode of care NOS or N/A**
- **1. Delivered**
- **3. Antepartum complication**

SUPERIOR

0 Cerebellar artery syndrome see 'Cerebrovascular', accident
902.25 Mesenteric artery (trunk) laceration (rupture) (hematoma) (avulsion) (aneurysm)
908.4 Mesenteric artery injury or laceration late effect
557.1 Mesenteric artery syndrome
902.31 Mesenteric vein injury (primary subdivisions)
908.4 Mesenteric vein injury or laceration late effect
902.31 Mesenteric vein laceration (rupture) (hematoma) (avulsion) (aneurysm) traumatic

SUPERIOR VENA CAVA

747.49 Absence (congenital)
747.40 Anomaly
901.2 Injury
908.4 Injury late effect
459.2 Obstruction
453.2 Occlusion
459.2 Syndrome
453.2 Thrombosis

SUPERNUMERARY

746.5 Cusps mitral valve (congenital)
755.00 Digits
755.01 Fingers
756.2 Rib cervical region
752.89 Testes congenital
755.02 Toes
520.1 Teeth
756.19 Vertebra

SUPERVISION

V20.1 Child (healthy)
V25.43 Contraceptive (subdermal implantable)
V20.0 Foundling
V20.1 Infant (healthy)
V24.1 Lactating mother

SUPERVISION OF PREGNANCY

V23.7 Prenatal care poor or none
V22.0 Normal (first)
V22.1 Normal (other than first)
V23.9 High risk
V23.2 High risk - abortion history
V23.49 High risk - difficult delivery history

Elderly multigravida:* *Second or more pregnancy in a woman who will be 35 years of age or older at expected date of delivery.

V23.82 High risk - elderly multigravida

Elderly primigravida:* *First pregnancy in a woman who will be 35 years of age or older at expected date of delivery.

V23.81 High risk - elderly primigravida
V23.49 High risk - forceps delivery history
V23.3 High risk - grand multiparity
V23.49 High risk - hemmorhage antepartum history
V23.49 High risk - hemmorhage postpartum history
V23.1 High risk - hydatidiform mole history
V23.0 High risk - infertility history
V23.89 High risk - mental disorder history
V23.5 High risk - neonatal death history
V23.49 High risk - poor obstetrical history
V23.7 High risk - prenatal care poor or none
V23.41 High risk - pre-term delivery history
V23.41 High risk - pre-term labor history
V23.5 High risk - stillbirth history
V23.1 High risk - trophoblastic disease history
V23.1 High risk - vesicular mole history

Young multigravida:* *Second or more pregnancy in a female who is less than 16 years old at expected date of delivery.

V23.84 High risk - young multigravida

Young primigravida:* *First pregnancy in a female who is less than 16 years old at expected date of delivery.

V23.83 High risk - young primigravida
V23.89 High risk - other specified

788.5 SUPPRESSION OF URINARY SECRETION
959.19 SUPRACLAVICULAR FOSSA INJURY NEC
738.8 SUPRACLAVICULAR RETRACTION
524.34 SUPRAERUPTION TEETH
478.6 SUPRAGLOTTIC EDEMA
464.5# SUPRAGLOTTITIS NOS

5th digit: 464.5
- **0. Without mention of obstruction**
- **1. With obstruction**

333.0 SUPRANUCLEAR OPHTHALMOPLEGIA PROGRESSIVE
333.0 SUPRANUCLEAR PALSY PROGRESSIVE
356.8 SUPRANUCLEAR PARALYSIS
959.09 SUPRAORBITAL INJURY

SUPRARENAL

902.49 Arteries laceration (rupture) (hematoma)(avulsion) (aneurysm) traumatic
902.49 Artery injury
908.4 Artery injury or laceration late effect
255.41 Atrophy with or without hypofunction (autoimmune) (capsule) (gland)
255.41 Calcification (capsule) (gland)
255.3 Cortical syndrome
255.8 Degeneration
255.41 Degeneration with hypofunction
255.41 Disease hypofunction
255.41 Hemorrhage
255.3 Hyperfunction
255.8 Hyperplasia
255.41 Hypofunction (capsule) (gland)
255.41 Infarction
868.01 Injury gland (multiple) traumatic
868.11 Injury gland (multiple) traumatic with open wound
255.41 Insufficiency
255.41 Melanosis
255.41 Melasma

SUPRASPINATUS

726.10 Impingement
840.6 Separation (rupture) (tear) (laceration)
840.6 Strain (sprain) (avulsion) (hemarthrosis)
726.10 Syndrome

427.61 SUPRAVENTRICULAR PREMATURE BEATS
427.89 SUPRAVENTRICULAR TACHYCARDIA
427.0 SUPRAVENTRICULAR TACHYCARDIA PAROXYSMAL
919.8 SURFER KNOTS
919.9 SURFER KNOTS INFECTED

When surgery is cancelled due to an unforseen problem, code the preoperative diagnosis first, then use a code from v 64.# to indicate that surgery was not carried out, and a third code to indicate the reason. (surgery re-scheduled, patient elects not to have the surgery, surgeon had an emergency.)

SURGERY

0 Aftercare see 'Aftercare'
V64.43 Arthroscopic converted to open procedure
V66.0 Convalescence
V67.00 Follow up exam unspecified
V67.09 Follow up exam other
V64.41 Laparoscopic converted to open procedure
760.6 Maternal affecting fetus or newborn
V64.1 Not carried out due to contraindication
V64.2 Not carried out patient decision
V62.6 Not carried out patient decision - conscience or religion based
V64.3 Not carried out for other reasons
V64.42 Thoracoscopic converted to open procedure

SURGERY ELECTIVE

V50.9 Unspecified
V50.1 Breast augmentation
V50.1 Breast reduction
V50.2 Circumcision routine or ritual
V50.1 Cosmetic
V50.3 Ear piercing
V50.1 Face lift
V50.0 Hair transplant
V50.8 Other

SUSCEPTIBILITY GENETIC

Code first any current malignant neoplasms. See 'Cancer', by site. Use an additional code, if applicable, for any personal history of malignant neoplasm. See 'History', CA, by site for those codes.

V84.0# Malignant neoplasm
5th digit: V84.0
1. Breast
2. Ovary
3. Prostate
4. Endometrium
9. Other site

Use an additional for any associated family history of the disease. See 'Family History.

V84.81 Multiple endocrine neoplasia (MEN)
V84.81 Neoplasia multiple endocrine (MEN)
V84.89 Other specified disease

709.09 SUTTON'S DISEASE

SUTURE

998.59 Abscess postoperative
998.32 Burst
674.1# Burst C section
674.2# Burst episiotomy
5th digit: 674.1-2
0. Episode of care NOS or N/A
2. Delivered with mention of postpartum complication
4. Postpartum condition or complication

998.32 Burst external
998.31 Burst internal
674.2# Burst perineal obstetrical
674.1# Burst uterine obstetrical
5th digit: 674.1-2
0. Episode of care NOS or N/A
2. Delivered with mention of postpartum complication
4. Postpartum condition or complication

998.89 Granuloma postoperative - external
998.89 Granuloma postoperative - internal
998.4 Inadvertently left in wound
998.89 Pain (wire)
V58.32 Removal

427.89 SVT (SUPRAVENTRICULAR TACHYCARDIA)
427.0 SVT PAROXYSMAL (SUPRAVENTRICULAR TACHYCARDIA PAROXYSMAL)
777.3 SWALLOWED BLOOD SYNDROME
787.20 SWALLOWING DIFFICULTY (DYSPHAGIA)
V41.6 SWALLOWING PROBLEMS
100.89 SWAMP FEVER
736.22 SWAN NECK DEFORMITY FINGER ACQUIRED

SWEAT, SWEATING

705.89 Colored
705.0 Deficiency
078.2 Disease
780.8 Excessive
705.21 Excessive hyperhidrosis - NOS (primary)
705.22 Excessive hyperhidrosis - secondary
705.89 Fetid
078.2 Fever

S

SWEAT, SWEATING (continued)

705.89 Foul smelling
705.9 Gland disorder NOS
705.89 Gland disorder other
705.83 Gland inflamed
238.2 Gland tumor site NOS
0 Gland tumor site specified see 'Neoplasm Uncertain Behavior', by site M8400/1
078.2 Miliary
780.8 Night
705.1 Retention syndrome
078.2 Sickness

272.4 SWEELEY-KLIONSKY DISEASE

695.89 SWEET'S SYNDROME (ACUTE FEBRILE NEUTROPHILIC DERMATOSIS)

SWELLING

782.3 NOS
789.3# Abdominal
5th digit: 789.3
0. Unspecified site
1. Upper right quadrant
2. Upper left quadrant
3. Lower right quadrant
4. Lower left quadrant
5. Periumbilic
6. Epigastric
7. Generalized
9. Other specified site (multiple)

789.59 Abdominal due to ascites
789.51 Abdominal due to ascites malignant
255.8 Adrenal gland, cloudy
0 Ankle see 'Swelling', joint
787.99 Anus
729.81 Arm
611.72 Breast
125.2 Calabar
785.6 Cervical gland
784.2 Cheek
786.6 Chest
388.8 Ear
789.36 Epigastric
729.81 Extremity (lower) (upper)
454.8 Extremity lower due to varicose vein
379.92 Eye
625.8 Female genital organ
729.81 Finger
729.81 Foot
785.6 Glands
784.2 Gum
729.81 Hand
784.2 Head
719.0# Joint
5th digit: 719.0
0. Site NOS
1. Shoulder region
2. Upper arm (elbow) (humerus)
3. Forearm (radius) (wrist) (ulna)
4. Hand (carpal) (metacarpal) (fingers)
5. Pelvic region and thigh (hip) (buttock) (femur)
6. Lower leg (fibula) (knee) (patella) (tibia)
7. Ankle and/or foot (metatarsals) (toes) (tarsals)
8. Other
9. Multiple

SWELLING (continued)

593.89 Kidney, cloudy
729.81 Leg
454.8 Leg due to varicose vein
729.81 Limb
573.8 Liver
786.6 Lung
785.6 Lymph nodes
197.6 Malignant
786.6 Mediastinal
784.2 Mouth
729.81 Muscle (limb)
784.2 Neck
784.2 Nose or sinus
729.81 Of limb
784.2 Palate
789.39 Pelvis
607.83 Penis
625.8 Perineum
787.99 Rectum
608.86 Scrotum
782.2 Skin
789.2 Spleen
786.6 Substernal
782.2 Superficial (skin)
608.86 Testicle
784.2 Throat
729.81 Toe
784.2 Tongue
593.9 Tubular NOS
789.35 Umbilicus
625.8 Uterus
625.8 Vagina
625.8 Vulva

985.0 SWIFT (-FEER) DISEASE
380.12 SWIMMERS' EAR ACUTE
120.3 SWIMMERS' ITCH CUTANEOUS
031.1 SWIMMING POOL BACILLUS
077.0 SWIMMING POOL CONJUNCTIVITIS

100.89 SWINEHERD'S DISEASE

785.6 SWOLLEN GLANDS

SWYER JAMES SYNDROME

492.8 NOS (unilateral hyperlucent lung)
752.7 Congenital (XY pure gonadal dysgenesis)
491.2# With bronchitis (chronic)
5th digit: 491.2
0. NOS
1. With (acute) exacerbation
2. With acute bronchitis

SYCOSIS

704.8 NOS
704.8 Barbae not parasitic
704.8 Lupoid
110.0 Mycotic
704.8 Vulgaris

392.9 SYDENHAM'S CHOREA
392.0 SYDENHAM'S CHOREA WITH HEART INVOLVEMENT

060.0 SYLVAN YELLOW FEVER
074.1 SYLVEST'S DISEASE (EPIDEMIC PLEURODYNIA)

372.63 SYMBLEPHARON

784.60 SYMBOLIC DYSFUNCTION

202.0# SYMMERS DISEASE (FOLLICULAR LYMPHOMA)

5th digit: 202.0

0. Unspecified site, extranodal and solid organ sites
1. Lymph nodes of head, face, neck
2. Lymph nodes intrathoracic
3. Lymph nodes abdominal
4. Lymph nodes axilla and upper limb
5. Lymph nodes inguinal region and lower limb
6. Lymph nodes intrapelvic
7. Spleen
8. Lymph nodes multiple sites

348.2 SYMOND'S SYNDROME

337.0 SYMPATHETIC CERVICAL PARALYSIS SYNDROME

337.9 SYMPATHETIC NERVE DISORDER NEC

625.5 SYMPATHETIC PELVIC SYNDROME

305.7# SYMPATHOMIMETIC ABUSE NONDEPENDENT

5th digit: 305.7

0. NOS
1. Continuous
2. Episodic
3. In remission

0 SYMPHALANGY/SYMPHALANGIA SEE 'SYNDACTYLY, SYNDACTYLIC'

959.19 SYMPHYSIS PUBIS INJURY

732.1 SYMPHYSIS PUBIS OSTEOCHONDROSIS

665.6# SYMPHYSIS PUBIS SEPARATION (OBSTETRICAL)

5th digit: 665.6

0. Episode of care NOS or N/A
1. Delivered
4. Postpartum complication

848.5 SYMPHYSIS PUBIS SPRAIN (STRAIN) (RUPTURE) (TEAR)

0 SYNARTHROSIS SEE 'JOINT', CALCIFICATION'

732.1 SYNCHONDROSIS ISCHIOPUBIC (OF VAN NECK)

379.22 SYNCHYSIS SCINTILLANS

780.2 SYNCOPE (NEAR) (-PRE) AND COLLAPSE UNKNOWN ETIOLOGY

337.0 SYNCOPE CAROTID SINUS

SYNDACTYLY, SYNDACTYLIC

755.10 Multiple and NOS sites
755.12 Fingers with fusion of bone
755.11 Fingers without fusion of bone
755.55 Oxycephaly
755.14 Toes with fusion of bone
755.13 Toes without fusion of bone

0 SYNDESMOSIS TIBIOFIBULAR JOINT SEE 'DISLOCATION', ANKLE

0 SYNDROME SEE BY SPECIFIC NAME

SYNECHIAE

364.70 NOS (eye)
364.72 Anterior (eye)
621.5 Intrauterine (traumatic)
364.70 Iris (eye)
478.19 Nasal or intranasal
364.73 Peripheral anterior (eye)
364.71 Posterior (eye)
752.49 Vulva congenital

752.89 SYNORCHIDISM

752.89 SYNORCHISM

0 SYNOVIAL SEE 'SYNOVIUM, SYNOVIAL'

215.# SYNOVIOMA BENIGN M9040/0

171.# SYNOVIOMA MALIGNANT M9040/3

4th digit: 171, 215

0. Head, face, neck
2. Upper limb including shoulder
3. Lower limb including hip
4. Thorax
5. Abdomen (wall), gastric, gastrointestinal, intestine, stomach
6. Pelvis, buttock, groin, inguinal region, perineum
7. Trunk NOS, back NOS, flank NOS
8. Other specified sites
9. Site NOS

SYNOVITIS

727.00 NOS
727.06 Ankle
275.49 Crystal induced - unspecified **[712.9#]**
0 Crystal induced - chondrocalcinosis see 'Chondrocalcinosis'
274.0 Crystal induced - gouty
275.49 Crystal induced - other specified **[712.8#]**

5th digit: 712.8-9

0. Site NOS
1. Shoulder region
2. Upper arm (elbow) (humerus)
3. Forearm (radius) (wrist) (ulna)
4. Hand (carpal) (metacarpal) (fingers)
5. Pelvic region and thigh (hip) (buttock) (femur)
6. Lower leg (fibula) (knee) (patella) (tibia)
7. Ankle and/or foot (metatarsals) (toes) (tarsals)
8. Other (head) (neck) (rib) (skull) (trunk) (vertebrae)
9. Multiple

727.05 Finger
727.06 Foot and ankle
098.51 Gonococcal
274.0 Gouty
727.05 Hand and wrist
095.7 Syphilitic
015.## Tuberculous [727.01]

4th digit: 015

0. Vertebral column
1. Hip
2. Knee
5. Limb bones
6. Mastoid
7. Other specified bone
8. Other specified joint
9. Unspecified bones and joints

5th digit: 015

0. NOS
1. Lab not done
2. Lab pending
3. Microscopy positive (in sputum)
4. Culture positive - microscopy negative
5. Culture negative - microscopy positive
6. Culture and microscopy negative confirmed by other methods

S

SYNOVITIS (continued)

719.2# Villonodular
5th digit: 719.2
0. Site NOS
1. Shoulder region
2. Upper arm (elbow) (humerus)
3. Forearm (radius) (wrist) (ulna)
4. Hand (carpal) (metacarpal) (fingers)
5. Pelvic region and thigh (hip) (buttock) (femur)
6. Lower leg (fibula) (knee) (patella) (tibia)
7. Ankle and/or foot (metatarsals) (toes) (tarsals)
8. Other
9. Multiple

727.05 Wrist
727.2 Wrist occupational
727.09 Other
0 See also 'Tenosynovitis'

SYNOVIUM, SYNOVIAL

727.40 Cyst
727.51 Cyst popliteal (Baker's)
0 Cyst see 'Ganglion'
727.9 Disorder
727.89 Disorder other specified
792.9 Fluid abnormal
727.83 Plica
727.50 Rupture
727.59 Rupture other

SYPHILIS

097.9 NOS
097.9 Acquired
093.9 Cardiovascular
093.89 Cardiovascular syndrome
093.89 Cardiovascular other
094.9 Central nervous system
0 Complicating pregnancy see 'Syphilis Complicating Pregnancy'
V65.45 Counseling
090.9 Death (from) unspecified (under two years of age)
094.1 Dementia [**294.1#**]
5th digit: 294.1
0. Without behavioral disturbance or NOS
1. With behavioral disturbance

093.22 Endocarditis aortic valve
093.21 Endocarditis mitral valve
093.24 Endocarditis pulmonary valve
093.23 Endocarditis tricuspid valve
093.20 Endocarditis valve unspecified
V01.6 Exposure
795.6 False positive serological test
091.0 Genital (primary)
097.0 Late NOS
096 Late latent
097.1 Latent NOS
092.9 Latent early NOS
092.0 Latent early serological relapse after treatment
096 Latent late
094.2 Meningitis
094.2 Meningovascular
093.82 Myocarditis

SYPHILIS (continued)

104.0 Nonvenereal endemic
093.20 Ostial coronary disease
093.81 Pericarditis
097.1 Positive serological reaction
091.0 Vulva

SYPHILIS COMPLICATING PREGNANCY

647.0#: Use an additional code to identify the maternal syphilis.

647.0# Maternal current (co-existent)
5th digit: 647.0
0. Episode of care NOS or N/A
1. Delivered
2. Delivered with postpartum complication
3. Antepartum complication
4. Postpartum complication

655.4# Maternal with known/suspected damage to fetus
5th digit: 655.4
0. Episode of care NOS or N/A
1. Delivered
3. Antepartum complication

SYPHILIS CONGENITAL

090.9 NOS
090.0 Choroiditis
090.0 Coryza (chronic)
090.1 Early latent
090.2 Early less than 2 years after birth
090.0 Early symptomatic
090.41 Encephalitis
090.0 Epiphysitis
090.0 Hepatomegaly
090.3 Keratitis interstitial
090.3 Keratitis parenchymatous
090.3 Keratitis punctata profunda
090.7 Late manifest 2 yrs. or more after birth
090.6 Latent manifest 2 yrs. or more after birth
090.42 Meningitis
090.0 Mucous patches
090.0 Pemphigus
090.0 Periostitis
090.0 Splenomegaly
090.49 Other
090.5 Other late symptomatic manifest 2 yrs. or more after birth

SYPHILIS PRIMARY

091.1 Anus
091.2 Breast
091.2 Fingers
091.0 Genital
091.2 Lip
091.2 Tonsils

SYPHILIS SECONDARY

091.9 NOS
091.4 Adenopathy
091.82 Alopecia
091.3 Anus
091.51 Chorioretinitis
091.62 Hepatitis
091.52 Iridocyclitis
091.62 Liver
091.4 Lymphadenitis

SYPHILIS SECONDARY (continued)

091.81 Meningitis acute
091.3 Mouth
091.3 Mucous membranes
091.61 Periostitis
091.3 Pharynx
091.7 Relapse
091.3 Skin
091.3 Tonsils
091.50 Uveitis
091.69 Viscera other
091.3 Vulva
091.89 Other

SYPHILIS TERTIARY

095.9 NOS
095.5 Bone
095.7 Bursitis
095.0 Episcleritis
095.4 Kidney
095.3 Liver
095.1 Lung
095.6 Muscle
095.2 Peritonitis
095.7 Synovitis
095.7 Synovium tendon and bursa
095.8 Other specified forms

SYPHILITIC

093.9 Angina
090.5 Angina congenital
091.51 Chorioretinitis secondary
090.41 Encephalitis congenital
091.52 Iridocyclitis secondary
091.4 Lymphadenitis (secondary)
090.5 Saddle nose manifest 2 yrs. or more after birth
091.50 Uveitis secondary

SYPHILITIC CNS

094.86 Acoustic neuritis
094.87 Cerebral aneurysm ruptured
094.83 Disseminated retinochoroiditis
094.81 Encephalitis
094.83 Neurorecidive retina
094.85 Neuroretinitis
094.84 Optic atrophy
094.82 Parkinsonism
094.85 Retrobulbar neuritis

094.89 SYPHILOMA CENTRAL NERVOUS SYSTEM
216.# SYRINGOADENOMA M8400/0
216.# SYRINGOMA M8407/0

4th digit: 216
0. Lip (skin of)
1. Eyelid including canthus
2. Ear (external) (auricle) (pinna)
3. Face (cheek) (nose) (eyebrow) (temple)
4. Scalp, neck
5. Trunk, back except scrotum
6. Upper limb including shoulder
7. Lower limb including hip
8. Other specified sites
9. Skin NOS

336.0 SYRINGOMYELIA

SYRINGOMYELOCELE

741.0# With hydrocephalus
741.9# Without hydrocephalus

5th digit: 741.0, 9
0. Region NOS
1. Cervical
2. Dorsal
3. Lumbar

SYSTEMIC

710.8 Fibrosclerosing
0 Inflammatory response syndrome see 'SIRS'
286.5 Lupus erythematosus inhibitor increase
0 Lupus erythematosus see 'Lupus', erythematosus
0 Sclerosis see 'Scleroderma'
202.6# Tissue mast cell disease M9740/3

5th digit: 202.6
0. Unspecified site, extranodal and solid organ sites
1. Lymph nodes of head, face, neck
2. Lymph nodes intrathoracic
3. Lymph nodes abdominal
4. Lymph nodes axilla and upper limb
5. Lymph nodes inguinal region and lower limb
6. Lymph nodes intrapelvic
7. Spleen
8. Lymph nodes multiple sites

785.2 SYSTOLIC CLICK (-MURMUR) SYNDROME
429.9 SYSTOLIC DYSFUNCTION

428.2# SYSTOLIC HEART FAILURE
428.4# SYSTOLIC AND DIASTOLIC HEART FAILURE

5th digit: 428.2, 4
0. NOS
1. Acute
2. Chronic
3. Acute on chronic

S

279.10 T-CELL DEFECT IMMUNODEFICIENCY PREDOMINANT
V03.1 TAB VACCINATION ALONE
305.1 TABAGISM SYNDROME

TABES

094.0 Dorsalis
094.0 Dorsalis with Charcot's [713.5]
090.40 Juvenile
799.89 Peripheral (nonsyphilitic)

094.1 TABOPARESIS
090.40 TABOPARESIS JUVENILE
923.20 TACHE NOIR
427.81 TACHYBRADY SYNDROME

TACHYCARDIA

785.0 NOS
427.89 Atrial
427.0 Atrial paroxysmal
426.89 AV
426.89 AV nodal re-entry (re-entrant)
427.0 AV paroxysmal
427.81 Bradycardia syndrome
659.7# Fetal affecting management of mother

5th digit: 659.7

0. Episode of care unspecified or N/A
1. Delivered
3. Antepartum complication

427.0 Junctional paroxysmal
779.82 Neonatal
779.82 Newborn
426.89 Nodal
427.2 Paroxysmal
427.89 Sinus
427.0 Supraventricular paroxysmal
427.42 Ventricular flutter
427.1 Ventricular paroxysmal

536.8 TACHYGASTRIA

TACHYPNEA

786.06 NOS
770.6 Idiopathic newborn
770.6 Newborn transitory

TAENIA

123.3 Infection
123.2 Saginata infection
123.0 Solium infection intestinal form

123.2 TAENIARHYNCHUS SAGINATUS INFECTION
123.3 TAENIASIS
757.4 TAENZER'S DISEASE

TAG (HYPERTROPHIED SKIN) (INFECTED)

701.9 NOS
474.8 Adenoid
474.01 Adenoid infected
455.9 Anus (skin) (hemorrhoidal)
455.9 Hemorrhoidal
623.8 Hymen
624.8 Perineum
744.1 Preauricular congenital
455.9 Rectal (skin) (hemorrhoidal)
455.9 Sentinel

TAG (HYPERTROPHIED SKIN) (INFECTED) (continued)

701.9 Skin
757.39 Skin accessory congenital
474.8 Tonsil
474.00 Tonsil infected
599.84 Urethra
624.8 Vulva

062.5 TAHYNA FEVER
0 TAIL BONE SEE 'COCCYX, COCCYGEAL'
446.7 TAKAYASU'S DISEASE OR SYNDROME (PULSELESS)
648.9# TAKAYASU'S DISEASE OR SYNDROME (PULSELESS) MATERNAL CURRENT (CO-EXISTENT) IN PREGNANCY [446.7]

5th digit: 648.9

0. Episode of care NOS or N/A
1. Delivered
2. Delivered with postpartum complication
3. Antepartum complication
4. Postpartum complication

429.83 TAKOTSUBO SYNDROME

TALIPES

754.70 NOS (congenital)
736.79 NEC acquired
754.62 Calcaneovalgus (congenital)
736.76 Calcaneovalgus acquired
754.59 Calcaneovarus (congenital)
736.76 Calcaneovarus acquired
754.79 Calcaneus (congenital)
736.76 Calcaneus acquired
754.71 Cavus (congenital)
736.73 Cavus acquired
754.69 Equinovalgus (congenital)
736.72 Equinovalgus acquired
754.51 Equinovarus (congenital)
736.71 Equinovarus acquired
754.79 Equinus (congenital)
736.72 Equinus acquired NEC
754.69 Planovalgus (congenital)
736.79 Planovalgus acquired
734 Planus (acquired)
754.61 Planus congenital
754.60 Valgus (congenital)
736.79 Valgus acquired
754.50 Varus (congenital)
736.79 Varus acquired

728.85 TALMA'S DISEASE
924.20 TALON NOIR NOS, HAND OR HEEL
924.3 TALON NOIR TOE
755.67 TALONAVICULAR SYNOSTOSIS
423.3 TAMPONADE CARDIAC (HEART)
078.89 TANAPOX
272.5 TANGIER DISEASE (FAMILIAL HIGH-DENSITY LIPOPROTEIN DEFICIENCY)
312.1# TANTRUMS

5th digit: 312.1

0. NOS
1. Mild
2. Moderate
3. Severe

692.4 TAPE DERMATITIS

T

TAPEWORM

123.9 NOS
123.2 Beef
123.1 Cysticerciasis (larvae form)
123.6 Dog
123.6 Dwarf
123.4 Fish
123.9 Infection (cestode)
123.0 Pork (intestinal)
123.6 Rat
123.5 Sparganum (Mansoni) (proliferum)
123.5 Spirometra
123.3 Taenia
123.3 Taeniasis NOS
123.8 Other specified cestode infection

352.6 TAPIA'S SYNDROME
747.41 TAPVR (TOTAL ANOMALOUS PULMONARY VENOUS RETURN) (SUBDIAPHRAGMATIC) (SUPRADIAPHRAGMATIC)
287.33 TAR SYNDROME (THROMBOCYTOPENIA WITH ABSENT RADII)

T

297.8 TARANTISM
989.5 TARANTULA BITE
995.0 TARANTULA BITE WITH ANAPHYLAXIS [989.5]
354.2 TARDY ULNAR NERVE PALSY
282.49 TARGET-OVAL CELL ANEMIA
355.9 TARLOV'S CYST
696.4 TARRAL-BESNIER DISEASE (PITYRIASIS RUBRA PILARIS)

TARSAL

755.38 Absence congenital with absence incomplete distal elements
755.67 Coalitions
755.38 Or metatarsals agenesis complete or partial
355.5 Tunnel syndrome

TARSOMETATARSAL

838.03 Joint dislocation closed
838.13 Joint dislocation open
845.11 Strain (sprain) (avulsion) (hemarthrosis)

743.66 TARSO-ORBITAL FASCIA ATROPHY CONGENITAL
306.7 TASTE DISORDER PSYCHOGENIC
438.6 TASTE DISTURBANCE LATE EFFECT OF CVA [781.1]
781.1 TASTE DISTURBANCE OF SENSATION
V41.5 TASTE PROBLEM
709.09 TATOO MARK
745.11 TAUSSIG BING SYNDROME OR DEFECT (TRANSPOSITION AORTA AND OVERRIDING PULMONARY ARTERY)
330.1 TAY SACHS DISEASE
759.89 TAYBI'S SYNDROME (OTOPALATODIGITAL) SYNDROME
701.8 TAYLOR'S DISEASE
625.5 TAYLOR'S SYNDROME
0 TB SEE 'TUBERCULOSIS'
246.8 TBG EXCESS OR DEFICIENCY (THYROID BINDING GLOBULIN)

375.69 TEAR DUCT DISEASE
0 TEAR DUCT SEE ALSO LACRIMAL
375.15 TEAR FILM INSUFFICIENCY
0 TEAR INTERNAL ORGAN SEE SPECIFIC ORGAN, INJURY
0 TEAR JOINT, LIGAMENT, MUSCLE OR TENDON SEE 'SPRAIN', BY SITE
0 TEAR LIGAMENT, MUSCLE OR TENDON WITH LACERATION SEE 'LACERATION', BY SITE
767.0 TEAR TENTORIAL BIRTH TRAUMA
375.20 TEARING EXCESSIVE
0 TEETH SEE 'TOOTH'
520.7 TEETHING SYNDROME
344.89 TEGMENTAL SYNDROME

TELANGIECTASIA

448.9 NOS
334.8 Ataxic (cerebellar)
448.0 Familial
448.0 Hereditary hemorrhagic

648.9#: Use an additional code to identify the specific telangiectasia.

648.9# Maternal current (co-existent) in pregnancy
5th digit: 648.9
0. Episode of care NOS or N/A
1. Delivered
2. Delivered with postpartum complication
3. Antepartum complication
4. Postpartum complication

757.33 Pigmentation-cataract syndrome
362.15 Retinal
362.15 Retinopathy
448.1 Spider

709.1 TELANGIECTODES
743.63 TELECANTHUS (CONGENITAL)
704.02 TELOGEN EFFLUVIUM
446.5 TEMPORAL ARTERITIS
310.0 TEMPORAL LOBECTOMY BEHAVIOR SYNDROME
959.09 TEMPORAL REGION INJURY
383.02 TEMPORAL SYNDROME
524.6# TEMPOROMANDIBULAR JOINT DISORDER OR SYNDROME
5th digit: 524.6
0. Unspecified
1. Adhesions and ankylosis
2. Arthralgia
3. Articular disc disorder (reducing or non reducing)
4. Sounds on opening and/or closing of jaw
9. Other specified joint disorder (malocclusion)

TENDINITIS

726.90 Site NOS
726.71 Achilles
726.70 Ankle and tarsus
726.12 Bicipital
727.82 Calcific

TENDINITIS (continued)

726.30 Elbow
726.5 Gluteal
726.64 Patellar
726.79 Peroneal
726.61 Pes anserinus
726.5 Psoas
726.11 Shoulder (calcific)
726.72 Tibialis
726.5 Trochanteric
0 See also 'Tenosynovitis', by site

TENDON

756.81 Absence (congenital)
727.82 Calcification
727.81 Contracture (achilles)
727.9 Disorder NOS
726.10 Disorder shoulder region
726.90 Inflammation NEC
905.8 Injury late effect (due to laceration, sprain or strain)
0 Laceration see 'Laceration', tendon
726.79 Peroneal dislocating
727.67 Rupture - achilles nontraumatic
727.62 Rupture - biceps (long head) nontraumatic
727.68 Rupture - foot and ankle nontraumatic
727.60 Rupture - nontraumatic
727.69 Rupture - nontraumatic NEC
727.66 Rupture - patellar nontraumatic
727.65 Rupture - quadriceps nontraumatic
727.61 Rupture - rotator cuff nontraumatic
0 Rupture - traumatic see 'Sprain'
0 Rupture - traumatic with laceration see 'Laceration', tendon
727.63 Rupture - wrist and hand extensor nontraumatic
727.64 Rupture - wrist and hand flexor nontraumatic
727.82 Sheath calcification
727.42 Sheath ganglion (any)
727.82 Sheath lesion (foot) (toes)
756.89 Shortening congenital
727.9 Slipping
727.89 Other disorder
0 Tear see 'Sprain', by site

787.99 TENESMUS
787.99 TENESMUS RECTAL
788.9 TENESMUS URINARY
726.32 TENNIS ELBOW
376.04 TENONITIS ORBIT

TENOSYNOVITIS

727.00 NOS
726.90 Adhesive
727.06 Ankle
726.12 Bicipital
727.09 Buttock

TENOSYNOVITIS (continued)

275.49 Crystal induced - unspecified [**712.9#**]
0 Crystal induced - chondrocalcinosis see 'Chondrocalcinosis'
274.0 Crystal induced - gouty
275.49 Crystal induced - other specified [**712.8#**]

5th digit: 712.8-9
0. Site NOS
1. Shoulder region
2. Upper arm (elbow) (humerus)
3. Forearm (radius) (wrist) (ulna)
4. Hand (carpal) (metacarpal) (fingers)
5. Pelvic region and thigh (hip) (buttock) (femur)
6. Lower leg (fibula) (knee) (patella) (tibia)
7. Ankle and/or foot (metatarsals) (toes) (tarsals)
8. Other (head) (neck) (rib) (skull) (trunk) (vertebrae)
9. Multiple

727.09 Elbow
727.05 Finger
727.06 Foot and ankle
098.51 Gonococcal
274.0 Gouty
727.05 Hand and wrist
727.09 Hip
727.09 Knee
727.04 Radial styloid
726.10 Shoulder
726.0 Shoulder adhesive
720.1 Spine
726.10 Supraspinatus
095.7 Syphilitic
727.06 Toe
015.## Tuberculous [727.01]

4th digit: 015
0. Vertebral column
1. Hip
2. Knee
5. Limb bones
6. Mastoid
7. Other specified bone
8. Other specified joint
9. Unspecified bones and joints

5th digit: 015
0. NOS
1. Lab not done
2. Lab pending
3. Microscopy positive (in sputum)
4. Culture positive - microscopy negative
5. Culture negative - microscopy positive
6. Culture and microscopy negative confirmed by other methods

727.05 Wrist
727.09 Other

307.81 TENSION HEADACHE PSYCHOGENIC
0 TENSION PNEUMOTHORAX SEE 'PNEUMOTHORAX'
352.3 TENTH CRANIAL NERVE ATROPHY
352.3 TENTH CRANIAL NERVE DISORDER
951.8 TENTH CRANIAL NERVE INJURY
352.3 TENTH NERVE PNEUMOGASTRIC DISORDERS

767.0 TENTORIAL TEAR BIRTH TRAUMA

199.1 TERATOCARCINOMA SITE NOS

0 TERATOCARCINOMA SITE SPECIFIED SEE 'CANCER', BY SITE M9081/3

TERATOMA

238.9 Site NOS

0 Site specified see 'Neoplasm Uncertain Behavior', by site M9080/1

211.5 Benign site NOS

0 Benign site specified see 'Benign Neoplasm', by site M9080/0

155.0 Malignant site NOS

0 Malignant site specified see 'Cancer', by site M9080/3

199.1 Malignant intermediate type site NOS

0 Malignant intermediate type site specified see 'Cancer', by site M9083/3

186.9 Malignant trophoblastic site NOS

0 Malignant trophoblastic site specified see 'Cancer', by site M9102/3

199.1 Malignant undifferentiated type site NOS

0 Malignant undifferentiated type site specified see 'Cancer', by site M9082/3

T

When using code V66.7, code the terminal illness first.

V66.7 TERMINAL CARE ENCOUNTER

127.7 TERNIDENS DIMINUTUS INFECTION

371.48 TERRIEN'S MARGINAL DEGENERATION OF CORNEA

362.21 TERRY'S SYNDROME

TESTIS, TESTICULAR

752.51 Aberrant (congenital)

752.51 Aberratio (congenital)

V45.77 Absence

752.89 Absence congenital

257.2 Androgen defective biosynthesis

752.9 Anomaly NOS

752.89 Anomaly congenital

752.89 Anomaly NEC

752.89 Appendage (organ of morgagni)

752.89 Aplasia congenital

608.23 Appendix torsion

608.3 Atrophy

V76.45 Cancer screening

608.4 Cellulitis (carbuncle) (boil)

752.51 Descended imperfectly

608.9 Disorder inflammatory

608.4 Disorder inflammatory other

608.89 Disorder other specified

257.9 Dysfunction NOS

752.51 Ectopic (congenital)

257.1 Failure iatrogenic (post irradiation) (postsurgical)

259.5 Feminization syndrome

608.89 Fibrosis (hypertrophy) (ulcer)

752.89 Fusion congenital

608.83 Hemorrhage (thrombosis) (hematoma) nontraumatic

257.2 Hormone deficiency

257.0 Hyperfunction

752.52 Hypermobility congenital

608.89 Hypertrophy

752.89 Hypertrophy congenital

TESTIS, TESTICULAR (continued)

257.1 Hypofunction iatrogenic

257.1 Hypofunction postablative

257.1 Hypofunction postirradiation

257.1 Hypofunction postsurgical

257.2 Hypofunction other

257.2 Hypogonadism

752.89 Hypoplasia congenital

752.51 Inguinal (congenital)

959.14 Injury NEC

911.8 Injury other and unspecified superficial

911.9 Injury other and unspecified superficial infected

752.51 Inversion (congenital)

752.51 Maldescended (congenital)

608.89 Mass

752.52 Migratory congenital

257.8 Nonvirilizing syndrome

608.9 Pain

752.52 Retractile (congenital)

752.51 Retroversion (congenital)

752.89 Supernumerary

016.5# TB [608.81]

5th digit: 016.5

0. NOS

1. Lab not done

2. Lab pending

3. Microscopy positive (in sputum)

4. Culture positive - microscopy negative

5. Culture negative - microscopy positive

6. Culture and microscopy negative confirmed by other methods

608.20 Torsion NOS

752.81 Transposed

752.51 Undescended congenital

TETANUS

037 NOS

V07.2 Antitoxin administration

670.0# Maternal due to pregnancy (puerperal) (major infection)

5th digit: 670.0

0. NOS

2. Delivered with postpartum complication

4. Postpartum complication

771.3 Neonatorum

771.3 Omphalitis perinatal

V74.8 Screening exam

V03.7 Toxoid vaccination (single)

TETANY

781.7 NOS

781.7 Hyperkinetic

300.11 Hysterical

771.3 Neonatorum

775.4 Newborn (hypocalcemic)

252.1 Parathyroid

252.1 Parathyroprival

306.0 Psychogenic

742.59 TETHERED SPINAL CORD SYNDROME

V09.3 TETRACYCLINE RESISTANT INFECTION (SEE 'DRUG RESISTANCE', FOR COMPLETE LISTING)

745.2 TETRALOGY FALLOT

338.0 THALAMIC PAIN SYNDROME (HYPERESTHETIC)

THALASSEMIA

282.49 NOS
282.49 Alpha
282.49 Beta
282.41 Hb-S disease (without crisis)

> *When coding Sickle cell thalassemia with crisis; it is necessary to report an additional code to indicate the manifestation of the crisis.*

282.42 Hb-S disease with acute chest syndrome [517.3]
282.42 Hb-S disease with crisis or vaso-occlusive pain
282.42 Hb-S disease with splenic sequestration [289.52]
282.49 High fetal gene
282.49 High fetal hemoglobin
282.49 Mixed
282.41 Sickle cell NOS (without crisis)
282.42 Sickle cell with acute chest syndrome [517.3]
282.42 Sickle cell with crisis or vaso-occlusive pain
282.42 Sickle cell with splenic sequestration [289.52]
282.49 Trait
282.49 Variants
282.49 Other

282.49 THALASSANEMIA
579.0 THAYSEN-GEE DISEASE (NONTROPICAL SPRUE)
183.0 THECA CELL CARCINOMA SITE NOS
0 THECA CELL CARCINOMA SITE SPECIFIED SEE 'CANCER', BY SITE M8600/3
620.2 THECA LUTEIN CYST OF OVARY
220 THECOMA SITE NOS
0 THECOMA SITE SPECIFIED SEE 'BENIGN NEOPLASM', BY SITE M8600/0
259.1 THELARCHE PREMATURE
354.0 THENAR ATROPHY, PARTIAL

THERAPY

V57.9 NOS
V57.0 Breathing exercise
V57.1 Exercise
V57.89 Multiple types
V57.21 Occupational
V57.4 Orthoptic
V57.81 Orthotic or gait
V57.1 Physical
V58.0 Radiation
V57.3 Speech
V57.22 Vocational
V46.2 Oxygen (supplemental) long term
V57.89 Other

793.#(#) THERMOGRAPHY ABNORMAL FINDINGS (NONSPECIFIC)
4th or 4th and 5th digit: 793
0. Skull and head
1. Lung field
2. Other intrathoracic
3. Biliary tract
4. Gastrointestinal tract
5. Genitourinary organs
6. Abdominal area including retroperitoneum
7. Musculoskeletal system
8#. Breast
80. Unspecified
81. Mammographic microcalcification
89. Other abnormal findings (calcification) (calculus)
9#. Other
91. Inconclusive due to excess body fat
99. Other abnormal findings (placenta) (skin) (subcutaneous)

> *When using code 793.91, Image test inconclusive due to excess body fat, use additional code to identify body mass index (BMI) which can be found at 'Body Mass Index'.*

992.0 THERMOPLEGIA
909.4 THERMOPLEGIA LATE EFFECT
277.39 THESAURISMOSIS AMYLOID
275.40 THESAURISMOSIS CALCIUM
255.41 THESAURISMOSIS MELANIN
710.1 THIBIERGE-WEISSENBACH SYNDROME (CUTANEOUS SYSTEMIC SCLEROSIS)
710.1 THIBIERGE-WEISSENBACH SYNDROME (CUTANEOUS SYSTEMIC SCLEROSIS) WITH LUNG INVOLVEMENT [517.2]
710.1 THIBIERGE-WEISSENBACH SYNDROME (CUTANEOUS SYSTEMIC SCLEROSIS) WITH MYOPATHY [359.6]
724.6 THIELE SYNDROME

THIGH

736.89 Absence acquired
904.8 Blood vessel NEC injury
904.7 Blood vessel NEC injury multiple
904.7 Blood vessel injury specified NEC
959.6 Injury
916.8 Injury other and unspecified superficial
916.9 Injury other and unspecified superficial infected
843.9 Separation (rupture) (tear) (laceration) unspecified site
843.9 Strain (sprain) (avulsion) (hemarthrosis) unspecified site

THIRD

426.0 Degree heart block
664.2# Degree laceration (perineal)
5th digit: 664.2
0. Episode of care NOS or N/A
1. Delivered
4. Postpartum complication

378.51 Nerve atrophy - partial
378.52 Nerve atrophy - total

T

THIRD (continued)

951.0	Nerve injury
378.51	Nerve palsy (disorder) - partial
378.52	Nerve palsy (disorder) - total
994.3	THIRST
783.5	THIRST EXCESSIVE
909.4	THIRST LATE EFFECT
359.22	THOMSEN'S DISEASE
757.33	THOMSON'S DISEASE (CONGENITAL POIKILODERMA)

> ***When coding back disorders due to degeneration, displacement or HNP of the intervertebral disc, it is important to distinguish whether these conditions are with or without myelopathy. Myelopathy refers to functional disturbances and/or pathological changes in the spinal cord that result from compression.***

THORACIC

901.0	Aorta injury
908.4	Aorta injury late effect
901.9	Blood vessel injury - NOS
901.83	Blood vessel injury - multiple
901.89	Blood vessel injury - specified NEC
722.92	Disc calcification or discitis
722.51	Disc disease/degeneration
722.72	Disc disease/degeneration - with myelopathy
722.92	Disc disorder
722.72	Disc disorder with myelopathy
722.11	Disc displacement
722.72	Disc displacement with myelopathy
722.11	Disc herniation
722.72	Disc herniation with myelopathy
457.1	Duct obstruction or occlusion
457.8	Duct rupture
959.11	Injury (external) NEC
722.11	Nerve compression - discogenic
722.72	Nerve compression - discogenic with myelopathy
724.4	Nerve compression - root (by scar tissue) NEC
722.82	Nerve compression - root postoperative
353.3	Nerve root disorder
353.0	Outlet syndrome (nondiscogenic)
724.4	Radiculitis (nonvertebral) (nondiscogenic)
739.2	Region segmental or somatic dysfunction
353.3	Root lesions NEC (nondiscogenic)
847.1	Separation (rupture) (tear) (laceration)
724.01	Spinal stenosis
724.1	Spine pain (nonvertebral) (nondiscogenic)
847.1	Strain (sprain) (avulsion) (hemarthrosis)

THORACIC SPONDYLOSIS: <u>WITH OSTEOPOROSIS</u> [733.0#]

721.2	Thoracic
721.41	Thoracic with myelopathy (cord compression)
721.7	Traumatic

WITH <u>OSTEOPOROSIS</u> [733.0#]
5th digit: 733.0
- **0. Unspecified**
- **1. Senile**
- **2. Idiopathic**
- **3. Disuse**
- **9. Drug induced**

0	THORACIC TRAUMA SEE 'CHEST', TRAUMA
0	THORACIC SEE ALSO 'DORSAL'
441.7	THORACOABDOMINAL ANEURYSM AORTIC
441.6	THORACOABDOMINAL ANEURYSM AORTIC RUPTURED
731.2	THORACOGENOUS RHEUMATIC SYNDROME (HYPERTROPHIC PULMONARY OSTEOARTHROPATHY)

THORACOLUMBAR

722.51	Disc disease/degeneration
722.72	Disc disease/degeneration with myelopathy
739.2	Region segmental or somatic dysfunction
759.4	THORACOPAGUS
V64.42	THORACOSCOPIC SURGICAL PROCEDURE CONVERTED TO OPEN PROCEDURE
593.9	THORN'S SYNDROME (RENAL DISEASE)
478.29	THORNWALDT'S DISEASE (PHARYNGEAL BURSITIS)
259.2	THORSON-BIORCK SYNDROME (MALIGNANT CARCINOID)
127.4	THREADWORM INFECTION
644.0#	THREATENED LABOR >22 <37 WEEKS
644.1#	THREATENED LABOR >37 WEEKS

5th digit: 644.0-1
- **0. Episode of care NOS or N/A**
- **3. Antepartum complication**

270.7	THREONINE METABOLISM DISTURBANCES

THROAT

478.29	Atrophy
795.39	Culture positive NEC
478.20	Disease NOS
034.0	Disease septic
959.09	Injury
910.8	Injury other and unspecified superficial
910.9	Injury other and unspecified superficial infected
784.1	Pain
0	Sore see 'Pharyngitis'
478.29	Ulcer
032.0	Ulcer diphtheritic
287.1	THROMBASTHENIA (HEMORRHAGIC) (HEREDITARY)
443.1	THROMBOANGIITIS OBLITERANS
<u>**648.9#**</u>	THROMBOANGIITIS OBLITERANS (PAROXYSMAL DIGITAL CYANOSIS) MATERNAL CURRENT (CO-EXISTENT) IN <u>PREGNANCY</u> [443.1]

5th digit: 648.9
- **0. Episode of care NOS or N/A**
- **1. Delivered**
- **2. Delivered with postpartum complication**
- **3. Antepartum complication**
- **4. Postpartum complication**

287.1	THROMBOCYTASTHENIA
238.71	THROMBOCYTHEMIA HEMORRHAGIC (ESSENTIAL) (IDIOPATHIC) (PRIMARY) M9962/1
207.2#	THROMBOCYTIC LEUKEMIA M9910/3

5th digit: 207.2
- **0. Without mention of remission**
- **1. In remission**

287.1	THROMBOCYTOPATHY (DYSTROPHIC)

THROMBOCYTOPENIA

287.5	NOS
287.33	Amegakaryocytic, congenital
287.33	Congenital
287.39	Cyclic
287.4	Dilutional
287.4	Due to dialysis
287.4	Due to drugs or transfusion
287.4	Due to platelet alloimmunization
287.30	Essential
287.4	Extracorporeal circulation of blood
287.33	Hereditary
287.39	Kasabach-Merritt
776.1	Neonatal transient
287.30	Primary NOS
287.39	Primary other
287.30	Purpura
287.39	Sex-linked
287.33	With absent radii (TAR) syndrome
287.39	With giant hemangioma

238.71 THROMBOCYTOSIS ESSENTIAL OR PRIMARY

444.9 THROMBOEMBOLIC DISEASE (SEE ALSO 'EMBOLISM')

287.1 THROMBOPATHY (BERNARD-SOULIER)

287.39 THROMBOPENIA-HEMANGIOMA SYNDROME

THROMBOPHLEBITIS LOWER EXTREMITIES

451.2	Unspecified deep or superficial
451.11	Femoral vein deep
451.11	Femoral vein superficial
451.19	Femoropopliteal (deep)
V12.52	History
451.11	Iliofemoral (deep)
453.1	Migrans (deep)
451.19	Popliteal vein deep
451.0	Popliteal vein superficial
451.0	Saphenous vein (greater) (lesser) superficial
451.0	Superficial vessels of lower extremities
451.19	Tibial vein (deep)
451.19	Other vessels (deep)

THROMBOPHLEBITIS UPPER EXTREMITIES

451.82	Antecubital vein (superficial)
451.84	Arm unspecified NEC
451.89	Axillary vein
451.82	Basilic vein (superficial)
451.83	Brachial vein (deep)
451.82	Cephalic vein (superficial)
451.83	Deep vessels
V12.52	History
451.89	Jugular vein
451.83	Radial vein (deep)
451.89	Subclavian vein
451.82	Superficial vessels
451.83	Ulnar vein (deep)
451.84	Upper extremities

THROMBOPHLEBITIS OTHER

451.9	Site unspecified
451.89	Breast
326	Cavernous sinus pyogenic late effect
451.89	Chest wall superficial
996.61	Due to cardiac device, implant, and graft
996.62	Due to other vascular device, implant, and graft
997.2	During or resulting from a procedure

THROMBOPHLEBITIS OTHER (continued)

639.8	Following abortion, ectopic or molar pregnancy
999.2	Following infusion perfusion or transfusion
274.89	Gouty [451.9]
451.89	Hepatic vein
V12.52	History
451.81	Iliac vein (deep)
325	Intracranial sinus (any)
326	Intracranial sinus (any) late effect
437.6	Nonpyogenic
572.1	Portal vein
997.2	Postoperative
362.18	Retina
451.9	Vein
451.89	Vein other specified site
453.2	Vena cava
451.89	Other specified site

THROMBOPHLEBITIS COMPLICATING ABORTION, PREGNANCY, OR PUERPERIUM

637.7# Abortion unspecified
638.7 Abortion failed attempted
636.7# Abortion illegally induced
635.7# Abortion legally induced
634.7# Abortion spontaneous
5th digit: 634.7, 635.7, 636.7, 637.7
0. Unspecified
1. Incomplete
2. Complete

639.8 Following abortion, ectopic or molar pregnancy

671.3# Maternal due to pregnancy antepartum - deep
5th digit: 671.3
0. Episode of care NOS or N/A
1. Delivered
3. Antepartum complication

671.4# Maternal due to pregnancy postpartum - deep
5th digit: 671.4
0. Episode of care NOS or N/A
2. Delivered with postpartum complication
4. Postpartum complication

671.2# Maternal due to pregnancy - superficial
5th digit: 671.2
0. Episode of care NOS or N/A
1. Delivered
2. Delivered with postpartum complication
3. Antepartum complication
4. Postpartum complication

> ***648.9#: Use an additional code to identify the specific thrombophlebitis.***

648.9# Maternal in pregnancy and puerperium current (co-existent)
5th digit: 648.9
0. Episode of care NOS or N/A
1. Delivered
2. Delivered with postpartum complication
3. Antepartum complication
4. Postpartum complication

287.39 THROMBOPOIETEN DEFICIENCY

THROMBOSIS

453.9 NOS
444.1 Aorta
444.0 Aorta abdominal
444.0 Aorta bifurcation
444.81 Aorta iliac
444.0 Aorta saddle
444.0 Aorta terminal
444.1 Aorta thoracic
434.0# Apoplexy
5th digit: 434.0
0. Without cerebral infarction
1. With cerebral infarction

0 Appendix, septic see 'appendicitis', acute
446.6 Arteriolar-capillary platelet disseminated
444.9 Artery NOS
433.8# Artery auditory internal
5th digit: 433.8
0. Without cerebral infarction
1. With cerebral infarction

444.22 Artery extremity lower
444.21 Artery extremity upper
433.3# Artery precerebral multiple and bilateral
5th digit: 433.3
0. Without cerebral infarction
1. With cerebral infarction

415.19 Artery pulmonary
415.11 Artery pulmonary iatrogenic
415.11 Artery pulmonary postoperative
415.12 Artery pulmonary septic
0 Artery traumatic see specified blood vessel, injury
444.89 Artery other specified NEC
424.90 Atrial (endocardial)
093.89 Atrial (endocardial) due to syphilis
429.89 Atrial without endocarditis
433.8# Auditory artery, internal
5th digit: 433.8
0. Without cerebral infarction
1. With cerebral infarction

0 Auricular heart see 'Myocardial Infarction Acute'
453.8 Axillary (vein)
433.0# Basilar artery
433.3# Basilar artery bilateral or multiple
5th digit: 433.0, 3
0. Without cerebral infarction
1. With cerebral infarction

453.9 Bland NEC
444.21 Brachial artery
434.0# Brain (artery) (stem)
5th digit: 434.0
0. Without cerebral infarction
1. With cerebral infarction

094.89 Brain due to syphilis
997.02 Brain iatrogenic
997.02 Brain postoperative
448.9 Capillary
446.6 Capillary arteriolar, generalized
093.89 Cardiac due to syphilis
0 Cardiac see 'Myocardial Infarction Acute'
433.1# Carotid artery
433.3# Carotid artery bilateral or multiple
5th digit: 433.1, 3
0. Without cerebral infarction
1. With cerebral infarction

THROMBOSIS (continued)

437.6 Cavernous sinus
325 Cavernous sinus pyogenic
433.8# Cerebellar artery (anterior inferior) (posterior inferior)
434.0# Cerebral artery
433.8# Choroidal artery (anterior)
433.8# Communicating posterior artery
5th digit: 433.8, 434.0
0. Without cerebral infarction
1. With cerebral infarction

411.81 Coronary artery acute without MI
093.89 Coronary artery due to syphilis
0 Coronary artery or vein with infarction see 'Myocardial Infarction Acute'
607.82 Corpus cavernosum
434.0# Cortical
5th digit: 434.0
0. Without cerebral infarction
1. With cerebral infarction

453.40 Deep vein (DVT) NOS
0 Due to a device see 'Complication Of A Device, Implant Or Graft - Other Specified'
453.8 Effort
0 Endocardial see 'Myocardial Infarction Acute'
444.22 Extremity artery NOS
444.22 Extremity artery lower
444.21 Extremity artery upper
0 Eye see 'Retinal Artery Occlusion'
444.22 Femoral artery
453.8 Femoral (vein)
453.41 Femoral (vein) deep
451.11 Femoral (vein) (deep) with inflammation or phlebitis
608.83 Genitalia male
0 Heart see 'Myocardial Infarction Acute'
444.89 Hepatic artery
572.1 Hepatic infectional or septic
453.0 Hepatic vein
V12.51 History vein
433.8# Hypophyseal artery
5th digit: 433.8
0. Without cerebral infarction
1. With cerebral infarction

444.81 Iliac artery
453.8 Iliac (vein)
453.41 Iliac (vein) deep
451.81 Iliac (vein) with inflammation or phlebitis
0 Inflammation vein see 'Thrombophlebitis Lower Extremities' or 'Thrombophlebitis Upper Extremities'
557.0 Intestine (with gangrene)
434.0# Intracranial
5th digit: 434.0
0. Without cerebral infarction
1. With cerebral infarction

325 Intracranial venous sinus (any)
326 Intracranial venous sinus (any) late effect
437.6 Intracranial venous sinus (any) nonpyogenic origin
0 Intramural see 'Myocardial Infarction Acute'
429.89 Intramural without cardiac condition, coronary artery disease or MI
453.8 Jugular (bulb)
593.81 Kidney (artery)

THROMBOSIS (continued)

453.4# Leg vessels deep
5th digit: 453.4
0. NOS
1. Proximal (femoral) (iliac) (popliteal) (thigh) (upper leg NOS)
2. Distal (calf) (peroneal) (tibial) (lower leg NOS)

453.8 Leg vessels superficial
0 Leg vessels superficial with inflammation or phlebitis see 'Thrombophlebitis'
453.0 Liver (venous)
444.89 Liver artery
572.1 Liver infectional or septic
444.22 Lower extremity artery
415.11 Lung iatrogenic
415.19 Lung other and unspecified
415.11 Lung postoperative
415.12 Lung septic
038.#(#) Lung septic with septicemia [415.12]
4th or 4th and 5th digit code for organism: 038
.9 NOS
.3 Anaerobic
.3 Bacteroides
.3 Clostridium
.42 E. coli
.49 Enterobacter aerogenes
.40 Gram negative
.49 Gram negative other
.41 Hemophilus influenzae
.2 Pneumococcal
.49 Proteus
.43 Pseudomonas
.44 Serratia
.10 Staphylococcal NOS
.11 Staphylococcal aureus
.19 Staphylococcal other
.0 Streptococcal (anaerobic)
.49 Yersinia enterocolitica
.8 Other specified

437.6 Marantic, dural sinus
433.8# Meningeal artery, anterior or posterior
434.0# Meninges (brain)
5th digit: 433.8, 434.0
0. Without cerebral infarction
1. With cerebral infarction

557.0 Mesenteric artery (with gangrene)
557.0 Mesenteric vein (with gangrene)
0 Mitral see 'Mitral Insufficiency'
0 Mural see 'Myocardial Infarction Acute'
093.89 Mural due to syphilis
429.79 Mural ischemic heart disease (due to) [414.8]
429.79 Mural post infarction [410.90]
429.89 Mural without cardiac condition, coronary artery disease or MI
0 Obstetric see 'Thrombosis Complicating Pregnancy'
557.0 Omentum (with gangrene)
0 Ophthalmic artery see 'Retinal Artery Occlusion'
620.8 Pampiniform plexus female
608.83 Pampiniform plexus male
0 Parietal see 'Myocardial Infarction Acute'
607.82 Penis
444.22 Peripheral arteries NOS
444.22 Peripheral arteries lower
444.21 Peripheral arteries upper

THROMBOSIS (continued)

453.42 Peroneal vein deep
446.6 Platelet
433.8# Pontine artery
5th digit: 433.8
0. Without cerebral infarction
1. With cerebral infarction

444.22 Popliteal artery
453.41 Popliteal vein deep
452 Portal
093.89 Portal due to syphilis
572.1 Portal infectional or septic
433.9# Precerebral artery NOS
433.3# Precerebral artery bilateral or multiple
433.8# Precerebral artery NEC
5th digit: 433.3, 8-9
0. Without cerebral infarction
1. With cerebral infarction

415.19 Pulmonary (artery) (vein)
415.11 Pulmonary (artery) (vein) iatrogenic
415.11 Pulmonary (artery) (vein) postoperative
415.12 Pulmonary septic
038.#(#) Pulmonary septic with septicemia [415.12]
4th or 4th and 5th digit code for organism: 038
.9 NOS
.3 Anaerobic
.3 Bacteroides
.3 Clostridium
.42 E. coli
.49 Enterobacter aerogenes
.40 Gram negative
.49 Gram negative other
.41 Hemophilus influenzae
.2 Pneumococcal
.49 Proteus
.43 Pseudomonas
.44 Serratia
.10 Staphylococcal NOS
.11 Staphylococcal aureus
.19 Staphylococcal other
.0 Streptococcal (anaerobic)
.49 Yersinia enterocolitica
.8 Other specified

446.6 Purpura
444.21 Radial artery
593.81 Renal (artery)
453.3 Renal vein
0 Retina (artery) see 'Retinal Artery Occlusion'
608.83 Scrotum
608.83 Seminal vesicle
325 Sigmoid (venous) sinus
437.6 Sigmoid (venous) sinus nonpyogenic origin
453.9 Silent NEC
434.0# Softening, brain
608.83 Spermatic cord
444.89 Spinal artery
433.8# Spinal artery, anterior or posterior
5th digit: 433.8, 434.0
0. Without cerebral infarction
1. With cerebral infarction

336.1 Spinal cord
094.89 Spinal cord due to syphilis
324.1 Spinal cord pyogenic origin
289.59 Spleen
444.89 Spleen artery

T

THROMBOSIS (continued)

608.83 Testes
453.42 Tibial vein deep
608.83 Tunica vaginalis
444.21 Ulnar artery
762.6 Umbilical cord affecting fetus or newborn
444.21 Upper extremity artery
608.83 Vas deferens
453.9 Vein unspecified
453.4# Vein lower extremity deep
5th digit: 453.4
0. NOS
1. Proximal (femoral) (iliac) (popliteal) (thigh) (upper leg NOS)
2. Distal (calf) (peroneal) (tibial) (lower leg NOS)

453.8 Vein other specified site
453.2 Vena cava
433.2# Vertebral artery
433.3# Vertebral artery bilateral or multiple
5th digit: 433.2-3
0. Without cerebral infarction
1. With cerebral infarction

453.8 Specified site NEC

THROMBOSIS COMPLICATING PREGNANCY

671.9# NOS maternal due to pregnancy
674.0# Brain (artery) (stem) maternal due to pregnancy
671.5# Brain venous maternal due to pregnancy
5th digit: 671.5, 9, 674.0
0. Episode of care NOS or N/A
1. Delivered
2. Delivered with mention of postpartum complication
3. Antepartum complication
4. Postpartum complication

> ***When coding a maternal cardiovascular disease complicating pregnancy, 648.6#, use an additional code to identify the condition.***

648.6# Cardiac maternal current (co-existent)
671.5# Cerebral vein or venous sinus maternal due to pregnancy
5th digit: 648.6, 671.5
0. Episode of care NOS or N/A
1. Delivered
2. Delivered with postpartum complication
3. Antepartum complication
4. Postpartum complication

671.3# Deep vein antepartum maternal due to pregnancy
5th digit: 671.3
0. Episode of care NOS or N/A
1. Delivered
3. Antepartum complication

671.4# Deep vein postpartum maternal due to pregnancy
5th digit: 671.4
0. Unspecified
2. Delivered with mention of postpartum complication
4. Postpartum condition or complication

THROMBOSIS COMPLICATING PREGNANCY (continued)

671.5# Intracranial venous sinus nonpyogenic maternal due to pregnancy
5th digit: 671.5
0. Episode of care NOS or N/A
1. Delivered
2. Delivered with mention of postpartum complication
3. Antepartum complication
4. Postpartum complication

671.4# Pelvic maternal due to pregnancy
5th digit: 671.4
0. Episode of care NOS or N/A
2. Delivered with mention of postpartum complication
4. Postpartum condition or complication

673.2# Pulmonary (artery) (vein) maternal due to pregnancy
671.5# Spinal cord maternal due to pregnancy
671.2# Superficial (vein) maternal due to pregnancy
5th digit: 671.2, 5, 673.2
0. Episode of care NOS or N/A
1. Delivered
2. Delivered with mention of postpartum complication
3. Antepartum complication
4. Postpartum complication

663.6# Umbilical cord (vessels)
5th digit: 663.6
0. Episode of care NOS or N/A
1. Delivered
3. Antepartum complication

671.5# Specified site NEC maternal due to pregnacy
5th digit: 671.5
0. Episode of care NOS or N/A
1. Delivered
2. Delivered with mention of postpartum complication
3. Antepartum complication
4. Postpartum complication

0 THROMBOTIC OBSTRUCTION SEE 'THROMBOSIS', BY SITE

446.6 THROMBOTIC PURPURA

446.6 THROMBOTIC THROMBOCYTOPENIC PURPURA

<u>**648.9#**</u> THROMBOTIC THROMBOCYTOPENIC PURPURA MATERNAL CURRENT (CO-EXISTENT) IN <u>PREGNANCY</u> [446.6]
5th digit: 648.9
0. Episode of care NOS or N/A
1. Delivered
2. Delivered with postpartum complication
3. Antepartum complication
4. Postpartum complication

0 THROMBOTIC TUMOR SEE 'NEOPLASM', BY SITE

0 THROMBUS SEE 'THROMBOSIS'

THRUSH

112.9 Candidal unspecified site
112.0 Mouth
771.7 Neonatal
112.0 Oral

THUMB

755.29 Absence congenital
V49.61 Amputation status
959.5 Injury
915.8 Injury other and unspecified superficial
915.9 Injury other and unspecified superficial infected
307.9 Sucking (child)

959.5 THUMBNAIL INJURY

370.21 THYGESON'S SUPERFICIAL PUNCTATE KERATITIS

0 THYMIC SEE 'THYMUS, THYMIC'

THYMOMA

212.6 Benign site NOS
0 Benign site specified see 'Benign Neoplasm', by site M8580/0
164.0 Malignant site NOS
0 Malignant site specified see 'Cancer', by site M8580/3

THYMUS, THYMIC

254.1 Abscess
759.2 Absence congenital
279.2 Alymphoplasia or dysplasia with immunodeficiency
254.8 Atrophy
254.8 Cyst
277.39 Degeneration lardaceous
254.9 Disease (gland)
254.8 Disease (gland) specified NEC
358.00 Disorder causing myasthenia gravis
358.01 Disorder causing myasthenia gravis with (acute) exacerbation (crisis)
254.8 Fibrosis
862.29 Gland injury
908.0 Gland injury late effect
862.39 Gland injury with open wound
254.0 Hyperplasia persistent
254.0 Hypertrophy
279.11 Hypoplasia
279.2 Hypoplasia with immunodeficiency
862.29 Injury
908.0 Injury late effect
862.39 Injury with open wound into cavity

246.0 THYROCALCITONIN SECRETION DISORDER

THYROGLOSSAL

759.2 Duct cyst congenital
759.2 Duct fistula congenital
759.2 Duct persistent

THYROID

245.0 Abscess
748.3 Absence - cartilage congenital
243 Absence - congenital (gland)
246.8 Absence - surgical
226 Adenoma
258.1 Adrenocortical insufficiency syndrome
246.8 Atrophy
243 Atrophy congenital
246.8 Binding globulin abnormality
748.3 Cartilage anomaly congenital
748.3 Cartilage cleft congenital
246.2 Cyst
226 Cystadenoma
277.39 Disease lardaceous

THYROID (continued)

246.9 Disorder (gland)
246.8 Disorder (gland) other specified
V77.0 Disorder screening

> ***Code the specific maternal thyroid dysfunction in addition to the 648.##.***

648.1# Dysfunction maternal current (co-existent) in pregnancy
5th digit: 648.1
0. Episode of care NOS or N/A
1. Delivered
2. Delivered with postpartum complication
3. Antepartum complication
4. Postpartum complication

759.2 Ectopic
0 Enlargement see 'Goiter'
794.5 Function abnormal finding
759.2 Gland accessory congenital
246.3 Hemorrhage
246.8 Hormone resistance
240.9 Hyperplasia (see also 'Goiter')
242.0# Hyperplasia primary
242.2# Hyperplasia secondary
5th digit: 242.0, 2
0. Without mention of thyrotoxic crisis or storm
1. With mention of thyrotoxic crisis or storm

246.8 Hyper-TBG-nemia
246.8 Hypo-TBG-nemia
246.3 Infarction or hemorrhage
959.09 Injury
244.# Insufficiency
4th digit: 244
0. Postsurgical
1. Postablative (irradiation)
2. Iodine ingestion
3. PAS, phenylbut, resorcinol
8. Secondary NEC
9. NOS

243 Insufficiency congenital
0 Nodule see 'Goiter'
794.5 Scan abnormal
848.2 Separation (rupture) (tear) (laceration)
848.2 Strain (sprain) (avulsion) (hemarthrosis)
794.5 Uptake abnormal

THYROIDITIS

245.9 NOS
245.0 Acute
245.0 Acute nonsuppurative
245.0 Acute pyogenic
245.0 Acute suppurative
245.3 Chronic fibrous (strumal) (ligneous) (invasive)
245.2 Chronic lymphocytic (Hashimoto's) (autoimmune) (strumal)
245.8 Chronic unspecified
245.1 De Quervain (giant cell) (granulomatous) (viral)
245.4 Iatrogenic
245.3 Riedel's
245.1 Subacute

759.2 THYROLINGUAL DUCT PERSISTENT

240.9 THYROMEGALY (SEE ALSO 'GOITER')

T

THYROTOXICOSIS

775.3 Neonatal
242.## Thyrotoxic exophthalmos [376.21]
242.## With myasthenic syndrome [358.1]
242.## With or without goiter

4th digit: 242
0. Diffuse
1. Uninodular
2. Multinodular
3. Nodular unspecified
4. Ectopic thyroid nodule
8. Other specified
9. NOS

5th digit: 242
0. Without mention of thyrotoxic crisis or storm
1. With mention of thyrotoxic crisis or storm

435.9 TIA (TRANSIENT ISCHEMIC ATTACK)
V12.54 TIA (TRANSIENT ISCHEMIC ATTACK) HISTORY

TIBIA

755.31 Absence congenital - with absence complete distal elements
755.36 Absence congenital - with absence incomplete distal elements
755.35 Absence congenital - with absence fibula with absence incomplete distal elements
755.36 Agenesis
754.43 And fibula bowing congenital
755.69 Angulation congenital
958.92 Compartment syndrome
736.89 Deformity acquired
733.90 Disorder
733.29 Disorder fibrocystic
733.99 Disorder other specified
755.69 Pseudoarthrosis congenital
736.89 Torsion acquired
732.4 Vara lower extremity excluding foot juvenile

TIBIAL

444.22 Artery (embolism) (thrombosis) (occlusion) (infarction)
904.50 Artery injury - NOS
904.51 Artery injury - anterior
908.3 Artery injury - late effect (anterior) (posterior)
904.53 Artery injury - posterior
355.5 Nerve posterior compression (disorder)
956.2 Nerve posterior injury
907.5 Nerve posterior injury late effect
736.89 Torsion
904.50 Vein injury - NOS
904.52 Vein injury - anterior
908.3 Vein injury - late effect (anterior) (posterior)
904.54 Vein injury - posterior
904.50 Vessel injury
908.3 Vessel injury late effect
908.3 Vessel laceration late effect
904.50 Vessel laceration (aneurysm) (avulsion) (hematoma) (rupture) traumatic

726.72 TIBIALIS TENDINITIS
844.3 TIBIOFIBULAR (JOINT) (LIGAMENT) SUPERIOR SPRAIN, STRAIN OR TEAR

TIC

307.20 NOS
307.22 Chronic motor or vocal habit
307.22 Chronic motor or vocal spasm
307.22 Chronic vocal
307.20 Disorder NOS
350.1 Douloureux
053.12 Douloureaux postherpetic
307.23 Gilles de la tourette's syndrome
307.20 Habit, spasm
307.22 Habit, spasm chronic (motor or vocal)
307.21 Habit, spasm transient (of childhood)
307.20 Lid, orbicularis
307.21 Lid, orbicularis transient (of childhood)
333.3 Organic origin
307.21 Transient (childhood)
307.23 Verbal motor
307.22 Verbal motor chronic

TICK

087.1 African tick-bite fever
066.1 American mountain tick-borne fever
0 Bite see 'Insect Bite', by site
082.#(#) Borne rickettsioses

4th or 4th and 5th digit: 082
0. Spotted fever
1. Boutonneuse fever
2. North asian tick fever
3. Queensland tick typhus
4#. Ehrlichiosis
40. NOS
41. E. Chaffeensis
49. Other
8. Other specified tick - borne rickettsiosis
9. Unspecified tick - borne rickettsiosis

066.1 Colorado (virus) tick-bite fever
066.1 Colorado tick-borne fever
0 Encephalitis (tick-borne) see 'Encephalitis'
066.1 Fever tick-borne NEC
065.0 Hemorrhagic Crimean tick-borne fever
065.2 Hemorrhagic Kyasanur forest tick-borne fever
065.1 Hemorrhagic Omsk tick-borne fever
065.3 Hemorrhagic tick-borne fever NEC
066.1 Kemerovo tick-borne fever
0 Lyme disease see 'Lyme Disease'
066.1 Mountain tick-borne fever
066.1 Nonexanthematous
989.5 Paralysis
066.1 Quaranfil tick-borne fever
082.0 Rocky mountain tick-bite fever

287.31 TIDAL PLATELET DYSGENESIS
733.6 TIETZE'S DISEASE OR SYNDROME
605 TIGHT FORESKIN
327.35 TIME-ZONE SYNDROME (RAPID)

TINEA

110.9 NOS
111.2 Blanca
110.# By site
4th digit: 110
0. Scalp and beard
1. Nail (unguium)
2. Hand (manuum)
3. Groin and perianal (cruris)
4. Foot (pedis)
5. Body (corporis)
6. Deep seated (granuloma trichophyticum)
8. Other specified site
9. Unspecified site

110.0 Capitis
110.5 Corporis
110.3 Cruris of groin and perianal area
111.0 Flava
110.5 Imbricata (Tokelau)
110.2 Manuum (of hand)
110.9 Microsporic
111.1 Nigra
110.0 Of scalp and beard kerion
111.1 Palmaris nigra
110.4 Pedis of foot athlete's foot
110.0 Trichophytic (black dot tinea), scalp
110.1 Unguium of nail
111.0 Versicolor

782.0 TINGLING OF SKIN

TINNITUS

388.30 NOS
388.32 Objective
388.31 Subjective

524.33 TIPPED TEETH

780.79 TIREDNESS

524.6# TMJ (TEMPOROMANDIBULAR JOINT) SYNDROME
5th digit: 524.6
0. Unspecified
1. Adhesions and ankylosis
2. Arthralgia
3. Articular disc disorder (reducing or non reducing)
4. Sounds on opening and/or closing of jaw
9. Other specified joint disorder (malocclusion)

305.1 TOBACCO USE (ABUSE) (DEPENDENCE)

649.0# TOBACCO USE DISORDER COMPLICATING PREGNANCY
5th digit: 649.0
0. Episode of care unspecified or N/A
1. Delivered
2. Delivered with postpartum complication
3. Antepartum complication
4. Postpartum complication

V15.82 TOBACCO USE HISTORY

162.3 TOBIAS' SYNDROME (CARCINOMA PULMONARY APEX) M8010/3

TOE

755.39 Absence congenital (partial) (complete)
755.31 Absence congenital all toes (complete)
V49.72 Amputation status
V49.71 Amputation status great toe
735.# Deformity
4th digit: 735
0. Hallux valgus (acquired)
1. Hallux varus (acquired)
2. Hallux rigidus
3. Hallux malleus
4. Other hammer toe (acquired)
5. Claw toe (acquired)
8. Other acquired deformity
9. NOS

755.66 Deformity congenital
755.39 Deformity congenital - reduction
735.8 Drop
917.8 Injury other and unspecified superficial
917.9 Injury other and unspecified superficial infected
718.17 Joint loose body
V54.81 Joint replacement aftercare [V43.69]
V43.69 Joint replacement status
703.8 Nail deformity (hypertrophy)
703.8 Nail discoloration
703.8 Nail disease other specified
110.1 Nail fungus
681.9 Nail infection
703.0 Nail infection ingrowing
681.11 Nail infection onychia or paronychia
703.0 Nail ingrown (infected)
959.7 Nail injury
110.1 Nail mycosis
703.8 Nail thickening
735.8 Overlapping
755.66 Overlapping congenital
729.5 Pain
0 See also 'Digital'

926.0 TOILET SEAT SYNDROME

378.55 TOLOSA-HUNT SYNDROME

TONGUE

0 See also 'Glottis, Glottic'
529.8 Atrophy (hypertrophy) (enlarged) (senile)
529.4 Atrophy papillae (senile)
474.00 Base lymphoid tissue infection
529.3 Coated
529.9 Disease unspecified
528.79 Dyskeratosis
478.6 Edema
528.79 Erythroplakia
528.8 Fibrosis
529.5 Fissured
529.5 Furrowed
529.1 Geographic
528.79 Hyperkeratosis
959.09 Injury
524.59 Lip or finger habits causing malocclusion
529.8 Other specified conditions
529.6 Pain glossodynia
529.4 Papillae atrophy
529.3 Papillae hypertrophy
529.8 Paralysis
529.5 Plicated
529.5 Scrotal

TONGUE (continued)

529.4 Smooth atrophic
478.75 Spasm
306.1 Spasm psychogenic
529.4 Ulceration
529.0 Ulceration traumatic

TONGUE CONGENITAL ANOMALY

750.10 Unspecified
750.11 Absence
750.12 Adhesions
750.13 Bifid
750.13 Double
750.13 Fissure
750.15 Hypertrophy
750.16 Hypoplasia
750.0 Tie
750.19 Other specified

270.0 TONI-FANCONI SYNDROME (CYSTINOSIS)

TONSIL, TONSILLAR

474.8 Amygdalolith
475 Angina
474.8 Calculus
474.8 Cicatrix
474.9 Disease (chronic)
474.8 Disease (chronic) specified NEC
474.11 Enlargement
474.01 Enlargement with chronic adenoiditis
474.02 Enlargement with chronic adenoiditis and tonsillitis
474.00 Enlargement with chronic tonsillitis
474.11 Hyperplasia (lymphoid)
474.10 Hyperplasia and adenoids hyperplasia (lymphoid)
474.11 Hypertrophy (hyperplasia)
474.10 Hypertrophy (hyperplasia) with adenoid hypertrophy
474.01 Hypertrophy (hyperplasia) with chronic adenoiditis
474.02 Hypertrophy (hyperplasia) with chronic adenoiditis and tonsillitis
474.00 Hypertrophy (hyperplasia) with chronic tonsillitis
959.09 Injury
474.8 Remnant
474.00 Remnant infected
474.8 Tag
474.00 Tag infected
474.8 Ulcer
474.10 With adenoids hypertrophy

If the diagnosis is not specified as acute on the record, select the chronic or NOS code. If the medical record indicates that the reason the patient sought care was due to an exacerbation of a chronic condition, consult the physician for further documentation.

TONSILLITIS

463 NOS
463 Acute
463 Acute follicular
463 Acute infective
463 Acute pneumococcal
463 Acute staphylococcal
034.0 Acute streptococcal
463 Acute viral

TONSILLITIS (continued)

474.00 Chronic
474.02 Chronic with chronic adenoiditis
474.00 Chronic with hypertrophy (adenoids) (tonsils)
474.02 Chronic with hypertrophy (adenoids) (tonsils) with chronic adenoiditis

475 Open peritonsillar abscess

465.8 TONSILLOPHARYNGITIS

TOOTH

520.2 Abnormal form
520.2 Abnormal size
520.0 Absence (complete) (partial) (congenital)
525.1# Absence acquired [**525.##**]

5th digit: 525.1
- **0. Unspecified**
- **1. Due to trauma**
- **2. Due to periodontal disease**
- **3. Due to caries**
- **9. Other**

4th digit: 525
- **4. Complete or NOS**
- **5. Partial**

5th digit: 525
- **0. Unspecified**
- **1. Class I**
- **2. Class II**
- **3. Class III**
- **4. Class IV**

524.3# Absence with malocclusion/abnormal spacing

5th digit: 524.3
- **0. Unspecified position**
- **1. Crowding**
- **2. Excessive spacing**
- **3. Horizontal displacement**
- **4. Vertical displacement**
- **5. Rotation of teeth**
- **6. Insufficient interocclusal distance**
- **7. Excessive interocclusal distance**
- **9. Other position**

523.6 Accretions
525.9 Ache
524.75 And alveolus extrusion
521.0# Ache due to dental caries

5th digit: 521.0
- **0. Unspecified**
- **1. Limited to enamel**
- **2. Extending into dentine**
- **3. Extending into pulp**
- **4. Arrested**
- **5. Odontoclasia**
- **6. Pit and fissure origin (primary)**
- **7. Smooth surface origin (primary)**
- **8. Root surface (primary)**
- **9. Other**

520.6 Ache due to obstructed or impacted tooth

TOOTH (continued)

524.3# Anomalies of position
5th digit: 524.3
0. Unspecified position
1. Crowding
2. Excessive spacing
3. Horizontal displacement
4. Vertical displacement
5. Rotation of teeth
6. Insufficient interocclusal distance
7. Excessive interocclusal distance
9. Other position

525.2# Atrophy of edentulous alveolar ridge
5th digit: 525.2
0. Unspecified (mandible) (maxilla)
1. Minimal of mandible
2. Moderate of mandible
3. Severe of mandible
4. Minimal of maxilla
5. Moderate of maxilla
6. Severe of maxilla

521.81 Broken nontraumatic
873.63 Broken traumatic
873.73 Broken traumatic complicated
524.55 Centric occlusion maximum intercuspation discrepancy
523.6 Color changes extrinsic due to deposits on teeth
521.7 Color changes intrinsic due to metals, drugs, bleeding or unspecified
521.7 Color changes intrinsic post-eruptive
520.8 Color changes pre-eruptive
520.2 Concrescence
520.2 Conical
521.81 Cracked
524.31 Crowding
521.89 Decalcification
523.6 Deposits betel
523.6 Deposits materia alba
523.6 Deposits soft
523.6 Deposits tartar
523.6 Deposits tobacco
524.30 Diastema NOS
520.4 Dilaceration developmental disorder
524.30 Direction abnormal
520.9 Disorder - development and eruption NOS
525.9 Disorder - teeth and supporting structures NOS
524.30 Displacement NOS
524.33 Displacement horizontal
524.34 Displacement vertical
520.6 Embedded

524.3# Embedded due to abnormal position of fully erupted teeth
5th digit: 524.3
0. Unspecified position
1. Crowding
2. Excessive spacing
3. Horizontal displacement
4. Vertical displacement
5. Rotation of teeth
6. Insufficient interocclusal distance
7. Excessive interocclusal distance
9. Other position

TOOTH (continued)

520.6 Eruption accelerated or neonatal
520.6 Eruption disorder
520.6 Eruption incomplete, delayed, difficult
520.6 Eruption late or premature
520.6 Eruption obstructed, persistent, primary
525.0 Exfoliation due to systemic causes
<u>525.10</u> <u>Extraction</u> <u>status</u> [**525.##**]
4th digit: 525
4. Complete or NOS
5. Partial
5th digit: 525
0. Unspecified
1. Class I
2. Class II
3. Class III
4. Class IV

524.34 Extruded
520.4 Formation disturbance
521.81 Fracture nontraumatic
873.63 Fracture traumatic
873.73 Fracture traumatic complicated
520.2 Fusion
520.2 Gemination
306.8 Grinding
524.39 Hag
520.4 Hypocalcification
520.6 Impacted

524.3# Impacted due to abnormal position of fully erupted teeth
5th digit: 524.3
0. Unspecified position
1. Crowding
2. Excessive spacing
3. Horizontal displacement
4. Vertical displacement
5. Rotation of teeth
6. Insufficient interocclusal distance
7. Excessive interocclusal distance
9. Other position

996.69 Implant complication - infection or inflammation
996.59 Implant complication - mechanical
996.79 Implant complication - other
523.30 Infection peridental
523.31 Infection periodontal
873.63 Injury
873.73 Injury complicated
521.20 Injury superficial
524.34 Intruded
521.89 Irradiated enamel
525.8 Loose
<u>525.1#</u> <u>Loss</u> [**525.##**]
5th digit: 525.1
0. Acquired, unspecified
1. Due to trauma
2. Due to periodontal disease
3. Due to caries
9. Other

4th digit: 525
4. Complete or NOS
5. Partial
5th digit: 525
0. Unspecified
1. Class I
2. Class II
3. Class III
4. Class IV

T

TOOTH (continued)

520.3 Mottled
524.29 Occlusion
520.2 Peg-shaped
520.6 Prenatal
524.39 Rake
V45.84 Restoration status
525.6# Restoration unsatisfactory
5th digit: 525.6
0. Unspecified
1. Open margins
2. Unrepairable overhanging materials
3. Fractured material without loss of material
4. Fractured material with loss of material
5. Contour incompatible with oral health
6. Allergy
7. Poor aesthetics
9. Other
525.3 Retained dental root
524.35 Rotation
V49.82 Sealant status
520.5 Shell
524.39 Snaggle
524.3# Spacing
5th digit: 524.3
0. Unspecified position
1. Crowding
2. Excessive spacing
3. Horizontal displacement
4. Vertical displacement
5. Rotation of teeth
6. Insufficient interocclusal distance
7. Excessive interocclusal distance
9. Other position
520.5 Structure disturbance hereditary
520.2 Supernumerary roots
520.1 Supernumerary teeth
520.1 Supplemental
524.33 Tipped
524.3# Transposition
5th digit: 524.3
0. Unspecified position
1. Crowding
2. Excessive spacing
3. Horizontal displacement
4. Vertical displacement
5. Rotation of teeth
6. Insufficient interocclusal distance
7. Excessive interocclusal distance
9. Other position
520.8 Other specified disorders of development and eruption
525.8 Other specified disorders of teeth and supporting structures

TOOTH DISORDER OF HARD TISSUE

521.9 NOS
521.2# Abrasion
5th digit: 521.2
0. Unspecified
1. Limited to enamel
2. Extending into dentine
3. Extending into pulp
4. Localized
5. Generalized
521.6 Ankylosis
521.1# Attrition
5th digit: 521.1
0. Unspecified
1. Limited to enamel
2. Extending into dentine
3. Extending into pulp
4. Localized
5. Generalized
521.81 Broken
873.63 Broken due to trauma
873.73 Broken due to trauma complicated
523.6 Color changes extrinsic due to deposits on teeth
521.7 Color changes intrinsic due to metals, drugs, bleeding or unspecified
521.7 Color changes intrinsic post-eruptive
520.8 Color changes pre-eruptive
521.81 Cracked
873.63 Cracked due to trauma
873.73 Cracked due to trauma complicated
521.20 Defect, wedge
521.0# Dental caries
5th digit: 521.0
0. Unspecified
1. Limited to enamel
2. Extending into dentine
3. Extending into pulp
4. Arrested
5. Odontoclasia
6. Pit and fissure origin (primary)
7. Smooth surface origin (primary)
8. Root surface (primary)
9. Other
521.9 Disease
521.89 Disease specified NEC
521.3# Erosion (due to medicine or vomiting) (idiopathic) (occupational)
5th digit: 521.3
0. Unspecified
1. Limited to enamel
2. Extending into dentine
3. Extending into pulp
4. Localized
5. Generalized
521.81 Fracture
873.63 Fracture due to trauma
873.73 Fracture due to trauma complicated
521.49 Granuloma internal of pulp
521.5 Hypercementosis
521.89 Irradiated enamel

TOOTH DISORDER OF HARD TISSUE (continued)

521.4# Pathological resorption
5th digit: 521.4
0. Unspecified
1. Internal
2. External
9. Other

521.89 Sensitive dentia
521.20 Wedge defect
521.01 White spot lesions
521.89 Other specified diseases (hard tissues)

TOOTH PULP AND PERIAPICAL DISORDERS

522.3 Abnormal hard tissue formation pulp
522.7 Abscess periapical with sinus
522.5 Abscess periapical without sinus
522.0 Abscess pulpal
522.8 Cyst apical, periapical or radicular
522.2 Degeneration of pulp
522.1 Necrosis of pulp
522.4 Periodontitis acute of pulpal origin
523.33 Periodontitis acute
523.30 Periodontitis aggressive
523.32 Periodontitis aggressive generalized
523.31 Periodontitis aggressive localized
523.40 Periodontitis chronic NOS
523.42 Periodontitis chronic generalized
523.41 Periodontitis chronic localized
522.0 Polyp pulpal
522.0 Pulpitis
522.9 Other and unspecified diseases of pulp or periapical tissue

TORCH SYNDROME

771.1 Cytomegalovirus
771.2 Herpes simplex
771.2 Listeriosis
771.2 Malaria
771.0 Rubella
771.2 Toxoplasmosis
771.2 Tuberculosis

008.69 TOROVIRUS ENTERITIS

TORSION

608.24 Appendix epididymis
608.23 Appendix testis
333.89 Dystonia (fragments) (other)
333.79 Dystonia acquired
333.6 Dystonia genetic
333.79 Dystonia symptomatic
608.24 Epididymis (appendix)
620.5 Hytadid of morgagni
560.2 Intestine
620.5 Ovary
752.0 Ovary congenital
608.22 Spermatic cord NOS
608.21 Spermatic cord extravaginal
608.22 Spermatic cord intravaginal
608.20 Testis NOS

TORTICOLLIS

723.5 NOS
754.1 Congenital
767.8 Due to birth injury
300.11 Hysterical
781.93 Ocular
306.0 Psychogenic
333.83 Spasmodic
306.0 Syndrome
847.0 Traumatic current

117.5 TORULA
0 TORUS FRACTURE SEE 'FRACTURE', (BONE) CLOSED OR OPEN
526.81 TORUS MANDIBULARIS
526.81 TORUS PALATINUS
747.41 TOTAL ANOMALOUS PULMONARY VENOUS CONNECTION
790.99 TOTAL PROTEINS ABNORMAL
756.89 TOURAINE'S SYNDROME (HEREDITARY OSTEO-ONYCHODYSPLASIA)
757.39 TOURAINE-SOLENTE-GOLE SYNDROME (ACROPACHYDERMA)
307.23 TOURETTE'S DISORDER
756.0 TOWER SKULL

TOXEMIA

799.89 NOS
0 Bacterial see 'Bacteremia' or 'Septicemia'
0 Eclampitc see 'Eclampsia' or 'Pre-eclampsia'
799.89 Fatigue
799.89 Stasis

TOXIC

377.34 Amblyopia
695.1 Epidermal necrolysis
695.0 Erythema
556.5 Megacolon
358.2 Myoneural disorders
357.7 Neuritis
710.5 Oil syndrome
799.89 Poisoning from disease
782.1 Rash

When coding an infection, use an additional code, [041.#(#)], to identify the organism. See 'Bacterial Infection'.

040.82 Shock syndrome
760.70 Substance NOS transmitted via placenta or breast milk affecting fetus or newborn
760.75 Substance cocaine transmitted via placenta or breast milk affecting fetus or newborn
760.79 Substance NEC transmitted via placenta or breast milk affecting fetus or newborn

796.0 TOXICITY DRUG - ASYMPTOMATIC
0 TOXICITY DRUG - SYMPTOMATIC SEE DRUGS AND CHEMICALS (APPENDIX B) OR 'POISONING MEDICINAL'
796.0 TOXICOLOGY FINDINGS ABNORMAL
0 TOXICOSIS SEE 'TOXEMIA'
799.89 TOXINFECTION
128.0 TOXOCARA CANIS CATI INFECTION
128.0 TOXOCARIASIS
0 TOXOPLASMA GONDII INFECTION SEE 'TOXOPLASMOSIS'

TOXOPLASMOSIS

130.9 NOS
130.2 Chorioretinitis
771.2 Congenital or perinatal
130.1 Conjunctivitis
130.5 Hepatitis
655.4# Maternal with suspected damage to fetus
5th digit: 655.4
0. Episode of care NOS or N/A
1. Delivered
3. Antepartum complication

130.0 Meningoencephalitis
130.8 Multiple sites
130.8 Multisystemic disseminated
130.3 Myocarditis
130.4 Pneumonia
130.7 Other specified sites

V07.8 TOXOXIFEN ADMINISTRATION DUE TO FAMILY HISTORY CANCER BREAST [V16.3]

TRACHEA

478.9 Abscess
519.19 Atrophy
519.19 Calcification
478.9 Cicatrix
519.19 Collapse
519.19 Compression
0 Complication following tracheostomy see 'Tracheostomy'
519.19 Deformity
519.19 Deviation
519.19 Disease
519.19 Diverticulum
874.02 Laceration
874.12 Laceration complicated
519.19 Obstruction
519.19 Ossification
519.19 Stenosis
519.19 Tracheomalacia
519.19 Ulcer

TRACHEA CONGENITAL

748.3 Absence or agenesis
748.3 Atresia
748.3 Cartilage anomaly
748.3 Dilation
748.3 Diverticulum
748.3 Stenosis
748.3 Tracheomalacia

464.4 TRACHEALIS ANGINA

TRACHEITIS

464.3# NOS
464.1# Acute
464.1# Acute viral
464.1# Acute with catarrh
464.2# Acute with laryngitis
5th digit: 464.1-3
1. With obstruction
0. NOS

034.0 Acute streptococcal
491.8 Chronic
476.1 Chronic with laryngitis
487.1 Viral influenza
0 With bronchitis see 'Bronchitis'

TRACHEOBRONCHITIS

490 NOS
466.0 Acute
493.## Acute asthmatic
4th or 4th and 5th digit: 493
0. Extrinsic (or allergic with stated cause)
1. Intrinsic
2. Chronic obstructive with COPD
8#. Other specified
81. Exercised induced bronchospasm
82. Cough variant
9. NOS (or allergic cause not stated)

5th digit: 493.0-2, 9
0. NOS
1. With status asthmaticus
2. With (acute) exacerbation

460 Acute due to RSV (respiratory syncytial virus) [079.6]
491.9 Chronic
493.2# Chronic asthmatic
5th digit: 493.2
0. NOS
1. With status asthmaticus
2. With (acute) exacerbation

491.20 Chronic obstructive
491.21 Chronic obstructive with exacerbation (acute)
491.2# With bronchitis (chronic)
5th digit: 491.2
0. NOS
1. With (acute) exacerbation
2. With acute bronchitis

0 See also 'Bronchitis'

748.3 TRACHEOBRONCHOMEGALY (CONGENITAL)
494.# TRACHEOBRONCHOMEGALY (CONGENITAL) WITH BRONCHIECTASIS
4th digit: 494
0. Without acute exacerbation
1. With acute exacerbation

519.19 TRACHEOBRONCHOMEGALY ACQUIRED
494.# TRACHEOBRONCHOMEGALY ACQUIRED WITH BRONCHIECTASIS
4th digit: 494
0. Without acute exacerbation
1. With acute exacerbation

519.19 TRACHEOCELE (EXTERNAL) (INTERNAL)
748.3 TRACHEOCELE CONGENITAL
750.3 TRACHEOESOPHAGEAL FISTULA CONGENITAL
519.19 TRACHEOMALACIA
748.3 TRACHEOMALACIA CONGENITAL
519.19 TRACHEOSTENOSIS

TRACHEOSTOMY

V55.0 Care
V55.0 Closure
519.00 Complication NOS
519.02 Complication mechanical
519.09 Complication other
519.09 Fistula
519.09 Granuloma
519.09 Hemorrhage

TRACHEOSTOMY (continued)

> *When coding an infection of an ostomy, use an additional code to specify the organism. See 'Bacterial Infection'*

519.01 Infection
519.01 Infection with cellulitis of neck [682.1]
519.01 Infection with septicemia [**038.#(#)**]

4th or 4th and 5th Digit Code for Organism: 038

.9 NOS
.3 Anaerobic
.3 Bacteroides
.3 Clostridium
.42 E. coli
.49 Enterobacter aerogenes
.40 Gram negative
.49 Gram negative other
.41 Hemophilus influenzae
.2 Pneumococcal
.49 Proteus
.43 Pseudomonas
.44 Serratia
.10 Staphylococcal NOS
.11 Staphylococcal aureus
.19 Staphylococcal other
.0 Streptococcal (anaerobic)
.49 Yersinia enterocolitica
.8 Other specified

519.02 Malfunction
519.09 Obstruction
V55.0 Removal or replacement
709.2 Scar (adherent, contracture, fibrosis)
V44.0 Status
519.02 Stenosis
V55.0 Toilet

TRACHOMA

076.9 NOS
076.1 Active stage
076.0 Dubium
076.0 Initial stage
139.1 Late effects
V73.6 Screening exam

V54.89 TRACTION DEVICE CHECKING CHANGE OR REMOVAL
744.1 TRAGUS ACCESSORY CONGENITAL
518.7 TRALI (TRANSFUSION RELATED ACUTE LUNG INJURY)
V60.0 TRAMP (HOMELESS PERSON)
780.09 TRANCE
305.4# TRANQUILIZER ABUSE (NONDEPENDENT)
304.1# TRANQUILIZER ADDICTION (DEPENDENT)

5th digit: 304.1, 305.4
0. NOS
1. Continuous
2. Episodic
3. In remission

763.5 TRANQUILIZER REACTION (MATERNAL) AFFECTING FETUS OR NEWBORN
790.4 TRANSAMINASE ABNORMAL (LEVEL)

TRANSFUSION

V58.2 Blood without reported diagnosis
772.0 Fetal-maternal syndrome
776.4 Maternal fetal with polycythemia

TRANSFUSION (continued)

999.8 Reaction
999.6 Reaction ABO incompatibility
999.7 Reaction RH incompatibility
518.7 Related acute lung injury (TRALI)
762.3 Twin donor syndrome (infant) [772.0]
762.3 Twin recipient syndrome (infant) [776.4]
762.3 Twin to twin syndrome (infant)

TRANSIENT

780.02 Alteration of consciousness
368.12 Blindness
388.02 Deafness (ischemic)
437.7 Global amnesia
435.9 Ischemic attack
V12.54 Ischemic attack history
429.83 Left ventricular apical ballooning syndrome
V60.0 Person (homeless) NEC
770.6 Tachypnea of newborn

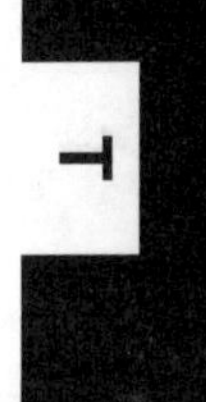

> *Carcinomas and neoplasms should be coded by site first, not cell type. If a site is not specified, then code by cell type. Code the 'site NOS' only if no site is mentioned. When no site is given, the code reverts to the histological origin.*

TRANSITIONAL CELL CARCINOMA

151.9 Site NOS
0 Site specified see 'Cancer', by site M8120/3
234.9 In situ site NOS
0 In situ site specified see 'CA In Situ', by site M8120/2
199.1 Papillary type site NOS
0 Papillary type site specified see 'Cancer', by site M8130/3
199.1 Spindle cell type site NOS
0 Spindle cell type site specified see 'Cancer', by site M8122/3

758.4 TRANSLOCATION AUTOSOMAL BALANCED IN NORMAL INDIVIDUAL

TRANSPLANT

V58.44 Aftercare [**V42.#(#)**]

4th or 4th and 5th digit: V42
0. Kidney
1. Heart
2. Heart valve
3. Skin
4. Bone
5. Cornea
6. Lung
7. Liver
8#. Other specified
81. Bone marrow
82. Peripheral stem cells
83. Pancreas
84. Intestine
89. Other specified
9. Unspecified

996.55 Allodermis decellularized failure or rejection (dislodgement) (displacement) (non-adherence) (poor incorporation) (shearing)
996.89 Failure organ NEC
V49.83 Organ – waiting status
996.80 Rejection (failure) organ unspecified
996.89 Rejection (failure) organ other specified

TRANSPLANT (continued)

996.55 Skin artificial failure or rejection (dislodgement) (displacement) (non-adherence) (poor incorporation) (shearing)
996.52 Skin failure
V42.#(#) Status
4th or 4th <u>and</u> 5th digit: V42
0. Kidney
1. Heart
2. Heart valve
3. Skin
4. Bone
5. Cornea
6. Lung
7. Liver
8#. Other specified
81. Bone marrow
82. Peripheral stem cells
83. Pancreas
84. Intestine
89. Other specified
9. Unspecified
V43.83 Status skin artificial

TRANSPOSITION

745.11 Aorta (dextra)
751.5 Appendix
751.5 Colon
745.10 Great vessels - classical
745.12 Great vessels - corrected
745.11 Great vessels - incomplete
745.19 Great vessels - other NEC
746.87 Heart
751.5 Intestines
747.49 Pulmonary veins
750.7 Stomach
524.3# Teeth
5th digit: 524.3
0. Unspecified position
1. Crowding
2. Excessive spacing
3. Horizontal displacement
4. Vertical displacement
5. Rotation of teeth
6. Insufficient interocclusal distance
7. Excessive interocclusal distance
9. Other position
759.3 Viscera (abdominal) (thoracic)

302.5# TRAN-SEXUALISM (SEX REASSIGNMENT SURGERY STATUS)
5th digit; 302.5
0. With unspecified sexual history
1. With asexual history
2. With homosexual history
3. With heterosexual history

660.3# TRANSVERSE ARREST OF FETAL HEAD
5th digit: 660.3
0. Episode of care NOS or N/A
1. Delivered
3. Antepartum complication

TRANSVERSE LIE

761.7 Affecting fetus or newborn - before labor
763.1 Affecting fetus or newborn - during labor
652.3# Complicating pregnancy
<u>660.0#</u> <u>Obstructing</u> <u>labor</u> **[652.3#]**
652.6# With multiple gestation
<u>660.0#</u> With multiple gestation <u>obstructing</u> <u>labor</u> **[652.6#]**
652.1# With version
<u>660.0#</u> With version <u>obstructing</u> <u>labor</u> **[652.1#]**
5th digit: 652.1, 3, 6, 660.0
0. Episode of care NOS or N/A
1. Delivered
3. Antepartum complication

302.3 TRANSVESTIC FETISHISM

TRAUMA

0 Blunt see anatomical site, injury
958.8 Complication (early) other specified
908.6 Late effect (complications of)
0 Obstetrical see 'Labor and Delivery Complications Trauma Obstetrical'
V15.4# Psychological history
5th digit: V15.4
1. Physical abuse, rape
2. Emotional abuse, neglect
9. Other
V66.6 Treatment convalescence combined
V62.6 Treatment refusal - religion based

756.0 TREACHER COLLINS' SYNDROME (INCOMPLETE MANDIBULOFACIAL DYSOSTOSIS)
V66.6 TREATMENT CONVALESCENCE COMBINED
V62.6 TREATMENT REFUSAL RELIGION BASED (REASON FOR ENCOUNTER)
121.9 TREMATODE INFECTION
121.8 TREMATODE INFECTION OTHER SPECIFIED

TREMOR

781.0 NOS
333.1 Benign essential
333.1 Familial
333.1 Postural medication-induced

083.1 TRENCH FEVER
991.4 TRENCH FOOT
909.4 TRENCH FOOT LATE EFFECT
101 TRENCH MOUTH
0 TREPONEMA (DENTICOLA) (MACRODENTICUM) SEE 'BACTERIAL INFECTION' OR SPECIFIED CONDITION
097.9 TREPONEMA PALLIDUM INFECTION

TRICHIASIS

704.2 NOS
704.2 Cicatrical
374.05 Eyelid
374.05 Without entropion (eyelid)

842.01 TRIANGULAR FIBROCARTILAGE COMPLEX SPRAIN (STRAIN) (TEAR)
719.83 TRIANGULAR FIBROCARTILAGE COMPLEX SPRAIN (STRAIN) (TEAR) - OLD

124 TRICHINELLA SPIRALIS INFECTION
124 TRICHINELLOSIS
124 TRICHINIASIS
124 TRICHINOSIS
127.3 TRICHOCEPHALIASIS
216.# TRICHOEPITHELIOMA M8100/0
216.# TRICHOFOLLICULOMA M8101/0
216.# TRICHOLEMMOMA M8102/0

4th digit: 216
0. Lip (skin of)
1. Eyelid including canthus
2. Ear (external) (auricle) (pinna)
3. Face (cheek) (nose) (eyebrow) (temple)
4. Scalp, neck
5. Trunk, back except scrotum
6. Upper limb including shoulder
7. Lower limb including hip
8. Other specified sites
9. Skin NOS

TRICHOMONAS
V01.89 Exposure
007.3 Gastroenteritis
131.9 Infection NOS
007.3 Intestinal infection
131.03 Prostatitis
131.02 Urethritis
131.00 Urogenital NOS
131.09 Urogenital other specified site
131.01 Vaginitis
131.01 Vulvovaginitis
131.8 Other specified sites - non urogenital

039.0 TRICHOMYCOSIS AXILLARIS
110.0 TRICHOPHYTIC TINEA
110.6 TRICHOPHYTICUM GRANULOMA
0 TRICHOPHYTON INFECTIONS SEE 'DERMATOPHYTOSIS'
704.2 TRICHORRHEXIS (NODOSA)
111.2 TRICHOSPORON (BEIGELII) CUTANEUM INFECTION
127.6 TRICHOSTRONGYLIASIS
127.6 TRICHOSTRONGYLUS SPECIES INFECTION
312.39 TRICHOTILLOMANIA
127.3 TRICHURIASIS
127.3 TRICHURIS TRICHIURIA INFECTION

TRICUSPID
746.1 Absence congenital
0 Incompetence see 'Tricuspid', insufficiency
424.2 Insufficiency
421.0 Insufficiency - bacterial (acute) (chronic)
397.0 Insufficiency - rheumatic
093.23 Insufficiency - syphilitic
0 Regurgitation see 'Tricuspid', insufficiency
424.2 Stenosis
421.0 Stenosis - bacterial
746.1 Stenosis - congenital
397.0 Stenosis - rheumatic
093.23 Stenosis - syphilitic
421.0 Stenosis - with insufficiency bacterial (acute) (chronic)
093.23 Stenosis - with insufficiency syphilitic
746.1 Stenosis and atresia congenital

TRICUSPID (continued)
746.1 Valve atresia (congenital)
424.2 Valve disorder nonrheumatic

426.54 TRIFASCICULAR BLOCK
753.3 TRIFID KIDNEY (PELVIS) CONGENITAL

TRIGEMINAL NERVE
350.8 Atrophy
350.9 Disorder
350.8 Disorders other specified
951.2 Injury
350.1 Neuralgia
053.12 Neuralgia postherpetic
350.9 Paralysis
350.1 Spasm

259.8 TRIGEMINAL PLATE SYNDROME
727.03 TRIGGER FINGER
756.89 TRIGGER FINGER CONGENITAL
272.9 TRIGLYCERIDE ABNORMAL FINDINGS
272.1 TRIGLYCERIDE ELEVATION
272.2 TRIGLYCERIDE ELEVATION WITH CHOLESTEROL
272.7 TRIGLYCERIDE STORAGE TYPE I, II OR III DISEASE
595.3 TRIGONITIS
756.0 TRIGONOCEPHALY
270.8 TRIMETHYLAMINURIA
344.89 TRIPLEGIA
758.81 TRIPLE X (FEMALE) SYNDROME
651.1# TRIPLET GESTATION
651.7# TRIPLET GESTATION FOLLOWING (ELECTIVE) FETAL REDUCTION
651.4# TRIPLET GESTATION WITH ONE OR MORE LOSSES

5th digit: 651.1, 4, 7
0. Episode of care NOS or N/A
1. Delivered
3. Antepartum complication

761.5 TRIPLET PREGNANCY AFFECTING FETUS OR NEWBORN
781.0 TRISMUS

TRISOMY
758.5 NOS
758.1 13
758.1 14
758.2 16-18
758.5 20
758.0 21 OR 22 (mongolism)
758.1 D1
758.2 E (3)
758.0 G (mongolism)

368.53 TRITAN DEFECT
368.53 TRITANOMALY
368.53 TRITANOPIA
726.5 TROCHANTERIC BURSITIS
726.5 TROCHANTERIC TENDINITIS

TROCHLEAR NERVE
378.53 Atrophy
378.53 Disorder
951.1 Injury
378.53 Palsy
378.53 Paralysis

T

275.0 TROISIER-HANOT-CHAUFFARD SYNDROME (BRONZE DIABETES)
133.8 TROMBICULA INFESTATION
757.0 TROPHEDEMA HEREDITARY
707.9 TROPHIC ULCER CHRONIC (SKIN) (SEE ALSO 'ULCER, ULCERATION SKIN')

TROPHOBLASTIC DISEASE

0 See also 'Hydatidiform Mole'
630 NOS
630 NOS with complication during treatment [639.#]
639.# NOS with complication following treatment

4th digit: 639
0. Genital tract and pelvic infection
1. Delayed or excessive hemorrhage
2. Damage to pelvic organs and tissue
3. Renal failure
4. Metabolic disorders
5. Shock
6. Embolism
8. Other specified complication
9. Unspecified complication

V13.1 History (nongravid)
V23.1 History maternal affecting pregnancy supervision

TROPICAL

099.1 Bubo
040.81 Pyomyositis
579.1 Sprue
579.1 Steatorrhea
707.9 Ulcer chronic (skin) (see also 'Ulcer, Ulceration Skin')
991.4 Wet feet syndrome

453.1 TROUSSEAU'S SYNDROME (THROMBOPHLEBITIS MIGRANS VISCERAL CANCER)
312.2# TRUANCY (CHILDHOOD) SOCIALIZED
312.1# TRUANCY (CHILDHOOD) UNSOCIALIZED

5th digit: 312.1-2
0. NOS
1. Mild
2. Moderate
3. Severe

745.0 TRUNCUS ARTERIOSUS PERSISTENT CONGENITAL

TRUNK

V48.1 Deficiency
V48.7 Disfigurement
959.19 Injury NOS/NEC
911.8 Injury other and unspecified superficial
911.9 Injury other and unspecified superficial infected
907.3 Injury nerve root(s) late effect, (spinal plexus and other nerves of trunk)
954.9 Nerve injury nerve unspecified
954.8 Nerve injury other specified nerve
V48.9 Problem
V48.3 Problem mechanical and motor
V48.5 Problem sensory
V48.8 Problem other

0 TRYPANOSOMA INFECTION SEE 'TRYPANOSOMIASIS'

TRYPANOSOMIASIS

086.# NOS
086.# Encephalitis [323.2]
086.# Meningitis [321.3]

4th digit: 086
0. Chagas' (American) with heart involvement
1. Chagas' (American) with involvement of organ other than heart
2. Chagas' (American) NOS
3. Gambian
4. Rhodesian
5. African NOS
9. Unspecified

V75.3 Screening exam - Chagas disease (sleeping sickness)

270.2 TRYPTOPHAN DISTURBANCES OF METABOLISM
242.8# TSH OVERPRODUCTION

5th digit: 242.8
0. Without thyrotoxic crisis or storm
1. With mention of throtoxic crisis or storm

081.2 TSUTSUGAMUSHI FEVER (SCRUB TYPHUS)
770.6 TTN (TRANSIENT TACHYPNEA OF NEWBORN)

TUBAL

633.10 Abortion
633.10 Abortion with complication during treatment [639.#]
639.# Abortion with complication following treatment
633.11 Abortion with intrauterine pregnancy
633.11 Abortion with intrauterine pregnancy with complication during treatment [639.#]
639.# Abortion with intrauterine pregnancy with complication following treatment

4th digit: 639
0. Genital tract and pelvic infection
1. Delayed or excessive hemorrhage
2. Damage to pelvic organs and tissue
3. Renal failure
4. Metabolic disorders
5. Shock
6. Embolism
8. Other specified complication
9. Unspecified complication

V25.2 Ligation encounter
998.89 Ligation failure
V26.51 Ligation status
628.2 Occlusion
633.10 Pregnancy
761.4 Pregnancy affecting fetus or newborn
633.10 Pregnancy with complication during treatment [639.#]
639.# Pregnancy with complication following treatment
633.11 Pregnancy with intrauterine pregnancy
633.11 Pregnancy with intrauterine pregnancy with complication during treatment [639.#]
639.# Pregnancy with intrauterine pregnancy with complication following treatment

4th digit: 639
0. Genital tract and pelvic infection
1. Delayed or excessive hemorrhage
2. Damage to pelvic organs and tissue
3. Renal failure
4. Metabolic disorders
5. Shock
6. Embolism
8. Other specified complication
9. Unspecified complication

A positive tuberculin test is not a diagnosis of tuberculosis, and should not be coded as such.

795.5 TUBERCULIN TEST POSITIVE (WITHOUT TB)

TUBERCULOSIS

011.9# Unspecified
013.3# Abscess brain
013.5# Abscess spinal cord
017.2# Adenitis
017.6# Adrenal glands
014.8# Anus
014.0# Ascites
016.1# Bladder
015.9# Bones and joints
015.5# Bones of limbs [727.01]
015.7# Bone other specified
013.2# Brain
013.3# Brain abscess
012.2# Bronchial isolated
011.5# Bronchiectasis
011.3# Bronchus
013.8# Central nervous system other specified
013.9# Central nervous system site NOS
016.7# Cervicitis
014.8# Colon
017.0# Colliquativa, cutis
771.2 Congenital or perinatal
795.5 Converter (without TB)
015.5# Dactylitis
018.9# Disseminated
018.0# Disseminated acute
018.8# Disseminated other specified
017.4# Ear
012.0# Empyema
013.6# Encephalitis or myelitis
016.7# Endometritis
014.8# Enteritis
016.4# Epididymis
017.1# Erythema nodosum w/hypersensitivity reaction
017.8# Esophagus
V01.1 Exposure
017.3# Eye
795.5 False positive serological test
014.8# Gastrocolic
018.9# Generalized
018.0# Generalized acute
018.8# Generalized other specified
016.7# Genital organs female other
016.5# Genital organs male other
016.9# Genitourinary
012.3# Glottis
015.1# Hip [727.01]

5th digit: 011, 012, 013, 014, 015, 016, 017, 018
0. NOS
1. Lab not done
2. Lab pending
3. Microscopy positive (in sputum)
4. Culture positive - microscopy negative
5. Culture negative - microscopy positive
6. Culture and microscopy negative confirmed by other methods

TUBERCULOSIS (continued)

V12.01 History personal
012.0# Hydrothorax
014.8# Ileum
017.1# Indurativia
014.8# Intestine (large) (small)
015.8# Joint other specified
016.0# Kidney
015.2# Knee [727.01]
012.3# Laryngitis
137.3 Late effects bones and joints
137.1 Late effects central nervous system
137.2 Late effects genitourinary
137.4 Late effects other specified organs
137.0 Late effects respiratory or unspecified
013.0# Leptomeningitis
017.0# Lichenoides
011.9# Lung NOS
011.4# Lung fibrosis
011.0# Lung infiltrative
011.1# Lung nodular
011.2# Lung with cavitation
012.1# Lymph nodes intrathoracic (hilar) (mediastinal) (tracheobronchial)
014.8# Lymph nodes mesenteric or retroperitoneal
017.2# Lymph nodes peripheral (cervical)
015.6# Mastoid

5th digit: 011, 012, 013, 014, 015, 016, 017
0. NOS
1. Lab not done
2. Lab pending
3. Microscopy positive (in sputum)
4. Culture positive - microscopy negative
5. Culture negative - microscopy positive
6. Culture and microscopy negative confirmed by other methods

647.3#: Use an additional code to identify the maternal tuberculosis.

647.3# Maternal current (co-existent) in pregnancy

5th digit: 647.3
0. Episode of care NOS or N/A
1. Delivered
2. Delivered with postpartum complication
3. Antepartum complication
4. Postpartum complication

012.8# Mediastinum
013.1# Meninges - tuberculoma
013.0# Meningitis, Meningoencephalitis
014.8# Mesenteric glands
018.9# Miliary
018.0# Miliary acute

5th digit: 012, 013, 014, 018
0. NOS
1. Lab not done
2. Lab pending
3. Microscopy positive (in sputum)
4. Culture positive - microscopy negative
5. Culture negative - microscopy positive
6. Culture and microscopy negative confirmed by other methods

T

TUBERCULOSIS (continued)

018.8# Miliary other specified
013.6# Myelitis
012.8# Nasopharynx
013.9# Nervous system (central)
012.8# Nose (septum)
016.6# Oophoritis
0 Osteomyelitis see 'Osteomyelitis', tuberculous
010.8# Other primary progressive
017.9# Other specified organs
017.0# Papulonecrotica
014.0# Peritonitis
012.0# Pleura, pleurisy
010.1# Pleurisy primary progressive TB
011.6# Pneumonia
011.7# Pneumothorax
018.9# Polyserositis
018.0# Polyserositis acute
018.8# Polyserositis other specified
010.0# Primary complex
010.9# Primary infection
016.5# Prostate [601.4]
011.9# Pulmonary
011.8# Pulmonary other specified
016.0# Pyelonephritis
014.8# Rectum
016.0# Renal
011.9# Respiratory NOS
012.8# Respiratory other specified
017.3# Retinalis (juvenilis) [362.18]
014.8# Retroperitoneal (lymph nodes)
016.6# Salpingitis oophoritis
V74.1 Screening exam
016.5# Seminal vesicle [608.81]
012.8# Sinus (any nasal)
017.0# Skin and subcutaneous cellular tissue
013.4# Spinal cord
017.7# Spleen
015.0# Spondylopathy [720.81]
0 Synovitis see 'Synovitis', tuberculous
0 Tenosynovitis see 'Tenosynovitis', tuberculous
795.5 Test nonspecific reaction (without active TB)
016.5# Testes [608.81]
017.5# Thyroid gland
012.2# Tracheal or bronchial isolated
012.1# Tracheobronchial adenopathy
013.1# Tuberculoma meninges
016.7# Ulcer vulva (nonobstetrical) [616.51]
016.2# Ureter
016.3# Urinary organs other
V03.2 Vaccination
017.0# Verrucosa cutis
015.0# Vertebral column

5th digit: 010, 012, 013, 014, 015, 016, 017, 018
0. NOS
1. Lab not done
2. Lab pending
3. Microscopy positive (in sputum)
4. Culture positive - microscopy negative
5. Culture negative - microscopy positive
6. Culture and microscopy negative confirmed by other methods

759.5 TUBEROUS SCLEROSIS
272.2 TUBO-ERUPTIVE XANTHOMA

TUBO OVARIAN

614.2 Abscess
614.0 Abscess acute
614.4 Abscess chronic
614.6 Adhesions (postoperative) (postinfection)
614.2 Disease - inflammatory
620.9 Disease - noninflammatory
620.8 Disease - noninflammatory specified NEC

TUBOPLASTY

V25.09 Counseling (proposed)
V25.2 Encounter
V26.0 Reversal after previous sterilization
V26.51 Status

382.1 TUBOTYMPANIC DISEASE CHRONIC (WITH ANTERIOR PERFORATION OF EAR DRUM)

TUBULAR (RENAL)

588.0 Disorder phosphate-losing
584.5 Necrosis
584.5 Necrosis acute
997.5 Necrosis acute specified as due to procedure
639.3 Necrosis following abortion/ectopic/molar pregnancy
0 Necrosis with SIRS see 'SIRS', renal failure

TULAREMIA

021.9 NOS
021.2 Bronchopneumonic
021.1 Cryptogenic
021.1 Enteric
V01.89 Exposure
021.8 Generalized or disseminated
021.8 Glandular
021.1 Intestinal
021.3 Oculoglandular
021.2 Pulmonary
021.1 Typhoidal
021.0 Ulceroglandular
V03.4 Vaccination
021.8 Other specified

TUMOR

239.# NOS (see also 'Neoplasm Unspecified Nature') M8001/1
4th digit: 239
0. Digestive system, anal
1. Respiratory system
2. Bone, soft tissue, skin, (anal skin margin)
3. Breast
4. Bladder
5. Other genitourinary
6. Brain
7. Endocrine glands and other parts of nervous system
8. Other specified sites
9. Site unspecified

229.9 Benign site NOS
0 Benign site specified see 'Benign Neoplasm', by site M8001/0
237.9 Cranial nerve (central)
199.1 Fusiform cell type - malignant site NOS
0 Fusiform cell type - malignant site specified see 'Cancer', by site M8004/3

TUMOR (continued)

0 Glomus see 'Hemangioma'
238.71 Hemorrhagic with thrombocythemia M9962/1
199.1 Malignant site NOS
0 Malignant site specified see 'Cancer', by site M8001/3
238.5 Mast cell NOS
199.1 Small cell type - malignant site NOS
0 Small cell type - malignant site specified see 'Cancer', by site M8041/3
215.9 Soft tissue - benign site NOS
0 Soft tissue - benign site specified see 'Benign Neoplasm', by site M8800/0
215.5 Stromal benign of digestive system (abdomen)
171.5 Stromal malignant of small intestine, duodenum (stomach)
238.1 Stromal uncertain behavior of digestive system
654.7# Vagina complicating pregnancy

5th digit: 654.7
0. Episode of care NOS or N/A
1. Delivered
2. Delivered with postpartum complication
3. Antepartum complication
4. Postpartum complication

238.9 TUMORLET SITE NOS
0 TUMORLET SITE SPECIFIED SEE 'NEOPLASM UNCERTAIN BEHAVIOR', BY SITE M8040/1
134.1 TUNGA PENETRANS INFESTATION
134.1 TUNGIASIS

TUNICA VAGINALIS

608.4 Abscess (cellulitis) (boil) (carbuncle)
608.89 Atrophy (fibrosis) (hypertrophy) (ulcer)
608.84 Chylocele
608.83 Hemorrhage (thrombosis) (hematoma) nontraumatic
603.9 Hydrocele
778.6 Hydrocele congenital
608.4 Infective
959.14 Injury NEC
608.85 Stricture

733.99 TURBINATES ATROPHY (BONE)
478.0 TURBINATES HYPERTROPHY NASAL
378.71 TURK'S SYNDROME (OCULAR RETRACTION SYNDROME)
758.6 TURNER'S SYNDROME
758.6 TURNER-VARNY SYNDROME
520.4 TURNER'S TOOTH
352.5 TWELFTH CRANIAL NERVE ATROPHY
352.5 TWELFTH CRANIAL NERVE DISORDERS
951.7 TWELFTH CRANIAL NERVE INJURY
352.5 TWELFTH NERVE HYPOGLOSSAL DISORDERS
298.2 TWILIGHT STATE PSYCHOGENIC
759.4 TWIN CONJOINED
651.0# TWIN PREGNANCY
651.7# TWIN PREGNANCY FOLLOWING (ELECTIVE) FETAL REDUCTION
651.3# TWIN PREGNANCY WITH ONE FETAL LOSS (ONE RETAINED)

5th digit: 651.0, 3, 7
0. Episode of care NOS or N/A
1. Delivered
3. Antepartum complication

761.5 TWIN PREGNANCY AFFECTING FETUS OR NEWBORN
762.3 TWIN-TO-TWIN TRANSFUSION SYNDROME NOS
762.3 TWIN-TO-TWIN TRANSFUSION SYNDROME-DONOR TWIN [772.0]
762.3 TWIN-TO-TWIN TRANSFUSION SYNDROME-RECIPIENT TWIN [776.4]
651.3# TWIN VANISHING

5th digit: 651.3
0. Episode of care NOS or N/A
1. Delivered
3. Antepartum complication

781.0 TWITCH

TYMPANIC MEMBRANE

744.29 Absence congenital
384.81 Atrophic flaccid
384.82 Atrophic nonflaccid
384.9 Disorder
959.09 Injury
384.82 Retracted

TYMPANIC MEMBRANE PERFORATION

384.20 Nontraumatic - NOS
384.22 Nontraumatic - attic
384.21 Nontraumatic - central
384.81 Nontraumatic - healed
384.24 Nontraumatic - multiple
384.22 Nontraumatic - pars flaccida
384.23 Nontraumatic - other marginal
384.25 Nontraumatic (posttraumatic) - total
872.61 Traumatic
872.71 Traumatic complicated
0 With otitis media see 'Otitis Media'

787.3 TYMPANITES (ABDOMINAL) (INTESTINAL)
384.00 TYMPANITIS ACUTE WITHOUT OTITIS MEDIA
384.1 TYMPANITIS CHRONIC WITHOUT OTITIS MEDIA

TYMPANOSCLEROSIS

385.00 NOS
385.09 Involving other combination structures
385.02 Involving tympanic membrane and ear ossicles
385.03 Involving tympanic membrane ear ossicles and middle ear
385.01 Involving tympanic membrane only

TYMPANOSTOMY TUBE

996.69 Complication - infection or inflammation
996.59 Complication - mechanical
996.79 Complication - other
V53.09 Removal
V53.09 Replacement

385.9 TYMPANUM DISEASE
786.7 TYMPANY CHEST
301.4 TYPE A PERSONALITY DISORDER

TYPHOID

V02.1	Carrier
002.0	Fever (infection) (any site)
002.0	Osteomyelitis [730.8#]
	5th digit: 730.8
	0. Site NOS
	1. Shoulder region
	2. Upper arm (elbow) (humerus)
	3. Forearm (radius) (wrist) (ulna)
	4. Hand (carpal) (metacarpal) (fingers)
	5. Pelvic region and thigh (hip) (buttock) (femur)
	6. Lower leg (fibula) (knee) (patella) (tibia)
	7. Ankle and/or foot (metatarsals) (toes) (tarsals)
	8. Other (head) (neck) (rib) (skull) (trunk) (vertebrae)
002.9	Paratyphoid
002.1	Paratyphoid A
002.2	Paratyphoid B
002.3	Paratyphoid C
V03.1	Vaccination

TYPHUS

082.9	NOS
082.1	African tick
081.1	Brill-Zinsser disease
080	Classical
081.0	Endemic
080	Epidemic
080	Exanthematic
081.9	Fever
081.0	Flea borne
082.1	India tick
082.1	Kenya tick
080	Louse borne
081.2	Mite borne
081.0	Murine (endemic)
081.1	Recrudescent
081.2	Scrub
082.2	Siberian tick
082.9	Tick borne

300.89	TYPIST'S CRAMP NEUROTIC
333.84	TYPIST'S CRAMP ORGANIC
270.2	TYROSINE DISTURBANCES OF METABOLISM
270.2	TYROSINEMIA
775.89	TYROSINEMIA NEONATAL
270.2	TYROSINOSIS
270.2	TYROSINURIA

T

757.39 UEHLINGER'S SYNDROME (ACROPACHYDERMA)

746.84 UHL'S DISEASE

ULCER

707.9 Unspecified site
707.9 Unspecified site with gangrene [785.4]
478.19 Ala, nose
526.5 Alveolar process
006.9 Amebic (intestine)
534.## Anastomotic

4th digit: 534
0. Acute with hemorrhage
1. Acute with perforation
2. Acute with hemorrhage and perforation
3. Acute
4. Chronic or NOS with hemorrhage
5. Chronic or NOS with perforation
6. Chronic or NOS with hemorrhage and perforation
7. Chronic
9. NOS as acute or chronic

5th digit: 534
0. Without obstruction
1. Obstructed

0 Antral see 'Ulcer', pyloric
569.41 Anus
569.41 Anus stercoral
455.8 Anus varicose
455.5 Anus varicose external
455.2 Anus varicose internal
0 Aorta see 'Aneurysm'
616.50 Aphthous genital organ female

When coding arteriosclerosis of the extremities use an additional code, if applicable to identify chronic complete or total occlusion of the artery of the extremities (440.4).

440.23 Arteriosclerotic lower limb **[707.1#]**

5th digit: 707.1
0. Unspecified
1. Thigh
2. Calf
3. Ankle
4. Heel and midfoot (plantar surface)
5. Other part of foot (toes)
9. Other part of lower limb

440.24 Arteriosclerotic lower limb with ischemic gangrene
447.2 Artery
447.8 Artery without rupture
530.85 Barrett's
576.8 Bile duct
596.8 Bladder
120.9 Bladder bilharzial [595.4]
595.1 Bladder submucosal
016.1# Bladder tuberculous [596.8]

5th digit: 016.1
0. NOS
1. Lab not done
2. Lab pending
3. Microscopy positive (in sputum)
4. Culture positive - microscopy negative
5. Culture negative - microscopy positive
6. Culture and microscopy negative confirmed by other methods

ULCER (continued)

730.9# Bone

5th digit: 730.9
0. Site NOS
1. Shoulder region
2. Upper arm (elbow) (humerus)
3. Forearm (radius) (wrist) (ulna)
4. Hand (carpal) (metacarpal) (fingers)
5. Pelvic region and thigh (hip) (buttock) (femur)
6. Lower leg (fibula) (knee) (patella) (tibia)
7. Ankle and/or foot (metatarsals) (toes) (tarsal)
8. Other (head) (neck) (rib) (skull) (trunk)
9. Multiple

519.19 Bronchus
031.1 Buruli
530.20 Cardio-esophageal (peptic)
530.21 Cardio-esophageal (peptic) with bleeding
622.0 Cervix
616.0 Cervix with cervicitis
099.0 Chancroidal
569.82 Colon
372.00 Conjunctiva

CORNEA

370.00 NOS
370.03 Central
054.42 Dendritic
264.3 Due to vitamin A deficiency
370.04 Hypopyon ulcer
370.01 Marginal (catarrhal)
370.07 Mooren's (rodent)
370.05 Mycotic
370.06 Perforated
370.02 Ring (annular)
370.04 Serpiginous
017.3# Tuberculous (phlyctenular) [370.31]

5th digit: 017.3
0. NOS
1. Lab not done
2. Lab pending
3. Microscopy positive (in sputum)
4. Culture positive - microscopy negative
5. Culture negative - microscopy positive
6. Culture and microscopy negative confirmed by other methods

ULCER (continued)

607.89 Corpus cavernosum chronic
575.8 Cystic duct
595.1 Cystitis (interstitial)
054.42 Dendritic
0 Dieulafoy's see 'Dieulafoy's Lesion'

ULCER (continued)

532.## Duodenal
532.## Duodenal due to helicobacter pylori [041.86]
316 Duodenal psychogenic [532.##]

4th digit: 532
0. Acute with hemorrhage
1. Acute with perforation
2. Acute with hemorrhage and perforation
3. Acute
4. Chronic or NOS with hemorrhage
5. Chronic or NOS with perforation
6. Chronic or NOS with hemorrhage and perforation
7. Chronic
9. NOS acute or chronic

5th digit: 532
0. Without obstruction
1. Obstructed

595.1 Elusive
478.79 Epiglottis
530.20 Esophagus
530.21 Esophagus with bleeding
530.85 Esophagus Barrett's
530.20 Esophagus due to ingestion of medicine/chemical agents
530.21 Esophagus due to ingestion of medicine/chemical agents with bleeding
530.20 Esophagus fungal
530.21 Esophagus fungal with bleeding
530.20 Esophagus infectional
530.21 Esophagus infectional with bleeding
360.00 Eye NEC
478.29 Fauces
575.8 Gallbladder
576.8 Gall duct
531.## Gastric
531.## Gastric due to helicobacter pylori [041.86]
316 Gastric psychogenic [531.##]
534.## Gastrocolic
533.## Gastroduodenal
533.## Gastroduodenal due to helicobacter pylori [041.86]
534.## Gastrointestinal
534.## Gastrojejunal

4th digit: 531, 533, 534
0. Acute with hemorrhage
1. Acute with perforation
2. Acute with hemorrhage and perforation
3. Acute
4. Chronic or NOS with hemorrhage
5. Chronic or NOS with perforation
6. Chronic or NOS with hemorrhage and perforation
7. Chronic
9. NOS acute or chronic

5th digit: 531, 533, 534
0. Without obstruction
1. Obstructed

629.89 Genital sites other female
616.89 Genital sites other female aphthous
608.89 Genital sites other male (aphthous)
523.8 Gingiva
523.10 Gingivitis
478.79 Glottis
523.8 Gum

ULCER (continued)

595.1 Hunner's
478.29 Hypopharynx
370.04 Hypopyon
569.82 Intestine (primary)
288.09 Intestine granulocytopenia
569.83 Intestine with perforation
478.79 Larynx
528.5 Lip
518.89 Lung
011.2# Lung tuberculous

5th digit: 011.2
0. NOS
1. Lab not done
2. Lab pending
3. Microscopy positive (in sputum)
4. Culture positive - microscopy negative
5. Culture negative - microscopy positive
6. Culture and microscopy negative confirmed by other methods

597.89 Meatus (urinarius)
528.9 Mouth (traumatic)
528.2 Mouth aphthous
031.1 Mycobacterium
478.19 Nasal septum
456.8 Nasal septum varicose
478.29 Nasopharynx
771.4 Navel cord (newborn)
528.9 Oral mucosa (traumatic)
528.9 Palate (hard) (soft)
533.## Peptic (syndrome)
533.## Peptic (syndrome) due to helicobacter pylori [041.86]
707.8 Perineum
474.8 Peritonsillar
478.29 Pharynx
601.8 Prostate
531.## Pyloric
531.## Pyloric due to helicobacter pylori [041.86]
569.41 Rectum
363.20 Retina (see also 'Chorioretinitis')
379.09 Sclera
608.89 Seminal vesicle
0 Skin see 'Ulcer, Ulceration Skin'
608.89 Spermatic cord
569.41 Stercoral anus or rectum
534.## Stomal or anastomotic
528.00 Stomatitis
533.## Stress (stress ulcer)

4th digit: 531, 533, 534
0. Acute with hemorrhage
1. Acute with perforation
2. Acute with hemorrhage and perforation
3. Acute
4. Chronic or NOS with hemorrhage
5. Chronic or NOS with perforation
6. Chronic or NOS with hemorrhage and perforation
7. Chronic
9. NOS as acute or chronic

5th digit: 531, 533, 534
0. Without obstruction
1. Obstructed

U-V-W

ULCER (continued)

608.89 Testis
478.29 Throat
529.0 Tongue (traumatic)
474.8 Tonsil
519.19 Trachea
608.89 Tunica vaginalis
597.89 Urethral meatus
131.02 Urethral meatus trichomonal
621.8 Uterus
622.0 Uterus neck
616.89 Vagina
421.0 Valve, heart
454.0 Varicose (skin)
454.2 Varicose (skin) with inflammation
608.89 Vas deferens

ULCER (ULCERATION) SKIN

707.9 NOS
707.9 NOS with gangrene [785.4]
707.8 Abdomen (wall)
006.6 Amebic
569.41 Anus
707.8 Arm
611.0 Breast
707.8 Buttock
707.05 Buttock decubitus
707.05 Buttock decubitus with gangrene [785.4]
707.9 Chronic NOS
707.8 Chronic other specified site
707.1# Crural (indolent) (non-healing) (perforating) (pyogenic) (trophic)

5th digit: 707.1
- **0. Unspecified**
- **1. Thigh**
- **2. Calf**
- **3. Ankle**
- **4. Heel and midfoot (plantar surface)**
- **5. Other part of foot (toes)**
- **9. Other part of lower limb**

707.0# Decubitus
707.0# Decubitus with gangrene [785.4]

5th digit: 707.0
- **0. NOS**
- **1. Elbow**
- **2. Upper back (shoulder blades)**
- **3. Lower back (sacrum)**
- **4. Hip**
- **5. Buttock**
- **6. Ankle**
- **7. Heel**
- **9. Other site (head)**

ULCER (ULCERATION) SKIN (continued)

250.8# Diabetic [707.#(#)]
250.6# Diabetic - neuropathic [707.#(#)]
250.7# Diabetic - peripheral vascular [707.#(#)]

5th digit: 250.6-8
- **0. Type II, adult-onset, non-insulin dependent (even if requiring insulin), or unspecified; controlled**
- **1. Type I, juvenile-onset or insulin-dependent; controlled**
- **2. Type II, adult-onset, non-insulin dependent (even if requiring insulin); uncontrolled**
- **3. Type I, juvenile-onset or insulin-dependent; uncontrolled**

4th or 4th and 5th digit: 707
- **1#. Lower limb except decubitus**
  - **10. Unspecified**
  - **11. Thigh**
  - **12. Calf**
  - **13. Ankle**
  - **14. Heel and midfoot**
  - **15. Other parts of foot, toes**
  - **19. Other**
- **8. Chronic of other specified site**
- **9. Chronic site NOS**

459.31 Due to chronic venous hypertension [707.1#]
459.33 Due to chronic venous hypertension with inflammation [707.1#]
459.11 Due to postphlebetic syndrome [707.1#]
459.13 Due to postphlebetic syndrome with inflammation [707.1#]

4th or 4th and 5th digit: 707
- **1#. Lower limb except decubitus**
  - **10. Unspecified**
  - **11. Thigh**
  - **12. Calf**
  - **13. Ankle**
  - **14. Heel and midfoot**
  - **15. Other parts of foot, toes**
  - **19. Other**

373.01 Eyelid (region)
707.8 Finger
707.15 Foot (indolent) (non-healing) (perforating) (pyogenic) (trophic)
629.89 Genital sites other female
616.89 Genital sites other female aphthous
608.89 Genital sites other male (aphthous)
707.#(#) Ischemic

4th or 4th and 5th digit: 707
- **1#. Lower limb except decubitus**
  - **10. Unspecified**
  - **11. Thigh**
  - **12. Calf**
  - **13. Ankle**
  - **14. Heel and midfoot**
  - **15. Other parts of foot, toes**
  - **19. Other**
- **8. Chronic of other specified site**
- **9. Chronic site NOS**

616.50 Labium (majus) (minus)

U-V-W

ULCER (ULCERATION) SKIN (continued)

707.1# Lower limb (trophic) (chronic) (neurogenic)

> ***When coding arteriosclerosis of the extremities use an additional code, if applicable to identify chronic complete or total occlusion of the artery of the extremities (440.4).***

440.23 Lower limb arteriosclerotic [707.1#]
440.24 Lower limb arteriosclerotic with ischemic gangrene [707.1#]
707.1# Lower limb chronic (indolent) (non-healing) (perforating) (pyogenic) (trophic)

5th digit: 707.1
0. Unspecified
1. Thigh
2. Calf
3. Ankle
4. Heel and midfoot (plantar surface)
5. Other part of foot (toes)
9. Other part of lower limb

250.8# Lower limb chronic (indolent) (non-healing) (perforating) (pyogenic) (trophic) diabetic [707.1#]
250.6# Lower limb chronic (indolent) (non-healing) (perforating) (pyogenic) (trophic) diabetic - neuropathic [707.1#]
250.7# Lower limb chronic (indolent) (nonhealing) (perforating) (pyogenic) (trophic) diabetic - peripheral vascular [707.1#]

5th digit: 250.6-8
0. Type II, adult-onset, non-insulin dependent (even if requiring insulin), or unspecified; controlled
1. Type I, juvenile-onset or insulin-dependent; controlled
2. Type II, adult-onset, non-insulin dependent (even if requiring insulin); uncontrolled
3. Type I, juvenile-onset or insulin-dependent; uncontrolled

5th digit: 707.1
0. Unspecified
1. Thigh
2. Calf
3. Ankle
4. Heel and midfoot (plantar surface)
5. Other part of foot (toes)
9. Other part of lower limb

707.1# Lower limb with gangrene [785.4]

4th digit: 707.1
0. Unspecified
1. Thigh
2. Calf
3. Ankle
4. Heel and midfoot (plantar surface)
5. Other part of foot (toes)
9. Other part of lower limb

686.09 Meleney's (chronic undermining)
031.1 Mycobacterium
707.8 Neurogenic chronic NEC
707.9 Non-healing
607.89 Penis chronic

ULCER (ULCERATION) SKIN (continued)

707.0# Plaster
607.89 Prepuce (chronic)
707.0# Pressure (due to cast)

5th digit: 707.0
0. NOS
1. Elbow
2. Upper back (shoulder blades)
3. Lower back (sacrum)
4. Hip
5. Buttock
6. Ankle
7. Heel
9. Other site (head)

608.89 Scrotum
016.5# Scrotum tuberculous [608.89]

5th digit: 016.5
0. NOS
1. Lab not done
2. Lab pending
3. Microscopy positive (in sputum)
4. Culture positive - microscopy negative
5. Culture negative - microscopy positive
6. Culture and microscopy negative confirmed by other methods

456.4 Scrotum varicose
707.9 Skin
454.0 Stasis lower extremity varicose
454.2 Stasis lower extremity varicose - infected
459.81 Stasis without varicose veins [707.1#]

5th digit: 707.1
0. Unspecified
1. Thigh
2. Calf
3. Ankle
4. Heel and midfoot (plantar surface)
5. Other part of foot (toes)
9. Other part of lower limb

091.3 Syphilitic
707.9 Trophic chronic
707.9 Tropical chronic
707.8 Upper limb
616.89 Vaginal (inflammatory) (nonobstetrical)
454.0 Varicose
454.2 Varicose with inflammation
616.50 Vulva
136.1 Vulva Behcet's [616.51]
098.0 Vulva gonococcal
054.12 Vulva herpes simplex
091.0 Vulva syphilitic (primary)
016.7# Vulva tuberculous (nonobstetrical) [616.51]

5th digit: 016.7
0. NOS
1. Lab not done
2. Lab pending
3. Microscopy positive (in sputum)
4. Culture positive - microscopy negative
5. Culture negative - microscopy positive
6. Culture and microscopy negative confirmed by other methods

616.50 Vulvobuccal
707.8 Other specified sites chronic (trophic) (neurogenic)

556.# ULCERATIVE COLITIS

316 ULCERATIVE COLITIS PSYCHOGENIC [556.#]

4th digit: 556

0. Enterocolitis (chronic)
1. Ileocolitis (chronic)
2. Proctitis (chronic)
3. Proctosigmoiditis (chronic)
4. Pseudopolyposis of colon
5. Left-sided (chronic)
6. Universal (chronic)
8. Other ulcerative colitis
9. Ulcerative colitis (enteritis) unspecified

099.0 ULCUS MOLLE (CUTIS) (SKIN)

742.4 ULEGYRIA CONGENITAL

758.6 ULLRICH (-BONNEVIE) (-TURNER) SYNDROME

759.89 ULLRICH-FEICHTIGER SYNDROME

755.21 ULNA AGENESIS CONGENITAL - WITH ABSENCE COMPLETE OF DISTAL ELEMENTS

755.27 ULNA AGENESIS CONGENITAL - WITH ABSENCE INCOMPLETE OF DISTAL ELEMENTS

736.00 ULNA DEFORMITY

755.50 ULNA DEFORMITY CONGENITAL

ULNAR

442.0 Artery aneurysm (ruptured) (cirsoid) (varix) (false)

440.2# Artery arteriosclerosis (degeneration) (occlusion)

440.2# Artery arteriosclerosis (degeneration) (occlusion) with chronic complete or total occlusion [440.4]

5th digit: 440.2

0. Unspecified
1. With intermittent claudication
2. With rest pain or rest pain and intermittent claudication
9. Other atherosclerosis extremities

> ***When coding arteriosclerosis of the extremities use an additional code, if applicable to identify chronic complete or total occlusion of the artery of the extremities (440.4).***

440.24 Artery arteriosclerosis (degeneration) (occlusion) with ischemic gangrene or ischemic gangrene ulceration, or ulceration and intermittent claudication, rest pain [707.8]

440.23 Artery arteriosclerosis (degeneration) (occlusion) with ulceration, or ulceration and intermittent claudication, rest pain [707.8]

440.3# Artery bypass graft arteriosclerosis

440.3# Artery bypass graft arteriosclerosis with chronic complete or total occlusion [440.4]

5th digit: 440.3

0. Unspecified graft
1. Autologous vein bypass graft
2. Nonautologous biological bypass graft

444.21 Artery embolism (thrombosis) (occlusion) (infarction)

903.3 Artery injury

908.3 Artery injury late effect

> ***Injury to nerve includes laceration, traumatic neuroma, or lesion in continuity. Use anatomical search (the name of the nerve) to find the specified injury.***

354.2 Nerve disorder

955.2 Nerve injury

907.4 Nerve injury late effect

ULNAR (continued)

354.2 Nerve lesion

723.4 Nerve neuralgia

723.4 Nerve neuritis non-paralytic

354.2 Nerve neuropathy

354.2 Nerve palsy (tardy)

354.2 Nerve paralysis

354.2 Nerve slipping

903.3 Vein injury

908.3 Vein injury late effect

451.83 Vein phlebitis

ULNOHUMERAL

841.3 Separation (rupture) (tear) (laceration)

841.3 Strain (sprain) (avulsion) (hemarthrosis)

ULTRASOUND STUDIES

793.#(#) Abnormal findings (nonspecific)

4th or 4th and 5th digit: 793

0. Skull and head
1. Lung field
2. Other intrathoracic
3. Biliary tract
4. Gastrointestinal tract
5. Genitourinary organs
6. Abdominal area including retroperitoneum
7. Musculoskeletal system
8#. Breast
80. Unspecified
81. Mammographic microcalcification
89. Other abnormal findings (calcification) (calculus)
9#. Other
91. Inconclusive due to excess body fat
99. Other abnormal findings (placenta) (skin) (subcutaneous)

> ***When using code 793.91, Image test inconclusive due to excess body fat, use additional code to identify body mass index (BMI) which can be found at 'Body Mass Index'.***

V28.3 Antenatal screening for malformation

793.2 Cardiogram abnormal

V28.4 For fetal growth retardation

UMBILICAL

747.5 Artery absence

747.5 Artery hypoplasia congenital

789.9 Bleeding

762.5 Cord - compression (around neck) (entanglement) (knot) (torsion) affecting fetus or newborn

771.4 Cord - infection affecting fetus or newborn

772.3 Cord - ligature slipped affecting fetus or newborn

762.4 Cord - prolapsed (presentation) affecting fetus or newborn

779.83 Cord - separation delayed

772.0 Cord - rupture affecting fetus or newborn

762.5 Cord - other entanglement of cord affecting fetus or newborn

762.6 Cord - other specified condition affecting fetus or newborn

789.9 Discharge

779.89 Disease newborn NEC

UMBILICAL (continued)

771.4 Granuloma newborn
686.1 Granuloma pyogenic
772.3 Hemorrhage after birth
771.4 Infection newborn
772.3 Ligature slipped
789.05 Pain
753.7 Sinus persistent congenital

UMBILICAL CORD COMPLICATIONS OF DELIVERY - MOTHER'S RECORD

663.9# Complication NOS
663.9# Abnormality complicating pregnancy
663.1# Around neck with compression
663.6# Bruising (hematoma) (thrombosis)
663.3# Entanglement NOS
663.2# Entanglement NOS - with compression
663.0# Prolapse
663.8# Rupture
663.4# Short
663.5# Vasa previa
663.6# Vascular lesions of cord

5th digit: 663.0-6, 8-9
0. Episode of care NOS or N/A
1. Delivered
3. Antepartum complication

663.8# Velamentous insertion
663.3# Other specified entanglement
663.2# Other specified entanglement - with compression
663.8# Other specified complications

5th digit: 663.2, 3, 8
0. Episode of care NOS or N/A
1. Delivered
3. Antepartum complication

996.1 UMBRELLA VENA CAVA COMPLICATION (MECHANICAL)
V60.4 UNABLE TO CARE FOR SELF
312.1# UNAGRESSIVE CONDUCT DISORDER

5th digit: 312.1
0. NOS
1. Mild
2. Moderate
3. Severe

0 UNCINARIASIS SEE 'ANCYLOSTOMA'
780.09 UNCONSCIOUS
313.83 UNDERACHIEVEMENT ACADEMIC DISORDER (CHILDHOOD) (ADOLESCENCE)
526.63 UNDERFILL, ENDODONTIC
868.00 UNDERWATER BLAST INJURY SYNDROME (ABDOMINAL)

783.22 Use an additional code to identify body mass index (BMI), if known. See 'Body Mass Index'.

783.22 UNDERWEIGHT
0 UNDERWEIGHT INFANT FOR GESTATIONAL AGE SEE 'LIGHT FOR DATES'
778.1 UNDERWOOD'S DISEASE (SCLEREMA NEONATORUM)
752.51 UNDESCENDED TESTIS CONGENITAL
V62.0 UNEMPLOYMENT AS CAUSE OF PROBLEM (REASON FOR ENCOUNTER)
703.0 UNGUIS INCARNATUS

313.1 UNHAPPINESS DISORDER CHILDHOOD AND ADOLESCENCE
620.6 UNIVERSAL JOINT SYNDROME-CERVIX
690.10 UNNA'S DISEASE (SEBORRHEIC DERMATITIS)
411.1 UNSTABLE ANGINA
652.0# UNSTABLE LIE COMPLICATING PREGNANCY
660.0# UNSTABLE LIE WITH OBSTRUCTED LABOR [652.0#]
652.6# UNSTABLE LIE WITH MULTIPLE GESTATION
660.0# UNSTABLE LIE WITH MULTIPLE GESTATION OBSTRUCTING LABOR [652.6#]

5th digit: 652.0, 6, 660.0
0. Episode of care NOS or N/A
1. Delivered
3. Antepartum complication

301.59 UNSTABLE PERSONALITY DISORDER
333.2 UNVERRICHT (-LUNDBORG) DISEASE OR SYNDROME
710.3 UNVERRICHT-WAGNER SYNDROME (DERMATOMYOSITIS)

UPPER ARM

912.8 Injury other and unspecified superficial
912.9 Injury other and unspecified superficial infected
840.8 Separation (rupture) (tear) (laceration) other specified sites
840.8 Strain (sprain) (avulsion) (hemarthrosis)

739.7 UPPER EXTREMITIES SEGMENTAL OR SOMATIC DYSFUNCTION
755.20 UPPER LIMB ECTROMELIA
755.20 UPPER LIMB HEMIMELIA

UPPER RESPIRATORY INFECTION

465.9 Acute
487.1 Acute influenzal
465.0 Acute laryngopharyngitis
465.8 Acute multiple sites NEC
034.0 Acute streptococcal chronic
519.8 Chronic

506.2 UPPER RESPIRATORY INFLAMMATION DUE TO FUMES AND VAPORS
478.9 UPPER RESPIRATORY TRACT ATROPHY
378.81 UPWARD GAZE SYNDROME
753.7 URACHUS CYST CONGENITAL
753.7 URACHUS FISTULA CONGENITAL
753.7 URACHUS PATENT CONGENITAL
250.8# URBACH-OPPENHEIM SYNDROME (NECROBIOSIS LIPOIDICA DIABETICORUM) [709.3]

5th digit: 250.8
0. Type II, adult-onset, non-insulin dependent (even if requiring insulin), or unspecified; controlled
1. Type I, juvenile-onset or insulin-dependent; controlled
2. Type II, adult-onset, non-insulin dependent (even if requiring insulin); uncontrolled
3. Type I, juvenile-onset or insulin-dependent; uncontrolled

272.8 URBACH-WIETHE DISEASE OR SYNDROME (LIPOID PROTEINOSIS)
270.6 UREA CYCLE METABOLISM DISORDER

UREMIA

586 NOS
586 NOS with neuropathy [357.4]
586 NOS with pericarditis [420.0]
586 NOS with polyneuropathy [357.4]
584.9 Acute
585.9 Chronic (syndrome)
585.9 Chronic with neuropathy [357.4]
585.9 Chronic with pericarditis [420.0]
585.9 Chronic with polyneuropathy [357.4]
779.89 Congenital
788.9 Extrarenal
403.91 Hypertensive
646.2# Maternal acute - without hypertension complicating pregnancy [584.9]
646.2# Maternal chronic - without hypertension complicating pregnancy [585.9]

5th digit: 646.2
0. Episode of care NOS or N/A
1. Delivered
2. Delivered with postpartum complication
3. Antepartum complication
4. Postpartum complication

639.3 Post (abortive) (ectopic) (molar) pregnancy
0 See also 'Renal Failure'

URETER, URETERAL

V45.74 Absence acquired
753.4 Absence congenital
753.4 Accessory congenital
593.89 Adhesions
753.22 Adynamic congenital
753.4 Anomalous implantation of ureter congenital
753.9 Anomaly NOS
753.20 Anomaly NOS obstructive
753.4 Anomaly NEC
753.29 Anomaly NEC obstructive
753.29 Atresia (congenital)
593.89 Calcification
592.1 Calculus
788.0 Colic
753.9 Defect congenital
753.29 Defect congenital obstructive
753.4 Deviation congenital
593.89 Dilatation (idiopathic)
753.20 Dilatation congenital
593.9 Disease (chronic)
593.89 Disorder NEC
753.4 Distortion congenital
753.20 Distortion congenital obstructive
593.89 Diverticulum
753.4 Diverticulum congenital
753.4 Double congenital
753.4 Ectopic congenital
593.89 Fibrosis
793.5 Filling defect
593.82 Fistula
593.5 Hydroureter
753.29 Hypoplasia congenital
753.29 Imperforate (congenital)
753.29 Impervious (congenital)
867.2 Injury (traumatic)
867.3 Injury (traumatic) with open wound into cavity
908.2 Injury late effect

URETER, URETERAL (continued)

593.3 Kinking
753.20 Kinking congenital
593.4 Obstruction
592.1 Obstruction calculus
753.20 Obstruction - defect NOS congenital
753.29 Obstruction - defect NEC congenital
593.4 Obstruction - ureteropelvic junction
753.21 Obstruction - ureteropelvic junction congenital
593.4 Obstruction - ureterovesical junction
753.22 Obstruction - ureterovesical junction congenital
593.4 Occlusion
753.29 Occlusion congenital
753.4 Orifice displaced congenital
593.89 Polyp
593.7# Reflux

5th digit: 593.7
0. Unspecified
1. With reflux nephropathy, unilateral
2. With reflux nephropathy, bilateral
3. With reflux nephropathy unspecified

753.4 Retrocaval congenital
V53.6 Stent removal
593.3 Stricture (postoperative)
753.29 Stricture congenital
753.29 Valve formation anomaly (congenital)

753.4 URETERIC ORIFICE DISPLACED CONGENITAL
590.3 URETERITIS CYSTICA
593.89 URETEROCELE
753.23 URETEROCELE CONGENITAL
753.23 URETEROCELE CONGENITAL CAUSING URINARY INCONTINENCE [788.3#]

5th digit: 788.3
0. Unspecified
1. Urge incontinence
2. Stress, male
3. Mixed urge and stress
4. Without sensory awareness
5. Post-void dribbling
6. Nocturnal enuresis
7. Continuous leakage
8. Overflow incontinence
9. Other

592.1 URETEROLITHIASIS
593.3 URETEROPELVIC JUNCTION STRICTURE (ATRESIA) (POST-OPERATIVE)
753.21 URETEROPELVIC JUNCTION STRICTURE (ATRESIA) CONGENITAL

When coding an infection of an ostomy, use an additional code to specify the organism. See 'Bacterial Infection'

URETEROSTOMY

V55.6 Care
V55.6 Catheter adjustment or repositioning
V55.6 Catheter removal or replacement
V55.6 Closure
996.39 Complication device mechanical
997.5 Complication stoma
997.5 Malfunction
V55.6 Removal or change
V44.6 Status
V55.6 Toilet stoma

593.3 URETEROVESICAL ORIFICE STRICTURE (ATRESIA) (POSTINFECTIONAL)
753.22 URETEROVESICAL ORIFICE STRICTURE (ATRESIA) CONGENITAL

URETHRA, URETHRAL

V45.74 Absence acquired
594.2 Calculus
599.3 Caruncle
0 Congenital disorder see 'Urethra, Urethral Congenital'
599.84 Cyst
599.84 Deformity (acquired)
599.84 Dilatation
788.7 Discharge
599.84 Discharge bloody
599.9 Disorder
599.84 Disorder specified type NEC
0 Disorders with incontinence see 'Urethra, Urethral Disorders With Incontinence'
599.2 Diverticulum
599.84 Ectropion
599.84 Eversion (meatus)
599.4 False passage
599.84 Fibrosis
599.1 Fistula
599.84 Granuloma
599.84 Hemorrhage (nontraumatic)
599.81 Hypermobility
599.84 Hypertrophy
996.64 Indwelling catheter complication - infection or inflammation
996.31 Indwelling catheter complication - mechanical
996.76 Indwelling catheter complication - other
665.5# Injury (obstetrical)

5th digit: 665.5

0. Episode of care NOS or N/A
1. Delivered
4. Postpartum complication

867.0 Injury (traumatic)
867.1 Injury (traumatic) with open wound into cavity
908.2 Injury (traumatic) late effect
599.82 Intrinsic sphincter deficiency (ISD)
599.83 Instability
599.84 Irritability
599.84 Laceration nontraumatic nonpuerperal
599.84 Leukoplakia
597.89 Meatitis
597.89 Meatus ulcer
131.02 Meatus ulcer trichomonal
599.5 Mucosa prolapsed

URETHRA, URETHRAL (continued)

599.84 Obliteration
599.60 Obstruction
598.9 Occlusion (see also 'Urethra', stricture)
599.3 Polyp
599.5 Prolapse
599.84 Relaxation
599.84 Rupture nontraumatic
599.84 Short
599.84 Spasm
0 Sphincter incontinence see 'Urinary', incontinence
599.84 Sphincter insufficiency
598.9 Stricture
598.00 Stricture due to unspecified infection
615.9 Stricture myometritis (due to) [598.01]
598.2 Stricture postoperative
598.1 Stricture posttraumatic
095.8 Stricture syphilitic [598.01]
098.2 Stricture gonococcal [598.01]
614.0 Stricture salpingo oophoritis (due to) [598.01]
120.9 Stricture schistosoma [598.01]
598.1 Stricture traumatic
598.8 Stricture other specified cause
597.81 Syndrome
599.84 Tag
599.84 Tortuous
599.89 Verumontanum
599.84 Other specified disorder urethra

URETHRA, URETHRAL CONGENITAL

753.8 Absence
753.8 Accessory
753.8 Diverticulum
753.8 Double
753.6 Impervious
753.6 Obstruction or occlusion
753.8 Pendulous
753.8 Prolapse
753.6 Stricture (meatus or bladder neck)
0 Stricture, obstruction, or impervious urethra with incontinence see 'Urethra, Urethral Disorders With Incontinence'
753.6 Valve formation

Urethral disorders with incontinence (retention): When coding the disorders below, code the disorder first, then the appropriate code for the incontinence (retention) (788.3# or 625.6). For example, the codes for urethral fibrosis with stress incontinence, female would be; 599.84 (urethral fibrosis) and 625.6, (stress incontinence). The disorder sequences before the incontinence (retention).

URETHRA, URETHRAL DISORDERS:
WITH INCONTINENCE, [788.3#]
WITH STRESS INCONTINENCE, FEMALE [625.6] WITH URINARY RETENTION [788.2#]

599.84 Cyst
599.84 Eversion (meatus)
599.84 Fibrosis
599.84 Granuloma
599.84 Hemorrhage (nontraumatic)
599.89 Hemorrhage genitourinary
599.84 Hydrourethra
599.81 Hypermobility
599.89 Hyperplasia urethrovaginal
599.84 Hypertrophy
599.89 Hypertrophy verumontanum
599.84 Incontinence urethral sphincter
599.83 Instability
599.82 Intrinsic sphincter deficiency (ISD)
599.84 Irritability
599.82 ISD - intrinsic (urethral) sphincter deficiency
599.84 Laceration nonpuerperal, nontraumatic
599.84 Leukoplakia (post infectional)
599.84 Malacoplakia
599.84 Obliteration
599.89 Other specified disorder urinary tract
599.84 Pneumaturia
599.84 Relaxation
599.84 Rupture
599.84 Short
599.84 Spasm
599.84 Sphincter insufficiency
599.84 Tag
599.84 Tortuous
599.89 Urinary tract disorder other specified
599.89 Verumontanum

WITH INCONTINENCE [788.3#]
5th digit: 788.3
0. Unspecified
1. Urge incontinence
2. Stress, male
3. Mixed urge and stress
4. Without sensory awareness
5. Post-void dribbling
6. Nocturnal enuresis
7. Continuous leakage
8. Overflow incontinence
9. Other

WITH URINARY RETENTION [788.2#]
5th digit: 788.2
0. Unspecified
1. Incomplete bladder emptying
9. Other specified retention

URETHRITIS

098.0 Acute gonococcal
098.2 Chronic gonococcal
646.6# Complicating pregnancy, childbirth or pueperium
5th digit: 646.6
0. Episode of care NOS or N/A
1. Delivered
2. Delivered with postpartum complication
3. Antepartum complication
4. Postpartum complication

099.4# Nongonococcal
5th digit: 099.4
0. Unspecified
1. Chlamydia trachomatis
9. Other specified organism

597.80 Nonspecific
099.40 Nonspecific venereal
131.02 Trichomonal

URETHROCELE

618.#(#) Female
618.#(#) Female with stress incontinence [625.6]
618.#(#) Female with other urinary incontinence **[788.3#]**
4th or 4th and 5th digit: 618
03. Without uterine prolapse
2. With incomplete uterine prolapse
3. With complete uterine prolapse
4. Uterine prolapse unspecified
5th digit: 788.3
1. Urge incontinence
3. Mixed urge and stress
4. Without sensory awareness
5. Post-void dribbling
6. Nocturnal enuresis
7. Continuous leakage
8. Overflow incontinence
9. Other

599.5 Male
599.5 Male with urinary incontinence **[788.3#]**
5th digit: 788.3
0. Unspecified
1. Urge incontinence
2. Stress, male
3. Mixed urge and stress
4. Without sensory awareness
5. Post-void dribbling
6. Nocturnal enuresis
7. Continuous leakage
8. Overflow incontinence
9. Other

099.3 URETHRO-OCULOARTICULAR SYNDROME
099.3 URETHRO-OCULOARTICULAR SYNDROME WITH ARTHROPATHY [711.1#]
5th digit: 711.1
0. Site NOS
1. Shoulder region
2. Upper arm (elbow) (humerus)
3. Forearm (radius) (wrist) (ulna)
4. Hand (carpal) (metacarpal) (fingers)
5. Pelvic region and thigh (hip) (buttock) (femur)
6. Lower leg (fibula) (knee) (patella) (tibia)
7. Ankle and/or foot (metatarsals) (toes) (tarsals)
8. Other (head) (neck) (rib) (skull) (trunk) (vertebrae)
9. Multiple

099.3 URETHRO-OCULOARTICULAR SYNDROME WITH CONJUNCTIVITIS [372.33]

099.3 URETHRO-OCULOSYNOVIAL SYNDROME
099.3 URETHRO-OCULOSYNOVIAL SYNDROME WITH ARTHROPATHY [711.1#]
5th digit: 711.1
0. Site NOS
1. Shoulder region
2. Upper arm (elbow) (humerus)
3. Forearm (radius) (wrist) (ulna)
4. Hand (carpal) (metacarpal) (fingers)
5. Pelvic region and thigh (hip) (buttock) (femur)
6. Lower leg (fibula) (knee) (patella) (tibia)
7. Ankle and/or foot (metatarsals) (toes) (tarsals)
8. Other (head) (neck) (rib) (skull) (trunk) (vertebrae)
9. Multiple

099.3 URETHRO-OCULOSYNOVIAL SYNDROME WITH CONJUNCTIVITIS [372.33]
599.1 URETHRORECTAL FISTULA
753.8 URETHRORECTAL FISTULA CONGENITAL
599.84 URETHRORRHAGIA
788.7 URETHRORRHEA

When coding an infection of an ostomy, use an additional code to specify the organism. See 'bacterial infection'

URETHROSTOMY

V55.6 Care
V55.6 Catheter adjustment or repositioning
V55.6 Catheter removal or replacement
V55.6 Closure
996.39 Complication device mechanical
997.5 Complication stoma
997.5 Malfunction
V55.6 Removal or change
V44.6 Status
V55.6 Toilet stoma

599.89 URETHROVAGINAL HYPERPLASIA
705.89 URHIDROSIS

URI (UPPER RESPIRATORY INFECTION)

465.9 Acute
487.1 Acute influenzal
465.0 Acute laryngopharyngitis
465.8 Acute multiple sites
034.0 Acute streptococcal
519.8 Chronic

790.6 URIC ACID BLOOD ABNORMAL

URINALYSIS ABNORMAL

791.4 Bilirubinuria
791.7 Cells, casts
791.1 Chyluria
791.9 Crystals
791.5 Glycosuria, glucose
791.2 Hemoglobinuria
791.6 Ketone acetone
791.3 Myoglobinuria
791.0 Proteinuria albuminuria Bence Jones
791.9 Pus in urine
796.0 Toxicology
791.9 Other

URINARY

592.9 Calculus
V13.01 Calculus history
V53.6 Catheter (fitting) (adjustment) (removal) (replacement)
0 Catheter of an ostomy see specific ostomy
791.9 Constituents abnormal
997.5 Cystitis due to a procedure
V53.6 Device fitting and adjustment
599.9 Disorder (tract)
V13.00 Disorder history
760.1 Disorder maternal affecting fetus or newborn
599.89 Disorder other specified
V13.09 Disorder other specified history
788.41 Frequency
788.43 Frequency nocturnal
788.64 Hesitancy
788.3# Incontinence
753.23 Incontinence with ureterocele congenital [788.3#]
625.6 Incontinence stress (female)
753.8 Meatus double - stricture congenital
753.6 Meatus imperforate congenital
599.60 Obstruction NOS
599.60 Obstruction with incontinence [788.3#]
5th digit: 788.3
0. Unspecified
1. Urge incontinence
2. Stress, male
3. Mixed urge and stress
4. Without sensory awareness
5. Post-void dribbling
6. Nocturnal enuresis
7. Continuous leakage
8. Overflow incontinence
9. Other

URINARY (continued)

599.60 Obstruction with stress incontinence (female) [625.6]
599.69 Obstruction NEC
752.69 Opening false - male
788.38 Overflow
V47.4 Problem NEC
788.2# Retention
997.5 Retention postoperative **[788.2#]**

5th digit: 788.2
0. Unspecified
1. Incomplete bladder emptying
9. Other specified retention

306.53 Retention psychogenic
788.5 Secretion suppression
788.65 Straining
788.61 Stream intermittent
788.62 Stream slowing
788.61 Stream splitting
788.62 Stream weak
788.69 Stream abnormality other
V45.74 System absence
753.8 System absence (part) congenital
753.9 System anomaly congenital
753.9 System deformity congenital
V13.00 System disorder history
788.9 System symptoms
753.29 Tract atresia congenital
760.1 Tract diseases maternal affecting fetus or newborn
599.9 Tract disorder
599.89 Tract disorder other specified
599.60 Tract obstruction NOS
599.69 Tract obstruction NEC
V44.6 Tract other artificial opening status
788.63 Urgency

> ***Urinary tract infection is a nonspecific diagnosis. Whenever possible be sure to code the specific condition such as cystitis, nephritis, or urethritis.***

URINARY TRACT INFECTION:
WITH KNOWN ORGANISM [041.#(#)]

599.0 Site not specified
112.2 Candidal
996.64 Due to indwelling foley
639.8 Following abortion/ectopic/molar pregnancy
V13.02 History
760.1 Maternal affecting fetus or newborn

> ***646.6#: Specify the maternal UTI with an additional code such as cystitis, urethritis.***

646.6# Maternal complicating pregnancy

5th digit: 646.6
0. Episode of care NOS or N/A
1. Delivered
2. Delivered with postpartum complication
3. Antepartum complication
4. Postpartum complication

771.82 Neonatal
997.5 Postoperative [599.0]
997.5 Specified as due to a procedure [599.0]

WITH KNOWN ORGANISM [041.#(#)]
4th or 4th and 5th digit code for organism: 041

.85 Aerobacter aerogenes
.84 Anaerobes other
.82 Bacteroides fragilis
.83 Clostridium perfringens
.4 E. coli (escherichia coli)
.81 Eaton's agent
.85 Enterobacter sakazakii
.04 Enterococcus
.3 Friedlander's bacillus
.84 Gram-negative anaerobes
.85 Gram-negative bacteria NOS
.5 H. influenzae
.86 H. pylori (helicobacter pylori)
.3 Klebsiella
.85 Mima polymorpha
.81 Mycoplasma
.81 Pleuropneumonia like organisms
.2 Pneumococcus
.6 Proteus (mirabilis) (morganii) (vulgaris)
.7 Pseudomonas
.85 Serratia (marcescens)
.10 Staphylococcus unspecified
.11 Staphylococcus aureus
.19 Staphylococcus other
.00 Streptococcus
.01 Streptococcus group A
.02 Streptococcus group B
.03 Streptococcus group C
.04 Streptococcus group D
.05 Streptococcus group G
.09 Streptococcus other
.89 Other specified bacteria

URINATION

788.4# Excessive
5th digit: 788.4
1. Urination frequency
2. Polyuria
3. Nocturia

788.1 Painful
788.2# Retention
5th digit: 788.2
0. Unspecified
1. Incomplete bladder emptying
9. Other specified retention

306.53 Retention psychogenic
788.6# Stream abnormality
5th digit: 788.6
1. Stream splitting, intermittent
2. Stream slowing, weak stream
4. Hesitancy
5. Straining
9. Other abnormality

788.63 Urgency

URINE

791.6 Acetone abnormal
791.0 Albumin abnormal
791.9 Bacteria abnormal findings
791.9 Bacteriuria
791.4 Bile abnormal
791.7 Casts abnormal
791.7 Cells abnormal
791.1 Chyluria abnormal
791.9 Culture positive abnormal findings
788.5 Deficient secretion
788.30 Enuresis
788.8 Extravasation
788.8 Extravasation unknown etiology
791.5 Glucose abnormal
791.2 Hemoglobin abnormal
0 Incontinence see 'Urinary', incontinence
791.6 Ketone abnormal
788.37 Leakage continuous
791.0 Protein abnormal
791.9 Pus
788.69 Residual
788.2# Retention
997.5 Retention postoperative [788.2#]
5th digit: 788.2
0. Unspecified
1. Incomplete bladder emptying
9. Other specified retention

306.53 Retention psychogenic
788.20 Stasis
791.5 Sugar abnormal
796.0 Toxicology abnormal

URINOMA

596.8 Bladder
998.2 Due to accidental puncture or laceration
593.89 Kidney
593.89 Ureter
599.84 Urethra

752.89 UROGENITAL SINUS (CONGENITAL)
572.4 UROHEPATIC SYNDROME
592.9 UROLITHIASIS
599.60 UROPATHY OBSTRUCTIVE NOS
599.69 UROPATHY OBSTRUCTIVE NEC
0 UROSEPSIS MEANING URINARY TRACT INFECTION SEE 'UTI'
0 UROSEPSIS MEANING SEPSIS SEE 'SEPSIS'

URTICARIA

708.9 NOS
708.0 Allergic
708.0 Angioedema (allergic)
277.6 Angioedema hereditary
995.1 Angioneurotic edema
909.9 Angioneurotic edema late effect
708.5 Cholinergic
708.8 Chronic
708.8 Chronic recurrent
708.3 Dermatographic
708.2 Due to cold and heat
995.1 Due to correctly administered substance
909.9 Due to correctly administered substance late effect
708.0 Due to drug allergy
999.5 Due to serum
909.3 Due to serum late effect
708.3 Factitial
708.0 Food allergy
995.1 Giant
909.9 Giant late effect
708.1 Idiopathic
778.8 Neonatorum
708.1 Nonallergic
698.2 Papulosa (Hebra)
757.33 Pigmentosa
708.8 Plant exposure
316 Psychogenic [708.8]
995.1 Quincke's
909.9 Quincke's late effect
708.8 Recurrent chronic
692.72 Solare
708.2 Thermal
708.4 Vibratory

URTICARIA (ANGIONEUROTIC EDEMA)

995.1 NOS
909.9 NOS late effect
999.5 Due to serum
909.3 Due to serum late effect
995.1 Giant
909.9 Giant late effect
995.1 Quincke's
909.9 Quincke's late effect

694.4 USHER-SENEAR DISEASE (PEMPHIGUS ERYTHEMATOSUS)
085.5 UTA
0 UTERINE SEE 'UTERUS, UTERINE'

U-V-W

UTERUS, UTERINE

615.9 Abscess
615.0 Abscess acute
615.1 Abscess chronic
V45.77 Absence acquired
752.3 Absence congenital
621.5 Adhesion
614.6 Adhesion to abdominal wall
752.3 Agenesis congenital
752.3 Anomaly congenital
621.6 Anteversion
752.3 Aplasia congenital
902.55 Artery injury
908.4 Artery injury late effect
902.55 Artery laceration (rupture) (hematoma) (avulsion) (aneurysm) traumatic
908.4 Artery laceration late effect
621.8 Atresia
752.3 Atresia congenital
621.8 Atrophy acquired
621.5 Bands
752.3 Bicornis (bicornuate) congenital
752.2 Bicornis (bicornuate) with cervix congenital
626.9 Bleeding (abnormal)
902.59 Blood vessel NEC injury
908.4 Blood vessel NEC injury late effect
621.8 Calcification
621.8 Contracture (non pregnant)
621.8 Cyst
752.2 Didelphic (congenital)
615.9 Disorder infective
621.9 Disorder noninflammatory
0 Disorders complicating pregnancy see 'Uterus, Uterine Disorders Complicating Pregnancy'
621.6 Displacement
752.3 Displacement congenital
752.2 Doubling congenital
621.2 Enlargement
618.1 Eversion - NOS (see also 'Uterus, Uterine Prolapse')
618.1 Eversion - with stress incontinence [625.6]
618.1 Eversion - with other urinary incontinence **[788.3#]**

5th digit: 788.3
- **1. Urge incontinence**
- **3. Mixed urge and stress**
- **4. Without sensory awareness**
- **5. Post-void dribbling**
- **6. Nocturnal enuresis**
- **7. Continuous leakage**
- **8. Overflow incontinence**
- **9. Other**

UTERUS, UTERINE (continued)

618.1 Extroversion
618.1 Extroversion with stress incontinence [625.6]
618.1 Extroversion with other urinary incontinence **[788.3#]**

5th digit: 788.3
- **1. Urge incontinence**
- **3. Mixed urge and stress**
- **4. Without sensory awareness**
- **5. Post-void dribbling**
- **6. Nocturnal enuresis**
- **7. Continuous leakage**
- **8. Overflow incontinence**
- **9. Other**

218.9 Fibroid - NOS
218.1 Fibroid - intramural
218.0 Fibroid - submucous
218.2 Fibroid - subserous
621.8 Fibrosis
621.6 Flexion
621.3# Hyperplasia endometrium

5th digit: 621.3
- **0. NOS**
- **1. Simple**
- **2. Complex**
- **3. With atypia**

621.2 Hyperplasia myometrium
621.2 Hypertrophy
763.7 Hypotonic congenital affecting fetus or newborn
621.8 Incarcerated
763.7 Inertia maternal affecting fetus or newborn
639.2 Injury post abortion/ectopic/molar pregnancy
867.4 Injury traumatic
867.5 Injury traumatic with open wound into cavity
908.2 Injury traumatic late effect
621.7 Inversion (chronic)
763.89 Inversion maternal affecting fetus newborn
621.8 Laceration (postpartum) old
621.6 Malposition
625.8 Mass
621.8 Metaplasia
621.8 Obstruction or occlusion
621.0 Polyp
0 Prolapse see 'Uterus, Uterine Prolapse'
621.6 Retraction
621.6 Retroflexion
621.6 Retroversion
621.8 Rupture (nonobstetrical) (nontraumatic)
763.89 Rupture maternal affecting fetus or newborn
763.1 Sacculation maternal affecting fetus or newborn
621.1 Subinvolution (chronic) (nonpuerperal)
621.5 Synechiae
621.8 Ulcer
752.3 Unicornis
902.56 Vein injury
908.4 Vein injury late effect
902.56 Vein laceration (rupture) (hematoma) (avulsion) (aneurysm) traumatic
908.4 Vein laceration late effect
752.3 With one functioning horn

UTERUS, UTERINE PROLAPSE:

WITH INCONTINENCE [788.3#]

WITH STRESS INCONTINENCE [625.6]

618.1 NOS
618.4 And vagina prolapse
618.3 And vagina prolapse complete
618.2 And vagina prolapse incomplete
618.1 Degree first
618.1 Degree second
618.1 Degree third
618.1 Descensus (first degree) (second degree) (third degree)
618.1 Procidentia

WITH INCONTINENCE [788.3#]
5th digit: 788.3
0. Unspecified
1. Urge incontinence
2. Stress, male
3. Mixed urge and stress
4. Without sensory awareness
5. Post-void dribbling
6. Nocturnal enuresis
7. Continuous leakage
8. Overflow incontinence
9. Other

UTERUS, UTERINE DISORDERS COMPLICATING PREGNANCY

763.89 Abnormalities shape or position affecting fetus or newborn
654.4# Abnormalities shape or position complicating childbirth
660.2# Abnormalities shape or position complicating childbirth obstructing labor [654.4#]
5th digit: 654.4
0. Episode of care NOS or N/A
1. Delivered
2. Delivered with postpartum complication
3. Antepartum complication
4. Postpartum complication

5th digit: 660.2
0. Episode of care NOS or N/A
1. Delivered
3. Antepartum complication

661.2# Atony (hypotonic) (inertia) without hemorrhage
5th digit: 661.2
0. Episode of care NOS or N/A
1. Delivered
3. Antepartum complication

669.8# Atony (hypotonic) (inertia) (postpartum)
5th digit: 669.8
0. Episode of care NOS or N/A
1. Delivered
2. Delivered with postpartum complication
3. Antepartum complication
4. Postpartum complication

666.1# Atony (hypotonic) (inertia) (postpartum) with hemorrhage
5th digit: 666.1
0. Episode of care NOS or N/A
2. Delivered with postpartum complication
4. Postpartum complication

UTERUS, UTERINE DISORDERS COMPLICATING PREGNANCY (continued)

654.0# Bicornis complicating childbirth
660.2# Bicornis complicating childbirth obstructing labor [654.0#]
5th digit: 654.0
0. Episode of care NOS or N/A
1. Delivered
2. Delivered with postpartum complication
3. Antepartum complication
4. Postpartum complication

5th digit: 660.2
0. Episode of care NOS or N/A
1. Delivered
3. Antepartum complication

661.4# Contractions hypertonic, incoordinate, prolonged or hourglass in labor
763.7 Dysfunction maternal affecting fetus or newborn
661.4# Dystocia NOS in labor
5th digit: 661.4
0. Episode of care NOS or N/A
1. Delivered
3. Antepartum complication

665.2# Eversion/inversion (obstetrical trauma)
763.89 Eversion/inversion affecting fetus newborn
665.2# Eversion/inversion complicating delivery
674.8# Eversion puerperal, postpartum maternal due to pregnancy
5th digit: 665.2, 674.8
0. Episode of care NOS or N/A
2. Delivered with postpartum complication
4. Postpartum complication

654.1# Fibroid complicating pregnancy
660.2# Fibroid complicating pregnancy obstructing labor [654.1#]
5th digit: 654.1
0. Episode of care NOS or N/A
1. Delivered
2. Delivered with postpartum complication
3. Antepartum complication
4. Postpartum complication

5th digit: 660.2
0. Episode of care NOS or N/A
1. Delivered
3. Antepartum complication

674.8# Hypertrophy postpartum maternal due to pregnancy
5th digit: 674.8
0. Episode of care NOS or N/A
2. Delivered with postpartum complication
4. Postpartum complication

UTERUS, UTERINE DISORDERS COMPLICATING PREGNANCY (continued)

763.7 Hypotonic congenital affecting fetus or newborn
0 Hypotonic see 'Uterus, Uterine Disorders Complicating Pregnancy', inertia
654.3# Incarcerated
660.2# Incarcerated obstructing labor **[654.3#]**
5th digit: 654.3
0. Episode of care NOS or N/A
1. Delivered
2. Delivered with postpartum complication
3. Antepartum complication
4. Postpartum complication

5th digit: 660.2
0. Episode of care NOS or N/A
1. Delivered
3. Antepartum complication

763.7 Inertia - or dysfunction affecting fetus or newborn
661.0# Inertia - primary
661.1# Inertia - secondary
661.2# Inertia - other and NOS
5th digit: 661.0-2
0. Episode of care NOS or N/A
1. Delivered
3. Antepartum complication

644.1# Irritability >37 weeks (threatened premature labor)
644.0# Irritability >22 and <37 weeks (threatened premature labor)
5th digit: 644.0-1
0. Episode of care unspecified or N/A
3. Antepartum complication

644.2# Irritability with premature onset of delivery <37 weeks
5th digit: 644.2
0. Episode of care unspecified or N/A
1. Delivered

654.4# Prolapse complicating pregnancy
660.2# Prolapse complicating pregnancy obstructing labor **[654.4#]**
654.3# Retroverted incarcerated complicating childbirth
660.2# Retroverted incarcerated complicating childbirth obstructing labor **[654.3#]**
5th digit: 654.3-4
0. Episode of care NOS or N/A
1. Delivered
2. Delivered with postpartum complication
3. Antepartum complication
4. Postpartum complication

5th digit: 660.2
0. Episode of care NOS or N/A
1. Delivered
3. Antepartum complication

UTERUS, UTERINE DISORDERS COMPLICATING PREGNANCY (continued)

763.89 Rupture affecting fetus or newborn
665.0# Rupture before onset of labor
5th digit: 665.0
0. Episode of care NOS or N/A
1. Delivered
3. Antepartum complication

665.1# Rupture during labor or NOS
5th digit: 665.1
0. Episode of care unspecified or N/A
1. Delivered

763.1 Sacculation affecting fetus or newborn
654.4# Sacculation complicating delivery
660.2# Sacculation complicating delivery obstructing labor **[654.4#]**
5th digit: 654.4
0. Episode of care NOS or N/A
1. Delivered
2. Delivered with postpartum complication
3. Antepartum complication
4. Postpartum complication

5th digit: 660.2
0. Episode of care NOS or N/A
1. Delivered
3. Antepartum complication

654.2# Scar from previous cesarean delivery complicating childbirth
660.2# Scar from previous cesarean delivery complicating childbirth obstructing labor **[654.2#]**
5th digit: 654.2, 660.2,
0. Episode of care unspecified or N/A
1. Delivered
3. Antepartum complication

649.6# Size-date discrepancy
5th digit: 649.6
0. Episode of care NOS or N/A
1. Delivered
2. Delivered with postpartum complication
3. Antepartum complication
4. Postpartum complication

661.4# Spasm in labor
5th digit: 661.4
0. Episode of care unspecified or N/A
1. Delivered
3. Antepartum complication

674.8# Subinvolution, postpartum maternal due to pregnancy
5th digit: 674.8
0. NOS
2. Delivered with postpartum complication
4. Postpartum complication

752.3 Unicornis congenital

> *Urinary tract infection is a nonspecific diagnosis. Whenever possible, be sure to code the specific condition such as cystitis, nephritis, or urethritis.*

UTI (URINARY TRACT INFECTION): WITH KNOWN ORGANISM [041.#(#)]

599.0 Site not specified
112.2 Candidal
996.64 Due to indwelling foley
639.8 Following abortion/ectopic/molar pregnancy
V13.02 History
646.6# Maternal complicating pregnancy

5th digit: 646.6
- **0. Episode of care NOS or N/A**
- **1. Delivered**
- **2. Delivered with postpartum complication**
- **3. Antepartum complication**
- **4. Postpartum complication**

771.82 Neonatal
997.5 Postoperative [599.0]
997.5 Specified as due to a procedure [599.0]

4th or 4th and 5th digit code for organism: 041
- **.85 Aerobacter aerogenes**
- **.84 Anaerobes other**
- **.82 Bacteroides fragilis**
- **.83 Clostridium perfringens**
- **.4 E. coli (escherichia coli)**
- **.81 Eaton's agent**
- **.85 Enterobacter sakazakii**
- **.04 Enterococcus**
- **.3 Friedlander's bacillus**
- **.84 Gram-negative anaerobes**
- **.85 Gram-negative bacteria NOS**
- **.5 H. influenzae**
- **.86 H. pylori (helicobacter pylori)**
- **.3 Klebsiella**
- **.85 Mima polymorpha**
- **.81 Mycoplasma**
- **.81 Pleuropneumonia like organisms**
- **.2 Pneumococcus**
- **.6 Proteus (mirabilis) (morganii) (vulgaris)**
- **.7 Pseudomonas**
- **.85 Serratia (marcescens)**
- **.10 Staphylococcus unspecified**
- **.11 Staphylococcus aureus**
- **.19 Staphylococcus other**
- **.00 Streptococcus**
- **.01 Streptococcus group A**
- **.02 Streptococcus group B**
- **.03 Streptococcus group C**
- **.04 Streptococcus group D**
- **.05 Streptococcus group G**
- **.09 Streptococcus other**
- **.89 Other specified bacteria**

364.9 UVEAL TRACT DISEASE – ANTERIOR
363.9 UVEAL TRACT DISEASE - POSTERIOR

UVEITIS

364.3 NOS
364.00 Anterior acute subacute
364.01 Anterior primary
364.02 Anterior recurrent
364.03 Anterior secondary infectious
364.04 Anterior secondary noninfectious
098.41 Gonococcal
054.44 Herpes simplex
053.22 Herpes zoster
363.20 Posterior
360.11 Sympathetic
091.50 Syphilitic secondary

364.24 UVEOCUTANEOUS SYNDROME
363.22 UVEOMENINGEAL, UVEOMENINGITIS SYNDROME
135 UVEOPAROTID FEVER

UVULA

750.26 Absence congenital
749.20 Bifid (with cleft lip)
0 Bifid see also 'Cleft Palate With Cleft Lip'
749.02 Cleft
528.9 Hypertrophy (elongation)
750.26 Hypertrophy (elongation) congenital
959.09 Injury

UVULITIS

528.9 NOS
528.3 Abscess cellulitis
462 Sore throat acute NOS (viral)
528.9 Other

427.1 V TACH
427.1 V TACH PAROXYSMAL

VACCINATION (NEED FOR)

V03.89 Against other single bacteria
V03.9 Bacterial
V03.89 Bacterial other specified
V03.2 BCG
V05.4 Chickenpox
V03.0 Cholera
V06.0 Cholera with typhoid paratyphoid
V04.7 Cold
V06.9 Combination
V06.8 Combination other specified
0 Complication see 'Complication of Medical Care Not Elsewhere Classified'
V03.5 Diphtheria
V06.5 Diphtheria-tetanus (TD)
V06.1 Diphtheria-tetanus-pertussis
V06.3 Diphtheria-tetanus-pertussis with polio
V06.2 Diphtheria-tetanus-pertussis with TAB
V05.9 Disease (single)
V05.8 Disease (single) other specified
V06.1 DPT (DTaP)
V06.3 DPT with polio
V06.2 DPT with TAB

VACCINATION (NEED FOR) (continued)

V06.5 DT (tetanus-diphtheria)
V06.1 DTaP (DPT)
V06.1 DTP
V06.3 DTP with polio
V06.2 DTP with TAB
V05.0 Encephalitis (viral/arthropod borne)
V04.81 Flu
V03.81 Hemophilus influenza, type B (HIB)
V05.3 Hepatitis viral (B, C, E)
V03.81 HIB (hemophilus influenza, type B)
V20.2 Infant or child routine appropriate for age
V04.81 Influenza
V05.2 Leishmaniasis
V03.89 Lyme's disease
V04.2 Measles alone
V06.4 Measles mumps rubella
V06.4 MMR
V04.6 Mumps (alone)
V64.0# Not carried out due to

5th digit: V64.0
0. Unspecified reason
1. Acute illness
2. Chronic illness or condition
3. Immune compromised state
4. Allergy to vaccine or component
5. Caregiver (guardian) (parent) refusal
6. Patient refusal
7. Religious reasons
8. Patient had disease being vaccinated against
9. Other reason

V03.6 Pertussis
V03.3 Plague
V03.82 Pneumococcus
V03.82 Pneumonia pneumococcal
V04.0 Polio
V03.82 PPV (pneumococcal polysaccharide vaccine)
V04.5 Rabies
V04.82 Respiratory syncytial virus (RSV)
V04.82 RSV (respiratory syncytial virus)
V04.3 Rubella (alone)
V04.1 Smallpox
V03.82 Streptococcus pneumoniae
V06.6 Streptococcus pneumoniae and influenza
V03.1 TAB
V03.2 TB
V06.5 TD
V06.5 Tetanus - diphtheria (TD)
V06.1 Tetanus - diphtheria with pertussis (DTP/DTaP)
V03.7 Tetanus toxoid
V03.4 Tularemia
V03.1 Typhoid-paratyphoid
V05.4 Varicella
V05.0 Viral arthropod borne encephalitis
V05.1 Viral arthropod borne other
V04.4 Yellow fever
V06.8 Other combination (prophylactic)
V04.89 Other viral diseases
V06.8 Other specified combination
V05.8 Other specified disease
V05.8 Other specified single disease

V14.7 VACCINE ALLERGY (HISTORY)

VACCINIA

999.0 NOS
771.2 Congenital

999.39 Other infection - Use an additional code to identify the specified infection such as septicemia, (038.#(#)).

999.39 Conjunctiva
999.0 Eyelids [373.5]
051.0 Eyelids not from vaccination [373.5]

999.39 Other infection - Use an additional code to identify the specified infection such as septicemia, (038.#(#)).

999.39 Localized

999.39 Other infection - Use an additional code to identify the specified infection such as septicemia, (038.#(#)).

999.39 Nose
051.0 Not from vaccination
051.0 Sine vaccinatione
051.0 Without vaccination

0 VACUUM EXTRACTION DELIVERY SEE ALSO 'DELIVERY', FORCEPS OR VACUUM
763.3 VACUUM EXTRACTOR DELIVERY AFFECTING FETUS OR NEWBORN
660.7# VACUUM EXTRACTOR FAILURE

5th digit: 660.7
0. Episode of care NOS or N/A
1. Delivered
3. Antepartum complication

V60.0 VAGABOND (HOMELESS PERSON)
132.1 VAGABOND'S DISEASE

VAGINA, VAGINAL

763.89 Abnormality affecting fetus or newborn
654.7# Abnormality complicating childbirth (tumor) (septate)
660.2# Abnormality (tumor) (septate) obstructing labor **[654.7#]**

5th digit: 654.7
0. Episode of care NOS or N/A
1. Delivered
2. Delivered with postpartum complication
3. Antepartum complication
4. Postpartum complication

5th digit: 660.2
0. Episode of care NOS or N/A
1. Delivered
3. Antepartum complication

V45.77 Absence acquired
752.49 Absence (agenesis) (stricture) congenital
623.2 Adhesions (postop) (postradiation)
752.40 Anomaly congenital
752.49 Anomaly congenital - other specified
V55.7 Artificial care (closure) (toilet) (attention)
V44.7 Artificial status
623.2 Atresia
752.49 Atresia congenital
098.2 Atresia postgonococcal (old)
623.2 Atresia postinfectional (senile)
627.3 Atrophy (senile)

U-V-W

VAGINA, VAGINAL (continued)

623.8 Bleeding
641.2# Bleeding abruptio placentae in pregnancy
640.9# Bleeding in pregnancy, antepartum (<22 weeks)
641.9# Bleeding in pregnancy, antepartum NOS
626.6 Bleeding irregular
626.7 Bleeding irregular postcoital
641.1# Bleeding placenta previa in pregnancy
5th digit: 640.9, 641.1-2, 9
0. Episode of care NOS or N/A
1. Delivered
3. Antepartum complication

V76.47 Cancer screening
V76.47 Cancer screening pap smear status post hysterectomy for nonmalignant condition [V45.77]
V67.01 Cancer screening pap smear status post hysterectomy for cancer **[V10.4#]** [V45.77]
5th digit: V10.4
0. Genital organ unspecified
1. Cervix uteri
2. Other part of uterus
3. Ovary
4. Genital organ other

623.8 Cyst
623.5 Discharge
616.10 Disorder inflammatory
623.9 Disorder noninflammatory
623.8 Disorder noninflammatory - specified NEC
752.2 Duplication (total) congenital
623.0 Dysplasia
623.0 Dysplasia VAIN I
623.0 Dysplasia VAIN II
233.31 Dysplasia VAIN III
618.6 Enterocele congenital or acquired
618.6 Enterocele congenital or acquired with stress incontinence [625.6]
618.6 Enterocele congenital or acquired with other urinary incontinence **[788.3#]**
5th digit: 788.3
1. Urge incontinence
3. Mixed urge and stress
4. Without sensory awareness
5. Post-void dribbling
6. Nocturnal enuresis
7. Continuous leakage
8. Overflow incontinence
9. Other

623.8 Fibrosis
792.9 Fluid abnormal
623.6 Hematoma
665.7# Hematoma obstetrical trauma
5th digit: 665.7
0. Episode of care NOS or N/A
1. Delivered
2. Delivered with postpartum complication
4. Postpartum complication

623.8 Hemorrhage
616.9 Inflammatory disease
616.89 Inflammatory disease other
959.14 Injury NEC
911.8 Injury other and unspecified superficial
911.9 Injury other and unspecified superficial infected
639.2 Injury post abortion/ectopic/molar pregnancy

VAGINA, VAGINAL (continued)

623.0 Intraepithelial neoplasia I (VAIN III)
623.0 Intraepithelial neoplasia II (VAIN III)
233.31 Intraepithelial neoplasia III (VAIN III)
623.1 Leukoplakia
625.8 Mass
616.81 Mucositis (ulcerative)
623.9 Noninflammatory disorder
623.2 Obstruction or occlusion
625.9 Pain
302.76 Pain psychogenic
623.7 Polyp
618.0# Prolapse
618.0# Prolapse with stress incontinence [625.6]
618.0# Prolapse with other urinary incontinence **[788.3#]**
5th digit: 618.0
0. Unspecified
1. Cystocele, midline
2. Cystocele, lateral (paravaginal)
3. Urethrocele
4. Rectocele (proctocele)
5. Perineocele
9. Other

5th digit: 788.3
1. Urge incontinence
3. Mixed urge and stress
4. Without sensory awareness
5. Post-void dribbling
6. Nocturnal enuresis
7. Continuous leakage
8. Overflow incontinence
9. Other

618.5 Prolapse after hysterectomy
618.5 Prolapse after hysterectomy with stress incontinence [625.6]
618.5 Prolapse after hysterectomy with other urinary incontinence **[788.3#]**
5th digit: 788.3
1. Urge incontinence
3. Mixed urge and stress
4. Without sensory awareness
5. Post-void dribbling
6. Nocturnal enuresis
7. Continuous leakage
8. Overflow incontinence
9. Other

618.4 Prolapse with uterine prolapse - NOS
618.3 Prolapse with uterine prolapse - complete
618.2 Prolapse with uterine prolapse - incomplete
618.89 Relaxation
618.89 Relaxation with stress incontinence [625.6]
618.89 Relaxation with other urinary incontinence **[788.3#]**
5th digit: 788.3
1. Urge incontinence
3. Mixed urge and stress
4. Without sensory awareness
5. Post-void dribbling
6. Nocturnal enuresis
7. Continuous leakage
8. Overflow incontinence
9. Other

VAGINA, VAGINAL (continued)

654.7# Rigid complicating pregnancy childbirth or puerperium
660.2# Rigid obstructing labor [**654.7#**]
5th digit: 654.7
0. Episode of care NOS or N/A
1. Delivered
2. Delivered with postpartum complication
3. Antepartum complication
4. Postpartum complication

5th digit: 660.2
0. Episode of care NOS or N/A
1. Delivered
3. Antepartum complication

623.4 Scarring
625.1 Spasms
623.2 Stenosis
623.2 Stricture or atresia
752.49 Stricture or atresia congenital
654.7# Tumor complicating pregnancy
660.2# Tumor obstructing labor [**654.7#**]
5th digit: 654.7
0. Episode of care NOS or N/A
1. Delivered
2. Delivered with postpartum complication
3. Antepartum complication
4. Postpartum complication

5th digit: 660.2
0. Episode of care NOS or N/A
1. Delivered
3. Antepartum complication

616.89 Ulcer (inflammatory)

625.1 VAGINISMUS
306.51 VAGINISMUS FUNCTIONAL PSYCHOGENIC
300.11 VAGINISMUS HYSTERICAL
306.51 VAGINISMUS PSYCHOGENIC

VAGINITIS

616.10 NOS
760.8 Affecting newborn or fetus
616.10 Bacterial
112.1 Candidal
099.53 Chlamydial

> ***646.6#: Specify the maternal vaginitis with an additional code.***

646.6# Complicating pregnancy, childbirth, or puerperium
5th digit: 646.6
0. Episode of care NOS or N/A
1. Delivered
2. Delivered with postpartum complication
3. Antepartum complication
4. Postpartum complication

616.10 E. coli [041.4]
639.0 Following ectopic molar or aborted pregnancy
616.10 Gardnerella [041.89]
098.0 Gonococcal acute
098.2 Gonococcal chronic
616.10 Hemophilus vaginalis [041.5]
054.11 Herpetic
112.1 Monilial
127.4 Pinworm [616.11]
616.10 Postirradiation

VAGINITIS (continued)

627.3 Postmenopausal
627.3 Senile (atrophic)
616.10 Staphylococcal [**041.1#**]
5th digit: 041.1
0. Unspecified
1. Aureus
9. Oher

616.10 Streptococcal [**041.0#**]
5th digit: 041.0
0. NOS
1. Group A
2. Group B
3. Group C
4. Group D (enterococcus)
5. Group G
9. Other strep

131.01 Trichomonal

0 VAGINOSIS SEE 'VAGINITIS'
352.6 VAGOHYPOGLOSSAL SYNDROME
780.2 VAGOVAGAL SYNDROME
352.3 VAGUS NERVE ATROPHY
951.8 VAGUS NERVE INJURY
352.3 VAGUS NERVE NEURITIS (DISORDER)
352.3 VAGUS NERVE PARALYSIS
623.0 VAIN I (VAGINAL INTRAEPITHELIAL NEOPLASIA I)
623.0 VAIN II (VAGINAL INTRAEPITHELIAL NEOPLASIA II)
233.31 VAIN III (VAGINAL INTRAEPITHELIAL NEOPLASIA III)
736.79 VALGUS DEFORMITY FOOT (ACQUIRED)
754.60 VALGUS DEFORMITY FOOT CONGENITAL
754.69 VALGUS DEFORMITY FOOT CONGENITAL OTHER NEC
736.03 VALGUS DEFORMITY WRIST
270.3 VALINE METABOLISM DISTURBANCES
304.1# VALIUM (VALMID) ADDICTION
5th digit: 304.1
0. NOS
1. Continuous
2. Episodic
3. In remission

648.2# VALSUANI'S DISEASE MATERNAL CURRENT (CO-EXISTENT) IN PREGNANCY (PROGRESSIVE PERNICIOUS ANEMIA) [**281.#**]
5th digit: 648.2
0. Episode of care NOS or N/A
1. Delivered
2. Delivered with postpartum complication
3. Antepartum complication
4. Postpartum complication

4th digit: 281
0. Pernicious (intrinsic factor) (castle's) deficiency
1. B12 deficiency
2. Folate deficiency
3. B12 with folate deficiency
4. Protein or amino acid deficiency
8. Nutritional (scorbutic)
9. NOS

U-V-W

046.2 VAN BOGAERT'S DISEASE (SCLEROSING LEUKOENCEPHALITIS)
330.0 VAN BOGAERT-NIJSSEN (-PFEIFFER) DISEASE (LEUKODYSTROPHY)
733.3 VAN BUCHEM'S SYNDROME (HYPEROSTOSIS CORTICALIS)
271.0 VAN CREVELD-VON GIERKE DISEASE (GLYCOGENOSIS I)
289.7 VAN DEN BERGH'S DISEASE (ENTEROGENOUS CYANOSIS)
756.51 VAN DER HOEVE'S SYNDROME (BRITTLE BONES AND BLUE SCLERA, DEAFNESS)
270.2 VAN DER HOEVE-HALBERTSMA-WAARDENBURG SYNDROME (PTOSIS-EPICANTHUS)
270.2 VAN DER HOEVE-WAARDENBURG-GUALDI SYNDROME (PTOSIS-EPICANTHUS)
V09.8 VANCOMYCIN (GLYCOPEPTIDE) INTERMEDIATE STAPHYLOCOCCUS AUREUS (VISA/GISA)
V09.8 VANCOMYCIN (GLYCOPEPTIDE) RESISTANT ENTEROCOCCUS (VRE)
V09.8 VANCOMYCIN (GLYCOPEPTIDE) RESISTANT STAPHYLOCOCCUS AUREUS (VRSA/GRSA)
791.9 VANILLYLMANDELIC ACID ELEVATION (URINARY)
651.3# VANISHING TWIN
5th digit: 651.3
0. Episode of care unspecified or N/A
1. Delivered
3. Antepartum complication

732.1 VAN NECK (-ODELBERG) DISEASE OR SYNDROME (JUVENILE OSTEOCHONDROSIS)
987.9 VAPORS INHALATION (NOXIOUS)
238.4 VAQUEZ (-OSLER) DISEASE (POLYCYTHEMIA VERA) M9950/1
413.1 VARIANT ANGINA

VARICELLA

052.9 NOS
052.8 Complication unspecified
052.7 Complication other specified
052.0 Encephalitis (post varicella)
V01.71 Exposure
052.7 Keratoconjunctivitis [370.44]
647.6# Maternal complicating pregnancy [052.#]
5th digit: 647.6
0. Episode of care unspecified or N/A
1. Delivered
2. Delivered with postpartum complication
3. Antepartum complication
4. Postpartum complication
5th digit: 052
0. Postvaricella encephalitis
1. Varicella pneumonia
7. Other specified complications
8. Unspecified complication
9. Without mention of complication

052.1 Pneumonitis hemorrhagic
V05.4 Vaccination
052.9 Without complication

VARICES

747.6# Arteriovenous peripheral vascular congenital
5th digit: 747.6
0. Peripheral vascular unspecified site
1. Gastrointestinal vessel
2. Renal vessel
3. Upper limb vessel
4. Lower limb vessel
9. Other specified site peripheral vascular

456.5 Broad ligament
456.1 Esophageal
747.69 Esophageal congenital
456.0 Esophageal with bleeding
456.8 Gastric

648.9#: Use an additional code to identify the varices.

648.9# Maternal current (co-existent) in pregnancy
5th digit: 648.9
0. Episode of NOS or N/A
1. Delivered
2. Delivered with postpartum complication
3. Antepartum complication
4. Postpartum complication

456.8 Nasal septum
747.69 Orbit congenital
456.5 Pelvic
456.6 Perineum
656.7# Placental affecting management of pregnancy
5th digit: 656.7
0. Episode of care NOS or N/A
1. Delivered
3. Antepartum complication

456.8 Prostate
362.17 Retinal
456.4 Scrotal
456.3 Sublingual
762.6 Umbilical cord affecting fetus or newborn
456.6 Vulval
456.8 Other sites

456.5 VARICOCELE OVARY
456.4 VARICOCELE SPERMATIC CORD (ULCERATED)

VARICOSE VEINS

454.9 NOS
454.9 Asymptomatic
747.6# Congenital (peripheral) NEC
5th digit: 747.6
0. Peripheral vascular unspecified site
1. Gastrointestinal vessel
2. Renal vessel
3. Upper limb vessel
4. Lower limb vessel
9. Other specified site peripheral vascular

454.9 Lower extremities
454.8 Lower extremities with complications
454.8 Lower extremities with edema
454.1 Lower extremities with inflammation
454.8 Lower extremities with pain
454.8 Lower extremities with swelling
454.0 Lower extremities with ulcer
454.2 Lower extremities with ulcer and inflammation

VARICOSE VEINS COMPLICATING PREGNANCY AND PUERPERIUM

671.0# Leg(s) maternal due to pregnancy

> ***648.9#:** Use an additional code to identify the specific type of varicose veins.*

648.9# Maternal current (co-existent)
671.1# Vulva and perineum maternal due to pregnancy
5th digit: 648.9, 671.0-1
0. Episode of care NOS or N/A
1. Delivered
2. Delivered with postpartum complication
3. Antepartum complication
4. Postpartum complication

050.0 VARIOLA MAJOR
050.1 VARIOLA MINOR
050.2 VARIOLOID
747.6# VARIX ARTERY PERIPHERAL VASCULAR CONGENITAL
5th digit: 747.6
0. Peripheral vascular unspecified site
1. Gastrointestinal vessel
2. Renal vessel
3. Upper limb vessel
4. Lower limb vessel
9. Other specified site peripheral vascular

736.79 VARUS DEFORMITY FOOT (ACQUIRED)
754.50 VARUS DEFORMITY FOOT CONGENITAL
754.59 VARUS DEFORMITY FOOT CONGENITAL OTHER NEC

VAS DEFERENS

V45.77 Absence acquired
752.89 Absence congenital
752.9 Anomaly NOS
752.89 Anomaly (congenital) NEC
752.89 Atresia congenital
608.89 Atrophy (fibrosis) (hypertrophy) (ulcer)
608.9 Disease
608.89 Disease other specified
752.89 Embryonic
608.83 Hemorrhage (thrombosis) (hematoma) nontraumatic
867.6 Injury (traumatic)
908.2 Injury late effect
867.7 Injury with open wound into cavity
996.65 Prosthetic reconstruction complication - infection or inflammation
996.39 Prosthetic reconstruction complication - mechanical
996.76 Prosthetic reconstruction complication - other
608.85 Stricture

663.5# VASA PREVIA
5th digit: 663.5
0. Episode of care NOS or N/A
1. Delivered
3. Antepartum complication

762.6 VASA PREVIA AFFECTING FETUS OR NEWBORN

VASCULAR

747.60 Atresia NEC
459.89 Atrophy
V58.81 Catheter care (removal) (replacement) (toilet) (cleansing)
785.59 Collapse
779.89 Collapse newborn
459.9 Disease NOS

> ***648.9#:** Use an additional code to identify the specific vascular disease.*

648.9# Disease maternal current (co-existent) in pregnancy
5th digit: 648.9
0. Episode of care NOS or N/A
1. Delivered
2. Delivered with postpartum complication
3. Antepartum complication
4. Postpartum complication

447.1 Disease - obliterative
443.9 Disease - obliterative (occlusive) peripheral
459.9 Disease - occlusive
443.9 Disease - peripheral (occlusive)
250.7# Disease - peripheral (occlusive) diabetic [443.81]
5th digit: 250.7
0. Type II, adult-onset, non-insulin dependent (even if requiring insulin), or unspecified; controlled
1. Type I, juvenile-onset or insulin-dependent; controlled
2. Type II, adult-onset, non-insulin dependent (even if requiring insulin); uncontrolled
3. Type I, juvenile-onset or insulin-dependent; uncontrolled

443.89 Disease - peripheral (occlusive) specified type NEC
459.3# Hypertension chronic
459.1# Hypertension chronic due to deep vein thrombosis
5th digit: 459.1, 3
0. NOS
1. With ulcer
2. With inflammation
3. With ulcer and inflammation
9. With other complication

443.9 Insufficiency - disease peripheral
996.1 Insufficiency - graft obstruction
286.4 Insufficiency - hemophilia
557.9 Insufficiency - intestine
557.0 Insufficiency - intestine acute
557.1 Insufficiency - intestine chronic

> ***648.9#:** Use an additional code to identify the specific vascular insufficiency.*

648.9# Insufficiency - maternal current (co-existent) in pregnancy
5th digit: 648.9
0. Episode of care NOS or N/A
1. Delivered
2. Delivered with postpartum complication
3. Antepartum complication
4. Postpartum complication

557.1 Insufficiency - mesenteric
443.89 Insufficiency - peripheral diseases other specified

VASCULAR (continued)

747.6# Insufficiency - peripheral system other anomalies congenital
5th digit: 747.6
0. Peripheral vascular unspecified site
1. Gastrointestinal vessel
2. Renal vessel
3. Upper limb vessel
4. Lower limb vessel
9. Other specified site peripheral vascular

743.57 Loop on papilla (optic)
459.9 Occlusion
557.0 Splanchnic syndrome

996.83 VASCULOPATHY CARDIAC ALLOGRAFT

VASCULITIS

447.6 NOS
287.0 Allergic
273.2 Cryoglobulinemic
446.29 Leukoclastic (leukocytoclastic)
695.2 Nodular
362.18 Retinal

VASECTOMY

V25.09 Counseling (proposed)
V25.2 Encounter
998.89 Failure
V26.0 Reversal after previous sterilization
V26.22 Sperm count – post reversal
V25.8 Sperm count – post vasectomy
V26.52 Status

443.9 VASOMOTOR DISEASE OR SYNDROME

0 VASOPLASTY SEE 'VASECTOMY'

253.5 VASOPRESSIN DEFICIENCY
588.1 VASOPRESSION DEFICIENCY NEPHROGENIC
413.1 VASOSPASM CORONARY
443.9 VASOSPASTIC PHENOMENON
780.2 VASOVAGAL ATTACK (SYNDROME)
780.2 VASOVAGAL PHENOMENON (VASOMOTOR)
576.8 VATER SPASM (AMPULLA OF VATER)
759.89 VATER SYNDROME
099.9 VD
V01.6 VD EXPOSURE
V74.5 VD SCREENING EXAM
0 VD SEE ALSO BY SPECIFIC DISEASE OR ORGANISM
0 VD SEE ALSO 'VENEREAL DISEASE'

VECTORCARDIOGRAM (VCG)

V72.85 NOS
794.39 Abnormal
V72.81 Preoperative
V71.7 Suspected MI

780.03 VEGETATIVE STATE PERSISTENT
0 VEILLONELLA SEE 'BACTERIAL INFECTION' OR SPECIFIED CONDITION

VEIN, VENOUS

747.81 Absence congenital - brain
747.49 Absence (atresia) congenital - great
747.49 Absence (atresia) congenital - portal
747.49 Absence (atresia) congenital - pulmonary
0 Access loss-code underlying disease
747.6# Anomaly other peripheral vascular (aberrant) (absence) (agenesis) (accessory) (aneurysm) (deformity) (hypoplasia) (malposition) (congenital)
5th digit: 747.6
0. Peripheral vascular unspecified site
1. Gastrointestinal vessel
2. Renal vessel
3. Upper limb vessel
4. Lower limb vessel
9. Other specified site peripheral vascular

> ***648.9#:** Use an additional code to identify the specific vein disorder.*

648.9# Disorder maternal current (co-existent) in pregnancy
5th digit: 648.9
0. Episode of care NOS or N/A
1. Delivered
2. Delivered with postpartum complication
3. Antepartum complication
4. Postpartum complication

459.89 Disorder other specified
0 Division see 'Blood Vessel Injury'
453.9 Embolism (thrombosis)
459.89 Fibrosis (lower extremities)
459.3# Hypertension chronic
459.1# Hypertension chronic due to deep vein thrombosis
5th digit: 459.1, 3
0. NOS
1. With ulcer
2. With inflammation
3. With ulcer and inflammation
9. With other complication

459.89 Hypertrophy
459.89 Increased pressure
459.81 Insufficiency NOS (chronic)
459.81 Insufficiency (chronic) ulcerated [**707.#(#)**]
4th or 4th and 5th digit: 707
1#. Lower limb except decubitus
10. Unspecified
11. Thigh
12. Calf
13. Ankle
14. Heel and midfoot
15. Other parts of foot, toes
19. Other
8. Chronic of other specified site
9. Chronic site NOS

459.2 Obstruction
0 Obstruction or occlusion thrombotic see 'Thrombosis', by site
459.81 Stasis
459.9 Stricture

762.6 VELAMENTOUS INSERTION UMBILICAL CORD AFFECTING FETUS OR NEWBORN

663.8# VELAMENTOUS INSERTION UMBILICAL CORD COMPLICATING PREGNANCY

5th digit: 663.8
0. Episode of care NOS or N/A
1. Delivered
3. Antepartum complication

758.32 VELO-CARDIO-FACIAL SYNDROME

VENA CAVA

902.10 Inferior injury NOS
908.4 Inferior injury late effect
902.19 Inferior injury other site
902.10 Inferior laceration site unspecified traumatic (rupture) (hematoma) (avulsion) (aneurysm)
908.4 Inferior laceration late effect
459.2 Obstruction
453.2 Occlusion
901.2 Superior injury
908.4 Superior injury late effect
908.4 Superior laceration late effect
901.2 Superior laceration traumatic (rupture) (hematoma) (avulsion) (aneurysm)
459.2 Syndrome (inferior) (superior) (obstruction)
453.2 Thrombosis (embolism)

VENA CAVA CONGENITAL

747.49 Absence
747.40 Anomaly
747.49 Atresia
747.49 Left superior persistent
747.49 Stenosis

VENEREAL DISEASE

099.9 NOS
V02.8 Carrier other specified
099.54 Due to chlamydia trachomatis pelvic inflammatory disease [614.9]
099.54 Due to chlamydia trachomatis orchitis and epididymis [604.91]
V01.6 Exposure

647.2#: Use an additional code to identify the maternal venereal disease.

647.2# Maternal current (co-existent) in pregnancy

5th digit: 647.2
0. Episode of care NOS or N/A
1. Delivered
2. Delivered with postpartum complication
3. Antepartum complication
4. Postpartum complication

099.8 Other specified
099.5# Other due to chlamydia trachomatis

5th digit: 099.5
0. Unspecified site
1. Pharynx
2. Anus and rectum
3. Lower genitourinary sites

V74.5 Screening exam

066.2 VENEZUELAN EQUINE FEVER
459.89 VENOFIBROSIS
0 VENOUS SEE VEIN, VENOUS
495.7 VENTILATION PNEUMONITIS
V46.1# VENTILATOR DEPENDENCE

5th digit: V46.1
1. Status
2. Encounter during power failure
3. Encounter for weaning from
4. Mechanical complication

794.2 VENTILATORY OR VITAL CAPACITY REDUCED

VENTRICLE, VENTRICULAR CARDIAC

414.10 Aneurysm
746.9 Anomaly developmental left congenital
745.3 Common congenital
429.9 Dysfunction
429.83 Dysfunction left, reversible following sudden emotional stress
428.0 Dysfunction with CHF
427.69 Escape beats
428.9 Failure NOS
402.91 Failure hypertensive **[428.#(#)]**
402.11 Failure hypertensive benign **[428.#(#)]**
402.01 Failure hypertensive malignant **[428.#(#)]**

4th digit: 428
0. Congestive
1. Left
2#. Systolic
3#. Diastolic
4#. Combined systolic and diastolic
9. NOS

5th digit: 428.2-4
0. NOS
1. Acute
2. Chronic
3. Acute on chronic

428.1 Failure left
391.8 Failure left active
392.0 Failure left active with chorea
398.91 Failure left inactive or quiescent
398.91 Failure left rheumatic
398.91 Failure rheumatic (chronic) (inactive)
391.8 Failure rheumatic active or acute
392.0 Failure rheumatic with active or acute chorea
428.0 Failure right with CHF
427.41 Fibrillation
427.42 Flutter
745.4 Fused congenital
429.3 Hypertrophy (left) (right)
746.89 Hypertrophy (left) (right) congenital
402.90 Hypertrophy hypertensive - NOS
402.10 Hypertrophy hypertensive - benign
402.00 Hypertrophy hypertensive - malignant
426.7 Pre-excitation
427.69 Premature beats contractions
427.69 Premature contractions
745.3 Septal absence congenital

VENTRICLE, VENTRICULAR CARDIAC (continued)

429.71 Septal defect acquired post MI acute (< 8 weeks) [410.##]
4th digit: 410
0. Anterolateral
1. Anterior (wall) anteroapical anteroseptal other anterior
2. Inferolateral
3. Inferoposterior
4. Inferior other
5. Lateral apical, basolateral, posterolateral, lateral other
6. Posterior (posterobasal)
7. Subendocardial
8. Atrium papillary or septum alone
9. Unspecified

5th digit: 410
0. Episode unspecified
1. Initial episode
2. Subsequent episode

429.71 Septal defect acquired following myocardial infarction (>8 weeks) [414.8]
745.4 Septal defect congenital
745.69 Septal defect congenital common atrioventricular canal type
429.71 Septal defect due to ischemic heart disease [414.8]
745.2 Septal defect hypertrophy of right ventricle
745.2 Septal defect in tetrology of fallot
745.2 Septal defect with pulmonary stenosis dextraposition of aorta
745.3 Single congenital
427.5 Standstill
427.1 Tachycardia
427.1 Tachycardia paroxysmal

VENTRICLE, VENTRICULAR CEREBRAL

431 Hemorrhage
331.4 Obstruction or occlusion
331.4 Obstruction or occlusion with dementia [294.1#]
5th digit: 294.1
0. Without behavioral disturbance or NOS
1. With behavioral disturbance

996.63 Shunt complication - infection or inflammation
996.2 Shunt complication - mechanical
996.75 Shunt complication - other
V53.01 Shunt fitting and adjustment
V45.2 Shunt in situ
793.0 Ventriculogram abnormal

793.0 VENTRICULOGRAM (CEREBRAL) ABNORMAL
435.1 VERBIEST'S SYNDROME (CLAUDICATIO INTERMITTENS SPINALIS)
742.2 VERMIS OF CEREBELLUM ABSENCE CONGENITAL
352.6 VERNET'S SYNDROME
095.7 VERNEUIL'S DISEASE (SYPHILITIC BURSITIS)
304.1# VERONAL ADDICTION
5th digit: 304.1
0. NOS
1. Continuous
2. Episodic
3. In remission

VERRUCA

078.11 Acuminata (any site)
078.10 Verruca
078.19 Plana juvenilis
078.19 Plantaris
078.19 Venereal
078.10 Viral NEC
078.10 Vulgaris

078.10 VERRUCOSITIES SEE 'VERRUCA'
199.1 VERRUCOUS CARCINOMA SITE NOS
0 VERRUCOUS CARCINOMA SITE SPECIFIED SEE 'CANCER', BY SITE M8051/3
088.0 VERRUGA PERUANA
275.49 VERSE'S DISEASE (CALCINOSIS INTERVERTEBRALIS) [722.9#]
5th digit: 722.9
0. Unspecified
1. Cervical
2. Thoracic
3. Lumbar

761.7 VERSION EXTERNAL OF MALPRESENTATION BEFORE L&D AFFECTING FETUS OR NEWBORN

VERTEBRA, VERTEBRAL

756.13 Absence congenital
433.2# Artery arteriosclerosis (degeneration) (deformans) (arteritis)
5th digit: 433.2
0. Without cerebral infarction
1. With cerebral infarction

721.1 Artery compression syndrome
443.24 Artery dissection
433.2# Artery occlusion (thrombosis) (obstruction) (embolism) (narrowing) (stenosis)
433.3# Artery occlusion bilateral or with basilar and/or carotid
5th digit: 433.2-3
0. Without cerebral infarction
1. With cerebral infarction

435.1 Artery spasm
721.1 Artery syndrome - compression
435.1 Artery syndrome (insufficiency)
733.99 Atrophy
724.4 Bodies impingement syndrome
722.90 Calcification (cartilage) (disc) - NOS
722.91 Calcification (cartilage) (disc) - cervical
722.93 Calcification (cartilage) (disc) - lumbar (lumbosacral)
722.92 Calcification (cartilage) (disc) - thoracic (thoracolumbar)
733.13 Collapse pathological
733.90 Disorder NEC
0 Disorder disc see 'Intervertebral Disc'
756.15 Fusion congenital
724.4 Lumbar syndrome
756.12 Slipping
435.1 Steal syndrome
756.19 Supernumerary
733.00 Wedging

435.3 VERTOBASILAR ARTERY SPASM

435.3 VERTEBROBASILAR ARTERY SYNDROME (INSUFFICIENCY) (SPASM)
724.5 VERTEBROGENIC (PAIN) SYNDROME
386.9 VERTIGINOUS SYNDROME (LABYRINTHINE)

U-V-W

VERTIGO

780.4 NOS
386.19 Aural
386.11 Benign paroxysmal positional
386.2 Central origin
780.4 Dizziness and giddiness
078.81 Epidemic
438.85 Late effect of CVA
386.2 Malignant positional
386.19 Otogenic
386.10 Peripheral
386.12 Vestibular (neuronitis)

VESICAL

596.0 Neck obstruction
753.6 Neck obstruction congenital
788.9 Pain
0 Retention see 'Urinary', retention
0 See also 'Bladder'
867.0 Sphincter injury traumatic
867.1 Sphincter injury traumatic with open wound
788.9 Tenesmus

593.7# VESICOURETERAL REFLUX
5th digit: 593.7
0. Unspecified
1. With reflux nephropathy, unilateral
2. With reflux nephropathy, bilateral
3. With reflux nephropathy unspecified

596.0 VESICOURETHRAL ORIFICE OBSTRUCTION
596.0 VESICOURETHRAL ORIFICE STRICTURE
753.6 VESICOURETHRAL ORIFICE STRICTURE CONGENITAL
0 VESICOURETHRAL ORIFICE STRICTURE WITH INCONTINENCE SEE 'URETHRA, URETHRAL DISORDERS WITH INCONTINENCE'
709.8 VESICULAR ERUPTION
V23.1 VESICULAR MOLE MATERNAL HISTORY AFFECTING PREGNANCY SUPERVISION
083.2 VESICULAR RICKETTSIOSIS
528.00 VESICULAR STOMATITIS

VESTIBULAR

386.50 Dsyfunction
386.58 Dsyfunction other
794.16 Function studies abnormal
386.12 Neuritis
386.12 Neuronitis

478.19 VESTIBULITIS NOSE (EXTERNAL)
616.10 VESTIBULITIS VULVAR
994.9 VIBRATION DISEASE
001.0 VIBRIO CHOLERA
001.1 VIBRIO CHOLERAE EL TOR
005.4 VIBRIO PARAHAEMOLYTICUS FOOD POISONING
0 VIBRIO VULNIFICUS SEE 'BACTERIAL INFECTION' OR SPECIFIED CONDITION
005.81 VIBRIO VULNIFICUS FOOD POISONING
698.3 VIDAL'S DISEASE (LICHEN SIMPLEX CHRONICUS)
723.8 VIDEO DISPLAY SYNDROME
352.6 VILLARET'S SYNDROME
624.01 VIN I (VULVAR INTRAEPITHELIAL NEOPLASIA I)
624.02 VIN II (VULVAR INTRAEPITHELIAL NEOPLASIA II)
233.32 VIN III (VULVAR INTRAEPITHELIAL NEOPLASIA III)
101 VINCENT'S ANGINA (TRENCH MOUTH)
101 VINCENT'S INFECTION (ANY SITE)
280.8 VINSON-PLUMMER SYNDROME (SIDEROPENIC DYSPHAGIA)
989.5 VIPER BITE
995.0 VIPER BITE WITH ANAPHYLAXIS [989.5]
0 VIRAL SEE 'VIRUS, VIRAL'
733.99 VIRCHOW'S DISEASE
790.8 VIREMIA
256.4 VIRILIZATION (FEMALE) ISOSEXUAL (STEIN LEVENTHAL)
255.2 VIRILIZATION (FEMALE) (SUPRARENAL)
255.2 VIRILIZING ADRENOCORTICAL HYPERPLASIA SYNDROME, CONGENITAL

VIRUS, VIRAL

077.99 Conjunctivitis NOS
079.89 Coronavirus
079.89 Coronavirus-SARS associated
078.89 Disease NEC
066.9 Disease arthropod borne
049.9 Disease central nervous system NEC
048 Disease central nervous system other enterovirus
049.8 Disease central nervous system other specified non arthropod borne
V01.79 Disease exposure other specified
V73.81 Disease human papillomavirus (HPV) screening
655.3# Disease maternal (with known/suspected damage to fetus)
5th digit: 655.3
0. Episode of care NOS or N/A
1. Delivered
3. Antepartum complication

> ***647.6#: Use an additional code to identify the maternal viral disease.***

647.6# Diseases maternal current (co-existent) in pregnancy
5th digit: 647.6
0. Episode of care NOS or N/A
1. Delivered
2. Delivered with postpartum complication
3. Antepartum complication
4. Postpartum complication

V73.99 Disease screening unspecified disease
V73.89 Disease screening other specified disease
049.9 Encephalitis
139.0 Encephalitis late effect
062.8 Encephalitis other specified mosquito-borne
063.9 Encephalitis tick borne
057.9 Exanthem
008.8 Gastroenteritis
079.99 Infection unspecified infecting agent
046.9 Infection central nervous system - slow virus
046.8 Infection central nervous system - other specified
079.89 Infection other specified

U-V-W

VIRUS, VIRAL (continued)

047.9 Meningitis
047.8 Meningitis other specified
079.99 Syndrome
066.40 West Nile NOS
066.42 West Nile with cranial nerve disorder
066.41 West Nile with encephalitis

Use an additional code with 066.42 to specify the neurologic manifestation.

066.42 West Nile with neurologic manifestation other
066.42 West Nile with optic neuritis
066.42 West Nile with polyradiculitis

Use an additional code with 066.49 to specify the other condition.

066.49 West Nile with other complications

V09.8 VISA (VANCOMYCIN (GLYCOPEPTIDE) INTERMEDIATE STAPHYLOCOCCUS AUREUS)

799.89 VISCERAL CONGESTION
128.0 VISCERAL LARVA MIGRANS SYNDROME
759.3 VISCERAL TRANSPOSITION (ABDOMINAL) (THORACIC) CONGENITAL
569.89 VISCEROPTOSIS INTESTINE
787.4 VISIBLE PERISTALSIS

VISION, VISUAL

368.34 Abnormal retinal correspondence
368.16 Agnosia
368.8 Blurred

CORTEX

377.73 Disorder
377.73 Disorder with inflammatory disorders
377.71 Disorder with neoplasms
377.72 Disorder with vascular disorders
950.3 Injury

VISION, VISUAL (continued)

368.13 Discomfort
368.30 Disorder (binocular)
306.7 Disorder psychogenic
368.16 Disorder psychophysical
368.16 Disorientation syndrome
368.14 Distortion shape and size
368.15 Distortion other (entoptic phenomena)
368.9 Disturbance

Use additional code to identify the visual disturbance.

438.7 Disturbance late effect of CVA
368.16 Disturbance psychophysical
368.10 Disturbance subjective
368.2 Double
794.13 Evoked potential abnormal
V72.0 Exam routine
V20.2 Exam routine infant or child

VISION, VISUAL (continued)

FIELD DEFECT

368.40 NOS
368.42 Angioscotoma enlarged
368.41 Central scotoma
368.41 Centrocecal scotoma
368.45 Generalized contraction or constriction
368.46 Hemianopsia (altitudinal) (homonymous)
368.47 Hemianopsia binasal
368.47 Heteronymous (bilateral)
368.44 Nasal step
368.44 Peripheral
368.46 Quadrant anopia
368.44 Scotoma
368.43 Scotoma arcuate
368.43 Scotoma bjerrum
368.42 Scotoma blind spot area
368.42 Scotoma paracecal
368.41 Scotoma paracentral
368.43 Scotoma seidel

VISION, VISUAL (continued)

368.33 Fusion with defective stereopsis
368.16 Hallucination psychophysical

Code first hearing and/or visual impairment.

V49.85 Impairment dual (combined visual hearing) (blindness with deafness)

LOSS

369.9 NOS
369.3 Both eyes unqualified
V19.0 Family history
369.4 Legal blindness as defined in U.S.A.
368.11 Sudden
V72.0 Test
368.12 Transient concentric fading
368.12 Transient scintillating scotoma
369.8 Unqualified one eye

PATHWAYS

377.9 Disorder
377.63 Disorder with inflammatory disorders
377.61 Disorder with neoplasms
377.62 Disorder with vascular disorders

VISION, VISUAL (continued)

V72.0 Screening exam
368.32 Simultaneous visual perception without fusion
V53.09 Substitution device fitting and adjustment
368.31 Suppression of binocular vision

VISION IMPAIRMENT COPYRIGHT 2004

BETTER EYE

FIRST DIGIT		Snellen Fraction	Visual Field in Degrees
0.	Vision unspecified	---------	--------
1.	Low vision NOS	---------	--------
2.	20/10 - 20/25 normal	2.0 -.80	--------
3.	20/30 - 20/60 near normal	.70 -.30	--------
4.	20/70 - 20/160 moderate	.25 -.12	--------
5.	20/200 - 20/400 severe	.10 -.05	<=20
6.	20/500 - 20/1000 profound	.04 - .02	<=10
7.	<20/1000 near total	<.02	<= 5
8.	Total blindness	----------	--------
9.	Blind NOS	----------	--------

LESSER EYE

SECOND DIGIT		Snellen Fraction	Visual Field in Degrees
0.	Vision unspecified	---------	--------
1.	Low vision NOS	---------	--------
2.	Moderate NOS	---------	--------
3.	Severe NOS	---------	--------
4.	20/70 - 20/400 moderate	.25 -.12	--------
5.	20/200 - 20/400 severe	.10 -.05	<=20
6.	20/500 - 20/1000 profound	.04 - .02	<=10
7.	<20/1000 near total	<.02	<= 5
8.	Total	----------	--------
9.	Blind NOS	----------	--------

Select the appropriate digit from the better eye, then select the second digit from the lesser eye. You now have a two digit key code which will correlate with the appropriate ICD-9 code listed in the table below.

VISION IMPAIRMENT (continued)

COPYRIGHT 2004

KEY CODE	ICD-9 CODE
01	369.70 Vision loss one eye moderate or severe impairment
04	369.74 Vision loss one eye moderate impairment other eye not specified
05	369.71 Vision loss one eye severe impairment other eye not specified
06	369.67 Vision loss one eye profound impairment other eye not specified
07	369.64 Vision loss one eye near total impairment other eye not specified
08	369.61 Vision loss one eye total impairment other eye not specified
09	369.60 Vision loss one eye profound impairment
11	369.20 Vision loss both eyes moderate or severe impairment
19	369.10 Better eye moderate or severe low vision lesser eye profound blind NOS
24	369.76 Vision loss one eye moderate impairment other eye normal vision
25	369.73 Vision loss one eye severe impairment other eye normal vision
26	369.69 Vision loss one eye profound impairment other eye normal
27	369.66 Vision loss one eye near total impairment other eye normal vision
28	369.63 Vision loss one eye total impairment other eye normal vision
34	369.75 Vision loss one eye moderate impairment other eye near normal vision
35	369.72 Vision loss one eye severe impairment other eye near normal vision
36	369.68 Vision loss one eye profound impairment other eye near normal vision

VISION IMPAIRMENT (continued)

COPYRIGHT 2004

KEY CODE	ICD-9 CODE
37	369.65 Vision loss one eye near total impairment other eye near normal vision
38	369.62 Vision loss one eye total impairment other eye near normal vision
43	369.23 Better eye moderate impairment lesser eye NOS
44	369.25 Better eye moderate impairment lesser eye moderate impairment
45	369.24 Better eye moderate impairment lesser eye severe impairment
46	369.18 Better eye moderate impairment lesser eye profound impairment
47	369.17 Better eye moderate impairment lesser eye near total impairment
48	369.16 Better eye moderate impairment lesser eye total impairment
49	369.15 Better eye moderate impairment lesser eye blind NOS
53	369.21 Vision loss better eye severe impairment lesser eye NOS
55	369.22 Vision loss better eye severe impairment lesser eye severe impairment
56	369.14 Better eye severe impairment lesser eye profound impairment
57	369.13 Better eye severe impairment lesser eye near total impairment
58	369.12 Better eye severe impairment lesser eye total impairment
59	369.11 Better eye severe impairment lesser eye blind NOS
66	369.08 Better eye profound impairment lesser eye profound impairment
67	369.07 Better eye profound impairment lesser eye near total impairment
68	369.06 Better eye profound impairment lesser eye total impairment
69	369.05 Better eye profound impairment lesser eye NOS
77	369.04 Better eye near total impairment lesser eye near total impairment
78	369.03 Better eye near total impairment lesser eye total impairment
79	369.02 Better eye near total impairment lesser eye NOS
88	369.01 Vision loss better eye total impairment lesser eye total impairment
99	369.00 Vision loss blindness both eyes NOS

0 VISUAL SEE 'VISION, VISUAL'

794.13 VISUALLY EVOKED POTENTIAL ABNORMAL
794.2 VITAL CAPACITY REDUCED
780.79 VITALITY, LACK OR WANT OF
779.89 VITALITY, LACK OR WANT OF, NEWBORN

VITAMIN

264.9 A deficiency-NOS
264.1 A deficiency-bitot's spot in young child
264.8 A deficiency-follicular keratosis
264.7 A deficiency-other ocular manifestations
264.0 A deficiency-with conjunctival xerosis
264.1 A deficiency-with conjunctival xerosis and bitot's spot
264.2 A deficiency-with corneal xerosis
264.3 A deficiency-with corneal ulceration and xerosis
264.4 A deficiency-with kerotomalacia
264.5 A deficiency-with night blindness
264.6 A deficiency-with xerophthalmic scars of cornea
264.8 A deficiency-xeroderma
278.2 A excess (hypervitaminosis)
266.9 B deficiency-NOS
266.9 B deficiency-NOS with polyneuropathy [357.4]
265.1 B1 deficiency
265.0 B1 deficiency with beriberi
266.0 B2 deficiency
266.1 B6 deficiency (syndrome)
266.1 B6 deficiency with polyneuropathy [357.4]
285.0 B6 deficiency with vitamin B6 responsive sideroblastic anemia
281.3 B12 and folic acid deficiency anemia
266.2 B12 deficiency
281.1 B12 deficiency anemia with myelopathy [336.2]
281.1 B12 deficiency anemia with subacute combined spinal cord degeneration [336.2]
266.2 B12 deficiency with cerebral degeneration [331.7]
266.2 B12 deficiency with myelopathy [336.2]
266.2 B12 deficiency with polyneuropathy [357.4]
281.1 B12 deficiency with anemia (dietary)
281.1 B12 malabsorption with proteinuria and anemia
267 C Deficiency
268.9 D Deficiency
275.3 D Deficiency causing rickets
278.4 D Excess hypervitaminosis
269.2 Deficiency NOS
269.2 Deficiency multiple
269.1 Deficiency other
269.1 E deficiency
266.0 G deficiency
269.0 K deficiency-NOS
286.7 K deficiency-causing deficiency of coagulation factor
286.7 K deficiency-coagulation defect acquired
286.7 K deficiency-due to liver disease
776.0 K deficiency-newborn
269.1 P deficiency
265.2 PP deficiency

362.76 VITELLIFORM DYSTROPHY HEREDITARY
751.0 VITELLINE DUCT PERSISTENT CONGENITAL
709.01 VITILIGO
374.53 VITILIGO EYELID
103.2 VITILIGO OF PINTA

VITREOUS

360.04 Abscess
379.29 Calcification
379.21 Cavitation
379.21 Degeneration
379.22 Deposits (crystalline)
379.21 Detachment
379.29 Disorder NOS
379.29 Disorder other
379.24 Floaters
379.23 Hemorrhage
743.51 Hyperplasia (humor) persistent congenital
379.29 Infiltrate (humor)
379.21 Liquefaction
379.25 Membranes and strands
379.24 Opacities
743.51 Opacity congenital
379.29 Other disorders
379.26 Prolapse
379.25 Strands
997.99 Touch syndrome

277.85 VLCAD, LCAD (LONG CHAIN/VERY LONG CHAIN ACYL COA DEHYDROGENASE DEFICIENCY)

272.1 VLDL ELEVATED (VERY LOW DENSITY LIPOID TYPE)

791.9 VMA (VANILLYLMANDELIC ACID) URINARY ELEVATED

VOCAL CORD

478.5 Abscess (cellulitis) (granuloma) (leukoplakia)
478.5 Chorditis
478.5 Disease NEC
478.5 Nodule
478.3# Paralysis
5th digit: 478.3
0. Unspecified
1. Unilateral partial
2. Unilateral complete
3. Bilateral partial
4. Bilateral complete
478.4 Polyp
0 See also 'Larynx, Laryngeal'

V57.22 VOCATIONAL REHABILITATION

333.71 VOGT'S DISEASE OR SYNDROME (CORPUS STRIATUM)

364.24 VOGT-KOYANAGI SYNDROME

330.1 VOGT-SPIELMEYER DISEASE

VOICE

784.49 Change
784.40 Disturbance
784.49 Hoarseness
784.41 Loss
V41.4 Problem (with production)

403.00 VOLHARD-FAHR DISEASE (MALIGNANT NEPHROSCLEROSIS)

958.6 VOLKMANN'S ISCHEMIC CONTRACTURE ACQUIRED (SYNDROME)

908.6 VOLKMANN'S ISCHEMIC CONTRACTURE LATE EFFECT

276.50 VOLUME DEPLETION NOS

276.52 VOLUME DEPLETION EXTRACELLULAR FLUID

276.52 VOLUME DEPLETION PLASMA

VOLVULUS

560.2 Colon
537.3 Duodenum
560.2 Intestine

VOMITING

787.03 NOS
787.01 NOS with nausea
0 Blood see 'Hematemesis'
779.3 Neonatal
536.2 Persistent nonpregnant
564.3 Post op GI surgery
307.54 Psychogenic
306.4 Psychogenic cyclical
536.2 Uncontrollable

VOMITING IN PREGNANCY

643.9# NOS
643.0# Hyperemesis gravidarum mild (<22 wks.)
643.1# Hyperemesis gravidarum with metabolic disturbance (<22 wks.)
643.2# Late (>22 wks.)
643.8# Due to disease or other cause
643.9# Mild
5th digit: 643.0-2, 8-9
0. Episode of care NOS or N/A
1. Delivered
3. Antepartum complication

720.0 VON BECHTEREW'S (STUMPELL) DISEASE OR SYNDROME (ANKYLOSING SPONDYLITIS)

049.8 VON ECONOMO'S DISEASE (ENCEPHALITIS LETHARGICA)

359.29 VON EULENBURG'S DISEASE (CONGENITAL PARAMYOTONIA)

271.0 VON GIERKE'S DISEASE (GLYCOGENOSIS I)

378.72 VON GRAEFE'S DISEASE OR SYNDROME

759.6 VON HIPPEL-LINDAU SYNDROME (ANGIOMATOSIS RETINOCEREBELLOSA)

285.8 VON JAKSCH'S DISEASE (PSEUDOLEUKEMIA INFANTUM)

237.71 VON RECKLINGHAUSEN'S DISEASE M9540/1

252.01 VON RECKLINGHAUSEN'S DISEASE OF BONE

275.0 VON RECKLINGHAUSEN-APPLEBAUM DISEASE (HEMOCHROMATOSIS)

453.8 VON SCHROETTER'S SYNDROME (INTERMITTENT VENOUS CLAUDICATION)

286.4 VON WILLEBRAND'S (-JURGENS) DISEASE OR SYNDROME (ANGIOHEMOPHILIA)

701.0 VON ZAMBUSCH'S DISEASE (LICHEN SCLEROSUS ET ATROPHICUS)

756.4 VOORHOEVE'S DISEASE (DYSCHONDROPLASIA)

366.21 VOSSIUS' RING TRAUMATIC

302.82 VOYEURISM

V09.8 VRE (VANCOMYCIN (GLYCOPEPTIDE) RESISTANT ENTEROCOCCUS)

756.51 VROLIK'S DISEASE (OSTEOGENESIS IMPERFECTA)

V09.8 VRSA (VANCOMYCIN (GLYCOPEPTIDE) RESISTANT STAPHYLOCOCCUS AUREUS)

745.4 VSD (VENTRICULAR SEPTAL DEFECT) CONGENITAL

684 VULGARIS IMPETIGO

VULVA, VULVAL

0	Abnormality complicating pregnancy, labor or delivery see 'Vulva, Vulval Disorders Complicating Childbirth'
752.49	Absence (agenesis) (stricture) congenital
624.8	Atresia
752.49	Atresia congenital
624.1	Atrophy
616.10	Bacterial infection NOS
233.32	Carcinoma in situ
624.8	Cyst
616.10	Disease inflammatory
0	Disorder complicating childbirth see 'Vulva, Vulval Disorders Complicating Childbirth'
616.10	Disorder inflammatory
624.10	Disorder noninflammatory
624.8	Dysplasia NOS
624.01	Dysplasia VIN I
624.02	Dysplasia VIN II
233.32	Dysplasia VIN III
624.09	Dystrophy noninflammatory
624.8	Edema
619.0	Fistula - urinary tract to vulva
619.1	Fistula - digestive to vulva
619.2	Fistula - genital tract to skin
619.8	Fistula - other
624.5	Hematoma nonobstetrical
624.8	Hemorrhage
624.09	Hyperkeratosis
624.3	Hyperplasia
624.3	Hypertrophy
959.14	Injury NEC
911.8	Injury other and unspecified superficial
911.9	Injury other and unspecified superficial infected
624.01	Intraepithelial neoplasia I (VIN I)
624.02	Intraepithelial neoplasia II (VIN II)
233.32	Intraepithelial neoplasia III (VIN III)
624.09	Kraurosis
624.4	Laceration old or scarring
624.09	Leukoplakia
624.09	Leukokraurosis
625.8	Mass
616.81	Mucositis (ulcerative)
624.8	Occlusion
624.6	Polyp
0	Previous surgery maternal see 'Vulva, Vulval Disorders Complicating Childbirth', abnormality
624.4	Scar (old)
624.8	Stricture
752.49	Stricture congenital
091.0	Syphilitic
616.50	Ulcer NOS (nonobstetrical)
136.1	Ulcer - Behcet's [616.51]
098.0	Ulcer - gonococcal
054.12	Ulcer - herpes simplex
091.0	Ulcer - syphilitic
016.7#	Ulcer - tuberculous [616.51]

5th digit: 016.7
- **0. Unspecified**
- **1. Lab not done**
- **2. Lab pending**
- **3. Microscopy positive (in sputum)**
- **4. Culture positive - microscopy negative**
- **5. Culture negative - microscopy positive**
- **6. Culture and microscopy negative confirmed by other methods**

VULVA, VULVAL (continued)

456.6	Varices
625.9	Vestibulitis

VULVA, VULVAL DISORDERS COMPLICATING CHILDBIRTH

763.89	Abnormality affecting fetus or newborn
654.8#	Abnormality complicating childbirth
660.2#	Abnormality obstructing labor **[654.8#]**
654.8#	Surgery previous complicating pregnancy childbirth or puerperium
660.2#	Surgery previous obstructing labor **[654.8#]**
654.8#	Tumor complicating childbirth
660.2#	Tumor obstructing labor **[654.8#]**

5th digit: 654.8
- **0. Episode of care NOS or N/A**
- **1. Delivered**
- **2. Delivered with postpartum complication**
- **3. Antepartum complication**
- **4. Postpartum complication**

5th digit: 660.2
- **0. Episode of care NOS or N/A**
- **1. Delivered**
- **3. Antepartum complication**

VULVITIS

616.10	NOS
752.49	Adhesive congenital
098.0	Blennorrhagic acute
098.2	Blennorrhagic chronic
099.53	Chlamydial

646.6#: Specify the maternal vulvitis with an additional code.

646.6#	Complicating pregnancy or puerperium

5th digit: 646.6
- **0. Episode of care NOS or N/A**
- **1. Delivered**
- **2. Delivered with postpartum complication**
- **3. Antepartum complication**
- **4. Postpartum complication**

098.0	Gonococcal acute
098.2	Gonococcal chronic
054.11	Herpetic
624.09	Leukoplakic
112.1	Monilial
091.0	Syphilitic early
095.8	Syphilitic late
131.01	Trichomonal

625.8	VULVODYNIA
0	VULVOVAGINITIS SEE 'VAGINITIS'

270.2	WAARDENBURG-KLEIN SYNDROME (PTOSIS EPICANTHUS)
709.3	WAGNER'S DISEASE (COLLOID MILIUM)
710.3	WAGNER (-UNVERRICHT) SYNDROME (DERMATOMYOSITIS)
780.54	WAKEFULNESS DISORDER (SEE ALSO 'HYPERSOMNIA')

732.1	WALDENSTROM'S DISEASE (OSTEOCHONDROSIS CAPITAL FEMORAL)
273.0	WALDENSTROM'S HYPERGAMMAGLOBULINEMIA
273.3	WALDENSTROM'S SYNDROME (MACROGLOBULINEMIA)
280.8	WALDENSTROM-KJELLBERG SYNDROME (SIDEROPENIC DYSPHAGIA)
719.7	WALKING DIFFICULTY
436	WALLENBERG'S SYNDROME (POSTERIOR INFERIOR CEREBELLAR ARTERY)
459.89	WALLGREN'S DISEASE (OBSTRUCTION OF SPLENIC VEIN WITH COLLATERAL CIRCULATION)
427.89	WANDERING (ATRIAL) PACEMAKER
681.9	WARDROP'S DISEASE (WITH LYMPHANGITIS)
681.02	WARDROP'S DISEASE (WITH LYMPHANGITIS) – FINGER
681.11	WARDROP'S DISEASE (WITH LYMPHANGITIS) – TOE

WARTS

078.10	NOS
078.11	Condyloma acuminatum
078.19	Fig
078.19	Genital
371.41	Hassall-Henle's of cornea
078.10	Infectious or viral
078.19	Juvenile
078.10	Moist
088.0	Peruvian
078.19	Plantar
702.0	Senile
702.1#	Seborrheic

5th digit: 702.1
1. Inflamed
9. Other

078.19	Venereal (male) (female)
078.19	Verruca (plana juvenilis) (plantaris)
078.10	Verruca vulgaris
078.10	Viral
078.19	Other specified
989.5	WASP STING
989.5	WASP STING WITH ANAPHYLAXIS [995.0]
097.1	WASSERMANN POSITIVE SCREENING EXAM
795.6	WASSERMANN REACTION FALSE POSITIVE
100.0	WASSILIEFF'S DISEASE (LEPTOSPIRAL JAUNDICE)

799.4 Wasting disease – Code first underlying condition, if known

799.4	WASTING DISEASE
366.12	WATER CLEFTS
994.3	WATER DEPRIVATION
909.4	WATER DEPRIVATION LATE EFFECT
989.5	WATER MOCCASIN BITE
995.0	WATER MOCCASIN BITE WITH ANAPHYLAXIS [989.5]
276.6	WATER OVERLOAD
276.6	WATER RETENTION SYNDROME
787.1	WATERBRASH
036.3	WATERHOUSE FRIDERICHSEN SYNDROME
537.83	WATERMELON STOMACH WITH HEMORRHAGE
537.82	WATERMELON STOMACH WITHOUT HEMORRHAGE
380.4	WAX IN EAR
277.39	WAXY DEGENERATION (DISEASE) ANY SITE
277.39	WAXY KIDNEY [583.81]

WEAK, WEAKNESS

734	Arches (foot)
754.61	Arches (foot) congenital
596.59	Bladder sphincter
781.94	Facial
780.79	Generalized
779.89	Generalized congenital
779.89	Generalized newborn
0	Leg see 'Limb Disorder'
728.87	Muscle (generalized)
618.81	Pelvic fundus - pubocervical tissue
618.81	Pelvic fundus - pubocervical tissue with stress incontinence [625.6]
618.81	Pelvic fundus - pubocervical tissue with other urinary incontinence **[788.3#]**
618.82	Pelvic fundus - rectovaginal tissue
618.82	Pelvic fundus - rectovaginal tissue with stress incontinence [625.6]
618.82	Pelvic fundus - rectovaginal tissue with other urinary incontinence **[788.3#]**

5th digit: 788.3
1. Urge incontinence
3. Mixed urge and stress
4. Without sensory awareness
5. Post-void dribbling
6. Nocturnal enuresis
7. Continuous leakage
8. Overflow incontinence
9. Other

785.9	Pulse
0	WEAKNESS SEE 'WEAK, WEAKNESS'
991.9	WEATHER EFFECT COLD
992.9	WEATHER EFFECT HEAT
909.4	WEATHER EFFECT LATE EFFECT COLD OR HEAT
692.74	WEATHERED SKIN
748.69	WEBBED ALVEOLI CONGENITAL
0	WEBBING OF DIGITS SEE 'SYNDACTYLY, SYNDACTYLIC'
729.30	WEBER-CHRISTIAN DISEASE OR SYNDROME (NODULAR NONSUPPURATIVE PANNICULITIS)
757.39	WEBER-COCKAYNE SYNDROME (EPIDERMOLYSIS BULLOSA)
759.6	WEBER-DIMITRI SYNDROME (ENCEPHALOCUTANEOUS ANGIOMATOSIS)
344.89	WEBER-GUBLER SYNDROME
344.89	WEBER-LEYDEN SYNDROME
448.0	WEBER-OSLER SYNDROME (FAMILIAL HEMORRHAGIC TELANGIECTASIA)
733.00	WEDGING OF VERTEBRA NOS

446.4 WEGENER'S SYNDROME (NECROTIZING RESPIRATORY GRANULOMATOSIS)

648.9# WEGENER'S SYNDROME (NECROTIZING RESPIRATORY GRANULOMATOSIS) MATERNAL CURRENT (CO-EXISTENT) IN PREGNANCY [446.4]

5th digit: 648.9

0. Episode of care NOS or N/A
1. Delivered
2. Delivered with postpartum complication
3. Antepartum complication
4. Postpartum complication

090.0 WEGNER'S DISEASE (SYPHILITIC OSTEOCHONDRITIS)

646.##: Specify the maternal weight gain with an additional code for the condition causing the abnormal weight.

WEIGHT

278.02 Excess
783.1 Gain abnormal

For codes 278.0, 278.02, 783.21 and 783.22, use an additional code to identify Body Mass Index if known. These codes can be found under 'Body Mass Index'.

278.00 Gain abnormal - obesity
278.01 Gain abnormal - obesity morbid (severe)
646.1# Gain excessive in pregnancy

5th digit: 646.1

0. Episode of care NOS or N/A
1. Delivered
2. Delivered with postpartum complication
3. Antepartum complication
4. Postpartum complication

642.## Gain excessive with pregnancy with hypertension

4th digit: 642

0. Benign essential
1. Secondary to renal disease
2. Other pre-existing
3. Transient

5th digit: 642

0. Episode of care NOS or N/A
1. Delivered
2. Delivered with postpartum complication
3. Antepartum complication
4. Postpartum complication

783.41 Gain failure in childhood
646.8# Gain insufficient in pregnancy

5th digit: 646.8

0. Episode of care NOS or N/A
1. Delivered
2. Delivered with postpartum complication
3. Antepartum complication
4. Postpartum complication

783.21 Loss abnormal (unknown cause)
783.22 Underweight

100.0 WEIL'S DISEASE (LEPTOSPIRAL JAUNDICE)
759.89 WEILL-MARCHESANI SYNDROME (BRACHYMORPHISM AND ECTOPIA LENTIS)

518.3 WEINGARTEN'S SYNDROME (TROPICAL EOSINOPHILIA)
443.82 WEIR MITCHELL'S DISEASE (ERYTHROMELALGIA)
337.0 WEISS-BAKER SYNDROME (CAROTID SINUS SYNCOPE)
710.1 WEISSENBACH-THIBIERGE SYNDROME (CUTANEOUS SYSTEMIC SCLEROSIS)
710.1 WEISSENBACH-THIBIERGE SYNDROME (CUTANEOUS SYSTEMIC SCLEROSIS) WITH LUNG INVOLVEMENT [517.2]
710.1 WEISSENBACH-THIBIERGE SYNDROME (CUTANEOUS SYSTEMIC SCLEROSIS) WITH MYOPATHY [359.6]
040.0 WELCHII BACILLUS INFECTION
370.24 WELDER'S FLASH
V20.2 WELL BABY CHECK
V20.2 WELL CHILD CHECK
V20.2 WELL NEWBORN CHECK INITIAL OR SUSEQUENT
V65.5 WELL-WORRIED EXAM
706.2 WEN
426.13 WENCKEBACK'S HEART BLOCK
335.0 WERDNIG-HOFFMANN DISEASE OR SYNDROME
287.39 WERLHOF'S DISEASE
287.39 WERLHOF-WICHMANN SYNDROME
258.01 WERMER'S SYNDROME (POLYGLANDULAR) (POLYENDOCRINE ADENOMATOSIS)
259.8 WERNER'S SYNDROME (PROGERIA ADULTORUM)
083.1 WERNER HIS DISEASE (TRENCH FEVER)
288.09 WERNER -SCHULTZ DISEASE (AGRANULOCYTOSIS)
291.1 WERNICKE SYNDROME (ALCOHOLIC) ACUTE
265.1 WERNICKE'S ENCEPHALOPATHY (SUPERIOR HEMORRHAGIC POLIOENCEPHALITIS)
291.1 WERNICKE-KORSAKOFF SYNDROME ALCOHOLIC
294.0 WERNICKE-KORSAKOFF SYNDROME NONALCOHOLIC
114.9 WERNICKE-POSADAS DISEASE
066.3 WESSELSBRON FEVER (VIRAL)

WEST NILE FEVER (VIRUS)

066.40 NOS
066.42 Cranial nerve disorder
066.41 Encephalitis

Use an additional code with 066.42 to specify the neurologic manifestation.

066.42 Neurologic manifestation other
066.42 Optic neuritis
066.42 Polyradiculitis

Use an additional code with 066.49 to specify the other condition.

066.49 Other complications

062.1 WESTERN EQUINE ENCEPHALITIS
275.1 WESTPHAL-STRUMPELL SYNDROME (HEPATOLENTICULAR DEGENERATION)

303.9#	WET BRAIN SYNDROME (ALCOHOLIC) **5th digit: 303.9** **0. NOS** **1. Continuous** **2. Episodic** **3. In remission**
991.4	WET FEET SYNDROME (MACERATION) (TROPICAL)
518.5	WET LUNG SYNDROME
770.6	WET LUNG SYNDROME NEWBORN
V53.8	WHEELCHAIR FITTING AND ADJUSTMENT
	WHEEZING
786.07	NOS
0	Asthmatic see 'Asthma, Asthmatic'
995.7	Due to adverse food reaction NEC [786.07]
847.0	WHIPLASH NECK (SYNDROME)
040.2	WHIPPLE'S DISEASE OR SYNDROME (INTESTINAL LIPODYSTROPHY)
127.3	WHIPWORM INFECTION
759.89	WHISTLING FACE SYNDROME (CRANIOCARPOTARSAL DYSTROPHY)
757.39	WHITE'S DISEASE (CONGENITAL) (KERATOSIS FOLLICULARIS)
	WHITE BLOOD CELL
288.60	Count elevated, abnormal findings
288.69	Count elevated, specified NEC, abnormal findings
288.50	Count low, abnormal findings
288.59	Count low, abnormal findings other specified
288.9	Differential, abnormal findings
288.9	Disease
288.8	Disease specified NEC
288.8	Granulocytic hyperplasia
288.9	Morphology, abnormal findings
518.82	WHITE LUNG SYNDROME
111.2	WHITE PIEDRA
521.01	WHITE SPOT LESION TEETH
681.01	WHITLOW
054.6	WHITLOW HERPES SIMPLEX
025	WHITMORE'S DISEASE (MELIOIDOSIS)
	WHOOPING COUGH
033.9	Unspecified organism
033.8	Bordetella bronchiseptica [B. bronchiseptica]
033.1	Bordetella parapertussis [B. parapertussis]
033.0	Bordetella pertussis [B. pertussis]
033.8	Due to other specified organism
V01.89	Exposure
033.#	Pneumonia [484.3] **4th digit: 033** **0. B. Pertussis** **1. B. Parapertussis** **8. B. Bronchiseptica** **9. Unspecified organism**
V74.8	Screening exam
283.9	WIDAL-ABRAMI DISEASE OR SYNDROME (ACQUIRED HEMOLYTIC JAUNDICE)
557.1	WILKIE'S DISEASE OR SYNDROME
694.1	WILKINSON-SNEDDON DISEASE OR SYNDROME (SUBCORNEAL PUSTULAR DERMATOSIS)
696.1	WILLAN-PLUMBE SYNDROME (PSORIASIS)
286.4	WILLEBRAND (-JURGENS) SYNDROME (ANGIOHEMOPHILIA)
759.81	WILLI-PRADER SYNDROME (HYPOGENITAL DYSTROPHY WITH DIABETIC TENDENCY)
189.0	WILM'S TUMOR M8960/3
695.89	WILSON-BROCQ DISEASE (DERMATITIS EXFOLIATIVA)
275.1	WILSON'S DISEASE OR SYNDROME (HEPATOLENTICULAR DEGENERATION)
275.1	WILSON'S DISEASE OR SYNDROME (HEPATOLENTICULAR DEGENERATION) WITH DEMENTIA [294.1#] **5th digit: 294.1** **0. Without behavioral disturbance or NOS** **1. With behavioral disturbance**
770.7	WILSON-MIKITY SYNDROME
380.00	WINKLER'S DISEASE
698.8	WINTER ITCH
078.82	WINTER VOMITING DISEASE
696.2	WISE'S DISEASE
279.12	WISKOTT-ALDRICH SYNDROME (ECZEMA-THROMBOCYTOPENIA)
	WITHDRAWAL
291.0	Alcohol - delirium (tremens)
291.3	Alcohol - hallucinosis (psychosis)
291.81	Alcohol - symptoms or syndrome
760.71	Alcohol - symptoms or syndrome newborn
292.0	Drug - symptoms or syndrome
779.5	Drug - symptoms or syndrome newborn or infant of dependent mother
313.22	Reaction of childhood or adolescence
255.41	Steroid - symptoms or syndrome correct substance properly administered NOS
471.1	WOAKE'S SYNDROME (ETHMOIDITIS)
335.11	WOHLFART-KUGELBERG-WELANDER DISEASE
518.5	WOILLEZ'S DISEASE (ACUTE IDIOPATHIC PULMONARY CONGESTION)
426.7	WOLFF-PARKINSON-WHITE SYNDROME (ANOMALOUS ATRIOVENTRICULAR EXCITATION)
752.89	WOLFFIAN DUCT PERSISTENCE (CONGENITAL)
083.1	WOLHYNIAN FEVER
272.7	WOLMAN'S DISEASE (PRIMARY FAMILIAL XANTHOMATOSIS)
0	WOMB SEE 'UTERUS, UTERINE'
495.8	WOOD ASTHMA
022.1	WOOL SORTER'S DISEASE
315.31	WORD DEAFNESS
V62.2	WORK DISSATISFACTION
V62.1	WORK PROBLEM (ADVERSE EFFECT OF WORK ENVIRONMENT)
102.3	WORM-EATEN SOLES
128.9	WORMS
127.9	WORMS INTESTINAL
780.79	WORN OUT (EXHAUSTION)

V65.5 WORRIED WELL EXAM

When coding an infection, use an additional code, [041.#], to identify the organism. See 'Bacterial Infection'.

WOUND

V58.3# Check (laceration)
5th digit: V58.3
0. NOS or nonsurgical wound dressing removal or change
1. Surgical wound dressing removal or change
2. Removal of sutures or staples

V58.41 Closure post op planned
674.3# Complication post op other specified maternal due to pregnancy
5th digit: 674.3
0. Episode of care unspecified or N/A
2. Delivered with postpartum complication
4. Postpartum complication

795.39 Culture abnormal
998.32 Dehiscence post op
674.1# Dehiscence post op C - section
674.2# Dehiscence post op episiotomy
5th digit: 674.1-2
0. NOS
2. Delivered with postpartum complication
4. Postpartum complication

998.32 Dehiscence post op external
998.31 Dehiscence post op internal
674.2# Dehiscence post op perineal first degree through fourth degree repair
674.2# Dehiscence post op perineal maternal due to pregnancy
674.1# Dehiscence post op uterine maternal due to pregnancy
5th digit: 674.1-2
0. NOS
2. Delivered with postpartum complication
4. Postpartum complication

998.12 Hematoma complicating a procedure
674.3# Hematoma or hemorrhage post op C-section or perineal procedure
5th digit: 674.3
0. Episode of care unspecified or N/A
2. Delivered with postpartum complication
4. Postpartum complication

998.59 Infection post op
909.3 Infection post op late effect
674.3# Infection post op C-section
674.3# Infection post op perineal procedure maternal due to pregnancy
5th digit: 674.3
0. Episode of care unspecified or N/A
2. Delivered with postpartum complication
4. Postpartum complication

958.3 Infection posttraumatic NEC
908.6 Infection posttraumatic NEC late effect
998.51 Infection post op seroma

WOUND (continued)

0 Open see 'Open Wound', by site
998.59 Operation granuloma
V58.3# Packing
5th digit: V58.3
0. NOS or nonsurgical wound dressing removal or change
1. Surgical wound dressing removal or change

767.8 Scalpel wound (birth trauma)
0 Superficial see 'Abrasion', by site
998.83 Surgical non-healing

447.8 WRIGHT'S SYNDROME (HYPERABDUCTION)
0 WRINGER INJURY SEE 'CRUSH INJURY'
701.8 WRINKLING SKIN

WRIST

V49.64 Amputation status
0 Bones see also 'Carpal'
726.4 Capsulitis
736.00 Deformity acquired
736.05 Drop (acquired)
959.3 Injury
913.8 Injury other and unspecified superficial
913.9 Injury other and unspecified superficial - infected
0 Joint see also 'Joint'
719.83 Joint calcification
718.93 Joint ligament relaxation
718.13 Joint loose body
V54.81 Joint replacement aftercare [V43.63]
V43.63 Joint replacement status
842.0# Sprain (strain) (avulsion) (hemarthrosis)
5th digit: 842.0
0. NOS site
1. Carpal (joint)
2. Radiocarpal (joint) (ligament)
9. Other or radioulnar joint (distal)

719.83 Triangular cartilage complex
736.03 Valgus deformity (acquired)
736.04 Varus deformity (acquired)

333.84 WRITERS' CRAMP ORGANIC
300.89 WRITERS' CRAMP PSYCHOGENIC
315.2 WRITTEN EXPRESSION DISORDER (LEARNING DIFFICULTY)
754.1 WRY NECK CONGENITAL
125.0 WUCHERERIASIS BANCROFTI
125.1 WUCHERERIASIS BRUGIA MALAYI

U-V-W

277.86	X- LINKED ADRENOLEUKODYSTROPHY
413.9	X SYNDROME

X-RAY STUDIES

793.#(#) Abnormal findings (nonspecific)

4th or 4th and 5th digit: 793
- **0. Skull and head**
- **1. Lung field**
- **2. Other intrathoracic**
- **3. Biliary tract**
- **4. Gastrointestinal tract**
- **5. Genitourinary organs**
- **6. Abdominal area including retroperitoneum**
- **7. Musculoskeletal system**
- **8#.Breast**
  - **80. Unspecified**
  - **81. Mammographic microcalcification**
  - **89. Other abnormal findings (calcification) (calculus)**
- **9#. Other**
  - **91. Inconclusive due to excess body fat**
  - **99. Other abnormal findings (placenta) (skin) (subcutaneous)**

> ***When using code 793.91, Image test inconclusive due to excess body fat, use additional code to identify body mass index (BMI) which can be found at 'Body Mass Index'.***

990	Adverse effects
909.2	Adverse effects late effect
V71.2	Chest for TB
V72.5	Chest (routine)
V72.5	Routine NEC
272.2	XANTHELASMA HYPERCHOLESTEROLEMIA [374.51]
272.2	XANTHELASMATOSIS ESSENTIAL
757.33	XANTHELASMOIDEA
277.2	XANTHINURIA
277.2	XANTHINURIA METABOLISM DISORDERS

XANTHOMA

272.7	Bone
277.89	Craniohypophyseal
272.7	Cutaneotendinous dissemination
272.2	Eyelid (planum) (tuberosum) [374.51]
272.0	Hypercholesterinemic
272.4	Hyperlipidemic
272.2	Tuberosum
272.7	XANTHOMATOSIS JUVENILE
272.7	XANTHOMATOSIS PRIMARY FAMILIAL
709.09	XANTHOSIS
998.81	XANTHOSIS SURGICAL
302.89	XENOPHILIA
300.29	XENOPHOBIA

XERODERMA

701.1	Acquired
757.39	Congenital
373.33	Eyelid
757.33	Pigmentosum congenital
264.8	Due to vitamin A deficiency
V72.5	XEROGRAM
V72.5	XEROMAMMOGRAPHY
793.8#	XEROGRAPHY ABNORMAL

5th digit: 793.8
- **0. Unspecified**
- **1. Mammographic microcalcification**
- **9. Other abnormal findings (calcification) (calculus)**

372.53	XEROPHTHALMIA
264.7	XEROPHTHALMIA DUE TO VITAMIN A DEFICIENCY

XEROSIS

372.53	Conjunctival
371.40	Cornea
370.00	Cornea (with ulceration)
706.8	Cutis
527.7	XEROSTOMIA
733.99	XIPHOIDITIS
733.99	XIPHOIDYNIA (XIPHOIDALGIA SYNDROME)
759.4	XIPHOPAGUS
758.6	XO SYNDROME
758.81	XXX SYNDROME (COMPLEMENT)
758.81	XXXXY SYNDROME
758.7	XXY SYNDROME
271.8	XYLOSURIA CARBOHYDRATE TRANSPORT DISORDERS
271.8	XYLULOSURIA CARBOHYDRATE TRANSPORT DISORDERS
758.81	XYY SYNDROME (COMPLEMENT)
306.1	YAWNING PSYCHOGENIC

YAWS

102.9	NOS
102.6	Bone and joint lesions
102.1	Butter
102.0	Chancre (initial lesion)
102.2	Cutaneous, less than five years after infection
102.2	Early (cutaneous) (macular) (papular) (maculopapular) (micropapular)
102.9	Eyelid dermatitis [373.4]
102.2	Frambeside
102.5	Gangosa
102.4	Gummata and ulcers
102.3	Hyperkeratosis (palmar or plantar)
102.7	Juxta articular nodules
102.8	Latent
102.7	Manifestation other
102.0	Mother
102.7	Mucosal
102.1	Multiple papillomata and wet crab
102.4	Nodular late (ulcerated)
102.1	Palmar papilloma
102.1	Plantar papilloma
102.8	Positive serology without clinical manifestations
V74.6	Screening exam
102.2	Skin lesions other early

112.9	YEAST INFECTION SITE UNSPECIFIED (SEE ALSO 'CANDIDIASIS')

YELLOW ATROPHY

571.5	Healed
570	Liver acute
571.8	Liver chronic
570	Liver postop

YELLOW FEVER

060.9	NOS
060.0	Jungle
V73.4	Screening exam
060.0	Sylvatic
060.1	Urban
V04.4	Vaccination

762.2	YELLOW VERNIX SYNDROME (PLACENTAL DYSFUNCTION)
008.44	YERSINIA ENTEROCOLITICA (INTESTINAL INFECTION)
0	YERSINIA (PATEURELLA) PESTIS INFECTION SEE 'PLAGUE'
027.8	YERSINIA SEPTICA
758.7	YXX SYNDROME
527.7	ZAGARI'S DISEASE (XEROSTOMIA)
058.10	ZAHORSKY'S DISEASE (EXANTHEM SUBITUM) NOS
058.11	ZAHORSKY'S DISEASE (EXANTHEM SUBITUM) DUE TO HUMAN HERPESVIRUS 6
058.12	ZAHORSKY'S DISEASE (EXANTHEM SUBITUM) DUE TO HUMAN HERPESVIRUS 7
277.86	ZELLWEGER SYNDROME
530.6	ZENKER'S DIVERTICULUM
333.6	ZIEHEN-OPPENHEIM (SCHWALBE-) DISEASE
571.1	ZIEVE'S SYNDROME (JAUNDICE, HYPERLIPEMIA AND HEMOLYTIC ANEMIA)
066.3	ZIKA FEVER (VIRAL)
790.6	ZINC ABNORMAL BLOOD LEVEL
251.5	ZOLLINGER-ELLISON SYNDROME (GASTRIC HYPERSECRETION WITH PANCREATIC ISLET CELL TUMOR)
0	ZONA SEE 'HERPES ZOSTER' FOR COMPLICATION
053.9	ZONA
027.9	ZOONOTIC BACTERIAL DISEASE
027.8	ZOONOTIC BACTERIAL DISEASES OTHER SPECIFIED
302.1	ZOOPHILIA
300.29	ZOOPHOBIA
117.4	ZOPFIA LEPTOSPHAERIAL SENEGALENSIS INFECTION
281.2	ZUELZER-OGDEN SYNDROME (NUTRITIONAL MEGALOBLASTIC ANEMIA)
755.10	ZYGODACTYLY
738.11	ZYGOMATIC HYPERPLASIA (ACQUIRED)
738.12	ZYGOMATIC HYPOPLASIA (ACQUIRED)
117.7	ZYGOMYCOSIS

APPENDIX A

E CODE DIRECTORY

ACCIDENT VEHICULAR

IN ORDER TO IDENTIFY VEHICLE ACCIDENTS WHERE A PATIENT IS ACCIDENTALLY STRUCK BY A FALLING OBJECT, USE CODE E916 STRUCK BY FALLING OBJECT AS AN ADDITIONAL CODE.

RAILWAY

0 DUE TO NATURAL CATACLYSM SEE 'NATURAL CATACLYSM'
E800.# COLLISION WITH OTHER MOVING RAILCAR
E801.# COLLISION WITH OTHER OBJECT
E802.# DERAILMENT WITHOUT COLLISION
E803.# EXPLOSION FIRE OR BURNING
E804.# FALL IN, ON, OR FROM
E805.# HIT BY TRAIN
E806.# HIT BY OBJECT SET IN MOTION BY TRAIN OR OTHER SPECIFIED
E807.# UNSPECIFIED

4th Digit: E800 - 807
- **0. RAILWAY EMPLOYEE**
- **1. PASSENGER ON TRAIN**
- **2. PEDESTRIAN**
- **3. BICYCLIST**
- **8. OTHER SPECIFIED PERSON**
- **9. UNSPECIFIED PERSON**

MOTOR VEHICLE ON PUBLIC ROADWAY

0 DUE TO NATURAL CATACLYSM SEE 'NATURAL CATACLYSM'
E810.# WITH TRAIN
E811.# RE-ENTRANT WITH ANOTHER MOTOR VEHICLE
E812.# WITH ANOTHER MOTOR VEHICLE
E813.# WITH ANOTHER VEHICLE
E814.# WITH PEDESTRIAN
E815.# WITH ANOTHER VEHICLE ON HIGHWAY
E816.# LOSS OF CONTROL WITHOUT COLLISION
E817.# GETTING INTO OR OUT OF VEHICLE
E818.# NON COLLISION ACCIDENT (FLYING OBJECTS SET IN MOTION BY VEHICLE)
E819.# UNSPECIFIED NATURE

4th Digit: E810 - 819
- **0. DRIVER**
- **1. PASSENGER**
- **2. MOTORCYCLIST**
- **3. PASSENGER ON MOTORCYCLE**
- **4. PASSENGER IN STREETCAR**
- **5. RIDER ON ANIMAL OR ANIMAL DRAWN VEHICLE**
- **6. BICYCLIST**
- **7. PEDESTRIAN**
- **8. OTHER SPECIFIED PERSON**
- **9. UNSPECIFIED PERSON**

ACCIDENT VEHICULAR (continued)

IN ORDER TO IDENTIFY VEHICLE ACCIDENTS WHERE A PATIENT IS ACCIDENTALLY STRUCK BY A FALLING OBJECT, USE CODE E916 STRUCK BY FALLING OBJECT AS AN ADDITIONAL CODE.

MOTOR VEHICLE NOT ON PUBLIC ROAD

0 DUE TO NATURAL CATACLYSM SEE 'NATURAL CATACLYSM'
E820.# SNOWMOBILE
E821.# OFF ROAD VEHICLE
E822.# COLLISION WITH MOVING OBJECT
E823.# COLLISION WITH STATIONARY OBJECT
E824.# WHILE GETTING ON OR OFF
E825.# OTHER AND UNSPECIFIED (CO) (STRUCK BY OBJECT)

4th Digit: E820 - 825
- **0. DRIVER**
- **1. PASSENGER**
- **2. MOTORCYCLIST**
- **3. PASSENGER ON MOTORCYCLE**
- **4. OCCUPANT OF STREETCAR**
- **5. RIDER OF ANIMAL OR ANIMAL DRAWN VEHICLE**
- **6. BICYCLIST**
- **7. PEDESTRIAN**
- **8. OTHER SPECIFIED PERSON**
- **9. UNSPECIFIED PERSON**

NON MOTOR VEHICLE

E826.# BICYCLE

4th Digit: E826
- **0. PEDESTRIAN**
- **1. BICYCLIST**
- **2. RIDER OF ANIMAL**
- **3. OCCUPANT OF ANIMAL DRAWN VEHICLE**
- **4. OCCUPANT OF STREETCAR**
- **8. OTHER SPECIFIED PERSON**
- **9. UNSPECIFIED PERSON**

E827.# ANIMAL DRAWN
E828.# ANIMAL RIDDEN
E829.# STREETCAR

4th Digit: E827 - 829
- **0. PEDESTRIAN**
- **2. RIDER OF ANIMAL**
- **3. OCCUPANT OF ANIMAL DRAWN VEHICLE**
- **4. OCCUPANT OF STREETCAR**
- **8. OTHER SPECIFIED PERSON**
- **9. UNSPECIFIED PERSON**

ACCIDENT VEHICULAR (continued)

IN ORDER TO IDENTIFY VEHICLE ACCIDENTS WHERE A PATIENT IS ACCIDENTALLY STRUCK BY A FALLING OBJECT, USE CODE E916 STRUCK BY FALLING OBJECT AS AN ADDITIONAL CODE.

WATERCRAFT

E830.# SINKING OR CAPSIZING
E831.# ANY INJURY WHETHER COLLISION OR NOT
E832.# FALLING OVERBOARD WHETHER DROWNED OR NOT
E833.# FALL FROM LADDER
E834.# FALL FROM UPPER LEVEL
E835.# OTHER AND UNSPECIFIED
E836.# MACHINERY ACCIDENT
E837.# EXPLOSION, FIRE, OR BURNING
E838.# OTHER AND UNSPECIFIED (BOAT ACCIDENT) (STRUCK BY BOAT)

4th Digit: E830 - 838

0. OCCUPANT OF SMALL BOAT - UNPOWERED
1. OCCUPANT OF SMALL BOAT - POWERED
2. OCCUPANT OF OTHER CRAFT - CREW
3. OCCUPANT OF OTHER CRAFT - NON CREW
4. WATER SKIER
5. SWIMMER
6. DOCKERS / STEVEDORE
8. OTHER SPECIFIED PERSON
9. UNSPECIFIED PERSON

AIRCRAFT OR SPACECRAFT

E840.# DURING TAKEOFF OR LANDING - POWERED AIRCRAFT
E841.# OTHER AND UNSPECIFIED - POWERED AIRCRAFT

4th Digit: E840 - 841

0. OCCUPANT OF SPACECRAFT
1. OCCUPANT OF MILITARY AIRCRAFT
2. CREW OF COMMERCIAL AIRCRAFT
3. OCCUPANT OF COMMERCIAL AIRCRAFT SURFACE TO SURFACE
4. OCCUPANT OF COMMERCIAL AIRCRAFT SURFACE TO AIR
5. OCCUPANT OF OTHER POWERED AIRCRAFT
6. OCCUPANT OF UNPOWERED AIRCRAFT
7. PARACHUTIST
8. GROUND CREW-AIRLINE EMPLOYEE
9. OTHER PERSON

E842.# UNPOWERED AIRCRAFT

4th Digit: E842

6. OCCUPANT OF UNPOWERED AIRCRAFT
7. PARACHUTIST
8. GROUND CREW-AIRLINE EMPLOYEE
9. OTHER PERSON

ACCIDENT VEHICULAR (continued)

E843.# FALL IN/OUT OF AIRCRAFT
E844.# OTHER SPECIFIED AIR TRANSPORT ACCIDENT

4th Digit: E843 - 844

0. OCCUPANT OF SPACECRAFT
1. OCCUPANT OF MILITARY AIRCRAFT
2. CREW OF COMMERCIAL AIRCRAFT
3. OCCUPANT OF COMMERCIAL AIRCRAFT SURFACE TO SURFACE
4. OCCUPANT OF COMMERCIAL AIRCRAFT SURFACE TO AIR
5. OCCUPANT OF OTHER POWERED AIRCRAFT
6. OCCUPANT OF UNPOWERED AIRCRAFT
7. PARACHUTIST
8. GROUND CREW-AIRLINE EMPLOYEE
9. OTHER PERSON

E845.# SPACECRAFT

4th Digit: E845

0. OCCUPANT OF SPACECRAFT
8. GROUND CREW-AIRLINE EMPLOYEE
9. OTHER PERSON

OTHER VEHICLES NEC

E846 POWERED VEHICLES USED SOLELY WITHIN BUILDINGS OR ESTABLISHMENTS
E847 CABLE CARS NOT RUNNING ON RAILS
E848 VEHICLES NEC

PLACE OF OCCURRENCE CODES [E849.#] ARE USED TO INDICATE THE PLACE WHERE THE INJURY OR POISONING OCCURRED.

PLACE OF OCCURRENCE

E849.# PLACE OF OCCURRENCE

4th Digit: E849

0. HOME
1. FARM
2. MINE OR QUARRY
3. INDUSTRIAL PLACE OR PREMISES
4. RECREATIONAL AREA
5. STREET OR HIGHWAY
6. PUBLIC BUILDING
7. INSTITUTION (HOSPITAL, DORM, PRISON, ETC.)
8. OTHER SPECIFIED PLACE
9. UNSPECIFIED PLACE

MISADVENTURES DURING SURGERY / PROCEDURE OR MEDICAL CARE

E870.# ACCIDENTAL CUT, PUNCTURE, PERFORATION, HEMORRHAGE DURING CARE

E870.7 ACCIDENTAL CUT, PUNCTURE, PERFORATION, HEMORRHAGE DURING ADMINISTRATION OF ENEMA

E871.# FOREIGN BODY LEFT IN BODY DURING A PROCEDURE

E871.7 FOREIGN BODY LEFT IN BODY DURING REMOVAL CATHETER / PACKING

E872.# FAILURE OF STERILE PRECAUTIONS DURING PROCEDURE

4th Digit: E870, E871, E872

0. SURGICAL OPERATION
1. INFUSION OR TRANSFUSION
2. KIDNEY DIALYSIS / OTHER PERFUSION
3. INJECTION / VACCINATION
4. ENDOSCOPIC EXAMINATION
5. ASPIRATION FLUID OR TISSUE, PUNCTURE, AND CATHETERIZATION
6. HEART CATHETERIZATION
8. OTHER SPECIFIED MEDICAL CARE
9. NOS MEDICAL CARE

E873.# FAILURE IN DOSAGE

4th Digit: E873

0. EXCESSIVE BLOOD OR OTHER FLUID DURING INFUSION / PERFUSION
1. INCORRECT DILUTION OF FLUID DURING INFUSION
2. OVERDOSE OF RADIATION IN THERAPY
3. INADVERTENT EXPOSURE OF PATIENT TO RADIATION
4. FAILURE IN DOSAGE ELECTROSHOCK OR INSULIN-SHOCK THERAPY
5. INAPPROPRIATE TEMPERATURE IN LOCAL APPLICATION AND PACKING
6. NONADMINISTRATION OF NECESSARY DRUG OR MEDICINAL SUBSTANCE
8. OTHER SPECIFIED FAILURE IN DOSAGE
9. NOS FAILURE IN DOSAGE

E874.# MECHANICAL FAILURE OF INSTRUMENT OR APPARATUS DURING PROCEDURE

4th Digit: E874

0. SURGICAL OPERATION
1. INFUSION OR TRANSFUSION
2. KIDNEY DIALYSIS / OTHER PERFUSION
3. ENDOSCOPIC EXAMINATION
4. ASPIRATION FLUID OR TISSUE, PUNCTURE, AND CATHETERIZATION
5. HEART CATHETERIZATION
8. OTHER SPECIFIED MEDICAL CARE
9. NOS MEDICAL CARE

MISADVENTURES DURING SURGERY / PROCEDURE OR MEDICAL CARE (continued)

E875.# CONTAMINATION OR INFECTED BLOOD, OTHER FLUID, DRUG, OR BIOLOGICAL SUBSTANCE

4th Digit: E875

0. CONTAMINATED SUBSTANCE TRANSFUSION / INFUSION
1. CONTAMINATED SUBSTANCE INJECTION / VACCINATION
2. CONTAMINATED DRUG / BIOLOGICAL SUBSTANCE ADMINISTERED OTHER MEANS
8. OTHER CONTAMINATED SUBSTANCE
9. UNSPECIFIED CONTAMINATED SUBSTANCE

E876.# OTHER AND UNSPECIFIED MISADVENTURES DURING MEDICAL CARE

4th Digit: E876

0. MISMATCHED BLOOD IN TRANSFUSION
1. WRONG FLUID IN INFUSION
2. FAILURE IN SUTURE AND LIGATURE DURING SURGERY
3. ENDOTRACHEAL TUBE WRONGLY PLACED DURING ANESTHESIA
4. FAILURE TO REMOVE TUBE OR OTHER TUBE / INSTRUMENT
5. PERFORMANCE OF INAPPROPRIATE OPERATION
8. OTHER SPECIFIED MISADVENTURES
9. NOS MISADVENTURE

SURGICAL/MEDICAL PROCEDURES CAUSING ABNORMAL REACTION OF PATIENT OR LATER COMPLICATION

E878.# DUE TO SURGICAL OPERATION

4th Digit: E878

0. TRANSPLANT WHOLE ORGAN
1. ARTIFICIAL IMPLANT, DEVICE
2. ANASTOMOSIS, BYPASS, OR GRAFT
3. OSTOMY
4. OTHER RESTORATIVE SURGERY
5. AMPUTATION LIMB(S)
6. ORGAN REMOVAL
8. OTHER SPECIFIED PROCEDURES
9. UNSPECIFIED PROCEDURE

E879.# DUE TO OTHER PROCEDURE

4th Digit: E879

0. CARDIAC CATHETERIZATION
1. KIDNEY DIALYSIS
2. RADIOLOGICAL PROCEDURE
3. SHOCK THERAPY
4. ASPIRATION OF FLUID
5. INSERTION OF GASTRIC OR DUODENAL SOUND
6. URINARY CATHETERIZATION
7. BLOOD SAMPLING
8. OTHER SPECIFIED, BLOOD TRANSFUSION
9. UNSPECIFIED PROCEDURE

FALLS

FROM/INTO DIFFERENT LEVELS

E880.0 ESCALATOR
E880.1 CURB/SIDEWALK - NONMOVING
E880.9 STAIRS/STEPS
E881.0 LADDER
E881.1 SCAFFOLDING
E882 BUILDING OR STRUCTURE (FIRE ESCAPE)
E883.0 WATER/SWIMMING POOL
E883.1 WELL
E883.2 STORM DRAIN OR MANHOLE
E883.9 OTHER HOLE
E884.0 PLAYGROUND EQUIPMENT
E884.1 CLIFF
E884.2 CHAIR
E884.3 WHEELCHAIR
E884.4 BED
E884.5 OTHER FURNITURE
E884.6 COMMODE/TOILET
E884.9 FROM ONE LEVEL TO ANOTHER

FROM/INTO SAME LEVEL

E885.0 SCOOTER (NON MOTORIZED)
E885.1 ROLLER SKATES OR INLINE SKATES
E885.2 SKATEBOARD
E885.3 SKIS
E885.4 SNOWBOARD
E885.9 SIDEWALK - MOVING
E885.9 SLIPPING ON ICE
E885.9 SLIPPING ON MUD
E885.9 SLIPPING ON OIL
E885.9 SLIPPING ON SLIPPERY SURFACE
E885.9 SLIPPING ON SNOW
E885.9 SLIPPING OR TRIPPING OTHER
E885.9 SLIPPING ON WET SURFACE
E885.9 STUMBLING OVER ANIMAL OR SMALL OBJECT
E885.9 TRIPPING OVER ANIMAL, CURB, RUG OR SMALL OBJECT
E886.0 SPORTS (COLLISION)
E886.9 OTHER AND UNSPECIFIED COLLISION

UNSPECIFIED

E887 RESULTING IN FRACTURE CAUSE UNSPECIFIED
E888.0 RESULTING IN STRIKING AGAINST SHARP OBJECT
E888.1 RESULTING IN STRIKING AGAINST OTHER OBJECT
E888.8 OTHER
E888.9 UNSPECIFIED

FIRE

CONFLAGRATION/UNCONTROLLED

IN ORDER TO IDENTIFY A CONFLAGRATION/ UNCONTROLLED FIRE IN A BUILDING WHERE A PATIENT IS ACCIDENTALLY STRUCK BY A FALLING OBJECT, USE CODE E916 STRUCK BY FALLING OBJECT AS AN ADDITIONAL CODE.

E890.# PRIVATE DWELLING
E891.# OTHER OR UNSPECIFIED BUILDING OR STRUCTURE

4th Digit: E890 - E891
0. EXPLOSION
1. FUMES FROM PVC (POLYVINYLCHLORIDE)
2. OTHER SMOKE AND FUMES
3. BURNING
8. OTHER ACCIDENT (FALL, COLLAPSE, NONTHERMAL INJURY)
9. UNSPECIFIED

E892 NOT IN BUILDING OR STRUCTURE

FIRE (continued)

CONTROLLED

E893.# IGNITION OF CLOTHING

4th Digit: E893
0. FIREPLACE, STOVE, FURNACE, ETC. IN PRIVATE DWELLING
1. FIREPLACE, STOVE, FURNACE, ETC. IN OTHER BUILDING OR STRUCTURE
2. BONFIRE, BRAZIER, TRASH FIRE, ETC. NOT IN BUILDING OR STRUCTURE
8. FROM OTHER SPECIFIED SOURCE
9. FROM UNSPECIFIED SOURCE

E894 IGNITION OF HIGHLY FLAMMABLE MATERIAL
E895 PRIVATE DWELLING - FIREPLACE, FURNACE, STOVE, ETC.
E896 OTHER BUILDING OR STRUCTURE - FIREPLACE, FURNACE, STOVE, ETC.
E897 NOT IN BUILDING OR STRUCTURE - BONFIRE, BRAZIER, TRASH FIRE ETC.

OTHER

E898.0 BURNING OF BEDCLOTHES
E898.1 OTHER FIRE (CIGARETTES, BLOWTORCH, LIGHTER,ETC.)
E899 UNSPECIFIED FIRE

ENVIRONMENTAL-EXPOSURE INJURIES

E900.# HEAT

4th Digit: E900
0. WEATHER
1. MAN MADE ORIGIN
9. UNSPECIFIED ORIGIN

E901.# COLD

4th Digit: E901
0. WEATHER
1. MAN MADE ORIGIN
8. OTHER SPECIFIED ORIGIN
9. UNSPECIFIED ORIGIN

E902.# AIR PRESSURE

4th Digit: E902
0. HIGH ALTITUDE
1. IN AIRCRAFT
2. DIVING
8. OTHER SPECIFIED CAUSES
9. UNSPECIFIED CAUSE

E903 TRAVEL AND MOTION
E904.# HUNGER, THIRST, EXPOSURE, NEGLECT

4th Digit: E904
0. ABANDONMENT/NEGLECT OF INFANT OR HELPLESS
1. LACK OF FOOD
2. LACK OF WATER
3. EXPOSURE TO WEATHER NEC
9. DESTITUTION OR ECONOMIC CIRCUMSTANCE

INJURIES CAUSED BY PLANTS OR ANIMALS

E905.# VENOMOUS

4th Digit: E905

0. SNAKES OR LIZARDS
1. SPIDERS
2. SCORPION
3. BEES, WASPS, HORNETS
4. CENTIPEDE OR MILLIPEDE
5. OTHER ARTHROPODS
6. MARINE ANIMALS OR PLANTS
7. POISONING OR TOXIC REACTION TO OTHER PLANTS
8. OTHER SPECIFIED
9. UNSPECIFIED

E906.# NONVENOMOUS

4th Digit: E906

0. DOG BITE
1. RAT BITE
2. SNAKES OR LIZARDS
3. ANIMAL-NON INSECT
4. ARTHROPOD (INSECT)
5. UNSPECIFIED ANIMAL (ANIMAL BITE NOS)
8. OTHER SPECIFIED INJURY CAUSED BY ANIMAL (FALL, BUTTED, ETC.)
9. UNSPECIFIED INJURY CAUSED BY ANIMAL

NATURAL CATACLYSMS

E907 LIGHTNING

> ***IN ORDER TO IDENTIFY STORMS OR EARTH SURFACE MOVEMENTS WHERE A PATIENT IS ACCIDENTALLY STRUCK BY A FALLING OBJECT, USE CODE E916 STRUCK BY FALLING OBJECT AS AN ADDITIONAL CODE.***

E908.# STORM OR FLOOD FROM STORM

4th Digit: E908

0. HURRICANE, STORM SURGE, TIDAL WAVE FROM STORM (TROPICAL), TYPHOON
1. TORNADO, CYCLONE, TWISTER
2. FLOODS, TORRENTIAL RAINFALL, FLASH FLOOD
3. BLIZZARD (SNOW) (ICE)
4. DUST STORM
8. OTHER STORM (CLOUDBURST)
9. UNSPECIFIED STORM OR FLOOD FROM STORM

E909.# EARTH SURFACE MOVEMENTS AND ERUPTIONS

4th Digit: E909

0. EARTHQUAKES
1. VOLCANIC ERUPTIONS, LAVA BURNS, ASH INHALATION
2. AVALANCHE (SNOW), LANDSLIDE, MUDSLIDE
3. COLLAPSE DAM OR MAN-MADE STRUCTURE CAUSING FLOOD
4. TIDALWAVE FROM EATHQUAKE, TIDALWAVE NOS, TSUNAMI
8. OTHER SPECIFIED EARTH MOVEMENTS AND ERUPTIONS
9. UNSPECIFIED EARTH MOVEMENTS AND ERUPTIONS

NATURAL CATACLYSMS (continued)

E910.# DROWNING SUBMERSION

4th Digit: E910

0. WATER SKIING
1. SCUBA OR SKIN DIVING (RECREATIONAL)
2. SWIMMING, FISHING, ETC.
3. SWIMMING/DIVING - COMMERCIALLY
4. IN BATHTUB
8. OTHER SPECIFIED (SWIMMING POOL OR FALL INTO WATER)
9. UNSPECIFIED (DROWNING NOS)

RESPIRATORY OBSTRUCTION

E911 FOOD
E912 OTHER OBJECT INHALED OR ASPIRATED
E913.# MECHANICAL SUFFOCATION

4th Digit: E913

0. BED OR CRADLE
1. PLASTIC BAG
2. ENCLOSURE OR INSUFFICIENT AIR SUPPLY (REFRIGERATOR OR DIVING WITH INSUFFICIENT AIR SUPPLY)
3. FALLING EARTH OR CAVE IN
8. OTHER MEANS OR HANGING
9. UNSPECIFIED (STRANGULATION, SUFFOCATION NOS)

FOREIGN BODY

E914 EYE OR ADNEXA
E915 OTHER ORIFICE

STRUCK BY

> ***WHEN USING CODE [E916] STRUCK BY FALLING OBJECT, CODE FIRST THE REASON FOR THE FALLING OBJECT, IE. COLLAPSE OF BUILDING ON FIRE, NATURAL CATACLYSMS OR OTHER ACCIDENTS.***

E916 FALLING OBJECT

OTHER ACCIDENTS

IN ORDER TO IDENTIFY AN ACCIDENT WHERE A PATIENT IS ACCIDENTALLY STRUCK BY A FALLING OBJECT USE CODE E916 STRUCK BY FALLING OBJECT AS AN ADDITIONAL CODE.

E917.# STRIKING AGAINST OR BY PERSONS OR OBJECTS (KICKING, THROWN, ETC.)
4th Digit: E917
0. SPORTS WITHOUT FALL
1. CAUSED BY CROWD OR PANIC WITHOUT FALL
2. RUNNING WATER WITHOUT FALL
3. FURNITURE WITHOUT FALL
4. OTHER STATIONARY OBJECT WITHOUT FALL
5. SPORTS WITH FALL
6. CAUSED BY CROWD OR PANIC WITH FALL
7. FURNITURE WITH FALL
8. OTHER STATIONARY OBJECT WITH FALL
9. OTHER STRIKING AGAINST WITH OR WITHOUT FALL

E918 CRUSHED OR CAUGHT BETWEEN OBJECTS

E919.# CAUSED BY MACHINERY
4th Digit: E919
0. AGRICULTURAL
1. MINING OR EARTH DRILLING
2. LIFTING MACHINES OR APPLIANCES
3. METALWORKING MACHINES
4. WOODWORKING MACHINES
5. NONELECTRIC MOTORS, TURBINES, OR ENGINES
6. TRANSMISSION MACHINERY (BELTS PULLEYS, GEARS, ETC.)
7. EARTH MOVING EQUIPMENT
8. OTHER SPECIFIED (MACHINES USED IN MANUFACTURING, PRINTING, ETC.)
9. UNSPECIFIED MACHINERY

E920.# CAUSED BY CUTTING OR PIERCING EQUIPMENT
4th Digit: E920
0. POWERED LAWNMOWER
1. POWERED HAND TOOLS
2. HOUSEHOLD APPLIANCES
3. KNIVES, SWORDS, DAGGERS
4. OTHER HAND TOOLS, NEEDLE (SEWING)
5. HYPODERMIC NEEDLE, CONTAMINATED NEEDLE, NEEDLE STICK
8. OTHER SPECIFIED (GLASS, NAIL, THORN, ETC.)
9. UNSPECIFIED CUTTING OR PIERCING INSTRUMENT

E921.# CAUSED BY EXPLOSION OF PRESSURE VESSEL
4th Digit: E921
0. BOILERS
1. GAS OR AIR TANKS
8. OTHER SPECIFIED (AEROSOL CAN, TIRE, PRESSURE COOKER)
9. UNSPECIFIED PRESSURE VESSEL

OTHER ACCIDENTS (continued)

E922.# FIREARM AND AIR GUN MISSILE
4th Digit: E922
0. HANDGUN
1. SHOTGUN
2. HUNTING RIFLE
3. MILITARY RIFLE
4. AIR GUN, BB GUN, PELLET GUN
5. PAINTBALL GUN
8. OTHER SPECIFIED FIREARM (FLAREGUN)
9. UNSPECIFIED (GUNSHOT NOS)

E923.# EXPLOSIVES
4th Digit: E923
0. FIREWORKS
1. BLASTING MATERIALS
2. EXPLOSIVE GASES
8. OTHER SPECIFIED (BOMBS, MINES, ETC.)
9. UNSPECIFIED EXPLOSION (EXPLOSION NOS)

E924.# CAUSED BY CAUSTICS, CORROSIVES, STEAM, HOT OBJECTS
4th Digit: E924
0. HOT VAPORS, LIQUIDS, STEAM
1. CAUSTICS, ACIDS, CORROSIVES
2. HOT (BOILING) TAP WATER
8. BURN BY OTHER HOT OBJECT
9. UNSPECIFIED

E925.# ELECTRICAL
4th Digit: E925
0. DOMESTIC WIRING
1. POWER LINES, GENERATORS, POWER STATIONS
2. INDUSTRIAL WIRING, APPLIANCES, ELECTRICAL MACHINERY
8. OTHER ELECTRICAL CURRENT (FARM, RESIDENTIAL, SCHOOL, PUBLIC BUILDINGS)
9. UNSPECIFIED (ELECTROCUTION NOS)

E926.# RADIATION
4th Digit: E926
0. RADIOFREQUENCY (MICROWAVE, RADAR, TRANSMITTERS)
1. INFRARED HEATERS AND LAMPS
2. VISIBLE AND ULTRAVIOLET LIGHT (ARC LAMP, WELDER, SUN, TANNING BED)
3. X-RAYS AND IONIZING RADIATION
4. LASERS
5. RADIOACTIVE ISOTOPES
8. OTHER SPECIFIED RADIATION (BETATRONS, SYNCHROTRONS)
9. UNSPECIFIED RADIATION

E927 OVEREXERTION AND STRENUOUS MOVEMENTS

E-CODES

OTHER ACCIDENTS (continued)

E928.# OTHER ENVIRONMENTAL CAUSES
4th Digit: E928
0. WEIGHTLESSNESS
1. NOISE EXPOSURE
2. VIBRATION
3. HUMAN BITE
4. CONSTRICTION BY HAIR EXTERNAL
5. CONSTRICTION BY OTHER EXTERNAL
6. EXPOSURE TO HARMFUL ALGAE AND TOXINS
8. OTHER SPECIFIED
9. UNSPECIFIED ACCIDENT (ACCIDENT NOS, NATURAL FACTOR NEC)

LATE EFFECTS

E929.# ACCIDENTAL INJURY
4th Digit: E929
0. MVA (MOTOR VEHICLE ACCIDENT)
1. OTHER TRANSPORT
2. POISONING
3. FALL
4. FIRE
5. NATURAL AND ENVIRONMENTAL FACTORS
8. OTHER ACCIDENTS
9. UNSPECIFIED ACCIDENT

E959 SELF INFLICTED INJURY
E969 ASSAULT INJURIES
E977 INJURIES DUE TO LEGAL INTERVENTION
E989 INJURY UNDETERMINED WHETHER SELF INFLICTED OR PURPOSELY
E999.0 WAR INJURIES
E999.1 TERRORISM INJURIES

ADVERSE EFFECT (DRUGS, MEDICINAL AND BIOLOGICAL SUBSTANCES - THERAPEUTIC USE)

E930.# ANTIBIOTICS
4th Digit: E930
0. PENICILLINS
1. ANTIFUNGAL ANTIBIOTICS
2. CHLORAMPHENICOL GROUP
3. ERYTHROMYCIN AND OTHER MACROLIDES
4. TETRACYCLINE GROUP
5. CEPHALOSPORIN GROUP
6. ANTIMYCOBACTERIAL ANTIBIOTICS
7. ANTINEOPLASTIC ANTIBIOTICS
8. OTHER SPECIFIED ANTIBIOTICS
9. UNSPECIFIED ANTIBIOTICS

E931.# OTHER ANTI-INFECTIVES
4th Digit: E931
0. SULFONAMIDES
1. ARSENICAL ANTI-INFECTIVES
2. HEAVY METAL ANTI-INFECTIVES
3. QUINOLINE AND HYDROXYQUINOLINE DERIVATIVES
4. ANTIMALARIALS AND DRUGS ACTING ON OTHER BLOOD PROTOZOA
5. OTHER ANTIPROTOZOAL
6. ANTIHELMINTICS
7. ANTIVIRAL DRUGS
8. OTHER ANTIMYCOBACTERIAL DRUGS
9. OTHER AND NOS ANTI-INFECTIVES

ADVERSE EFFECT (DRUGS, MEDICINAL AND BIOLOGICAL SUBSTANCES - THERAPEUTIC USE) (continued)

E932.# HORMONES AND SYNTHETIC SUBSTITUTES
4th Digit: E932
0. ADRENAL CORTICAL STEROIDS
1. ANDROGENS AND ANABOLIC CONGENERS
2. OVARIAN HORMONES AND SYNTHETIC SUBSTITUTES
3. INSULINS AND ANTIDIABETIC AGENTS
4. ANTERIOR PITUITARY HORMONES
5. POSTERIOR PITUITARY HORMONES
6. PARATHYROID/PARATHYROID DERIVATIVES
7. THYROID/THYROID DERIVATIVES
8. ANTITHYROID AGENTS
9. OTHER AND NOS HORMONES / SYNTHETIC SUBSTITUTES

E933.# SYSTEMIC AGENTS
4th Digit: E933
0. ANTIALLERGIC AND ANTIEMETIC DRUGS
1. ANTINEOPLASTIC AND IMMUNOSUPPRESSIVE DRUGS
2. ACIDIFYING AGENTS
3. ALKALIZING AGENTS
4. ENZYMES NEC
5. VITAMINS NEC
6. ORAL BISPHOSPHONATES
7. INTRAVENOUS BISPHOSPHONATES
8. OTHER SYSTEMIC AGENTS NEC
9. NOS SYSTEMIC AGENT

E934.# AGENTS AFFECTING BLOOD CONSTITUENTS
4th Digit: E934
0. IRON AND ITS COMPOUNDS
1. LIVER PREPARATIONS AND OTHER ANTIANEMIC AGENTS
2. ANTICOAGULANTS
3. VITAMIN K (PHYTONADIONE)
4. FIBRINOLYSIS-AFFECTING DRUGS
5. ANTICOAGULANT ANTAGONISTS AND OTHER COAGULANTS
6. GAMMA GLOBULIN
7. NATURAL BLOOD AND BLOOD PRODUCTS
8. OTHER AGENTS AFFECTING BLOOD CONSTITUENTS
9. NOS AGENT AFFECTING BLOOD CONSTITUENTS

E935.# ANALGESICS, ANTIPYRETICS, ANTIRHEUMATICS
4th Digit: E935
0. HEROIN
1. METHADONE
2. OTHER OPIATES AND RELATED NARCOTICS
3. SALICYLATES
4. AROMATIC ANALGESICS NEC
5. PYRAZOLE DERIVATIVES
6. ANTIRHEUMATICS (ANTIPHLOGISTICS)
7. OTHER NON-NARCOTIC
8. OTHER SPECIFIED
9. UNSPECIFIED

ADVERSE EFFECT (DRUGS, MEDICINAL AND BIOLOGICAL SUBSTANCES - THERAPEUTIC USE) (continued)

E936.# ANTICONVULSANTS ANTI-PARKINSONISM
4th Digit: E936
0. OXAZOLIDINE
1. HYDANTOIN
2. SUCCINIMIDES
3. OTHER AND NOS ANTICONVULSANTS
4. ANTI-PARKINSONISM

E937.# SEDATIVES AND HYPNOTICS
4th Digit: E937
0. BARBITURATES
1. CHLORAL HYDRATE
2. PARALDEHYDE
3. BROMINE COMPOUNDS
4. METHAQUALONE
5. GLUTETHIMIDE
6. MIXED SEDATIVES
8. OTHER SEDATIVES AND HYPNOTICS
9. UNSPECIFIED SEDATIVES

E938.# OTHER CENTRAL NERVOUS SYSTEM DEPRESSANTS AND ANESTHETICS
4th Digit: E938
0. MUSCLE-TONE DEPRESSANTS
1. HALOTHANE
2. OTHER GASEOUS ANESTHETICS
3. INTRAVENOUS ANESTHETICS
4. OTHER AND NOS GENERAL ANESTHETICS
5. SURFACE AND INFILTRATION ANESTHETICS
6. PERIPHERAL NERVE-PLEXUS BLOCKING ANESTHETICS
7. SPINAL ANESTHETICS
9. OTHER AND NOS LOCAL ANESTHETICS

E939.# PSYCHOTROPIC AGENTS
4th Digit: E939
0. ANTIDEPRESSANTS
1. PHENOTHIAZINE-BASED TRANQUILIZERS
2. BUTYROPHENONE-BASED TRANQUILIZERS
3. OTHER ANTIPSYCHOTICS, NEUROLEPTICS AND MAJOR TRANQUILIZERS
4. BENZODIAZEPINE-BASED TRANQUILIZERS
5. OTHER TRANQUILIZERS
6. PSYCHODYSLEPTICS (HALLUCINOGENS)
7. PSYCHOSTIMULANTS
8. OTHER PSYCHOTROPIC AGENTS
9. NOS PSYCHOTROPIC AGENT

E940.# CENTRAL NERVOUS STIMULANTS
4th Digit: E940
0. ANALEPTICS
1. OPIATE ANTAGONISTS
8. OTHER SPECIFIED CENTRAL NERVOUS SYSTEM STIMULANTS
9. NOS CENTRAL NERVOUS SYSTEM STIMULANT

ADVERSE EFFECT (DRUGS, MEDICINAL AND BIOLOGICAL SUBSTANCES - THERAPEUTIC USE) (continued)

E941.# AUTONOMIC NERVOUS SYSTEM
4th Digit: E941
0. PARASYMPATHOMIMETICS (CHOLINERGICS)
1. PARASYMPATHOLYTICS (ANTICHOLINERGICS AND ANTIMUSCARINICS) AND SPASMOLYTICS
2. SYMPATHOMIMETICS (ADRENERGICS)
3. SYMPATHOLYTICS (ANTIADRENERGICS)
9. NOS DRUG AFFECTING THE AUTONOMIC NERVOUS SYSTEM

E942.# AFFECTING CARDIOVASCULAR SYSTEM
4th Digit: E942
0. CARDIAC RHYTHM REGULATOR
1. CARDIOTONIC GLYCOSIDES AND DRUGS OF SIMILAR ACTION
2. ANTILIPEMIC AND ANTIARTERIOSCLEROTIC DRUGS
3. GANGLION-BLOCKING AGENTS
4. CORONARY VASODILATORS
5. OTHER VASODILATORS
6. OTHER ANTIHYPERTENSIVE AGENTS
7. ANTIVARICOSE DRUGS INCLUDING SCLEROSING AGENTS
8. CAPILLARY-ACTIVE DRUGS
9. OTHER AND NOS

E943.# AGENTS PRIMARILY AFFECTING GASTROINTESTINAL SYSTEM
4th Digit: E943
0. ANTACIDS AND ANTIGASTRIC SECRETION DRUGS
1. IRRITANT CATHARTICS
2. EMOLLIENT CATHARTICS
3. OTHER CATHARTICS, INCLUDING INTESTINAL ATONIA DRUGS
4. DIGESTANTS
5. ANTIDIARRHEAL DRUGS
6. EMETICS
8. OTHER SPECIFIED
9. UNSPECIFIED

E944.# WATER, MINERAL, AND URIC ACID METABOLISM DRUGS
4th Digit: E944
0. MERCURIAL DIURETICS
1. PURINE DERIVATIVE DIURETICS
2. CARBONIC ACID ANHYDRASE INHIBITORS
3. SALURETICS
4. OTHER DIURETICS
5. ELECTROLYTIC, CALORIC, AND WATER-BALANCE AGENTS
6. OTHER MINERAL SALTS, NEC
7. URIC ACID METABOLISM DRUGS

ADVERSE EFFECT (DRUGS, MEDICINAL AND BIOLOGICAL SUBSTANCES - THERAPEUTIC USE) (continued)

E945.# AGENTS PRIMARILY ACTING ON THE SMOOTH AND SKELETAL MUSCLES AND RESPIRATORY SYSTEM

4th Digit: E945

0. OXYTOCIC AGENTS
1. SMOOTH MUSCLE RELAXANTS
2. SKELETAL MUSCLE RELAXANTS
3. OTHER AND NOS DRUGS ACTING ON MUSCLES
4. ANTITUSSIVES
5. EXPECTORANTS
6. ANTI-COMMON COLD DRUGS
7. ANTIASTHMATICS
8. OTHER AND NOS RESPIRATORY DRUGS

E946.# AGENTS PRIMARILY AFFECTING SKIN AND MUCOUS MEMBRANE: OPHTHALMOLOGICAL, DENTAL , AND OTORHINOLARYNGOLOGICAL DRUGS

4th Digit: E946

0. LOCAL ANTI-INFECTIVES AND ANTI-INFLAMMATORY DRUGS
1. ANTIPRURITICS
2. LOCAL ASTRINGENTS AND LOCAL DETERGENTS
3. EMOLLIENTS, DEMULCENTS, AND PROTECTANTS
4. KERATOLYTICS, KERATOPLASTICS, OTHER HAIR TREATMENT DRUGS AND PREPARATIONS
5. EYE ANTI-INFECTIVES AND OTHER EYE DRUGS
6. ANTI-INFECTIVES AND OTHER DRUGS AND PREPARATIONS FOR EAR, NOSE, AND THROAT
7. DENTAL DRUGS TOPICALLY APPLIED
8. OTHER AGENTS PRIMARILY AFFECTING SKIN AND MUCOUS MEMBRANE
9. NOS AGENT PRIMARILY AFFECTING SKIN AND MUCOUS MEMBRANE

E947.# OTHER AND NOS DRUGS AND MEDICINAL SUBSTANCES

4th Digit: E947

0. DIETETICS
1. LIPOTROPIC DRUGS
2. ANTIDOTES AND CHELATING AGENTS, NEC
3. ALCOHOL DETERRENTS
4. PHARMACEUTICAL EXCIPIENTS
8. OTHER DRUGS AND MEDICINAL SUBSTANCES
9. NOS DRUG OR MEDICINAL SUBSTANCE

ADVERSE EFFECT (DRUGS, MEDICINAL AND BIOLOGICAL SUBSTANCES - THERAPEUTIC USE) (continued)

E948.# BACTERIAL VACCINES

4th Digit: E948

0. BCG VACCINE
1. TYPHOID AND PARATYPHOID
2. CHOLERA
3. PLAGUE
4. TETANUS
5. DIPHTHERIA
6. PERTUSSIS VACCINE, INCLUDING COMBINATIONS WITH A PERTUSSIS COMPONENT
8. OTHER AND NOS BACTERIAL VACCINES
9. MIXED BACTERIAL VACCINES, EXCEPT COMBINATIONS WITH A PERTUSSIS COMPONENT

E949.# OTHER VACCINES AND BIOLOGICAL SUBSTANCES

4th Digit: E949

0. SMALLPOX VACCINE
1. RABIES VACCINE
2. TYPHUS VACCINE
3. YELLOW FEVER VACCINE
4. MEASLES VACCINE
5. POLIOMYELITIS VACCINE
6. OTHER AND NOS VIRAL AND RICKETTSIAL VACCINES
7. MIXED VIRAL-RICKETTSIAL AND BACTERIAL VACCINES, EXCEPT COMBINATIONS WITH A PERTUSSIS COMPONENT
9. OTHER AND NOS VACCINES AND BIOLOGICAL SUBSTANCES

SUICIDE AND SELF INFLICTED INJURY

E950.# POISONING BY SOLID OR LIQUID SUBSTANCES

4th Digit: E950

0. ANALGESICS, ANTIPYRETICS, ANTIRHEUMATICS
1. BARBITURATES
2. SEDATIVES HYPNOTICS
3. TRANQUILIZERS OR OTHER PSYCHOTROPICS
4. OTHER DRUGS AND MEDICINE
5. UNSPECIFIED DRUG OR MEDICINE
6. AGRICULTURAL CHEMICALS AND PHARMACEUTICALS OTHER THAN FERTILIZERS AND PLANT FOODS
7. CORROSIVES AND CAUSTICS
8. ARSENIC OR ARSENIC COMPOUNDS
9. OTHER AND UNSPECIFIED SOLID AND LIQUID COMPOUNDS

E951.# POISONING GASES IN DOMESTIC USE

4th Digit: E951

0. DISTRIBUTED BY PIPELINE
1. IN MOBILE CONTAINERS
8. OTHER UTILITY GAS

SUICIDE AND SELF INFLICTED INJURY (continued)

E952.# POISONING BY OTHER GASES AND VAPORS
4th Digit: E952
0. MOTOR VEHICLE EXHAUST
1. OTHER CARBON MONOXIDE
8. OTHER SPECIFIED GASES AND VAPORS
9. UNSPECIFIED GASES AND VAPORS

E953.# HANGING, STRANGULATION, SUFFOCATION
4th Digit: E953
0. HANGING
1. BY PLASTIC BAG
8. OTHER SPECIFIED MEANS
9. UNSPECIFIED MEANS

E954 DROWNING OR SUBMERSION

E955.# FIREARMS, AIR GUNS OR EXPLOSIVES
4th Digit: E955
0. HANDGUN
1. SHOTGUN
2. HUNTING RIFLE
3. MILITARY FIREARM
4. OTHER AND UNSPECIFIED FIREARM
5. EXPLOSIVES
6. AIR GUN, BB GUN, PELLET GUN
7. PAINTBALL GUN
9. UNSPECIFIED

E956 CUTTING OR PIERCING INSTRUMENT

E957.# JUMPING FROM HIGH PLACE
4th Digit: E957
0. RESIDENTIAL
1. OTHER MAN MADE STRUCTURE
2. NATURAL SITES
9. UNSPECIFIED

E958.# OTHER OR UNSPECIFIED MEANS
4th Digit: E958
0. JUMPING BEFORE MOVING OBJECT
1. FIRE
2. SCALD
3. EXTREMES OF COLD
4. ELECTROCUTION
5. CRASHING MOTOR VEHICLE
6. CRASHING AIRCRAFT
7. CAUSTICS (EXCEPT POISONING)
8. OTHER SPECIFIED MEANS
9. UNSPECIFIED MEANS

ASSAULT

E960.0 FIGHT OR BRAWL
E960.1 RAPE OR SODOMY
E961 ASSAULT BY CAUSTIC OR CORROSIVES EXCEPT POISONING

E962.# POISONING
4th Digit: E962
0. DRUGS OR MEDICINE
1. OTHER SOLID OR LIQUIDS
2. OTHER GASES OR VAPORS
9. UNSPECIFIED POISONING

E963 HANGING OR STRANGULATION
E964 DROWNING

ASSAULT (continued)

E965.# FIREARMS OR EXPLOSIVES
4th Digit: E965
0. HANDGUN
1. SHOTGUN
2. HUNTING RIFLE
3. MILITARY FIREARM
4. OTHER AND UNSPECIFIED FIREARM
5. ANTIPERSONNEL BOMB
6. GASOLINE BOMB
7. LETTER BOMB
8. OTHER EXPLOSIVE
9. UNSPECIFIED EXPLOSIVE

E966 CUTTING OR PIERCING INSTRUMENT

SELECTION OF THE CORRECT PERPETRATOR CODE IS BASED ON THE RELATIONSHIP BETWEEN THE PERPETRATOR AND THE VICTIM.

E967.# PERPETRATOR OF CHILD AND ADULT ABUSE
4th Digit: E967
0. BY FATHER, STEPFATHER OR BOYFRIEND (MALE PARTNER OF CHILD'S PARENT OR GUARDIAN)
1. BY OTHER SPECIFIED PERSON
2. BY MOTHER, STEPMOTHER OR GIRLFRIEND (FEMALE PARTNER OF CHILD'S PARENT OF GUARDIAN))
3. BY SPOUSE OR PARTNER (ABUSE OF SPOUSE OR PARTNER BY EX-SPOUSE OR OR EX-PARTNER)
4. BY CHILD
5. BY SIBLING
6. BY GRANDPARENT
7. BY OTHER RELATIVE (GRANDCHILD)
8. BY NON-RELATED CAREGIVER
9. BY UNSPECIFIED PERSON

E968.# BY OTHER SPECIFIED MEANS
4th Digit: E968
0. FIRE
1. PUSHED FROM HIGH PLACE
2. STRUCK BY BLUNT OR THROWN OBJECT
3. HOT LIQUID
4. CRIMINAL NEGLECT
5. TRANSPORT VEHICLE PUSHED IN FRONT OF, THROWN FROM, DRAGGED OR RUN DOWN BY, OR COLLIDING WITH A MOVING VEHICLE
6. AIR GUN, BB GUN, PELLET GUN
7. HUMAN BITE
8. OTHER SPECIFIED MEANS
9. UNSPECIFIED MEANS

INJURY DUE TO LEGAL INTERVENTION

E970 FIREARMS
E971 EXPLOSIVES
E972 GAS
E973 BLUNT TRAUMA
E974 CUTTING OR PIERCING INSTRUMENT
E975 OTHER SPECIFIED (BLOW OR MANHANDLING)
E976 UNSPECIFIED MEANS
E978 EXECUTION

INJURY UNDETERMINED WHETHER ACCIDENTAL

E980.# POISONING SOLIDS OR LIQUID SUBSTANCES
4th Digit: E980
0. ANALGESICS, ANTIPYRETICS, AND ANTIRHEUMATICS
1. BARBITURATES
2. OTHER SEDATIVES AND HYPNOTICS
3. TRANQUILIZERS AND OTHER PSYCHOTROPIC AGENTS
4. OTHER SPECIFIED DRUGS AND MEDICINE
5. NOS DRUG OR MEDICINE
6. CORROSIVE AND CAUSTIC SUBSTANCES
7. AGRICULTURAL CHEMICALS AND PHARMACEUTICALS OTHER THAN FERTILIZERS AND PLANT FOODS
8. ARSENIC AND ITS COMPOUNDS
9. OTHER AND NOS SOLIDS AND LIQUIDS

E981.# POISONING GASES IN DOMESTIC USE
4th Digit: E981
0. PIPELINE GAS
1. LIQUEFIED PETROLEUM GAS DISTRIBUTED IN MOBILE CONTAINERS
8. OTHER UTILITY GAS

E982.# POISONING OTHER GASES
4th Digit: E982
0. MOTOR VEHICLE EXHAUST GAS
1. OTHER CARBON MONOXIDE
8. OTHER SPECIFIED GASES / VAPORS
9. UNSPECIFIED GASES / VAPORS

E983.# HANGING, STRANGULATION, SUFFOCATION
4th Digit: E983
0. HANGING
1. SUFFOCATION BY PLASTIC BAG
8. OTHER SPECIFIED MEANS
9. UNSPECIFIED MEANS

E984 DROWNING OR SUBMERSION

E985.# FIREARMS OR EXPLOSIVES
4th Digit: E985
0. HANDGUN
1. SHOTGUN
2. HUNTING RIFLE
3. MILITARY FIREARM
4. OTHER AND UNSPECIFIED FIREARM
5. EXPLOSIVES
6. AIR GUN, BB GUN, PELLET GUN
7. PAINTBALL GUN

E986 CUTTING OR PIERCING INSTRUMENTS

E987.# FALL FROM HIGH PLACE
4th Digit: E987
0. RESIDENTIAL
1. OTHER MAN MADE STRUCTURE
2. NATURAL SITES
9. UNSPECIFIED

INJURY UNDETERMINED WHETHER ACCIDENTAL (continued)

E988.# OTHER OR UNSPECIFIED MEANS
4th Digit: E988
0. JUMPING BEFORE MOVING OBJECT
1. FIRE
2. SCALD
3. EXTREMES OF COLD
4. ELECTROCUTION
5. CRASHING MOTOR VEHICLE
6. CRASHING AIRCRAFT
7. CAUSTICS (EXCEPT POISONING)
8. OTHER SPECIFIED MEANS
9. UNSPECIFIED MEANS

WAR, INSURRECTION, MILITARY ACTION

E990.# AS A RESULT OF FIRE
4th Digit: E990
0. FROM GASOLINE BOMB
9. FROM OTHER OR UNSPECIFIED SOURCE

E991.# FROM BULLETS OR FRAGMENTS
4th Digit: E991
0. RUBBER BULLETS
1. PELLETS (RIFLE)
2. OTHER BULLETS
3. ANTIPERSONNEL BOMB (FRAGMENTS)
4. OTHER AND NOS FRAGMENTS

E992 FROM EXPLOSION OF MARINE WEAPONS
E993 OTHER EXPLOSIONS
E994 DESTRUCTION OF AIRCRAFT
E995 OTHER AND UNSPECIFIED CONVENTIONAL WARFARE
E996 NUCLEAR WEAPONS

E997.# OTHER UNCONVENTIONAL WEAPONS
4th Digit: E997
0. LASERS
1. BIOLOGICAL
2. GAS OR CHEMICALS
8. OTHER SPECIFIED UNCONVENTIONAL WARFARE
9. UNSPECIFIED UNCONVENTIONAL WARFARE

E998 INJURIES AFTER CESSATION OF HOSTILITIES

TERRORISM

E979.0 MARINE WEAPON EXPLOSION
E979.1 AIRCRAFT DESTRUCTION
E979.2 OTHER EXPLOSIONS AND FRAGMENTS
E979.3 FIRES, CONFLAGRATION AND HOT SUBSTANCES
E979.4 FIREARMS
E979.5 NUCLEAR WEAPONS (RADIATION)
E979.6 BIOLOGICAL WEAPONS
E979.7 CHEMICAL WEAPONS
E979.8 OTHER MEANS
E979.9 SECONDARY EFFECTS

POISONING - ACCIDENTAL

E850.# ANALGESICS, ANTIPYRETICS, AND ANTIRHEUMATICS
4th Digit: E850
- **0. HEROIN**
- **1. METHADONE**
- **2. OTHER OPIATES AND RELATED NARCOTICS**
- **3. SALICYLATES**
- **4. AROMATIC ANALGESICS, NEC**
- **5. PYRAZOLE DERIVATIVES**
- **6. ANTIRHEUMATICS (ANTIPHLOGISTICS)**
- **7. OTHER NON-NARCOTIC ANALGESICS**
- **8. OTHER SPECIFIED ANALGESICS AND ANTIPYRETICS**
- **9. NOS ANALGESICS AND ANTIPYRETICS**

E851 BARBITURATES

E852.# OTHER SEDATIVES / HYPNOTICS
4th Digit: E852
- **0. CHLORAL HYDRATE GROUP**
- **1. PARALDEHYDE**
- **2. BROMINE COMPOUNDS**
- **3. METHAQUALONE COMPOUNDS**
- **4. GLUTETHIMIDE GROUP**
- **5. MIXED SEDATIVES, NEC**
- **8. OTHER SPECIFIED SEDATIVES / HYPNOTICS**
- **9. NOS SEDATIVE / HYPNOTIC**

E853.# TRANQUILIZERS
4th Digit: E853
- **0. PHENOTHIAZINE-BASED TRANQUILIZERS**
- **1. BUTYROPHENONE-BASED TRANQUILIZERS**
- **2. BENZODIAZEPINE-BASED TRANQUILIZERS**
- **8. OTHER SPECIFIED TRANQUILIZERS**
- **9. NOS TRANQUILIZER**

E854.# OTHER PSYCHOTROPIC AGENTS
4th Digit: E854
- **0. ANTIDEPRESSANTS**
- **1. PSYCHODYSLEPTICS (HALLUCINOGENS)**
- **2. PSYCHOSTIMULANTS**
- **3. CENTRAL NERVOUS SYSTEM STIMULANTS**
- **8. OTHER PSYCHOTROPIC AGENTS**

POISONING - ACCIDENTAL (continued)

E855.# OTHER DRUGS ACTING ON CENTRAL AND AUTONOMIC NERVOUS SYSTEM
4th Digit: E855
- **0. ANTICONVULSANT AND ANTI-PARKINSONISM DRUGS**
- **1. OTHER CNS DEPRESSANTS**
- **2. LOCAL ANESTHETICS**
- **3. PARASYMPATHOMIMETICS (CHOLINERGICS)**
- **4. PARASYMPATHOLYTICS (ANTICHOLINERGICS AND ANTIMUSCARINICS) AND SPASMOLYTICS**
- **5. SYMPATHOMIMETICS (ADRENERGICS)**
- **6. SYMPATHOLYTICS (ANTIADRENERGICS)**
- **8. OTHER SPECIFIED DRUGS ACTING ON CENTRAL AND AUTONOMIC NERVOUS SYSTEMS**
- **9. NOS DRUG ACTING ON CENTRAL AND AUTONOMIC NERVOUS SYSTEMS**

E856 ANTIBIOTICS
E857 OTHER ANTI-INFECTIVES

E858.# OTHER DRUGS
4th Digit: E858
- **0. HORMONES AND SYNTHETIC SUBSTITUTES**
- **1. PRIMARILY SYSTEMIC AGENTS**
- **2. AGENTS PRIMARILY AFFECTING BLOOD CONSTITUENTS**
- **3. AGENTS PRIMARILY AFFECTING CARDIOVASCULAR SYSTEM**
- **4. AGENTS PRIMARILY AFFECTING GASTROINTESTINAL SYSTEM**
- **5. WATER, MINERAL, AND URIC ACID MATABOLISM DRUGS**
- **6. AGENTS PRIMARILY ACTING ON THE SMOOTH AND SKELETAL MUSCLES AND RESPIRATORY SYSTEM**
- **7. AGENTS PRIMARILY AFFECTING SKIN AND MUCOUS MEMBRANE OPHTHALMOLOGICAL, OTORHINOLARYNGOLOGICAL, AND DENTAL DRUGS**
- **8. OTHER SPECIFIED DRUGS**
- **9. NOS DRUG**

E860.# ALCOHOL NEC
4th Digit: E860
- **0. ALCOHOLIC BEVERAGES**
- **1. OTHER AND NOS ETHYL ALCOHOL AND ITS PRODUCTS**
- **2. METHYL ALCOHOL**
- **3. ISOPROPYL ALCOHOL**
- **4. FUSEL ALCOHOL**
- **8. OTHER SPECIFIED ALCOHOLS**
- **9. NOS ALCOHOL**

POISONING - ACCIDENTAL (continued)

E861.# CLEANSERS, POLISHES, DISINFECTANTS, PAINTS, VARNISHES
4th Digit: E861
0. SYNTHETIC DETERGENTS / SHAMPOOS
1. SOAP PRODUCTS
2. POLISHES
3. OTHER CLEANSERS, POLISHES
4. DISINFECTANTS
5. LEAD PAINTS
8. OTHER PAINTS / VARNISHES
9. UNSPECIFIED

E862.# PETROLEUM PRODUCTS OTHER SOLVENTS AND THEIR VAPORS NEC
4th Digit: E862
0. PETROLEUM SOLVENTS
1. PETROLEUM FUELS AND CLEANERS
2. LUBRICATING OILS
3. PETROLEUM SOLIDS
4. OTHER SPECIFIED SOLVENTS
9. UNSPECIFIED SOLVENT

E863.# AGRICULTURAL, HORTICULTURAL CHEMICAL AND PHARMACEUTICAL PREPARATIONS OTHER THAN PLANT FOODS AND FERTILIZERS
4th Digit: E863
0. INSECTICIDES OF ORGANOCHLORINE COMPOUNDS
1. INSECTICIDES OF ORGANOPHOSPHORUS COMPOUNDS
2. CARBAMATES
3. MIXTURES OF INSECTICIDES
4. OTHER AND NOS INSECTICIDES
5. HERBICIDES
6. FUNGICIDES
7. RODENTICIDES
8. FUMIGANTS
9. OTHER AND NOS

E864.# CORROSIVES AND CAUSTICS, NEC
4th Digit: E864
0. CORROSIVE AROMATICS
1. ACIDS
2. CAUSTIC ALKALIS
3. OTHER SPECIFIED CORROSIVES AND CAUSTICS
4. NOS CORROSIVES AND CAUSTICS

E865.# POISONOUS FOODSTUFFS AND POISONOUS PLANTS
4th Digit: E865
0. MEAT
1. SHELLFISH
2. OTHER FISH
3. BERRIES AND SEEDS
4. OTHER SPECIFIED PLANTS
5. MUSHROOMS AND OTHER FUNGI
8. OTHER SPECIFIED FOODS
9. NOS FOODSTUFF OR POISONOUS PLANT

POISONING - ACCIDENTAL (continued)

E866.# OTHER AND NOS SOLID / LIQUID SUBSTANCES
4th Digit: E866
0. LEAD AND ITS COMPOUNDS AND FUMES
1. MERCURY AND ITS COMPOUNDS AND FUMES
2. ANTIMONY AND ITS COMPOUNDS AND FUMES
3. ARSENIC AND ITS COMPOUNDS AND FUMES
4. OTHER METALS AND THEIR COMPOUNDS AND FUMES
5. PLANT FOODS AND FERTILIZERS
6. GLUES AND ADHESIVES
7. COSMETICS
8. OTHER SPECIFIED SOLID OR LIQUID SUBSTANCES
9. NOS SOLID OR LIQUID SUBSTANCE

E867 GAS DISTRIBUTED BY PIPELINE

E868.# OTHER UTILITY GAS AND OTHER CARBON MONOXIDE
4th Digit: E868
0. LIQUEFIED PETROLEUM GAS DISTRIBUTED IN MOBILE CONTAINERS
1. OTHER AND NOS UTILITY GAS
2. MOTOR VEHICLE EXHAUST GAS
3. CARBON MONOXIDE FROM INCOMPLETE COMBUSTION OTHER DOMESTIC FUELS
8. CARBON MONOXIDE OTHER SOURCES
9. NOS CARBON MONOXIDE

E869.# OTHER GASES AND VAPORS
4th Digit: E869
0. NITROGEN OXIDES
1. SULFUR DIOXIDE
2. FREON
3. LACRIMOGENIC GAS (TEAR GAS)
4. TOBACCO SMOKE SECOND-HAND
8. OTHER SPECIFIED GASES AND VAPORS
9. NOS GASES AND VAPORS

E-CODES

POISONING - ASSAULT

E962.# ASSAULT
4th Digit: E962
0. DRUGS OR MEDICINE
1. OTHER SOLID OR LIQUIDS
2. OTHER GASES OR VAPORS
9. UNSPECIFIED POISONING

POISONING - SUICIDE AND SELF INFLICTED INJURY

E950.# BY SOLID OR LIQUID SUBSTANCES
4th Digit: E950
0. ANALGESICS, ANTIPYRETICS, ANTIRHEUMATICS
1. BARBITURATES
2. SEDATIVES / HYPNOTICS
3. TRANQUILIZERS OR OTHER PSYCHOTROPICS
4. OTHER DRUGS AND MEDICINE
5. UNSPECIFIED DRUG OR MEDICINE
6. AGRICULTURAL CHEMICALS AND PHARMACEUTICALS OTHER THAN FERTILIZERS AND PLANT FOODS
7. CORROSIVES AND CAUSTICS
8. ARSENIC OR ARSENIC COMPOUNDS
9. OTHER AND UNSPECIFIED SOLID AND LIQUID COMPOUNDS

E951.# GASES IN DOMESTIC USE
4th Digit: E951
0. DISTRIBUTED BY PIPELINE
1. IN MOBILE CONTAINERS
8. OTHER UTILITY GAS

E952.# BY OTHER GASES AND VAPORS
4th Digit: E952
0. MOTOR VEHICLE EXHAUST
1. OTHER CARBON MONOXIDE
8. OTHER SPECIFIED GASES AND VAPORS
9. UNSPECIFIED GASES AND VAPORS

POISONING - UNDETERMINED

E980.# SOLIDS OR LIQUID SUBSTANCES
4th Digit: E980
0. ANALGESICS, ANTIPYRETICS, AND ANTIRHEUMATICS
1. BARBITURATES
2. OTHER SEDATIVES AND HYPNOTICS
3. TRANQUILIZERS AND OTHER PSYCHOTROPIC AGENTS
4. OTHER SPECIFIED DRUGS AND MEDICINE
5. NOS DRUG OR MEDICINE
6. CORROSIVE AND CAUSTIC SUBSTANCES
7. AGRICULTURAL CHEMICALS AND PHARMACEUTICALS OTHER THAN FERTILIZERS AND PLANT FOODS
8. ARSENIC AND ITS COMPOUNDS
9. OTHER AND NOS SOLIDS AND LIQUIDS

E981.# GASES IN DOMESTIC USE
4th Digit: E981
0. PIPELINE GAS
1. LIQUEFIED PETROLEUM GAS DISTRIBUTED IN MOBILE CONTAINERS
8. OTHER UTILITY GAS

E982.# OTHER GASES
4th Digit: E982
0. MOTOR VEHICLE EXHAUST GAS
1. OTHER CARBON MONOXIDE
8. OTHER SPECIFIED GASES / VAPORS
9. UNSPECIFIED GASES / VAPORS

NOTES

NOTES

APPENDIX B

DRUGS AND CHEMICALS

POISON	THERA-PEUTIC	ACCIDENT	SUICIDE	ASSAULT	UNDETER-MINED	SUBSTANCE
961.7	E931.7	E857	E950.4	E962.0	E980.4	ABOB
988.2		E865.3	E950.9	E962.1	E980.9	ABRUS SEED
980.0		E860.1	E950.9	E962.1	E980.9	ABSINTHE
980.0		E860.0	E950.9	E962.1	E980.9	ABSINTHE BEVERAGE
964.2	E934.2	E858.2	E950.4	E962.0	E980.4	ACENOCOUMARIN ACENOCOUMAROL
969.1	E939.1	E853.0	E950.3	E962.0	E980.3	ACEPROMAZINE
982.8		E862.4	E950.9	E962.1	E980.9	ACETAL
989.89		E866.5	E950.9	E962.1	E980.9	ACETALDEHYDE LIQUID
987.8		E869.8	E952.8	E962.2	E982.8	ACETALDEHYDE VAPOR
965.4		E850.4	E950.0	E962.0	E980.0	ACETAMINOPHEN
965.1	E935.3	E850.3	E950.0	E962.0	E980.0	ACETAMINOSALOL
965.4	E935.4	E850.4	E950.0	E962.0	E980.0	ACETANILID(E)
961.1	E931.1	E857	E950.4	E962.0	E980.4	ACETARSOL ACETARSONE
974.2	E944.2	E858.5	E950.4	E962.0	E980.4	ACETAZOLAMIDE
983.1		E864.1	E950.7	E962.1	E980.6	ACETIC ACID
974.5	E944.5	E858.5	E950.4	E962.0	E980.4	ACETIC ACID IRRIGATING SOLUTION
976.2	E946.2	E858.7	E950.4	E962.0	E980.4	ACETIC ACID LOTION
976.3	E946.3	E858.7	E950.4	E962.0	E980.4	ACETIC ACID WITH SODIUM ACETATE OINTMENT
983.1		E864.1	E950.7	E962.1	E980.6	ACETIC ANHYDRIDE
982.8		E862.4	E950.9	E962.1	E980.9	ACETIC ETHER VAPOR
962.3	E932.3	E858.0	E950.4	E962.0	E980.4	ACETOHEXAMIDE
964.3	E934.3	E858.2	E950.4	E962.0	E980.4	ACETOMENAPHTHONE
965.01	E935.0	E850.0	E950.0	E962.0	E980.0	ACETOMORPHINE
982.8		E862.4	E950.9	E962.1	E980.9	ACETONE OILS VAPOR
969.1	E939.1	E853.0	E950.3	E962.0	E980.3	ACETOPHENAZINE MALEATE
965.4	E935.4	E850.4	E950.0	E962.0	E980.0	ACETOPHENETIDIN
982.0		E862.4	E950.9	E962.1	E980.9	ACETOPHENONE
965.09	E935.2	E850.2	E950.0	E962.0	E980.0	ACETORPHINE
961.8	E931.8	E857	E950.4	E962.0	E980.4	ACETOSULFONE SODIUM
977.8	E947.8	E858.8	E950.4	E962.0	E980.4	ACETRIZOATE SODIUM
967.3	E937.3	E852.2	E950.2	E962.0	E980.2	ACETYLCARBROMAL
971.0	E941.0	E855.3	E950.4	E962.0	E980.4	ACETYLCHOLINE (CHLORIDE)
975.5	E945.5	E858.6	E950.4	E962.0	E980.4	ACETYLCYSTEINE
972.1	E942.1	E858.3	E950.4	E962.0	E980.4	ACETYLDIGITOXIN
965.09	E935.2	E850.2	E950.0	E962.0	E980.0	ACETYLDIHYDROCODEINE
965.09	E935.2	E850.2	E950.0	E962.0	E980.0	ACETYLDIHYDROCODEINONE
987.1		E868.1	E951.8	E962.2	E981.8	ACETYLENE GAS INDUSTRIAL
0						ACETYLENE GAS INDUSTRIAL INCOMPLETE COMBUSTION SEE CARBON MONOXIDE FUEL
982.3		E862.4	E950.9	E962.1	E980.9	ACETYLENE TETRACHLORIDE VAPOR
965.1	E935.3	E850.3	E950.0	E962.0	E980.0	ACETYLIODOSALICYLIC ACID
965.8	E935.8	E850.8	E950.0	E962.0	E980.0	ACETYLPHENYLHYDRAZINE
965.1	E935.3	E850.3	E950.0	E962.0	E980.0	ACETYLSALICYLIC ACID (ASPIRIN)
960.4	E930.4	E856	E950.4	E962.0	E980.4	ACHROMYCIN
976.5	E946.5	E858.7	E950.4	E962.0	E980.4	ACHROMYCIN OPHTHALMIC PREPARATION
976.0	E946.0	E858.7	E950.4	E962.0	E980.4	ACHROMYCIN TOPICAL NEC
963.2	E933.2	E858.1	E950.4	E962.0	E980.4	ACIDIFYING AGENTS
983.1		E864.1	E950.7	E962.1	E980.6	ACIDS CORROSIVE NEC
988.2	E865.4	E950.9	E962.1	E980.9		ACONITE WILD
976.8	E946.8	E858.7	E950.4	E962.0	E980.4	ACONITINE LINIMENT
988.2		E865.4	E950.9	E962.1	E980.9	ACONITUM FEROX
983.0		E864.0	E950.7	E962.1	E980.6	ACRIDINE
987.8		E869.8	E952.8	E962.2	E982.8	ACRIDINE VAPOR
961.9	E931.9	E857	E950.4	E962.0	E980.4	ACRIFLAVINE
976.0	E946.0	E858.7	E950.4	E962.0	E980.4	ACRISORCIN
987.8		E869.8	E952.8	E962.2	E982.8	ACROLEIN GAS
989.89		E866.8	E950.9	E962.1	E980.9	ACROLEIN LIQUID
988.2		E865.4	E950.9	E962.1	E980.9	ACTAEA SPICATA
961.5	E931.5	E857	E950.4	E962.0	E980.4	ACTEROL
962.4	E932.4	E858.0	E950.4	E962.0	E980.4	ACTH
962.4	E932.4	E858.0	E950.4	E962.0	E980.4	ACTHAR
960.7	E930.7	E856	E950.4	E962.0	E980.4	ACTINOMYCIN (C) (D)
967.3	E937.3	E852.2	E950.2	E962.0	E980.2	ADALIN ACETYL
977.8	E947.8	E858.8	E950.4	E962.0	E980.4	ADENOSINE PHOSPHATE
962.5	E932.5	E858.0	E950.4	E962.0	E980.4	ADH
989.89		E866.6	E950.9	E962.1	E980.9	ADHESIVES
960.0	E930.0	E856	E950.4	E962.0	E980.4	ADICILLIN
975.1	E945.1	E855.6	E950.4	E962.0	E980.4	ADIPHENINE
977.4	E947.4	E858.8	E950.4	E962.0	E980.4	ADJUNCT PHARMACEUTICAL
962.0	E932.0	E858.0	E950.4	E962.0	E980.4	ADRENAL CORTICAL STEROIDS

POISON	THERA-PEUTIC	ACCIDENT	SUICIDE	ASSAULT	UNDETER-MINED	SUBSTANCE
976.6	E946.6	E858.7	E950.4	E962.0	E980.4	ADRENAL ENT AGENT
976.5	E946.5	E858.7	E950.4	E962.0	E980.4	ADRENAL OPHTHALMIC PREPARATION
976.0	E946.0	E858.7	E950.4	E962.0	E980.4	ADRENAL TOPICAL NEC
971.2	E941.2	E855.5	E950.4	E962.0	E980.4	ADRENALIN
971.3	E941.3	E855.6	E950.4	E962.0	E980.4	ADRENERGIC BLOCKING AGENTS
971.2	E941.2	E855.5	E950.4	E962.0	E980.4	ADRENERGICS
972.8	E942.8	E858.3	E950.4	E962.0	E980.4	ADRENOCHROME DERIVATIVES
962.4	E932.4	E858.0	E950.4	E962.0	E980.4	ADRENOCORTICOTROPIC HORMONE
962.4	E932.4	E858.0	E950.4	E962.0	E980.4	ADRENOCORTICOTROPIN
960.7	E930.7	E856	E950.4	E962.0	E980.4	ADRIAMYCIN
989.89		E866.8	E950.9	E962.1	E980.9	AEROSOL SPRAY
960.8	E930.8	E856	E950.4	E962.0	E980.4	AEROSPORIN
976.6	E946.6	E858.7	E950.4	E962.0	E980.4	AEROSPORIN ENT AGENT
976.5	E946.5	E858.7	E950.4	E962.0	E980.4	AEROSPORIN OPHTHALMIC PREPARATION
976.0	E946.0	E858.7	E950.4	E962.0	E980.4	AEROSPORIN TOPICAL NEC
988.2		E865.4	E950.9	E962.1	E980.9	AETHUSA CYNAPIUM
969.6	E939.6	E854.1	E950.3	E962.0	E980.3	AFGHANISTAN BLACK
989.7		E865.9	E950.9	E962.1	E980.9	AFLATOXIN
988.2		E865.4	E950.9	E962.1	E980.9	AFRICAN BOXWOOD
973.3	E943.3	E858.4	E950.4	E962.0	E980.4	AGAR (-AGAR)
989.89		E863.9	E950.6	E962.1	E980.7	AGRICULTURAL AGENT NEC
967.0	E937.0	E851	E950.1	E962.0	E980.1	AGRYPNAL
0						AIR CONTAMINANT(S) SPECIFIED TYPE SEE SPECIFIC SUBSTANCE
987.9		E869.9	E952.9	E962.2	E982.9	AIR CONTAMINANT(S) SOURCE OR TYPE NOS
988.2		E865.4	E950.9	E962.1	E980.9	AKEE
976.0	E946.0	E858.7	E950.4	E962.0	E980.4	AKRINOL
961.6	E931.6	E857	E950.4	E962.0	E980.4	ALANTOLACTONE
960.8	E930.8	E856	E950.4	E962.0	E980.4	ALBAMYCIN
964.7	E934.7	E858.2	E950.4	E962.0	E980.4	ALBUMIN NORMAL HUMAN SERUM
975.7	E945.7	E858.6	E950.4	E962.0	E980.4	ALBUTEROL
980.0		E860.1	E950.9	E962.1	E980.9	ALCOHOL ABSOLUTE
980.0	E947.8	E860.0	E950.9	E962.1	E980.9	ALCOHOL ABSOLUTE BEVERAGE
980.3		E860.4	E950.9	E962.1	E980.9	ALCOHOL AMYL
980.1		E860.2	E950.9	E962.1	E980.9	ALCOHOL ANTIFREEZE
980.3		E860.4	E950.9	E962.1	E980.9	ALCOHOL BUTYL
980.0		E860.1	E950.9	E962.1	E980.9	ALCOHOL DEHYDRATED BEVERAGE
980.0		E860.1	E950.9	E962.1	E980.9	ALCOHOL DENATURED
977.3	E947.3	E858.8	E950.4	E962.0	E980.4	ALCOHOL DETERRENTS
977.8	E947.8	E858.8	E950.4	E962.0	E980.4	ALCOHOL DIAGNOSTIC GASTRIC FUNCTION
980.0		E860.1	E950.9	E962.1	E980.9	ALCOHOL ETHYL
980.0	E947.8	E860.0	E950.9	E962.1	E980.9	ALCOHOL ETHYL BEVERAGE
980.0		E860.1	E950.9	E962.1	E980.9	ALCOHOL GRAIN
980.0	E947.8	E860.0	E950.9	E962.1	E980.9	ALCOHOL GRAIN BEVERAGE
980.9		E860.9	E950.9	E962.1	E980.9	ALCOHOL INDUSTRIAL
980.2		E860.3	E950.9	E962.1	E980.9	ALCOHOL ISOPROPYL
980.1		E860.2	E950.9	E962.1	E980.9	ALCOHOL METHYL
980.0	E947.8	E860.2	E950.9	E962.1	E980.9	ALCOHOL PREPARATION FOR CONSUMPTION
980.3		E860.4	E950.9	E962.1	E980.9	ALCOHOL PROPYL
980.2		E860.3	E950.9	E962.1	E980.9	ALCOHOL PROPYL SECONDARY
980.1		E860.2	E950.9	E962.1	E980.9	ALCOHOL RADIATOR
980.2		E860.3	E950.9	E962.1	E980.9	ALCOHOL RUBBING
980.8		E860.8	E950.9	E962.1	E980.9	ALCOHOL SPECIFIED TYPE NEC
980.9		E860.9	E950.9	E962.1	E980.9	ALCOHOL SURGICAL
980.9		E860.9	E950.9	E962.1	E980.9	ALCOHOL UNSPECIFIED
987.8		E869.8	E952.8	E962.2	E982.8	ALCOHOL VAPOR FROM ANY TYPE OF ALCOHOL
980.1		E860.2	E950.9	E962.1	E980.9	ALCOHOL WOOD
975.2	E945.2	E858.6	E950.4	E962.0	E980.4	ALCURONIUM CHLORIDE
974.4	E944.4	E858.5	E950.4	E962.0	E980.4	ALDACTONE
989.3		E863.2	E950.6	E962.1	E980.7	ALDICARB
972.6	E942.6	E858.3	E950.4	E962.0	E980.4	ALDOMET
962.0	E932.0	E858.0	E950.4	E962.0	E980.4	ALDOSTERONE
989.2		E863.0	E950.6	E962.1	E980.7	ALDRIN DUST
973.0	E943.0	E858.4	E950.4	E962.0	E980.4	ALGELDRATE
963.4	E933.4	E858.1	E950.4	E962.0	E980.4	ALIDASE

POISON	THERA-PEUTIC	ACCIDENT	SUICIDE	ASSAULT	UNDETER-MINED	SUBSTANCE
989.0		E866.8	E950.9	E962.1	E980.9	ALIPHATIC THIOCYANATES
965.1	E935.3	E850.3	E950.0	E962.0	E980.0	ALKA SELTZER
976.6	E946.6	E858.7	E950.4	E962.0	E980.4	ALKALINE ANTISEPTIC SOLUTION AROMATIC
983.2		E864.2	E950.7	E962.1	E980.6	ALKALIS CAUSTIC
963.3	E933.3	E858.1	E950.4	E962.0	E980.4	ALKALIZING AGENTS MEDICINAL
972.6	E942.6	E858.3	E950.4	E962.0	E980.4	ALKAVERVIR
969.0	E939.0	E854.0	E950.3	E962.0	E980.3	ALLEGRON
967.0	E937.0	E851	E950.1	E962.0	E980.1	ALLOBARBITAL ALLOBARBITONE
974.7	E944.7	E858.5	E950.4	E962.0	E980.4	ALLOPURINOL
962.2	E932.2	E858.0	E950.4	E962.0	E980.4	ALLYLESTRENOL
967.8	E937.8	E852.8	E950.2	E962.0	E980.2	ALLYLISO PROPYLACETYLUREA
967.0	E937.0	E851	E950.1	E962.0	E980.1	ALLYLISOPROPYLMALONYLUREA
967.3	E937.3	E852.2	E950.2	E962.0	E980.2	ALLYLTRIBROMIDE
973.1	E943.1	E858.4	E950.4	E962.0	E980.4	ALOE ALOES ALOIN
973.8	E943.8	E858.4	E950.4	E962.0	E980.4	ALOSETRON
966.0	E936.0	E855.0	E950.4	E962.0	E980.4	ALOXIDONE
965.1	E935.3	E850.3	E950.0	E962.0	E980.0	ALOXIPRIN
963.4	E933.4	E858.1	E950.4	E962.0	E980.4	ALPHA AMYLASE
963.5	E933.5	E858.1	E950.4	E962.0	E980.4	ALPHA TOCOPHEROL
971.3	E855.6	E941.3	E950.4	E962.0	E980.4	ALPHA-1 BLOCKERS
965.09	E935.2	E850.2	E950.0	E962.0	E980.0	ALPHAPRODINE HYDROCHLORIDE
972.6	E942.6	E858.3	E950.4	E962.0	E980.4	ALSEROXYLON
983.2		E864.2	E950.7	E962.1	E980.6	ALUM AMMONIUM POTASSIUM
976.2	E946.2	E858.7	E950.4	E962.0	E980.4	ALUM MEDICINAL ASTRINGENT NEC
976.2	E946.2	E858.7	E950.4	E962.0	E980.4	ALUMINIUM ACETATE SOLUTION
973.0	E943.0	E858.4	E950.4	E962.0	E980.4	ALUMINIUM (GEL) (HYDROXIDE)
965.1	E935.3	E850.3	E950.0	E962.0	E980.0	ALUMINIUM ASPIRIN
973.0	E943.0	E858.4	E950.4	E962.0	E980.4	ALUMINIUM CARBONATE
973.0	E943.0	E858.4	E950.4	E962.0	E980.4	ALUMINIUM GLYCINATE
973.0	E943.0	E858.4	E950.4	E962.0	E980.4	ALUMINIUM HYDROXIDE
972.2	942.2	E858.3	E950.4	E962.0	E980.4	ALUMINIUM NICOTINATE
976.3	E946.3	E858.7	E950.4	E962.0	E980.4	ALUMINIUM OINTMENT SURGICAL TOPICAL
973.0	E943.0	E858.4	E950.4	E962.0	E980.4	ALUMINIUM PHOSPHATE
976.2	E946.2	E858.7	E950.4	E962.0	E980.4	ALUMINIUM SUBACETATE
976.3	E946.3	E858.7	E950.4	E962.0	E980.4	ALUMINIUM TOPICAL NEC
967.0	E937.0	E851	E950.1	E962.0	E980.1	ALURATE
975.1	E945.1	E855.6	E950.4	E962.0	E980.4	ALVERINE CITRATE
965.09	E935.2	E850.2	E950.0	E962.0	E980.0	ALVODINE
988.1		E865.5	E950.9	E962.1	E980.9	AMANITA PHALLOIDES
966.4	E936.4	E855.0	E950.4	E962.0	E980.4	AMANTADINE (HYDROCHLORIDE)
961.9	E931.9	E857	E950.4	E962.0	E980.4	AMBAZONE
971.0	E941.0	E855.3	E950.4	E962.0	E980.4	AMBENONIUM
971.1	E941.1	E855.4	E950.4	E962.0	E980.4	AMBUTONIUM BROMIDE
977.8	E947.8	E858.8	E950.4	E962.0	E980.4	AMETAZOLE
968.5	E938.5	E855.2	E950.4	E962.0	E980.4	AMETHOCAINE INFILTRATION TOPICAL
968.6	E938.6	E855.2	E950.4	E962.0	E980.4	AMETHOCAINE NERVE BLOCK PERIPHERAL LEXUS
968.7	E938.7	E855.2	E950.4	E962.0	E980.4	AMETHOCAINE SPINAL
963.1	E933.1	E858.1	E950.4	E962.0	E980.4	AMETHOPTERIN
977.0	E947.0	E858.8	E950.4	E962.0	E980.4	AMFEPRAMONE
965.02	E935.1	E850.1	E950.0	E962.0	E980.0	AMIDON
965.5	E935.5	E850.5	E950.0	E962.0	E980.0	AMIDOPYRINE
976.0	E946.0	E858.7	E950.4	E962.0	E980.4	AMINACRINE
961.5	E931.5	E857	E950.4	E962.0	E980.4	AMINITROZOLE
974.5	E944.5	E858.5	E950.4	E962.0	E980.4	AMINO ACIDS
974.5	E944.5	E858.5	E950.4	E962.0	E980.4	AMINOACETIC ACID
964.4	E934.4	E858.2	E950.4	E962.0	E980.4	AMINOCAPROIC ACID
963.8	E933.8	E858.1	E950.4	E962.0	E980.4	AMINOETHYL-ISOTHIOURIUM
966.3	E936.3	E855.0	E950.4	E962.0	E980.4	AMINOGLUTETHIMIDE
974.3	E944.3	E858.5	E950.4	E962.0	E980.4	AMINOMETRADINE
971.1	E941.1	E855.4	E950.4	E962.0	E980.4	AMINOPENTAMIDE
965.5	E935.5	E850.5	E950.0	E962.0	E980.0	AMINOPHENAZONE (AMINOPYRINE)
983.0		E864.0	E950.7	E962.1	E980.6	AMINOPHENOL
969.5	E939.5	E853.8	E950.3	E962.0	E980.3	AMINOPHENYLPYRIDONE
975.7	E945.7	E858.6	E950.4	E962.0	E980.4	AMINOPHYLLINE (THEOPHYLLINE ETHYLENE DIAMINE)
963.1	E933.1	E858.1	E950.4	E962.0	E980.4	AMINOPTERIN
965.5	E935.5	E850.5	E950.0	E962.0	E980.0	AMINOPYRINE
961.8	E931.8	E857	E950.4	E962.0	E980.4	AMINOSALICYLIC ACID
970.1	E940.1	E854.3	E950.4	E962.0	E980.4	AMIPHENAZOLE
972.6	E942.6	E858.3	E950.4	E962.0	E980.4	AMIQUINSIN
974.3	E944.3	E858.5	E950.4	E962.0	E980.4	AMISOMETRADINE

POISON	THERA-PEUTIC	ACCIDENT	SUICIDE	ASSAULT	UNDETER-MINED	SUBSTANCE
969.0	E939.0	E854.0	E950.3	E962.0	E980.3	AMITRIPTYLINE
987.8		E869.8	E952.8	E962.8	E982.8	AMMONIA FUMES GAS VAPOR
983.2		E861.4	E950.7	E962.1	E980.6	AMMONIA LIQUID HOUSEHOLD NEC
970.8	E940.8	E854.3	E950.4	E962.0	E980.4	AMMONIA SPIRIT AROMATIC
976.0	E946.0	E858.7	E950.4	E962.0	E980.4	AMMONIATED MERCURY
983.2		E864.2	E950.7	E962.1	E980.6	AMMONIUM CARBONATE
975.5	E945.5	E858.6	E950.4	E962.0	E980.4	AMMONIUM CHLORIDE EXPECTORANT
963.2	E933.2	E858.1	E950.4	E962.0	E980.4	AMMONIUM CHLORIDE ACIDIFYING AGENT
987.8		E869.8	E952.8	E962.2	E982.8	AMMONIUM COMPOUNDS FUMES ANY USAGE
983.2		E861.4	E950.7	E962.1	E980.6	AMMONIUM COMPOUNDS HOUSEHOLD NEC
983.2		E864.2	E950.7	E962.1	E980.6	AMMONIUM COMPOUNDS INDUSTRIAL
976.4	E946.4	E858.7	E950.4	E962.0	E980.4	AMMONIUM ICHTHYOSULFONATE
961.9	E931.9	E857	E950.4	E962.0	E980.4	AMMONIUM MANDELATE
967.0	E937.0	E851	E950.1	E962.0	E980.1	AMOBARBITAL (AMYLOBARBITONE)
961.4	E931.4	E857	E950.4	E962.0	E980.4	AMODIAQUIN(E)
961.4	E931.4	E857	E950.4	E962.0	E980.4	AMOPYROQUIN(E)
969.5	E939.5	E853.8	E950.3	E962.0	E980.3	AMPHENIDONE
969.7	E939.7	E854.2	E950.3	E962.0	E980.3	AMPHETAMINE
960.8	E930.8	E856	E950.4	E962.0	E980.4	AMPHOMYCIN
960.1	E930.1	E856	E950.4	E962.0	E980.4	AMPHOTERICIN B
976.0	E946.0	E858.7	E950.4	E962.0	E980.4	AMPHOTERICIN TOPICAL
960.0	E930.0	E856	E950.4	E962.0	E980.4	AMPICILLIN
971.1	E941.1	E855.4	E950.4	E962.0	E980.4	AMPROTROPINE
977.8	E947.8	E858.8	E950.4	E962.0	E980.4	AMYGADALIN
982.8		E862.4	E950.9	E962.1	E980.9	AMYL ACETATE VAPOR
980.3		E860.4	E950.9	E962.1	E980.9	AMYL ALCOHOL
972.4	E942.4	E858.3	E950.4	E962.0	E980.4	AMYL NITRITE MEDICINAL
963.4	E933.4	E858.1	E950.4	E962.0	E980.4	AMYLASE ALPHA
980.8		E860.8	E950.9	E962.1	E980.9	AMYLENE HYDRATE
967.0	E937.0	E851	E950.1	E962.0	E980.1	AMYLOBARBITONE
968.9	E938.9	E855.2	E950.4	E962.0	E980.4	AMYLOCAINE
968.5	E938.5	E855.2	E950.4	E962.0	E980.4	AMYLOCAINE INFILTRATION SUBCUTANEOUS
968.6	E938.6	E855.2	E950.4	E962.0	E980.4	AMYLOCAINE NERVE BLOCK PERIPHERAL PLEXUS
968.7	E938.7	E855.2	E950.4	E962.0	E980.4	AMYLOCAINE SPINAL
968.5	E938.5	E855.2	E950.4	E962.0	E980.4	AMYLOCAINE TOPICAL SURFACE
967.0	E937.0	E851	E950.1	E962.0	E980.1	AMYTAL SODIUM
970.0	E940.0	E854.3	E950.4	E962.0	E980.4	ANALEPTICS
965.9	E935.9	E850.9	E950.0	E962.0	E980.0	ANALGESIC AND ANTIPYRETIC NOS
965.4	E935.4	E850.4	E950.0	E962.0	E980.0	ANALGESICS AROMATIC NEC
965.7	E935.7	E850.7	E950.0	E962.0	E980.0	ANALGESICS NON NARCOTIC NEC
965.8	E935.8	E850.8	E950.0	E962.0	E980.0	ANALGESICS SPECIFIED NEC
988.2		E865.3	E950.9	E962.1	E980.9	ANAMIRTA COCCULUS
960.0	E930.0	E856	E950.4	E962.0	E980.4	ANCILLIN
962.1	E932.1	E858.0	E950.4	E962.0	E980.4	ANDROGENS ANABOLIC CONGENERS
962.1	E932.1	E858.0	E950.4	E962.0	E980.4	ANDROSTALONE
962.1	E932.1	E858.0	E950.4	E962.0	E980.4	ANDROSTERONE
988.2		E865.4	E950.9	E962.1	E980.9	ANEMONE PULSATILLA
968.2	E938.2	E855.1	E950.4	E962.0	E980.4	ANESTHESIA HALOGENATED HYDROCARBON DERIVATIVES NEC
968.2	E938.2	E855.1	E950.4	E962.0	E980.4	ANESTHESIA GASEOUS NEC
968.5	E938.5	E855.2	E950.4	E962.0	E980.4	ANESTHESIA INFILTRATION INTRADERMAL SUBCUTANEOUS SUBMUCOSAL
968.3	E938.3	E855.1	E950.4	E962.0	E980.4	ANESTHESIA INTRAVENOUS
968.3	E938.3	E855.1	E950.4	E962.0	E980.4	ANESTHESIA RECTAL NEC
968.5	E938.5	E855.2	E950.4	E962.0	E980.4	ANESTHESIA SURFACE
968.5	E938.5	E855.2	E950.4	E962.0	E980.4	ANESTHESIA TOPICAL
968.4	E938.4	E855.1	E950.4	E962.0	E980.4	ANESTHETICS (GENERAL OTHER AND NOS)
968.9	E938.9	E855.2	E950.4	E962.0	E980.4	ANESTHETICS LOCAL OTHER AND NOS
968.6	E938.6	E855.2	E950.4	E962.0	E980.4	ANESTHETICS PERIPHERAL NERVE- AND PLEXUS- BLOCKING
968.7	E938.7	E855.2	E950.4	E962.0	E980.4	ANESTHETICS SPINAL
963.5	E933.5	E858.1	E950.4	E962.0	E980.4	ANEURINE
977.8	E947.8	E858.8	E950.4	E962.0	E980.4	ANGIO-CONRAY

DRUGS & CHEMICALS

POISON	THERA-PEUTIC	ACCIDENT	SUICIDE	ASSAULT	UNDETER-MINED	SUBSTANCE
971.2	E941.2	E855.5	E950.4	E962.0	E980.4	ANGIOTENSIN
962.2	E932.2	E858.0	E950.4	E962.0	E980.4	ANHYDROHYDROXPRO-GESTERONE
974.3	E944.3	E858.5	E950.4	E962.0	E980.4	ANHYDRON
965.09	E935.2	E850.2	E950.0	E962.0	E980.0	ANILERIDINE
965.4	E935.4	E850.4	E950.0	E962.0	E980.0	ANILINE ANALGESIC
965.4	E935.4	E850.4	E950.0	E962.0	E980.0	ANILINE DERIVATIVES THERAPEUTIC NEC
983.0		E864.0	E950.7	E962.1	E980.6	ANILINE DYE LIQUID
987.8		E869.8	E952.8	E962.2	E982.8	ANILINE VAPOR
964.2	E934.2	E858.2	E950.4	E962.0	E980.4	ANISINDIONE
971.1	E941.1	E855.4	E950.4	E962.0	E980.4	ANISOTROPINE
977.0	E947.0	E858.8	E950.4	E962.0	E980.4	ANOREXIC AGENTS
989.5		E905.5	E950.9	E962.1	E980.9	ANT BITE STING
0						ANT POISONS SEE PESTICIDES
977.3	E947.3	E858.8	E950.4	E962.0	E980.4	ANTABUSE
973.0	E943.0	E858.4	E950.4	E962.0	E980.4	ANTACIDS
963.0	E933.0	E858.1	E950.4	E962.0	E980.4	ANTAZOLINE
961.6	E931.6	E857	E950.4	E962.0	E980.4	ANTHELMINTICS
976.4	E946.4	E858.7	E950.4	E962.0	E980.4	ANTHRALIN
960.7	E930.7	E856	E950.4	E962.0	E980.4	ANTHRAMYCIN
975.6	945.6	E858.6	E950.4	E962.0	E980.4	ANTI-COMMON COLD AGENTS NEC
960.9	E930.9	E856	E950.4	E962.0	E980.4	ANTI-INFECTIVES ANTIBIOTICS
960.8	E930.8	E856	E950.4	E962.0	E980.4	ANTI-INFECTIVES ANTIBIOTICS SPECIFIED NEC
961.4	E931.4	E857	E950.4	E962.0	E980.4	ANTI-INFECTIVES ANTIMALARIAL
960.6	E930.6	E856	E950.4	E962.0	E980.4	ANTI-INFECTIVES ANTIMYCOBACTERIAL ANTIBIOTICS
961.8	E931.8	E857	E950.4	E962.0	E980.4	ANTI-INFECTIVES ANTIMYCOBACTERIAL NEC
961.4	E931.4	E857	E950.4	E962.0	E980.4	ANTI-INFECTIVES ANTIPROTOZOAL BLOOD
961.4	E931.4	E857	E950.4	E962.0	E980.4	ANTI-INFECTIVES ANTIPROTOZOAL BLOOD NEC
961.5	E931.5	E857	E950.4	E962.0	E980.4	ANTI-INFECTIVES ANTIPROTOZOAL NEC
961.7	E931.7	E857	E950.4	E962.0	E980.4	ANTI-INFECTIVES ANTIVIRAL NEC
961.6	E931.6	E857	E950.4	E962.0	E980.4	ANTI-INFECTIVES ANTHELMINTIC
961.1	E931.1	E857	E950.4	E962.0	E980.4	ANTI-INFECTIVES ARSENICAL
976.6	E946.6	E858.7	E950.4	E962.0	E980.4	ANTI-INFECTIVES ENT AGENTS
961.2	E931.2	E857	E950.4	E962.0	E980.4	ANTI-INFECTIVES HEAVY METALS NEC
976.0	E946.0	E858.7	E950.4	E962.0	E980.4	ANTI-INFECTIVES LOCAL
961.9	E931.9	E857	E950.4	E962.0	E980.4	ANTI-INFECTIVES NEC
976.5	E946.5	E858.7	E950.4	E962.0	E980.4	ANTI-INFECTIVES OPHTHALMIC PREPARATION
976.0	E946.0	E858.7	E950.4	E962.0	E980.4	ANTI-INFECTIVES TOPICAL NEC
976.0	E946.0	E858.7	E950.4	E962.0	E980.4	ANTI-INFLAMMATORY AGENTS TOPICAL
966.4	E936.4	E855.0	E950.4	E962.0	E980.4	ANTI-PARKINSONISM AGENTS
971.3	E941.3	E855.6	E950.4	E962.0	E980.4	ANTIADRENERGICS
963.0	E933.0	E858.1	E950.4	E962.0	E980.4	ANTIALLERGIC AGENTS
964.1	E934.1	E858.2	E950.4	E962.0	E980.4	ANTIANEMIC AGENTS NEC
988.2		E865.4	E950.9	E962.1	E980.9	ANTIARIS TOXICARIA
972.2	E942.2	E858.3	E950.4	E962.0	E980.4	ANTIARTERIOSCLEROTIC AGENTS
975.7	E945.7	E858.6	E950.4	E962.0	E980.4	ANTIASTHMATICS
960.8	E930.8	E856	E950.4	E962.0	E980.4	ANTIBIOTICS (OTHER SPECIFIED)
960.1	E930.1	E856	E950.4	E962.0	E980.4	ANTIBIOTICS ANTI-FUNGAL
960.9	E930.9	E856	E950.4	E962.0	E980.4	ANTIBIOTIC
960.6	E930.6	E856	E950.4	E962.0	E980.4	ANTIBIOTICS ANTIMY-COBACTERIAL
960.7	E930.7	E856	E950.4	E962.0	E980.4	ANTIBIOTICS ANTINEO-PLASTIC
960.5	E930.5	E856	E950.4	E962.0	E980.4	ANTIBIOTICS CEPHALOSPORIN GROUP
960.2	E930.2	E856	E950.4	E962.0	E980.4	ANTIBIOTICS CHLORAMPHENICOL GROUP
960.3	E930.3	E856	E950.4	E962.0	E980.4	ANTIBIOTICS MACROLIDES
960.4	E930.4	E856	E950.4	E962.0	E980.4	ANTIBIOTICS TETRACYCLINE GROUP
960.7	E930.7	E856	E950.4	E962.0	E980.4	ANTICANCER AGENTS ANTIBIOTICS
963.1	E933.1	E858.1	E950.4	E962.0	E980.4	ANTICANCER AGENTS NEC
971.1	E941.1	E855.4	E950.4	E962.0	E980.4	ANTICHOLINERGICS
971.0	E941.0	E855.3	E950.4	E962.0	E980.4	ANTICHOLINESTERASE ORGANOPHOSPHORUS REVERSIBLE

POISON	THERA-PEUTIC	ACCIDENT	SUICIDE	ASSAULT	UNDETER-MINED	SUBSTANCE
964.2	E934.2	E858.2	E950.4	E962.0	E980.4	ANTICOAGULANTS
964.5	E934.5	E858.2	E950.4	E962.0	E980.4	ANTICOAGULANTS ANTAGONISTS
966.3	E936.3	E855.0	E950.4	E962.0	E980.4	ANTICONVULSANTS NEC
969.0	E939.0	E854.0	E950.3	E962.0	E980.3	ANTIDEPRESSANTS
962.3	E932.3	E858.0	E950.4	E962.0	E980.4	ANTIDIABETIC AGENTS
973.5	E943.5	E858.4	E950.4	E962.0	E980.4	ANTIDIARRHEAL AGENTS
962.5	E932.5	E858.0	E950.4	E962.0	E980.4	ANTIDIURETIC HORMONE
977.2	E947.2	E858.8	E950.4	E962.0	E980.4	ANTIDOTES NEC
963.0	E933.0	E858.1	E950.4	E962.0	E980.4	ANTIEMETIC AGENTS
966.3	E936.3	E855.0	E950.4	E962.0	E980.4	ANTIEPILEPSY AGENT NEC
962.2	E932.2	E858.0	E950.4	E962.0	E980.4	ANTIFERTILITY PILLS
973.8	E943.8	E858.4	E950.4	E962.0	E980.4	ANTIFLATULENTS
989.89		E866.8	E950.9	E962.1	E980.9	ANTIFREEZE
980.1		E860.2	E950.9	E962.1	E980.9	ANTIFREEZE ALCOHOL
982.8		E862.4	E950.9	E962.1	E980.9	ANTIFREEZE ETHYLENE GLYCOL
960.1	E930.1	E856	E950.4	E962.0	E980.4	ANTIFUNGALS MEDICINAL ANTIBIOTIC
961.9	E931.9	E857	E950.4	E962.0	E980.4	ANTIFUNGALS MEDICINAL NEC
976.0	E946.0	E858.7	E950.4	E962.0	E980.4	ANTIFUNGALS MEDICINAL TOPICAL
989.4		E863.6	E950.6	E962.1	E980.7	ANTIFUNGALS NONMEDICINAL SPRAYS
973.0	E943.0	E858.4	E950.4	E962.0	E980.4	ANTIGASTRIC SECRETION AGENTS
961.6	E931.6	E857	E950.4	E962.0	E980.4	ANTIHELMINTICS
964.7	E934.7	E858.2	E950.4	E962.0	E980.4	ANTIHEMOPHILIC FACTOR HUMAN
963.0	E933.0	E858.1	E950.4	E962.0	E980.4	ANTIHISTAMINE
972.6	E942.6	E858.3	E950.4	E962.0	E980.4	ANTIHYPERTENSIVE AGENTS NEC
984.1	E862.1	E950.9	E962.1		E980.9	ANTIKNOCK TETRAETHYL LEAD
972.2	E942.2	E858.3	E950.4	E962.0	E980.4	ANTILIPEMICS
961.4	E931.4	E857	E950.4	E962.0	E980.4	ANTIMALARIALS
961.2	E931.2	E857	E950.4	E962.0	E980.4	ANTIMONY ANTI-INFECTIVES
985.4		E866.2	E950.9	E962.1	E980.9	ANTIMONY COMPOUNDS VAPOR NEC
985.4		E863.4	E950.6	E962.2	E980.7	ANTIMONY PESTICIDES VAPOR
961.2	E931.2	E857	E950.4	E962.0	E980.4	ANTIMONY POTASSIUM TARTRATE
961.2	E931.2	E857	E950.4	E962.0	E980.4	ANTIMONY TARTRATED
971.1	E941.1	E855.4	E950.4	E962.0	E980.4	ANTIMUSCARINIC AGENTS
960.6	E930.6	E856	E950.4	E962.0	E980.4	ANTIMYCOBACTERIALS ANTIBIOTICS
961.8	E931.8	E857	E950.4	E962.0	E980.4	ANTIMYCOBACTERIALS NEC
960.7	E930.7	E856	E950.4	E962.0	E980.4	ANTINEOPLASTIC AGENTS ANTIBIOTICS
963.1	E933.1	E858.1	E950.4	E962.0	E980.4	ANTINEOPLASTIC AGENTS IMMUNOSUPPRESIVES
965.69	E935.6	E850.6	E950.0	E962.0	E980.0	ANTIPHLOGISTICS
961.4	E931.4	E857	E950.4	E962.0	E980.4	ANTIPROTOZOALS BLOOD
961.5	E931.5	E857	E950.4	E962.0	E980.4	ANTIPROTOZOALS NEC
976.1	E946.1	E858.7	E950.4	E962.0	E980.4	ANTIPRURITICS LOCAL
969.3	E939.3	E853.8	E950.3	E962.0	E980.3	ANTIPSYCHOTIC AGENTS NEC
965.9	E935.9	E850.9	E950.0	E962.0	E980.0	ANTIPYRETICS
965.8	E935.8	E850.8	E950.0	E962.0	E980.0	ANTIPYRETICS SPECIFIED NEC
965.5	E935.5	E850.5	E950.0	E962.0	E980.0	ANTIPYRINE
979.9	E949.9	E858.8	E950.4	E962.0	E980.4	ANTIRABIES SERUM EQUINE
965.69	E935.6	E850.6	E950.0	E962.0	E980.0	ANTIRHEUMATICS
976.4	E946.4	E858.7	E950.4	E962.0	E980.4	ANTISEBORRHEICS
976.0	E946.0	E858.7	E950.4	E962.0	E980.4	ANTISEPTICS EXTERNAL MEDICINAL
963.0	E933.0	E858.1	E950.4	E962.0	E980.4	ANTISTINE
962.8	E932.8	E858.0	E950.4	E962.0	E980.4	ANTITHYROID AGENTS
979.9	E949.9	E858.8	E950.4	E962.0	E980.4	ANTITOXIN ANY
961.8	E931.8	E857	E950.4	E962.0	E980.4	ANTITUBERCULARS
960.6	E930.6	E856	E950.4	E962.0	E980.4	ANTITUBERCULARS ANTIBIOTICS
975.4	E945.4	E858.6	E950.4	E962.0	E980.4	ANTITUSSIVES
972.7	E942.7	E858.3	E950.4	E962.0	E980.4	ANTIVARICOSE AGENTS SCLEROSING
979.9	E949.9	E858.8	E950.4	E962.0	E980.4	ANTIVENIN CROTALINE SPIDER-BITE
963.0	E933.0	E858.1	E950.4	E962.0	E980.4	ANTIVERT
961.7	E931.7	E857	E950.4	E962.0	E980.4	ANTIVIRALS NEC
989.4		E863.4	E950.6	E962.1	E980.7	ANTROL
989.4		E863.6	E950.6	E962.1	E980.7	ANTROL FUNGICIDE
973.6	E943.6	E858.4	E950.4	E962.0	E980.4	APOMORPHINE HYDROCHLORIDE EMETIC
977.0	E947.0	E858.8	E950.4	E962.0	E980.4	APPETITE DEPRESSANTS CENTRAL
972.6	E942.6	E858.3	E950.4	E962.0	E980.4	APRESOLINE
967.0	E937.0	E851	E950.1	E962.0	E980.1	APROBARBITAL APROBARBITONE

POISON	THERA-PEUTIC	ACCIDENT	SUICIDE	ASSAULT	UNDETER-MINED	SUBSTANCE
967.8	E937.8	E852.8	E950.2	E962.0	E980.2	APRONALIDE
983.1		E864.1	E950.7	E962.1	E980.6	AQUA FORTIS
973.2	E943.2	E858.4	E950.4	E962.0	E980.4	ARACHIS OIL CATHARTIC
976.3	E946.3	E858.7	E950.4	E962.0	E980.4	ARACHIS OIL TOPICAL
961.4	E931.4	E857	E950.4	E962.0	E980.4	ARALEN
974.5	E944.5	E858.5	E950.4	E962.0	E980.4	ARGININE SALTS
976.0	E946.0	E858.7	E950.4	E962.0	E980.4	ARGYROL
976.6	E946.6	E858.7	E950.4	E962.0	E980.4	ARGYROL ENT AGENT
976.5	E946.5	E858.7	E950.4	E962.0	E980.4	RGYROL OPHTHALMIC PREPARATION
962.0	E932.0	E858.0	E950.4	E962.0	E980.4	ARISTOCORT
976.6	E946.6	E858.7	E950.4	E962.0	E980.4	ARISTOCORT ENT AGENT
976.5	E946.5	E858.7	E950.4	E962.0	E980.4	ARISTOCORT OPHTHALMIC PREPARATION
976.0	E946.0	E858.7	E950.4	E962.0	E980.4	ARISTOCORT TOPICAL NEC
983.0		E864.0	E950.7	E962.1	E980.6	AROMATICS CORROSIVE
983.0		E864.0	E950.7	E962.1	E980.6	AROMATICS CORROSIVE DISINFECTANTS
985.1		E866.3	E950.8	E962.1	E980.8	ARSENIC COMPOUNDS DUST FUMES VAPOR NEC
985.1		E863.4	E950.8	E962.1	E980.8	ARSENIC PESTICIDE DUST FUMES
961.1	E931.1	E857	E950.4	E962.0	E980.4	ARSENICAL ANTI-INFECTIVES
985.1		E866.3	E950.8	E962.1	E980.8	ARSINE GAS
961.1	E931.1	E857	E950.4	E962.0	E980.4	ARSPHENAMINE SILVER
961.1	E931.1	E857	E950.4	E962.0	E980.4	ARSTHINOL
971.1	E941.1	E855.4	E950.4	E962.0	E980.4	ARTANE
989.5		E905.5	E950.9	E962.1	E980.9	ARTHROPOD VENOMOUS NEC
989.81		E866.8	E950.9	E962.1	E980.9	ASBESTOS
961.6	E931.6	E857	E950.4	E962.0	E980.4	ASCARIDOLE
963.5	E933.5	E858.1	E950.4	E962.0	E980.4	ASCORBIC ACID
976.0	E946.0	E858.7	E950.4	E962.0	E980.4	ASIATICOSIDE
961.6	E931.6	E857	E950.4	E962.0	E980.4	ASPIDIUM OLEORESIN
965.1	E935.3	E850.3	E950.0	E962.0	E980.0	ASPIRIN
976.2	E946.2	E858.7	E950.4	E962.0	E980.4	ASTRINGENTS LOCAL
961.3	E931.3	E857	E950.4	E962.0	E980.4	ATABRINE
969.5	E939.5	E853.8	E950.3	E962.0	E980.3	ATARACTICS
973.3	E943.3	E858.4	E950.4	E962.0	E980.4	ATONIA DRUG INTESTINAL
974.7	E944.7	E858.5	E950.4	E962.0	E980.4	ATOPHAN
971.1	E941.1	E855.4	E950.4	E962.0	E980.4	ATROPINE
973.5	E943.5	E858.4	E950.4	E962.0	E980.4	ATTAPULGITE
979.4	E949.4	E858.8	E950.4	E962.0	E980.4	ATTENUVAX
960.4	E930.4	E856	E950.4	E962.0	E980.4	AUREOMYCIN
976.5	E946.5	E858.7	E950.4	E962.0	E980.4	AUREOMYCIN OPHTHALMIC PREPARATION
976.0	E946.0	E858.7	E950.4	E962.0	E980.4	AUREOMYCIN TOPICAL NEC
965.69	E935.6	E850.6	E950.0	E962.0	E980.0	AUROTHIOGLUCOSE
965.69	E935.6	E850.6	E950.0	E962.0	E980.0	AUROTHIOGLYCANIDE
965.69	E935.6	E850.6	E950.0	E962.0	E980.0	AUROTHIOMALATE
981		E862.1	E950.9	E962.1	E980.9	AUTOMOBILE FUEL
971.9	E941.9	E855.9	E950.4	E962.0	E980.4	AUTONOMIC NERVOUS SYSTEM AGENTS NEC
961.8	E931.8	E857	E950.4	E962.0	E980.4	AVLOSULFON
967.8	E937.8	E852.8	E950.2	E962.0	E980.2	AVOMINE
969.5	E939.5	E853.8	E950.3	E962.0	E980.3	AZACYCLONOL
971.3	E941.3	E855.6	E950.4	E962.0	E980.4	AZAPETINE
963.1	E933.1	E858.1	E950.4	E962.0	E980.4	AZARIBINE
960.7	E930.7	E856	E950.4	E962.0	E980.4	AZASERINE
963.1	E933.1	E858.1	E950.4	E962.0	E980.4	AZATHIOPRINE
961.0	E931.0	E857	E950.4	E962.0	E980.4	AZOSULFAMIDE
961.0	E931.0	E857	E950.4	E962.0	E980.4	AZULFIDINE
977.8	E947.8	E858.8	E950.4	E962.0	E980.4	AZURESIN
976.0	E946.0	E858.7	E950.4	E962.0	E980.4	BACIMYCIN
976.5	E946.5	E858.7	E950.4	E962.0	E980.4	BACIMYCIN OPHTHALMIC PREPARATION
960.8	E930.8	E856	E950.4	E962.0	E980.4	BACITRACIN
976.6	E946.6	E858.7	E950.4	E962.0	E980.4	BACITRACIN ENT AGENT
976.5	E946.5	E858.7	E950.4	E962.0	E980.4	BACITRACIN OPHTHALMIC PREPARATION
976.0	E946.0	E858.7	E950.4	E962.0	E980.4	BACITRACIN TOPICAL NEC
963.3	E933.3	E858.1	E950.4	E962.0	E980.4	BAKING SODA
963.8	E933.8	E858.1	E950.4	E962.0	E980.4	BAL
972.5	E942.5	E858.3	E950.4	E962.0	E980.4	BAMETHAN SULFATE
963.0	E933.0	E858.1	E950.4	E962.0	E980.4	BAMIPINE
988.2	E865.4	E950.9	E962.1		E980.9	BANEBERRY
988.2	E866.0	E950.9	E962.1		E980.9	BANEWORT

POISON	THERA-PEUTIC	ACCIDENT	SUICIDE	ASSAULT	UNDETER-MINED	SUBSTANCE
967.0	E937.0	E851	E950.1	E962.0	E980.1	BARBENYL
967.0	E937.0	E851	E950.1	E962.0	E980.1	BARBITAL (BARBITONE)
968.3	E938.3	E855.1	E950.4	E962.0	E980.4	BARBITURATES ANESTHETIC INTRAVENOUS
967.0	E937.0	E851	E950.1	E962.0	E980.1	BARBITURATES BARBITURIC ACID
985.8		E866.4	E950.9	E962.1	E980.9	BARIUM CARBONATE CHLORIDE SULFATE
977.8	E947.8	E858.8	E950.4	E962.0	E980.4	BARIUM DIAGNOSTIC AGENT
985.8	E863.4	E950.6	E962.1		E980.7	BARIUM PESTICIDE
985.8	E863.7	E950.6	E962.1		E980.7	BARIUM RODENTICIDE
976.3	E946.3	E858.7	E950.4	E962.0	E980.4	BARRIER CREAM
983.1	E864.1	E950.7	E962.1		E980.6	BATTERY ACID OR FLUID
980.8	E860.8	E950.9	E962.1		E980.9	BAY RUM
978.0	E948.0	E858.8	E950.4	E962.0	E980.4	BCG VACCINE
988.2	E865.4	E950.9	E962.1		E980.9	BEARSFOOT
966.3	E936.3	E855.0	E950.4	E962.0	E980.4	BECLAMIDE
989.5	E905.3	E950.9	E962.1		E980.9	BEE STING VENOM
971.1	E941.1	E855.4	E950.4	E962.0	E980.4	BELLADONNA ALKALOIDS
970.0	E940.0	E854.3	E950.4	E962.0	E980.4	BEMEGRIDE
969.8	E939.8	E855.8	E950.3	E962.0	E980.3	BENACTYZINE
963.0	E933.0	E858.1	E950.4	E962.0	E980.4	BENADRYL
974.3	E944.3	E858.5	E950.4	E962.0	E980.4	BENDROFLUAZIDE
974.3	E944.3	E858.5	E950.4	E962.0	E980.4	BENDROFLUMETHIAZIDE
974.7	E944.7	E858.5	E950.4	E962.0	E980.4	BENEMID
960.0	E930.0	E856	E950.4	E962.0	E980.4	BENETHAMINE PENICILLIN G
976.0	E946.0	E858.7	E950.4	E962.0	E980.4	BENISONE
976.8	E946.8	E858.7	E950.4	E962.0	E980.4	BENOQUIN
968.5	E938.5	E855.2	E950.4	E962.0	E980.4	BENOXINATE
976.3	E946.3	E858.7	E950.4	E962.0	E980.4	BENTONITE
976.0	E946.0	E858.7	E950.4	E962.0	E980.4	BENZALKONIUM CHLORIDE
976.5	E946.5	E858.7	E950.4	E962.0	E980.4	BENZALKONIUM OPHTHALMIC PREPARATION
961.8	E931.8	E857	E950.4	E962.0	E980.4	BENZAMIDOSALICYLATE CALCIUM
960.0	E930.0	E856	E950.4	E962.0	E980.4	BENZATHINE PENICILLIN
963.1	E933.1	E858.1	E950.4	E962.0	E980.4	BENZCARBIMINE
971.2	E941.2	E855.5	E950.4	E962.0	E980.4	BENZEDREX
969.7	E939.7	E854.2	E950.3	E962.0	E980.3	BENZEDRINE AMPHETAMINE
982.0		E862.4	E950.9	E962.1	E980.9	BENZENE ACETYL DIMETHYL METHYL SOLVENT VAPOR
989.2		E863.0	E950.6	E962.1	E980.7	BENZENE HEXACHLORIDEGAMMA INSECTICIDE VAPOR
976.0	E946.0	E858.7	E950.4	E962.0	E980.4	BENZETHONIUM
966.4	E936.4	E855.0	E950.4	E962.0	E980.4	BENZHEXOL CHLORIDE
971.1	E941.1	E855.4	E950.4	E962.0	E980.4	BENZILONIUM
981	E862.0	E950.9	E962.1	E980.9		BENZIN(E) SOLVENT
987.1	E869.8	E952.8	E962.2	E982.8		BENZIN(E) VAPOR
972.4	E942.4	E858.3	E950.4	E962.0	E980.4	BENZIODARONE
968.5	E938.5	E855.2	E950.4	E962.0	E980.4	BENZOCAINE
969.4	E939.4	E853.2	E950.3	E962.0	E980.3	BENZODIAZEPINES (TRANQUILIZERS) NEC
976.0	E946.0	E858.7	E950.4	E962.0	E980.4	BENZOIC ACID WITH SALICYLIC ACID ANTI-INFECTIVE
976.3	E946.3	E858.7	E950.4	E962.0	E980.4	BENZOIN
982.0		E862.4	E950.9	E962.1	E980.9	BENZOL VAPOR
965.09	E935.2	E850.2	E950.0	E962.0	E980.0	BENZOMORPHAN
975.4	E945.4	E858.6	E950.4	E962.0	E980.4	BENZONATATE
974.3	E944.3	E858.5	E950.4	E962.0	E980.4	BENZOTHIADIAZIDES
961.8	E931.8	E857	E950.4	E962.0	E980.4	BENZOYLPAS
969.5	E939.5	E853.8	E950.3	E962.0	E980.3	BENZPERIDOL
977.0	E947.0	E858.8	E950.4	E962.0	E980.4	BENZPHETAMINE
971.0	E941.0	E855.3	E950.4	E962.0	E980.4	BENZPYRINIUM
963.0	E933.0	E858.1	E950.4	E962.0	E980.4	BENZQUINAMIDE
974.3	E944.3	E858.5	E950.4	E962.0	E980.4	BENZTHIAZIDE
971.1	E941.1	E855.4	E950.4	E962.0	E980.4	BENZTROPINE
982.8		E862.4	E950.9	E962.1	E980.9	BENZYL ACETATE
976.0	E946.0	E858.7	E950.4	E962.0	E980.4	BENZYL BENZOATE ANTI-INFECTIVE
965.09	E935.2	E850.2	E950.0	E962.0	E980.0	BENZYL MORPHINE
960.0	E930.0	E856	E950.4	E962.0	E980.4	BENZYL PENICILLIN
961.6	E931.6	E857	E950.4	E962.0	E980.4	BEPHENIUM HYDROXYNAPTHOATE
989.89		E866.8	E950.9	E962.1	E980.9	BERGAMOT OIL
988.2		E865.3	E950.9	E962.1	E980.9	BERRIES POISONOUS
985.3		E866.4	E950.9	E962.1	E980.9	BERYLLIUM COMPOUNDS FUMES
976.3	E946.3	E858.7	E950.4	E962.0	E980.4	BETA-CAROTENE
967.1	E937.1	E852.0	E950.2	E962.0	E980.2	BETA-CHLOR
962.0	E932.0	E858.0	E950.4	E962.0	E980.4	BETAMETHASONE

POISON	THERA-PEUTIC	ACCIDENT	SUICIDE	ASSAULT	UNDETER-MINED	SUBSTANCE
976.0	E946.0	E858.7	E950.4	E962.0	E980.4	BETAMETHASONE TOPICAL
977.8	E947.8	E858.8	E950.4	E962.0	E980.4	BETAZOLE
971.0	E971.0	E855.3	E950.4	E962.0	E980.4	BETHANECHOL
972.6	E942.6	E858.3	E950.4	E962.0	E980.4	BETHANIDINE
976.3	E946.3	E858.7	E950.4	E962.0	E980.4	BETULA OIL
969.6	E939.6	E854.1	E950.3	E962.0	E980.3	BHANG
961.5	E931.5	E857	E950.4	E962.0	E980.4	BIALAMICOL
0						BICHLORIDE OF MERCURY SEE MERCURY CHLORIDE
983.9		E864.3	E950.7	E962.1	E980.6	BICHROMATES CALCIUM CRYSTALS POTASSIUM SODIUM
987.8		E869.8	E952.8	E962.2	E982.8	BICHROMATES FUMES
962.3	E932.3	E858.0	E950.4	E962.0	E980.4	BIGUANIDE DERIVATIVES ORAL
977.8	E947.8	E858.8	E950.4	E962.0	E980.4	BILIGRAFIN
977.8	E947.8	E858.8	E950.4	E962.0	E980.4	BILOPAQUE
972.8	E942.8	E858.3	E950.4	E962.0	E980.4	BIOFLAVONOIDS
979.9	E949.9	E858.8	E950.4	E962.0	E980.4	BIOLOGICAL SUBSTANCENEC
966.4	E936.4	E855.0	E950.4	E962.0	E980.4	BIPERIDEN
973.1	E943.1	E858.4	E950.4	E962.0	E980.4	BISACODYL
964.2	E934.2	E858.2	E950.4	E962.0	E980.4	BISHYDROXYCOUMARIN
961.1	E931.1	E857	E950.4	E962.0	E980.4	BISMARSEN
985.8		E866.4	E950.9	E962.1	E980.9	BISMUTH COMPOUNDS NEC
961.2	E931.2	E857	E950.4	E962.0	E980.4	BISMUTH COMPOUNDS NEC ANTI-INFECTIVES
973.5	E943.5	E858.4	E950.4	E962.0	E980.4	BISMUTH COMPOUNDS SUBCARBONATE NEC
961.1	E931.1	E857	E950.4	E962.0	E980.4	BISMUTH COMPOUNDS SULFARSPHENAMINE NEC
963.1	E858.1	E933.7	E950.4	E962.0	E980.4	BISPHOSPHONATES INTRAVENOUS
963.1	E858.1	E933.6	E950.4	E962.0	E980.4	BISPHOSPHONATES ORAL
961.6	E931.6	E857	E950.4	E962.0	E980.4	BITHIONOL
989.0		E866.8	E950.9	E962.1	E980.9	BITTER ALMOND OIL
988.2		E865.4	E950.9	E962.1	E980.9	BITTERSWEET
989.4		E863.4	E950.6	E962.1	E980.7	BLACK FLAG
988.2		E865.4	E950.9	E962.1	E980.9	BLACK HENBANE
989.4		E863.4	E950.6	E962.1	E980.7	BLACK LEAF 40
989.5		E905.1	E950.9	E962.1	E980.9	BLACK WIDOW SPIDER BITE
979.9	E949.9	E858.8	E950.4	E962.0	E980.4	BLACK WIDOW SPIDER BITE ANTIVENIN
986		E868.8	E952.1	E962.2	E982.1	BLAST FURNACE GAS CARBON MONOXIDE FROM
983.9		E864.3	E950.7	E962.1	E980.6	BLEACH NEC
983.9		E864.3	E950.7	E962.1	E980.6	BLEACHING SOLUTIONS
960.7	E930.7	E856	E950.4	E962.0	E980.4	BLEOMYCIN (SULFATE)
968.9	E938.9	E855.2	E950.4	E962.0	E980.4	BLOCKAIN
968.5	E938.5	E855.2	E950.4	E962.0	E980.4	BLOCKAIN INFILTRATION SUBCUTANEOUS
968.6	E938.6	E855.2	E950.4	E962.0	E980.4	BLOCKAIN NERVE BLOCK PERIPHERAL PLEXUS
968.5	E938.5	E855.2	E950.4	E962.0	E980.4	BLOCKAIN TOPICAL SURFACE
964.8	E934.8	E858.2	E950.4	E962.0	E980.4	BLOOD AFFECTING AGENT SPECIFIED NEC
964.9	E934.9	E858.2	E950.4	E962.0	E980.4	BLOOD CONSTITUENTS AGENT AFFECTING NOS
964.7	E934.7	E858.2	E950.4	E962.0	E980.4	BLOOD DERIVATIVES
964.7	E934.7	E858.2	E950.4	E962.0	E980.4	BLOOD NATURAL
964.7	E934.7	E858.2	E950.4	E962.0	E980.4	BLOOD PLASMA
964.8	E934.8	E858.2	E950.4	E962.0	E980.4	BLOOD SUBSTITUTE MACROMOLECULAR
964.7	E934.7	E858.2	E950.4	E962.0	E980.4	BLOOD WHOLE
965.09	E935.2	E850.2	E950.0	E962.0	E980.0	BLUE VELVET
989.89	E866.5	E950.9	E962.1	E980.9		BONE MEAL
963.0	E933.0	E858.1	E950.4	E962.0	E980.4	BONINE
976.0	E946.0	E858.7	E950.4	E962.0	E980.4	BORACIC ACID
976.6	E946.6	E858.7	E950.4	E962.0	E980.4	BORACIC ACID ENT AGENT
976.5	E946.5	E858.7	E950.4	E962.0	E980.4	BORACIC ACID OPHTHALMIC PREPARATION
989.6		E861.3	E950.9	E962.1	E980.9	BORATE CLEANSER SODIUM
989.6		E861.3	E950.9	E962.1	E980.9	BORAX CLEANSER
976.0	E946.0	E858.7	E950.4	E962.0	E980.4	BORIC ACID
976.5	E946.5	E858.7	E950.4	E962.0	E980.4	BORIC ACID OPHTHALMIC PREPARATION
976.6	E946.6	E858.7	E950.4	E962.0	E980.4	BORIC ACID ENT AGENT
987.8		E869.8	E952.8	E962.2	E982.8	BORON HYDRIDE FUMES OR GAS
989.89		E866.8	E950.9	E962.1	E980.9	BORON HYDRIDE NEC
975.3	E945.3	E858.6	E950.4	E962.0	E980.4	BOTOX
987.8		E869.8	E952.8	E962.2	E982.8	BRAKE FLUID VAPOR
985.8		E866.4	E950.9	E962.1	E980.9	BRASS COMPOUNDS FUMES
981		E861.3	E950.9	E962.1	E980.9	BRASSO

POISON	THERA-PEUTIC	ACCIDENT	SUICIDE	ASSAULT	UNDETER-MINED	SUBSTANCE
972.6	E942.6	E858.3	E950.4	E962.0	E980.4	BRETYLIUM TOSYLATE
968.3	E938.3	E855.1	E950.4	E962.0	E980.4	BREVITAL SODIUM
963.8	E933.8	E858.1	E950.4	E962.0	E980.4	BRITISH ANTILEWISITE
967.3	E937.3	E852.2	E950.2	E962.0	E980.2	BROMAL HYDRATE
963.4	E933.4	E858.1	E950.4	E962.0	E980.4	BROMELAINS
967.3	E937.3	E852.1	E950.2	E962.0	E980.2	BROMIDES NEC
967.3	E937.3	E852.2	E950.2	E962.0	E980.2	BROMINE COMPOUNDS MEDICINAL
987.8		E869.8	E952.8	E962.2	E982.8	BROMINE VAPOR
967.3	E937.3	E852.2	E950.2	E962.0	E980.2	BROMISOVALUM
965.4	E935.4	E850.4	E950.0	E962.0	E980.0	BROMOSELTZER
987.5		E869.3	E952.8	E962.2	E982.8	BROMOBENZYL CYANIDE
963.0	E933.0	E858.1	E950.4	E962.0	E980.4	BROMODIPHENHYDRAMINE
967.3	E937.3	E852.2	E950.2	E962.0	E980.2	BROMOFORM
977.8	E947.8	E858.8	E950.4	E962.0	E980.4	BROMOPHENOL BLUE REAGENT
961.8	E931.8	E857	E950.4	E962.0	E980.4	BROMOSALICYLHYDRO-XAMIC ACID
963.0	E933.0	E858.1	E950.4	E962.0	E980.4	BROMPHENIRAMINE
967.3	E937.3	E852.2	E950.2	E962.0	E980.2	BROMURAL
989.5		E905.1	E950.9	E962.1	E980.9	BROWN SPIDER BITE VENOM
988.2		E865.3	E950.9	E962.1	E980.9	BRUCIA
989.1		E863.7	E950.6	E962.1	E980.7	BRUCINE
0						BRUNSWICK GREEN SEE COPPER
988.2		E865.4	E950.9	E962.1	E980.9	BRYONIA ALBA DIOICA
969.5	E939.5	E853.8	E950.3	E962.0	E980.3	BUCLIZINE
965.1	E935.3	E850.3	E950.0	E962.0	E980.0	BUFFERIN
969.6	E939.6	E854.1	E950.3	E962.0	E980.3	BUFOTENINE
971.2	E941.2	E855.5	E950.4	E962.0	E980.4	BUPHENINE
968.5	E938.5	E855.2	E950.4	E962.0	E980.4	BUPIVACAINE INFILTRATION SUBCUTANEOUS
968.6	E938.6	E855.2	E950.4	E962.0	E980.4	BUPIVACAINE NERVE BLOCK PERIPHERAL PLEXUS
963.1	E933.1	E858.1	E950.4	E962.0	E980.4	BUSULFAN
967.0	E937.0	E851	E950.1	E962.0	E980.1	BUTABARBITAL (SODIUM)
967.0	E937.0	E851	E950.1	E962.0	E980.1	BUTABARBITONE
967.0	E937.0	E851	E950.1	E962.0	E980.1	BUTABARPAL
968.5	E938.5	E855.2	E950.4	E962.0	E980.4	BUTACAINE
967.0	E937.0	E851	E950.1	E962.0	E980.1	BUTALLYLONAL
987.0		E868.0	E951.1	E962.2	E981.1	BUTANE DISTRIBUTED IN MOBILE CONTAINER
987.0		E867	E951.0	E962.2	E981.0	BUTANE DISTRIBUTED THROUGH PIPES
0						BUTANE INCOMPLETE COMBUSTION OF SEE CARBON MONOXIDE
980.3		E860.4	E950.9	E962.1	E980.9	BUTANOL
982.8		E862.4	E950.9	E962.1	E980.9	BUTANONE
969.1	E939.1	E853.0	E950.3	E962.0	E980.3	BUTAPERAZINE
965.5	E935.5	E850.5	E950.0	E962.0	E980.0	BUTAZOLIDIN
967.0	E937.0	E851	E950.1	E962.0	E980.1	BUTETHAL
971.1	E941.1	E855.4	E950.4	E962.0	E980.4	BUTETHAMATE
968.3	E938.3	E855.1	E950.4	E962.0	E980.4	BUTHALITONE SODIUM
967.0	E937.0	E851	E950.1	E962.0	E980.1	BUTISOL SODIUM
967.0	E937.0	E851	E950.1	E962.0	E980.1	BUTOBARBITAL BUTOBARBITONE
969.0	E939.0	E854.0	E950.3	E962.0	E980.3	BUTRIPTYLINE
0						BUTTER OF ANTIMONY SEE ANTIMONY
988.2		E865.4	E950.9	E962.1	E980.9	BUTTERCUPS
982.8		E862.4	E950.9	E962.1	E980.9	BUTYL ACETATE SECONDARY
980.3		E860.4	E950.9	E962.1	E980.9	BUTYL ALCOHOL
980.8		E860.8	E950.9	E962.1	E980.9	BUTYL CARBINOL
982.8		E862.4	E950.9	E962.1	E980.9	BUTYL CARBITOL
982.8		E862.4	E950.9	E962.1	E980.9	BUTYL CELLOSOLVE
967.1	E937.1	E852.0	E950.2	E962.0	E980.2	BUTYL CHLORAL HYDRATE
982.8		E862.4	E950.9	E962.1	E980.9	BUTYL FORMATE
968.5	E938.5	E855.2	E950.4	E962.0	E980.4	BUTYN
969.2	E939.2	E853.1	E950.3	E962.0	E980.3	BUTYROPHENONE (-BASED TRANQUILIZERS)
985.1		E866.3	E950.8	E962.1	E980.8	CACODYL (CACODYLIC ACID)
961.1	E931.1	E857	E950.4	E962.0	E980.4	CACODYL (CACODYLIC ACID) ANTI-INFECTIVE
960.7	E930.7	E856	E950.4	E962.0	E980.4	CACTINOMYCIN
976.4	E946.4	E858.7	E950.4	E962.0	E980.4	CADE OIL
985.5		E866.4	E950.9	E962.1	E980.9	CADMIUM CHLORIDE COMPOUNDS DUST FUMES OXIDE
976.4	E946.4	E858.7	E950.4	E962.0	E980.4	CADMIUM SULFIDE MEDICINAL NEC
969.7	E939.7	E854.2	E950.3	E962.0	E980.3	CAFFEINE
988.2		E865.4	E950.9	E962.1	E980.9	CALABAR BEAN
988.2		E865.4	E950.9	E962.1	E980.9	CALADIUM SEGUINIUM
976.3	E946.3	E858.7	E950.4	E962.0	E980.4	CALAMINE LINIMENT LOTION
963.5	E933.5	E858.1	E950.4	E962.0	E980.4	CALCIFEROL

DRUGS & CHEMICALS

POISON	THERA-PEUTIC	ACCIDENT	SUICIDE	ASSAULT	UNDETER-MINED	SUBSTANCE
965.1	E935.3	E850.3	E950.0	E962.0	E980.0	CALCIUM ACETYLSALICYLATE
961.8	E931.8	E857	E950.4	E962.0	E980.4	CALCIUM BENZAMIDOSALICYLATE
963.8	E933.8	E858.1	E950.4	E962.0	E980.4	CALCIUM DISODIUM EDETATE
965.1	E935.3	E850.3	E950.0	E962.0	E980.0	CALCIUM CARBASPIRIN
977.3	E947.3	E858.8	E950.4	E962.0	E980.4	CALCIUM CARBIMIDE CITRATED
973.0	E943.0	E858.4	E950.4	E962.0	E980.4	CALCIUM CARBONATE ANTACID
977.3	E947.3	E858.8	E950.4	E962.0	E980.4	CALCIUM CYANIDE CITRATED
973.2	E943.2	E858.4	E950.4	E962.0	E980.4	CALCIUM DIOCTYL SULFOSUCCINATE
963.8	E933.8	E858.1	E950.4	E962.0	E980.4	CALCIUM DISODIUM EDATHAMIL
963.8	E933.8	E858.1	E950.4	E962.0	E980.4	CALCIUM EDTA
983.2		E864.2	E950.7	E962.1	E980.6	CALCIUM HYDRATE HYDROXIDE
961.9	E931.9	E857	E950.4	E962.0	E980.4	CALCIUM MANDELATE
983.2		E864.2	E950.7	E962.1	E980.6	CALCIUM OXIDE
974.5	E944.5	E858.5	E950.4	E962.0	E980.4	CALCIUM SALTS NEC
0						CALOMEL SEE MERCURY CHLORIDE
974.5	E944.5	E858.5	E950.4	E962.0	E980.4	CALORIC AGENTS NEC
963.1	E933.1	E858.1	E950.4	E962.0	E980.4	CALUSTERONE
961.4	E931.4	E857	E950.4	E962.0	E980.4	CAMOQUIN
976.1	E946.1	E858.7	E950.4	E962.0	E980.4	CAMPHOR OIL
976.0	E946.0	E858.7	E950.4	E962.0	E980.4	CANDEPTIN
976.0	E946.0	E858.7	E950.4	E962.0	E980.4	CANDICIDIN
969.6	E939.6	E854.1	E950.3	E962.0	E980.3	CANNABIS (DERIVATIVES) (INDICA) (SATIVA)
980.1		E860.2	E950.9	E962.1	E980.9	CANNED HEAT
976.8	E946.8	E858.7	E950.4	E962.0	E980.4	CANTHARIDES CANTHARIDIN CANTHARIS
972.8	E942.8	E858.3	E950.4	E962.0	E980.4	CAPILLARY AGENTS
960.6	E930.6	E856	E950.4	E962.0	E980.4	CAPREOMYCIN
969.5	E939.5	E853.8	E950.3	E962.0	E980.3	CAPTODIAME CAPTODIAMINE
971.1	E941.1	E855.4	E950.4	E962.0	E980.4	CARAMIPHEN HYDROCHLORIDE
971.0	E941.0	E855.3	E950.4	E962.0	E980.4	CARBACHOL
974.5	E944.5	E858.5	E950.4	E962.0	E980.4	CARBACRYLAMINE RESINS
989.3		E863.2	E950.6	E962.1	E980.7	CARBAMATE INSECTICIDE
989.3		E863.5	E950.6	E962.1	E980.7	CARBAMATE HERBICIDE
967.8	E937.8	E852.8	E950.2	E962.0	E980.2	CARBAMATE SEDATIVE
966.3	E936.3	E855.0	E950.4	E962.0	E980.4	CARBAMAZEPINE
967.8	E937.8	E852.8	E950.2	E962.0	E980.2	CARBAMIC ESTERS
974.4	E944.4	E858.5	E950.4	E962.0	E980.4	CARBAMIDE
976.8	E946.8	E858.7	E950.4	E962.0	E980.4	CARBAMIDE TOPICAL
971.0	E941.0	E855.3	E950.4	E962.0	E980.4	CARBAMYLCHOLINE CHLORIDE
961.1	E931.1	E857	E950.4	E962.0	E980.4	CARBARSONE
989.3		E863.2	E950.6	E962.1	E980.7	CARBARYL
965.1	E935.3	E850.3	E950.0	E962.0	E980.0	CARBASPIRIN
972.8	E942.8	E858.3	E950.4	E962.0	E980.4	CARBAZOCHROME
960.0	E930.0	E856	E950.4	E962.0	E980.4	CARBENICILLIN
973.8	E943.8	E858.4	E950.4	E962.0	E980.4	CARBENOXOLONE
975.4	E945.4	E858.6	E950.4	E962.0	E980.4	CARBETAPENTANE
962.8	E932.8	E858.0	E950.4	E962.0	E980.4	CARBIMAZOLE
980.1		E860.2	E950.9	E962.1	E980.9	CARBINOL
963.0	E933.0	E858.1	E950.4	E962.0	E980.4	CARBINOXAMINE
982.8		E862.4	E950.9	E962.1	E980.9	CARBITOL
968.9	E938.9	E855.2	E950.4	E962.0	E980.4	CARBOCAINE
968.5	E938.5	E855.2	E950.4	E962.0	E980.4	CARBOCAINE INFILTRATION SUBCUTANEOUS
968.6	E938.6	E855.2	E950.4	E962.0	E980.4	CARBOCAINE NERVE BLOCK PERIPHERAL PLEXUS
968.5	E938.5	E855.2	E950.4	E962.0	E980.4	CARBOCAINE TOPICAL SURFACE
976.0	E946.0	E858.7	E950.4	E962.0	E980.4	CARBOL-FUCHSIN SOLUTION
983.0		E864.0	E950.7	E962.1	E980.6	CARBOLIC ACID
960.8	E930.8	E856	E950.4	E962.0	E980.4	CARBOMYCIN
982.2		E862.4	E950.9	E962.1	E980.9	CARBON BISULFIDE LIQUID VAPOR
987.8		E869.8	E952.8	E962.2	E982.8	CARBON DIOXIDE GAS
982.2		E862.4	E950.9	E962.1	E980.9	CARBON DISULFIDE LIQUID VAPOR
986		E868.0	E951.1	E962.2	E981.1	CARBON MONOXIDE BUTANE DISTRIBUTED IN MOBILE CONTAINER
986		E867	E951.0	E962.2	E981.0	CARBON MONOXIDE BUTANE DISTRIBUTED THROUGH PIPES
986		E868.3	E952.1	E962.2	E982.1	CARBON MONOXIDE CHARCOAL FUMES
986		E868.3	E952.1	E962.2	E982.1	CARBON MONOXIDE COAL SOLID IN DOMESTIC STOVES FIREPLACES
986		E867	E952.0	E962.2	E982.0	CARBON MONOXIDE COAL GAS PIPED
986		E868.3	E952.1	E962.2	E982.1	CARBON MONOXIDE COKE IN DOMESTIC STOVES FIREPLACES
986		E868.2	E952.0	E962.2	E982.0	CARBON MONOXIDE EXHAUST GAS MOTOR NOT IN TRANSIT

POISON	THERA-PEUTIC	ACCIDENT	SUICIDE	ASSAULT	UNDETER-MINED	SUBSTANCE
986		E868.9	E952.1	E962.2	E982.1	CARBON MONOXIDE FROM INCOMPLETE COMBUSTION OF IN NEC
982.1		E862.4	E950.9	E962.1	E980.9	CARBON TETRACHLORIDE LIQUID CLEANSING AGENT NEC
982.1		E862.4	E950.9	E962.1	E980.9	CARBON TETRACHLORIDE SOLVENT
987.8		E869.8	E952.8	E962.2	E982.8	CARBON TETRACHLORIDEVAPOR NEC
987.8		E869.8	E952.8	E962.2	E982.8	CARBONIC ACID GAS
974.2	E944.2	E858.5	E950.4	E962.0	E980.4	CARBONIC ACID GAS ANHYDRASE INHIBITORS
974.2	E944.2	E858.5	E950.4	E962.0	E980.4	CARBONIC ACID HYDRASE INHIBITORS
976.3	E946.3	E858.7	E950.4	E962.0	E980.4	CARBOWAX
967.0	E937.0	E851	E950.1	E962.0	E980.1	CARBRITAL
967.3	E937.3	E852.2	E950.2	E962.0	E980.2	CARBROMAL (DERIVATIVES)
972.0	E942.0	E858.3	E950.4	E962.0	E980.4	CARDIAC DEPRESSANTS
972.0	E942.0	E858.3	E950.4	E962.0	E980.4	CARDIAC RHYTHM REGULATORS
977.8	E947.8	E858.8	E950.4	E962.0	E980.4	CARDIOGRAFIN
977.8	E947.8	E858.8	E950.4	E962.0	E980.4	CARDIOGREEN
972.1	942.1	E858.3	E950.4	E962.0	E980.4	CARDIOTONIC GLYCOSIDES
972.9	E942.9	E858.3	E950.4	E962.0	E980.4	CARDIOVASCULAR AGENTS OTHER AND NOS
974.2	E944.2	E858.5	E950.4	E962.0	E980.4	CARDRASE
976.0	E946.0	E858.7	E950.4	E962.0	E980.4	CARFUSIN
968.0	E938.0	E855.1	E950.4	E962.0	E980.4	CARISOPRODOL
963.1	E933.1	E858.1	E950.4	E962.0	E980.4	CARMUSTINE
963.5	E933.5	E858.1	E950.4	E962.0	E980.4	CAROTENE
969.1	E939.1	E853.0	E950.3	E962.0	E980.3	CARPHENAZINE MALEATE
973.1	E943.1	E858.4	E950.4	E962.0	E980.4	CARTER'S LITTLE PILLS
973.1	E943.1	E858.4	E950.4	E962.0	E980.4	CASCARA SAGRADA
988.2		E865.4	E950.9	E962.1	E980.9	CASSAVA
976.0	E946.0	E858.7	E950.4	E962.0	E980.4	CASTELLANI'S PAINT
988.2		E865.3	E950.9	E962.1	E980.9	CASTOR BEAN
973.1	E943.1	E858.4	E950.4	E962.0	E980.4	CASTOR OIL
989.5		E905.5	E950.9	E962.1	E980.9	CATERPILLAR STING
970.8	E940.8	E854.3	E950.4	E962.0	E980.4	CATHA EDULIS
973.1	E943.1	E858.4	E950.4	E962.0	E980.4	CATHARTICS CONTACT
973.2	E943.2	E858.4	E950.4	E962.0	E980.4	CATHARTICS EMOLLIENT
973.1	E943.1	E858.4	E950.4	E962.0	E980.4	CATHARTICS INTESTINAL IRRITANTS
973.3	E943.3	E858.4	E950.4	E962.0	E980.4	CATHARTICS NEC
973.3	E943.3	E858.4	E950.4	E962.0	E980.4	CATHARTICS SALINE
960.8	E930.8	E856	E950.4	E962.0	E980.4	CATHOMYCIN
983.2		E864.2	E950.7	E962.1	E980.6	CAUSTIC ALKALI
983.2		E864.2	E950.7	E962.1	E980.6	CAUSTIC HYDROXIDE
983.2		E864.2	E950.7	E962.1	E980.6	CAUSTIC POTASH
983.2		E864.2	E950.7	E962.1	E980.6	CAUSTIC SODA
983.9		E864.3	E950.7	E962.1	E980.6	CAUSTIC SPECIFIED NEC
983.9		E864.4	E950.7	E962.1	E980.6	CAUSTICS UNSPECIFIED
976.0	E946.0	E858.7	E950.4	E962.0	E980.4	CEEPRYN
976.6	E946.6	E858.7	E950.4	E962.0	E980.4	CEEPRYN ENT AGENT
976.6	E946.6	E858.7	E950.4	E962.0	E980.4	CEEPRYN LOZENGES
962.0	E932.0	E858.0	E950.4	E962.0	E980.4	CELESTONE
976.0	E946.0	E858.7	E950.4	E962.0	E980.4	CELESTONE TOPICAL
976.8	E946.8	E858.7	E950.4	E962.0	E980.4	CELL STIMULANTS AND PROLIFERANTS
982.8		E862.4	E950.9	E962.1	E980.9	CELLOSOLVE
973.3	E943.3	E858.4	E950.4	E962.0	E980.4	CELLULOSE DERIVATIVES CATHARTIC
976.3	E946.3	E858.7	E950.4	E962.0	E980.4	CELLULOSE NITRATES TOPICAL
989.5		E905.4	E950.9	E962.1	E980.9	CENTIPEDE BITE
968.4	E938.4	E855.1	E950.4	E962.0	E980.4	CENTRAL NERVOUS SYSTEM DEPRESSANTS NEC
968.2	E938.2	E855.1	E950.4	E962.0	E980.4	CENTRAL NERVOUS SYSTEM DEPRESSANTS ANESTHETIC GASES NEC
968.4	E938.4	E855.1	E950.4	E962.0	E980.4	CENTRAL NERVOUS SYSTEM DEPRESSANTS ANESTHETIC GENERAL NEC
968.3	E938.3	E855.1	E950.4	E962.0	E980.4	CENTRAL NERVOUS SYSTEM DEPRESSANTS ANESTHETIC INTRAVENOUS
967.0	E937.0	E851	E950.1	E962.0	E980.1	CENTRAL NERVOUS SYSTEM DEPRESSANTS BARBITURATES
967.3	E937.3	E852.2	E950.2	E962.0	E980.2	CENTRAL NERVOUS SYSTEM DEPRESSANTS BROMIDES
969.6	E939.6	E854.1	E950.3	E962.0	E980.3	CENTRAL NERVOUS SYSTEM DEPRESSANTS CANNABIS SATIVA
967.1	E937.1	E852.0	E950.2	E962.0	E980.2	CENTRAL NERVOUS SYSTEM DEPRESSANTS CHLORAL HYDRATE

POISON	THERA-PEUTIC	ACCIDENT	SUICIDE	ASSAULT	UNDETER-MINED	SUBSTANCE
969.6	E939.6	E854.1	E950.3	E962.0	E980.3	CENTRAL NERVOUS SYSTEM DEPRESSANTS HALLUCINOGENICS
967.8	E937.8	E852.8	E950.2	E962.0	E980.2	CENTRAL NERVOUS SYSTEM DEPRESSANTS HYPNOTICS SPECIFIED NEC
967.9	E937.9	E852.9	E950.2	E962.0	E980.2	CENTRAL NERVOUS SYSTEM DEPRESSANTS HYPNOTICS
968.0	E938.0	E855.1	E950.4	E962.0	E980.4	CENTRAL NERVOUS SYSTEM DEPRESSANTS MUSCLE RELAXANTS
968.0	E938.0	E855.1	E950.4	E962.0	E980.4	CENTRAL NERVOUS SYSTEM DEPRESSANTS MUSCLE TONE
967.2	E937.2	E852.1	E950.2	E962.0	E980.2	CENTRAL NERVOUS SYSTEM DEPRESSANTS PARALDEHYDE
967.9	E937.9	E852.9	E950.2	E962.0	E980.2	CENTRAL NERVOUS SYSTEM DEPRESSANTS SEDATIVES
967.6	E937.6	E852.5	E950.2	E962.0	E980.2	CENTRAL NERVOUS SYSTEM DEPRESSANTS SEDATIVES MIXED NEC
967.8	E937.8	E852.8	E950.2	E962.0	E980.2	CENTRAL NERVOUS SYSTEM DEPRESSANTS SEDATIVES SPECIFIED NEC
970.9	E940.9	E854.3	E950.4	E962.0	E980.4	CENTRAL NERVOUS SYSTEM STIMULANTS
969.0	E939.0	E854.0	E950.3	E962.0	E980.3	CENTRAL NERVOUS SYSTEM STIMULANTS ANTIDEPRESSANTS
969.7	E939.7	E854.2	E950.3	E962.0	E980.3	CENTRAL NERVOUS SYSTEM STIMULANTS AMPHETAMINES
970.0	E940.0	E854.3	E950.4	E962.0	E980.4	CENTRAL NERVOUS SYSTEM STIMULANTS ANALEPTICS
970.1	E940.0	E854.3	E950.4	E962.0	E980.4	CENTRAL NERVOUS SYSTEM STIMULANTS OPIATE ANTAGONISTS
970.8	E940.8	E854.3	E950.4	E962.0	E980.4	CENTRAL NERVOUS SYSTEM STIMULANTS OTHER SPECIFIED NEC
970.9	E940.9	E854.3	E950.4	E962.0	E980.4	CENTRAL NERVOUS SYSTEM STIMULANTS NOS
960.5	E930.5	E856	E950.4	E962.0	E980.4	CEPHALEXIN
960.5	E930.5	E856	E950.4	E962.0	E980.4	CEPHALOGLYCIN
960.5	E930.5	E856	E950.4	E962.0	E980.4	CEPHALORIDINE
960.5	E930.5	E856	E950.4	E962.0	E980.4	CEPHALOSPORINS 8:12.06
960.0	E930.0	E856	E950.4	E962.0	E980.4	CEPHALOSPORINS N ADICILLIN
960.5	E930.5	E856	E950.4	E962.0	E980.4	CEPHALOSPORINS NEC
960.5	E930.5	E856	E950.4	E962.0	E980.4	CEPHALOTHIN
988.2		E865.4	E950.9	E962.1	E980.9	CERBERA ODALLAM
972.1	E942.1	E858.3	E950.4	E962.0	E980.4	CERBERIN
970.9	E940.9	E854.3	E950.4	E962.0	E980.4	CEREBRAL STIMULANTS
969.7	E939.7	E854.2	E950.3	E962.0	E980.3	CEREBRAL STIMULANTS PSYCHOTHERAPEUTIC
970.8	E940.8	E854.3	E950.4	E962.0	E980.4	CEREBRAL STIMULANTS SPECIFIED NEC
976.0	E946.0	E858.7	E950.4	E962.0	E980.4	CETALKONIUM CHLORIDE
963.0	E933.0	E858.1	E950.4	E962.0	E980.4	CETOXIME
976.2	E946.2	E858.7	E950.4	E962.0	E980.4	CETRIMIDE
976.0	E946.0	E858.7	E950.4	E962.0	E980.4	CETYLPYRIDINIUM
976.6	E946.6	E858.7	E950.4	E962.0	E980.4	CETYLPYRIDINIUM ENT AGENT
976.6	E946.6	E858.7	E950.4	E962.0	E980.4	CETYLPYRIDINIUM LOZENGES
0						CEVADILLA SEE SABADILLA
963.5	E933.5	E858.1	E950.4	E962.0	E980.4	CEVITAMIC ACID
973.0	E943.0	E858.4	E950.4	E962.0	E980.4	CHALK PRECIPITATED
986		E868.3	E952.1	E962.2	E982.1	CHARCOAL FUMES CARBON MONOXIDE
986		E868.8	E952.1	E962.2	E982.1	CHARCOAL FUMES CARBON MONOXIDE INDUSTRIAL
973.0	E943.0	E858.4	E950.4	E962.0	E980.4	CHARCOAL MEDICINAL ACTIVATED
977.2	E947.2	E858.8	E950.4	E962.0	E980.4	CHELATING AGENTS ANTIDOTES NEC
988.2		E865.4	E950.9	E962.1	E980.9	CHELIDONIUM MAJUS
989.9		E866.9	E950.9	E962.1	E980.9	CHEMICAL SUBSTANCE UNSPECIFIED (NONMEDICAL)
989.89		E866.8	E950.9	E962.1	E980.9	CHEMICAL SUBSTANCE SPECIFIED NEC (NONMEDICAL)
963.1	E933.1	E858.1	E950.4	E962.0	E980.4	CHEMOTHERAPY, ANTINEOPLASTIC
961.6	E931.6	E857	E950.4	E962.0	E980.4	CHENOPODIUM OIL
988.2		E865.4	E950.9	E962.1	E980.9	CHERRY LAUREL
961.3	E931.3	E857	E950.4	E962.0	E980.4	CHINIOFON
975.4	E945.4	E858.6	E950.4	E962.0	E980.4	CHLOPHEDIANOL
960.4	E930.4	E856	E950.4	E962.0	E980.4	CHLOR-METHYLENECYCLINE
963.0	E933.0	E858.1	E950.4	E962.0	E980.4	CHLOR-TRIMETON
967.1	E937.1	E852.0	E950.2	E962.0	E980.2	CHLORAL HYDRATE GROUP
967.1	E937.1	E852.0	E950.2	E962.0	E980.2	CHLORALAMIDE
963.1	E933.1	E858.1	E950.4	E962.0	E980.4	CHLORAMBUCIL
960.2	E930.2	E856	E950.4	E962.0	E980.4	CHLORAMPHENICOL

POISON	THERA-PEUTIC	ACCIDENT	SUICIDE	ASSAULT	UNDETER-MINED	SUBSTANCE
976.6	E946.6	E858.7	E950.4	E962.0	E980.4	CHLORAMPHENICOL ENT AGENT
976.5	E946.5	E858.7	E950.4	E962.0	E980.4	CHLORAMPHENICOL OPHTHALMIC PREPARATION
976.0	E946.0	E858.7	E950.4	E962.0	E980.4	CHLORAMPHENICOL TOPICAL NEC
989.4		E863.5	E950.6	E962.1	E980.7	CHLORATE HERBICIDES
983.9		E864.3	E950.7	E962.1	E980.6	CHLORATE(S) POTASSIUM SODIUM NEC
963.0	E933.0	E858.1	E950.4	E962.0	E980.4	CHLORCYLIZINE
989.2		E863.0	E950.6	E962.1	E980.7	CHLORDAN(E) DUST
976.0	E946.0	E858.7	E950.4	E962.0	E980.4	CHLORDANTOIN
969.4	E939.4	E853.2	E950.3	E962.0	E980.3	CHLORDIAZEPOXIDE
976.8	E946.8	E858.7	E950.4	E962.0	E980.4	CHLORESIUM
967.1	E937.1	E852.0	E950.2	E962.0	E980.2	CHLORETHIAZOL
0						CHLORETHYL SEE ETHYL CHLORIDE
967.1	E937.1	E852.0	E950.2	E962.0	E980.2	CHLORETONE
982.3		E862.4	E950.9	E962.1	E980.9	CHLOREX
967.1	E937.1	E852.0	E950.2	E962.0	E980.2	CHLORHEXADOL
976.0	E946.0	E858.7	E950.4	E962.0	E980.4	CHLORHEXIDINE HYDROCHLORIDE
976.0	E946.0	E858.7	E950.4	E962.0	E980.4	CHLORHYDROXYQUINOLIN
983.9		E864.3	E950.7	E962.1	E980.6	CHLORIDE OF LIME BLEACH
989.2		E863.0	E950.6	E962.1	E980.7	CHLORINATED CAMPHENE
989.89		E866.8	E950.9	E962.1	E980.9	CHLORINATED DIPHENYL
989.2		E863.0	E950.6	E962.1	E980.7	CHLORINATED HYDROCARBONS NEC
982.3		E862.4	E950.9	E962.1	E980.9	CHLORINATED HYDROCARBONS SOLVENT
983.9		E864.3	E950.7	E962.1	E980.6	CHLORINATED LIME BLEACH
989.2		E863.0	E950.6	E962.1	E980.7	CHLORINATED PESTICIDES NEC
983.9		E864.3	E950.7	E962.1	E980.6	CHLORINE BLEACH
983.9		E864.3	E950.7	E962.1	E980.6	CHLORINE COMPOUNDS NEC
983.9		E861.4	E950.7	E962.1	E980.6	CHLORINE DISINFECTANT
987.6		E869.8	E952.8	E962.2	E982.8	CHLORINE FUMES GAS
983.9		E864.3	E950.7	E962.1	E980.6	CHLORINE RELEASING AGENTS NEC
972.3	E942.3	E858.3	E950.4	E962.0	E980.4	CHLORISONDAMINE
962.2	E932.2	E858.0	E950.4	E962.0	E980.4	CHLORMADINONE
974.0	E944.0	E858.5	E950.4	E962.0	E980.4	CHLORMERODRIN
967.1	E937.1	E852.0	E950.2	E962.0	E980.2	CHLORMETHIAZOLE
969.5	E939.5	E853.8	E950.3	E962.0	E980.3	CHLORMEZANONE
987.5		E869.3	E952.8	E962.2	E982.8	CHLOROACETOPHENONE
983.0		E864.0	E950.7	E962.1	E980.6	CHLOROANILINE
982.0		E862.4	E950.9	E962.1	E980.9	CHLOROBENZENE CHLOROBENZOL
967.1	E937.1	E852.0	E950.2	E962.0	E980.2	CHLOROBUTANOL
983.0		E864.0	E950.7	E962.1	E980.6	CHLORODINITROBENZENE
987.8		E869.8	E952.8	E962.2	E982.8	CHLORODINITROBENZENE DUST OR VAPOR
0						CHLOROETHANE SEE ETHYL CHLORIDE
968.2	E938.2	E855.1	E950.4	E962.0	E980.4	CHLOROFORM ANESTHETIC GAS
987.8		E869.8	E952.8	E962.2	E982.8	CHLOROFORM FUMES VAPOR
968.4	E938.4	E855.1	E950.4	E962.0	E980.4	CHLOROFORM LIQUID NEC
982.3		E862.4	E950.9	E962.1	E980.9	CHLOROFORM SOLVENT
961.4	E931.4	E857	E950.4	E962.0	E980.4	CHLOROGUANIDE
960.2	E930.2	E856	E950.4	E962.0	E980.4	CHLOROMYCETIN
976.6	E946.6	E858.7	E950.4	E962.0	E980.4	CHLOROMYCETIN ENT AGENT
976.5	E946.5	E858.7	E950.4	E962.0	E980.4	CHLOROMYCETIN OPHTHALMIC PREPARATION
976.6	E946.6	E858.7	E950.4	E962.0	E980.4	CHLOROMYCETIN OTIC SOLUTION
976.0	E946.0	E858.7	E950.4	E962.0	E980.4	CHLOROMYCETIN TOPICAL NEC
983.0		E864.0	E950.7	E962.1	E980.6	CHLORONITROBENZENE
987.8		E869.8	E952.8	E962.2	E982.8	CHLORONITROBENZENE DUST OR VAPOR
983.0		E864.0	E950.7	E962.1	E980.6	CHLOROPHENOL
989.2		E863.0	E950.6	E962.1	E980.7	CHLOROPHENOTHANE
976.8	E946.8	E858.7	E950.4	E962.0	E980.4	CHLOROPHYLL DERIVATIVES
987.8		E869.8	E952.8	E962.2	E982.8	CHLOROPICRIN FUMES
989.4		E863.8	E950.6	E962.1	E980.7	CHLOROPICRIN FUMIGANT
989.4		E863.6	E950.6	E962.1	E980.7	CHLOROPICRIN FUNGICIDE
989.4		E863.4	E950.6	E962.1	E980.7	CHLOROPICRIN PESTICIDE FUMES
968.9	E938.9	E855.2	E950.4	E962.0	E980.4	CHLOROPROCAINE
968.5	E938.5	E855.2	E950.4	E962.0	E980.4	CHLOROPROCAINE INFILTRATION SUBCUTANEOUS
968.6	E938.6	E855.2	E950.4	E962.0	E980.4	CHLOROPROCAINE NERVE BLOCK PERIPHERAL PLEXUS
976.5	E946.5	E858.7	E950.4	E962.0	E980.4	CHLOROPTIC
963.1	E933.1	E858.1	E950.4	E962.0	E980.4	CHLOROPURINE
961.4	E931.4	E857	E950.4	E962.0	E980.4	CHLOROQUINE
961.4	E931.4	E857	E950.4	E962.0	E980.4	CHLOROQUINE (HYDROCHLORIDE) (PHOSPHATE)

POISON	THERA-PEUTIC	ACCIDENT	SUICIDE	ASSAULT	UNDETER-MINED	SUBSTANCE
963.0	E933.0	E858.1	E950.4	E962.0	E980.4	CHLOROTHEN
974.3	E944.3	E858.5	E950.4	E962.0	E980.4	CHLOROTHIAZIDE GROUP
962.2	E932.2	E858.0	E950.4	E962.0	E980.4	CHLOROTRIANISENE
985.1		E866.3	E950.8	E962.1	E980.8	CHLOROVINYLDICHLOROARSINE
976.0	E946.0	E858.7	E950.4	E962.0	E980.4	CHLOROXYLENOL
968.0	E938.0	E855.1	E950.4	E962.0	E980.4	CHLORPHENESIN (CARBAMATE)
976.0	E946.0	E858.7	E950.4	E962.0	E980.4	CHLORPHENESIN TOPICAL ANTIFUNGAL
963.0	E933.0	E858.1	E950.4	E962.0	E980.4	CHLORPHENIRAMINE
966.4	E936.4	E855.0	E950.4	E962.0	E980.4	CHLORPHENOXAMINE
977.0	E947.0	E858.8	E950.4	E962.0	E980.4	CHLORPHENTERMINE
961.4	E931.4	E857	E950.4	E962.0	E980.4	CHLORPROGUANIL
969.1	E939.1	E853.0	E950.3	E962.0	E980.3	CHLORPROMAZINE
962.3	E932.3	E858.0	E950.4	E962.0	E980.4	CHLORPROPAMIDE
969.3	E939.3	E853.8	E950.3	E962.0	E980.3	CHLORPROTHIXENE
976.0	E946.0	E858.7	E950.4	E962.0	E980.4	CHLORQUINALDOL
960.4	E930.4	E856	E950.4	E962.0	E980.4	CHLORTETRACYCLINE
974.4	E944.4	E858.5	E950.4	E962.0	E980.4	CHLORTHALIDONE
962.2	E932.2	E858.0	E950.4	E962.0	E980.4	CHLORTRIANISENE
968.0	E938.0	E855.1	E950.4	E962.0	E980.4	CHLORZOXAZONE
987.8		E869.8	E952.8	E962.2	E982.8	CHOKE DAMP
977.8	E947.8	E858.8	E950.4	E962.0	E980.4	CHOLEBRINE
978.2	E948.2	E858.8	E950.4	E962.0	E980.4	CHOLERA VACCINE
972.2	E942.2	E858.3	E950.4	E962.0	E980.4	CHOLESTEROL-LOWERING AGENTS
972.2	E942.2	E858.3	E950.4	E962.0	E980.4	CHOLESTYRAMINE RESIN
973.4	E943.4	E858.4	E950.4	E962.0	E980.4	CHOLIC ACID
977.1	E947.1	E858.8	E950.4	E962.0	E980.4	CHOLINE DIHYDROGEN CITRATE
965.1	E935.3	E850.3	E950.0	E962.0	E980.0	CHOLINE SALICYLATE
974.1	E944.1	E858.5	E950.4	E962.0	E980.4	CHOLINE THEOPHYLLINATE
971.0	E941.0	E855.3	E950.4	E962.0	E980.4	CHOLINERGICS
977.8	E947.8	E858.8	E950.4	E962.0	E980.4	CHOLOGRAFIN
962.4	E932.4	E858.0	E950.4	E962.0	E980.4	CHORIONIC GONADOTROPIN
983.9		E864.3	E950.7	E962.1	E980.6	CHROMATES
987.8		E869.8	E952.8	E962.2	E982.8	CHROMATES DUST OR MIST
984.0		E866.0	E950.9	E962.1	E980.9	CHROMATES LEAD
984.0		E861.5	E950.9	E962.1	E980.9	CHROMATES LEAD PAINT
983.9		E864.3	E950.7	E962.1	E980.6	CHROMIC ACID
987.8		E869.8	E952.8	E962.2	E982.8	CHROMIC ACID DUST OR MIST
985.6		E866.4	E950.9	E962.1	E980.9	CHROMIUM
0						CHROMIUM COMPOUNDS SEE CHROMATES
983.9		E864.3	E950.7	E962.1	E980.6	CHROMYL CHLORIDE
976.4	E946.4	E858.7	E950.4	E962.0	E980.4	CHRYSAROBIN OINTMENT
973.1	E943.1	E858.4	E950.4	E962.0	E980.4	CHRYSAZIN
963.4	E933.4	E858.1	E950.4	E962.0	E980.4	CHYMAR
976.5	E946.5	E858.7	E950.4	E962.0	E980.4	CHYMAR OPHTHALMIC PREPARATION
963.4	E933.4	E858.1	E950.4	E962.0	E980.4	CHYMOTRYPSIN
976.5	E946.5	E858.7	E950.4	E962.0	E980.4	CHYMOTRYPSIN OPHTHALMIC PREPARATION
988.2		E865.4	E950.9	E962.1	E980.9	CICUTA MACULATA OR VIROSA
981		E862.1	E950.9	E962.1	E980.9	CIGARETTE LIGHTER FLUID
968.7	E938.7	E855.2	E950.4	E962.0	E980.4	CINCHOCAINE SPINAL
968.5	E938.5	E855.2	E950.4	E962.0	E980.4	CINCHOCAINE TOPICAL SURFACE
961.4	E931.4	E857	E950.4	E962.0	E980.4	CINCHONA
961.4	E931.4	E857	E950.4	E962.0	E980.4	CINCHONINE ALKALOIDS
974.7	E944.7	E858.5	E950.4	E962.0	E980.4	CINCHOPHEN
963.0	E933.0	E858.1	E950.4	E962.0	E980.4	CINNARIZINE
968.5	E938.5	E855.2	E950.4	E962.0	E980.4	CITANEST INFILTRATION SUBCUTANEOUS
968.6	E938.6	E855.2	E950.4	E962.0	E980.4	CITANEST NERVE BLOCK PERIPHERAL PLEXUS
968.9	E938.9	E855.2	E950.4	E962.0	E980.4	CITANEST
989.89		E866.8	E950.9	E962.1	E980.9	CITRIC ACID
964.1	E934.1	E858.2	E950.4	E962.0	E980.4	CITROVORUM FACTOR
988.2		E865.4	E950.9	E962.1	E980.9	CLAVICEPS PURPUREA
989.89		E861.3	E950.9	E962.1	E980.9	CLEANER CLEANSING AGENT NEC
982.8		E862.9	E950.9	E962.1	E980.9	CLEANER OF PAINT OR VARNISH
988.2		E865.4	E950.9	E962.1	E980.9	CLEMATIS VITALBA
963.0	E933.0	E858.1	E950.4	E962.0	E980.4	CLEMIZOLE
960.0	E930.0	E856	E950.4	E962.0	E980.4	CLEMIZOLE PENICILLIN
971.1	E941.1	E855.4	E950.4	E962.0	E980.4	CLIDINIUM
960.8	E930.8	E856	E950.4	E962.0	E980.4	CLINDAMYCIN
965.09	E935.2	E850.2	E950.0	E962.0	E980.0	CLIRADON
962.0	E932.0	E858.0	E950.4	E962.0	E980.4	CLOCORTOLONE
975.4	E945.4	E858.6	E950.4	E962.0	E980.4	CLOFEDANOL
972.2	E942.2	E858.3	E950.4	E962.0	E980.4	CLOFIBRATE

DRUGS & CHEMICALS

POISON	THERA-PEUTIC	ACCIDENT	SUICIDE	ASSAULT	UNDETER-MINED	SUBSTANCE
967.1	E937.1	E852.0	E950.2	E962.0	E980.2	CLOMETHIAZOLE
977.8	E947.8	E858.8	E950.4	E962.0	E980.4	CLOMIPHENE
969.4	E939.4	E853.2	E950.3	E962.0	E980.3	CLONAZEPAM
972.6	E942.6	E858.3	E950.4	E962.0	E980.4	CLONIDINE
974.3	E944.3	E858.5	E950.4	E962.0	E980.4	CLOPAMIDE
969.4	E939.4	E853.2	E950.3	E962.0	E980.3	CLORAZEPATE
974.4	E944.4	E858.5	E950.4	E962.0	E980.4	CLOREXOLONE
983.9		E864.3	E950.7	E962.1	E980.6	CLOROX BLEACH
977.0	E947.0	E858.8	E950.4	E962.0	E980.4	CLORTERMINE
976.0	E946.0	E858.7	E950.4	E962.0	E980.4	CLOTRIMAZOLE
960.0	E930.0	E856	E950.4	E962.0	E980.4	CLOXACILLIN
964.5	E934.5	E858.2	E950.4	E962.0	E980.4	COAGULANTS NEC
0						COAL CARBON MONOXIDE FROM SEE ALSO CARBON MONOXIDE COAL
0						COAL OIL SEE KEROSENE
987.8		E869.8	E952.8	E962.2	E982.8	COAL TAR FUMES
965.5	E935.5	E850.5	E950.0	E962.0	E980.0	COAL TAR MEDICINAL ANALGESICS NEC
976.4	E946.4	E858.7	E950.4	E962.0	E980.4	COAL TAR MEDICINAL OINTMENT
981		E862.0	E950.9	E962.1	E980.9	COAL TAR NAPHTHA SOLVENT
983.0		E864.0	E950.7	E962.1	E980.6	COAL TAR NEC
985.8		E866.4	E950.9	E962.1	E980.9	COBALT FUMES INDUSTRIAL
989.5		E905.0	E950.9	E962.1	E980.9	COBRA VENOM
970.8	E940.8	E854.3	E950.4	E962.0	E980.4	COCA LEAF
970.8	E940.8	E854.3	E950.4	E962.0	E980.4	COCAINE (HYDROCHLORIDE) (SALT)
968.5	E938.5	E855.2	E950.4	E962.0	E980.4	COCAINE (HYDROCHLORIDE) (SALT) TOPICAL ANESTHETIC
977.8	E947.8	E858.8	E950.4	E962.0	E980.4	COCCIDIOIDIN
988.2		E865.3	E950.9	E962.1	E980.9	COCCULUS INDICUS
989.89		E866.8	E950.9	E962.1	E980.9	COCHINEAL
977.4	E947.4	E858.8	E950.4	E962.0	E980.4	COCHINEAL MEDICINAL PRODUCTS
965.09	E935.2	E850.2	E950.0	E962.0	E980.0	CODEINE (METHYLMORPHINE)
989.89		E866.8	E950.9	E962.1	E980.9	COFFEE
971.1	E941.1	E855.4	E950.4	E962.0	E980.4	COGENTIN
986		E868.8	E952.1	E962.2	E982.1	COKE FUMES OR GAS INDUSTRIAL USE
986		E868.3	E952.1	E962.2	E982.1	COKE FUMES OR GAS CARBON MONOXIDE
973.2	E943.2	E858.4	E950.4	E962.0	E980.4	COLACE
974.7	E944.7	E858.5	E950.4	E962.0	E980.4	COLCHICINE
988.2		E865.3	E950.9	E962.1	E980.9	COLCHICUM
976.3	E946.3	E858.7	E950.4	E962.0	E980.4	COLD CREAM
975.6	945.6	E858.6	E950.9	E962.0	E980.4	COLD DRUGS
972.2	E942.2	E858.3	E950.4	E962.0	E980.4	COLESTIPOL
960.8	E930.8	E856	E950.4	E962.0	E980.4	COLISTIMETHATE
960.8	E930.8	E856	E950.4	E962.0	E980.4	COLISTIN
976.8	E946.8	E858.7	E950.4	E962.0	E980.4	COLLAGENASE
976.3	E946.3	E858.7	E950.4	E962.0	E980.4	COLLODION FLEXIBLE
973.1	E943.1	E858.4	E950.4	E962.0	E980.4	COLOCYNTH
0						COLORING MATTER SEE DYE(S)
0						COMBUSTION GAS SEE CARBON MONOXIDE
969.1	E939.1	E853.0	E950.3	E962.0	E980.3	COMPAZINE
962.0	E932.0	E858.0	E950.4	E962.0	E980.4	COMPOUND E CORTISONE
989.4		E863.4	E950.6	E962.1	E980.7	COMPOUND 4124 DICAPTHON
989.2		E863.0	E950.6	E962.1	E980.7	COMPOUND 497 DIELDRIN
989.2		E863.0	E950.6	E962.1	E980.7	COMPOUND 269 ENDRIN
962.0	E932.0	E858.0	E950.4	E962.0	E980.4	COMPOUND F HYDROCORTISONE
989.3		E863.1	E950.6	E962.1	E980.7	COMPOUND 4049 MALATHION
989.3		E863.1	E950.6	E962.1	E980.7	COMPOUND 3422 PARATHION
989.3		E863.1	E950.6	E962.1	E980.7	COMPOUND 3911 PHORATE
989.4		E863.7	E950.6	E962.1	E980.7	COMPOUND 1080 SODIUM FLUOROACETATE
989.2		E863.0	E950.6	E962.1	E980.7	COMPOUND 3956 TOXAPHENE
989.4		E863.7	E950.6	E962.1	E980.7	COMPOUND 42 WARFARIN
977.8	E947.8	E858.8	E950.4	E962.0	E980.4	CONGO RED
965.7	E935.7	E850.7	E950.0	E962.0	E980.0	CONIINE CONINE
988.2		E865.4	E950.9	E962.1	E980.9	CONIUM MACULATUM
962.2	E932.2	E858.0	E950.4	E962.0	E980.4	CONJUGATED ESTROGENSE QUINE
975.6	E945.6	E858.6	E950.4	E962.0	E980.4	CONTAC
976.5	E946.5	E858.7	E950.4	E962.0	E980.4	CONTACT LENS SOLUTION
962.2	E932.2	E858.0	E950.4	E962.0	E980.4	CONTRACEPTIVES ORAL
976.8	E946.8	E858.7	E950.4	E962.0	E980.4	CONTRACEPTIVES VAGINAL
977.8	E947.8	E858.8	E950.4	E962.0	E980.4	CONTRAST MEDIA (USED FOR DIAGNOSTIC X-RAY PROCEDURES) (ROENTGENOGRAPHIA)

POISON	THERA-PEUTIC	ACCIDENT	SUICIDE	ASSAULT	UNDETER-MINED	SUBSTANCE
988.2		E865.4	E950.9	E962.1	E980.9	CONVALLARIA MAJALIS
985.1		E866.3	E950.8	E962.1	E980.8	COPPER ARSENATE ARSENITE
985.1		E863.4	E950.8	E962.1	E980.8	COPPER ARSENATE INSECTICIDE
985.8		E866.4	E950.9	E962.1	E980.9	COPPER DUST FUMES SALTS NEC
973.6	E943.6	E858.4	E950.4	E962.0	E980.4	COPPER EMETIC
985.8		E863.6	E950.6	E962.1	E980.7	COPPER FUNGICIDE
985.8		E863.4	E950.6	E962.1	E980.7	COPPER INSECTICIDE
976.0	E946.0	E858.7	E950.4	E962.0	E980.4	COPPER OLEATE
983.9		E864.3	E950.7	E962.1	E980.6	COPPER SULFATE
973.6	E943.6	E858.4	E950.4	E962.0	E980.4	COPPER SULFATE CUPRIC
983.9		E864.3	E950.7	E962.1	E980.6	COPPER SULFATE CUPROUS
983.9		E863.6	E950.7	E962.1	E980.6	COPPER SULFATE FUNGICIDE
989.5		E905.0	E950.9	E962.1	E980.9	COPPERHEAD SNAKE BITE VENOM
989.5		E905.0	E950.9	E962.1	E980.9	CORAL SNAKE BITE VENOM
989.5		E905.6	E950.9	E962.1	E980.9	CORAL STING
976.0	E946.0	E858.7	E950.4	E962.0	E980.4	CORDRAN
976.4	E946.4	E858.7	E950.4	E962.0	E980.4	CORN CURES
976.3	E946.3	E858.7	E950.4	E962.0	E980.4	CORN STARCH
976.3	E946.3	E858.7	E950.4	E962.0	E980.4	CORNHUSKER'S LOTION
983.9		E864.4	E950.7	E962.1	E980.6	CORROSIVE
983.1		E864.1	E950.7	E962.1	E980.6	CORROSIVE ACIDS NEC
983.0		E864.0	E950.7	E962.1	E980.6	CORROSIVE AROMATICS
983.0		E861.4	E950.7	E962.1	E980.6	CORROSIVE AROMATICS DISINFECTANT
987.9		E869.8	E952.9	E962.2	E982.9	CORROSIVE FUMES NEC
983.9		E864.3	E950.7	E962.1	E980.6	CORROSIVE SPECIFIED NEC
0						CORROSIVE SUBLIMATE SEE MERCURY CHLORIDE
962.0	E932.0	E858.0	E950.4	E962.0	E980.4	CORT-DOME
976.6	E946.6	E858.7	E950.4	E962.0	E980.4	CORT-DOME ENT AGENT
976.5	E946.5	E858.7	E950.4	E962.0	E980.4	CORT-DOME OPHTHALMIC PREPARATION
976.0	E946.0	E858.7	E950.4	E962.0	E980.4	CORT-DOME TOPICAL NEC
962.0	E932.0	E858.0	E950.4	E962.0	E980.4	CORTATE
962.0	E932.0	E858.0	E950.4	E962.0	E980.4	CORTEF
976.6	E946.6	E858.7	E950.4	E962.0	E980.4	CORTEF ENT AGENT
976.5	E946.5	E858.7	E950.4	E962.0	E980.4	CORTEF OPHTHALMIC PREPARATION
976.0	E946.0	E858.7	E950.4	E962.0	E980.4	CORTEF TOPICAL NEC
976.6	E946.6	E858.7	E950.4	E962.0	E980.4	CORTICOSTEROIDS ENT AGENT
962.0	E932.0	E858.0	E950.4	E962.0	E980.4	CORTICOSTEROIDS FLUORINATED
976.5	E946.5	E858.7	E950.4	E962.0	E980.4	CORTICOSTEROIDS OPHTHALMIC PREPARATION
976.0	E946.0	E858.7	E950.4	E962.0	E980.4	CORTICOSTEROIDS TOPICAL NEC
962.4	E932.4	E858.0	E950.4	E962.0	E980.4	CORTICOTROPIN
962.0	E932.0	E858.0	E950.4	E962.0	E980.4	CORTISOL
976.6	E946.6	E858.7	E950.4	E962.0	E980.4	CORTISOL ENT AGENT
976.5	E946.5	E858.7	E950.4	E962.0	E980.4	CORTISOL OPHTHALMIC PREPARATION
976.0	E946.0	E858.7	E950.4	E962.0	E980.4	CORTISOL TOPICAL NEC
962.0	E932.0	E858.0	E950.4	E962.0	E980.4	CORTISONE DERIVATIVES (ACETATE)
976.6	E946.6	E858.7	E950.4	E962.0	E980.4	CORTISONE DERIVATIVES ENT AGENT
976.5	E946.5	E858.7	E950.4	E962.0	E980.4	CORTISONE DERIVATIVES OPHTHALMIC PREPARATION
976.0	E946.0	E858.7	E950.4	E962.0	E980.4	CORTISONE DERIVATIVES TOPICAL NEC
962.0	E932.0	E858.0	E950.4	E962.0	E980.4	CORTOGEN
976.6	E946.6	E858.7	E950.4	E962.0	E980.4	CORTOGEN ENT AGENT
976.5	E946.5	E858.7	E950.4	E962.0	E980.4	CORTOGEN OPHTHALMIC PREPARATION
962.0	E932.0	E858.0	E950.4	E962.0	E980.4	CORTONE
976.6	E946.6	E858.7	E950.4	E962.0	E980.4	CORTONE ENT AGENT
976.5	E946.5	E858.7	E950.4	E962.0	E980.4	CORTONE OPHTHALMIC PREPARATION
962.0	E932.0	E858.0	E950.4	E962.0	E980.4	CORTRIL
976.6	E946.6	E858.7	E950.4	E962.0	E980.4	CORTRIL ENT AGENT
976.5	E946.5	E858.7	E950.4	E962.0	E980.4	CORTRIL OPHTHALMIC PREPARATION
976.0	E946.0	E858.7	E950.4	E962.0	E980.4	CORTRIL TOPICAL NEC
989.89		E866.7	E950.9	E962.1	E980.9	COSMETICS
977.8	E947.8	E858.8	E950.4	E962.0	E980.4	COSYNTROPIN
964.5	E934.5	E858.2	E950.4	E962.0	E980.4	COTARNINE
976.3	E946.3	E858.7	E950.4	E962.0	E980.4	COTTONSEED OIL
975.4	E945.4	E858.6	E950.4	E962.0	E980.4	COUGH MIXTURES (ANTITUSSIVES)
965.09	E935.2	E850.2	E950.0	E962.0	E980.0	COUGH MIXTURES CONTAINING OPIATES
975.5	E945.5	E858.6	E950.4	E962.0	E980.4	COUGH MIXTURES EXPECTORANTS
964.2	E934.2	E858.2	E950.4	E962.0	E980.4	COUMADIN
989.4		E863.7	E950.6	E962.1	E980.7	COUMADIN RODENTICIDE
964.2	E934.2	E858.2	E950.4	E962.0	E980.4	COUMARIN
964.2	E934.2	E858.2	E950.4	E962.0	E980.4	COUMETAROL
988.2		E865.4	E950.9	E962.1	E980.9	COWBANE

DRUGS & CHEMICALS

POISON	THERA-PEUTIC	ACCIDENT	SUICIDE	ASSAULT	UNDETER-MINED	SUBSTANCE
963.5	E933.5	E858.1	E950.4	E962.0	E980.4	COZYME
970.8	E940.8	E854.3	E950.4	E962.0	E980.4	CRACK
983.0		E864.0	E950.7	E962.1	E980.6	CREOLIN
983.0		E861.4	E950.7	E962.1	E980.6	CREOLIN DISINFECTANT
983.0		E864.0	E950.7	E962.1	E980.6	CREOSOL (COMPOUND)
983.0		E864.0	E950.7	E962.1	E980.6	CREOSOTE (BEECHWOOD) (COAL TAR)
975.5	E945.5	E858.6	E950.4	E962.0	E980.4	CREOSOTE MEDICINAL (EXPECTORANT)
975.5	E945.5	E858.6	E950.4	E962.0	E980.4	CREOSOTE SYRUP
983.0		E864.0	E950.7	E962.1	E980.6	CRESOL
983.0		E861.4	E950.7	E962.1	E980.6	CRESOL DISINFECTANT
983.0		E864.0	E950.7	E962.1	E980.6	CRESYLIC ACID
965.7	E935.7	E850.7	E950.0	E962.0	E980.0	CROPROPAMIDE
970.0	E940.0	E854.3	E950.4	E962.0	E980.4	CROPROPAMIDE WITH CROTEHAMIDE
976.0	E946.0	E858.7	E950.4	E962.0	E980.4	CROTAMITON
965.7	E935.7	E850.7	E950.0	E962.0	E980.0	CROTETHAMIDE
970.0	E940.0	E854.3	E950.4	E962.0	E980.4	CROTETHAMIDE WITH CROPROPAMIDE
973.1	E943.1	E858.4	E950.4	E962.0	E980.4	CROTON (OIL)
967.1	E937.1	E852.0	E950.2	E962.0	E980.2	CROTON CHLORAL
981		E862.1	E950.9	E962.1	E980.9	CRUDE OIL
965.8	E935.8	E850.8	E950.0	E962.0	E980.0	CRYOGENINE
989.4		E863.4	E950.6	E962.1	E980.7	CRYOLITE (PESTICIDE)
972.6	E942.6	E858.3	E950.4	E962.0	E980.4	CRYPTENAMINE
976.0	E946.0	E858.7	E950.4	E962.0	E980.4	CRYSTAL VIOLET
988.2		E865.4	E950.9	E962.1	E980.9	CUCKOOPINT
964.2	E934.2	E858.2	E950.4	E962.0	E980.4	CUMETHAROL
973.6	E943.6	E858.4	E950.4	E962.0	E980.4	CUPRIC SULFATE
983.9		E864.3	E950.7	E962.1	E980.6	CUPROUS SULFATE
975.2	E945.2	E858.6	E950.4	E962.0	E980.4	CURARE
975.2	E945.2	E858.6	E950.4	E962.0	E980.4	CURARINE
0						CYANIC ACID SEE CYANIDE(S)
989.0		E866.8	E950.9	E962.1	E980.9	CYANIDE(S) (COMPOUNDS) (HYDROGEN) (POTASSIUM) (SODIUM) NEC
987.7		E869.8	E952.8	E962.2	E982.8	CYANIDE(S) DUST OR GAS (INHALATION) NEC
989.0		E863.8	E950.6	E962.1	E980.7	CYANIDE(S) FUMIGANT
0						CYANIDE(S) MERCURIC SEE MERCURY
989.0		E863.4	E950.6	E962.1	E980.7	CYANIDE(S) PESTICIDE(DUST) (FUMES)
964.1	E934.1	E858.2	E950.4	E962.0	E980.4	CYANOCOBALAMIN
987.8		E869.8	E952.8	E962.2	E982.8	CYANOGEN (CHLORIDE) (GAS) NEC
968.5	E938.5	E855.2	E950.4	E962.0	E980.4	CYCLAINE
988.2		E865.4	E950.9	E962.1	E980.9	CYCLAMEN EUROPAEUM
972.5	E942.5	E858.3	E950.4	E962.0	E980.4	CYCLANDELATE
965.09	E935.2	E850.2	E950.0	E962.0	E980.0	CYCLAZOCINE
963.0	E933.0	E858.1	E950.4	E962.0	E980.4	CYCLIZINE
967.0	E937.0	E851	E950.1	E962.0	E980.1	CYCLOBARBITAL
967.0	E937.0	E851	E950.1	E962.0	E980.1	CYCLOBARBITONE
961.4	E931.4	E857	E950.4	E962.0	E980.4	CYCLOGUANIL
982.0		E862.4	E950.9	E962.1	E980.9	CYCLOHEXANE
980.8		E860.8	E950.9	E962.1	E980.9	CYCLOHEXANOL
982.8		E862.4	E950.9	E962.1	E980.9	CYCLOHEXANONE
968.5	E938.5	E855.2	E950.4	E962.0	E980.4	CYCLOMETHYCAINE
971.2	E941.2	E855.5	E950.4	E962.0	E980.4	CYCLOPENTAMINE
974.3	E944.3	E858.5	E950.4	E962.0	E980.4	CYCLOPENTHIAZIDE
971.1	E941.1	E855.4	E950.4	E962.0	E980.4	CYCLOPENTOLATE
963.1	E933.1	E858.1	E950.4	E962.0	E980.4	CYCLOPHOSPHAMIDE
968.2	E938.2	E855.1	E950.4	E962.0	E980.4	CYCLOPROPANE
960.6	E930.6	E856	E950.4	E962.0	E980.4	CYCLOSERINE
974.3	E944.3	E858.5	E950.4	E962.0	E980.4	CYCLOTHIAZIDE
966.4	E936.4	E855.0	E950.4	E962.0	E980.4	CYCRIMINE
972.1	E942.1	E858.3	E950.4	E962.0	E980.4	CYMARIN
963.0	E933.0	E858.1	E950.4	E962.0	E980.4	CYPROHEPTADINE
969.0	E939.0	E854.0	E950.3	E962.0	E980.3	CYPROLIDOL
963.1	E933.1	E858.1	E950.4	E962.0	E980.4	CYTARABINE
988.2		E865.4	E950.9	E962.1	E980.9	CYTISUS LABURNUM
988.2		E865.4	E950.9	E962.1	E980.9	CYTISUS SCOPARIUS
962.7	E932.7	E858.0	E950.4	E962.0	E980.4	CYTOMEL
963.1	E933.1	E858.1	E950.4	E962.0	E980.4	CYTOSINE (ANTINEOPLASTIC)
963.1	E933.1	E858.1	E950.4	E962.0	E980.4	CYTOXAN
989.4		E863.7	E950.6	E962.1	E980.7	D-CON (RODENTICIDE)
969.6	E939.6	E854.1	E950.3	E962.0	E980.3	D-LYSERGIC ACID DIETHYLAMIDE
963.1	E933.1	E858.1	E950.4	E962.0	E980.4	DACARBAZINE
960.7	E930.7	E856	E950.4	E962.0	E980.4	DACTINOMYCIN
961.8	E931.8	E857	E950.4	E962.0	E980.4	DADPS
976.0	E946.0	E858.7	E950.4	E962.0	E980.4	DAKIN'S SOLUTION (EXTERNAL)

POISON	THERA-PEUTIC	ACCIDENT	SUICIDE	ASSAULT	UNDETER-MINED	SUBSTANCE
969.4	E939.4	E853.2	E950.3	E962.0	E980.3	DALMANE
977.2	E947.2	E858.8	E950.4	E962.0	E980.4	DAM
964.2	E934.2	E858.2	E950.4	E962.0	E980.4	DANILONE
973.1	E943.1	E858.4	E950.4	E962.0	E980.4	DANTHRON
975.2	E945.2	E858.6	E950.4	E962.0	E980.4	DANTROLENE
988.2		E865.4	E950.9	E962.1	E980.9	DAPHNE (GNIDIUM) (MEZEREUM)
988.2		E865.3	E950.9	E962.1	E980.9	DAPHNE BERRY
961.8	E931.8	E857	E950.4	E962.0	E980.4	DAPSONE
961.4	E931.4	E857	E950.4	E962.0	E980.4	DARAPRIM
988.2		E865.3	E950.9	E962.1	E980.9	DARNEL
965.8	E935.8	E850.8	E950.0	E962.0	E980.0	DARVON
960.7	E930.7	E856	E950.4	E962.0	E980.4	DAUNORUBICIN
962.3	E932.3	E858.0	E950.4	E962.0	E980.4	DBI
961.8	E931.8	E857	E950.4	E962.0	E980.4	DDS
989.2		E863.0	E950.6	E962.1	E980.7	DDT
988.2		E865.4	E950.9	E962.1	E980.9	DEADLY NIGHTSHADE
988.2		E865.3	E950.9	E962.1	E980.9	DEADLY NIGHTSHADE BERRY
969.7	E939.7	E854.2	E950.3	E962.0	E980.3	DEANOL
972.6	E942.6	E858.3	E950.4	E962.0	E980.4	DEBRISOQUINE
989.89		E866.8	E950.9	E962.1	E980.9	DECABORANE
987.8		E869.8	E952.8	E962.2	E982.8	DECABORANE FUMES
962.0	E932.0	E858.0	E950.4	E962.0	E980.4	DECADRON
976.6	E946.6	E858.7	E950.4	E962.0	E980.4	DECADRON ENT AGENT
976.5	E946.5	E858.7	E950.4	E962.0	E980.4	DECADRON OPHTHALMIC PREPARATION
976.0	E946.0	E858.7	E950.4	E962.0	E980.4	DECADRON TOPICAL NEC
982.0		E862.4	E950.9	E962.1	E980.9	DECAHYDRONAPHTHALENE
982.0		E862.4	E950.9	E962.1	E980.9	DECALIN
975.2	E945.2	E858.6	E950.4	E962.0	E980.4	DECAMETHONIUM
963.1	E933.1	E858.1	E950.4	E962.0	E980.4	DECARBAZINE
973.4	E943.4	E858.4	E950.4	E962.0	E980.4	DECHOLIN
977.8	E947.8	E858.8	E950.4	E962.0	E980.4	DECHOLIN SODIUM (DIAGNOSTIC)
960.4	E930.4	E856	E950.4	E962.0	E980.4	DECLOMYCIN
963.8	E933.8	E858.1	E950.4	E962.0	E980.4	DEFEROXAMINE
980.0		E860.1	E950.9	E962.1	E980.9	DEHYDRATED ALCOHOL
973.4	E943.4	E858.4	E950.4	E962.0	E980.4	DEHYDROCHOLIC ACID
982.0		E862.4	E950.9	E962.1	E980.9	DEKALIN
962.2	E932.2	E858.0	E950.4	E962.0	E980.4	DELALUTIN
988.2		E865.3	E950.9	E962.1	E980.9	DELPHINIUM
962.0	E932.0	E858.0	E950.4	E962.0	E980.4	DELTASONE
962.0	E932.0	E858.0	E950.4	E962.0	E980.4	DELTRA
967.0	E937.0	E851	E950.1	E962.0	E980.1	DELVINAL
971.0	E941.0	E855.3	E950.4	E962.0	E980.4	DEMECARIUM (BROMIDE)
960.4	E930.4	E856	E950.4	E962.0	E980.4	DEMECLOCYCLINE
963.1	E933.1	E858.1	E950.4	E962.0	E980.4	DEMECOLCINE
976.8	E946.8	E858.7	E950.4	E962.0	E980.4	DEMELANIZING AGENTS
965.09	E935.2	E850.2	E950.0	E962.0	E980.0	DEMEROL
960.4	E930.4	E856	E950.4	E962.0	E980.4	DEMETHYLCHLORTETRACYCLINE
960.4	E930.4	E856	E950.4	E962.0	E980.4	DEMETHYLTETRACYCLINE
989.3		E863.1	E950.6	E962.1	E980.7	DEMETON
976.3	E946.3	E858.7	E950.4	E962.0	E980.4	DEMULCENTS
962.2	E932.2	E858.0	E950.4	E962.0	E980.4	DEMULEN
980.0		E860.1	E950.9	E962.1	E980.9	DENATURED ALCOHOL
976.5	E946.5	E858.7	E950.4	E962.0	E980.4	DENDRID
976.7	E946.7	E858.7	E950.4	E962.0	E980.4	DENTAL AGENTS TOPICAL
976.8	E946.8	E858.7	E950.4	E962.0	E980.4	DEODORANT SPRAY (FEMININE HYGIENE)
963.4	E933.4	E858.1	E950.4	E962.0	E980.4	DEOXYRIBONUCLEASE
977.0	E947.0	E858.8	E950.4	E962.0	E980.4	DEPRESSANTS APPETITE CENTRAL
972.0	E942.0	E858.3	E950.4	E962.0	E980.4	DEPRESSANTS CARDIAC
968.4	E938.4	E855.1	E950.4	E962.0	E980.4	DEPRESSANTS CENTRAL NERVOUS SYSTEM (ANESTHETIC)
969.5	E939.5	E853.9	E950.9	E962.0	E980.3	DEPRESSANTS PSYCHOTHERAPEUTIC
976.0	E946.0	E858.7	E950.4	E962.0	E980.4	DEQUALINIUM
976.2	E946.2	E858.7	E950.4	E962.0	E980.4	DERMOLATE
962.2	E932.2	E858.0	E950.4	E962.0	E980.4	DES
976.0	E946.0	E858.7	E950.4	E962.0	E980.4	DESENEX
972.6	E942.6	E858.3	E950.4	E962.0	E980.4	DESERPIDINE
969.0	E939.0	E854.0	E950.3	E962.0	E980.3	DESIPRAMINE
972.1	E942.1	E858.3	E950.4	E962.0	E980.4	DESLANOSIDE
965.09	E935.2	E850.2	E950.0	E962.0	E980.0	DESOCODEINE
965.09	E935.2	E850.2	E950.0	E962.0	E980.0	DESOMORPHINE
976.0	E946.0	E858.7	E950.4	E962.0	E980.4	DESONIDE
962.0	E932.0	E858.0	E950.4	E962.0	E980.4	DESOXYCORTICOSTERONE DERIVATIVES
969.7	E939.7	E854.2	E950.3	E962.0	E980.3	DESOXYEPHEDRINE

DRUGS & CHEMICALS

POISON	THERA-PEUTIC	ACCIDENT	SUICIDE	ASSAULT	UNDETER-MINED	SUBSTANCE
969.6	E939.6	E854.1	E950.3	E962.0	E980.3	DET
989.6		E861.0	E950.9	E962.1	E980.9	DETERGENTS (INGESTED) (SYNTHETIC)
976.2	E946.2	E858.7	E950.4	E962.0	E980.4	DETERGENTS EXTERNAL MEDICATION
977.3	E947.3	E858.8	E950.4	E962.0	E980.4	DETERRENT ALCOHOL
962.7	E932.7	E858.0	E950.4	E962.0	E980.4	DETROTHYRONINE
976.0	E946.0	E858.7	E950.4	E962.0	E980.4	DETTOL (EXTERNAL MEDICATION)
962.0	E932.0	E858.0	E950.4	E962.0	E980.4	DEXAMETHASONE
976.6	E946.6	E858.7	E950.4	E962.0	E980.4	DEXAMETHASONE ENT AGENT
976.5	E946.5	E858.7	E950.4	E962.0	E980.4	DEXAMETHASONE OPHTHALMIC PREPARATION
976.0	E946.0	E858.7	E950.4	E962.0	E980.4	DEXAMETHASONE TOPICAL NEC
969.7	E939.7	E854.2	E950.3	E962.0	E980.3	DEXAMPHETAMINE
969.7	E939.7	E854.2	E950.3	E962.0	E980.3	DEXEDRINE
963.5	E933.5	E858.1	E950.4	E962.0	E980.4	DEXPANTHENOL
964.8	E934.8	E858.2	E950.4	E962.0	E980.4	DEXTRAN
964.0	E934.0	E858.2	E950.4	E962.0	E980.4	DEXTRIFERRON
963.5	E933.5	E858.1	E950.4	E962.0	E980.4	DEXTRO CALCIUM PANTOTHENATE
963.5	E933.5	E858.1	E950.4	E962.0	E980.4	DEXTRO PANTOTHENYL ALCOHOL
976.8	E946.8	E858.7	E950.4	E962.0	E980.4	DEXTRO PANTOTHENYL ALCOHOL TOPICAL
969.7	E939.7	E854.2	E950.3	E962.0	E980.3	DEXTROAMPHETAMINE
975.4	E945.4	E858.6	E950.4	E962.0	E980.4	DEXTROMETHORPHAN
965.09	E935.2	E850.2	E950.0	E962.0	E980.0	DEXTROMORAMIDE
965.8	E935.8	E850.8	E950.0	E962.0	E980.0	DEXTROPROPOXYPHENE (HYDROCHLORIDE)
965.09	E935.2	E850.2	E950.0	E962.0	E980.0	DEXTRORPHAN
974.5	E944.5	E858.5	E950.4	E962.0	E980.4	DEXTROSE NEC
962.7	E932.7	E858.0	E950.4	E962.0	E980.4	DEXTROTHYROXIN
971.0	E941.0	E855.3	E950.4	E962.0	E980.4	DFP
972.9	E942.9	E858.3	E950.4	E962.0	E980.4	DHE-45
962.3	E932.3	E858.0	E950.4	E962.0	E980.4	DIABINESE
977.2	E947.2	E858.8	E950.4	E962.0	E980.4	DIACETYL MONOXIME
965.01	E935.0	E850.0	E950.4	E962.0	E980.0	DIACETYLMORPHINE
977.8	E947.8	E858.8	E950.4	E962.0	E980.4	DIAGNOSTIC AGENTS AND KITS
976.2	E946.2	E858.7	E950.4	E962.0	E980.4	DIAL (SOAP)
967.0	E937.0	E851	E950.1	E962.0	E980.1	DIAL SEDATIVE
967.0	E937.0	E851	E950.1	E962.0	E980.1	DIALLYLBARBITURIC ACID
961.8	E931.8	E857	E950.4	E962.0	E980.4	DIAMINODIPHENYLSULFONE
965.01	E935.0	E850.0	E950.0	E962.0	E980.0	DIAMORPHINE
974.2	E944.2	E858.5	E950.4	E962.0	E980.4	DIAMOX
976.0	E946.0	E858.7	E950.4	E962.0	E980.4	DIAMTHAZOLE
961.8	E931.8	E857	E950.4	E962.0	E980.4	DIAPHENYLSULFONE
961.8	E931.8	E857	E950.4	E962.0	E980.4	DIASONE (SODIUM)
969.4	E939.4	E853.2	E950.3	E962.0	E980.3	DIAZEPAM
989.3		E863.1	E950.6	E962.1	E980.7	DIAZINON
987.8		E869.8	E952.8	E962.2	E982.8	DIAZOMETHANE (GAS)
972.5	E942.5	E858.3	E950.4	E962.0	E980.4	DIAZOXIDE
971.3	E941.3	E855.6	E950.4	E962.0	E980.4	DIBENAMINE
963.0	E933.0	E858.1	E950.4	E962.0	E980.4	DIBENZHEPTROPINE
971.3	E941.3	E855.6	E950.4	E962.0	E980.4	DIBENZYLINE
987.8		E869.8	E952.8	E962.2	E982.8	DIBORANE (GAS)
963.1	E933.1	E858.1	E950.4	E962.0	E980.4	DIBROMOMANNITOL
968.7	E938.7	E855.2	E950.4	E962.0	E980.4	DIBUCAINE (SPINAL)
968.5	E938.5	E855.2	E950.4	E962.0	E980.4	DIBUCAINE TOPICAL (SURFACE)
975.4	E945.4	E858.6	E950.4	E962.0	E980.4	DIBUNATE SODIUM
971.1	E941.1	E855.4	E950.4	E962.0	E980.4	DIBUTOLINE
989.4		E863.4	E950.6	E962.1	E980.7	DICAPTHON
967.1	E937.1	E852.0	E950.2	E962.0	E980.2	DICHLORALPHENAZONE
987.4		E869.2	E952.8	E962.2	E982.8	DICHLORODIFLUOROMETHANE
982.3		E862.4	E950.9	E962.1	E980.9	DICHLOROETHANE
987.8		E869.8	E952.8	E962.2	E982.8	DICHLOROETHYL SULFIDE
982.3		E862.4	E950.9	E962.1	E980.9	DICHLOROETHYLENE
982.3		E862.4	E950.9	E962.1	E980.9	DICHLOROHYDRIN
982.3		E862.4	E950.9	E962.1	E980.9	DICHLOROMETHANE (SOLVENT) (VAPOR)
961.6	E931.6	E857	E950.4	E962.0	E980.4	DICHLOROPHEN(E)
989.4		E863.4	E950.6	E962.1	E980.7	DICHLOROPHENOXYACETIC ACID (2 4D)
974.2	E944.2	E858.5	E950.4	E962.0	E980.4	DICHLORPHENAMIDE
989.3		E863.1	E950.6	E962.1	E980.7	DICHLORVOS
965.69	E935.6	E850.6	E950.0	E962.0	E980.0	DICLOFENAC SODIUM (ANTIRHEUMATICS)
969.4	E939.4	E853.2	E950.3	E962.0	E980.3	DICLOFENAC SODIUM TRANQUILIZERS
964.2	E934.2	E858.2	E950.4	E962.0	E980.4	DICOUMARIN DICUMAROL
987.8		E869.8	E952.8	E962.2	E982.8	DICYANOGEN (GAS)
971.1	E941.1	E855.4	E950.4	E962.0	E980.4	DICYCLOMINE

POISON	THERA-PEUTIC	ACCIDENT	SUICIDE	ASSAULT	UNDETER-MINED	SUBSTANCE
989.2		E863.0	E950.6	E962.1	E980.7	DIELDRIN (VAPOR)
962.2	E932.2	E858.0	E950.4	E962.0	E980.4	DIENESTROL
977.0	E947.0	E858.8	E950.4	E962.0	E980.4	DIETETICS CENTRAL APPETITIE DEPRESSANTS
966.4	E936.4	E855.0	E950.4	E962.0	E980.4	DIETHAZINE
967.0	E937.0	E851	E950.1	E962.0	E980.1	DIETHYL BARBITURIC ACID
961.6	E931.6	E857	E950.4	E962.0	E980.4	DIETHYL CARBAMAZINE
980.8		E860.8	E950.9	E962.1	E980.9	DIETHYL CARBINOL
982.8		E862.4	E950.9	E962.1	E980.9	DIETHYL CARBONATE
0						DIETHYL ETHER (VAPOR) SEE ETHER(S)
977.0	E947.0	E858.8	E950.4	E962.0	E980.4	DIETHYL PROPION
962.2	E932.2	E858.0	E950.4	E962.0	E980.4	DIETHYL STILBESTROL
982.8		E862.4	E950.9	E962.1	E980.9	DIETHYLENE DIOXIDE
982.8		E862.4	E950.9	E962.1	E980.9	DIETHYLENE GLYCOL (MONOACETATE) (MONOETHYL ETHER)
967.8	E937.8	E852.8	E950.2	E962.0	E980.2	DIETHYLSULFONEDIETHYLMETHANE
965.09	E935.2	E850.2	E950.0	E962.0	E980.0	DIFENCLOXAZINE
963.4	E933.4	E858.1	E950.4	E962.0	E980.4	DIFFUSIN
971.0	E941.0	E855.3	E950.4	E962.0	E980.4	DIFLOS
973.4	E943.4	E858.4	E950.4	E962.0	E980.4	DIGESTANTS
972.1	E942.1	E858.3	E950.4	E962.0	E980.4	DIGITALIN(E)
972.1	E942.1	E858.3	E950.4	E962.0	E980.4	DIGITALIS GLYCOSIDES
972.1	E942.1	E858.3	E950.4	E962.0	E980.4	DIGITOXIN
972.1	E942.1	E858.3	E950.4	E962.0	E980.4	DIGOXIN
965.09	E935.2	E850.2	E950.0	E962.0	E980.0	DIHYDROCODEINE
965.09	E935.2	E850.2	E950.0	E962.0	E980.0	DIHYDROCODEINONE
972.9	E942.9	E858.3	E950.4	E962.0	E980.4	DIHYDROERGOCRISTINE
972.9	E942.9	E858.3	E950.4	E962.0	E980.4	DIHYDROERGOTAMINE
972.9	E942.9	E858.3	E950.4	E962.0	E980.4	DIHYDROERGOTOXINE
965.09	E935.2	E850.2	E950.0	E962.0	E980.0	DIHYDROHYDRO-XYMORPHINONE
965.09	E935.2	E850.2	E950.0	E962.0	E980.0	DIHYDROHYDROXY-CODEINONE
965.09	E935.2	E850.2	E950.0	E962.0	E980.0	DIHYDROISOCODEINE
965.09	E935.2	E850.2	E950.0	E962.0	E980.0	DIHYDROMORPHINE
965.09	E935.2	E850.2	E950.0	E962.0	E980.0	DIHYDROMORPHINONE
960.6	E930.6	E856	E950.4	E962.0	E980.4	DIHYDROSTREPTOMYCIN
962.6	E932.6	E858.0	E950.4	E962.0	E980.4	DIHYDROTACHYSTEROL
973.1	E943.1	E858.4	E950.4	E962.0	E980.4	DIHYDROXYANTHRA-QUINONE
965.09	E935.2	E850.2	E950.0	E962.0	E980.0	DIHYDROXYCODEINONE
961.3	E931.3	E857	E950.4	E962.0	E980.4	DIIODOHYDRO-XYQUINOLINE
961.3	E931.3	E857	E950.4	E962.0	E980.4	DIIODOHYDROXYQUIN
976.0	E946.0	E858.7	E950.4	E962.0	E980.4	DIIODOHYDROXYQUIN TOPICAL
983.0		E864.0	E950.7	E962.1	E980.6	DIISOCYANATE 2 4-TOLUENE
966.1	E936.1	E855.0	E950.4	E962.0	E980.4	DILANTIN
965.09	E935.2	E850.2	E950.0	E962.0	E980.0	DILAUDID
961.5	E931.5	E857	E950.4	E962.0	E980.4	DILOXANIDE
970.0	E940.0	E854.3	E950.4	E962.0	E980.4	DIMEFLINE
963.0	E933.0	E858.1	E950.4	E962.0	E980.4	DIMENHYDRINATE
963.8	E933.8	E858.1	E950.4	E962.0	E980.4	DIMERCAPROL
963.8	E933.8	E858.1	E950.4	E962.0	E980.4	DIMERCAPTOPROPANOL
963.0	E933.0	E858.1	E950.4	E962.0	E980.4	DIMETANE
976.3	E946.3	E858.7	E950.4	E962.0	E980.4	DIMETHICONE
963.0	E933.0	E858.1	E950.4	E962.0	E980.4	DIMETHINDENE
968.5	E938.5	E855.2	E950.4	E962.0	E980.4	DIMETHISOQUIN
962.2	E932.2	E858.0	E950.4	E962.0	E980.4	DIMETHISTERONE
975.4	E945.4	E858.6	E950.4	E962.0	E980.4	DIMETHOXANATE
0						DIMETHYL ARSINE ARSINIC ACID SEE ARSENIC
980.2		E860.3	E950.9	E962.1	E980.9	DIMETHYL CARBINOL
962.3	E932.3	E858.0	E950.4	E962.0	E980.4	DIMETHYL DIGUANIDE
982.8		E862.4	E950.9	E962.1	E980.9	DIMETHYL KETONE
987.8		E869.8	E952.8	E962.2	E982.8	DIMETHYL KETONE VAPOR
965.09	E935.2	E850.2	E950.0	E962.0	E980.0	DIMETHYL MEPERIDINE
973.8	E943.8	E858.4	E950.4	E962.0	E980.4	DIMETHYL POLYSILOXANE
987.8		E869.8	E952.8	E962.2	E982.8	DIMETHYL SULFATE (FUMES)
983.9		E864.3	E950.7	E962.1	E980.6	DIMETHYL SULFATE LIQUID
976.4	E946.4	E858.7	E950.4	E962.0	E980.4	DIMETHYL SULFOXIDE MEDICINAL
982.8		E862.4	E950.9	E962.1	E980.9	DIMETHYL SULFOXIDE NEC
969.6	E939.6	E854.1	E950.3	E962.0	E980.3	DIMETHYL TRIPTAMINE
975.2	E945.2	E858.6	E950.4	E962.0	E980.4	DIMETHYL TUBOCURARINE
964.2	E934.2	E858.2	E950.4	E962.0	E980.4	DINDEVAN
989.4		E863.5	E950.6	E962.1	E980.7	DINITRO (-ORTHO-) CRESOL (HERBICIDE) (SPRAY)
989.4		E863.4	E950.6	E962.1	E980.7	DINITRO INSECTICIDE
989.4		E863.4	E950.6	E962.1	E980.7	DINITROORTHOCRESOL INSECTICIDE
989.4		E863.5	E950.6	E962.1	E980.7	DINITROORTHOCRESOL (HERBICIDE)

DRUGS & CHEMICALS

DRUGS & CHEMICALS

POISON	THERA-PEUTIC	ACCIDENT	SUICIDE	ASSAULT	UNDETER-MINED	SUBSTANCE
983.0		E864.0	E950.7	E962.1	E980.6	DINITROBENZENE
987.8		E869.8	E952.8	E962.2	E982.8	DINITROBENZENE VAPOR
989.4		E863.5	E950.6	E962.1	E980.7	DINITROPHENOL (HERBICIDE) (SPRAY)
989.4		E863.4	E950.6	E962.1	E980.7	DINITROPHENOL INSECTICIDE
975.0	E945.0	E858.6	E950.4	E962.0	E980.4	DINOPROST
973.2	E943.2	E858.4	E950.4	E962.0	E980.4	DIOCTYL SULFOSUCCINATE (CALCIUM) (SODIUM)
961.3	E931.3	E857	E950.4	E962.0	E980.4	DIODOQUIN
966.3	E936.3	E855.0	E950.4	E962.0	E980.4	DIONE DERIVATIVES NEC
965.09	E935.2	E850.2	E950.0	E962.0	E980.0	DIONIN
982.8		E862.4	E950.9	E962.1	E980.9	DIOXANE
972.5	E942.5	E858.3	E950.4	E962.0	E980.4	DIOXYLINE
982.8		E862.4	E950.9	E962.1	E980.9	DIPENTENE
971.1	E941.1	E855.4	E950.4	E962.0	E980.4	DIPHEMANIL
964.2	E934.2	E858.2	E950.4	E962.0	E980.4	DIPHENADIONE
963.0	E933.0	E858.1	E950.4	E962.0	E980.4	DIPHENHYDRAMINE
963.0	E933.0	E858.1	E950.4	E962.0	E980.4	DIPHENIDOL
973.5	E943.5	E858.4	E950.4	E962.0	E980.4	DIPHENOXYLATE
985.1		E866.3	E950.8	E962.1	E980.8	DIPHENYLCHLOROARSINE
966.1	E936.1	E855.0	E950.4	E962.0	E980.4	DIPHENYLHYDRANTOIN (SODIUM)
963.0	E933.0	E858.1	E950.4	E962.0	E980.4	DIPHENYLPYRALINE
979.9	E949.9	E858.8	E950.4	E962.0	E980.4	DIPHTHERIA ANTITOXIN
978.5	E948.5	E858.8	E950.4	E962.0	E980.4	DIPHTHERIA TOXOID
978.9	E948.9	E858.8	E950.4	E962.0	E980.4	DIPHTHERIA TOXOID WITH TETANUS TOXOID
978.6	E948.6	E858.8	E950.4	E962.0	E980.4	DIPHTHERIA TOXOID WITH TETANUS TOXOID WITH PERTUSSIS COMPONENT
978.5	E948.5	E858.8	E950.4	E962.0	E980.4	DIPHTHERIA VACCINE
965.09	E935.2	E850.2	E950.0	E962.0	E980.0	DIPIPANONE
979.5	E949.5	E858.8	E950.4	E962.0	E980.4	DIPLOVAX
975.1	E945.1	E858.6	E950.4	E962.0	E980.4	DIPROPHYLLINE
972.4	E942.4	E858.3	E950.4	E962.0	E980.4	DIPYRIDAMOLE
965.5	E935.5	E850.5	E950.0	E962.0	E980.0	DIPYRONE
989.4		E863.5	E950.6	E962.1	E980.7	DIQUAT
983.2		E861.4	E950.7	E962.1	E980.6	DISINFECTANT ALKALINE
983.0		E861.4	E950.7	E962.1	E980.6	DISINFECTANT AROMATIC
983.9		E861.4	E950.7	E962.1	E980.6	DISINFECTANT NEC
966.4	E936.4	E855.0	E950.4	E962.0	E980.4	DISIPAL
963.8	E933.8	E858.1	E950.4	E962.0	E980.4	DISODIUM EDETATE
974.4	E944.4	E858.5	E950.4	E962.0	E980.4	DISULFAMIDE
961.0	E931.0	E857	E950.4	E962.0	E980.4	DISULFANILAMIDE
977.3	E947.3	E858.8	E950.4	E962.0	E980.4	DISULFIRAM
961.6	E931.6	E857	E950.4	E962.0	E980.4	DITHIAZANINE
963.8	E933.8	E858.1	E950.4	E962.0	E980.4	DITHIOGLYCEROL
976.4	E946.4	E858.7	E950.4	E962.0	E980.4	DITHRANOL
974.3	E944.3	E858.5	E950.4	E962.0	E980.4	DIUCARDIN
974.3	E944.3	E858.5	E950.4	E962.0	E980.4	DIUPRES
974.2	E944.2	E858.5	E950.4	E962.0	E980.4	DIURETICS CARBONIC ACID ANHYDRASE INHIBITORS
974.0	E944.0	E858.5	E950.4	E962.0	E980.4	DIURETICS MERCURIAL
974.4	E944.4	E858.5	E950.4	E962.0	E980.4	DIURETICS NEC
974.4	E944.4	E858.5	E950.4	E962.0	E980.4	DIURETICS OSMOTIC
974.1	E944.1	E858.5	E950.4	E962.0	E980.4	DIURETICS PURINE DERIVATIVES
974.3	E944.3	E858.5	E950.4	E962.0	E980.4	DIURETICS SALURETIC
974.3	E944.3	E858.5	E950.4	E962.0	E980.4	DIURIL
968.2	E938.2	E855.1	E950.4	E962.0	E980.4	DIVINYL ETHER
960.4	E930.4	E856	E950.4	E962.0	E980.4	DMCT
982.8		E862.4	E950.9	E962.1	E980.9	DMSO
969.6	E939.6	E854.1	E950.3	E962.0	E980.3	DMT
989.4		E863.4	E950.6	E962.1	E980.7	DNOC
962.0	E932.0	E858.0	E950.4	E962.0	E980.4	DOCA
965.02	E935.0	E850.1	E950.0	E962.0	E980.0	DOLOPHINE
965.8	E935.8	E850.8	E950.0	E962.0	E980.0	DOLOXENE
969.6	E939.6	E854.1	E950.3	E962.0	E980.3	DOM
0						DOMESTIC GAS SEE GAS UTILITY
976.6	E946.6	E858.7	E950.4	E962.0	E980.4	DOMIPHEN (BROMIDE) (LOZENGES)
966.4	E936.4	E855.0	E950.4	E962.0	E980.4	DOPA (LEVO)
971.2	E941.2	E855.5	E950.4	E962.0	E980.4	DOPAMINE
967.5	E937.5	E852.4	E950.2	E962.0	E980.2	DORIDEN
967.0	E937.0	E851	E950.1	E962.0	E980.1	DORMIRAL
967.8	E937.8	E852.8	E950.2	E962.0	E980.2	DORMISON
963.4	E933.4	E858.1	E950.4	E962.0	E980.4	DORNASE
968.5	E938.5	E855.2	E950.4	E962.0	E980.4	DORSACAINE
970.0	E940.0	E854.3	E950.4	E962.0	E980.4	DOXAPRAM
969.0	E939.0	E854.0	E950.3	E962.0	E980.3	DOXEPIN

POISON	THERA-PEUTIC	ACCIDENT	SUICIDE	ASSAULT	UNDETER-MINED	SUBSTANCE
960.7	E930.7	E856	E950.4	E962.0	E980.4	DOXORUBICIN
960.4	E930.4	E856	E950.4	E962.0	E980.4	DOXYCYCLINE
963.0	E933.0	E858.1	E950.4	E962.0	E980.4	DOXYLAMINE
963.0	E933.0	E858.1	E950.4	E962.0	E980.4	DRAMAMINE
983.2	E864.2	E864.2	E950.7	E962.1	E980.6	DRANO (DRAIN CLEANER)
965.09	E935.2	E850.2	E950.0	E962.0	E980.0	DROMORAN
962.1	E932.1	E858.0	E950.4	E962.0	E980.4	DROMOSTANOLONE
969.2	E939.2	E853.1	E950.3	E962.0	E980.3	DROPERIDOL
964.2	E934.2	E858.2	E950.4	E962.0	E980.4	DROTRECOGIN ALFA
977.9	E947.9	E858.9	E950.5	E962.0	E980.5	DRUG
963.2	E933.2	E858.1	E950.4	E962.0	E980.4	DRUG ACIDIFYING AGENTS (40:04)
962.0	E932.0	E858.0	E950.4	E962.0	E980.4	DRUG ADRENALS (68:04)
963.3	E933.3	E858.1	E950.4	E962.0	E980.4	DRUG ALKALINIZING AGENTS (40:08)
961.5	E931.5	E857	E950.4	E962.0	E980.4	DRUG AMEBACIDES (8:04)
961.1	E931.1	E857	E950.4	E962.0	E980.4	DRUG AMEBACIDES ARSENICAL ANTI-INFECTIVES (8:04)
961.3	E931.3	E857	E950.4	E962.0	E980.4	DRUG AMEBACIDES QUINOLINE DERIVATIVES (8:04)
974.5	E944.5	E858.5	E950.4	E962.0	E980.4	DRUG AMMONIA DETOXICANTS (40:10)
965.9	E935.9	E850.9	E950.0	E962.0	E980.0	DRUG ANALGESICS AND ANTIPYRETICS (28:08)
965.8	E935.8	E850.8	E950.0	E962.0	E980.0	DRUG ANALGESICS AND ANTIPYRETICS SPECIFIED NEC (28:08)
973.0	E943.0	E858.4	E950.4	E962.0	E980.4	DRUG ANTACIDS AND ABSORBENTS (56:04)
961.6	E931.6	E857	E950.4	E962.0	E980.4	DRUG ANTHELMINTICS (8:08)
961.3	E931.3	E857	E950.4	E962.0	E980.4	DRUG ANTHELMINTICS QUINOLINE DERIVATIVES (8:08)
976.5	E946.5	E858.7	E950.4	E962.0	E980.4	DRUG ANTI INFECTIVES (EENT) OPHTHALMIC PREPARATION (52:04)
976.6	E946.6	E858.7	E950.4	E962.0	E980.4	DRUG ANTI INFECTIVES (EENT) ENT AGENT (52:04)
976.5	E946.5	E858.7	E950.4	E962.0	E980.4	DRUG ANTI INFLAMMATORY AGENTS (EENT) OPHTHALMIC PREPARATION (52:08)
976.6	E946.6	E858.7	E950.4	E962.0	E980.4	DRUG ANTI INFLAMMATORY AGENTS (EENT) ENT AGENTS (52:08)
976.0	E946.0	E858.7	E950.4	E962.0	E980.4	DRUG ANTI INFLAMMATORY AGENTS (SKIN AND MUCOUS MEMBRANE) (84:06)
962.2	E932.2	E858.0	E950.4	E962.0	E980.4	DRUG ANTI NEOPLASTIC AGENTS PROGESTOGENS (10:00)
964.1	E934.1	E858.2	E950.4	E962.0	E980.4	DRUG ANTIANEMIA DRUGS (20:04)
960.6	E930.6	E856	E950.4	E962.0	E980.4	DRUG ANTIBIOTICS (8:16)
976.5	E946.5	E858.7	E950.4	E962.0	E980.4	DRUG ANTIBIOTICS (EENT) OPHTHALMIC PREPARATION (52:04.04)
976.6	E946.6	E858.7	E950.4	E962.0	E980.4	DRUG ANTIBIOTICS (EENT) ENT AGENT (52:04.04)
976.0	E946.0	E858.7	E950.4	E962.0	E980.4	DRUG ANTIBIOTICS (SKIN AND MUCOUS MEMBRANES) (84:04.04)
964.2	E934.2	E858.2	E950.4	E962.0	E980.4	DRUG ANTICOAGULANTS (20:12.04)
966.3	E936.3	E855.0	E950.4	E962.0	E980.4	DRUG ANTICONVULSANTS(28:12)
967.0	E937.0	E851	E950.1	E962.0	E980.1	DRUG ANTICONVULSANTS BARBITURATES (28:12)
969.4	E939.4	E853.4	E950.3	E962.0	E980.3	DRUG ANTICONVULSANTS BENZODIAZEPINE BASED TRANQUILIZERS
967.3	E937.3	E852.2	E950.2	E962.0	E980.2	DRUG ANTICONVULSANTS BROMIDES (28:12)
966.1	E936.1	E855.0	E950.4	E962.0	E980.4	DRUG ANTICONVULSANTSHYDANTOIN DERIVATIVES (28:12)
966.0	E936.0	E855.0	E950.4	E962.0	E980.4	DRUG ANTICONVULSANTSOXAZOLIDINE (DERIVATIVES) (28:12)
966.2	E936.2	E855.0	E950.4	E962.0	E980.4	DRUG ANTICONVULSANTS SUCCINIMIDES (28:12)
969.0	E939.0	E854.0	E950.3	E962.0	E980.3	DRUG ANTIDEPRESSANTS(28:16.04)
973.5	E943.5	E858.4	E950.4	E962.0	E980.4	DRUG ANTIDIARRHEA AGENTS (56:08)
973.8	E943.8	E858.4	E950.4	E962.0	E980.4	DRUG ANTIFLATULENTS (56:10)
960.1	E930.1	E856	E950.4	E962.0	E980.4	DRUG ANTIFUNGAL ANTIBIOTICS (8:12.04)
964.5	E934.5	E858.2	E950.4	E962.0	E980.4	DRUG ANTIHEPARIN AGENTS (20:12.08)
963.0	E933.0	E858.1	E950.4	E962.0	E980.4	DRUG ANTIHISTAMIN DRUGS (4:00)
962.7	E932.7	E858.0	E950.4	E962.0	E980.4	DRUG ANTILIPEMIC AGENTS THYROID DERIVATIVES (24:06)
972.2	E942.2	E858.3	E950.4	E962.0	E980.4	DRUG ANTILIPEMIC AGENTS (24:06)
960.6	E930.6	E856	E950.4	E962.0	E980.4	DRUG ANTIMYCO-BACTERIAL (8:12.28)

POISON	THERA-PEUTIC	ACCIDENT	SUICIDE	ASSAULT	UNDETER-MINED	SUBSTANCE
963.1	E933.1	E858.1	E950.4	E962.0	E980.4	DRUG ANTINEOPLASTIC AGENTS (10:00)
960.7	E930.7	E856	E950.4	E962.0	E980.4	DRUG ANTINEOPLASTIC AGENTS ANTIBIOTICS (10:10)
976.1	E946.1	E858.7	E950.4	E962.0	E980.4	DRUG ANTIPRURITICS (84:08)
965.69	E935.6	E850.6	E950.0	E962.0	E980.0	DRUG ANTI RHEUMATICS(28:08)
961.8	E931.8	E857	E950.4	E962.0	E980.4	DRUG ANTITUBERCULARS(8:16)
961.7	E931.7	E857	E950.4	E962.0	E980.4	DRUG ANTIVIRALS (8:18)
976.6	E946.6	E858.7	E950.4	E962.0	E980.4	DRUG ANTIVIRALS ENT AGENT (52:04.06)
976.5	E946.5	E858.7	E950.4	E962.0	E980.4	DRUG ANTIVIRALS OPHTHALMIC PREPARATION (52:04.06)
965.4	E935.4	E850.4	E950.0	E962.0	E980.0	DRUG AROMATIC ANALGESICS (28:08)
976.2	E946.2	E858.7	E950.4	E962.0	E980.4	DRUG ASTRINGENTS (84:12)
964.7	E934.7	E858.2	E950.4	E962.0	E980.4	DRUG BLOOD DERIVATIVES (16:00)
979.6	E949.6	E858.8	E950.4	E962.0	E980.4	DRUG CACCINES RICKETTSIAL NEC (80:12)
974.5	E944.5	E858.5	E950.4	E962.0	E980.4	DRUG CALORIC AGENTS (40:20)
974.2	E944.2	E858.5	E950.4	E962.0	E980.4	DRUG CARBONIC ANHYDRASE INHIBITORS (52:10)
972.9	E942.9	E858.3	E950.4	E962.0	E980.4	DRUG CARDIAC DRUGS (24:04)
972.1	E942.1	E858.3	E950.4	E962.0	E980.4	DRUG CARDIAC DRUGS CARDIOTONIC AGENTS (24:04)
972.0	E942.0	E858.3	E950.4	E962.0	E980.4	DRUG CARDIAC DRUGS RHYTHM REGULATORS (24:04)
973.2	E943.2	E858.4	E950.4	E962.0	E980.4	DRUG CATHARTICS EMOLLIENTS (56:12)
973.1	E943.1	E858.4	E950.4	E962.0	E980.4	DRUG CATHARTICS IRRITANTS (56:12)
973.3	E943.3	E858.4	E950.4	E962.0	E980.4	DRUG CATHARTICS NEC (56:12)
976.8	E946.8	E858.7	E950.4	E962.0	E980.4	DRUG CELL STIMULANTS AND PROLIFERANTS (84:16)
960.2	E930.2	E856	E950.4	E962.0	E980.4	DRUG CHLORAMPHENICOL (8:12.08)
964.5	E934.5	E858.2	E950.4	E962.0	E980.4	DRUG COAGULANTS (20:12.12)
976.5	E946.5	E858.7	E950.4	E962.0	E980.4	DRUG CONTACT LENS SOLUTIONS (52:12)
962.2	E932.2	E858.0	E950.4	E962.0	E980.4	DRUG CONTRACEPTIVES ORAL (68:12)
976.2	E946.2	E858.7	E950.4	E962.0	E980.4	DRUG DETERGENTS (84:20)
977.8	E947.8	E858.8	E950.4	E962.0	E980.4	DRUG DIAGNOSTIC AGENTS (36:04 TO 36:88)
973.4	E943.4	E858.4	E950.4	E962.0	E980.4	DRUG DIGESTANTS (56:16)
974.2	E944.2	E858.5	E950.4	E962.0	E980.4	DRUG DIURETICS CARBONIC ACID ANHYDRASE INHIBITORS (40:28)
974.0	E944.0	E858.5	E950.4	E962.0	E980.4	DRUG DIURETICS MERCURIALS (40:28)
974.4	E944.4	E858.5	E950.4	E962.0	E980.4	DRUG DIURETICS NEC (40:28)
974.1	E944.1	E858.5	E950.4	E962.0	E980.4	DRUG DIURETICS PURINE DERIVATIVES (40:28)
974.3	E944.3	E858.5	E950.4	E962.0	E980.4	DRUG DIURETICS SALURETICS (40:28)
974.3	E944.3	E858.5	E950.4	E962.1	E980.4	DRUG DIURETICS THIAZIDES (40:28)
968.5	E938.5	E855.2	E950.4	E962.0	E980.4	DRUG DYCLONINE
974.5	E944.5	E858.5	E950.4	E962.0	E980.4	DRUG ELECTROLYTE CALORIC AND WATER BALANCE AGENTS NEC (40:00)
963.0	E933.0	E858.1	E950.4	E962.0	E980.4	DRUG EMETICS AND ANTIEMETICS (56:20)
973.6	E943.6	E858.4	E950.4	E962.0	E980.4	DRUG EMETICS AND ANTIEMETICS EMETICS (56:20)
976.3	E946.3	E858.7	E950.4	E962.0	E980.4	DRUG EMOLLIENTS DEMULCENTS AND PROTECTANTS (84:24)
963.4	E933.4	E858.1	E950.4	E962.0	E980.4	DRUG ENZYMES (44:00)
964.4	E934.4	E858.2	E950.4	E962.0	E980.4	DRUG ENZYMES FIBRINOLYSIS AFFECTING AGENTS (44:00)
973.4	E943.4	E858.4	E950.4	E962.0	E980.4	DRUG ENZYMES GASTRIC AGENTS (44:00)
960.3	E930.3	E856	E950.4	E962.0	E980.4	DRUG ERYTHROMYCINS (8:12.12)
962.2	E932.2	E858.0	E950.4	E962.0	E980.4	DRUG ESTROGENS (68:16)
963.0	E933.0	E858.1	E950.4	E962.0	E980.4	DRUG EXPECTORANTS AND COUGH PREPARATIONS ANTIHISTAMINE AGENTS (48:00)
975.4	E945.4	E858.6	E950.4	E962.0	E980.4	DRUG EXPECTORANTS AND COUGH PREPARATIONS ANTITUSSIVES (48:00)
965.09	E935.2	E850.2	E950.0	E962.0	E980.0	DRUG EXPECTORANTS AND COUGH PREPARATIONS CODEINE DERIVATIVES (48:00)
975.5	E945.5	E858.6	E950.4	E962.0	E980.4	DRUG EXPECTORANTS AND COUGH PREPARATIONS EXPECTORANTS (48:00)
965.09	E935.2	E850.2	E950.0	E962.0	E980.0	DRUG EXPECTORANTS AND COUGH PREPARATIONS NARCOTIC AGENTS NEC (48:00)
976.0	E946.0	E858.7	E950.4	E962.0	E980.4	DRUG FUNGICIDES (SKIN AND MUCOUS MEMBRANES) (84:04.08)

POISON	THERA-PEUTIC	ACCIDENT	SUICIDE	ASSAULT	UNDETER-MINED	SUBSTANCE
968.2	E938.2	E855.1	E950.4	E962.0	E980.4	DRUG GASEOUS ANESTHETICS (28:04)
968.1	E938.1	E855.1	E950.4	E962.0	E980.4	DRUG GASEOUS ANESTHETICS HALOTHANE (28:04)
968.4	E938.4	E855.1	E950.4	E962.0	E980.4	DRUG GENERAL ANESTHETICS (28:04)
965.69	E935.6	E850.6	E950.0	E962.0	E980.0	DRUG GOLD COMPOUNDS (60:00)
962.4	E932.4	E858.0	E950.4	E962.0	E980.4	DRUG GONADOTROPINS (68:18)
963.8	E933.8	E858.1	E950.4	E962.0	E980.4	DRUG HEAVY METAL ANTAGONISTS (64:00)
972.8	E942.8	E858.3	E950.4	E962.0	E980.4	DRUG HEMOSTATICS CAPILLARY ACTIVE DRUGS (20:12.16)
964.5	E934.5	E858.2	E950.4	E962.0	E980.4	DRUG HEMOSTATICS NEC (20:12.16)
965.01	E935.0	E850.0	E950.0	E962.0	E980.0	DRUG HEROIN (28:08)
972.6	E942.6	E858.3	E950.4	E962.0	E980.4	DRUG HYPOTENSIVE AGENTS (24:08)
971.3	E941.3	E855.6	E950.4	E962.0	E980.4	DRUG HYPOTENSIVE AGENTS ADRENERGIC BLOCKING AGENTS (24:08)
972.3	E942.3	E858.3	E950.4	E962.0	E980.4	DRUG HYPOTENSIVE AGENTS GANGLION BLOCKING AGENTS (24:08)
972.5	E942.5	E858.3	E950.4	E962.0	E980.4	DRUG HYPOTENSIVE AGENTS VASODILATORS (24:08)
962.3	E932.3	E858.0	E950.4	E962.0	E980.4	DRUG INSULINS (68:20.08)
962.3	E932.3	E858.0	E950.4	E962.0	E980.4	DRUG INSULINS AND ANTIDIABETIC AGENTS (68:20)
968.3	E938.3	E855.1	E950.4	E962.0	E980.4	DRUG INTRAVENOUS ANESTHETICS (28:04)
964.0	E934.0	E858.2	E950.4	E962.0	E980.4	DRUG IRON PREPARATIONS (20:04.04)
974.5	E944.5	E858.5	E950.4	E962.0	E980.4	DRUG IRRIGATING SOLUTIONS (40:36)
976.4	E946.4	E858.7	E950.4	E962.0	E980.4	DRUG KERATOLYTIC AGENTS (84:28)
976.4	E946.4	E858.7	E950.4	E962.0	E980.4	DRUG KERATOPLASTIC AGENTS (84:32)
977.1	E947.1	E858.8	E950.4	E962.0	E980.4	DRUG LIPOTROPIC AGENTS (56:24)
964.1	E934.1	E858.2	E950.4	E962.0	E980.4	DRUG LIVER AND STOMACH PREPARATIONS (20:04.08)
968.5	E938.5	E855.2	E950.4	E962.0	E980.4	DRUG LOCAL ANESTHETICS (84:08)
968.5	E938.5	E855.2	E950.4	E962.0	E980.4	DRUG LOCAL ANESTHETICS (EENT) (52:16)
968.5	E938.5	E855.2	E950.4	E962.0	E980.4	DRUG LOCAL ANESTHETICS INFILTRATION (INTRADER-MAL)\ (SUBCUTANEOUS) (72:00)
968.9	E938.9	E855.2	E950.4	E962.0	E980.4	DRUG LOCAL ANESTHETICS NEC (72:00)
968.6	E938.6	E855.2	E950.4	E962.0	E980.4	DRUG LOCAL ANESTHETICS NERVE BLOCKING (PERIPHERAL) (PLEXUS) (72:00)
968.7	E938.7	E855.2	E950.4	E962.0	E980.4	DRUG LOCAL ANESTHETICS SPINAL (72:00)
968.5	E938.5	E855.2	E950.4	E962.0	E980.4	DRUG LOCAL ANESTHETICS TOPICAL (SURFACE) (72:00)
960.3	E930.3	E856	E950.4	E962.0	E980.4	DRUG MACROLIDES (8:12.28)
965.02	E935.0	E850.1	E950.0	E962.0	E980.0	DRUG METHADONE (28:08)
971.0	E941.0	E855.3	E950.4	E962.0	E980.4	DRUG MIOTICS (52:20)
976.8	E946.8	E858.7	E950.4	E962.0	E980.4	DRUG MISCELLANEOUS AGENTS (SKIN AND MUCOUS MEMBRANE) (84:36)
976.6	E946.6	E858.7	E950.4	E962.0	E980.4	DRUG MISCELLANEOUS ANTI-INFECTIVES ENT AGENT (52:04.12)
976.5	E946.5	E858.7	E950.4	E962.0	E980.4	DRUG MISCELLANEOUS ANTI-INFECTIVES OPHTH-ALMIC PREPARATION (52:04.12)
973.8	E943.8	E858.4	E950.4	E962.0	E980.4	DRUG MISCELLANEOUS GI DRUGS (56:40)
976.0	E946.0	E858.7	E950.4	E962.0	E980.4	DRUG MISCELLANEOUS LOCAL ANTI-INFECTIVES (SKIN/MUCOUS MEMBRANE) (84:04.16)
976.6	E946.6	E858.7	E950.4	E962.0	E980.4	DRUG MOUTH WASHES AND GARGLES (52:28)
963.5	E933.5	E858.1	E950.4	E962.0	E980.4	DRUG MULTI-VITAMIN PREPARATIONS (88:28)
971.2	E941.2	E855.5	E950.4	E962.0	E980.4	DRUG MYDRIATICS ADRENERGICS (52:24)
971.1	E941.1	E855.4	E950.4	E962.0	E980.4	DRUG MYDRIATICS ANTICHOLINERGICS (52:24)
971.1	E941.1	E855.4	E950.4	E962.0	E980.4	DRUG MYDRIATICS ANTIMUSCARINICS (52:24)
971.1	E941.1	E855.4	E950.4	E962.0	E980.4	DRUG MYDRIATICS PARASYMPATHOLYTICS (52:24)
971.1	E941.1	E855.4	E950.4	E962.0	E980.4	DRUG MYDRIATICS SPASMOLYTICS (52:24)
971.2	E941.2	E855.5	E950.4	E962.0	E980.4	DRUG MYDRIATICS SYMPATHOMIMETICS (52:24)
970.1	E940.1	E854.3	E950.4	E962.0	E980.4	DRUG NARCOTIC ANTAGONISTS (28:10)

POISON	THERA-PEUTIC	ACCIDENT	SUICIDE	ASSAULT	UNDETER-MINED	SUBSTANCE
965.7	E935.7	E850.7	E950.0	E962.0	E980.0	DRUG NONNARCOTIC NEC (28:08)
965.00	E935.2	E850.2	E950.0	E962.0	E980.0	DRUG OPIUM ALKALOIDS (28:08)
965.09	E935.2	E850.2	E950.0	E962.0	E980.0	DRUG OPIUM ALKALOIDS SPECIFIED TYPE NEC (28:08)
977.9	E947.9	E858.9	E950.5	E962.0	E980.5	DRUG OR MEDICINAL SUBSTANCE NOS
961.9	E931.9	E857	E950.4	E962.0	E980.4	DRUG OTHER ANTI-INFECTIVES (8:40)
960.8	E930.8	E856	E950.4	E962.0	E980.4	DRUG OTHER ANTIBIOTICS (8:12.28)
962.2	E932.2	E858.0	E950.4	E962.0	E980.4	DRUG OTHER CORPUS LUTEUM HORMONES NEC (68:34)
969.8	E939.8	E855.8	E950.3	E962.0	E980.3	DRUG OTHER PSYCHOTHERAPEUTIC AGENTS (28:16.12)
975.0	E945.0	E858.6	E950.4	E962.0	E980.4	DRUG OXYTOCICS (76:00)
971.0	E941.0	E855.3	E950.4	E962.0	E980.4	DRUG PARA-SYMPATHOMIMETIC (CHOLINERGIC) AGENTS (12:04)
962.6	E932.6	E858.0	E950.4	E962.0	E980.4	DRUG PARATHYROID (68:24)
960.0	E930.0	E856	E950.4	E962.0	E980.4	DRUG PENICILLINS (8:12.16)
962.4	E932.4	E858.0	E950.4	E962.0	E980.4	DRUG PITUITARY ANTERIOR (68:28)
962.5	E932.5	E858.0	E950.4	E962.0	E980.4	DRUG PITUITARY (POSTERIOR) (68:28)
961.4	E931.4	E857	E950.4	E962.0	E980.4	DRUG PLASMODICIDES (ANTIMALARIALS) (8:20)
974.5	E944.5	E858.5	E950.4	E962.0	E980.4	DRUG POTASSIUM REMOVING RESINS (40:18)
971.9	E941.9	E855.9	E950.4	E962.0	E980.4	DRUG PRIMARILY AFFECTING AUTONOMIC NERVOUS SYSTEM NOS
962.2	E932.2	E858.0	E950.4	E962.0	E980.4	DRUG PROGESTOGENS (68:32)
965.5	E935.5	E850.5	E950.0	E962.0	E980.0	DRUG PYRAZOLE DERIVATIVES (28:08)
990						DRUG RADIOACTIVE AGENTS (78:00)
974.5	E944.5	E858.5	E950.4	E962.0	E980.4	DRUG REPLACEMENT SOLUTIONS (40:12)
964.8	E934.8	E858.2	E950.4	E962.0	E980.4	DRUG REPLACEMENT SOLUTIONS PLASMA EXPANDERS (40:12)
970.9	E940.9	E854.3	E950.4	E962.0	E980.4	DRUG RESPIRATORY AND CEREBRAL STIMULANTS (28:20)
970.0	E940.0	E854.3	E950.4	E962.0	E980.4	DRUG RESPIRATORY AND CEREBRAL STIMULANTS ANALEPTICS (28:20)
977.0	E947.0	E858.8	E950.4	E962.0	E980.4	DRUG RESPIRATORY AND CEREBRAL STIMULANTS ANOREXIGENIC AGENTS (28:20)
969.7	E939.7	E854.2	E950.3	E962.0	E980.3	DRUG RESPIRATORY AND CEREBRAL STIMULANTS PSYCHOSTIMULANTS (28:20)
970.8	E940.8	E854.3	E950.4	E962.0	E980.4	DRUG RESPIRATORY AND CEREBRAL STIMULANTS SPECIFIED NEC (28:20)
965.1	E935.3	E850.3	E950.0	E962.0	E980.0	DRUG SALICYLATES (28:08)
974.5	E944.5	E858.5	E950.4	E962.0	E980.4	DRUG SALT AND SUGAR SUBSTITUTES (40:24)
976.0	E946.0	E858.7	E950.4	E962.0	E980.4	DRUG SCABICIDES AND PEDICULICIDES (SKIN AND MUCOUS MEMBRANES) (84:04.12)
972.7	E942.7	E858.3	E950.4	E962.0	E980.4	DRUG SCLEROSING AGENTS (24:16)
967.9	E937.9	E852.9	E950.2	E962.0	E980.2	DRUG SEDATIVES AND HYPNOTICS (28:24)
967.0	E937.0	E851	E950.1	E962.0	E980.1	DRUG SEDATIVES AND HYPNOTICS BARBITURATES (28:24)
969.4	E939.4	E853.2	E950.3	E962.0	E980.3	DRUG SEDATIVES AND HYPNOTICS BENZODIAZEPINE BASED RANQUILIZERS (28:24)
967.1	E937.1	E852.0	E950.2	E962.0	E980.2	DRUG SEDATIVES AND HYPNOTICS CHLORAL HYDRATE (GROUP) (28:24)
967.5	E937.5	E852.4	E950.2	E962.0	E980.2	DRUG SEDATIVES AND HYPNOTICS GLUTETHAMIDE GROUP (28:24)
968.3	E938.3	E855.1	E950.4	E962.0	E980.4	DRUG SEDATIVES AND HYPNOTICS INTRAVENOUS ANESTHETICS (28:24)
967.4	E937.4	E852.3	E950.2	E962.0	E980.2	DRUG SEDATIVES AND HYPNOTICS METHAQUALONE (COMPOUNDS) (28:24)
967.2	E937.2	E852.1	E950.2	E962.0	E980.2	DRUG SEDATIVES AND HYPNOTICS PARALDEHYDE (28:24)
969.1	E939.1	E853.0	E950.3	E962.0	E980.3	DRUG SEDATIVES AND HYPNOTICS PHENOTHIAZINE BASED TRANQUILIZERS (28:24)
967.8	E937.8	E852.8	E950.2	E962.0	E980.2	DRUG SEDATIVES AND HYPNOTICS SPECIFIED NEC (28:24)
968.3	E938.3	E855.1	E950.4	E962.0	E980.4	DRUG SEDATIVES AND HYPNOTICS THIOBARBITURATES (28:24)
969.5	E939.5	E853.9	E950.3	E962.0	E980.3	DRUG SEDATIVES AND HYPNOTICS TRANQUILIZER NEC (28:24)
964.6	E934.6	E858.2	E950.4	E962.0	E980.4	DRUG SERUMS IMMUNE GAMMA GLOBULIN (HUMAN) (80:04)

POISON	THERA-PEUTIC	ACCIDENT	SUICIDE	ASSAULT	UNDETER-MINED	SUBSTANCE
979.9	E949.9	E858.8	E950.4	E962.0	E980.4	DRUG SERUMS NEC (80:04)
968.0	E938.0	E855.1	E950.4	E962.0	E980.4	DRUG SKELETAL MUSCLE RELAXANTS CNS MUSCLE-TONE DEPRESSANTS (12:20)
975.2	E945.2	E858.6	E950.4	E962.0	E980.4	DRUG SKELETAL MUSCLE RELAXANTS MYONEURAL BLOCKING AGENTS (12:20)
974.5	E944.5	E858.5	E950.4	E962.0	E980.4	DRUG SODIUM REMOVING RESINS (40:16)
975.1	E945.1	E858.6	E950.4	E962.0	E980.4	DRUG SPASMOLYTIC AGENTS (86:00)
975.7	E945.7	E858.6	E950.4	E962.0	E980.4	DRUG SPASMOLYTIC AGENTS ANTIASTHMATICS (86:00)
972.5	E942.5	E858.3	E950.4	E962.0	E980.4	DRUG SPASMOLYTIC AGENTS PAPAVERINE (86:00)
974.1	E944.1	E858.5	E950.4	E962.0	E980.4	DRUG SPASMOLYTIC AGENTS THEOPHYLLINE (86:00)
977.8	E947.8	E858.8	E950.4	E962.0	E980.4	DRUG SPECIFIED NEC
960.6	E930.6	E856	E950.4	E962.0	E980.4	DRUG STREPTOMYCINS (8:12.20)
961.0	E931.0	E857	E950.4	E962.0	E980.4	DRUG SULFONAMIDES (8:24)
976.6	E946.6	E858.7	E950.4	E962.0	E980.4	DRUG SULFONAMIDES ENT AGENT (52:04.08)
976.5	E946.5	E858.7	E950.4	E962.0	E980.4	DRUG SULFONAMIDES OPHTHALMIC PREPARATION (52:04.08)
961.8	E931.8	E857	E950.4	E962.0	E980.4	DRUG SULFONES (8:26)
971.3	E941.3	E855.6	E950.4	E962.0	E980.4	DRUG SYMPATHOLYTIC (ADRENERGIC-BLOCKING) AGENTS (12:16)
971.1	E941.1	E855.4	E950.4	E962.0	E980.4	DRUG SYMPATHOLYTIC (CHOLINERGIC-BLOCKING) AGENTS (12:08)
971.2	E941.2	E855.5	E950.4	E962.0	E980.4	DRUG SYMPATHOMIMETIC (ADRENERGIC) AGENTS (12:12)
960.4	E930.4	E856	E950.4	E962.0	E980.4	DRUG TETRACYCLINES (8:12.24)
962.7	E932.7	E858.0	E950.4	E962.0	E980.4	DRUG THYROID (DERIVATIVES) (68:36)
962.8	E932.8	E858.0	E950.4	E962.0	E980.4	DRUG THYROID AND ANTITHYROID ANTITHYROID (68:36)
978.9	E948.9	E858.8	E950.4	E962.0	E980.4	DRUG TOXOID TETANUS AND DIPHTHERIA (80:08)
978.6	E948.6	E858.8	E950.4	E962.0	E980.4	DRUG TOXOID TETANUS AND DIPHTHERIA WITH PERTUSSIS COMPONENT (80:08)
978.5	E948.5	E858.8	E950.4	E962.0	E980.4	DRUG TOXOIDS DIPHTHERIA (80:08)
978.9	E948.9	E858.8	E950.4	E962.0	E980.4	DRUG TOXOIDS DIPHTHERIA AND TETANUS (80:08)
978.6	E948.6	E858.8	E950.4	E962.0	E980.4	DRUG TOXOIDS DIPHTHERIA AND TETANUS WITH PERTUSSIS COMPONENT (80:08)
978.8	E948.8	E858.8	E950.4	E962.0	E980.4	DRUG TOXOIDS NEC (80:08)
978.4	E948.4	E858.8	E950.4	E962.0	E980.4	DRUG TOXOIDS TETANUS (80:08)
969.5	E939.5	E853.9	E950.3	E962.0	E980.3	DRUG TRANQUILIZERS (28:16.08)
969.4	E939.4	E853.2	E950.3	E962.0	E980.3	DRUG TRANQUILIZERS BENZODIAZEPINE BASED (28:16.08)
969.2	E939.2	E853.1	E950.3	E962.0	E980.3	DRUG TRANQUILIZERS BUTYROPHENONE BASED (28:16.08)
969.3	E939.3	E853.8	E950.3	E962.0	E980.3	DRUG TRANQUILIZERS MAJOR NEC (28:16.08)
969.1	E939.1	E853.0	E950.3	E962.0	E980.3	DRUG TRANQUILIZERS PHENOTHIAZINE BASED (28:16.08)
961.2	E931.2	E857	E950.4	E962.0	E980.4	DRUG TREPONEMICIDES (8:28)
961.5	E931.5	E857	E950.4	E962.0	E980.4	DRUG TRICHOMONACIDES (8:32)
961.9	E931.9	E857	E950.4	E962.0	E980.4	DRUG TRICHOMONACIDES NITROFURAN DERIVATIVES (8:32)
961.3	E931.3	E857	E950.4	E962.0	E980.4	DRUG TRICHOMONACIDES QUINOLINE DERIVATIVES (8:32)
976.6	E946.6	E858.7	E950.4	E962.0	E980.4	DRUG UNCLASSIFIED AGENTS (EENT) ENT AGENT (52:36)
976.5	E946.5	E858.7	E950.4	E962.0	E980.4	DRUG UNCLASSIFIED AGENTS (EENT) OPHTHALMIC PREPARATION (52:36)
977.8	E947.8	E858.8	E950.4	E962.0	E980.4	DRUG UNCLASSIFIED THERAPEUTIC AGENTS (92:00)
974.7	E944.7	E858.5	E950.4	E962.0	E980.4	DRUG URICOSURIC AGENTS (40:40)
961.9	E931.9	E857	E950.4	E962.0	E980.4	DRUG URINARY GERMICIDES (8:36)
961.3	E931.3	E857	E950.4	E962.0	E980.4	DRUG URINARY GERMICIDES QUINOLINE DERIVATIVES (8:36)
979.9	E949.9	E858.8	E950.4	E962.0	E980.4	DRUG VACCINES (80:12)
978.8	E948.8	E858.8	E950.4	E962.0	E980.4	DRUG VACCINES BACTERIAL NEC (80:12)
978.6	E948.6	E858.8	E950.4	E962.0	E980.4	DRUG VACCINES BACTERIAL WITH PERTUSSIS COMPONENTS (80:12)

POISON	THERA-PEUTIC	ACCIDENT	SUICIDE	ASSAULT	UNDETER-MINED	SUBSTANCE
978.9	E948.9	E858.8	E950.4	E962.0	E980.4	DRUG VACCINES BACTERIAL WITH OTHER BACTERIAL COMPONENTS 80:12)
979.7	E949.7	E858.8	E950.4	E962.0	E980.4	DRUG VACCINES BACTERIAL WITH VIRAL AND RICKETTSIAL (80:12)
979.7	E949.7	E858.8	E950.4	E962.0	E980.4	DRUG VACCINES RICKETTSIAL WITH BACTERIAL COMPONENT (80:12)
978.6	E948.6	E858.8	E950.4	E962.0	E980.4	DRUG VACCINES RICKETTSIAL WITH PERTUSSIS COMPONENT (80:12)
979.7	E949.7	E858.8	E950.4	E962.0	E980.4	DRUG VACCINES RICKETTSIAL WITH VIRAL COMPONENT (80:12)
979.6	E949.6	E858.8	E950.4	E962.0	E980.4	DRUG VACCINES VIRAL NEC (80:12)
979.7	E949.7	E858.8	E950.4	E962.0	E980.4	DRUG VACCINES VIRAL WITH BACTERIAL COMPONENT (80:12)
978.6	E948.6	E858.8	E950.4	E962.0	E980.4	DRUG VACCINES VIRAL WITH PERTUSSIS COMPONENT (80:12)
971.2	E941.2	E855.5	E950.4	E962.0	E980.4	DRUG VASO-CONSTRICTORS (EENT) (52:32)
972.4	E942.4	E858.3	E950.4	E962.0	E980.4	DRUG VASODILATING AGENTS CORONARY (24:12)
972.5	E942.5	E858.3	E950.4	E962.0	E980.4	DRUG VASODILATING AGENTS NEC (24:12)
972.2	E942.2	E858.3	E950.4	E962.0	E980.4	DRUG VASODILATING AGENTS NICOTINIC ACID DERIVATIVES (24:12)
963.5	E933.5	E858.1	E950.4	E962.0	E980.4	DRUG VITAMIN A (88:04)
963.5	E933.5	E858.1	E950.4	E962.0	E980.4	DRUG VITAMIN B COMPLEX (88:08)
964.1	E934.1	E858.2	E950.4	E962.0	E980.4	DRUG VITAMIN B COMPLEX HEMATOPOIETIC VITAMIN (88:08)
972.2	E942.2	E858.3	E950.4	E962.0	E980.4	DRUG VITAMIN B COMPLEX NICOTINIC ACID DERIVATIVES (88:08)
963.5	E933.5	E858.1	E950.4	E962.0	E980.4	DRUG VITAMIN C (88:12)
963.5	E933.5	E858.1	E950.4	E962.0	E980.4	DRUG VITAMIN D (88:16)
963.5	E933.5	E858.1	E950.4	E962.0	E980.4	DRUG VITAMIN E (88:20)
964.3	E934.3	E858.2	E950.4	E962.0	E980.4	DRUG VITAMIN K ACTIVITY (88:24)
971.1	E941.1	E855.4	E950.4	E962.0	E980.4	DUBOISINE
973.1	E943.1	E858.4	E950.4	E962.0	E980.4	DULCOLAX
976.2	E946.2	E858.7	E950.4	E962.0	E980.4	DUPONOL (C) (EP)
962.1	E932.1	E858.0	E950.4	E962.0	E980.4	DURABOLIN
968.5	E938.5	E855.2	E950.4	E962.0	E980.4	DYCLONE
968.5	E938.5	E855.2	E950.4	E962.0	E980.4	DYCLONINE
962.2	E932.2	E858.0	E950.4	E962.0	E980.4	DYDROGESTERONE
977.8	E947.8	E858.8	E950.4	E962.0	E980.4	DYES DIAGNOSTIC AGENTS
989.89		E866.8	E950.9	E962.1	E980.9	DYES NEC
977.4	E947.4	E858.8	E950.4	E962.0	E980.4	DYES PHARMACEUTICAL NEC
971.0	E941.0	E855.3	E950.4	E962.0	E980.4	DYFOLS
962.3	E932.3	E858.0	E950.4	E962.0	E980.4	DYMELOR
989.89		E866.8	E950.9	E962.1	E980.9	DYNAMITE
987.8		E869.8	E952.8	E962.2	E982.8	DYNAMITE FUMES
975.1	E945.1	E858.6	E950.4	E962.0	E980.4	DYPHYLLINE
976.6	E946.6	E858.7	E950.4	E962.0	E980.4	EAR PREPARATIONS
971.0	E941.0	E855.3	E950.4	E962.0	E980.4	ECHOTHIOPATE ECOTHIOPATE
969.7	E939.7	E854.2	E950.3	E962.0	E980.3	ECSTASY
967.8	E937.8	E852.8	E950.2	E962.0	E980.2	ECTYLUREA
963.8	E933.8	E858.1	E950.4	E962.0	E980.4	EDATHAMIL DISODIUM
974.4	E944.4	E858.5	E950.4	E962.0	E980.4	EDECRIN
963.8	E933.8	E858.1	E950.4	E962.0	E980.4	EDETATE DISODIUM (CALCIUM)
971.0	E941.0	E855.3	E950.4	E962.0	E980.4	EDROPHONIUM
976.8	E946.8	E858.7	E950.4	E962.0	E980.4	ELASE
973.1	E943.1	E858.4	E950.4	E962.0	E980.4	ELATERIUM
988.2		E865.4	E950.9	E962.1	E980.9	ELDER
988.2		E865.3	E950.9	E962.1	E980.9	ELDER BERRY (UNRIPE)
974.5	E944.5	E858.5	E950.4	E962.0	E980.4	ELECTROLYTES NEC
974.5	E944.5	E858.5	E950.4	E962.0	E980.4	ELECTROLYTIC AGENT NEC
974.5	E944.5	E858.5	E950.4	E962.0	E980.4	ELECTROLYTIC CALORIC AND WATER-BALANCE AGENTS
963.0	E933.0	E858.1	E950.4	E962.0	E980.4	EMBRAMINE
973.6	E943.6	E858.4	E950.4	E962.0	E980.4	EMETICS
961.5	E931.5	E857	E950.4	E962.0	E980.4	EMETINE (HYDROCHLORIDE)
976.3	E946.3	E858.7	E950.4	E962.0	E980.4	EMOLLIENTS
969.5	E939.5	E853.8	E950.3	E962.0	E980.3	EMYLCAMATE
969.0	E939.0	E854.0	E950.3	E962.0	E980.3	ENCYPRATE
968.5	E938.5	E855.2	E950.4	E962.0	E980.4	ENDOCAINE
989.2		E863.0	E950.6	E962.1	E980.7	ENDRIN
968.2	E938.2	E855.1	E950.4	E962.0	E980.4	ENFLURANE
962.2	E932.2	E858.0	E950.4	E962.0	E980.4	ENOVID
976.6	E946.6	E858.7	E950.4	E962.0	E980.4	ENT AGENTS ANTI-INFECTIVES NEC

POISON	THERA-PEUTIC	ACCIDENT	SUICIDE	ASSAULT	UNDETER-MINED	SUBSTANCE
976.6	E946.6	E858.7	E950.4	E962.0	E980.4	ENT PREPARATIONS (ANTI-INFECTIVES)
963.4	E933.4	E858.1	E950.4	E962.0	E980.4	ENZODASE
963.4	E933.4	E858.1	E950.4	E962.0	E980.4	ENZYMES NEC
966.1	E936.1	E855.0	E950.4	E962.0	E980.4	EPANUTIN
971.2	E941.2	E855.5	E950.4	E962.0	E980.4	EPHEDRA (TINCTURE)
971.2	E941.2	E855.5	E950.4	E962.0	E980.4	EPHEDRINE
962.2	E932.2	E858.0	E950.4	E962.0	E980.4	EPIESTRIOL
971.2	E941.2	E855.5	E950.4	E962.0	E980.4	EPINEPHRINE (ADRENALIN)
973.3	E943.3	E858.4	E950.4	E962.0	E980.4	EPSOM SALT
969.5	E939.5	E853.8	E950.3	E962.0	E980.3	EQUANIL
974.4	E944.4	E858.5	E950.4	E962.0	E980.4	EQUISETUM (DIURETIC)
975.0	E945.0	E858.6	E950.4	E962.0	E980.4	ERGOMETRINE
975.0	E945.0	E858.6	E950.4	E962.0	E980.4	ERGONOVINE
975.0	E945.0	E858.6	E950.4	E962.0	E980.4	ERGOT ALKALOIDS
975.0	E945.0	E858.6	E950.4	E962.0	E980.4	ERGOT MEDICINAL (ALKALOIDS)
988.2		E865.4	E950.9	E962.1	E980.9	ERGOT NEC
972.9	E942.9	E858.3	E950.4	E962.0	E980.4	ERGOTAMINE (TARTRATE) (FOR MIGRAINE) NEC
975.0	E945.0	E858.6	E950.4	E962.0	E980.4	ERGOTRATE
972.4	E942.4	E858.3	E950.4	E962.0	E980.4	ERYTHRITYL TETRANITRATE
972.4	E942.4	E858.3	E950.4	E962.0	E980.4	ERYTHROL TETRANITRATE
960.3	E930.3	E856	E950.4	E962.0	E980.4	ERYTHROMYCIN
976.5	E946.5	E858.7	E950.4	E962.0	E980.4	ERYTHROMYCIN OPHTHALMIC PREPARATION
976.0	E946.0	E858.7	E950.4	E962.0	E980.4	ERYTHROMYCIN TOPICAL NEC
971.0	E941.0	E855.3	E950.4	E962.0	E980.4	ESERINE
967.0	E937.0	E851	E950.1	E962.0	E980.1	ESKABARB
969.8	E939.8	E855.8	E950.3	E962.0	E980.3	ESKALITH
962.2	E932.2	E858.0	E950.4	E962.0	E980.4	ESTRADIOL (CYPIONATE) (DIPROPIONATE) (VALERATE)
962.2	E932.2	E858.0	E950.4	E962.0	E980.4	ESTRIOL
962.2	E932.2	E858.0	E950.4	E962.0	E980.4	ESTROGENS (WITH PROGESTOGENS)
962.2	E932.2	E858.0	E950.4	E962.0	E980.4	ESTROGENS AND PROGESTOGENS COMBINED
962.2	E932.2	E858.0	E950.4	E962.0	E980.4	ESTRONE
971.2	E941.2	E855.5	E950.4	E962.0	E980.4	ETAFEDRINE
974.4	E944.4	E858.5	E950.4	E962.0	E980.4	ETHACRYNATE SODIUM
974.4	E944.4	E858.5	E950.4	E962.0	E980.4	ETHACRYNIC ACID
961.8	E931.8	E857	E950.4	E962.0	E980.4	ETHAMBUTOL
974.2	E944.2	E858.5	E950.4	E962.0	E980.4	ETHAMIDE
970.0	E940.0	E854.3	E950.4	E962.0	E980.4	ETHAMIVAN
964.5	E934.5	E858.2	E950.4	E962.0	E980.4	ETHAMSYLATE
980.0		E860.1	E950.9	E962.1	E980.9	ETHANOL
980.0		E860.0	E950.9	E962.1	E980.9	ETHANOL BEVERAGE
967.8	E937.8	E852.8	E950.2	E962.0	E980.2	ETHCHLORVYNOL
974.7	E944.7	E858.5	E950.4	E962.0	E980.4	ETHEBENECID
968.2	E938.2	E855.1	E950.4	E962.0	E980.4	ETHER (ANESTHETIC)
0						ETHER PETROLEUM SEE LIGROIN
982.8		E862.4	E950.9	E962.1	E980.9	ETHER SOLVENT
987.8		E869.8	E952.8	E962.2	E982.8	ETHER(S) (DIETHYL) (ETHYL) (VAPOR)
987.8		E869.8	E952.8	E962.2	E982.8	ETHIDINE CHLORIDE (VAPOR)
982.3		E862.4	E950.9	E962.1	E980.9	ETHIDINE CHLORIDE LIQUID (SOLVENT)
967.8	E937.8	E852.8	E950.2	E962.0	E980.2	ETHINAMATE
962.2	E932.2	E858.0	E950.4	E962.0	E980.4	ETHINYLESTRADIOL
961.8	E931.8	E857	E950.4	E962.0	E980.4	ETHIONAMIDE
962.2	E932.2	E858.0	E950.4	E962.0	E980.4	ETHISTERONE
967.0	E937.0	E851	E950.1	E962.0	E980.1	ETHOBRAL
968.5	E938.5	E855.2	E950.4	E962.0	E980.4	ETHOCAINE (INFILTRATION) (TOPICAL)
968.6	E938.6	E855.2	E950.4	E962.0	E980.4	ETHOCAINE NERVE BLOCK (PERIPHERAL) (PLEXUS)
968.7	E938.7	E855.2	E950.4	E962.0	E980.4	ETHOCAINE SPINAL
965.7	E935.7	E850.7	E950.0	E962.0	E980.0	ETHOHEPTAZINE (CITRATE)
966.4	E936.4	E855.0	E950.4	E962.0	E980.4	ETHOPROPAZINE (PROFENAMINE)
966.2	E936.2	E855.0	E950.4	E962.0	E980.4	ETHOSUXIMIDE
966.1	E936.1	E855.0	E950.4	E962.0	E980.4	ETHOTOIN
961.9	E931.9	E857	E950.4	E962.0	E980.4	ETHOXAZENE
974.2	E944.2	E858.5	E950.4	E962.0	E980.4	ETHOXZOLAMIDE
982.8		E862.4	E950.9	E962.1	E980.9	ETHYL ACETATE (VAPOR)
980.0		E860.1	E950.9	E962.1	E980.9	ETHYL ALCOHOL
980.0		E860.0	E950.9	E962.1	E980.9	ETHYL ALCOHOL BEVERAGE
987.8		E869.8	E952.8	E962.2	E982.8	ETHYL ALDEHYDE (VAPOR)
989.89		E866.8	E950.9	E962.1	E980.9	ETHYL ALDEHYDE LIQUID
968.5	E938.5	E855.2	E950.4	E962.0	E980.4	ETHYL AMINOBENZOATE
964.2	E934.2	E858.2	E950.4	E962.0	E980.4	ETHYL BISCOUMACETATE
968.2	E938.2	E855.1	E950.4	E962.0	E980.4	ETHYL BROMIDE (ANESTHETIC)

POISON	THERA-PEUTIC	ACCIDENT	SUICIDE	ASSAULT	UNDETER-MINED	SUBSTANCE
963.1	E933.1	E858.1	E950.4	E962.0	E980.4	ETHYL CARBAMATE (ANTINEOPLASTIC)
980.3		E860.4	E950.9	E962.1	E980.9	ETHYL CARBINOL
961.8	E931.8	E857	E950.4	E962.0	E980.4	ETHYL CHAULMOOGRATE
987.8		E869.8	E952.8	E962.2	E982.8	ETHYL CHLORIDE (VAPOR)
968.5	E938.5	E855.2	E950.4	E962.0	E980.4	ETHYL CHLORIDE ANESTHETIC (LOCAL)
968.2	E938.2	E855.1	E950.4	E962.0	E980.4	ETHYL CHLORIDE ANESTHETIC INHALED
982.3		E862.4	E950.9	E962.1	E980.9	ETHYL CHLORIDE SOLVENT
962.1	E932.1	E858.0	E950.4	E962.0	E980.4	ETHYL ESTRANOL
0						ETHYL ETHER SEE ETHER(S)
982.8		E862.4	E950.9	E962.1	E980.9	ETHYL FORMATE (SOLVENT) NEC
987.5		E869.3	E952.8	E962.2	E982.8	ETHYL IODOACETATE
982.8		E862.4	E950.9	E962.1	E980.9	ETHYL LACTATE (SOLVENT) NEC
980.8		E860.8	E950.9	E962.1	E980.9	ETHYL METHYLCARBINOL
965.09	E935.2	E850.2	E950.0	E962.0	E980.0	ETHYL MORPHINE
982.3		E862.4	E950.9	E962.1	E980.9	ETHYLENE CHLOROHYDRIN (VAPOR)
987.1		E869.8	E952.8	E962.2	E982.8	ETHYLENE (GAS)
968.2	E938.2	E855.1	E950.4	E962.0	E980.4	ETHYLENE ANESTHETIC (GENERAL)
982.3		E862.4	E950.9	E962.1	E980.9	ETHYLENE DICHLORIDE (VAPOR)
982.8		E862.4	E950.9	E962.1	E980.9	ETHYLENE GLYCOL(S) (ANY) (VAPOR)
982.3		E862.4	E950.9	E962.1	E980.9	ETHYLIDENE CHLORIDE NEC
982.8		E862.4	E950.9	E962.1	E980.9	ETHYLIDENE DIETHYL ETHER
962.2	E932.2	E858.0	E950.4	E962.0	E980.4	ETHYNODIOL
968.5	E938.5	E855.2	E950.4	E962.0	E980.4	ETIDOCAINE INFILTRATION (SUBCUTANEOUS)
968.9	E938.9	E855.2	E950.4	E962.0	E980.4	ETIDOCAINE
968.6	E938.6	E855.2	E950.4	E962.0	E980.4	ETIDOCAINE NERVE (PERIPHERAL) (PLEXUS)
967.0	E937.0	E851	E950.1	E962.0	E980.1	ETILFEN
965.7	E935.7	E850.7	E950.0	E962.0	E980.0	ETOMIDE
965.09	E935.2	E850.2	E950.0	E962.0	E980.0	ETORPHINE
967.0	E937.0	E851	E950.1	E962.0	E980.1	ETOVAL
969.0	E939.0	E854.0	E950.3	E962.0	E980.3	ETRYPTAMINE
968.5	E938.5	E855.2	E950.4	E962.0	E980.4	EUCAINE
975.5	E945.5	E858.6	E950.4	E962.0	E980.4	EUCALYPTUS (OIL) NEC
971.1	E941.1	E855.4	E950.4	E962.0	E980.4	EUCATROPINE
965.09	E935.2	E850.2	E950.0	E962.0	E980.0	EUCODAL
967.0	E937.0	E851	E950.1	E962.0	E980.1	EUNERYL
971.1	E941.1	E855.4	E950.4	E962.0	E980.4	EUPHTHALMINE
976.0	E946.0	E858.7	E950.4	E962.0	E980.4	EURAX
976.4	E946.4	E858.7	E950.4	E962.0	E980.4	EURESOL
962.7	E932.7	E858.0	E950.4	E962.0	E980.4	EUTHROID
977.8	E947.8	E858.8	E950.4	E962.0	E980.4	EVANS BLUE
967.0	E937.0	E851	E950.1	E962.0	E980.1	EVIPAL
968.3	E938.3	E855.1	E950.4	E962.0	E980.4	EVIPAL SODIUM
967.0	E937.0	E851	E950.1	E962.0	E980.1	EVIPAN
968.3	E938.3	E855.1	E950.4	E962.0	E980.4	EVIPAN SODIUM
973.1	E943.1	E858.4	E950.4	E962.0	E980.4	EX-LAX (PHENOLPHTHALEIN)
965.4	E935.4	E850.4	E950.0	E962.0	E980.0	EXALGIN
977.4	E947.4	E858.8	E950.4	E962.0	E980.4	EXCIPIENTS PHARMACEUTICAL
0						EXHAUST GAS SEE CARBON MONOXIDE
975.5	E945.5	E858.6	E950.4	E962.0	E980.4	EXPECTORANTS
976.9	E946.9	E858.7	E950.4	E962.0	E980.4	EXTERNAL MEDICATIONS (SKIN) (MUCOUS MEMBRANE)
976.7	E946.7	E858.7	E950.4	E962.0	E980.4	EXTERNAL MEDICATIONS DENTAL AGENT
976.6	E946.6	E858.7	E950.4	E962.0	E980.4	EXTERNAL MEDICATIONS ENT AGENT
976.5	E946.5	E858.7	E950.4	E962.0	E980.4	EXTERNAL MEDICATIONS OPHTHALMIC PREPARATION
976.8	E946.8	E858.7	E950.4	E962.0	E980.4	EXTERNAL MEDICATIONS SPECIFIED NEC
976.5	E946.5	E858.7	E950.4	E962.0	E980.4	EYE AGENTS (ANTI-INFECTIVE)
964.5	E934.5	E858.2	E950.4	E962.0	E980.4	FACTOR IX COMPLEX (HUMAN)
973.2	E943.2	E858.4	E950.4	E962.0	E980.4	FECAL SOFTENERS
977.0	E947.0	E858.8	E950.4	E962.0	E980.4	FENBUTRAZATE
970.8	E940.8	E854.3	E950.4	E962.0	E980.4	FENCAMFAMIN
977.0	E947.0	E858.8	E950.4	E962.0	E980.4	FENFLURAMINE
965.61	E935.6	E850.6	E950.0	E962.0	E980.0	FENOPROFEN
965.09	E935.2	E850.2	E950.0	E962.0	E980.0	FENTANYL
969.1	E939.1	E853.0	E950.3	E962.0	E980.3	FENTAZIN
976.0	E946.0	E858.7	E950.4	E962.0	E980.4	FENTICLOR FENTICHLOR
989.5		E905.0	E950.9	E962.1	E980.9	FER DE LANCE (BITE) (VENOM)
964.0	E934.0	E858.2	E950.4	E962.0	E980.4	FERRIC SALTS
0						FERRIC SEE IRON
964.0	E934.0	E858.2	E950.4	E962.0	E980.4	FERROCHOLINATE

POISON	THERAPEUTIC	ACCIDENT	SUICIDE	ASSAULT	UNDETERMINED	SUBSTANCE
964.0	E934.0	E858.2	E950.4	E962.0	E980.4	FERROUS SULFATE AND OTHER FERROUS SALTS
0						FERRUM SEE IRON
989.89		E866.5	E950.9	E962.1	E980.4	FERTILIZERS NEC
989.4		E863.5	E950.6	E962.1	E980.7	FERTILIZERS WITH HERBICIDE MIXTURE
964.7	E934.7	E858.2	E950.4	E962.0	E980.4	FIBRINOGEN (HUMAN)
964.4	E934.4	E858.2	E950.4	E962.0	E980.4	FIBRINOLYSIN
964.4	E934.4	E858.2	E950.4	E962.0	E980.4	FIBRONOLYSIS-AFFECTING AGENTS
961.6	E931.6	E857	E950.4	E962.0	E980.4	FILIX MAS
965.1	E935.3	E850.3	E950.0	E962.0	E980.0	FIORINAL
987.1		E869.8	E952.8	E962.2	E982.8	FIRE DAMP
988.0		E865.2	E950.9	E962.1	E980.9	FISH NONBACTERIAL ORNOXIOUS
988.0		E865.1	E950.9	E962.1	E980.9	FISH SHELL
961.5	E931.5	E857	E950.4	E962.0	E980.4	FLAGYL
975.1	E945.1	E858.6	E950.4	E962.0	E980.4	FLAVOXATE
975.2	E945.2	E858.6	E950.4	E962.0	E980.4	FLAXEDIL
976.3	E946.3	E858.7	E950.4	E962.0	E980.4	FLAXSEED (MEDICINAL)
971.3	E855.9	E941.3	E950.4	E962.0	E980.4	FLOMAX
973.4	E943.4	E858.4	E950.4	E962.0	E980.4	FLORANTYRONE
961.3	E931.3	E857	E950.4	E962.0	E980.4	FLORAQUIN
962.0	E932.0	E858.0	E950.4	E962.0	E980.4	FLORINEF
976.6	E946.6	E858.7	E950.4	E962.0	E980.4	FLORINEF ENT AGENT
976.5	E946.5	E858.7	E950.4	E962.0	E980.4	FLORINEF OPHTHALMIC PREPARATION
976.0	E946.0	E858.7	E950.4	E962.0	E980.4	FLORINEF TOPICAL NEC
976.4	E946.4	E858.7	E950.4	E962.0	E980.4	FLOWERS OF SULFUR
963.1	E933.1	E858.1	E950.4	E962.0	E980.4	FLOXURIDINE
961.9	E931.9	E857	E950.4	E962.0	E980.4	FLUCYTOSINE
962.0	E932.0	E858.0	E950.4	E962.0	E980.4	FLUDROCORTISONE
976.6	E946.6	E858.7	E950.4	E962.0	E980.4	FLUDROCORTISONE ENT AGENT
976.5	E946.5	E858.7	E950.4	E962.0	E980.4	FLUDROCORTISONE OPHTHALMIC PREPARATION
976.0	E946.0	E858.7	E950.4	E962.0	E980.4	FLUDROCORTISONE TOPICAL NEC
976.0	E946.0	E858.7	E950.4	E962.0	E980.4	FLUMETHASONE
974.3	E944.3	E858.5	E950.4	E962.0	E980.4	FLUMETHIAZIDE
961.7	E931.7	E857	E950.4	E962.0	E980.4	FLUMIDIN
969.4	E939.4	E853.2	E950.3	E962.0	E980.3	FLUNITRAZEPAM
976.0	E946.0	E858.7	E950.4	E962.0	E980.4	FLUOCINOLONE
962.0	E932.0	E858.0	E950.4	E962.0	E980.4	FLUOCORTOLONE
962.0	E932.0	E858.0	E950.4	E962.0	E980.4	FLUOHYDROCORTISONE
976.6	E946.6	E858.7	E950.4	E962.0	E980.4	FLUOHYDROCORTISONE ENT AGENT
976.5	E946.5	E858.7	E950.4	E962.0	E980.4	FLUOHYDROCORTISONE OPHTHALMIC PREPARATION
976.0	E946.0	E858.7	E950.4	E962.0	E980.4	FLUOHYDROCORTISONE TOPICAL NEC
976.0	E946.0	E858.7	E950.4	E962.0	E980.4	FLUONID
969.1	E939.1	E853.0	E950.3	E962.0	E980.3	FLUOPROMAZINE
989.4		E863.7	E950.6	E962.1	E980.7	FLUORACETATE
977.8	E947.8	E858.8	E950.4	E962.0	E980.4	FLUORESCEIN (SODIUM)
0						FLUORIDE HYDROGEN SEE HYDROFLUORIC ACID
976.7	E946.7	E858.7	E950.4	E962.0	E980.4	FLUORIDE MEDICINAL
983.9		E864.4	E950.7	E962.1	E980.6	FLUORIDE NOT PESTICIDE NEC
976.7	E946.7	E858.7	E950.4	E962.0	E980.4	FLUORIDE STANNOUS
989.4		E863.4	E950.6	E962.1	E980.7	FLUORIDE(S) (PESTICIDES) (SODIUM) NEC
962.0	E932.0	E858.0	E950.4	E962.0	E980.4	FLUORINATED CORTICOSTEROIDS
987.8		E869.8	E952.8	E962.2	E982.8	FLUORINE (COMPOUNDS)(GAS)
0						FLUORINE SALT SEE FLUORIDE(S)
976.7	E946.7	E858.7	E950.4	E962.0	E980.4	FLUORISTAN
989.4		E863.7	E950.6	E962.1	E980.7	FLUOROACETATE
963.1	E933.1	E858.1	E950.4	E962.0	E980.4	FLUORODEOXYURIDINE
976.5	E946.5	E858.7	E950.4	E962.0	E980.4	FLUOROMETHOLONE OPHTHALMIC PREPARATION
976.0	E946.0	E858.7	E950.4	E962.0	E980.4	FLUOROMETHOLONE TOPICAL NEC
963.1	E933.1	E858.1	E950.4	E962.0	E980.4	FLUOROURACIL
968.1	E938.1	E855.1	E950.4	E962.0	E980.4	FLUOTHANE
962.1	E932.1	E858.0	E950.4	E962.0	E980.4	FLUOXYMESTERONE
969.1	E939.1	E853.0	E950.3	E962.0	E980.3	FLUPHENAZINE
962.0	E932.0	E858.0	E950.4	E962.0	E980.4	FLUPREDNISOLONE
976.0	E946.0	E858.7	E950.4	E962.0	E980.4	FLURANDRENOLIDE
969.4	E939.4	E853.2	E950.3	E962.0	E980.3	FLURAZEPAM (HYDROCHLORIDE)
965.61	E935.6	E850.6	E950.0	E962.0	E980.0	FLURBIPROFEN
976.0	E946.0	E858.7	E950.4	E962.0	E980.4	FLUROBATE
969.8	E939.8	E855.8	E950.3	E962.0	E980.3	FLUROTHYL
968.2	E938.2	E855.1	E950.4	E962.0	E980.4	FLUROXENE
964.1	E934.1	E858.2	E950.4	E962.0	E980.4	FOLACIN

DRUGS & CHEMICALS

DRUGS & CHEMICALS

POISON	THERA-PEUTIC	ACCIDENT	SUICIDE	ASSAULT	UNDETER-MINED	SUBSTANCE
987.0		E867	E951.0	E962.2	E981.0	FOLEUM DISTRIBUTED THROUGH PIPE (PURE OR MIXED WITH AIR)
964.1	E934.1	E858.2	E950.4	E962.0	E980.4	FOLIC ACID
962.4	E932.4	E858.0	E950.4	E962.0	E980.4	FOLLICLE STIMULATING HORMONE
988.2		E865.3	E950.9	E962.1	E980.9	FOOD BERRIES SEEDS
988.0		E865.2	E950.9	E962.1	E980.9	FOOD FISH
988.9		E865.9	E950.9	E962.1	E980.9	FOOD FOODSTUFFS NONBACTRIAL OR NOXIOUS
988.1		E865.5	E950.9	E962.1	E980.9	FOOD MUSHROOMS
988.2		E865.9	E950.9	E962.1	E980.9	FOOD PLANTS
988.2		E865.4	E950.9	E962.1	E980.9	FOOD PLANTS SPECIFIED TYPE NEC
988.0		E865.1	E950.9	E962.1	E980.9	FOOD SHELLFISH
988.8		E865.8	E950.9	E962.1	E980.9	FOOD SPECIFIED NEC
988.2		E865.4	E950.9	E962.1	E980.9	FOOL'S PARSLEY
989.89		E861.4	E950.9	E962.1	E980.9	FORMALDEHYDE (SOLUTION)
989.4		E863.6	E950.6	E962.1	E980.7	FORMALDEHYDE FUNGICIDE
987.8		E869.8	E952.8	E962.2	E982.8	FORMALDEHYDE GAS OR VAPOR
989.89		E861.4	E950.9	E962.1	E980.9	FORMALIN
989.4		E863.6	E950.6	E962.1	E980.7	FORMALIN FUNGICIDE
987.8		E869.8	E952.8	E962.2	E982.8	FORMALIN VAPOR
983.1		E864.1	E950.7	E962.1	E980.6	FORMIC ACID
987.8		E869.8	E952.8	E962.2	E982.8	FORMIC ACID VAPOR
985.1		E866.3	E950.8	E962.1	E980.8	FOWLER'S SOLUTION
977.8	E947.8	E858.8	E950.4	E962.0	E980.4	FOX GREEN
988.2		E865.4	E950.9	E962.1	E980.9	FOXGLOVE
960.8	E930.8	E856	E950.4	E962.0	E980.4	FRAMYCETIN
973.1	E943.1	E858.4	E950.4	E962.0	E980.4	FRANGULA (EXTRACT)
977.8	E947.8	E858.8	E950.4	E962.0	E980.4	FREI ANTIGEN
987.4		E869.2	E952.8	E962.2	E982.8	FREONS
974.5	E944.5	E858.5	E950.4	E962.0	E980.4	FRUCTOSE
974.4	E944.4	E858.5	E950.4	E962.0	E980.4	FRUSEMIDE
962.4	E932.4	E858.0	E950.4	E962.0	E980.4	FSH
981		E862.1	E950.9	E962.1	E980.9	FUEL AUTOMOBILE
986		E868.2	E952.0	E962.2	E982.0	FUEL AUTOMOBILE EXHAUST GAS NOT IN TRANSIT
987.1		E869.8	E952.8	E962.2	E982.8	FUEL AUTOMOBILE VAPOR NEC
0						FUEL GAS (DOMESTIC USE) SEE ALSO CARBON MONOXIDE FUEL
987.1		E868.1	E951.8	E962.2	E981.8	FUEL GAS UTILITY
987.0		E868.0	E951.1	E962.2	E981.1	FUEL GAS UTILITY IN MOBILE CONTAINER
0						FUEL GAS UTILITY INCOMPLETE COMBUSTION OF SEE CARBON MONOXIDE FUEL UTILITY
986		E868.3	E952.1	E962.2	E982.1	FUEL INDUSTRIAL INCOMPLETE COMBUSTION
960.8	E930.8	E856	E950.4	E962.0	E980.4	FUGILLIN
985.0		E866.1	E950.9	E962.1	E980.9	FULMINATE OF MERCURY
960.1	E930.1	E856	E950.4	E962.0	E980.4	FULVICIN
960.8	E930.8	E856	E950.4	E962.0	E980.4	FUMADIL
960.8	E930.8	E856	E950.4	E962.0	E980.4	FUMAGILLIN
0						FUMES (FROM) CARBON MONOXIDE SEE CARBON MONOXIDE
986		E868.3	E952.1	E962.2	E982.1	FUMES (FROM) CHARCOAL (DOMESTIC USE)
0						FUMES (FROM) CHLOROFORM SEE CHLOROFORM
986		E868.3	E952.1	E962.2	E982.1	FUMES (FROM) COKE (IN DOMESTIC STOVES FIREPLACES)
987.8		E869.8	E952.8	E962.2	E982.8	FUMES (FROM) CORROSIVE NEC
987.8		E869.8	E952.8	E962.2	E982.8	FUMES (FROM) ETHER SEE ETHER(S)
987.4		E869.2	E952.8	E962.2	E982.8	FUMES (FROM) FREONS
987.9		E869.9	E952.9	E962.2	E982.9	FUMES (FROM) GAS VAPOR UNSPECIFIED
987.1		E869.8	E952.8	E962.2	E982.8	FUMES (FROM) HYDROCARBONS
987.0		E868.0	E951.1	E962.2	E981.1	FUMES (FROM) HYDROCARBONS PETROLEUM (LIQUEFIED)
987.0		E867	E951.0	E962.2	E981.0	FUMES (FROM) HYDROCARBONS PETROLEUM (LIQUEFIED) DISTRIBUTED THROUGH PIPES (PURE OR MIXED WITH AIR)
0						FUMES (FROM) LEAD SEE LEAD
0						FUMES (FROM) METALS SEE SPECIFIED METALS
987.2		E869.0	E952.8	E962.2	E982.8	FUMES (FROM) NITROGEN DIOXIDE
0						FUMES (FROM) PESTICIDES SEE PESTICIDES

POISON	THERA-PEUTIC	ACCIDENT	SUICIDE	ASSAULT	UNDETER-MINED	SUBSTANCE
987.0		E868.0	E951.1	E962.2	E981.1	FUMES (FROM) PETROLEUM (LIQUEFIED)
987.0		E867	E951.0	E962.2	E981.0	FUMES (FROM) PETROLEUM DISTRIBUTED THROUGH PIPES (PURE OR MIXED WITH AIR)
987.8		E869.8	E952.8	E962.2	E982.8	FUMES (FROM) POLYESTER
987.8		E869.8	E952.8	E962.2	E982.8	FUMES (FROM) SPECIFIED SOURCE OTHER
987.3		E869.1	E952.8	E962.2	E982.8	FUMES (FROM) SULFUR DIOXIDE
989.4		E863.8	E950.6	E962.1	E980.7	FUMIGANTS
988.1		E865.5	E950.9	E962.1	E980.9	FUNGI NOXIOUS USED AS FOOD
989.4		E863.6	E950.6	E962.1	E980.7	FUNGICIDES
960.1	E930.1	E856	E950.4	E962.0	E980.4	FUNGIZONE
976.0	E946.0	E858.7	E950.4	E962.0	E980.4	FUNGIZONE TOPICAL
976.0	E946.0	E858.7	E950.4	E962.0	E980.4	FURACIN
961.9	E931.9	E857	E950.4	E962.0	E980.4	FURADANTIN
961.9	E931.9	E857	E950.4	E962.0	E980.4	FURAZOLIDONE
986		E868.3	E952.1	E962.2	E982.1	FURNACE (COAL BURNING) (DOMESTIC) GAS FROM
986		E868.8	E952.1	E962.2	E982.1	FURNACE INDUSTRIAL
989.89		E861.2	E950.9	E962.1	E980.9	FURNITURE POLISH
974.4	E944.4	E858.5	E950.4	E962.0	E980.4	FUROSEMIDE
961.9	E931.9	E857	E950.4	E962.0	E980.4	FUROXONE
980.3		E860.4	E950.9	E962.1	E980.9	FUSEL OIL (AMYL) (BUTYL) (PROPYL)
960.8	E930.8	E856	E950.4	E962.0	E980.4	FUSIDIC ACID
975.2	E945.2	E858.6	E950.4	E962.0	E980.4	GALLAMINE
976.2	E946.2	E858.7	E950.4	E962.0	E980.4	GALLOTANNIC ACID
973.1	E943.1	E858.4	E950.4	E962.0	E980.4	GAMBOGE
964.6	E934.6	E858.2	E950.4	E962.0	E980.4	GAMIMUNE
964.6	E934.6	E858.2	E950.4	E962.0	E980.4	GAMMA GLOBULIN
989.2		E863.0	E950.6	E962.1	E980.7	GAMMA BENZENE HEXACHLORIDE (VAPOR)
968.4	E938.4	E855.1	E950.4	E962.0	E980.4	GAMMA HYDROXY BUTYRATE (GHB)
964.6	E934.6	E858.2	E950.4	E962.0	E980.4	GAMULIN
972.3	E942.3	E858.3	E950.4	E962.0	E980.4	GANGLIONIC BLOCKING AGENTS
969.6	E939.6	E854.1	E950.3	E962.0	E980.3	GANJA
960.8	E930.8	E856	E950.4	E962.0	E980.4	GARAMYCIN
976.5	E945.5	E858.7	E950.4	E962.0	E980.4	GARAMYCIN OPHTHALMIC PREPARATION
976.0	E946.0	E858.7	E950.4	E962.0	E980.4	GARAMYCIN TOPICAL NEC
967.0	E937.0	E851	E950.1	E962.0	E980.1	GARDENAL
967.0	E937.0	E851	E950.1	E962.0	E980.1	GARDEPANYL
987.9		E869.9	E952.9	E962.2	E982.9	GAS
0						GAS ACETYLENE INCOMPLETE COMBUSTION OF SEE CARBON MONOXIDE FUEL UTILITY
987.1		E868.1	E951.8	E962.2	E981.8	GAS ACETYLENE UNSPECIFIED
987.9		E869.9	E952.9	E962.2	E982.9	GAS AIR CONTAMINANTS SOURCE OR TYPE NOT SPECIFIED
968.2	E938.2	E855.1	E950.4	E962.0	E980.4	GAS ANESTHETIC (GENERAL) NEC
986		E868.8	E952.1	E962.2	E982.1	GAS BLAST FURNACE
0						GAS BUTANE SEE BUTANE
0						GAS CARBON MONOXIDE SEE CARBON MONOXIDE
987.6		E869.8	E952.8	E962.2	E982.8	GAS CHLORINE
0						GAS COAL SEE CARBON MONOXIDE COAL
987.7		E869.8	E952.8	E962.2	E982.8	GAS CYANIDE
987.8		E869.8	E952.8	E962.2	E982.8	GAS DICYANOGEN
0						GAS DOMESTIC SEE GAS UTILITY
0						GAS EXHAUST SEE CARBON MONOXIDE EXHAUST GAS
986		E868.3	E952.1	E962.2	E982.1	GAS FROM WOOD- OR COAL-BURNING STOVE OR FIREPLACE
0						GAS FUEL (DOMESTIC USE) SEE ALSO CARBON MONOXIDE FUEL
987.0		E868.0	E951.1	E962.2	E981.1	GAS FUEL (DOMESTIC USE) UTILITY IN MOBILE CONTAINER
986		E868.8	E952.1	E962.2	E982.1	GAS FUEL INDUSTRIAL USE
987.1		E868.1	E951.8	E962.2	E981.8	GAS FUEL UTILITY
0						GAS FUEL UTILITY INCOMPLETE COMBUSTION OF SEE CARBON MONOXIDE FUEL UTILITY
986		E868.2	E952.0	E962.2	E982.0	GAS GARAGE
0						GAS HYDROCARBON INCOMPLETE COMBUSTION OF SEE CARBON MONOXIDE FUEL UTILITY

DRUGS & CHEMICALS

POISON	THERA- PEUTIC	ACCIDENT	SUICIDE	ASSAULT	UNDETER- MINED	SUBSTANCE
987.0		E867	E951.0	E962.2	E981.0	GAS HYDROCARBON LIQUEFIED PIPED
987.0		E868.0	E951.1	E962.2	E981.1	GAS HYDROCARBON LIQUEFIED (MOBILE CONTAINER)
987.1		E869.8	E952.8	E962.2	E982.8	GAS HYDROCARBON NEC
987.7		E869.8	E952.8	E962.2	E982.8	GAS HYDROCYANIC ACID
0						GAS ILLUMINATING SEE GAS UTILITY
0						GAS INCOMPLETE COMBUSTION ANY SEE CARBON MONOXIDE
986		E868.8	E952.1	E962.2	E982.1	GAS KILN
987.5		E869.3	E952.8	E962.2	E982.8	GAS LACRIMOGENIC
987.1		E869.8	E952.8	E962.2	E982.8	GAS MARSH
986		E868.8	E952.1	E962.2	E982.0	GAS MOTOR EXHAUST NOT IN TRANSIT
0						GAS MUSTARD SEE MUSTARD GAS
987.1		E867	E951.0	E962.2	E981.0	GAS NATURAL
987.9		E869.9	E952.9	E962.2	E982.9	GAS NERVE (WAR)
981		E862.1	E950.9	E962.1	E980.9	GAS OILS
987.0		E868.0	E951.1	E962.2	E981.1	GAS PETROLEUM (LIQUEFIED) (DISTRIBUTED IN MOBILE CONTAINERS)
987.0		E867	E951.1	E962.2	E981.1	GAS PETROLEUM PIPED (PURE OR MIXED WITH AIR)
987.1		E867	E951.0	E962.2	E981.0	GAS PIPED (MANUFACTURERED) (NATURAL) NEC
986		E868.8	E952.1	E962.2	E982.1	GAS PRODUCER
0						GAS PROPANE SEE PROPANE
987.4		E869.2	E952.8	E962.2	E982.8	GAS REFRIGERANT (FREON)
987.9		E869.9	E952.9	E962.2	E982.9	GAS REFRIGERANT NOT FREON
987.8		E869.8	E952.8	E962.2	E982.8	GAS SEWER
987.8		E869.8	E952.8	E962.2	E982.8	GAS SPECIFIED SOURCE NEC
0						GAS STOVE SEE GAS UTILITY
987.5		E869.3	E952.8	E962.2	E982.8	GAS TEAR
987.1		E868.1	E951.8	E962.2	E981.8	GAS UTILITY (FOR COOKING HEATING OR LIGHTING) (PIPED) NEC
987.0		E868.0	E951.1	E962.2	E981.1	GAS UTILITY IN MOBILE CONTAINER
0						GAS UTILITY INCOMPLETE COMBUSTION OF SEE CARBON MONOXIDE FUEL UTILITY
987.1		E867	E951.0	E962.2	E981.0	GAS UTILITY PIPED (NATURAL)
987.1		E868.1	E951.8	E962.2	E981.8	GAS WATER
0						GAS WATER INCOMPLETE COMBUSTION OF SEE CARBON MONOXIDE FUEL UTILITY
0						GASEOUS SUBSTANCE SEE GAS
981		E862.1	E950.9	E962.1	E980.9	GASOLINE
987.1		E869.8	E952.8	E962.2	E982.8	GASOLINE VAPOR
973.4	E943.4	E858.4	E950.4	E962.0	E980.4	GASTRIC ENZYMES
977.8	E947.8	E858.8	E950.4	E962.0	E980.4	GASTROGRAFIN
973.9	E943.9	E858.4	E950.4	E962.0	E980.4	GASTROINTESTINAL AGENT NOS
973.8	E943.8	E858.4	E950.4	E962.0	E980.4	GASTROINTESTINAL AGENTS OTHER SPECIFIED
988.2		E865.4	E950.9	E962.1	E980.9	GAULTHERIA PROCUMBENS
964.8	E934.8	E858.2	E950.4	E962.0	E980.4	GELATIN (INTRAVENOUS)
964.5	E934.5	E858.2	E950.4	E962.0	E980.4	GELATIN ABSORBABLE (SPONGE)
976.8	E946.8	E858.7	E950.4	E962.0	E980.4	GELFILM
964.5	E934.5	E858.2	E950.4	E962.0	E980.4	GELFOAM
970.8	E940.8	E854.3	E950.4	E962.0	E980.4	GELSEMINE
988.2		E865.4	E950.9	E962.1	E980.9	GELSEMIUM (SEMPERVIRENS)
967.0	E937.0	E851	E950.1	E962.0	E980.1	GEMONIL
960.8	E930.8	E856	E950.4	E962.0	E980.4	GENTAMICIN
976.5	E946.5	E858.7	E950.4	E962.0	E980.4	GENTAMICIN OPHTHALMIC PREPARATION
976.0	E946.0	E858.7	E950.4	E962.0	E980.4	GENTAMICIN TOPICAL NEC
976.0	E946.0	E858.7	E950.4	E962.0	E980.4	GENTIAN VIOLET
976.0	E946.0	E858.7	E950.4	E962.0	E980.4	GEXANE
989.5		E905.0	E950.9	E962.1	E980.9	GILA MONSTER (VENOM)
989.89		E866.8	E950.9	E962.1	E980.9	GINGER JAMAICA
972.1	E942.1	E858.3	E950.4	E962.0	E980.4	GITALIN
972.1	E942.1	E858.3	E950.4	E962.0	E980.4	GITOXIN
977.9	E947.9	E858.9	E950.5	E962.0	E980.5	GLANDULAR EXTRACT (MEDICINAL) NEC
961.5	E931.5	E857	E950.4	E962.0	E980.4	GLAUCARUBIN
962.3	E932.3	E858.0	E950.4	E962.0	E980.4	GLOBIN ZINC INSULIN
962.3	E932.3	E858.0	E950.4	E962.0	E980.4	GLUCAGON
967.1	E937.1	E852.0	E950.2	E962.0	E980.2	GLUCOCHLORAL
962.0	E932.0	E858.0	E950.4	E962.0	E980.4	GLUCOCORTICOIDS
974.5	E944.5	E858.5	E950.4	E962.0	E980.4	GLUCOSE
977.8	E947.8	E858.8	E950.4	E962.0	E980.4	GLUCOSE OXIDASE REAGENT
961.8	E931.8	E857	E950.4	E962.0	E980.4	GLUCOSULFONE SODIUM

POISON	THERA-PEUTIC	ACCIDENT	SUICIDE	ASSAULT	UNDETER-MINED	SUBSTANCE
989.89		E866.6	E950.9	E962.1	E980.9	GLUE(S)
989.89		E861.4	E950.9	E962.1	E980.9	GLUTARALDEHYDE
963.8	E933.8	E858.1	E950.4	E962.0	E980.4	GLUTATHIONE
967.5	E937.5	E852.4	E950.2	E962.0	E980.2	GLUTETHIMIDE (GROUP)
976.3	E946.3	E858.7	E950.4	E962.0	E980.4	GLYCERIN (LOTION)
976.3	E946.3	E858.7	E950.4	E962.0	E980.4	GLYCEROL (TOPICAL)
975.5	E945.5	E858.6	E950.4	E962.0	E980.4	GLYCERYL GUAIACOLATE
976.0	E946.0	E858.7	E950.4	E962.0	E980.4	GLYCERYL TRIACETATE (TOPICAL)
972.4	E942.4	E858.3	E950.4	E962.0	E980.4	GLYCERYL TRINITRATE
974.5	E944.5	E858.5	E950.4	E962.0	E980.4	GLYCINE
961.1	E931.1	E857	E950.4	E962.0	E980.4	GLYCOBIARSOL
982.8		E862.4	E950.9	E962.1	E980.9	GLYCOLS (ETHER)
971.1	E941.1	E855.4	E950.4	E962.0	E980.4	GLYCOPYRROLATE
962.3	E932.3	E858.0	E950.4	E962.0	E980.4	GLYMIDINE
965.69	E935.6	E850.6	E950.0	E962.0	E980.0	GOLD (COMPOUNDS) (SALTS)
985.4		E866.2	E950.9	E962.1	E980.9	GOLDEN SULFIDE OF ANTIMONY
988.2		E865.4	E950.9	E962.1	E980.9	GOLDYLOCKS
962.9	E932.9	E858.0	E950.4	E962.0	E980.4	GONADAL TISSUE EXTRACT
962.2	E932.2	E858.0	E950.4	E962.0	E980.4	GONADAL TISSUE EXTRACT FEMALE
962.1	E932.1	E858.0	E950.4	E962.0	E980.4	GONADAL TISSUE EXTRACT MALE
962.4	E932.4	E858.0	E950.4	E962.0	E980.4	GONADOTROPIN
980.0		E860.1	E950.9	E962.1	E980.9	GRAIN ALCOHOL
980.0		E860.0	E950.9	E962.1	E980.9	GRAIN ALCOHOL BEVERAGE
960.8	E930.8	E856	E950.4	E962.0	E980.4	GRAMICIDIN
988.2		E865.4	E950.9	E962.1	E980.9	GRATIOLA OFFICINALIS
989.89		E866.8	E950.9	E962.1	E980.9	GREASE
988.2		E865.4	E950.9	E962.1	E980.9	GREEN HELLEBORE
976.2	E946.2	E858.7	E950.4	E962.0	E980.4	GREEN SOAP
960.1	E930.1	E856	E950.4	E962.0	E980.4	GRIFULVIN
960.1	E930.1	E856	E950.4	E962.0	E980.4	GRISEOFULVIN
962.4	E932.4	E858.0	E950.4	E962.0	E980.4	GROWTH HORMONE
977.8	E947.8	E858.8	E950.4	E962.0	E980.4	GUAIAC REAGENT
975.5	E945.5	E858.6	E950.4	E962.0	E980.4	GUAIACOL
975.5	E945.5	E858.6	E950.4	E962.0	E980.4	GUAIFENESIN
975.5	E945.5	E858.6	E950.4	E962.0	E980.4	GUAIPHENESIN
961.4	E931.4	E857	E950.4	E962.0	E980.4	GUANATOL
972.6	E942.6	E858.3	E950.4	E962.0	E980.4	GUANETHIDINE
989.89		E866.5	E950.9	E962.1	E980.9	GUANO
972.6	E942.6	E858.3	E950.4	E962.0	E980.4	GUANOCHLOR
972.6	E942.6	E858.3	E950.4	E962.0	E980.4	GUANOCTINE
972.6	E942.6	E858.3	E950.4	E962.0	E980.4	GUANOXAN
976.4	E946.4	E858.7	E950.4	E962.0	E980.4	HAIR TREATMENT AGENT NEC
976.0	E946.0	E858.7	E950.4	E962.0	E980.4	HALCINONIDE
976.0	E946.0	E858.7	E950.4	E962.0	E980.4	HALETHAZOLE
969.6	E939.6	E854.1	E950.3	E962.0	E980.3	HALLUCINOGENS
968.2	E938.2	E855.1	E950.4	E962.0	E980.4	HALOGENATED HYDROCARBON DERIVATIVES EXCEPT HALOTHANE
969.2	E939.2	E853.1	E950.3	E962.0	E980.3	HALOPERIDOL
976.0	E946.0	E858.7	E950.4	E962.0	E980.4	HALOPROGIN
976.0	E946.0	E858.7	E950.4	E962.0	E980.4	HALOTEX
968.1	E938.1	E855.1	E950.4	E962.0	E980.4	HALOTHANE
976.0	E946.0	E858.7	E950.4	E962.0	E980.4	HALQUINOLS
972.6	E942.6	E858.3	E950.4	E962.0	E980.4	HARMONYL
974.5	E944.5	E858.5	E950.4	E962.0	E980.4	HARTMANN'S SOLUTION
969.6	E939.6	E854.1	E950.3	E962.0	E980.3	HASHISH
969.6	E939.6	E854.1	E950.3	E962.0	E980.3	HAWAIIAN WOOD ROSE SEEDS
977.9	E947.9	E858.9	E950.5	E962.0	E980.9	HEADACHE CURES DRUGS POWDERS NEC
969.6	E939.6	E854.1	E950.3	E962.0	E980.3	HEAVENLY BLUE (MORNING GLORY)
963.8	E933.8	E858.1	E950.4	E962.0	E980.4	HEAVY METAL ANTAGONISTS
961.2	E931.2	E857	E950.4	E962.0	E980.4	HEAVY METALS ANTI-INFECTIVES
976.0	E946.0	E858.7	E950.4	E962.0	E980.4	HEDAQUINIUM
988.2		E865.4	E950.9	E962.1	E980.9	HEDGE HYSSOP
976.8	E946.8	E858.7	E950.4	E962.0	E980.4	HEET
961.6	E931.6	E857	E950.4	E962.0	E980.4	HELENIN
988.2		E865.4	E950.9	E962.1	E980.9	HELLEBORE (BLACK) (GREEN) (WHITE)
988.2		E865.4	E950.9	E962.1	E980.9	HEMLOCK
964.5	E934.5	E858.2	E950.4	E962.0	E980.4	HEMOSTATICS
972.8	E942.8	E858.3	E950.4	E962.0	E980.4	HEMOSTATICS CAPILLARY ACTIVE DRUGS
988.2		E865.4	E950.9	E962.1	E980.9	HENBANE
964.2	E934.2	E858.2	E950.4	E962.0	E980.4	HEPARIN
967.0	E937.0	E851	E950.1	E962.0	E980.1	HEPTABARBITAL HEPTABARBITONE
989.2		E863.0	E950.6	E962.1	E980.7	HEPTACHLOR
965.09	E935.2	E850.2	E950.0	E962.0	E980.0	HEPTALGIN

DRUGS & CHEMICALS

POISON	THERA-PEUTIC	ACCIDENT	SUICIDE	ASSAULT	UNDETER-MINED	SUBSTANCE
989.4		E863.5	E950.6	E962.1	E980.7	HERBICIDES
965.01	E935.0	E850.0	E950.0	E962.0	E980.0	HEROIN (DIACETYLMORPHINE)
976.5	E946.5	E858.7	E950.4	E962.0	E980.4	HERPLEX
964.8	E934.8	E858.2	E950.4	E962.0	E980.4	HES
964.8	E934.8	E858.2	E950.4	E962.0	E980.4	HETASTARCH
989.2		E863.0	E950.6	E962.1	E980.7	HEXA-CHLOROCYCLOHEXANE
976.2	E946.2	E858.7	E950.4	E962.0	E980.4	HEXA-GERM
976.2	E946.2	E858.7	E950.4	E962.0	E980.4	HEXACHLOROPHENE
964.5	E934.5	E858.2	E950.4	E962.0	E980.4	HEXADIMETHRINE (BROMIDE)
975.2	E945.2	E858.6	E950.4	E962.0	E980.4	HEXAFLUORENIUM
980.8		E860.8	E950.9	E962.1	E980.9	HEXAHYDROPHENOL
980.8		E860.8	E950.9	E962.1	E980.9	HEXALIN
972.3	E942.3	E858.3	E950.4	E962.0	E980.4	HEXAMETHONIUM
961.9	E931.9	E857	E950.4	E962.0	E980.4	HEXAMETHYLENEAMINE
961.9	E931.9	E857	E950.4	E962.0	E980.4	HEXAMINE
982.8		E862.4	E950.9	E962.1	E980.9	HEXANONE
967.8	E937.8	E852.8	E950.2	E962.0	E980.2	HEXAPROPYMATE
962.2	E932.2	E858.0	E950.4	E962.0	E980.4	HEXESTROL
967.0	E937.0	E851	E950.1	E962.0	E980.1	HEXETHAL (SODIUM)
976.0	E946.0	E858.7	E950.4	E962.0	E980.4	HEXETIDINE
967.0	E937.0	E851	E950.1	E962.0	E980.1	HEXOBARBITAL
968.3	E938.3	E855.1	E950.4	E962.0	E980.4	HEXOBARBITAL SODIUM (ANESTHETIC)
968.3	E938.3	E855.1	E950.4	E962.0	E980.4	HEXOBARBITAL SOLUBLE
971.1	E941.1	E855.4	E950.4	E962.0	E980.4	HEXOCYCLIUM
962.2	E932.2	E858.0	E950.4	E962.0	E980.4	HEXOESTROL
982.8		E862.4	E950.9	E962.1	E980.9	HEXONE
968.5	E938.5	E855.2	E950.4	E962.0	E980.4	HEXYLCAINE
961.6	E931.6	E857	E950.4	E962.0	E980.4	HEXYLRESORCINOL
973.1	E943.1	E858.4	E950.4	E962.0	E980.4	HINKLE'S PILLS
977.8	E947.8	E858.8	E950.4	E962.0	E980.4	HISTALOG
972.5	E942.5	E858.3	E950.4	E962.0	E980.4	HISTAMINE (PHOSPHATE)
977.8	E947.8	E858.8	E950.4	E962.0	E980.4	HISTOPLASMIN
988.2		E865.3	E950.9	E962.1	E980.9	HOLLY BERRIES
971.1	E941.1	E855.4	E950.4	E962.0	E980.4	HOMATROPINE
964.6	E934.6	E858.2	E950.4	E962.0	E980.4	HOMO-TET
962.9	E932.9	E858.0	E950.4	E962.0	E980.4	HORMONES (SYNTHETIC SUBSTITUTES) NEC
962.0	E932.0	E858.0	E950.4	E962.0	E980.4	HORMONES ADRENAL CORTICAL STEROIDS
962.3	E932.3	E858.0	E950.4	E962.0	E980.4	HORMONES ANTI-DIABETIC AGENTS
962.4	E932.4	E858.0	E950.4	E962.0	E980.4	HORMONES FOLLICLE STIMULATING
962.4	E932.4	E858.0	E950.4	E962.0	E980.4	HORMONES GONADO-TROPIC
962.4	E932.4	E858.0	E950.4	E962.0	E980.4	HORMONES GROWTH
962.2	E932.2	E858.0	E950.4	E962.0	E980.4	HORMONES OVARIAN (SUBSTITUTES)
962.6	E932.6	E858.0	E950.4	E962.0	E980.4	HORMONES PARATHYROID(DERIVATIVES)
962.5	E932.5	E858.0	E950.4	E962.0	E980.4	HORMONES PITUITARY (POSTERIOR)
962.4	E932.4	E858.0	E950.4	E962.0	E980.4	HORMONES PITUITARY ANTERIOR
962.7	E932.7	E858.0	E950.4	E962.0	E980.4	HORMONES THYROID (DERIVATIVES)
989.5		E905.3	E950.9	E962.1	E980.9	HORNET (STING)
989.4		E863.9	E950.6	E962.1	E980.7	HORTICULTURE AGENT NEC
964.7	E934.7	E858.2	E950.4	E962.0	E980.4	HUMAN FIBRINOGEN
963.4	E933.4	E858.1	E950.4	E962.0	E980.4	HYALURONIDASE
963.4	E933.4	E858.1	E950.4	E962.0	E980.4	HYAZYME
965.09	E935.2	E850.2	E950.0	E962.0	E980.0	HYCODAN
966.1	E936.1	E855.0	E950.4	E962.0	E980.4	HYDANTOIN DERIVATIVES
962.0	E932.0	E858.0	E950.4	E962.0	E980.4	HYDELTRA
971.3	E941.3	E855.6	E950.4	E962.0	E980.4	HYDERGINE
960.0	E930.0	E856	E950.4	E962.0	E980.4	HYDRABAMINE PENICILLIN
972.6	E942.6	E858.3	E950.4	E962.0	E980.4	HYDRALAZINE
976.0	E946.0	E858.7	E950.4	E962.0	E980.4	HYDRARGAPHEN
983.9		E864.3	E950.7	E962.1	E980.6	HYDRAZINE
975.5	E945.5	E858.6	E950.4	E962.0	E980.4	HYDRIODIC ACID
965.09	E935.2	E850.2	E950.0	E962.0	E980.0	HYDRO-XYDIHYDROCODEINONE
965.5	E935.5	E850.5	E950.0	E962.0	E980.0	HYDRO-XYPHENYLBUTAZONE
987.1		E869.8	E952.8	E962.2	E982.8	HYDROCARBON GAS
0						HYDROCARBON GAS INCOMPLETE COMBUSTION OF SEE CARBON MONOXIDE FUEL UTILITY
987.0		E867	E951.0	E962.2	E981.0	HYDROCARBON GAS LIQUEFIED PIPED (NATURAL)
983.1		E864.1	E950.7	E962.1	E980.6	HYDROCLORIC ACID (LIQUID)
973.4	E943.4	E858.4	E950.4	E962.0	E980.4	HYDROCHLORIC ACID MEDICINAL
987.8		E869.8	E952.8	E962.2	E982.8	HYDROCHLORIC ACID VAPOR
973.6	E943.6	E858.4	E950.4	E962.0	E980.4	HYDROCHLORIDE (EMETIC)

POISON	THERA-PEUTIC	ACCIDENT	SUICIDE	ASSAULT	UNDETER-MINED	SUBSTANCE
974.3	E944.3	E858.5	E950.4	E962.0	E980.4	HYDROCHLOROTHIAZIDE
965.09	E935.2	E850.2	E950.0	E962.0	E980.0	HYDROCODONE
962.0	E932.0	E858.0	E950.4	E962.0	E980.4	HYDROCORTISONE
976.6	E946.6	E858.7	E950.4	E962.0	E980.4	HYDROCORTISONE ENT AGENT
976.5	E946.5	E858.7	E950.4	E962.0	E980.4	HYDROCORTISONE OPHTHALMIC PREPARATION
976.0	E946.0	E858.7	E950.4	E962.0	E980.4	HYDROCORTISONE TOPICAL NEC
962.0	E932.0	E858.0	E950.4	E962.0	E980.4	HYDROCORTONE
976.6	E946.6	E858.7	E950.4	E962.0	E980.4	HYDROCORTONE ENT AGENT
976.5	E946.5	E858.7	E950.4	E962.0	E980.4	HYDROCORTONE OPHTHALMIC PREPARATION
976.0	E946.0	E858.7	E950.4	E962.0	E980.4	HYDROCORTONE TOPICAL NEC
0						HYDROCYANIC ACID SEE CYANIDE(S)
974.3	E944.3	E858.5	E950.4	E962.0	E980.4	HYDROFLUMETHIAZIDE
983.1		E864.1	E950.7	E962.1	E980.6	HYDROFLUORIC ACID (LIQUID)
987.8		E869.8	E952.8	E962.2	E982.8	HYDROFLUORIC ACID VAPOR
987.8		E869.8	E952.8	E962.2	E982.8	HYDROGEN
985.1		E866.3	E950.8	E962.1	E980.8	HYDROGEN ARSENIDE
985.1		E866.3	E950.8	E962.1	E980.8	HYDROGEN ARSENIURETED
989.0		E866.8	E950.9	E962.1	E980.9	HYDROGEN CYANIDE (SALTS)
987.7		E869.8	E952.8	E962.2	E982.8	HYDROGEN CYANIDE GAS
983.1		E864.1	E950.7	E962.1	E980.6	HYDROGEN FLUORIDE (LIQUID)
987.8		E869.8	E952.8	E962.2	E982.8	HYDROGEN FLUORIDE VAPOR
976.6	E946.6	E858.7	E950.4	E962.0	E980.4	HYDROGEN PEROXIDE (SOLUTION)
987.8		E869.8	E952.8	E962.2	E982.8	HYDROGEN PHOS-PHURETED
985.1		E866.3	E950.8	E962.1	E980.8	HYDROGEN SULFIDE ARSENIURETED
987.8		E869.8	E952.8	E962.2	E982.8	HYDROGEN SULFIDE (GAS)
987.8		E869.8	E952.8	E962.2	E982.8	HYDROGEN SULFURETED
965.09	E935.2	E850.2	E950.0	E962.0	E980.0	HYDROMORPHINOL
965.09	E935.2	E850.2	E950.0	E962.0	E980.0	HYDROMORPHINONE
965.09	E935.2	E850.2	E950.0	E962.0	E980.0	HYDROMORPHONE
974.3	E944.3	E858.5	E950.4	E962.0	E980.4	HYDROMOX
976.3	E946.3	E858.7	E950.4	E962.0	E980.4	HYDROPHILIC LOTION
983.0		E864.0	E950.7	E962.1	E980.6	HYDROQUINONE
987.8		E869.8	E952.8	E962.2	E982.8	HYDROQUINONE VAPOR
987.8		E869.8	E952.8	E962.2	E982.8	HYDROSULFURIC ACID (GAS)
976.3	E946.3	E858.7	E950.4	E962.0	E980.4	HYDROUS WOOL FAT (LOTION)
983.2		E864.2	E950.7	E962.1	E980.6	HYDROXIDE CAUSTIC
964.1	E934.1	E858.2	E950.4	E962.0	E980.4	HYDROXOCOBALAMIN
971.2	E941.2	E855.5	E950.4	E962.0	E980.4	HYDROXYAMPHETAMINE
961.4	E931.4	E857	E950.4	E962.0	E980.4	HYDROXYCHLOROQUINE
965.09	E935.2	E850.2	E950.0	E962.0	E980.0	HYDROXYDIHYDRO-MORPHINONE 14
964.8	E934.8	E858.2	E950.4	E962.0	E980.4	HYDROXYETHYL STARCH
969.5	E939.5	E853.8	E950.3	E962.0	E980.3	HYDROXYPHENAMATE
962.2	E932.2	E858.0	E950.4	E962.0	E980.4	HYDROXYPROGESTERONE
961.3	E931.3	E857	E950.4	E962.0	E980.4	HYDROXYQUINOLINE DERIVATIVES
961.5	E931.5	E857	E950.4	E962.0	E980.4	HYDROXYSTILBAMIDINE
963.1	E933.1	E858.1	E950.4	E962.0	E980.4	HYDROXYUREA
969.5	E939.5	E853.8	E950.3	E962.0	E980.3	HYDROXYZINE
971.1	E941.1	E855.4	E950.4	E962.0	E980.4	HYOSCINE (HYDROBROMIDE)
971.1	E941.1	E855.4	E950.4	E962.0	E980.4	HYOSCYAMINE
988.2		E865.4	E950.9	E962.1	E980.9	HYOSCYAMUS (ALBUS) (NIGER)
977.8	E947.8	E858.8	E950.4	E962.0	E980.4	HYPAQUE
964.6	E934.6	E858.2	E950.4	E962.0	E980.4	HYPERTUSSIS
967.9	E937.9	E852.9	E950.2	E962.0	E980.2	HYPNOTICS NEC
0						HYPOCHLORITES SEE SODIUM HYPOCHLORITE
972.6	E942.6	E858.3	E950.4	E962.0	E980.4	HYPOTENSIVE AGENTS NEC
962.7	E932.7	E858.0	E950.4	E962.0	E980.4	I-THYROXINE SODIUM
965.69	E935.6	E850.6	E950.0	E962.0	E980.0	IBUFENAC
965.61	E935.6	E850.6	E950.0	E962.0	E980.0	IBUPROFEN
977.8	E947.8	E858.8	E950.4	E962.0	E980.4	ICG
976.4	E946.4	E858.7	E950.4	E962.0	E980.4	ICHTHAMMOL
976.4	E946.4	E858.7	E950.4	E962.0	E980.4	ICHTHYOL
976.5	E946.5	E858.7	E950.4	E962.0	E980.4	IDOXURIDINE
976.5	E946.5	E858.7	E950.4	E962.0	E980.4	IDU
962.3	E932.3	E858.0	E950.4	E962.0	E980.4	ILETIN
988.2		E865.4	E950.9	E962.1	E980.9	ILEX
0						ILLUMINATING GAS SEE GAS UTILITY
963.5	E933.5	E858.1	E950.4	E962.0	E980.4	ILOPAN
960.3	E930.3	E856	E950.4	E962.0	E980.4	ILOTYCIN
976.5	E946.5	E858.7	E950.4	E962.0	E980.4	ILOTYCIN OPHTHALMIC PREPARATION
976.0	E946.0	E858.7	E950.4	E962.0	E980.4	ILOTYCIN TOPICAL NEC
969.0	E939.0	E854.0	E950.3	E962.0	E980.3	IMIPRAMINE
964.6	E934.6	E858.2	E950.4	E962.0	E980.4	IMMU-G

POISON	THERA-PEUTIC	ACCIDENT	SUICIDE	ASSAULT	UNDETER-MINED	SUBSTANCE
964.6	E934.6	E858.2	E950.4	E962.0	E980.4	IMMU-TETANUS
964.6	E934.6	E858.2	E950.4	E962.0	E980.4	IMMUGLOBIN
964.6	E934.6	E858.2	E950.4	E962.0	E980.4	IMMUNE SERUM GLOBULIN
963.1	E933.1	E858.1	E950.4	E962.0	E980.4	IMMUNOSUPPRESSIVE AGENTS
964.2	E934.2	E858.2	E950.4	E962.0	E980.4	INDANDIONE (DERIVATIVES)
972.0	E942.0	E858.3	E950.4	E962.0	E980.4	INDERAL
969.6	E939.6	E854.1	E950.3	E962.0	E980.3	INDIAN HEMP
988.2		E865.4	E950.9	E962.1	E980.9	INDIAN TOBACCO
977.8	E947.8	E858.8	E950.4	E962.0	E980.4	INDIGO CARMINE
965.69	E935.6	E850.6	E950.0	E962.0	E980.0	INDOCIN
977.8	E947.8	E858.8	E950.4	E962.0	E980.4	INDOCYANINE GREEN
965.69	E935.6	E850.6	E950.0	E962.0	E980.0	INDOMETHACIN
980.9		E860.9	E950.9	E962.1	E980.9	INDUSTRIAL ALCOHOL
987.8		E869.8	E952.8	E962.2	E982.8	INDUSTRIAL FUMES
982.8		E862.9	E950.9	E962.1	E980.9	INDUSTRIAL SOLVENTS (FUMES) (VAPORS)
979.6	E949.6	E858.8	E950.4	E962.0	E982.8	INFLUENZA VACCINE
989.9		E866.9	E950.9	E962.1	E980.9	INGESTED SUBSTANCES NEC
961.8	E931.8	E857	E950.4	E962.0	E980.4	INH (ISONIAZID)
0						INHALATION GAS (NOXIOUS) SEE GAS
989.89		E866.8	E950.9	E962.1	E980.9	INK
967.6	E937.6	E852.5	E950.2	E962.0	E980.2	INNOVAR
972.2	E942.2	E858.3	E950.4	E962.0	E980.4	INOSITOL NIACINATE
963.1	E933.1	E858.1	E950.4	E962.0	E980.4	INPROQUONE
989.5		E905.5	E950.9	E962.1	E980.9	INSECT (STING) VENOMOUS
989.4		E863.4	E950.6	E962.1	E980.7	INSECTICIDES
989.2		E863.0	E950.6	E962.1	E980.7	INSECTICIDES CHLORINATED
989.4		E863.3	E950.6	E962.1	E980.7	INSECTICIDES MIXTURES
989.2		E863.0	E950.6	E962.1	E980.7	INSECTICIDES ORGANO-CHLORINE (COMPOUNDS)
989.3		E863.1	E950.6	E962.1	E980.7	INSECTICIDES ORGANOPHOSPHORUS (COMPOUNDS)
962.3	E932.3	E858.0	E950.4	E962.0	E980.4	INSULAR TISSUE EXTRACT
962.3	E932.3	E858.0	E950.4	E962.0	E980.4	INSULIN
968.3	E938.3	E855.1	E950.4	E962.0	E980.4	INTRANARCON
977.8	E947.8	E858.8	E950.4	E962.0	E980.4	INULIN
974.5	E944.5	E858.5	E950.4	E962.0	E980.4	INVERT SUGAR
976.0	E946.0	E858.7	E950.4	E962.0	E980.4	IODIDE MERCURY (OINTMENT)
976.0	E946.0	E858.7	E950.4	E962.0	E980.4	IODIDE METHYLATE
976.0	E946.0	E858.7	E950.4	E962.0	E980.4	IODIDE NEC
975.5	E945.5	E858.6	E950.4	E962.0	E980.4	IODIDE POTASSIUM (EXPECTORANT) NEC
962.8	E932.8	E858.0	E950.4	E962.0	E980.4	IODIDES OTHER
975.5	E945.5	E858.6	E950.4	E962.0	E980.4	IODINATED GLYCEROL
976.0	E946.0	E858.7	E950.4	E962.0	E980.4	IODINE (ANTISEPTIC EXTERNAL) (TINCTURE) NEC
977.8	E947.8	E858.8	E950.4	E962.0	E980.4	IODINE DIAGNOSTIC
962.8	E932.8	E858.0	E950.4	E962.0	E980.4	IODINE FOR THYROID CONDITIONS (ANTITHYROID)
987.8		E869.8	E952.8	E962.2	E982.8	IODINE VAPOR
977.8	E947.8	E858.8	E950.4	E962.0	E980.4	IODIZED OIL
961.2	E931.2	E857	E950.4	E962.0	E980.4	IODOBISMITOL
961.3	E931.3	E857	E950.4	E962.0	E980.4	IODOCHLORHYDROXYQUIN
976.0	E946.0	E858.7	E950.4	E962.0	E980.4	IODOCHLORHYDROXYQUIN TOPICAL
976.0	E946.0	E858.7	E950.4	E962.0	E980.4	IODOFORM
977.8	E947.8	E858.8	E950.4	E962.0	E980.4	IODOPANOIC ACID
977.8	E947.8	E858.8	E950.4	E962.0	E980.4	IODOPHTHALEIN
974.5	E944.5	E858.5	E950.4	E962.0	E980.4	ION EXCHANGE RESINS
977.8	E947.8	E858.8	E950.4	E962.0	E980.4	IOPANOIC ACID
977.8	E947.8	E858.8	E950.4	E962.0	E980.4	IOPHENDYLATE
962.8	E932.8	E858.0	E950.4	E962.0	E980.4	IOTHIOURACIL
973.6	E943.6	E858.4	E950.4	E962.0	E980.4	IPECAC
973.6	E943.6	E858.4	E950.4	E962.0	E980.4	IPECACUANHA
977.8	E947.8	E858.8	E950.4	E962.0	E980.4	IPODATE
967.0	E937.0	E851	E950.1	E962.0	E980.1	IPRAL
975.1	E945.1	E858.6	E950.4	E962.0	E980.4	IPRATROPIUM
969.0	E939.0	E854.0	E950.3	E962.0	E980.3	IPRONIAZID
964.0	E934.0	E858.2	E950.4	E962.0	E980.4	IRON AND ITS COMPOUNDS
964.0	E934.0	E858.2	E950.4	E962.0	E980.4	IRON DEXTRAN
985.8		E866.4	E950.9	E962.1	E980.9	IRON NONMEDICINAL (DUST) (FUMES) NEC
977.9	E947.9	E858.9	E950.5	E962.0	E980.5	IRRITANT DRUG
972.6	E942.6	E858.3	E950.4	E962.0	E980.4	ISMELIN
972.4	E942.4	E858.3	E950.4	E962.0	E980.4	ISOAMYL NITRITE
982.8		E862.4	E950.9	E962.1	E980.9	ISOBUTYL ACETATE
969.0	E939.0	E854.0	E950.3	E962.0	E980.3	ISOCARBOXAZID
971.2	E941.2	E855.5	E950.4	E962.0	E980.4	ISOEPHEDRINE

POISON	THERAPEUTIC	ACCIDENT	SUICIDE	ASSAULT	UNDETERMINED	SUBSTANCE
971.2	E941.2	E855.5	E950.4	E962.0	E980.4	ISOETHARINE
971.0	E941.0	E855.3	E950.4	E962.0	E980.4	ISOFLUOROPHATE
961.8	E931.8	E857	E950.4	E962.0	E980.4	ISONIAZID (INH)
961.4	E931.4	E857	E950.4	E962.0	E980.4	ISOPENTAQUINE
962.3	E932.3	E858.0	E950.4	E962.0	E980.4	ISOPHANE INSULIN
962.2	E932.2	E858.0	E950.4	E962.0	E980.4	ISOPREGNENONE
971.2	E941.2	E855.5	E950.4	E962.0	E980.4	ISOPRENALINE
971.1	E941.1	E855.4	E950.4	E962.0	E980.4	ISOPROPAMIDE
980.2		E860.3	E950.9	E962.1	E980.9	ISOPROPANOL
976.0	E946.0	E858.7	E950.4	E962.0	E980.4	ISOPROPANOL TOPICAL (GERMICIDE)
982.8		E862.4	E950.9	E962.1	E980.9	ISOPROPYL ACETATE
980.2		E860.3	E950.9	E962.1	E980.9	ISOPROPYL ALCOHOL
976.0	E946.0	E858.7	E950.4	E962.0	E980.4	ISOPROPYL ALCOHOL TOPICAL (GERMICIDE)
982.8		E862.4	E950.9	E962.1	E980.9	ISOPROPYL ETHER
971.2	E941.2	E855.5	E950.4	E962.0	E980.4	ISOPROTERENOL
972.4	E942.4	E858.3	E950.4	E962.0	E980.4	ISOSORBIDE DINITRATE
963.0	E933.0	E858.1	E950.4	E962.0	E980.4	ISOTHIPENDYL
960.0	E930.0	E856	E950.4	E962.0	E980.4	ISOXAZOLYL PENICILLIN
972.5	E942.5	E858.3	E950.4	E962.0	E980.4	ISOXSUPRINE HYDROCHLORIDE
971.0	E941.0	E855.3	E950.4	E962.0	E980.4	JABORANDI (PILOCARPUS) (EXTRACT)
973.1	E943.1	E858.4	E950.4	E962.0	E980.4	JALAP
965.7	E935.7	E850.7	E950.0	E962.0	E980.0	JAMAICA DOGWOOD (BARK)
989.89		E866.8	E950.9	E962.1	E980.9	JAMAICA GINGER
988.2		E865.4	E950.9	E962.1	E980.9	JATROPHA
988.2		E865.3	E950.9	E962.1	E980.9	JATROPHA CURCAS
964.0	E934.0	E858.2	E950.4	E962.0	E980.4	JECTOFER
989.5		E905.6	E950.9	E962.1	E980.9	JELLYFISH (STING)
988.2		E865.3	E950.9	E962.1	E980.9	JEQUIRITY (BEAN)
988.2		E865.4	E950.9	E962.1	E980.9	JIMSON WEED
988.2		E865.3	E950.9	E962.1	E980.9	JIMSON WEED SEEDS
976.4	E946.4	E858.7	E950.4	E962.0	E980.4	JUNIPER TAR (OIL) (OINTMENT)
972.5	E942.5	E858.3	E950.4	E962.0	E980.4	KALLIKREIN
960.6	E930.6	E856	E950.4	E962.0	E980.4	KANAMYCIN
960.6	E930.6	E856	E950.4	E962.0	E980.4	KANTREX
973.5	E943.5	E858.4	E950.4	E962.0	E980.4	KAOLIN
973.3	E943.3	E858.4	E950.4	E962.0	E980.4	KARAYA (GUM)
968.3	E938.3	E855.1	E950.4	E962.0	E980.4	KEMITHAL
962.0	E932.0	E858.0	E950.4	E962.0	E980.4	KENACORT
976.4	E946.4	E858.7	E950.4	E962.0	E980.4	KERATOLYTICS
976.4	E946.4	E858.7	E950.4	E962.0	E980.4	KERATOPLASTICS
981		E862.1	E950.9	E962.1	E980.9	KEROSENE (FUEL) (SOLVENT) NEC
981		E863.4	E950.6	E962.1	E980.7	KEROSENE INSECTICIDE
987.1		E869.8	E952.8	E962.2	E982.8	KEROSENE VAPOR
968.3	E938.3	E855.1	E950.4	E962.0	E980.4	KETAMINE
965.09	E935.2	E850.2	E950.0	E962.0	E980.0	KETOBEMIDONE
982.8		E862.4	E950.9	E962.1	E980.9	KETOLS
982.8		E862.4	E950.9	E962.1	E980.9	KETONE OILS
965.61	E935.6	E850.6	E950.0	E962.0	E980.0	KETOPROFEN
973.3	E943.3	E858.4	E950.4	E962.0	E980.4	KETOPROFEN CELLULOSE
986		E868.8	E952.1	E962.2	E982.1	KILN GAS OR VAPOR (CARBON MONOXIDE)
973.3	E943.3	E858.4	E950.4	E962.0	E980.4	KONSYL
988.2		E865.3	E950.9	E962.1	E980.9	KOSAM SEED
989.5		E905.0	E950.9	E962.1	E980.9	KRAIT (VENOM)
989.2		E863.0	E950.6	E962.1	E980.7	KWELL (INSECTICIDE)
976.0	E946.0	E858.7	E950.4	E962.0	E980.4	KWELL ANTI-INFECTIVE(TOPICAL)
966.4	E936.4	E855.0	E950.4	E962.0	E980.4	L-DOPA
988.2		E865.3	E950.9	E962.1	E980.9	LABURNUM (FLOWERS) (SEEDS)
988.2		E865.4	E950.9	E962.1	E980.9	LABURNUM LEAVES
989.89		E861.6	E950.9	E962.1	E980.9	LACQUERS
987.5		E869.3	E952.8	E962.2	E982.8	LACRIMOGENIC GAS
983.1		E864.1	E950.7	E962.1	E980.6	LACTIC ACID
973.5	E943.5	E858.4	E950.4	E962.0	E980.4	LACTOBACILLUS ACIDOPHILUS
963.5	E933.5	E858.1	E950.4	E962.0	E980.4	LACTOFLAVIN
967.8	E937.8	E852.8	E950.2	E962.0	E980.2	LACTUCA (VIROSA) (EXTRACT)
967.8	E937.8	E852.8	E950.2	E962.0	E980.2	LACTUCARIUM
974.5	E944.5	E858.5	E950.4	E962.0	E980.4	LAEVULOSE
972.1	E942.1	E858.3	E950.4	E962.0	E980.4	LANATOSIDE(C)
976.3	E946.3	E858.7	E950.4	E962.0	E980.4	LANOLIN (LOTION)
969.1	E939.1	E853.0	E950.3	E962.0	E980.3	LARGACTIL
988.2		E865.3	E950.9	E962.1	E980.9	LARKSPUR
969.0	E939.0	E854.0	E950.3	E962.0	E980.3	LAROXYL

POISON	THERA-PEUTIC	ACCIDENT	SUICIDE	ASSAULT	UNDETER-MINED	SUBSTANCE
974.4	E944.4	E858.5	E950.4	E962.0	E980.4	LASIX
909.0						LATE EFFECT DRUG MEDICINAL OR BIOLOGICAL SUBSTANCE
989.82		E866.8	E950.9	E962.1	E980.9	LATEX
988.2		E865.3	E950.9	E962.1	E980.9	LATHYRUS (SEED)
965.09	E935.2	E850.2	E950.0	E962.0	E980.0	LAUDANUM
975.2	E945.2	E858.6	E950.4	E962.0	E980.4	LAUDEXIUM
988.2		E865.4	E950.9	E962.1	E980.9	LAUREL BLACK OR CHERRY
976.0	E946.0	E858.7	E950.4	E962.0	E980.4	LAUROLINIUM
976.2	E946.2	E858.7	E950.4	E962.0	E980.4	LAURYL SULFOACETATE
973.2	E943.2	E858.4	E950.4	E962.0	E980.4	LAXATIVES EMOLLIENT
973.3	E943.3	E858.4	E950.4	E962.0	E980.4	LAXATIVES NEC
984.9		E866.0	E950.9	E962.1	E980.9	LEAD (DUST) (FUMES) (VAPOR) NEC
984.1		E866.0	E950.9	E962.1	E980.9	LEAD ACETATE (DUST)
961.2	E931.2	E857	E950.4	E962.0	E980.4	LEAD ANTI-INFECTIVES
984.1		E862.1	E950.9	E962.1	E980.9	LEAD ANTIKNOCK COMPOUND (TETRAETHYL)
985.1		E863.4	E950.8	E962.1	E980.8	LEAD ARSENATE (DUST)(INSECTICIDE) (VAPOR)
985.1		E863.5	E950.8	E962.1	E980.8	LEAD ARSENATE HERBICIDE
984.0		E866.0	E950.9	E962.1	E980.9	LEAD CARBONATE
984.0		E861.5	E950.9	E962.1	E980.9	LEAD CARBONATE PAINT
984.0		E866.0	E950.9	E962.1	E980.9	LEAD CHROMATE
984.0		E861.5	E950.9	E962.1	E980.9	LEAD CHROMATE PAINT
984.0		E866.0	E950.9	E962.1	E980.9	LEAD DIOXIDE
984.0		E866.0	E950.9	E962.1	E980.9	LEAD INORGANIC (COMPOUND)
984.0		E861.5	E950.9	E962.1	E980.9	LEAD INORGANIC PAINT
984.0		E866.0	E950.9	E962.1	E980.9	LEAD IODIDE
984.0		E861.5	E950.9	E962.1	E980.9	LEAD IODIDE PIGMENT (PAINT)
984.0		E866.0	E950.9	E962.1	E980.9	LEAD MONOXIDE (DUST)
984.0		E861.5	E950.9	E962.1	E980.9	LEAD MONOXIDE PAINT
984.1		E866.0	E950.9	E962.1	E980.9	LEAD ORGANIC
984.0		E866.0	E950.9	E962.1	E980.9	LEAD OXIDE
984.0		E861.5	E950.9	E962.1	E980.9	LEAD OXIDE PAINT
984.0		E861.5	E950.9	E962.1	E980.9	LEAD PAINT
984.0		E866.0	E950.9	E962.1	E980.9	LEAD SALTS
984.8		E866.0	E950.9	E962.1	E980.9	LEAD SPECIFIED COMPOUND NEC
984.1		E862.1	E950.9	E962.1	E980.9	LEAD TETRA-ETHYL
969.6	E939.6	E854.1	E950.3	E962.0	E980.3	LEBANESE RED
962.3	E932.3	E858.0	E950.4	E962.0	E980.4	LENTE ILETIN (INSULIN)
970.0	E940.0	E854.3	E950.4	E962.0	E980.4	LEPTAZOL
965.09	E935.2	E850.2	E950.0	E962.0	E980.0	LERITINE
962.7	E932.7	E858.0	E950.4	E962.0	E980.4	LETTER
967.8	E937.8	E852.8	E950.2	E962.0	E980.2	LETTUCE OPIUM
964.1	E934.1	E858.2	E950.4	E962.0	E980.4	LEUCOVORIN (FACTOR)
963.1	E933.1	E858.1	E950.4	E962.0	E980.4	LEUKERAN
975.7	E945.7	E858.6	E950.4	E962.0	E980.4	LEVALBUTEROL
970.1	E940.1	E854.3	E950.4	E962.0	E980.4	LEVALLORPHAN
967.8	E937.8	E852.8	E950.2	E962.0	E980.2	LEVANIL
971.2	E941.2	E855.5	E950.4	E962.0	E980.4	LEVARTERENOL (NORADRENALIN)
965.09	E935.2	E850.2	E950.0	E962.0	E980.0	LEVO-DROMORAN
965.02	E935.1	E850.1	E950.0	E962.0	E980.0	LEVO-ISO-METHADONE
966.4	E936.4	E855.0	E950.4	E962.0	E980.4	LEVODOPA (L-DOPA)
962.7	E932.7	E858.0	E950.4	E962.0	E980.4	LEVOID
967.8	E937.8	E852.8	E950.2	E962.0	E980.2	LEVOMEPROMAZINE
967.8	E937.8	E852.8	E950.2	E962.0	E980.2	LEVOPROME
975.4	E945.4	E858.6	E950.4	E962.0	E980.4	LEVOPROPOXYPHENE
965.09	E935.2	E850.2	E950.0	E962.0	E980.0	LEVORPHAN
962.7	E932.7	E858.0	E950.4	E962.0	E980.4	LEVOTHYROXINE (SODIUM)
971.1	E941.1	E855.4	E950.4	E962.0	E980.4	LEVSIN
974.5	E944.5	E858.5	E950.4	E962.0	E980.4	LEVULOSE
985.1		E866.3	E950.8	E962.1	E980.8	LEWISITE (GAS)
969.4	E939.4	E853.2	E950.3	E962.0	E980.3	LIBRIUM
976.0	E946.0	E858.7	E950.4	E962.0	E980.4	LIDEX
968.5	E938.5	E855.2	E950.4	E962.0	E980.4	LIDOCAINE (LIGNOCAINE)
968.5	E938.5	E855.2	E950.4	E962.0	E980.4	LIDOCAINE (INFILTRATION) (TOPICAL)
968.6	E938.6	E855.2	E950.4	E962.0	E980.4	LIDOCAINE NERVE BLOCK (PERIPHERAL) (PLEXUS)
968.7	E938.7	E855.2	E950.4	E962.0	E980.4	LIDOCAINE SPINAL
981		E862.1	E950.9	E962.1	E980.9	LIGHTER FLUID
968.5	E938.5	E855.2	E950.4	E962.0	E980.4	LIGNOCAINE
968.5	E938.5	E855.2	E950.4	E962.0	E980.4	LIGNOCAINE (INFILTRATION) (TOPICAL)
968.6	E938.6	E855.2	E950.4	E962.0	E980.4	LIGNOCAINE NERVE BLOCK (PERIPHERAL) (PLEXUS)
968.7	E938.7	E855.2	E950.4	E962.0	E980.4	LIGNOCAINE SPINAL

POISON	THERA-PEUTIC	ACCIDENT	SUICIDE	ASSAULT	UNDETER-MINED	SUBSTANCE
981		E862.0	E950.9	E962.1	E980.9	LIGROIN(E) SOLVENT
987.1		E869.8	E952.8	E962.2	E982.8	LIGROIN(E) VAPOR
988.2		E865.3	E950.9	E962.1	E980.9	LIGUSTRUM VULGARE
988.2		E865.4	E950.9	E962.1	E980.9	LILY OF THE VALLEY
983.2		E864.2	E950.7	E962.1	E980.6	LIME (CHLORIDE)
976.4	E946.4	E858.7	E950.4	E962.0	E980.4	LIME SOLUTION SULFERATED
982.8		E862.4	E950.9	E962.1	E980.9	LIMONENE
960.8	E930.8	E856	E950.4	E962.0	E980.4	LINCOMYCIN
989.2		E863.0	E950.6	E962.1	E980.7	LINDANE (INSECTICIDE) (VAPOR)
976.0	E946.0	E858.7	E950.4	E962.0	E980.4	LINDANE ANTI-INFECTIVE (TOPICAL)
976.9	E946.9	E858.7	E950.4	E962.0	E980.4	LINIMENTS NEC
972.2	E942.2	E858.3	E950.4	E962.0	E980.4	LINOLEIC ACID
962.7	E932.7	E858.0	E950.4	E962.0	E980.4	LIOTHYRONINE
962.7	E932.7	E858.0	E950.4	E962.0	E980.4	LIOTRIX
973.4	E943.4	E858.4	E950.4	E962.0	E980.4	LIPANCREATIN
962.2	E932.2	E858.0	E950.4	E962.0	E980.4	LIPO-LUTIN
977.1	E947.1	E858.8	E950.4	E962.0	E980.4	LIPOTROPIC DRUGS
987.0		E867	E951.0	E962.2	E981.0	LIQUEFIED PETROLEUM GASES PIPED (PURE OR MIXED WITH AIR)
987.0		E868.0	E951.1	E962.2	E981.1	LIQUEFIED PETROLEUM GASES
973.2	E943.2	E858.4	E950.4	E962.0	E980.4	LIQUID PETROLATUM
989.89		E866.8	E950.9	E962.1	E980.9	LIQUID SUBSTANCE SPECIFIED NEC
989.9		E866.9	E950.9	E962.1	E980.9	LIQUID SUBSTANCE
979.4	E949.4	E858.8	E950.4	E962.0	E980.4	LIRUGEN
969.8	E939.8	E855.8	E950.3	E962.0	E980.3	LITHANE
985.8		E866.4	E950.9	E962.1	E980.9	LITHIUM
969.8	E939.8	E855.8	E950.3	E962.0	E980.3	LITHIUM CARBONATE
969.8	E939.8	E855.8	E950.3	E962.0	E980.3	LITHONATE
964.1	E934.1	E858.2	E950.4	E962.0	E980.4	LIVER (EXTRACT) (INJECTION) (PREPARATIONS)
989.5		E905.0	E950.9	E962.1	E980.9	LIZARD (BITE) (VENOM)
964.8	E934.8	E858.2	E950.4	E962.0	E980.4	LMD
988.2		E865.4	E950.9	E962.1	E980.9	LOBELIA
970.0	E940.0	E854.3	E950.4	E962.0	E980.4	LOBELINE
976.0	E946.0	E858.7	E950.4	E962.0	E980.4	LOCAL ANTI-INFECTIVES NEC
976.0	E946.0	E858.7	E950.4	E962.0	E980.4	LOCORTEN
988.2		E865.3	E950.9	E962.1	E980.9	LOLIUM TEMULENTUM
973.5	E943.5	E858.4	E950.4	E962.0	E980.4	LOMOTIL
963.1	E933.1	E858.1	E950.4	E962.0	E980.4	LOMUSTINE
969.6	E939.6	E854.1	E950.3	E962.0	E980.3	LOPHOPHORA WILLIAMSII
969.4	E939.4	E853.2	E950.3	E962.0	E980.3	LORAZEPAM
976.9	E946.9	E858.7	E950.4	E962.0	E980.4	LOTIONS NEC
973.8	E943.8	E858.4	E950.4	E962.0	E980.4	LOTRONEX
967.0	E937.0	E851	E950.1	E962.0	E980.1	LOTUSATE
976.2	E946.2	E858.7	E950.4	E962.0	E980.4	LOWILA
969.3	E939.3	E853.8	E950.3	E962.0	E980.3	LOXAPINE
976.6	E946.6	E858.7	E950.4	E962.0	E980.4	LOZENGES (THROAT)
969.6	E939.6	E854.1	E950.3	E962.0	E980.3	LSD (25)
981		E862.2	E950.9	E962.1	E980.9	LUBRICATING OIL NEC
961.6	E931.6	E857	E950.4	E962.0	E980.4	LUCANTHONE
967.0	E937.0	E851	E950.1	E962.0	E980.1	LUMINAL
987.9		E869.9	E952.9	E962.2	E982.9	LUNG IRRITANT (GAS) NEC
962.2	E932.2	E858.0	E950.4	E962.0	E980.4	LUTOCYLOL
962.2	E932.2	E858.0	E950.4	E962.0	E980.4	LUTROMONE
975.0	E945.0	E858.6	E950.4	E962.0	E980.4	LUTUTRIN
983.2		E864.2	E950.7	E962.1	E980.6	LYE (CONCENTRATED)
977.8	E947.8	E858.8	E950.4	E962.0	E980.4	LYGRANUM (SKIN TEST)
960.4	E930.4	E856	E950.4	E962.0	E980.4	LYMECYCLINE
977.8	E947.8	E858.8	E950.4	E962.0	E980.4	LYMPHOGRANULOMA VENEREUM ANTIGEN
962.2	E932.2	E858.0	E950.4	E962.0	E980.4	LYNESTRENOL
974.4	E944.4	E858.5	E950.4	E962.0	E980.4	LYOVAC SODIUM EDECRIN
962.5	E932.5	E858.0	E950.4	E962.0	E980.4	LYPRESSIN
969.6	E939.6	E854.1	E950.3	E962.0	E980.3	LYSERGIC ACID (AMIDE) (DIETHYLAMIDE)
969.6	E939.6	E854.1	E950.3	E962.0	E980.3	LYSERGIDE (LSD)
962.5	E932.5	E858.0	E950.4	E962.0	E980.4	LYSINE VASOPRESSIN
983.0		E864.0	E950.7	E962.1	E980.6	LYSOL
976.8	E946.8	E858.7	E950.4	E962.0	E980.4	LYTTA (VITATTA)
979.4	E949.4	E858.8	E950.4	E962.0	E980.4	M-VAC
987.5		E869.3	E952.8	E962.2	E982.8	MACE
960.3	E930.3	E856	E950.4	E962.0	E980.4	MACROLIDES (ANTIBIOTICS)
964.8	E934.8	E858.2	E950.4	E962.0	E980.4	MACROMOLECULAR BLOOD SUBSTITUTES
976.0	E946.0	E858.7	E950.4	E962.0	E980.4	MAFENIDE
973.0	E943.0	E858.4	E950.4	E962.0	E980.4	MAGALDRATE

DRUGS & CHEMICALS

POISON	THERA-PEUTIC	ACCIDENT	SUICIDE	ASSAULT	UNDETER-MINED	SUBSTANCE
969.6	E939.6	E854.1	E950.3	E962.0	E980.3	MAGIC MUSHROOM
960.8	E930.8	E856	E950.4	E962.0	E980.4	MAGNAMYCIN
973.0	E943.0	E858.4	E950.4	E962.0	E980.4	MAGNESIA MAGMA
985.8		E866.4	E950.9	E962.1	E980.9	MAGNESIUM (COMPOUNDS) (FUMES) NEC
973.0	E943.0	E858.4	E950.4	E962.0	E980.4	MAGNESIUM ANTACID
973.0	E943.0	E858.4	E950.4	E962.0	E980.4	MAGNESIUM CARBONATE
973.3	E943.3	E858.4	E950.4	E962.0	E980.4	MAGNESIUM CATHARTIC
973.3	E943.3	E858.4	E950.4	E962.0	E980.4	MAGNESIUM CITRATE
973.0	E943.0	E858.4	E950.4	E962.0	E980.4	MAGNESIUM HYDROXIDE
973.0	E943.0	E858.4	E950.4	E962.0	E980.4	MAGNESIUM OXIDE
973.3	E943.3	E858.4	E950.4	E962.0	E980.4	MAGNESIUM SULFATE (ORAL)
966.3	E936.3	E855.0	E950.4	E962.0	E980.4	MAGNESIUM SULFATE INTRAVENOUS
973.0	E943.0	E858.4	E950.4	E962.0	E980.4	MAGNESIUM TRISILICATE
989.3		E863.1	E950.6	E962.1	E980.7	MALATHION (INSECTICIDE)
961.6	E931.6	E857	E950.4	E962.0	E980.4	MALE FERN (OLEORESIN)
961.9	E931.9	E857	E950.4	E962.0	E980.4	MANDELIC ACID
985.2		E866.4	E950.9	E962.1	E980.9	MANGANESE COMPOUNDS (FUMES) NEC
974.4	E944.4	E858.5	E950.4	E962.0	E980.4	MANNITOL (DIURETIC) (MEDICINAL) NEC
972.4	E942.4	E858.3	E950.4	E962.0	E980.4	MANNITOL HEXANITRATE
963.1	E933.1	E858.1	E950.4	E962.0	E980.4	MANNITOL MUSTARD
963.1	E933.1	E858.1	E950.4	E962.0	E980.4	MANNOMUSTINE
969.0	E939.0	E854.0	E950.3	E962.0	E980.3	MAO INHIBITORS
961.1	E931.1	E857	E950.4	E962.0	E980.4	MAPHARSEN
968.9	E938.9	E855.2	E950.4	E962.0	E980.4	MARCAINE
968.5	E938.5	E855.2	E950.4	E962.0	E980.4	MARCAINE INFILTRATION (SUBCUTANEOUS)
968.6	E938.6	E855.2	E950.4	E962.0	E980.4	MARCAINE NERVE BLOCK (PERIPHERAL) (PLEXUS)
963.0	E933.0	E858.1	E950.4	E962.0	E980.4	MAREZINE
969.6	E939.6	E854.1	E950.3	E962.0	E980.3	MARIHUANA (DERIVATIVES)
989.5		E905.6	E950.9	E962.1	E980.9	MARINE ANIMALS OR PLANTS (STING)
969.0	E939.0	E854.0	E950.3	E962.0	E980.3	MARPLAN
987.1		E869.8	E952.8	E962.2	E982.8	MARSH GAS
969.0	E939.0	E854.0	E950.3	E962.0	E980.3	MARSILID
963.1	E933.1	E858.1	E950.4	E962.0	E980.4	MATULANE
977.0	E947.0	E858.8	E950.4	E962.0	E980.4	MAZINDOL
969.7	E939.7	E854.2	E950.3	E962.0	E980.3	MDMA
988.2		E865.3	E950.9	E962.1	E980.9	MEADOW SAFFRON
979.4	E949.4	E858.8	E950.4	E962.0	E980.4	MEASLES VACCINE
988.8		E865.0	E950.9	E962.1	E980.9	MEAT NOXIOUS OR NONBACTERIAL
969.0	E939.0	E854.0	E950.3	E962.0	E980.3	MEBANAZINE
967.0	E937.0	E851	E950.1	E962.0	E980.1	MEBARAL
961.6	E931.6	E857	E950.4	E962.0	E980.4	MEBENDAZOLE
975.1	E945.1	E858.6	E950.4	E962.0	E980.4	MEBEVERINE
963.0	E933.0	E858.1	E950.4	E962.0	E980.4	MEBHYDROLINE
963.0	E933.0	E858.1	E950.4	E962.0	E980.4	MEBROPHENHYDRAMINE
969.5	E939.5	E853.8	E950.3	E962.0	E980.3	MEBUTAMATE
972.3	E942.3	E858.3	E950.4	E962.0	E980.4	MECAMYLAMINE (CHLORIDE)
963.1	E933.1	E858.1	E950.4	E962.0	E980.4	MECHLORETHAMINE HYDROCHLORIDE
963.0	E933.0	E858.1	E950.4	E962.0	E980.4	MECLIZENE (HYDROCHLORIDE)
970.0	E940.0	E854.3	E950.4	E962.0	E980.4	MECLOFENOXATE
963.0	E933.0	E858.1	E950.4	E962.0	E980.4	MECLOZINE (HYDROCHLORIDE)
969.4	E939.4	E853.2	E950.3	E962.0	E980.3	MEDAZEPAM
977.9	E947.9	E858.9	E950.5	E962.0	E980.5	MEDICINE UNSPECIFIED
977.8	E947.8	E858.8	E950.4	E962.0	E980.4	MEDICINE SPECIFIED NEC
967.0	E937.0	E851	E950.1	E962.0	E980.1	MEDINAL
967.0	E937.0	E851	E950.1	E962.0	E980.1	MEDOMIN
962.2	E932.2	E858.0	E950.4	E962.0	E980.4	MEDROXYPROGESTERONE
976.5	E946.5	E858.7	E950.4	E962.0	E980.4	MEDRYSONE
965.7	E935.7	E850.7	E950.0	E962.0	E980.0	MEFENAMIC ACID
969.6	E939.6	E854.1	E950.3	E962.0	E980.3	MEGAHALLUCINOGEN
962.2	E932.2	E858.0	E950.4	E962.0	E980.4	MEGESTROL
977.8	E947.8	E858.8	E950.4	E962.0	E980.4	MEGLUMINE
976.3	E946.3	E858.7	E950.4	E962.0	E980.4	MELANIZING AGENTS
961.1	E931.1	E857	E950.4	E962.0	E980.4	MELARSOPROL
988.2		E865.3	E950.9	E962.1	E980.9	MELIA AZEDARACH
969.1	E939.1	E853.0	E950.3	E962.0	E980.3	MELLARIL
976.3	E946.3	E858.7	E950.4	E962.0	E980.4	MELOXINE
963.1	E933.1	E858.1	E950.4	E962.0	E980.4	MELPHALAN
964.3	E934.3	E858.2	E950.4	E962.0	E980.4	MENADIOL SODIUM DIPHOSPHATE
964.3	E934.3	E858.2	E950.4	E962.0	E980.4	MENADIONE (SODIUM BISULFITE)
964.3	E934.3	E858.2	E950.4	E962.0	E980.4	MENAPHTHONE
978.8	E948.8	E858.8	E950.4	E962.0	E980.4	MENINGOCOCCAL VACCINE
978.8	E948.8	E858.8	E950.4	E962.0	E980.4	MENNINGOVAX-C

POISON	THERA-PEUTIC	ACCIDENT	SUICIDE	ASSAULT	UNDETER-MINED	SUBSTANCE
962.4	E932.4	E858.0	E950.4	E962.0	E980.4	MENOTROPINS
976.1	E946.1	E858.7	E950.4	E962.0	E980.4	MENTHOL NEC
961.3	E931.3	E857	E950.4	E962.0	E980.4	MEPACRINE
967.8	E937.8	E852.8	E950.2	E962.0	E980.2	MEPARFYNOL
969.1	E939.1	E853.0	E950.3	E962.0	E980.3	MEPAZINE
971.1	E941.1	E855.4	E950.4	E962.0	E980.4	MEPENZOLATE
965.09	E935.2	E850.2	E950.0	E962.0	E980.0	MEPERIDINE (PETHIDINE)
966.4	E936.4	E855.0	E950.4	E962.0	E980.4	MEPHENAMIN(E)
968.0	E938.0	E855.1	E950.4	E962.0	E980.4	MEPHENESIN (CARBAMATE)
969.5	E939.5	E853.8	E950.3	E962.0	E980.3	MEPHENOXALONE
971.2	E941.2	E855.5	E950.4	E962.0	E980.4	MEPHENTERMINE
966.1	E936.1	E855.0	E950.4	E962.0	E980.4	MEPHENYTOIN
967.0	E937.0	E851	E950.1	E962.0	E980.1	MEPHOBARBITAL
971.1	E941.1	E855.4	E950.4	E962.0	E980.4	MEPIPERPHENIDOL
968.9	E938.9	E855.2	E950.4	E962.0	E980.4	MEPIVACAINE
968.5	E938.5	E855.2	E950.4	E962.0	E980.4	MEPIVACAINE INFILTRATION (SUBCUTANEOUS)
968.6	E938.6	E855.2	E950.4	E962.0	E980.4	MEPIVACAINE NERVE BLOCK (PERIPHERAL) (PLEXUS)
968.5	E938.5	E855.2	E950.4	E962.0	E980.4	MEPIVACAINE TOPICAL (SURFACE)
962.0	E932.0	E858.0	E950.4	E962.0	E980.4	MEPREDNISONE
969.5	E939.5	E853.8	E950.3	E962.0	E980.3	MEPROBAM
969.5	E939.5	E853.8	E950.3	E962.0	E980.3	MEPROBAMATE
963.0	E933.0	E858.1	E950.4	E962.0	E980.4	MEPYRAMINE (MALEATE)
974.0	E944.0	E858.5	E950.4	E962.0	E980.4	MERALLURIDE
974.0	E944.0	E858.5	E950.4	E962.0	E980.4	MERBAPHEN
976.0	E946.0	E858.7	E950.4	E962.0	E980.4	MERBROMIN
974.0	E944.0	E858.5	E950.4	E962.0	E980.4	MERCAPTOMERIN
963.1	E933.1	E858.1	E950.4	E962.0	E980.4	MERCAPTOPURINE
974.0	E944.0	E858.5	E950.4	E962.0	E980.4	MERCUMATILIN
974.0	E944.0	E858.5	E950.4	E962.0	E980.4	MERCURAMIDE
976.0	E946.0	E858.7	E950.4	E962.0	E980.4	MERCURANIN
976.0	E946.0	E858.7	E950.4	E962.0	E980.4	MERCUROCHROME
985.0		E866.1	E950.9	E962.1	E980.9	MERCURY (COMPOUNDS) (CYANIDE) (FUMES) (NONMEDICI-NAL) (VAPOR) NEC
976.0	E946.0	E858.7	E950.4	E962.0	E980.4	MERCURY AMMONIATED
961.2	E931.2	E857	E950.4	E962.0	E980.4	MERCURY ANTI-INFECTIVE
976.0	E946.0	E858.7	E950.4	E962.0	E980.4	MERCURY ANTI-INFECTIVE TOPICAL
976.0	E946.0	E858.7	E950.4	E962.0	E980.4	MERCURY CHLORIDE (ANTISEPTIC) NEC
985.0		E863.6	E950.6	E962.1	E980.7	MERCURY CHLORIDE FUNGICIDE
974.0	E944.0	E858.5	E950.4	E962.0	E980.4	MERCURY DIURETIC COMPOUNDS
985.0		E863.6	E950.6	E962.1	E980.7	MERCURY FUNGICIDE
985.0		E863.6	E950.6	E962.1	E980.7	MERCURY ORGANIC (FUNGICIDE)
974.0	E944.0	E858.5	E950.4	E962.0	E980.4	MERETHOXYLLINE
974.0	E944.0	E858.5	E950.4	E962.0	E980.4	MERSALYL
976.0	E946.0	E858.7	E950.4	E962.0	E980.4	MERTHIOLATE (TOPICAL)
976.5	E946.5	E858.7	E950.4	E962.0	E980.4	MERTHIOLATE OPHTHALMIC PREPARATION
979.4	E949.4	E858.8	E950.4	E962.0	E980.4	MERUVAX
969.6	E939.6	E854.1	E950.3	E962.0	E980.3	MESCAL BUTTONS
969.6	E939.6	E854.1	E950.3	E962.0	E980.3	MESCALINE (SALTS)
969.1	E939.1	E853.0	E950.3	E962.0	E980.3	MESORIDAZINE BESYLATE
962.1	E932.1	E858.0	E950.4	E962.0	E980.4	MESTANOLONE
962.2	E932.2	E858.0	E950.4	E962.0	E980.4	MESTRANOL
976.0	E946.0	E858.7	E950.4	E962.0	E980.4	METACRESYLACETATE
989.4		E863.4	E950.6	E962.1	E980.7	METALDEHYDE (SNAIL KILLER) NEC
985.9		E866.4	E950.9	E962.1	E980.9	METALS (HEAVY) (NONMEDICINAL) NEC
985.9		E866.4	E950.9	E962.1	E980.9	METALS DUST FUMES OR VAPOR NEC
985.9		E866.4	E950.9	E962.1	E980.9	METALS LIGHT DUST FUMES OR VAPOR NEC
985.9		E866.4	E950.9	E962.1	E980.9	METALS LIGHT NEC
985.9		E863.4	E950.6	E962.1	E980.7	METALS PESTICIDES (DUST) (VAPOR)
973.3	E943.3	E858.4	E950.4	E962.0	E980.4	METAMUCIL
976.0	E946.0	E858.7	E950.4	E962.0	E980.4	METAPHEN
975.1	E945.1	E858.6	E950.4	E962.0	E980.4	METAPROTERENOL (ORCIPRENALINE)
972.8	E942.8	E858.3	E950.4	E962.0	E980.4	METARAMINOL
968.0	E938.0	E855.1	E950.4	E962.0	E980.4	METAXALONE
962.3	E932.3	E858.0	E950.4	E962.0	E980.4	METFORMIN
960.4	E930.4	E856	E950.4	E962.0	E980.4	METHACYCLINE
965.02	E935.1	E850.1	E950.0	E962.0	E980.0	METHADONE
962.2	E932.2	E858.0	E950.4	E962.0	E980.4	METHALLENESTRIL
969.7	E939.7	E854.2	E950.3	E962.0	E980.3	METHAMPHETAMINE
962.1	E932.1	E858.0	E950.4	E962.0	E980.4	METHANDIENONE
962.1	E932.1	E858.0	E950.4	E962.0	E980.4	METHANDRIOL

POISON	THERA-PEUTIC	ACCIDENT	SUICIDE	ASSAULT	UNDETER-MINED	SUBSTANCE
962.1	E932.1	E858.0	E950.4	E962.0	E980.4	METHANDROSTENOLONE
987.1		E869.8	E952.8	E962.2	E982.8	METHANE GAS
980.1		E860.2	E950.9	E962.1	E980.9	METHANOL
987.8		E869.8	E952.8	E962.2	E982.8	METHANOL VAPOR
971.1	E941.1	E855.4	E950.4	E962.0	E980.4	METHANTHELINE
963.0	E933.0	E858.1	E950.4	E962.0	E980.4	METHAPHENILENE
963.0	E933.0	E858.1	E950.4	E962.0	E980.4	METHAPYRILENE
967.4	E937.4	E852.3	E950.2	E962.0	E980.2	METHAQUALONE (COMPOUNDS)
967.0	E937.0	E851	E950.1	E962.0	E980.1	METHARBITAL
974.2	E944.2	E858.5	E950.4	E962.0	E980.4	METHAZOLAMIDE
963.0	E933.0	E858.1	E950.4	E962.0	E980.4	METHDILAZINE
969.7	E939.7	E854.2	E950.3	E962.0	E980.3	METHEDRINE
961.9	E931.9	E857	E950.4	E962.0	E980.4	METHENAMINE (MANDELATE)
962.1	E932.1	E858.0	E950.4	E962.0	E980.4	METHENOLONE
975.0	E945.0	E858.6	E950.4	E962.0	E980.4	METHERGINE
962.8	E932.8	E858.0	E950.4	E962.0	E980.4	METHIACIL
960.0	E930.0	E856	E950.4	E962.0	E980.4	METHICILLIN (SODIUM)
962.8	E932.8	E858.0	E950.4	E962.0	E980.4	METHIMAZOLE
977.1	E947.1	E858.8	E950.4	E962.0	E980.4	METHIONINE
961.7	E931.7	E857	E950.4	E962.0	E980.4	METHISAZONE
967.0	E937.0	E851	E950.1	E962.0	E980.1	METHITURAL
971.1	E941.1	E855.4	E950.4	E962.0	E980.4	METHIXENE
967.0	E937.0	E851	E950.1	E962.0	E980.1	METHOBARBITAL
968.0	E938.0	E855.1	E950.4	E962.0	E980.4	METHOCARBAMOL
968.3	E938.3	E855.1	E950.4	E962.0	E980.4	METHOHEXITAL (METHOHEXITONE)
966.1	E936.1	E855.0	E950.4	E962.0	E980.4	METHOIN
965.7	E935.7	E850.7	E950.0	E962.0	E980.0	METHOPHOLINE
975.4	E945.4	E858.6	E950.4	E962.0	E980.4	METHORATE
972.6	E942.6	E858.3	E950.4	E962.0	E980.4	METHOSERPIDINE
963.1	E933.1	E858.1	E950.4	E962.0	E980.4	METHOTREXATE
967.8	E937.8	E852.8	E950.2	E962.0	E980.2	METHOTRIMEPRAZINE
976.3	E946.3	E858.7	E950.4	E962.0	E980.4	METHOXA-DOME
971.2	E941.2	E855.5	E950.4	E962.0	E980.4	METHOXAMINE
976.3	E946.3	E858.7	E950.4	E962.0	E980.4	METHOXSALEN
960.0	E930.0	E856	E950.4	E962.0	E980.4	METHOXYBENZYL PENICILLIN
989.2		E863.0	E950.6	E962.1	E980.7	METHOXYCHLOR
968.2	E938.2	E855.1	E950.4	E962.0	E980.4	METHOXYFLURANE
971.2	E941.2	E855.5	E950.4	E962.0	E980.4	METHOXYPHENAMINE
969.1	E939.1	E853.0	E950.3	E962.0	E980.3	METHOXYPROMAZINE
976.3	E946.3	E858.7	E950.4	E962.0	E980.4	METHOXYPSORALEN
971.1	E941.1	E855.4	E950.4	E962.0	E980.4	METHSCOPOLAMINE (BROMIDE)
966.2	E936.2	E855.0	E950.4	E962.0	E980.4	METHSUXIMIDE
974.3	E944.3	E858.5	E950.4	E962.0	E980.4	METHYCLOTHIAZIDE
982.8		E862.4	E950.9	E962.1	E980.9	METHYL ACETATE
982.8		E862.4	E950.9	E962.1	E980.9	METHYL ACETONE
980.1		E860.2	E950.9	E962.1	E980.9	METHYL ALCOHOL
969.7	E939.7	E854.2	E950.3	E962.0	E980.3	METHYL AMPHETAMINE
962.1	E932.1	E858.0	E950.4	E962.0	E980.4	METHYL ANDROSTANOLONE
971.1	E941.1	E855.4	E950.4	E962.0	E980.4	METHYL ATROPINE
982.0		E862.4	E950.9	E962.1	E980.9	METHYL BENZENE
987.8		E869.8	E952.8	E962.2	E982.8	METHYL BROMIDE (GAS)
987.8		E863.8	E950.6	E962.2	E980.7	METHYL BROMIDE FUMIGANT
980.8		E860.8	E950.9	E962.1	E980.9	METHYL BUTANOL
980.1		E860.2	E950.9	E962.1	E980.9	METHYL CARBINOL
982.8		E862.4	E950.9	E962.1	E980.9	METHYL CELLOSOLVE
973.3	E943.3	E858.4	E950.4	E962.0	E980.4	METHYL CELLULOSE
987.8		E869.8	E952.8	E962.2	E982.8	METHYL CHLORIDE (GAS)
982.8		E862.4	E950.9	E962.1	E980.9	METHYL CYCLOHEXANE
982.8		E862.4	E950.9	E962.1	E980.9	METHYL CYCLOHEXANONE
965.09	E935.2	E850.2	E950.0	E962.0	E980.0	METHYL DIHYDROMORPHINONE
975.0	E945.0	E858.6	E950.4	E962.0	E980.4	METHYL ERGOMETRINE
975.0	E945.0	E858.6	E950.4	E962.0	E980.4	METHYL ERGONOVINE
982.8		E862.4	E950.9	E962.1	E980.9	METHYL ETHYL KETONE
983.9		E864.3	E950.7	E962.1	E980.6	METHYL HYDRAZINE
982.8		E862.4	E950.9	E962.1	E980.9	METHYL ISOBUTYL KETONE
965.09	E935.2	E850.2	E950.0	E962.0	E980.0	METHYL MORPHINE NEC
967.8	E937.8	E852.8	E950.2	E962.0	E980.2	METHYL PARAFYNOL
989.3		E863.1	E950.6	E962.1	E980.7	METHYL PARATHION
967.8	E937.8	E852.8	E950.2	E962.0	E980.2	METHYL PENTYNOL NEC
969.2	E939.2	E853.1	E950.3	E962.0	E980.3	METHYL PERIDOL
969.7	E939.7	E854.2	E950.3	E962.0	E980.3	METHYL PHENIDATE
962.0	E932.0	E858.0	E950.4	E962.0	E980.4	METHYL PREDNISOLONE
976.6	E946.6	E858.7	E950.4	E962.0	E980.4	METHYL PREDNISOLONE ENT AGENT
976.5	E946.5	E858.7	E950.4	E962.0	E980.4	METHYL PREDNISOLONE OPHTHALMIC PREPARATION

POISON	THERA-PEUTIC	ACCIDENT	SUICIDE	ASSAULT	UNDETER-MINED	SUBSTANCE
976.0	E946.0	E858.7	E950.4	E962.0	E980.4	METHYL PREDNISOLONE TOPICAL NEC
980.8		E860.8	E950.9	E962.1	E980.9	METHYL PROPYLCARBINOL
976.0	E946.0	E858.7	E950.4	E962.0	E980.4	METHYL ROSANILINE NEC
976.3	E946.3	E858.7	E950.4	E962.0	E980.4	METHYL SALICYLATE NEC
987.8		E869.8	E952.8	E962.2	E982.8	METHYL SULFATE (FUMES)
983.9		E864.3	E950.7	E962.1	E980.6	METHYL SULFATE LIQUID
967.8	E937.8	E852.8	E950.2	E962.0	E980.2	METHYL SULFONAL
962.1	E932.1	E858.0	E950.4	E962.0	E980.4	METHYL TESTOSTERONE
962.8	E932.8	E858.0	E950.4	E962.0	E980.4	METHYL THIOURACIL
980.0		E860.1	E950.9	E962.1	E980.9	METHYLATED SPIRIT
972.6	E942.6	E858.3	E950.4	E962.0	E980.4	METHYLDOPA
961.9	E931.9	E857	E950.4	E962.0	E980.4	METHYLENE BLUE
982.3		E862.4	E950.9	E962.1	E980.9	METHYLENE CHLORIDE OR DICHLORIDE (SOLVENT) NEC
967.0	E937.0	E851	E950.1	E962.0	E980.1	METHYLHEXABITAL
976.5	E946.5	E858.7	E950.4	E962.0	E980.4	METHYLPARABEN (OPHTHALMIC)
967.5	E937.5	E852.4	E950.2	E962.0	E980.2	METHYPRYLON
971.3	E941.3	E855.6	E950.4	E962.0	E980.4	METHYSERGIDE
963.0	E933.0	E858.1	E950.4	E962.0	E980.4	METOCLOPRAMIDE
965.7	E935.7	E850.7	E950.0	E962.0	E980.0	METOFOLINE
965.09	E935.2	E850.2	E950.0	E962.0	E980.0	METOPON
961.5	E931.5	E857	E950.4	E962.0	E980.4	METRONIDAZOLE
968.9	E938.9	E855.2	E950.4	E962.0	E980.4	METYCAINE
968.5	E938.5	E855.2	E950.4	E962.0	E980.4	METYCAINE INFILTRATION (SUBCUTANEOUS)
968.6	E938.6	E855.2	E950.4	E962.0	E980.4	METYCAINE NERVE BLOCK (PERIPHERAL) (PLEXUS)
968.5	E938.5	E855.2	E950.4	E962.0	E980.4	METYCAINE TOPICAL (SURFACE)
977.8	E947.8	E858.8	E950.4	E962.0	E980.4	METYRAPONE
989.3		E863.1	E950.6	E962.1	E980.7	MEVINPHOS
988.2		E865.3	E950.9	E962.1	E980.9	MEZEREON (BERRIES)
976.0	E946.0	E858.7	E950.4	E962.0	E980.4	MICATIN
976.0	E946.0	E858.7	E950.4	E962.0	E980.4	MICONAZOLE
965.1	E935.3	E850.3	E950.0	E962.0	E980.0	MIDOL
962.9	E932.9	E858.0	E950.4	E962.0	E980.4	MIFEPRISTONE
973.0	E943.0	E858.4	E950.4	E962.0	E980.4	MILK OF MAGNESIA
989.5		E905.4	E950.9	E962.1	E980.9	MILLIPEDE (TROPICAL) (VENOMOUS)
969.5	E939.5	E853.8	E950.3	E962.0	E980.3	MILTOWN
981		E862.1	E950.9	E962.1	E980.9	MINERAL NONMEDICINAL
973.2	E943.2	E858.4	E950.4	E962.0	E980.4	MINERAL OIL (MEDICINAL)
976.3	E946.3	E858.7	E950.4	E962.0	E980.4	MINERAL OIL TOPICAL
974.6	E944.6	E858.5	E950.4	E962.0	E980.4	MINERAL SALTS NEC OTHER
981		E862.0	E950.9	E962.1	E980.9	MINERAL SPIRITS
960.4	E930.4	E856	E950.4	E962.0	E980.4	MINOCYCLINE
960.7	E930.7	E856	E950.4	E962.0	E980.4	MITHRAMYCIN (ANTINEOPLASTIC)
963.1	E933.1	E858.1	E950.4	E962.0	E980.4	MITOBRONITOL
960.7	E930.7	E856	E950.4	E962.0	E980.4	MITOMYCIN (ANTINEOPLASTIC)
963.1	E933.1	E858.1	E950.4	E962.0	E980.4	MITOTANE
972.6	E942.6	E858.3	E950.4	E962.0	E980.4	MODERIL
969.3	E939.3	E853.8	E950.3	E962.0	E980.3	MOLINDONE
976.0	E946.0	E858.7	E950.4	E962.0	E980.4	MONISTAT
988.2		E865.4	E950.9	E962.1	E980.9	MONKSHOOD
969.0	E939.0	E854.0	E950.3	E962.0	E980.3	MONOAMINE OXIDASE (MAO) INHIBITORS
982.0		E862.4	E950.9	E962.1	E980.9	MONOCHLOROBENZENE
989.89		E866.8	E950.9	E962.1	E980.9	MONOSODIUM GLUTAMATE
0						MONOXIDE CARBON SEE CARBON MONOXIDE
969.2	E939.2	E853.1	E950.3	E962.0	E980.3	MOPERONE
969.6	E939.6	E854.1	E950.3	E962.0	E980.3	MORNING GLORY SEEDS
961.7	E931.7	E857	E950.4	E962.0	E980.4	MOROXYDINE (HYDROCHLORIDE)
961.8	E931.8	E857	E950.4	E962.0	E980.4	MORPHAZINAMIDE
965.09	E935.2	E850.2	E950.0	E962.0	E980.0	MORPHINANS
970.1	E940.1	E854.3	E950.4	E962.0	E980.4	MORPHINE ANTAGONISTS
965.09	E935.2	E850.2	E950.0	E962.0	E980.0	MORPHINE NEC
965.09	E935.2	E850.2	E950.0	E962.0	E980.0	MORPHOLINYLETHYL-MORPHINE
972.7	E942.7	E858.3	E950.4	E962.0	E980.4	MORRHUATE SODIUM
989.4		E863.4	E950.6	E962.1	E980.7	MOTH BALLS
983.0		E863.4	E950.7	E962.1	E980.6	MOTH BALLS NAPHTHALENE
0						MOTOR EXHAUST GAS SEE CARBON MONOXIDE EXHAUST GAS
976.6	E946.6	E858.7	E950.4	E962.0	E980.4	MOUTH WASH
975.5	E945.5	E858.6	E950.4	E962.0	E980.4	MUCOLYTIC AGENT
975.5	E945.5	E858.6	E950.4	E962.0	E980.4	MUCOMYST

DRUGS & CHEMICALS

POISON	THERA-PEUTIC	ACCIDENT	SUICIDE	ASSAULT	UNDETER-MINED	SUBSTANCE
976.9	E946.9	E858.7	E950.4	E962.0	E980.4	MUCOUS MEMBRANE AGENTS (EXTERNAL)
976.8	E946.8	E858.7	E950.4	E962.0	E980.4	MUCOUS MEMBRANE AGENTS SPECIFIED NEC
964.6	E934.6	E858.2	E950.4	E962.0	E980.4	MUMPS IMMUNE GLOBULIN (HUMAN)
977.8	E947.8	E858.8	E950.4	E962.0	E980.4	MUMPS SKIN TEST ANTIGEN
979.6	E949.6	E858.8	E950.4	E962.0	E980.4	MUMPS VACCINE
979.6	E949.6	E858.8	E950.4	E962.0	E980.4	MUMPSVAX
0						MURIATIC ACID SEE HYDROCHLORIC ACID
971.0	E941.0	E855.3	E950.4	E962.0	E980.4	MUSCARINE
975.3	E945.3	E858.6	E950.4	E962.0	E980.4	MUSCLE AFFECTING AGENTS NEC
975.0	E945.0	E858.6	E950.4	E962.0	E980.4	MUSCLE AFFECTING AGENTS OXYTOCIC
975.3	E945.3	E858.6	E950.4	E962.0	E980.4	MUSCLE AFFECTING AGENTS RELAXANTS
975.3	E945.3	E858.6	E950.4	E962.0	E980.4	MUSCLE RELAXANTS
975.1	E945.1	E858.6	E950.4	E962.0	E980.4	MUSCLE RELAXANTS (SMOOTH)
968.0	E938.0	E855.1	E950.4	E962.0	E980.4	MUSCLE RELAXANTS CENTRAL NERVOUS SYSTEM
975.2	E945.2	E858.6	E950.4	E962.0	E980.4	MUSCLE RELAXANTS SKELETAL
988.1		E865.5	E950.9	E962.1	E980.9	MUSHROOMS NOXIOUS
988.0		E865.1	E950.9	E962.1	E980.9	MUSSEL NOXIOUS
973.6	E943.6	E858.4	E950.4	E962.0	E980.4	MUSTARD (EMETIC)
987.8		E869.8	E952.8	E962.2	E982.8	MUSTARD GAS
963.1	E933.1	E858.1	E950.4	E962.0	E980.4	MUSTARD NITROGEN
963.1	E933.1	E858.1	E950.4	E962.0	E980.4	MUSTINE
960.8	E930.8	E856	E950.4	E962.0	E980.4	MYCIFRADIN
976.0	E946.0	E858.7	E950.4	E962.0	E980.4	MYCIFRADIN TOPICAL
960.8	E930.8	E856	E950.4	E962.0	E980.4	MYCITRACIN
976.5	E946.5	E858.7	E950.4	E962.0	E980.4	MYCITRACIN OPHTHALMIC PREPARATION
960.1	E930.1	E856	E950.4	E962.0	E980.4	MYCOSTATIN
976.0	E946.0	E858.7	E950.4	E962.0	E980.4	MYCOSTATIN TOPICAL
971.1	E941.1	E855.4	E950.4	E962.0	E980.4	MYDRIACYL
963.1	E933.1	E858.1	E950.4	E962.0	E980.4	MYELOBROMAL
963.1	E933.1	E858.1	E950.4	E962.0	E980.4	MYLERAN
965.69	E935.6	E850.6	E950.0	E962.0	E980.0	MYOCHRYSIN(E)
975.2	E945.2	E858.6	E950.4	E962.0	E980.4	MYONEURAL BLOCKING AGENTS
988.2		E865.3	E950.9	E962.1	E980.9	MYRISTICA FRAGRANS
988.2		E865.3	E950.9	E962.1	E980.9	MYRISTICIN
966.3	E936.3	E855.0	E950.4	E962.0	E980.4	MYSOLINE
960.0	E930.0	E856	E950.4	E962.0	E980.4	NAFCILLIN (SODIUM)
961.9	E931.9	E857	E950.4	E962.0	E980.4	NALIDIXIC ACID
970.1	E940.1	E854.3	E950.4	E962.0	E980.4	NALORPHINE
970.1	E940.1	E854.3	E950.4	E962.0	E980.4	NALOXONE
962.1	E932.1	E858.0	E950.4	E962.0	E980.4	NANDROLONE (DECANOATE) (PHENPROPRIOATE)
971.2	E941.2	E855.5	E950.4	E962.0	E980.4	NAPHAZOLINE
981		E862.0	E950.9	E962.1	E980.9	NAPHTHA (PAINTER'S) (PETROLEUM)
981		E862.0	E950.9	E962.1	E980.9	NAPHTHA SOLVENT
987.1		E869.8	E952.8	E962.2	E982.8	NAPHTHA VAPOR
983.0		E864.0	E950.7	E962.1	E980.6	NAPHTHALENE (CHLORINATED)
983.0		E863.4	E950.7	E962.1	E980.6	NAPHTHALENE INSECTICIDE OR MOTH REPELLENT
0						NAPHTHALENE SEE NAPHTHALENE
987.8		E869.8	E952.8	E962.2	E982.8	NAPHTHALENE VAPOR
983.0		E864.0	E950.7	E962.1	E980.6	NAPHTHOL
983.0		E864.0	E950.7	E962.1	E980.6	NAPHTHYLAMINE
965.61	E935.6	E850.6	E950.0	E962.0	E980.0	NAPROXEN
967.9	E937.9	E852.9	E950.2	E962.0	E980.2	NARCOTIC (DRUG)
965.8	E935.8	E850.8	E950.0	E962.0	E980.0	NARCOTIC ANALGESIC NEC
970.1	E940.1	E854.3	E950.4	E962.0	E980.4	NARCOTIC ANTAGONIST
967.8	E937.8	E852.8	E950.2	E962.0	E980.2	NARCOTIC SPECIFIED NEC
975.4	E945.4	E858.6	E950.4	E962.0	E980.4	NARCOTINE
969.0	E939.0	E854.0	E950.3	E962.0	E980.3	NARDIL
0						NATRIUM CYANIDE SEE CYANIDE(S)
964.7	E934.7	E858.2	E950.4	E962.0	E980.4	NATURAL BLOOD (PRODUCT)
987.1		E867	E951.0	E962.2	E981.0	NATURAL GAS (PIPED)
986		E867	E951.0	E962.2	E981.0	NATURAL GAS INCOMPLETE COMBUSTION
967.0	E937.0	E851	E950.1	E962.0	E980.1	NEALBARBITAL
975.4	E945.4	E858.6	E950.4	E962.0	E980.4	NECTADON
989.5		E905.6	E950.9	E962.1	E980.9	NEMATOCYST (STING)
967.0	E937.0	E851	E950.1	E962.0	E980.1	NEMBUTAL
961.1	E931.1	E857	E950.4	E962.0	E980.4	NEOARSPHENAMINE

POISON	THERA-PEUTIC	ACCIDENT	SUICIDE	ASSAULT	UNDETER-MINED	SUBSTANCE
974.7	E944.7	E858.5	E950.4	E962.0	E980.4	NEOCINCHOPHEN
960.8	E930.8	E856	E950.4	E962.0	E980.4	NEOMYCIN
976.6	E946.6	E858.7	E950.4	E962.0	E980.4	NEOMYCIN ENT AGENT
976.5	E946.5	E858.7	E950.4	E962.0	E980.4	NEOMYCIN OPHTHALMIC PREPARATION
976.0	E946.0	E858.7	E950.4	E962.0	E980.4	NEOMYCIN TOPICAL NEC
967.0	E937.0	E851	E950.1	E962.0	E980.1	NEONAL
961.0	E931.0	E857	E950.4	E962.0	E980.4	NEOPRONTOSIL
961.1	E931.1	E857	E950.4	E962.0	E980.4	NEOSALVARSAN
961.1	E931.1	E857	E950.4	E962.0	E980.4	NEOSILVERSALVARSAN
960.8	E930.8	E856	E950.4	E962.0	E980.4	NEOSPORIN
976.6	E946.6	E858.7	E950.4	E962.0	E980.4	NEOSPORIN ENT AGENT
976.5	E946.5	E858.7	E950.4	E962.0	E980.4	NEOSPORIN OPHTHALMIC PREPARATION
976.0	E946.0	E858.7	E950.4	E962.0	E980.4	NEOSPORIN TOPICAL NEC
971.0	E941.0	E855.3	E950.4	E962.0	E980.4	NEOSTIGMINE
967.0	E937.0	E851	E950.1	E962.0	E980.1	NERAVAL
967.0	E937.0	E851	E950.1	E962.0	E980.1	NERAVAN
988.2		E865.4	E950.9	E962.1	E980.9	NERIUM OLEANDER
987.9		E869.9	E952.9	E962.2	E982.9	NERVE GASES (WAR)
968.5	E938.5	E855.2	E950.4	E962.0	E980.4	NESACAINE INFILTRATION (SUBCUTANEOUS)
968.9	E938.9	E855.2	E950.4	E962.0	E980.4	NESACAINE
968.6	E938.6	E855.2	E950.4	E962.0	E980.4	NESACAINE NERVE BLOCK (PERIPHERAL) (PLEXUS)
967.0	E937.0	E851	E950.1	E962.0	E980.1	NEUROBARB
969.3	E939.3	E853.8	E950.3	E962.0	E980.3	NEUROLEPTICS NEC
977.8	E947.8	E858.8	E950.4	E962.0	E980.4	NEUROPROTECTIVE AGENT
980.0		E860.1	E950.9	E962.1	E980.9	NEUTRAL SPIRITS
980.0		E860.0	E950.9	E962.1	E980.9	NEUTRAL SPIRITS BEVERAGE
972.2	E942.2	E858.3	E950.4	E962.0	E980.4	NIACIN
969.0	E939.0	E854.0	E950.3	E962.0	E980.3	NIALAMIDE
985.8		E866.4	E950.9	E962.1	E980.9	NICKLE (CARBONYL) (COMPOUNDS) (FUMES) (TETRACARBONYL) (VAPOR)
961.6	E931.6	E857	E950.4	E962.0	E980.4	NICLOSAMIDE
965.09	E935.2	E850.2	E950.0	E962.0	E980.0	NICOMORPHINE
972.2	E942.2	E858.3	E950.4	E962.0	E980.4	NICOTINAMIDE
989.4		E863.4	E950.6	E962.1	E980.7	NICOTINE (INSECTICIDE) (SPRAY) (SULFATE) NEC
989.89		E866.8	E950.9	E962.1	E980.9	NICOTINE NOT INSECTICIDE
972.2	E942.2	E858.3	E950.4	E962.0	E980.4	NICOTINIC ACID (DERIVATIVES)
972.2	E942.2	E858.3	E950.4	E962.0	E980.4	NICOTINYL ALCOHOL
964.2	E934.2	E858.2	E950.4	E962.0	E980.4	NICOUMALONE
965.5	E935.5	E850.5	E950.0	E962.0	E980.0	NIFENAZONE
961.9	E931.9	E857	E950.4	E962.0	E980.4	NIFURALDEZONE
988.2		E865.4	E950.9	E962.1	E980.9	NIGHTSHADE (DEADLY)
970.0	E940.0	E854.3	E950.4	E962.0	E980.4	NIKETHAMIDE
960.1	E930.1	E856	E950.4	E962.0	E980.4	NILSTAT
976.0	E946.0	E858.7	E950.4	E962.0	E980.4	NILSTAT TOPICAL
977.8	E947.8	E858.8	E950.4	E962.0	E980.4	NIMODIPINE
961.6	E931.6	E857	E950.4	E962.0	E980.4	NIRIDAZOLE
965.09	E935.2	E850.2	E950.0	E962.0	E980.0	NISENTIL
972.4	E942.4	E858.3	E950.4	E962.0	E980.4	NITRATES {NITROGLYCERIN}
969.4	E939.4	E853.2	E950.3	E962.0	E980.3	NITRAZEPAM
983.1		E864.1	E950.7	E962.1	E980.6	NITRIC ACID (LIQUID)
987.8		E869.8	E952.8	E962.2	E982.8	NITRIC ACID VAPOR
987.2		E869.0	E952.8	E962.2	E982.8	NITRIC OXIDE (GAS)
972.4	E942.4	E858.3	E950.4	E962.0	E980.4	NITRITE AMYL (MEDICINAL) (VAPOR)
983.0		E864.0	E950.7	E962.1	E980.6	NITROANILINE
987.8		E869.8	E952.8	E962.2	E982.8	NITROANILINE VAPOR
983.0		E864.0	E950.7	E962.1	E980.6	NITROBENZENE
987.8		E869.8	E952.8	E962.2	E982.8	NITROBENZENE VAPOR
976.3	E946.3	E858.7	E950.4	E962.0	E980.4	NITROCELLULOSE
961.9	E931.9	E857	E950.4	E962.0	E980.4	NITROFURAN DERIVATIVES
961.9	E931.9	E857	E950.4	E962.0	E980.4	NITROFURANTOIN
976.0	E946.0	E858.7	E950.4	E962.0	E980.4	NITROFURAZONE
987.2		E869.0	E952.8	E962.2	E982.8	NITROGEN (DIOXIDE) (GAS) (OXIDE)
963.1	E933.1	E858.1	E950.4	E962.0	E980.4	NITROGEN MUSTARD (ANTINEOPLASTIC)
972.4	E942.4	E858.3	E950.4	E962.0	E980.4	NITROGLYCERIN (MEDICINAL)
989.89		E866.8	E950.9	E962.1	E980.9	NITROGLYCERIN NONMEDICINAL
987.8		E869.8	E952.8	E962.2	E982.8	NITROGLYCERIN NONMEDICINAL FUMES
983.1		E864.1	E950.7	E962.1	E980.6	NITROHYDROCHLORIC ACID
976.0	E946.0	E858.7	E950.4	E962.0	E980.4	NITROMERSOL
983.0		E864.0	E950.7	E962.1	E980.6	NITRONAPHTHALENE
983.0		E864.0	E950.7	E962.1	E980.6	NITROPHENOL
961.6	E931.6	E857	E950.4	E962.0	E980.4	NITROTHIAZOL

POISON	THERA-PEUTIC	ACCIDENT	SUICIDE	ASSAULT	UNDETER-MINED	SUBSTANCE
983.0		E864.0	E950.7	E962.1	E980.6	NITROTOLUENE
987.8		E869.8	E952.8	E962.2	E982.8	NITROTOLUENE VAPOR
968.2	E938.2	E855.1	E950.4	E962.0	E980.4	NITROUS
983.1		E864.1	E950.7	E962.1	E980.6	NITROUS ACID (LIQUID)
987.2		E869.0	E952.8	E962.2	E982.8	NITROUS ACID FUMES
968.2	E938.2	E855.1	E950.4	E962.0	E980.4	NITROUS OXIDE (ANESTHETIC) NEC
976.0	E946.0	E858.7	E950.4	E962.0	E980.4	NITROZONE
967.1	E937.1	E852.0	E950.2	E962.0	E980.2	NOCTEC
967.5	E937.5	E852.4	E950.2	E962.0	E980.2	NOLUDAR
967.0	E937.0	E851	E950.1	E962.0	E980.1	NOPTIL
971.2	E941.2	E855.5	E950.4	E962.0	E980.4	NORADRENALIN
965.5	E935.5	E850.5	E950.0	E962.0	E980.0	NORAMIDOPYRINE
971.2	E941.2	E855.5	E950.4	E962.0	E980.4	NOREPINEPHRINE
962.1	E932.1	E858.0	E950.4	E962.0	E980.4	NORETHANDROLONE
962.2	E932.2	E858.0	E950.4	E962.0	E980.4	NORETHINDRONE
962.2	E932.2	E858.0	E950.4	E962.0	E980.4	NORETHISTERONE
962.2	E932.2	E858.0	E950.4	E962.0	E980.4	NORETHYNODREL
962.2	E932.2	E858.0	E950.4	E962.0	E980.4	NORLESTRIN
962.2	E932.2	E858.0	E950.4	E962.0	E980.4	NORLUTIN
965.09	E935.2	E850.2	E950.0	E962.0	E980.0	NORMORPHINE
969.0	E939.0	E854.0	E950.3	E962.0	E980.3	NORTRIPTYLINE
963.9	E933.9	E858.1	E950.4	E962.0	E980.4	NOS SYSTEMIC AGENT NOS
975.4	E945.4	E858.6	E950.4	E962.0	E980.4	NOSCAPINE
976.6	E946.6	E858.7	E950.4	E962.0	E980.4	NOSE PREPARATIONS
960.8	E930.8	E856	E950.4	E962.0	E980.4	NOVOBIOCIN
968.5	E938.5	E855.2	E950.4	E962.0	E980.4	NOVOCAIN (INFILTRATION) (TOPICAL)
968.6	E938.6	E855.2	E950.4	E962.0	E980.4	NOVOCAIN NERVE BLOCK (PERIPHERAL) (PLEXUS)
968.7	E938.7	E855.2	E950.4	E962.0	E980.4	NOVOCAIN SPINAL
961.9	E931.9	E857	E950.4	E962.0	E980.4	NOXYTHIOLIN
962.3	E932.3	E858.0	E950.4	E962.0	E980.4	NPH ILETIN (INSULIN)
965.09	E935.2	E850.2	E950.0	E962.0	E980.0	NUMORPHAN
967.0	E937.0	E851	E950.1	E962.0	E980.1	NUNOL
968.7	E938.7	E855.2	E950.4	E962.0	E980.4	NUPERCAINE (SPINAL ANESTHETIC)
968.5	E938.5	E855.2	E950.4	E962.0	E980.4	NUPERCAINE TOPICAL (SURFACE)
976.3	E946.3	E858.7	E950.4	E962.0	E980.4	NUTMEG OIL (LINIMENT)
989.1		E863.7	E950.6	E962.1	E980.7	NUX VOMICA
961.8	E931.8	E857	E950.4	E962.0	E980.4	NYDRAZID
971.2	E941.2	E855.5	E950.4	E962.0	E980.4	NYLIDRIN
960.1	E930.1	E856	E950.4	E962.0	E980.4	NYSTATIN
976.0	E946.0	E858.7	E950.4	E962.0	E980.4	NYSTATIN TOPICAL
963.0	E933.0	E858.1	E950.4	E962.0	E980.4	NYTOL
967.8	E937.8	E852.8	E950.2	E962.0	E980.2	OBLIVION
972.4	E942.4	E858.3	E950.4	E962.0	E980.4	OCTYL NITRITE
962.2	E932.2	E858.0	E950.4	E962.0	E980.4	OESTRADIOL (CYPIONATE) (DIPROPIONATE) (VALERATE)
962.2	E932.2	E858.0	E950.4	E962.0	E980.4	OESTRIOL
962.2	E932.2	E858.0	E950.4	E962.0	E980.4	OESTRONE
989.89		E866.8	E950.9	E962.1	E980.9	OIL NEC
989.0		E866.8	E950.9	E962.1	E980.9	OIL BITTER ALMOND
976.1	E946.1	E858.7	E950.4	E962.0	E980.4	OIL CAMPHOR
989.89		E861.6	E950.9	E962.1	E980.9	OIL COLORS
987.8		E869.8	E952.8	E962.2	E982.8	OIL FUMES
981		E862.2	E950.9	E962.1	E980.9	OIL LUBRICATING
0						OIL SPECIFIED SOURCE OTHER SEE SUBSTANCE SPECIFIED
983.1		E864.1	E950.7	E962.1	E980.6	OIL VITRIOL (LIQUID)
987.8		E869.8	E952.8	E962.2	E982.8	OIL VITRIOL FUMES
976.3	E946.3	E858.7	E950.4	E962.0	E980.4	OIL WINTERGREEN (BITTER) NEC
976.9	E946.9	E858.7	E950.4	E962.0	E980.4	OINTMENTS NEC
988.2		E865.4	E950.9	E962.1	E980.9	OLEANDER
960.3	E930.3	E856	E950.4	E962.0	E980.4	OLEANDOMYCIN
963.5	E933.5	E858.1	E950.4	E962.0	E980.4	OLEOVITAMIN A
973.1	E943.1	E858.4	E950.4	E962.0	E980.4	OLEUM RICINI
973.2	E943.2	E858.4	E950.4	E962.0	E980.4	OLIVE OIL (MEDICINAL) NEC
989.3		E863.1	E950.6	E962.1	E980.7	OMPA
963.1	E933.1	E858.1	E950.4	E962.0	E980.4	ONCOVIN
968.5	E938.5	E855.2	E950.4	E962.0	E980.4	OPHTHAINE
968.5	E938.5	E855.2	E950.4	E962.0	E980.4	OPHTHETIC
970.1	E940.1	E854.3	E950.4	E962.0	E980.4	OPIATES ANTAGONISTS
965.00	E935.2	E850.2	E950.0	E962.0	E980.0	OPIUM NEC
962.2	E932.2	E858.0	E950.4	E962.0	E980.4	ORACON
977.8	E947.8	E858.8	E950.4	E962.0	E980.4	ORAGRAFIN
962.2	E932.2	E858.0	E950.4	E962.0	E980.4	ORAL CONTRACEPTIVES
975.1	E945.1	E858.6	E950.4	E962.0	E980.4	ORCIPRENALINE

POISON	THERA-PEUTIC	ACCIDENT	SUICIDE	ASSAULT	UNDETER-MINED	SUBSTANCE
975.5	E945.5	E858.6	E950.4	E962.0	E980.4	ORGANIDIN
989.3		E863.1	E950.6	E962.1	E980.7	ORGANOPHOSPHATES
979.5	E949.5	E858.8	E950.4	E962.0	E980.4	ORIMUNE
962.3	E932.3	E858.0	E950.4	E962.0	E980.4	ORINASE
966.4	E936.4	E855.0	E950.4	E962.0	E980.4	ORPHENADRINE
967.0	E937.0	E851	E950.1	E962.0	E980.1	ORTAL (SODIUM)
962.2	E932.2	E858.0	E950.4	E962.0	E980.4	ORTHO-NOVUM
976.0	E946.0	E858.7	E950.4	E962.0	E980.4	ORTHOBORIC ACID
976.6	E946.6	E858.7	E950.4	E962.0	E980.4	ORTHOBORIC ACID ENT AGENT
976.5	E946.5	E858.7	E950.4	E962.0	E980.4	ORTHOBORIC ACID OPHTHALMIC PREPARATION
968.5	E938.5	E855.2	E950.4	E962.0	E980.4	ORTHOCAINE
977.8	E947.8	E858.8	E950.4	E962.0	E980.4	ORTHOTOLIDINE (REAGENT)
983.1		E864.1	E950.7	E962.1	E980.6	OSMIC ACID (LIQUID)
987.8		E869.8	E952.8	E962.2	E982.8	OSMIC ACID FUMES
974.4	E944.4	E858.5	E950.4	E962.0	E980.4	OSMOTIC DIURETICS
975.3	E945.3	E858.6	E950.4	E962.0	E980.4	OTHER AND NOS DRUGS ACTING ON MUSCLES
972.1	E942.1	E858.3	E950.4	E962.0	E980.4	OUABAIN
962.2	E932.2	E858.0	E950.4	E962.0	E980.4	OVARIAN HORMONES (SYNTHETIC SUBSTITUTES)
962.2	E932.2	E858.0	E950.4	E962.0	E980.4	OVRAL
962.2	E932.2	E858.0	E950.4	E962.0	E980.4	OVULATION SUPPRESSANTS
962.2	E932.2	E858.0	E950.4	E962.0	E980.4	OVULEN
973.4	E943.4	E858.4	E950.4	E962.0	E980.4	OX BILE EXTRACT
960.0	E930.0	E856	E950.4	E962.0	E980.4	OXACILLIN (SODIUM)
983.1		E864.1	E950.7	E962.1	E980.6	OXALIC ACID
969.5	E939.5	E853.8	E950.3	E962.0	E980.3	OXANAMIDE
962.1	E932.1	E858.0	E950.4	E962.0	E980.4	OXANDROLONE
965.61	E935.6	E850.6	E950.0	E962.0	E980.0	OXAPROZIN
969.4	E939.4	E853.2	E950.3	E962.0	E980.3	OXAZEPAM
966.0	E936.0	E855.0	E950.4	E962.0	E980.4	OXAZOLIDINE DERIVATIVES
975.1	E945.1	E855.6	E950.4	E962.0	E980.4	OXBUTYNIN
971.2	E941.2	E855.5	E950.4	E962.0	E980.4	OXEDRINE
975.4	E945.4	E858.6	E950.4	E962.0	E980.4	OXELADIN
968.5	E938.5	E855.2	E950.4	E962.0	E980.4	OXETHAZAINE NEC
983.9		E864.3	E950.7	E962.1	E980.6	OXIDIZING AGENTS NEC
961.3	E931.3	E857	E950.4	E962.0	E980.4	OXOLINIC ACID
961.1	E931.1	E857	E950.4	E962.0	E980.4	OXOPHENARSINE
976.3	E946.3	E858.7	E950.4	E962.0	E980.4	OXSORALEN
975.7	E945.7	E858.6	E950.4	E962.0	E980.4	OXTRIPHYLLINE
968.5	E938.5	E855.2	E950.4	E962.0	E980.4	OXYBUPROCAINE
965.09	E935.2	E850.2	E950.0	E962.0	E980.0	OXYCODONE
987.8		E869.8	E952.8	E962.2	E982.8	OXYGEN
976.0	E946.0	E858.7	E950.4	E962.0	E980.4	OXYLONE
976.5	E946.5	E858.7	E950.4	E962.0	E980.4	OXYLONE OPHTHALMIC PREPARATION
962.1	E932.1	E858.0	E950.4	E962.0	E980.4	OXYMESTERONE
971.2	E941.2	E855.5	E950.4	E962.0	E980.4	OXYMETAZOLINE
962.1	E932.1	E858.0	E950.4	E962.0	E980.4	OXYMETHOLONE
965.09	E935.2	E850.2	E950.0	E962.0	E980.0	OXYMORPHONE
969.0	E939.0	E854.0	E950.3	E962.0	E980.3	OXYPERTINE
965.5	E935.5	E850.5	E950.0	E962.0	E980.0	OXYPHENBUTAZONE
971.1	E941.1	E855.4	E950.4	E962.0	E980.4	OXYPHENCYCLIMINE
973.1	E943.1	E858.4	E950.4	E962.0	E980.4	OXYPHENISATIN
971.1	E941.1	E855.4	E950.4	E962.0	E980.4	OXYPHENONIUM
961.3	E931.3	E857	E950.4	E962.0	E980.4	OXYQUINOLINE
960.4	E930.4	E856	E950.4	E962.0	E980.4	OXYTETRACYCLINE
975.0	E945.0	E858.6	E950.4	E962.0	E980.4	OXYTOCICS
975.0	E945.0	E858.6	E950.4	E962.0	E980.4	OXYTOCIN
987.8		E869.8	E952.8	E962.2	E982.8	OZONE
976.3	E946.3	E858.7	E950.4	E962.0	E980.4	PABA
964.7	E934.7	E858.2	E950.4	E962.0	E980.4	PACKED RED CELLS
982.8		E862.9	E950.9	E962.1	E980.9	PAINT CLEANER
987.8		E869.8	E952.8	E962.1	E982.8	PAINT FUMES NEC
984.0		E861.5	E950.9	E962.1	E980.9	PAINT LEAD (FUMES)
989.89		E861.6	E950.9	E962.1	E980.9	PAINT NEC
982.8		E862.9	E950.9	E962.1	E980.9	PAINT SOLVENT NEC
982.8		E862.9	E950.9	E962.1	E980.9	PAINT STRIPPER
965.09	E935.2	E850.2	E950.0	E962.0	E980.0	PALFIUM
979.9	E949.6	E858.8	E950.4	E962.0	E980.4	PALIVIZUMAB
961.4	E931.4	E857	E950.4	E962.0	E980.4	PALUDRINE
977.2	E947.2	E855.8	E950.4	E962.0	E980.4	PAM
961.4	E931.4	E857	E950.4	E962.0	E980.4	PAMAQUINE (NAPHTHOATE)
965.1	E935.3	E850.3	E950.0	E962.0	E980.0	PAMPRIN
965.4	E935.4	E850.4	E950.0	E962.0	E980.0	PANADOL

DRUGS & CHEMICALS

POISON	THERA-PEUTIC	ACCIDENT	SUICIDE	ASSAULT	UNDETER-MINED	SUBSTANCE
963.4	E933.4	E858.1	E950.4	E962.0	E980.4	PANCREATIC DORNASE (MUCOLYTIC)
973.4	E943.4	E858.4	E950.4	E962.0	E980.4	PANCREATIN
973.4	E943.4	E858.4	E950.4	E962.0	E980.4	PANCRELIPASE
963.5	E933.5	E858.1	E950.4	E962.0	E980.4	PANGAMIC ACID
963.5	E933.5	E858.1	E950.4	E962.0	E980.4	PANTHENOL
976.8	E946.8	E858.7	E950.4	E962.0	E980.4	PANTHENOL TOPICAL
977.8	E947.8	E858.8	E950.4	E962.0	E980.4	PANTOPAQUE
965.00	E935.2	E850.2	E950.0	E962.0	E980.0	PANTOPON
963.5	E933.5	E858.1	E950.4	E962.0	E980.4	PANTOTHENIC ACID
964.2	E934.2	E858.2	E950.4	E962.0	E980.4	PANWARFIN
973.4	E943.4	E858.4	E950.4	E962.0	E980.4	PAPAIN
972.5	E942.5	E858.3	E950.4	E962.0	E980.4	PAPAVERINE
976.3	E946.3	E858.7	E950.4	E962.0	E980.4	PARA-AMINOBENZOIC ACID
965.4	E935.4	E850.4	E950.0	E962.0	E980.0	PARA-AMINOPHENOL DERIVATIVES
961.8	E931.8	E857	E950.4	E962.0	E980.4	PARA-AMINOSALICYLIC ACID (DERIVATIVES)
967.2	E937.2	E852.1	E950.2	E962.0	E980.2	PARACETALDEHYDE (MEDICINAL)
965.4	E935.4	E850.4	E950.0	E962.0	E980.0	PARACETAMOL (ACETAMINOPHEN)
965.09	E935.2	E850.2	E950.0	E962.0	E980.0	PARACODIN
966.0	E936.0	E855.0	E950.4	E962.0	E980.4	PARADIONE
973.2	E943.2	E858.4	E950.4	E962.0	E980.4	PARAFFIN LIQUID (MEDICINAL)
981		E862.1	E950.9	E962.1	E980.9	PARAFFIN LIQUID NONMEDICINAL (OIL)
981		E862.3	E950.9	E962.1	E980.9	PARAFFIN(S) (WAX)
967.2	E937.2	E852.1	E950.2	E962.0	E980.2	PARALDEHYDE (MEDICINAL)
966.0	E936.0	E855.0	E950.4	E962.0	E980.4	PARAMETHADIONE
962.0	E932.0	E858.0	E950.4	E962.0	E980.4	PARAMETHASONE
989.4		E863.5	E950.6	E962.1	E980.7	PARAQUAT
971.1	E941.1	E855.4	E950.4	E962.0	E980.4	PARASYMPATHOLYTICS
971.0	E941.0	E855.3	E950.4	E962.0	E980.4	PARASYMPATHOMIMETICS
989.3		E863.1	E950.6	E962.1	E980.7	PARATHION
962.6	E932.6	E858.0	E950.4	E962.0	E980.4	PARATHORMONE
962.6	E932.6	E858.0	E950.4	E962.0	E980.4	PARATHYROID (DERIVATIVES)
962.6	E932.6	E858.0	E950.4	E962.0	E980.4	PARATHYROID AND PARATHYROID DERIVATIVES
978.1	E948.1	E858.8	E950.4	E962.0	E980.4	PARATYPHOID VACCINE
971.2	E941.2	E855.5	E950.4	E962.0	E980.4	PAREDRINE
965.00	E935.2	E850.2	E950.0	E962.0	E980.0	PAREGORIC
972.3	E942.3	E858.3	E950.4	E962.0	E980.4	PARGYLINE
985.1		E866.3	E950.8	E962.1	E980.8	PARIS GREEN
985.1		E863.4	E950.8	E962.1	E980.8	PARIS GREEN INSECTICIDE
969.0	E939.0	E854.0	E950.3	E962.0	E980.3	PARNATE
960.8	E930.8	E856	E950.4	E962.0	E980.4	PAROMOMYCIN
963.1	E933.1	E858.1	E950.4	E962.0	E980.4	PAROXYPROPIONE
965.09	E935.2	E850.2	E950.0	E962.0	E980.0	PARZONE
961.8	E931.8	E857	E950.4	E962.0	E980.4	PAS
989.4		E863.6	E950.6	E962.1	E980.7	PCP (PENTACHLOROPHENOL)
989.4		E863.5	E950.6	E962.1	E980.7	PCP HERBICIDE
989.4		E863.4	E950.6	E962.1	E980.7	PCP INSECTICIDE
968.3	E938.3	E855.1	E950.4	E962.0	E980.4	PCP PHENCYCLIDINE
973.2	E943.2	E858.4	E950.4	E962.0	E980.4	PEACH KERNEL OIL (EMULSION)
973.2	E943.2	E858.4	E950.4	E962.0	E980.4	PEANUT OIL (EMULSION) NEC
976.3	E946.3	E858.7	E950.4	E962.0	E980.4	PEANUT OIL TOPICAL
969.6	E939.6	E854.1	E950.3	E962.0	E980.3	PEARLY GATES (MORNING GLORY SEEDS)
969.1	E939.1	E853.0	E950.3	E962.0	E980.3	PECAZINE
960.1	E930.1	E856	E950.4	E962.0	E980.4	PECILOCIN
973.5	E943.5	E858.4	E950.4	E962.0	E980.4	PECTIN (WITH KAOLIN) NEC
961.6	E931.6	E857	E950.4	E962.0	E980.4	PELLETIERINE TANNATE
969.7	E939.7	E854.2	E950.3	E962.0	E980.3	PEMOLINE
972.3	E942.3	E858.3	E950.4	E962.0	E980.4	PEMPIDINE
960.0	E930.0	E856	E950.4	E962.0	E980.4	PENAMECILLIN
960.0	E930.0	E856	E950.4	E962.0	E980.4	PENETHAMATE HYDRIODIDE
963.8	E933.8	E858.1	E950.4	E962.0	E980.4	PENICILLAMINE
960.0	E930.0	E856	E950.4	E962.0	E980.4	PENICILLIN (ANY TYPE)
960.0	E930.0	E856	E950.4	E962.0	E980.4	PENICILLIN G
963.4	E933.4	E858.1	E950.4	E962.0	E980.4	PENICILLINASE
972.4	E942.4	E858.3	E950.4	E962.0	E980.4	PENTAERYTHRITOL TETRANITRATE NEC
989.4		E863.6	E950.6	E962.1	E980.7	PENTACHLOROPHENOL (FUNGICIDE)
989.4		E863.4	E950.6	E962.1	E980.7	PENTACHLOROPHENOL INSECTICIDE
989.4		E863.5	E950.6	E962.1	E980.7	PENTACHLOROPHENOL HERBICIDE
967.1	E937.1	E852.0	E950.2	E962.0	E980.2	PENTAERYTHRITOL CHLORAL
972.4	E942.4	E858.3	E950.4	E962.0	E980.4	PENTAERYTHRITOL
977.8	E947.8	E858.8	E950.4	E962.0	E980.4	PENTAGASTRIN
982.3		E862.4	E950.9	E962.1	E980.9	PENTALIN
972.3	E942.3	E858.3	E950.4	E962.0	E980.4	PENTAMETHONIUM (BROMIDE)

POISON	THERA-PEUTIC	ACCIDENT	SUICIDE	ASSAULT	UNDETER-MINED	SUBSTANCE
961.5	E931.5	E857	E950.4	E962.0	E980.4	PENTAMIDINE
980.8		E860.8	E950.9	E962.1	E980.9	PENTANOL
961.4	E931.4	E857	E950.4	E962.0	E980.4	PENTAQUINE
965.8	E935.8	E850.8	E950.0	E962.0	E980.0	PENTAZOCINE
971.1	E941.1	E855.4	E950.4	E962.0	E980.4	PENTHIENATE
967.0	E937.0	E851	E950.1	E962.0	E980.1	PENTOBARBITAL (PENTOBARBITONE)
972.3	E942.3	E858.3	E950.4	E962.0	E980.4	PENTOLINIUM (TARTRATE)
968.3	E938.3	E855.1	E950.4	E962.0	E980.4	PENTOTHAL
970.0	E940.0	E854.3	E950.4	E962.0	E980.4	PENTYLENETETRAZOL
961.8	E931.8	E857	E950.4	E962.0	E980.4	PENTYLSALICYLAMIDE
973.4	E943.4	E858.4	E950.4	E962.0	E980.4	PEPSIN
977.8	E947.8	E858.8	E950.4	E962.0	E980.4	PEPTAVLON
968.7	E938.7	E855.2	E950.4	E962.0	E980.4	PERCAINE (SPINAL)
968.5	E938.5	E855.2	E950.4	E962.0	E980.4	PERCAINE TOPICAL (SURFACE)
982.3		E862.4	E950.9	E962.1	E980.9	PERCHLOROETHYLENE (VAPOR)
961.6	E931.6	E857	E950.4	E962.0	E980.4	PERCHLOROETHYLENE MEDICINAL
965.09	E935.2	E850.2	E950.0	E962.0	E980.0	PERCODAN
965.09	E935.2	E850.2	E950.0	E962.0	E980.0	PERCOGESIC
962.0	E932.0	E858.0	E950.4	E962.0	E980.4	PERCORTEN
962.4	E932.4	E858.0	E950.4	E962.0	E980.4	PERGONAL
972.4	E942.4	E858.3	E950.4	E962.0	E980.4	PERHEXILINE
963.0	E933.0	E858.1	E950.4	E962.0	E980.4	PERIACTIN
967.1	E937.1	E852.0	E950.2	E962.0	E980.2	PERICLOR
969.1	E939.1	E853.0	E950.3	E962.0	E980.3	PERICYAZINE
972.4	E942.4	E858.3	E950.4	E962.0	E980.4	PERITRATE
976.0	E946.0	E858.7	E950.4	E962.0	E980.4	PERMANGANATES POTASSIUM (TOPICAL)
983.9		E864.4	E950.7	E962.1	E980.6	PERMANGANATES NEC
967.0	E937.0	E851	E950.1	E962.0	E980.1	PERNOSTON
965.09	E935.2	E850.2	E950.0	E962.0	E980.0	PERONIN(E)
969.1	E939.1	E853.0	E950.3	E962.0	E980.3	PERPHENAZINE
969.0	E939.0	E854	E950.3	E962.0	E980.3	PERTOFRANE
964.6	E934.6	E858.2	E950.4	E962.0	E980.4	PERTUSSIS IMMUNE SERUM (HUMAN)
978.6	E948.6	E858.8	E950.4	E962.0	E980.4	PERTUSSIS VACCINE (WITH DIPHTHERIA TOXOID) (WITH TETANUS TOXOID)
976.8	E946.8	E858.7	E950.4	E962.0	E980.4	PERUVIAN BALSAM
989.4		E863.4	E950.6	E962.1	E980.7	PESTICIDES (DUST) (FUMES) (VAPOR)
985.1		E863.4	E950.8	E962.1	E980.8	PESTICIDES ARSENIC
989.2		E863.0	E950.6	E962.1	E980.7	PESTICIDES CHLORINATED
989.0		E863.4	E950.6	E962.1	E980.7	PESTICIDES CYANIDE
981		E863.4	E950.6	E962.1	E980.7	PESTICIDES KEROSENE
989.4		E863.3	E950.6	E962.1	E980.7	PESTICIDES MIXTURE (OF COMPOUNDS)
983.0		E863.4	E950.7	E962.1	E980.6	PESTICIDES NAPHTHALENE
989.2		E863.0	E950.6	E962.1	E980.7	PESTICIDES ORGANO-CHLORINE (COMPOUNDS)
981		E863.4	E950.6	E962.1	E980.7	PESTICIDES PETROLEUM (DISTILLATE) (PRODUCTS) NEC
989.4		E863.4	E950.6	E962.1	E980.7	PESTICIDES SPECIFIED INGREDIENT NEC
989.1		E863.4	E950.6	E962.1	E980.7	PESTICIDES STRYCHNINE
985.8		E863.7	E950.6	E962.1	E980.7	PESTICIDES THALLIUM
965.09	E935.2	E850.2	E950.0	E962.0	E980.0	PETHIDINE (HYDROCHLORIDE)
967.1	E937.1	E852.0	E950.2	E962.0	E980.2	PETRICHLORAL
981		E862.1	E950.9	E962.1	E980.9	PETROL
987.1		E869.8	E952.8	E962.2	E982.8	PETROL VAPOR
976.3	E946.3	E858.7	E950.4	E962.0	E980.4	PETROLATUM (JELLY) (OINTMENT)
976.3	E946.3	E858.7	E950.4	E962.0	E980.4	PETROLATUM HYDROPHILIC
973.2	E943.2	E858.4	E950.4	E962.0	E980.4	PETROLATUM LIQUID
981		E862.1	E950.9	E962.1	E980.9	PETROLATUM NON-MEDICINAL
976.3	E946.3	E858.7	E950.4	E962.0	E980.4	PETROLATUM TOPICAL
981		E862.1	E950.9	E962.1	E980.9	PETROLEUM (CLEANERS)(FUELS) (PRODUCTS) NEC
0						PETROLEUM BENZIN(E) SEE LIGROIN
0						PETROLEUM ETHER SEE LIGROIN
987.0		E867	E951.0	E962.2	E981.0	PETROLEUM GASES PIPED (PURE OR MIXED WITH AIR)
0						PETROLEUM JELLY SEE PETROLATUM
0						PETROLEUM NAPHTHA SEE LIGROIN
981		E863.4	E950.6	E962.1	E980.7	PETROLEUM PESTICIDE
981		E862.3	E950.9	E962.1	E980.9	PETROLEUM SOLIDS
981		E862.0	E950.9	E962.1	E980.9	PETROLEUM SOLVENTS
987.1		E869.8	E952.8	E962.2	E982.8	PETROLEUM VAPOR
969.6	E939.6	E854.1	E950.3	E962.0	E980.3	PEYOTE
967.0	E937.0	E851	E950.1	E962.0	E980.1	PHANODORM

POISON	THERA-PEUTIC	ACCIDENT	SUICIDE	ASSAULT	UNDETER-MINED	SUBSTANCE
961.5	E931.5	E857	E950.4	E962.0	E980.4	PHANQUINONE
977.4	E947.4	E858.8	E950.4	E962.0	E980.4	PHARMACEUTICAL EXCIPIENT OR ADJUNCTS
966.3	E936.3	E855.0	E950.4	E962.0	E980.4	PHENACEMIDE
965.4	E935.4	E850.4	E950.0	E962.0	E980.0	PHENACETIN (ACETOPHENETIDIN)
965.09	E935.2	E850.2	E950.0	E962.0	E980.0	PHENADOXONE
969.5	E939.5	E853.8	E950.3	E962.0	E980.3	PHENAGLYCODOL
966.1	E936.1	E855.0	E950.4	E962.0	E980.4	PHENANTOIN
977.8	E947.8	E858.8	E950.4	E962.0	E980.4	PHENAPHTHAZINE REAGENT
965.09	E935.2	E850.2	E950.0	E962.0	E980.0	PHENAZOCINE
965.5	E935.5	E850.5	E950.0	E962.0	E980.0	PHENAZONE
976.1	E946.1	E858.7	E950.4	E962.0	E980.4	PHENAZOPYRIDINE
960.0	E930.0	E856	E950.4	E962.0	E980.4	PHENBENICILLIN
977.0	E947.0	E858.8	E950.4	E962.0	E980.4	PHENBUTRAZATE
968.3	E938.3	E855.1	E950.4	E962.0	E980.4	PHENCYCLIDINE
977.0	E947.0	E858.8	E950.4	E962.0	E980.4	PHENDIMETRAZINE
969.0	E939.0	E854.0	E950.3	E962.0	E980.3	PHENELZINE
967.8	E937.8	E852.8	E950.2	E962.0	E980.2	PHENERGAN
960.0	E930.0	E856	E950.4	E962.0	E980.4	PHENETHICILLIN (POTASSIUM)
965.1	E935.3	E850.3	E950.0	E962.0	E980.0	PHENETSAL
966.3	E936.3	E855.0	E950.4	E962.0	E980.4	PHENETURIDE
962.3	E932.3	E858.0	E950.4	E962.0	E980.4	PHENFORMIN
971.1	E941.1	E855.4	E950.4	E962.0	E980.4	PHENGLUTARIMIDE
965.8	E935.8	E850.8	E950.0	E962.0	E980.0	PHENICARBAZIDE
963.0	E933.0	E858.1	E950.4	E962.0	E980.4	PHENINDAMINE (TARTRATE)
964.2	E934.2	E858.2	E950.4	E962.0	E980.4	PHENINDIONE
969.0	E939.0	E854.0	E950.3	E962.0	E980.3	PHENIPRAZINE
963.0	E933.0	E858.1	E950.4	E962.0	E980.4	PHENIRAMINE (MALEATE)
977.0	E947.0	E858.8	E950.4	E962.0	E980.4	PHENMETRAZINE
967.0	E937.0	E851	E950.1	E962.0	E980.1	PHENOBAL
967.0	E937.0	E851	E950.1	E962.0	E980.1	PHENOBARBITAL (PHENOBARBITONE) (SODIUM)
967.0	E937.0	E851	E950.1	E962.0	E980.1	PHENOBARBITONE
976.0	E946.0	E858.7	E950.4	E962.0	E980.4	PHENOCTIDE
983.0		E864.0	E950.7	E962.1	E980.6	PHENOL (DERIVATIVES) NEC
983.0		E864.0	E950.7	E962.1	E980.6	PHENOL DISINFECTANT
989.4		E863.4	E950.6	E962.1	E980.7	PHENOL PESTICIDE
977.8	E947.8	E858.8	E950.4	E962.0	E980.4	PHENOL RED
973.1	E943.1	E858.4	E950.4	E962.0	E980.4	PHENOLPHTHALEIN
977.8	E947.8	E858.8	E950.4	E962.0	E980.4	PHENOLSULFON-PHTHALEIN
965.09	E935.2	E850.2	E950.0	E962.0	E980.0	PHENOMORPHAN
967.0	E937.0	E851	E950.1	E962.0	E980.1	PHENONYL
965.09	E935.2	E850.2	E950.0	E962.0	E980.0	PHENOPERIDINE
974.7	E944.7	E858.5	E950.4	E962.0	E980.4	PHENOQUIN
969.1	E939.1	E853.0	E950.3	E962.0	E980.3	PHENOTHIAZINES (TRANQUILIZERS) NEC
989.3		E863.4	E950.6	E962.1	E980.7	PHENOTHIAZINES INSECTICIDE
971.3	E941.3	E855.6	E950.4	E962.0	E980.4	PHENOXYBENZAMINE
960.0	E930.0	E856	E950.4	E962.0	E980.4	PHENOXYMETHYL PENICILLIN
964.2	E934.2	E858.2	E950.4	E962.0	E980.4	PHENPROCOUMON
966.2	E936.2	E855.0	E950.4	E962.0	E980.4	PHENSUXIMIDE
977.0	E947.0	E858.8	E950.4	E962.0	E980.4	PHENTERMINE
971.3	E941.3	E855.6	E950.4	E962.0	E980.4	PHENTOLAMINE
965.5	E935.5	E850.5	E950.0	E962.0	E980.0	PHENYL BUTAZONE
983.0		E864.0	E950.7	E962.1	E980.6	PHENYL ENEDIAMINE
983.0		E864.0	E950.7	E962.1	E980.6	PHENYL HYDRAZINE
963.1	E933.1	E858.1	E950.4	E962.0	E980.4	PHENYL HYDRAZINE ANTINEOPLASTIC
0						PHENYL MERCURIC COMPOUNDS SEE MERCURY
976.3	E946.3	E858.7	E950.4	E962.0	E980.4	PHENYL SALICYLATE
971.2	E941.2	E855.5	E950.4	E962.0	E980.4	PHENYLEPHRIN
962.3	E932.3	E858.0	E950.4	E962.0	E980.4	PHENYLETHYLBIGUANIDE
971.2	E941.2	E855.5	E950.4	E962.0	E980.4	PHENYLPROPANOLAMINE
989.3		E863.1	E950.6	E962.1	E980.7	PHENYLSULFTHION
965.7	E935.7	E850.7	E950.0	E962.0	E980.0	PHENYRAMIDOL
966.1	E936.1	E855.0	E950.4	E962.0	E980.4	PHENYTOIN
976.2	E946.2	E858.7	E950.4	E962.0	E980.4	PHISOHEX
965.09	E935.2	E850.2	E950.0	E962.0	E980.0	PHOLCODINE
989.3		E863.1	E950.6	E962.1	E980.7	PHORATE
989.3		E863.1	E950.6	E962.1	E980.7	PHOSDRIN
987.8		E869.8	E952.8	E962.2	E982.8	PHOSGENE (GAS)
989.89		E866.8	E950.9	E962.1	E980.9	PHOSPHATE (TRICRESYL)
989.3		E863.1	E950.6	E962.1	E980.7	PHOSPHATE ORGANIC
982.8		E862.4	E950.9	E962.1	E980.9	PHOSPHATE SOLVENT
987.8		E863.8	E950.6	E962.2	E980.7	PHOSPHINE (FUMIGANT)
971.0	E941.0	E855.3	E950.4	E962.0	E980.4	PHOSPHOLINE

POISON	THERA-PEUTIC	ACCIDENT	SUICIDE	ASSAULT	UNDETER-MINED	SUBSTANCE
983.1		E864.1	E950.7	E962.1	E980.6	PHOSPHORIC ACID
983.9		E864.3	E950.7	E962.1	E980.6	PHOSPHORUS (COMPOUNDS) NEC
983.9		E863.7	E950.7	E962.1	E980.6	PHOSPHORUS RODENTICIDE
967.8	E937.8	E852.8	E950.2	E962.0	E980.2	PHTHALIMIDO-GLUTARIMIDE
961.0	E931.0	E857	E950.4	E962.0	E980.4	PHTHALYL-SULFATHIAZOLE
964.3	E934.3	E858.2	E950.4	E962.0	E980.4	PHYLLOQUINONE
965.02	E935.1	E850.1	E950.0	E962.0	E980.0	PHYSEPTONE
988.2		E865.4	E950.9	E962.1	E980.9	PHYSOSTIGMA VENENOSUM
971.0	E941.0	E855.3	E950.4	E962.0	E980.4	PHYSOSTIGMINE
988.2		E865.4	E950.9	E962.1	E980.9	PHYTOLACCA DECANDRA
964.3	E934.3	E858.2	E950.4	E962.0	E980.4	PHYTOMENADIONE
964.3	E934.3	E858.2	E950.4	E962.0	E980.4	PHYTONADIONE
983.0		E864.0	E950.7	E962.1	E980.6	PICRIC (ACID)
970.0	E940.0	E854.3	E950.4	E962.0	E980.4	PICROTOXIN
971.0	E941.0	E855.3	E950.4	E962.0	E980.4	PILOCARPINE
971.0	E941.0	E855.3	E950.4	E962.0	E980.4	PILOCARPUS (JABORANDI) EXTRACT
960.1	E930.1	E856	E950.4	E962.0	E980.4	PIMARICIN
965.09	E935.2	E850.2	E950.0	E962.0	E980.0	PIMINODINE
983.9		E861.4	E950.7	E962.1	E980.6	PINE OIL PINESOL (DISINFECTANT)
961.6	E931.6	E857	E950.4	E962.0	E980.4	PINKROOT
965.09	E935.2	E850.2	E950.0	E962.0	E980.0	PIPADONE
963.0	E933.0	E858.1	E950.4	E962.0	E980.4	PIPAMAZINE
975.4	E945.4	E858.6	E950.4	E962.0	E980.4	PIPAZETHATE
971.1	E941.1	E855.4	E950.4	E962.0	E980.4	PIPENZOLATE
988.2		E865.4	E950.9	E962.1	E980.9	PIPER CUBEBA
969.1	E939.1	E853.0	E950.3	E962.0	E980.3	PIPERACETAZINE
962.2	E932.2	E858.0	E950.4	E962.0	E980.4	PIPERAZINE ESTRONE SULFATE
961.6	E931.6	E857	E950.4	E962.0	E980.4	PIPERAZINE NEC
975.4	E945.4	E858.6	E950.4	E962.0	E980.4	PIPERIDIONE
971.1	E941.1	E855.4	E950.4	E962.0	E980.4	PIPERIDOLATE
968.9	E938.9	E855.2	E950.4	E962.0	E980.4	PIPEROCAINE
968.5	E938.5	E855.2	E950.4	E962.0	E980.4	PIPEROCAINE INFILTRATION (SUBCUTANEOUS)
968.6	E938.6	E855.2	E950.4	E962.0	E980.4	PIPEROCAINE NERVE BLOCK (PERIPHERAL) (PLEXUS)
968.5	E938.5	E855.2	E950.4	E962.0	E980.4	PIPEROCAINE TOPICAL (SURFACE)
963.1	E933.1	E858.1	E950.4	E962.0	E980.4	PIPOBROMAN
970.8	E940.8	E854.3	E950.4	E962.0	E980.4	PIPRADROL
965.7	E935.7	E850.7	E950.0	E962.0	E980.0	PISCIDIA (BARK) (ERYTHRINA)
983.0		E864.0	E950.7	E962.1	E980.6	PITCH
968.7	E938.7	E855.2	E950.4	E962.0	E980.4	PITKIN'S SOLUTION
975.0	E945.0	E858.6	E950.4	E962.0	E980.4	PITOCIN
962.5	E932.5	E858.0	E950.4	E962.0	E980.4	PITRESSIN (TANNATE)
962.5	E932.5	E858.0	E950.4	E962.0	E980.4	PITUITARY EXTRACTS (POSTERIOR)
962.4	E932.4	E858.0	E950.4	E962.0	E980.4	PITUITARY EXTRACTS ANTERIOR
962.5	E932.5	E858.0	E950.4	E962.0	E980.4	PITUITRIN
962.9	E932.9	E858.0	E950.4	E962.0	E980.4	PLACENTAL EXTRACT
967.8	E937.8	E852.8	E950.2	E962.0	E980.2	PLACIDYL
978.3	E948.3	E858.8	E950.4	E962.0	E980.4	PLAGUE VACCINE
989.4		E863.5	E950.6	E962.1	E980.7	PLANT FOODS OR FERTILIZERS MIXED WITH HERBICIDES
989.89		E866.5	E950.9	E962.1	E980.9	PLANT FOODS OR FERTILIZERS NEC
988.2		E865.3	E950.9	E962.1	E980.9	PLANTS NOXIOUS BERRIES AND SEEDS
988.2		E865.4	E950.9	E962.1	E980.9	PLANTS NOXIOUS SPECIFIED TYPE NEC
988.2		E865.9	E950.9	E962.1	E980.9	PLANTS NOXIOUS USED AS FOOD
964.7	E934.7	E858.2	E950.4	E962.0	E980.4	PLASMA (BLOOD)
964.8	E934.8	E858.2	E950.4	E962.0	E980.4	PLASMA EXPANDERS
964.7	E934.7	E858.2	E950.4	E962.0	E980.4	PLASMANATE
969.1	E939.1	E853.0	E950.3	E962.0	E980.3	PLEGICIL
976.4	E946.4	E858.7	E950.4	E962.0	E980.4	PODOPHYLLIN
976.4	E946.4	E858.7	E950.4	E962.0	E980.4	PODOPHYLLUM RESIN
989.9		E866.9	E950.9	E962.1	E980.9	POISON NEC
988.2		E865.3	E950.9	E962.1	E980.9	POISONOUS BERRIES
988.2		E865.4	E950.9	E962.1	E980.9	POKEWEED (ANY PART)
971.1	E941.1	E855.4	E950.4	E962.0	E980.4	POLDINE
979.5	E949.5	E858.8	E950.4	E962.0	E980.4	POLIOMYELITIS VACCINE
979.5	E949.5	E858.8	E950.4	E962.0	E980.4	POLIOVIRUS VACCINE
989.89		E861.2	E950.9	E962.1	E980.9	POLISH (CAR) (FLOOR) (FURNITURE) (METAL) (SILVER)
989.89		E861.3	E950.9	E962.1	E980.9	POLISH ABRASIVE
989.89		E861.3	E950.9	E962.1	E980.9	POLISH PORCELAIN
973.2	E943.2	E858.4	E950.4	E962.0	E980.4	POLOXALKOL
974.5	E944.5	E858.5	E950.4	E962.0	E980.4	POLYAMINOSTYRENE RESINS
960.4	E930.4	E856	E950.4	E962.0	E980.4	POLYCYCLINE
987.8		E869.8	E952.8	E962.2	E982.8	POLYESTER FUMES

DRUGS & CHEMICALS

POISON	THERA-PEUTIC	ACCIDENT	SUICIDE	ASSAULT	UNDETER-MINED	SUBSTANCE
982.8		E862.4	E950.9	E962.1	E980.9	POLYESTER RESIN HARDENER
962.2	E932.2	E858.0	E950.4	E962.0	E980.4	POLYESTRADIOL (PHOSPHATE)
976.2	E946.2	E858.7	E950.4	E962.0	E980.4	POLYETHANOLAMINE ALKYL SULFATE
976.3	E946.3	E858.7	E950.4	E962.0	E980.4	POLYETHYLENE GLYCOL
964.0	E934.0	E858.2	E950.4	E962.0	E980.4	POLYFEROSE
960.8	E930.8	E856	E950.4	E962.0	E980.4	POLYMYXIN B
976.6	E946.6	E858.7	E950.4	E962.0	E980.4	POLYMYXIN B ENT AGENT
976.5	E946.5	E858.7	E950.4	E962.0	E980.4	POLYMYXIN B OPHTHALMIC PREPARATION
976.0	E946.0	E858.7	E950.4	E962.0	E980.4	POLYMYXIN B TOPICAL NEC
976.0	E946.0	E858.7	E950.4	E962.0	E980.4	POLYNOXYLIN(E)
976.0	E946.0	E858.7	E950.4	E962.0	E980.4	POLYOXYMETHYLENEUREA
987.8		E869.8	E952.8	E962.2	E982.8	POLYTETRA-FLUOROETHYLENE (INHALED)
974.3	E944.3	E858.5	E950.4	E962.0	E980.4	POLYTHIAZIDE
964.8	E934.8	E858.2	E950.4	E962.0	E980.4	POLYVINYLPYRROLIDONE
968.5	E938.5	E855.2	E950.4	E962.0	E980.4	PONTOCAINE (HYDROCHLORIDE) (INFILTRATION) (TOPICAL)
968.6	E938.6	E855.2	E950.4	E962.0	E980.4	PONTOCAINE NERVE BLOCK (PERIPHERAL) (PLEXUS)
968.7	E938.7	E855.2	E950.4	E962.0	E980.4	PONTOCAINE SPINAL
969.6	E939.6	E854.1	E950.3	E962.0	E980.3	POT
983.2		E864.2	E950.7	E962.1	E980.6	POTASH (CAUSTIC)
974.5	E944.5	E858.5	E950.4	E962.0	E980.4	POTASSIC SALINE INJECTION (LACTATED)
974.5	E944.5	E858.5	E950.4	E962.0	E980.4	POTASSIUM (SALTS) NEC
961.8	E931.8	E857	E950.4	E962.0	E980.4	POTASSIUM AMINOSALICYLATE
985.1		E866.3	E950.8	E962.1	E980.8	POTASSIUM ARSENITE (SOLUTION)
983.9		E864.3	E950.7	E962.1	E980.6	POTASSIUM BICHROMATE
983.9		E864.3	E950.7	E962.1	E980.6	POTASSIUM BISULFATE
967.3	E937.3	E852.2	E950.2	E962.0	E980.2	POTASSIUM BROMIDE (MEDICINAL) NEC
983.2		E864.2	E950.7	E962.1	E980.6	POTASSIUM CARBONATE
983.9		E864.3	E950.7	E962.1	E980.6	POTASSIUM CHLORATE NEC
983.2		E864.2	E950.7	E962.1	E980.6	POTASSIUM HYDROXIDE
975.5	E945.5	E858.6	E950.4	E962.0	E980.4	POTASSIUM IODIDE (EXPECTORANT) NEC
989.89		E866.8	E950.9	E962.1	E980.9	POTASSIUM NITRATE
983.9		E864.3	E950.7	E962.1	E980.6	POTASSIUM OXALATE
962.8	E932.8	E858.0	E950.4	E962.0	E980.4	POTASSIUM PERCHLORATE ANTITHYROID
977.8	E947.8	E858.8	E950.4	E962.0	E980.4	POTASSIUM PERCHLORATE NEC
976.0	E946.0	E858.7	E950.4	E962.0	E980.4	POTASSIUM PERMANGANATE
983.9		E864.3	E950.7	E962.1	E980.6	POTASSIUM PERMANGANATE NONMEDICINAL
976.0	E946.0	E858.7	E950.4	E962.0	E980.4	POVIDONE-IODINE (ANTI-INFECTIVE) NEC
972.0	E942.0	E858.3	E950.4	E962.0	E980.4	PRACTOLOL
977.2	E947.2	E858.8	E950.4	E962.0	E980.4	PRALIDOXIME (CHLORIDE)
968.5	E938.5	E855.2	E950.4	E962.0	E980.4	PRAMOXINE
972.6	E942.6	E858.3	E950.4	E962.0	E980.4	PRAZOSIN
962.0	E932.0	E858.0	E950.4	E962.0	E980.4	PREDNISOLONE
976.6	E946.6	E858.7	E950.4	E962.0	E980.4	PREDNISOLONE ENT AGENT
976.5	E946.5	E858.7	E950.4	E962.0	E980.4	PREDNISOLONE OPHTHALMIC PREPARATION
976.0	E946.0	E858.7	E950.4	E962.0	E980.4	PREDNISOLONE TOPICALNEC
962.0	E932.0	E858.0	E950.4	E962.0	E980.4	PREDNISONE
962.2	E932.2	E858.0	E950.4	E962.0	E980.4	PREGNANEDIOL
962.2	E932.2	E858.0	E950.4	E962.0	E980.4	PREGNENINOLONE
977.0	E947.0	E858.8	E950.4	E962.0	E980.4	PRELUDIN
962.2	E932.2	E858.0	E950.4	E962.0	E980.4	PREMARIN
972.4	E942.4	E858.3	E950.4	E962.0	E980.4	PRENYLAMINE
976.8	E946.8	E858.7	E950.4	E962.0	E980.4	PREPARATION H
989.89		E866.8	E950.9	E962.1	E980.9	PRESERVATIVES
988.2		E865.3	E950.9	E962.1	E980.9	PRIDE OF CHINA
968.9	E938.9	E855.2	E950.4	E962.0	E980.4	PRILOCAINE
968.5	E938.5	E855.2	E950.4	E962.0	E980.4	PRILOCAINE INFILTRATION (SUBCUTANEOUS)
968.6	E938.6	E855.2	E950.4	E962.0	E980.4	PRILOCAINE NERVE BLOCK (PERIPHERAL) (PLEXUS)
961.4	E931.4	E857	E950.4	E962.0	E980.4	PRIMAQUINE
966.3	E936.3	E855.0	E950.4	E962.0	E980.4	PRIMIDONE
988.2		E865.4	E950.9	E962.1	E980.9	PRIMULA (VERIS)
965.09	E935.2	E850.2	E950.0	E962.0	E980.0	PRINADOL
971.3	E941.3	E855.6	E950.4	E962.0	E980.4	PRISCOL
988.2		E865.4	E950.9	E962.1	E980.9	PRIVET
971.2	E941.2	E855.5	E950.4	E962.0	E980.4	PRIVINE
971.1	E941.1	E855.4	E950.4	E962.0	E980.4	PRO-BANTHINE

DRUGS & CHEMICALS

POISON	THERA-PEUTIC	ACCIDENT	SUICIDE	ASSAULT	UNDETER-MINED	SUBSTANCE
967.0	E937.0	E851	E950.1	E962.0	E980.1	PROBARBITAL
974.7	E944.7	E858.5	E950.4	E962.0	E980.4	PROBENECID
972.0	E942.0	E858.3	E950.4	E962.0	E980.4	PROCAINAMIDE (HYDROCHLORIDE)
968.5	E938.5	E855.2	E950.4	E962.0	E980.4	PROCAINE (HYDROCHLORIDE) (INFILTRATION) (TOPICAL)
968.6	E938.6	E855.2	E950.4	E962.0	E980.4	PROCAINE NERVE BLOCK (PERIPHERAL) (PLEXUS)
960.0	E930.0	E856	E950.4	E962.0	E980.4	PROCAINE PENICILLIN G
968.7	E938.7	E855.2	E950.4	E962.0	E980.4	PROCAINE SPINAL
969.5	E939.5	E853.8	E950.3	E962.0	E980.3	PROCALMIDOL
963.1	E933.1	E858.1	E950.4	E962.0	E980.4	PROCARBAZINE
969.1	E939.1	E853.0	E950.3	E962.0	E980.3	PROCHLORPERAZINE
966.4	E936.4	E855.0	E950.4	E962.0	E980.4	PROCYCLIDINE
986		E868.8	E952.1	E962.2	E982.1	PRODUCER GAS
966.4	E936.4	E855.0	E950.4	E962.0	E980.4	PROFENAMINE
975.1	E945.1	E858.6	E950.4	E962.0	E980.4	PROFENIL
962.2	E932.2	E858.0	E950.4	E962.0	E980.4	PROGESTIN
962.2	E932.2	E858.0	E950.4	E962.0	E980.4	PROGESTOGENS (WITH ESTROGENS)
962.2	E932.2	E858.0	E950.4	E962.0	E980.4	PROGESTONE
961.4	E931.4	E857	E950.4	E962.0	E980.4	PROGUANIL (CHLOROGUANIDE)
962.4	E932.4	E858.0	E950.4	E962.0	E980.4	PROLACTIN
962.7	E932.7	E858.0	E950.4	E962.0	E980.4	PROLOID
962.2	E932.2	E858.0	E950.4	E962.0	E980.4	PROLUTON
961.8	E931.8	E857	E950.4	E962.0	E980.4	PROMACETIN
969.1	E939.1	E853.0	E950.3	E962.0	E980.3	PROMAZINE
965.09	E935.2	E850.2	E950.0	E962.0	E980.0	PROMEDOL
967.8	E937.8	E852.8	E950.2	E962.0	E980.2	PROMETHAZINE
961.8	E931.8	E857	E950.4	E962.0	E980.4	PROMIN
972.0	E942.0	E858.3	E950.4	E962.0	E980.4	PRONESTYL (HYDROCHLORIDE)
972.0	E942.0	E858.3	E950.4	E962.0	E980.4	PRONETALOL
961.0	E931.0	E857	E950.4	E962.0	E980.4	PRONTOSIL
961.5	E931.5	E857	E950.4	E962.0	E980.4	PROPAMIDINE ISETHIONATE
967.8	E937.8	E852.8	E950.2	E962.0	E980.2	PROPANAL (MEDICINAL)
987.0		E868.0	E951.1	E962.2	E981.1	PROPANE (GAS) (DISTRIBUTED IN MOBILE CONTAINER)
987.0		E867	E951.0	E962.2	E981.0	PROPANE DISTRIBUTED THROUGH PIPES
0						PROPANE INCOMPLETE COMBUSTION OF SEE CARBON MONOXIDE PROPANE
968.3	E938.3	E855.1	E950.4	E962.0	E980.4	PROPANIDID
980.3		E860.4	E950.9	E962.1	E980.9	PROPANOL
980.3		E860.4	E950.9	E962.1	E980.9	PROPANOL 1
980.2		E860.3	E950.9	E962.1	E980.9	PROPANOL 2
971.1	E941.1	E855.4	E950.4	E962.0	E980.4	PROPANTHELINE
968.5	E938.5	E855.2	E950.4	E962.0	E980.4	PROPARACAINE
972.4	E942.4	E858.3	E950.4	E962.0	E980.4	PROPATYL NITRATE
960.0	E930.0	E856	E950.4	E962.0	E980.4	PROPICILLIN
987.8		E869.8	E952.8	E962.2	E982.8	PROPIOLACTONE (VAPOR)
967.8	E937.8	E852.8	E950.2	E962.0	E980.2	PROPIOMAZINE
976.0	E946.0	E858.7	E950.4	E962.0	E980.4	PROPION GEL
967.8	E937.8	E852.8	E950.2	E962.0	E980.2	PROPIONALDEHYDE (MEDICINAL)
976.0	E946.0	E858.7	E950.4	E962.0	E980.4	PROPIONATE COMPOUND
968.9	E938.9	E855.2	E950.4	E962.0	E980.4	PROPITOCAINE
968.5	E938.5	E855.2	E950.4	E962.0	E980.4	PROPITOCAINE INFILTRATION (SUBCUTANEOUS)
968.6	E938.6	E855.2	E950.4	E962.0	E980.4	PROPITOCAINE NERVE BLOCK (PERIPHERAL) (PLEXUS)
989.3		E863.2	E950.6	E962.1	E980.7	PROPOXUR
968.9	E938.9	E855.2	E950.4	E962.0	E980.4	PROPOXYCAINE
968.5	E938.5	E855.2	E950.4	E962.0	E980.4	PROPOXYCAINE INFILTRATION (SUBCUTANEOUS)
968.6	E938.6	E855.2	E950.4	E962.0	E980.4	PROPOXYCAINE NERVE BLOCK (PERIPHERAL) (PLEXUS)
968.5	E938.5	E855.2	E950.4	E962.0	E980.4	PROPOXYCAINE TOPICAL (SURFACE)
965.8	E935.8	E850.8	E950.0	E962.0	E980.0	PROPOXYPHENE (HYDROCHLORIDE)
972.0	E942.0	E858.3	E950.4	E962.0	E980.4	PROPRANOLOL
980.3		E860.4	E950.9	E962.1	E980.9	PROPYL ALCOHOL
980.3		E860.4	E950.9	E962.1	E980.9	PROPYL CARBINOL
971.2	E941.2	E855.5	E950.4	E962.0	E980.4	PROPYL HEXADRINE
977.8	E947.8	E858.8	E950.4	E962.0	E980.4	PROPYL IODONE
962.8	E932.8	E858.0	E950.4	E962.0	E980.4	PROPYL THIOURACIL
987.1		E869.8	E952.8	E962.2	E982.8	PROPYLENE
976.5	E946.5	E858.7	E950.4	E962.0	E980.4	PROPYLPARABEN (OPHTHALMIC)
972.1	E942.1	E858.3	E950.4	E962.0	E980.4	PROSCILLARIDIN
975.0	E945.0	E858.6	E950.4	E962.0	E980.4	PROSTAGLANDINS

POISON	THERA-PEUTIC	ACCIDENT	SUICIDE	ASSAULT	UNDETER-MINED	SUBSTANCE
971.0	E941.1	E855.3	E950.4	E962.0	E980.4	PROSTIGMIN
964.5	E934.5	E858.2	E950.4	E962.0	E980.4	PROTAMINE (SULFATE)
962.3	E932.3	E858.0	E950.4	E962.0	E980.4	PROTAMINE ZINC INSULIN
976.3	E946.3	E858.7	E950.4	E962.0	E980.4	PROTECTANTS (TOPICAL)
974.5	E944.5	E858.5	E950.4	E962.0	E980.4	PROTEIN HYDROLYSATE
961.8	E931.8	E857	E950.4	E962.0	E980.4	PROTHIONAMIDE
969.5	E939.5	E853.8	E950.3	E962.0	E980.3	PROTHIPENDYL
971.2	E941.2	E855.5	E950.4	E962.0	E980.4	PROTOKYLOL
977.2	E947.2	E858.8	E950.4	E962.0	E980.4	PROTOPAM
972.6	E942.6	E858.3	E950.4	E962.0	E980.4	PROTOVERATRINE(S) (A) (B)
969.0	E939.0	E854.0	E950.3	E962.0	E980.3	PROTRIPTYLINE
962.2	E932.2	E858.0	E950.4	E962.0	E980.4	PROVERA
963.5	E933.5	E858.1	E950.4	E962.0	E980.4	PROVITAMIN A
968.5	E938.5	E855.2	E950.4	E962.0	E980.4	PROXYMETACAINE
975.1	E945.1	E858.6	E950.4	E962.0	E980.4	PROXYPHYLLINE
988.2		E865.4	E950.9	E962.1	E980.9	PRUNUS LAUROCERASUS
988.2		E865.4	E950.9	E962.1	E980.9	PRUNUS VIRGINIANA
989.0		E866.8	E950.9	E962.1	E980.9	PRUSSIC ACID
987.7		E869.8	E952.8	E962.2	E982.8	PRUSSIC ACID VAPOR
971.2	E941.2	E855.5	E950.4	E962.0	E980.4	PSEUDOEPHEDRINE
969.6	E939.6	E854.1	E950.3	E962.0	E980.3	PSILOCIN
969.6	E939.6	E854.1	E950.3	E962.0	E980.3	PSILOCYBIN
977.8	E947.8	E858.8	E950.4	E962.0	E980.4	PSP
969.6	E939.6	E854.1	E950.3	E962.0	E980.3	PSYCHEDELIC AGENTS
969.6	E939.6	E854.1	E950.3	E962.0	E980.3	PSYCHODYSLEPTICS
969.7	E939.7	E854.2	E950.3	E962.0	E980.3	PSYCHOSTIMULANTS
969.9	E939.9	E855.9	E950.3	E962.0	E980.3	PSYCHOTHERAPEUTIC AGENTS
969.0	E939.0	E854.0	E950.3	E962.0	E980.3	PSYCHOTHERAPEUTIC AGENTS ANTIDEPRESSANTS
969.5	E939.5	E853.9	E950.3	E962.0	E980.3	PSYCHOTHERAPEUTIC AGENTS TRANQUILIZERS NEC
969.8	E939.8	E855.8	E950.3	E962.0	E980.3	PSYCHOTHERAPEUTIC AGENTS SPECIFIED NEC
969.6	E939.6	E854.1	E950.3	E962.0	E980.3	PSYCHOTOMIMETIC AGENTS
969.9	E939.9	E855.9	E950.3	E962.0	E980.3	PSYCHOTROPIC AGENTS NOS
969.8	E939.8	E855.8	E950.3	E962.0	E980.3	PSYCHOTROPIC AGENTS OTHER SPECIFIED
969.8	E939.8	E855.8	E950.3	E962.0	E980.3	PSYCHOTROPIC AGENTS SPECIFIED NEC
973.3	E943.3	E858.4	E950.4	E962.0	E980.4	PSYLLIUM
964.1	E934.1	E858.2	E950.4	E962.0	E980.4	PTEROYLGLUTAMIC ACID
963.1	E933.1	E858.1	E950.4	E962.0	E980.4	PTEROYLTRIGLUTAMATE
987.8		E869.8	E952.8	E962.2	E982.8	PTFE
988.2		E865.4	E950.9	E962.1	E980.9	PULSATILLA
983.9		E864.3	E950.7	E962.1	E980.6	PUREX (BLEACH)
974.1	E944.1	E858.5	E950.4	E962.0	E980.4	PURINE DIURETICS
963.1	E933.1	E858.1	E950.4	E962.0	E980.4	PURINETHOL
964.8	E934.8	E858.2	E950.4	E962.0	E980.4	PVP
965.7	E935.7	E850.7	E950.0	E962.0	E980.0	PYRABITAL
965.5	E935.5	E850.5	E950.0	E962.0	E980.0	PYRAMIDON
961.6	E931.6	E857	E950.4	E962.0	E980.4	PYRANTEL (PAMOATE)
963.0	E933.0	E858.1	E950.4	E962.0	E980.4	PYRATHIAZINE
961.8	E931.8	E857	E950.4	E962.0	E980.4	PYRAZINAMIDE
961.8	E931.8	E857	E950.4	E962.0	E980.4	PYRAZINOIC ACID (AMIDE)
965.5	E935.5	E850.5	E950.0	E962.0	E980.0	PYRAZOLE (DERIVATIVES)
965.5	E935.5	E850.5	E950.0	E962.0	E980.0	PYRAZOLONE (ANALGESICS)
989.4		E863.4	E950.6	E962.1	E980.7	PYRETHRINS
963.0	E933.0	E858.1	E950.4	E962.0	E980.4	PYRIBENZAMINE
982.0		E862.4	E950.9	E962.1	E980.9	PYRIDINE (LIQUID) (VAPOR)
977.2	E947.2	E858.8	E950.4	E962.0	E980.4	PYRIDINE ALDOXIME CHLORIDE
976.1	E946.1	E858.7	E950.4	E962.0	E980.4	PYRIDIUM
971.0	E941.0	E855.3	E950.4	E962.0	E980.4	PYRIDOSTIGMINE
963.5	E933.5	E858.1	E950.4	E962.0	E980.4	PYRIDOXINE
963.0	E933.0	E858.1	E950.4	E962.0	E980.4	PYRILAMINE
961.4	E931.4	E857	E950.4	E962.0	E980.4	PYRIMETHAMINE
983.0		E864.0	E950.7	E962.1	E980.6	PYROGALLIC ACID
976.3	E946.3	E858.7	E950.4	E962.0	E980.4	PYROXYLIN
963.0	E933.0	E858.1	E950.4	E962.0	E980.4	PYRROBUTAMINE
968.5	E938.5	E855.2	E950.4	E962.0	E980.4	PYRROCAINE
961.6	E931.6	E857	E950.4	E962.0	E980.4	PYRVINIUM (PAMOATE)
962.3	E932.3	E858.0	E950.4	E962.0	E980.4	PZI
967.4	E937.4	E852.3	E950.2	E962.0	E980.2	QUAALUDE
971.1	E941.1	E855.4	E950.4	E962.0	E980.4	QUATERNARY AMMONIUM DERIVATIVES
983.2		E864.2	E950.7	E962.1	E980.6	QUICKLIME
961.3	E931.3	E857	E950.4	E962.0	E980.4	QUINACRINE

POISON	THERA-PEUTIC	ACCIDENT	SUICIDE	ASSAULT	UNDETER-MINED	SUBSTANCE
972.0	E942.0	E858.3	E950.4	E962.0	E980.4	QUINAGLUTE
967.0	E937.0	E851	E950.1	E962.0	E980.1	QUINALBARBITONE
962.2	E932.2	E858.0	E950.4	E962.0	E980.4	QUINESTRADIOL
974.3	E944.3	E858.5	E950.4	E962.0	E980.4	QUINETHAZONE
972.0	E942.0	E858.3	E950.4	E962.0	E980.4	QUINIDINE (GLUCONATE) (POLYGALACTURO-NATE) (SALTS) (SULFATE)
961.4	E931.4	E857	E950.4	E962.0	E980.4	QUININE
961.3	E931.3	E857	E950.4	E962.0	E980.4	QUINIOBINE
961.3	E931.3	E857	E950.4	E962.0	E980.4	QUINOLINES
968.5	E938.5	E855.2	E950.4	E962.0	E980.4	QUOTANE
964.6	E934.6	E858.2	E950.4	E962.0	E980.4	RABIES IMMUNE GLOBULIN (HUMAN)
979.1	E949.1	E858.8	E950.4	E962.0	E980.4	RABIES VACCINE
965.09	E935.2	E850.2	E950.0	E962.0	E980.0	RACEMORAMIDE
965.09	E935.2	E850.2	E950.0	E962.0	E980.0	RACEMORPHAN
980.1		E860.2	E950.9	E962.1	E980.9	RADIATOR ALCOHOL
977.8	E947.8	E858.8	E950.4	E962.0	E980.4	RADIO-OPAQUE (DRUGS) (MATERIAL)
988.2		E865.4	E950.9	E962.1	E980.9	RANUNCULUS
989.4		E863.7	E950.6	E962.1	E980.7	RAT POISON
989.5		E905.0	E950.9	E962.1	E980.9	RATTLESNAKE (VENOM)
972.6	E942.6	E858.3	E950.4	E962.0	E980.4	RAUDIXIN
972.6	E942.6	E858.3	E950.4	E962.0	E980.4	RAUTENSIN
972.6	E942.6	E858.3	E950.4	E962.0	E980.4	RAUTINA
972.6	E942.6	E858.3	E950.4	E962.0	E980.4	RAUTOTAL
972.6	E942.6	E858.3	E950.4	E962.0	E980.4	RAUWILOID
972.6	E942.6	E858.3	E950.4	E962.0	E980.4	RAUWOLDIN
972.6	E942.6	E858.3	E950.4	E962.0	E980.4	RAUWOLFIA (ALKALOIDS)
985.1		E866.3	E950.8	E962.1	E980.8	REALGAR
964.7	E934.7	E858.2	E950.4	E962.0	E980.4	RED CELLS PACKED
983.9		E864.3	E950.7	E962.1	E980.6	REDUCING AGENTS INDUSTRIAL NEC
987.4		E869.2	E952.8	E962.2	E982.8	REFRIGERANT GAS (FREON)
987.9		E869.9	E952.9	E962.2	E982.9	REFRIGERANT GAS NOT FREON
974.4	E944.4	E858.5	E950.4	E962.0	E980.4	REGROTON
968.0	E938.0	E855.1	E950.4	E962.0	E980.4	RELA
968.0	E938.0	E855.1	E950.4	E962.0	E980.4	RELAXANTS CENTRAL NERVOUS SYSTEM
975.2	E945.2	E858.6	E950.4	E962.0	E980.4	RELAXANTS SKELETAL MUSCLE (AUTONOMIC)
974.3	E944.3	E858.5	E950.4	E962.0	E980.4	RENESE
977.8	E947.8	E858.8	E950.4	E962.0	E980.4	RENOGRAFIN
974.5	E944.5	E858.5	E950.4	E962.0	E980.4	REPLACEMENT SOLUTIONS
972.6	E942.6	E858.3	E950.4	E962.0	E980.4	RESCINNAMINE
972.6	E942.6	E858.3	E950.4	E962.0	E980.4	RESERPINE
976.4	E946.4	E858.7	E950.4	E962.0	E980.4	RESORCIN
975.5	E945.5	E858.6	E950.4	E962.0	E980.4	RESPAIRE
975.8	E945.8	E858.6	E950.4	E962.0	E980.4	RESPIRATORY AGENTS NEC
975.8	E945.8	E858.6	E950.4	E962.0	E980.4	RESPIRATORY DRUGS OTHER AND NOS
979.6	E949.6	E858.8	E950.4	E962.0	E980.4	RESPIRATORY SYNCYTIAL VIRUS
976.8	E946.8	E858.7	E950.4	E962.0	E980.4	RETINOIC ACID
963.5	E933.5	E858.1	E950.4	E962.0	E980.4	RETINOL
964.6	E934.6	E858.2	E950.4	E962.0	E980.4	RH (D) IMMUNE GLOBULIN (HUMAN)
965.1	E935.3	E850.3	E950.0	E962.0	E980.0	RHODINE
964.6	E934.6	E858.2	E950.4	E962.0	E980.4	RHOGAM
963.5	E933.5	E858.1	E950.4	E962.0	E980.4	RIBOFLAVIN
989.89		E866.8	E950.9	E962.1	E980.9	RICIN
988.2		E865.3	E950.9	E962.1	E980.9	RICINUS COMMUNIS
979.6	E949.6	E858.8	E950.4	E962.0	E980.4	RICKETTSIAL VACCINE NEC
979.7	E949.7	E858.8	E950.4	E962.0	E980.4	RICKETTSIAL VACCINE WITH VIRAL AND BACTERIAL VACCINE
979.7	E949.7	E858.8	E950.4	E962.0	E980.4	RICKETTSIAL WITH BACTERIAL COMPONENT
960.6	E930.6	E856	E950.4	E962.0	E980.4	RIFAMPIN
961.8	E931.8	E857	E950.4	E962.0	E980.4	RIMIFON
974.5	E944.5	E858.5	E950.4	E962.0	E980.4	RINGER'S INJECTION (LACTATED)
960.8	E930.8	E856	E950.4	E962.0	E980.4	RISTOCETIN
969.7	E939.7	E854.2	E950.3	E962.0	E980.3	RITALIN
0						ROACH KILLERS SEE PESTICIDES
979.6	E949.6	E858.8	E950.4	E962.0	E980.4	ROCKY MOUNTAIN SPOTTED FEVER VACCINE
989.4		E863.7	E950.6	E962.1	E980.7	RODENTICIDES
969.4	E939.4	E853.2	E950.3	E962.0	E980.3	ROHYPNOL
973.0	E943.0	E858.4	E950.4	E962.0	E980.4	ROLAIDS
960.4	E930.4	E856	E950.4	E962.0	E980.4	ROLITETRACYCLINE
975.4	E945.4	E858.6	E950.4	E962.0	E980.4	ROMILAR
976.3	E946.3	E858.7	E950.4	E962.0	E980.4	ROSE WATER OINTMENT

POISON	THERAPEUTIC	ACCIDENT	SUICIDE	ASSAULT	UNDETERMINED	SUBSTANCE
979.6	E949.6	E858.8	E950.4	E962.0	E980.4	ROTAVIRUS VACCINE
989.4		E863.4	E950.6	E962.1	E980.7	ROTENONE
963.0	E933.0	E858.1	E950.4	E962.0	E980.4	ROTOXAMINE
989.4		E863.7	E950.6	E962.1	E980.7	ROUGH-ON-RATS
962.9	E932.9	E858.0	E950.4	E962.0	E980.4	RU486
980.2		E860.3	E950.9	E962.1	E980.9	RUBBING ALCOHOL
979.4	E949.4	E858.8	E950.4	E962.0	E980.4	RUBELLA VIRUS VACCINE
979.4	E949.4	E858.8	E950.4	E962.0	E980.4	RUBELOGEN
979.4	E949.4	E858.8	E950.4	E962.0	E980.4	RUBEOVAX
960.7	E930.7	E856	E950.4	E962.0	E980.4	RUBIDOMYCIN
988.2		E865.4	E950.9	E962.1	E980.9	RUE
988.2		E865.4	E950.9	E962.1	E980.9	RUTA
976.0	E946.0	E858.7	E950.4	E962.0	E980.4	SABADILLA (MEDICINAL)
989.4		E863.4	E950.6	E962.1	E980.7	SABADILLA PESTICIDE
979.5	E949.5	E858.8	E950.4	E962.0	E980.4	SABIN ORAL VACCINE
964.0	E934.0	E858.2	E950.4	E962.0	E980.4	SACCHARATED IRON OXIDE
974.5	E944.5	E858.5	E950.4	E962.0	E980.4	SACCHARIN
972.2	E942.2	E858.3	E950.4	E962.0	E980.4	SAFFLOWER OIL
965.1	E935.3	E850.3	E950.0	E962.0	E980.0	SALICYLAMIDE
974.1	E944.1	E858.5	E950.4	E962.0	E980.4	SALICYLATE THEOBROMINE CALCIUM
976.3	E946.3	E858.7	E950.4	E962.0	E980.4	SALICYLATE METHYL
965.1	E935.3	E850.3	E950.0	E962.0	E980.0	SALICYLATE(S)
961.0	E931.0	E857	E950.4	E962.0	E980.4	SALICYLAZOSULFA-PYRIDINE
976.0	E946.0	E858.7	E950.4	E962.0	E980.4	SALICYLHYDROXAMIC ACID
965.1	E935.3	E850.3	E950.0	E962.0	E980.0	SALICYLIC ACID CONGENERS
976.4	E946.4	E858.7	E950.4	E962.0	E980.4	SALICYLIC ACID (KERATOLYTIC) NEC
965.1	E935.3	E850.3	E950.0	E962.0	E980.0	SALICYLIC ACID SALTS
961.8	E931.8	E857	E950.4	E962.0	E980.4	SALINIAZID
976.3	E946.3	E858.7	E950.4	E962.0	E980.4	SALOL
974.5	E944.5	E858.5	E950.4	E962.0	E980.4	SALT (SUBSTITUTE) NEC
974.3	E944.3	E858.5	E950.4	E962.0	E980.4	SALURETICS
974.3	E944.3	E858.5	E950.4	E962.0	E980.4	SALURON
961.1	E931.1	E857	E950.4	E962.0	E980.4	SALVARSAN 606 (NEOSILVER) (SILVER)
988.2		E865.4	E950.9	E962.1	E980.9	SAMBUCUS CANADENSIS
988.2		E865.3	E950.9	E962.1	E980.9	SAMBUCUS CANADENSIS BERRY
972.6	E942.6	E858.3	E950.4	E962.0	E980.4	SANDRIL
988.2		E865.4	E950.9	E962.1	E980.9	SANGUINARIA CANADENSIS
983.9		E861.3	E950.7	E962.1	E980.6	SANIFLUSH (CLEANER)
961.6	E931.6	E857	E950.4	E962.0	E980.4	SANTONIN
976.8	E946.8	E858.7	E950.4	E962.0	E980.4	SANTYL
960.7	E930.7	E856	E950.4	E962.0	E980.4	SARKOMYCIN
969.0	E939.0	E854.0	E950.3	E962.0	E980.3	SAROTEN
0						SATURNINE SEE LEAD
976.4	E946.4	E858.7	E950.4	E962.0	E980.4	SAVIN (OIL)
973.1	E943.1	E858.4	E950.4	E962.0	E980.4	SCAMMONY
976.8	E946.8	E858.7	E950.4	E962.0	E980.4	SCARLET RED
985.1		E866.3	E950.8	E962.1	E980.8	SCHEELE'S GREEN
985.1		E863.4	E950.8	E962.1	E980.8	SCHEELE'S GREEN INSECTICIDE
985.1		E863.4	E950.8	E962.1	E980.8	SCHWEINFURT GREEN INSECTICIDE
985.1		E866.3	E950.8	E962.1	E980.8	SCHWEINFURT(H) GREEN
0						SCILLA SEE SQUILL
972.7	E942.7	E858.3	E950.4	E962.0	E980.4	SCLEROSING AGENTS
971.1	E941.1	E855.4	E950.4	E962.0	E980.4	SCOPOLAMINE
971.1	E941.1	E855.4	E950.4	E962.0	E980.4	SCOPOLAMMONIUM BROMIDE
989.5		E905.2	E950.9	E962.1	E980.9	SCORPION VENOM
989.89		E861.3	E950.9	E962.1	E980.9	SCOURING POWDER
989.5		E905.6	E950.9	E962.1	E980.9	SEA ANEMONE (STING)
989.5		E905.6	E950.9	E962.1	E980.9	SEA CUCUMBER (STING)
989.5		E905.0	E950.9	E962.1	E980.9	SEA SNAKE (BITE) (VENOM)
989.5		E905.6	E950.9	E962.1	E980.9	SEA URCHIN SPINE (PUNCTURE)
967.0	E937.0	E851	E950.1	E962.0	E980.1	SECBUTABARBITAL
967.0	E937.0	E851	E950.1	E962.0	E980.1	SECBUTABARITONE
967.0	E937.0	E851	E950.1	E962.0	E980.1	SECOBARBITAL (QUINALBARBITONE)
967.0	E937.0	E851	E950.1	E962.0	E980.1	SECONAL
977.8	E947.8	E858.8	E950.4	E962.0	E980.4	SECRETIN
967.9	E937.9	E852.9	E950.2	E962.0	E980.2	SEDATIVE OR HYPNOTIC NOS
967.8	E937.8	E852.8	E950.2	E962.0	E980.2	SEDATIVES AND HYPNOTICS OTHER
967.6	E937.6	E852.5	E950.2	E962.0	E980.2	SEDATIVES MIXED NEC
967.9	E937.9	E852.9	E950.2	E962.0	E980.2	SEDATIVES NONBARBITURATE
967.8	E937.8	E852.8	E950.2	E962.0	E980.2	SEDATIVES NONBARBITURATE SPECIFIED NEC
967.8	E937.8	E852.8	E950.2	E962.0	E980.2	SEDORMID
988.2		E865.3	E950.9	E962.1	E980.9	SEED (PLANT)
989.89		E866.5	E950.9	E962.1	E980.9	SEED DISINFECTANT OR DRESSING
985.8		E866.4	E950.9	E962.1	E980.9	SELENIUM (FUMES) NEC

POISON	THERA-PEUTIC	ACCIDENT	SUICIDE	ASSAULT	UNDETER-MINED	SUBSTANCE
976.4	E946.4	E858.7	E950.4	E962.0	E980.4	SELENIUM DISULFIDE OR SULFIDE
976.4	E946.4	E858.7	E950.4	E962.0	E980.4	SELSUN
973.1	E943.1	E858.4	E950.4	E962.0	E980.4	SENNA
976.2	E946.2	E858.7	E950.4	E962.0	E980.4	SEPTISOL
969.4	E939.4	E853.2	E950.3	E962.0	E980.3	SERAX
967.8	E937.8	E852.8	E950.2	E962.0	E980.2	SERENESIL
961.9	E931.9	E857	E950.4	E962.0	E980.4	SERENIUM (HYDROCHLORIDE)
968.3	E938.3	E855.1	E950.4	E962.0	E980.4	SERNYL
977.8	E947.8	E858.8	E950.4	E962.0	E980.4	SEROTONIN
972.6	E942.6	E858.3	E950.4	E962.0	E980.4	SERPASIL
987.8		E869.8	E952.8	E962.2	E982.8	SEWER GAS
989.6		E861.0	E950.9	E962.1	E980.9	SHAMPOO
988.0		E865.1	E950.9	E962.1	E980.9	SHELLFISH NONBACTERIAL OR NOXIOUS
989.83	E947.8	E866.8	E950.9	E962.1	E980.9	SILICONES NEC
976.0	E946.0	E858.7	E950.4	E962.0	E980.4	SILVADENE
976.0	E946.0	E858.7	E950.4	E962.0	E980.4	SILVER (COMPOUND) (MEDICINAL) NEC
976.0	E946.0	E858.7	E950.4	E962.0	E980.4	SILVER ANTI-INFECTIVES
961.1	E931.1	E857	E950.4	E962.0	E980.4	SILVER ARSPHENAMINE
976.0	E946.0	E858.7	E950.4	E962.0	E980.4	SILVER NITRATE
976.5	E946.5	E858.7	E950.4	E962.0	E980.4	SILVER NITRATE OPHTHALMIC PREPARATION
976.4	E946.4	E858.7	E950.4	E962.0	E980.4	SILVER NITRATE TOUGHENED (KERATOLYTIC)
985.8		E866.4	E950.9	E962.1	E980.9	SILVER NONMEDICINAL (DUST)
976.0	E946.0	E858.7	E950.4	E962.0	E980.4	SILVER PROTEIN (MILD) (STRONG)
961.1	E931.1	E857	E950.4	E962.0	E980.4	SILVER SALVARSAN
973.8	E943.8	E858.4	E950.4	E962.0	E980.4	SIMETHICONE
969.0	E939.0	E854.0	E950.3	E962.0	E980.3	SINEQUAN
972.6	E942.6	E858.3	E950.4	E962.0	E980.4	SINGOSERP
964.2	E934.2	E858.2	E950.4	E962.0	E980.4	SINTROM
972.2	E942.2	E858.3	E950.4	E962.0	E980.4	SITOSTEROLS
975.2	E945.2	E858.6	E950.4	E962.0	E980.4	SKELETAL MUSCLE RELAXANTS
976.8	E946.8	E858.7	E950.4	E962.0	E980.4	SKIN AGENTS SPECIFIED NEC
976.9	E946.9	E858.7	E950.4	E962.0	E980.4	SKIN AGENTS (EXTERNAL)
977.8	E947.8	E858.8	E950.4	E962.0	E980.4	SKIN TEST ANTIGEN
963.0	E933.0	E858.1	E950.4	E962.0	E980.4	SLEEP-EZE
967.9	E937.9	E852.9	E950.2	E962.0	E980.2	SLEEPING DRAUGHT (DRUG) (PILL) (TABLET)
979.0	E949.0	E858.8	E950.4	E962.0	E980.4	SMALLPOX VACCINE
985.9		E866.4	E950.9	E962.1	E980.9	SMELTER FUMES NEC
987.3		E869.1	E952.8	E962.2	E982.8	SMOG
987.9		E869.9	E952.9	E962.2	E982.9	SMOKE NEC
975.1	E945.1	E858.6	E950.4	E962.0	E980.4	SMOOTH MUSCLE RELAXANT
989.4		E863.4	E950.6	E962.1	E980.7	SNAIL KILLER
989.5		E905.0	E950.9	E962.1	E980.9	SNAKE (BITE) (VENOM)
989.89		E866.8	E950.9	E962.1	E980.9	SNUFF
989.6		E861.1	E950.9	E962.1	E980.9	SOAP (POWDER) (PRODUCT)
976.2	E946.2	E858.7	E950.4	E962.0	E980.4	SOAP MEDICINAL SOFT
983.2		E864.2	E950.7	E962.1	E980.6	SODA (CAUSTIC)
963.3	E933.3	E858.1	E950.4	E962.0	E980.4	SODA BICARB
0						SODA CHLORINATED SEE SODIUM HYPOCHLORITE
0						SODA SEE SODIUM HYPOCHLORITE
961.8	E931.8	E857	E950.4	E962.0	E980.4	SODIUM ACETOSULFONE
977.8	E947.8	E858.8	E950.4	E962.0	E980.4	SODIUM ACETRIZOATE
967.0	E937.0	E851	E950.1	E962.0	E980.1	SODIUM AMYTAL
0						SODIUM AMYTAL ARSENATE SEE ARSENIC
963.3	E933.3	E858.1	E950.4	E962.0	E980.4	SODIUM BICARBONATE
983.9		E864.3	E950.7	E962.1	E980.6	SODIUM BICHROMATE
963.2	E933.2	E858.1	E950.4	E962.0	E980.4	SODIUM BIPHOSPHATE
983.9		E864.3	E950.7	E962.1	E980.6	SODIUM BISULFATE
989.6		E861.3	E950.9	E962.1	E980.9	SODIUM BORATE (CLEANSER)
967.3	E937.3	E852.2	E950.2	E962.0	E980.2	SODIUM BROMIDE NEC
978.8	E948.8	E858.8	E950.4	E962.0	E980.4	SODIUM CACODYLATE (NONMEDICINAL) NEC
961.1	E931.1	E857	E950.4	E962.0	E980.4	SODIUM CACODYLATE ANTI-INFECTIVE
989.4		E863.5	E950.6	E962.1	E980.7	SODIUM CACODYLATE HERBICIDE
963.8	E933.8	E858.1	E950.4	E962.0	E980.4	SODIUM CALCIUM EDETATE
983.2		E864.2	E950.7	E962.1	E980.6	SODIUM CARBONATE NEC
983.9		E863.5	E950.7	E962.1	E980.6	SODIUM CHLORATE HERBICIDE
983.9		E864.3	E950.7	E962.1	E980.6	SODIUM CHLORATE NEC
974.5	E944.5	E858.5	E950.4	E962.0	E980.4	SODIUM CHLORIDE NEC
983.9		E864.3	E950.7	E962.1	E980.6	SODIUM CHROMATE
963.3	E933.3	E858.1	E950.4	E962.0	E980.4	SODIUM CITRATE

DRUGS & CHEMICALS

POISON	THERA-PEUTIC	ACCIDENT	SUICIDE	ASSAULT	UNDETER-MINED	SUBSTANCE
0						SODIUM CYANIDE CYANIDE(S)
974.5	E944.5	E858.5	E950.4	E962.0	E980.4	SODIUM CYCLAMATE
977.8	E947.8	E858.8	E950.4	E962.0	E980.4	SODIUM DIATRIZOATE
975.4	E945.4	E858.6	E950.4	E962.0	E980.4	SODIUM DIBUNATE
973.2	E943.2	E858.4	E950.4	E962.0	E980.4	SODIUM DIOCTYL SULFOSUCCINATE
963.8	E933.8	E858.1	E950.4	E962.0	E980.4	SODIUM EDETATE
974.4	E944.4	E858.5	E950.4	E962.0	E980.4	SODIUM ETHACRYNATE
989.4		E863.7	E950.6	E962.1	E980.7	SODIUM FLUORACETATE (DUST) (RODENTICIDE)
0						SODIUM FLUORIDE SEE FLUORIDE(S)
974.5	E944.5	E858.5	E950.4	E962.0	E980.4	SODIUM FREE SALT
961.8	E931.8	E857	E950.4	E962.0	E980.4	SODIUM GLUCOSULFONE
983.2		E864.2	E950.7	E962.1	E980.6	SODIUM HYDROXIDE
983.9		E864.3	E950.7	E962.1	E980.6	SODIUM HYPOCHLORITE (BLEACH) NEC
983.9		E861.4	E950.7	E962.1	E980.6	SODIUM HYPOCHLORITE DISINFECTANT
976.0	E946.0	E858.7	E950.4	E962.0	E980.4	SODIUM HYPOCHLORITE MEDICINAL (ANTI-INFECTIVE) (EXTERNAL)
987.8		E869.8	E952.8	E962.2	E982.8	SODIUM HYPOCHLORITE VAPOR
976.0	E946.0	E858.7	E950.4	E962.0	E980.4	SODIUM HYPOSULFITE
977.8	E947.8	E858.8	E950.4	E962.0	E980.4	SODIUM INDIGOTIN-DISULFONATE
977.8	E947.8	E858.8	E950.4	E962.0	E980.4	SODIUM IODIDE
977.8	E947.8	E858.8	E950.4	E962.0	E980.4	SODIUM IOTHALAMATE
964.0	E934.0	E858.2	E950.4	E962.0	E980.4	SODIUM IRON EDETATE
962.7	E932.7	E858.0	E950.4	E962.0	E980.4	SODIUM L-TRIIODO-THYRONINE
963.3	E933.3	E858.1	E950.4	E962.0	E980.4	SODIUM LACTATE
976.2	E946.2	E858.7	E950.4	E962.0	E980.4	SODIUM LAURYL SULFATE
977.8	E947.8	E858.8	E950.4	E962.0	E980.4	SODIUM METRIZOATE
989.4		E863.7	E950.6	E962.1	E980.7	SODIUM MONO-FLUORACETATE (DUST) (RODENTICIDE)
972.7	E942.7	E858.3	E950.4	E962.0	E980.4	SODIUM MORRHUATE
960.0	E930.0	E856	E950.4	E962.0	E980.4	SODIUM NAFCILLIN
983.9		E864.3	E950.7	E962.1	E980.6	SODIUM NITRATE (OXIDIZING AGENT)
972.4	E942.4	E858.3	E950.4	E962.0	E980.4	SODIUM NITRITE (MEDICINAL)
972.6	E942.6	E858.3	E950.4	E962.0	E980.4	SODIUM NITRO-FERRICYANIDE
972.6	E942.6	E858.3	E950.4	E962.0	E980.4	SODIUM NITROPRUSSIDE
977.8	E947.8	E858.8	E950.4	E962.0	E980.4	SODIUM PARA-AMINOHIPPURATE
976.6	E946.6	E858.7	E950.4	E962.0	E980.4	SODIUM PERBORATE MEDICINAL
989.6		E861.1	E950.9	E962.1	E980.9	SODIUM PERBORATE SOAP
989.89		E866.8	E950.9	E962.1	E980.9	SODIUM PERBORATE (NONMEDICINAL) NEC
0						SODIUM PERCARBONATE SEE SODIUM PERBORATE
973.3	E943.3	E858.4	E950.4	E962.0	E980.4	SODIUM PHOSPHATE
974.5	E944.5	E858.5	E950.4	E962.0	E980.4	SODIUM POLYSTYRENE SULFONATE
976.0	E946.0	E858.7	E950.4	E962.0	E980.4	SODIUM PROPIONATE
972.7	E942.7	E858.3	E950.4	E962.0	E980.4	SODIUM PSYLLIATE
974.5	E944.5	E858.5	E950.4	E962.0	E980.4	SODIUM REMOVING RESINS
965.1	E935.3	E850.3	E950.0	E962.0	E980.0	SODIUM SALICYLATE
973.3	E943.3	E858.4	E950.4	E962.0	E980.4	SODIUM SULFATE
961.8	E931.8	E857	E950.4	E962.0	E980.4	SODIUM SULFOXONE
972.7	E942.7	E858.3	E950.4	E962.0	E980.4	SODIUM TETRADECYL SULFATE
968.3	E938.3	E855.1	E950.4	E962.0	E980.4	SODIUM THIOPENTAL
965.1	E935.3	E850.3	E950.0	E962.0	E980.0	SODIUM THIOSALICYLATE
976.0	E946.0	E858.7	E950.4	E962.0	E980.4	SODIUM THIOSULFATE
977.8	E947.8	E858.8	E950.4	E962.0	E980.4	SODIUM TOLBUTAMIDE
977.8	E947.8	E858.8	E950.4	E962.0	E980.4	SODIUM TYROPANOATE
977.8	E947.8	E858.8	E950.4	E962.0	E980.4	SOLANINE
988.2		E865.4	E950.9	E962.1	E980.9	SOLANUM DULCAMARA
961.8	E931.8	E857	E950.4	E962.0	E980.4	SOLAPSONE
961.8	E931.8	E857	E950.4	E962.0	E980.4	SOLASULFONE
983.1		E864.1	E950.7	E962.1	E980.6	SOLDERING FLUID
989.9		E866.8	E950.9	E962.1	E980.9	SOLID SUBSTANCE SPECIFIED NEC
982.8		E862.9	E950.9	E962.1	E980.9	SOLVENTS INDUSTRIAL
981		E862.0	E950.9	E962.1	E980.9	SOLVENTS NAPHTHA
981		E862.0	E950.9	E962.1	E980.9	SOLVENTS PETROLEUM
982.8		E862.4	E950.9	E962.1	E980.9	SOLVENTS SPECIFIED NEC
968.0	E938.0	E855.1	E950.4	E962.0	E980.4	SOMA
962.4	E932.4	E858.0	E950.4	E962.0	E980.4	SOMATOTROPIN (GROWTH HORMONE)
963.0	E933.0	E858.1	E950.4	E962.0	E980.4	SOMINEX
967.1	E937.1	E852.0	E950.2	E962.0	E980.2	SOMNOS
967.0	E937.0	E851	E950.1	E962.0	E980.1	SOMONAL
967.0	E937.0	E851	E950.1	E962.0	E980.1	SONERYL
977.9	E947.9	E858.9	E950.5	E962.0	E980.5	SOOTHING SYRUP
967.4	E937.4	E852.3	E950.2	E962.0	E980.2	SOPOR
967.9	E937.9	E852.9	E950.2	E962.0	E980.2	SOPORIFIC DRUG

POISON	THERA-PEUTIC	ACCIDENT	SUICIDE	ASSAULT	UNDETER-MINED	SUBSTANCE
967.8	E937.8	E852.8	E950.2	E962.0	E980.2	SOPORIFIC DRUG SPECIFIED TYPE NEC
977.4	E947.4	E858.8	E950.4	E962.0	E980.4	SORBITOL NEC
972.7	E942.7	E858.3	E950.4	E962.0	E980.4	SOTRADECOL
975.1	E945.1	E858.6	E950.4	E962.0	E980.4	SPACOLINE
976.8	E946.8	E858.7	E950.4	E962.0	E980.4	SPANISH FLY
969.1	E939.1	E853.0	E950.3	E962.0	E980.3	SPARINE
975.0	E945.0	E858.6	E950.4	E962.0	E980.4	SPARTEINE
975.1	E945.1	E855.6	E950.4	E962.0	E980.4	SPASMOLYTICS
971.1	E941.1	E855.4	E950.4	E962.0	E980.4	SPASMOLYTICS ANTICHOLINERGICS
960.8	E930.8	E856	E950.4	E962.0	E980.4	SPECTINOMYCIN
969.7	E939.7	E854.2	E950.3	E962.0	E980.3	SPEED
976.8	E946.8	E858.7	E950.4	E962.0	E980.4	SPERMICIDES
989.5		E905.1	E950.9	E962.1	E980.9	SPIDER (BITE) (VENOM)
979.9	E949.9	E858.8	E950.4	E962.0	E980.4	SPIDER ANTIVENIN
961.6	E931.6	E857	E950.4	E962.0	E980.4	SPIGELIA (ROOT)
969.2	E939.2	E853.1	E950.3	E962.0	E980.3	SPIPERONE
960.3	E930.3	E856	E950.4	E962.0	E980.4	SPIRAMYCIN
969.5	E939.5	E853.8	E950.3	E962.0	E980.3	SPIRILENE
980.0		E860.0	E950.9	E962.1	E980.9	SPIRIT BEVERAGE
980.9		E860.9	E950.9	E962.1	E980.9	SPIRIT INDUSTRIAL
981		E862.0	E950.9	E962.1	E980.9	SPIRIT MINERAL
0						SPIRIT OF SALT SEE HYDROCHLORIC ACID
980.9		E860.9	E950.9	E962.1	E980.9	SPIRIT SURGICAL
980.0		E860.1	E950.9	E962.1	E980.9	SPIRIT(S) (NEUTRAL) NEC
974.4	E944.4	E858.5	E950.4	E962.0	E980.4	SPIRONOLACTONE
964.5	E934.5	E858.2	E950.4	E962.0	E980.4	SPONGE ABSORBABLE (GELATIN)
976.0	E946.0	E858.7	E950.4	E962.0	E980.4	SPOROSTACIN
989.89		E866.8	E950.9	E962.1	E980.9	SPRAYS (AEROSOL)
989.89		E866.7	E950.9	E962.1	E980.9	SPRAYS COSMETIC
977.9	E947.9	E858.9	E950.5	E962.0	E980.5	SPRAYS MEDICINAL NEC
0						SPRAYS PESTICIDES SEE PESTICIDES
0						SPRAYS SPECIFIED CONTENT SEE SUBSTANCE SPECIFIED
988.2		E865.4	E950.9	E962.1	E980.9	SPURGE FLAX
988.2		E865.4	E950.9	E962.1	E980.9	SPURGES
975.5	E945.5	E858.6	E950.4	E962.0	E980.4	SQUILL (EXPECTORANT) NEC
989.4		E863.7	E950.6	E962.1	E980.7	SQUILL RAT POISON
973.1	E943.1	E858.4	E950.4	E962.0	E980.4	SQUIRTING CUCUMBER (CATHARTIC)
989.89		E866.8	E950.9	E962.1	E980.9	STAINS
976.7	E946.7	E858.7	E950.4	E962.0	E980.4	STANNOUS FLUORIDE
0						STANNOUS SEE ALSO TIN
962.1	E932.1	E858.0	E950.4	E962.0	E980.4	STANOLONE
962.1	E932.1	E858.0	E950.4	E962.0	E980.4	STANOZOLOL
976.0	E946.0	E858.7	E950.4	E962.0	E980.4	STAPHISAGRIA OR STAVESACRE (PEDICULICIDE)
969.1	E939.1	E853.0	E950.3	E962.0	E980.3	STELAZINE
969.1	E939.1	E853.0	E950.3	E962.0	E980.3	STEMETIL
973.3	E943.3	E858.4	E950.4	E962.0	E980.4	STERCULIA (CATHARTIC) (GUM)
987.8		E869.8	E952.8	E962.2	E982.8	STERNUTATOR GAS
976.6	E946.6	E858.7	E950.4	E962.0	E980.4	STEROIDS ENT AGENT
962.0	E932.0	E858.0	E950.4	E962.0	E980.4	STEROIDS NEC
976.5	E946.5	E858.7	E950.4	E962.0	E980.4	STEROIDS OPHTHALMIC PREPARATION
976.0	E946.0	E858.7	E950.4	E962.0	E980.4	STEROIDS TOPICAL NEC
985.8		E866.4	E950.9	E962.1	E980.9	STIBINE
961.2	E931.2	E857	E950.4	E962.0	E980.4	STIBOPHEN
961.5	E931.5	E857	E950.4	E962.0	E980.4	STILBAMIDE
962.2	E932.2	E858.0	E950.4	E962.0	E980.4	STILBESTROL
969.0	E939.0	E854.0	E950.3	E962.0	E980.3	STIMULANTS PSYCHOTHERAPEUTIC NEC
970.9	E940.9	E854.3	E950.4	E962.0	E980.4	STIMULANTS (CENTRAL NERVOUS SYSTEM)
970.0	E940.0	E854.3	E950.4	E962.0	E980.4	STIMULANTS ANALEPTICS
970.1	E940.1	E854.3	E950.4	E962.0	E980.4	STIMULANTS OPIATE ANTAGONIST
970.8	E940.8	E854.3	E950.4	E962.0	E980.4	STIMULANTS SPECIFIED NEC
983.1		E864.1	E950.7	E962.1	E980.6	STORAGE BATTERIES (ACID) (CELLS)
968.9	E938.9	E855.2	E950.4	E962.0	E980.4	STOVAINE
968.5	E938.5	E855.2	E950.4	E962.0	E980.4	STOVAINE INFILTRATION (SUBCUTANEOUS)
968.6	E938.6	E855.2	E950.4	E962.0	E980.4	STOVAINE NERVE BLOCK (PERIPHERAL) (PLEXUS)
968.7	E938.7	E855.2	E950.4	E962.0	E980.4	STOVAINE SPINAL
968.5	E938.5	E855.2	E950.4	E962.0	E980.4	STOVAINE TOPICAL (SURFACE)
961.1	E931.1	E857	E950.4	E962.0	E980.4	STOVARSAL
0						STOVE GAS SEE GAS UTILITY

DRUGS & CHEMICALS

POISON	THERA-PEUTIC	ACCIDENT	SUICIDE	ASSAULT	UNDETER-MINED	SUBSTANCE
976.5	E946.5	E858.7	E950.4	E962.0	E980.4	STOXIL
969.6	E939.6	E854.1	E950.3	E962.0	E980.3	STP
971.1	E941.1	E855.4	E950.4	E962.0	E980.4	STRAMONIUM (MEDICINAL) NEC
988.2		E865.4	E950.9	E962.1	E980.9	STRAMONIUM NATURAL STATE
964.4	E934.4	E858.2	E950.4	E962.0	E980.4	STREPTODORNASE
960.6	E930.6	E856	E950.4	E962.0	E980.4	STREPTODUOCIN
964.4	E934.4	E858.2	E950.4	E962.0	E980.4	STREPTOKINASE
960.6	E930.6	E856	E950.4	E962.0	E980.4	STREPTOMYCIN
960.7	E930.7	E856	E950.4	E962.0	E980.4	STREPTOZOCIN
982.8		E862.9	E950.9	E962.1	E980.9	STRIPPER (PAINT) (SOLVENT)
989.2		E863.0	E950.6	E962.1	E980.7	STROBANE
972.1	E942.1	E858.3	E950.4	E962.0	E980.4	STROPHANTHINS
988.2		E865.4	E950.9	E962.1	E980.9	STROPHANTHUS HISPIDUS OR KOMBE
989.1		E863.7	E950.6	E962.1	E980.7	STRYCHNINE (RODENTICIDE) (SALTS)
970.8	E940.8	E854.3	E950.4	E962.0	E980.4	STRYCHNINE MEDICINALNEC
0						STRYCHNOS (IGNATII) SEE STRYCHNINE
968.0	E938.0	E855.1	E950.4	E962.0	E980.4	STYRAMATE
983.0		E864.0	E950.7	E962.1	E980.6	STYRENE
966.2	E936.2	E855.0	E950.4	E962.0	E980.4	SUCCINIMIDE (ANTICONVULSANT)
0						SUCCINIMIDE MERCURICSEE MERCURY
975.2	E945.2	E858.6	E950.4	E962.0	E980.4	SUCCINYLCHOLINE
961.0	E931.0	E857	E950.4	E962.0	E980.4	SUCCINYLSULFA-THIAZOLE
974.5	E944.5	E858.5	E950.4	E962.0	E980.4	SUCROSE
961.0	E931.0	E857	E950.4	E962.0	E980.4	SULFACETAMIDE
976.5	E946.5	E858.7	E950.4	E962.0	E980.4	SULFACETAMIDE OPHTHALMIC PREPARATION
961.0	E931.0	E857	E950.4	E962.0	E980.4	SULFACHLORPYRIDAZINE
961.0	E931.0	E857	E950.4	E962.0	E980.4	SULFACYTINE
961.0	E931.0	E857	E950.4	E962.0	E980.4	SULFADIAZINE
976.0	E946.0	E858.7	E950.4	E962.0	E980.4	SULFADIAZINE SILVER (TOPICAL)
961.0	E931.0	E857	E950.4	E962.0	E980.4	SULFADIMETHOZINE
961.0	E931.0	E857	E950.4	E962.0	E980.4	SULFADIMIDINE
961.0	E931.0	E857	E950.4	E962.0	E980.4	SULFAETHIDOLE
961.0	E931.0	E857	E950.4	E962.0	E980.4	SULFAFURAZOLE
961.0	E931.0	E857	E950.4	E962.0	E980.4	SULFAGUANIDINE
961.0	E931.0	E857	E950.4	E962.0	E980.4	SULFAMERAZINE
961.0	E931.0	E857	E950.4	E962.0	E980.4	SULFAMETER
961.0	E931.0	E857	E950.4	E962.0	E980.4	SULFAMETHIZOLE
961.0	E931.0	E857	E950.4	E962.0	E980.4	SULFAMETHO-XYPYRIDAZINE
961.0	E931.0	E857	E950.4	E962.0	E980.4	SULFAMETHOXAZOLE
961.0	E931.0	E857	E950.4	E962.0	E980.4	SULFAMETHOXYDIAZINE
961.0	E931.0	E857	E950.4	E962.0	E980.4	SULFAMETHYLTHIAZOLE
976.0	E946.0	E858.7	E950.4	E962.0	E980.4	SULFAMYLON
977.8	E947.8	E858.8	E950.4	E962.0	E980.4	SULFAN BLUE (DIAGNOSTIC DYE)
961.0	E931.0	E857	E950.4	E962.0	E980.4	SULFANILAMIDE
961.0	E931.0	E857	E950.4	E962.0	E980.4	SULFANILYLGUANIDINE
961.0	E931.0	E857	E950.4	E962.0	E980.4	SULFAPHENAZOLE
961.0	E931.0	E857	E950.4	E962.0	E980.4	SULFAPHENYLTHIAZOLE
961.0	E931.0	E857	E950.4	E962.0	E980.4	SULFAPROXYLINE
961.0	E931.0	E857	E950.4	E962.0	E980.4	SULFAPYRIDINE
961.0	E931.0	E857	E950.4	E962.0	E980.4	SULFAPYRIMIDINE
961.1	E931.1	E857	E950.4	E962.0	E980.4	SULFARSPHENAMINE
961.0	E931.0	E857	E950.4	E962.0	E980.4	SULFASALAZINE
961.0	E931.0	E857	E950.4	E962.0	E980.4	SULFASOMIZOLE
961.0	E931.0	E857	E950.4	E962.0	E980.4	SULFASUXIDINE
987.8		E869.8	E952.8	E962.2	E982.8	SULFATE (FUMES)
976.6	E946.6	E858.7	E950.4	E962.0	E980.4	SULFATE ENT AGENT
974.7	E944.7	E858.5	E950.4	E962.0	E980.4	SULFINPYRAZONE
961.0	E931.0	E857	E950.4	E962.0	E980.4	SULFISOXAZOLE
976.5	E946.5	E858.7	E950.4	E962.0	E980.4	SULFISOXAZOLE OPHTHALMIC PREPARATION
960.8	E930.8	E856	E950.4	E962.0	E980.4	SULFOMYXIN
967.8	E937.8	E852.8	E950.2	E962.0	E980.2	SULFONAL
961.0	E931.0	E857	E950.4	E962.0	E980.4	SULFONAMIDES
961.8	E931.8	E857	E950.4	E962.0	E980.4	SULFONES
967.8	E937.8	E852.8	E950.2	E962.0	E980.2	SULFONETHYLMETHANE
967.8	E937.8	E852.8	E950.2	E962.0	E980.2	SULFONMETHANE
977.8	E947.8	E858.8	E950.4	E962.0	E980.4	SULFONPHTHAL
962.3	E932.3	E858.0	E950.4	E962.0	E980.4	SULFONYLUREA DERIVATIVES ORAL
961.8	E931.8	E857	E950.4	E962.0	E980.4	SULFOXONE
989.89		E866.8	E950.9	E962.1	E980.9	SULFUR (COMPOUNDS) NEC
983.1		E864.1	E950.7	E962.1	E980.6	SULFUR ACID
987.3		E869.1	E952.8	E962.2	E982.8	SULFUR DIOXIDE
0						SULFUR ETHER SEE ETHER(S)

POISON	THERAPEUTIC	ACCIDENT	SUICIDE	ASSAULT	UNDETERMINED	SUBSTANCE
987.8		E869.8	E952.8	E962.2	E982.8	SULFUR HYDROGEN
976.4	E946.4	E858.7	E950.4	E962.0	E980.4	SULFUR MEDICINAL (KERATOLYTIC) (OINTMENT) NEC
989.4		E863.4	E950.6	E962.1	E980.7	SULFUR PESTICIDE (VAPOR)
987.8		E869.8	E952.8	E962.2	E982.8	SULFUR VAPOR NEC
977.8	E947.8	E858.8	E950.4	E962.0	E980.4	SULKOWITCH'S REAGENT
961.8	E931.8	E857	E950.4	E962.0	E980.4	SULPHADIONE
966.3	E936.3	E855.0	E950.4	E962.0	E980.4	SULTHIAME
975.5	E945.5	E858.6	E950.4	E962.0	E980.4	SUPERINONE
961.5	E931.5	E857	E950.4	E962.0	E980.4	SURAMIN
968.5	E938.5	E855.2	E950.4	E962.0	E980.4	SURFACAINE
968.3	E938.3	E855.1	E950.4	E962.0	E980.4	SURITAL
976.8	E946.8	E858.7	E950.4	E962.0	E980.4	SUTILAINS
975.2	E945.2	E858.6	E950.4	E962.0	E980.4	SUXAMETHONIUM (BROMIDE) (CHLORIDE)
975.2	E945.2	E858.6	E950.4	E962.0	E980.4	SUXETHONIUM (BROMIDE)
975.2	E945.2	E858.6	E950.4	E962.0	E980.4	SUXETHONIUM (IODIDE)
976.3	E946.3	E858.7	E950.4	E962.0	E980.4	SWEET OIL (BIRCH)
982.3		E862.4	E950.9	E962.1	E980.9	SYM-DICHLOROETHYL ETHER
971.3	E941.3	E855.6	E950.4	E962.0	E980.4	SYMPATHOLYTICS
971.2	E941.2	E855.5	E950.4	E962.0	E980.4	SYMPATHOMIMETICS
979.6	E949.6	E858.8	E950.4	E962.0	E980.4	SYNAGIS
976.0	E946.0	E858.7	E950.4	E962.0	E980.4	SYNALAR
962.7	E932.7	E858.0	E950.4	E962.0	E980.4	SYNTHROID
975.0	E945.0	E858.6	E950.4	E962.0	E980.4	SYNTOCINON
972.6	E942.6	E858.3	E950.4	E962.0	E980.4	SYROSINGOPINE
963.9	E933.9	E858.1	E950.4	E962.0	E980.4	SYSTEMIC AGENTS (PRIMARILY)
963.8	E933.8	E858.1	E950.4	E962.0	E980.4	SYSTEMIC AGENTS SPECIFIED NEC
977.9	E947.9	E858.9	E950.5	E962.0	E980.5	TABLETS
962.2	E932.2	E858.0	E950.4	E962.0	E980.4	TACE
971.0	941.0	E855.3	E950.4	E962.0	E980.4	TACRINE
967.0	E937.0	E851	E950.1	E962.0	E980.1	TALBUTAL
976.3	E946.3	E858.7	E950.4	E962.0	E980.4	TALC
976.3	E946.3	E858.7	E950.4	E962.0	E980.4	TALCUM
971.3	E855.6	E941.3	E950.4	E962.0	E980.4	TAMSULOSIN
965.5	E935.5	E850.5	E950.0	E962.0	E980.0	TANDEARIL
983.1		E864.1	E950.7	E962.1	E980.6	TANNIC ACID
976.2	E946.2	E858.7	E950.4	E962.0	E980.4	TANNIC ACID MEDICINAL (ASTRINGENT)
0						TANNIN SEE TANNIC ACID
988.2		E865.4	E950.9	E962.1	E980.9	TANSY
960.3	E930.3	E856	E950.4	E962.0	E980.4	TAO
962.8	E932.8	E858.0	E950.4	E962.0	E980.4	TAPAZOLE
0						TAR CAMPHOR SEE NAPHTHALENE
987.8		E869.8	E952.8	E962.2	E982.8	TAR FUMES
983.0		E864.0	E950.7	E962.1	E980.6	TAR NEC
969.3	E939.3	E853.8	E950.3	E962.0	E980.3	TARACTAN
989.5		E905.1	E950.9	E962.1	E980.9	TARANTULA (VENOMOUS)
961.2	E931.2	E857	E950.4	E962.0	E980.4	TARTAR EMETIC (ANTI-INFECTIVE)
983.1		E864.1	E950.7	E962.1	E980.6	TARTARIC ACID
961.2	E931.2	E857	E950.4	E962.0	E980.4	TARTRATED ANTIMONY (ANTI-INFECTIVE)
0						TCA SEE TRICHLOROACETIC ACID
983.0		E864.0	E950.7	E962.1	E980.6	TDI
987.8		E869.8	E952.8	E962.2	E982.8	TDI VAPOR
987.5		E869.3	E952.8	E962.2	E982.8	TEAR GAS
974.3	E944.3	E858.5	E950.4	E962.0	E980.4	TECLOTHIAZIDE
966.3	E936.3	E855.0	E950.4	E962.0	E980.4	TEGRETOL
977.8	E947.8	E858.8	E950.4	E962.0	E980.4	TELEPAQUE
985.8		E866.4	E950.9	E962.1	E980.9	TELLURIUM
985.8		E866.4	E950.9	E962.1	E980.9	TELLURIUM FUMES
963.1	E933.1	E858.1	E950.4	E962.0	E980.4	TEM
963.1	E933.1	E858.1	E950.4	E962.0	E980.4	TEPA
989.3		E863.1	E950.6	E962.1	E980.7	TEPP
971.2	E941.2	E855.5	E950.4	E962.0	E980.4	TERBUTALINE
961.6	E931.6	E857	E950.4	E962.0	E980.4	TEROXALENE
975.5	E945.5	E858.6	E950.4	E962.0	E980.4	TERPIN HYDRATE
960.4	E930.4	E856	E950.4	E962.0	E980.4	TERRAMYCIN
975.4	E945.4	E858.6	E950.4	E962.0	E980.4	TESSALON
962.1	E932.1	E858.0	E950.4	E962.0	E980.4	TESTOSTERONE
978.4	E948.4	E858.8	E950.4	E962.0	E980.4	TETANUS (VACCINE)
979.9	E949.9	E858.8	E950.4	E962.0	E980.4	TETANUS ANTITOXIN
964.6	E934.6	E858.2	E950.4	E962.0	E980.4	TETANUS IMMUNE GLOBULIN (HUMAN)
978.4	E948.4	E858.8	E950.4	E962.0	E980.4	TETANUS TOXOID
978.9	E948.9	E858.8	E950.4	E962.0	E980.4	TETANUS TOXOID WITH DIPHTHERIA TOXOID

DRUGS & CHEMICALS

POISON	THERA-PEUTIC	ACCIDENT	SUICIDE	ASSAULT	UNDETER-MINED	SUBSTANCE
978.6	E948.6	E858.8	E950.4	E962.0	E980.4	TETANUS TOXOID WITH DIPHTHERIA TOXOID WITH PERTUSSIS
982.0		E862.4	E950.9	E962.1	E980.9	TETRA HYDRONAPHTHALENE
982.3		E861.6	E950.9	E962.1	E980.9	TETRA-CHLOROETHANE PAINT OR VARNISH
969.5	E939.5	E853.8	E950.3	E962.0	E980.3	TETRABENAZINE
968.5	E938.5	E855.2	E950.4	E962.0	E980.4	TETRACAINE
968.6	E938.6	E855.2	E950.4	E962.0	E980.4	TETRACAINE NERVE BLOCK (PERIPHERAL) (PLEXUS)
968.7	E938.7	E855.2	E950.4	E962.0	E980.4	TETRACAINE SPINAL
0						TETRACHLORETHYLENE SEE TETRACHLOROETHYLENE
974.3	E944.3	E858.5	E950.4	E962.0	E980.4	TETRACHLORMETHIAZIDE
982.3		E861.6	E950.9	E962.1	E980.9	TETRACHLOROE-THANE PAINT OR VARNISH
982.3		E862.4	E950.9	E962.1	E980.9	TETRACHLOROETHANE (LIQUID) (VAPOR)
982.3		E862.4	E950.9	E962.1	E980.9	TETRACHLOROETHYLENE (LIQUID) (VAPOR)
961.6	E931.6	E857	E950.4	E962.0	E980.4	TETRACHLOROETHYLENE MEDICINAL
0						TETRACHLOROMETHANE SEE CARBON TETRACHLORIDE
960.4	E930.4	E856	E950.4	E962.0	E980.4	TETRACYCLINE
976.5	E946.5	E858.7	E950.4	E962.0	E980.4	TETRACYCLINE OPHTHALMIC PREPARATION
976.0	E946.0	E858.7	E950.4	E962.0	E980.4	TETRACYCLINE TOPICAL NEC
989.3		E863.1	E950.6	E962.1	E980.7	TETRAETHYL PYROPHOSPHATE
984.1		E862.1	E950.9	E962.1	E980.9	TETRAETHYL LEAD (ANTIKNOCK COMPOUND)
972.3	E942.3	E858.3	E950.4	E962.0	E980.4	TETRAETHYLAMMONIUM CHLORIDE
977.3	E947.3	E858.8	E950.4	E962.0	E980.4	TETRAETHYLTHIURAM DISULFIDE
982.0		E862.4	E950.9	E962.1	E980.9	TETRAHYDRO-NAPHTHALENE
971.0	941.0	E855.3	E950.4	E962.0	E980.4	TETRAHYDROAMINO-ACRIDINE
969.6	E939.6	E854.1	E950.3	E962.0	E980.3	TETRAHYDROCANNABINOL
971.2	E941.2	E855.5	E950.4	E962.0	E980.4	TETRAHYDROZOLINE
982.0		E862.4	E950.9	E962.1	E980.9	TETRALIN
989.4		E863.6	E950.6	E962.1	E980.7	TETRAMETHYLTHIURAM (DISULFIDE) NEC
976.2	E946.2	E858.7	E950.4	E962.0	E980.4	TETRAMETHYLTHIURAM MEDICINAL
967.8	E937.8	E852.8	E950.2	E962.0	E980.2	TETRONAL
983.0		E864.0	E950.7	E962.1	E980.6	TETRYL
967.8	E937.8	E852.8	E950.2	E962.0	E980.2	THALIDOMIDE
985.8		E866.4	E950.9	E962.1	E980.9	THALLIUM (COMPOUNDS) (DUST) NEC
985.8		E863.7	E950.6	E962.1	E980.7	THALLIUM PESTICIDE (RODENTICIDE)
969.6	E939.6	E854.1	E950.3	E962.0	E980.3	THC
965.09	E935.2	E850.2	E950.0	E962.0	E980.0	THEBACON
965.09	E935.2	E850.2	E950.0	E962.0	E980.0	THEBAINE
974.1	E944.1	E858.5	E950.4	E962.0	E980.4	THEOBROMINE
974.1	E944.1	E858.5	E950.4	E962.0	E980.4	THEOBROMINE (CALCIUMSALICYLATE)
974.1	E944.1	E858.5	E950.4	E962.0	E980.4	THEOPHYLLINE (DIURETIC)
975.7	E945.7	E858.6	E950.4	E962.0	E980.4	THEOPHYLLINE ETHYLENEDIAMINE
961.6	E931.6	E857	E950.4	E962.0	E980.4	THIABENDAZOLE
968.3	E938.3	E855.1	E950.4	E962.0	E980.4	THIALBARBITAL
963.5	E933.5	E858.1	E950.4	E962.0	E980.4	THIAMINE
960.2	E930.2	E856	E950.4	E962.0	E980.4	THIAMPHENICOL
968.3	E938.3	E855.1	E950.4	E962.0	E980.4	THIAMYLAL (SODIUM)
969.0	E939.0	E854.0	E950.3	E962.0	E980.3	THIAZESIM
974.3	E944.3	E858.5	E950.4	E962.0	E980.4	THIAZIDES (DIURETICS)
963.0	E933.0	E858.1	E950.4	E962.0	E980.4	THIETHYLPERAZINE
976.5	E946.5	E858.7	E950.4	E962.0	E980.4	THIMEROSAL OPHTHALMIC PREPARATION
976.0	E946.0	E858.7	E950.4	E962.0	E980.4	THIMEROSAL (TOPICAL)
963.1	E933.1	E858.1	E950.4	E962.0	E980.4	THIO-TEPA
961.8	E931.8	E857	E950.4	E962.0	E980.4	THIOACETAZONE
968.3	E938.3	E855.1	E950.4	E962.0	E980.4	THIOBARBITURATES SUCH AS THIOPENTAL SODIUM
961.2	E931.2	E857	E950.4	E962.0	E980.4	THIOBISMOL
962.8	E932.8	E858.0	E950.4	E962.0	E980.4	THIOCARBAMIDE
961.1	E931.1	E857	E950.4	E962.0	E980.4	THIOCARBARSONE
961.8	E931.8	E857	E950.4	E962.0	E980.4	THIOCARLIDE
963.1	E933.1	E858.1	E950.4	E962.0	E980.4	THIOGUANINE
974.0	E944.0	E858.5	E950.4	E962.0	E980.4	THIOMERCAPTOMERIN
974.0	E944.0	E858.5	E950.4	E962.0	E980.4	THIOMERIN
968.3	E938.3	E855.1	E950.4	E962.0	E980.4	THIOPENTAL THIOPENTONE (SODIUM)
969.1	E939.1	E853.0	E950.3	E962.0	E980.3	THIOPROPAZATE
969.1	E939.1	E853.0	E950.3	E962.0	E980.3	THIOPROPERAZINE

POISON	THERA-PEUTIC	ACCIDENT	SUICIDE	ASSAULT	UNDETER-MINED	SUBSTANCE
969.1	E939.1	E853.0	E950.3	E962.0	E980.3	THIORIDAZINE
969.3	E939.3	E853.8	E950.3	E962.0	E980.3	THIOTHIXENE
962.8	E932.8	E858.0	E950.4	E962.0	E980.4	THIOURACIL
962.8	E932.8	E858.0	E950.4	E962.0	E980.4	THIOUREA
971.1	E941.1	E855.4	E950.4	E962.0	E980.4	THIPHENAMIL
976.2	E946.2	E858.7	E950.4	E962.0	E980.4	THIRAM MEDICINAL
989.4		E863.6	E950.6	E962.1	E980.7	THIRAM NEC
963.0	E933.0	E858.1	E950.4	E962.0	E980.4	THONZYLAMINE
969.1	E939.1	E853.0	E950.3	E962.0	E980.3	THORAZINE
988.2		E865.4	E950.9	E962.1	E980.9	THORNAPPLE
976.6	E946.6	E858.7	E950.4	E962.0	E980.4	THROAT PREPARATION (LOZENGES) NEC
964.5	E934.5	E858.2	E950.4	E962.0	E980.4	THROMBIN
964.4	E934.4	E858.2	E950.4	E962.0	E980.4	THROMBOLYSIN
983.0		E864.0	E950.7	E962.1	E980.6	THYMOL
962.9	E932.9	E858.0	E950.4	E962.0	E980.4	THYMUS EXTRACT
962.7	E932.7	E858.0	E950.4	E962.0	E980.4	THYROGLOBULIN
962.7	E932.7	E858.0	E950.4	E962.0	E980.4	THYROID AND THYROID (DERIVATIVES) (EXTRACT)
962.7	E932.7	E858.0	E950.4	E962.0	E980.4	THYROLAR
977.8	E947.8	E858.8	E950.4	E962.0	E980.4	THYROTHROPHIN
962.7	E932.7	E858.0	E950.4	E962.0	E980.4	THYROXIN(E)
963.0	E933.0	E858.1	E950.4	E962.0	E980.4	TIGAN
968.0	E938.0	E855.1	E950.4	E962.0	E980.4	TIGLOIDINE
985.8		E866.4	E950.9	E962.1	E980.9	TIN (CHLORIDE) (DUST) (OXIDE) NEC
961.2	E931.2	E857	E950.4	E962.0	E980.4	TIN ANTI-INFECTIVES
976.0	E946.0	E858.7	E950.4	E962.0	E980.4	TINACTIN
0						TINCTURE IODINE SEE IODINE
969.1	E939.1	E853.0	E950.3	E962.0	E980.3	TINDAL
985.8		E866.4	E950.9	E962.1	E980.9	TITANIUM (COMPOUNDS) (VAPOR)
976.3	E946.3	E858.7	E950.4	E962.0	E980.4	TITANIUM OINTMENT
962.7	E932.7	E858.0	E950.4	E962.0	E980.4	TITROID
0						TMTD SEE TETRAMETHYLTHIURAM
989.89		E866.8	E950.9	E962.1	E980.9	TNT
987.8		E869.8	E952.8	E962.2	E982.8	TNT FUMES
988.1		E865.5	E950.9	E962.1	E980.9	TOADSTOOL
988.2		E865.4	E950.9	E962.1	E980.9	TOBACCO INDIAN
987.8		E869.4				TOBACCO SMOKE SECOND-HAND
989.84		E866.8	E950.9	E962.1	E980.9	TOBACCO NEC
963.5	E933.5	E858.1	E950.4	E962.0	E980.4	TOCOPHEROL
975.0	E945.0	E858.6	E950.4	E962.0	E980.4	TOCOSAMINE
969.0	E939.0	E854.0	E950.3	E962.0	E980.3	TOFRANIL
989.89		E866.8	E950.9	E962.1	E980.9	TOILET DEODORIZER
962.3	E932.3	E858.0	E950.4	E962.0	E980.4	TOLAZAMIDE
971.3	E941.3	E855.6	E950.4	E962.0	E980.4	TOLAZOLINE HYDROCHLORIDE
962.3	E932.3	E858.0	E950.4	E962.0	E980.4	TOLBUTAMIDE
977.8	E947.8	E858.8	E950.4	E962.0	E980.4	TOLBUTAMIDE SODIUM
965.69	E935.6	E850.6	E950.0	E962.0	E980.0	TOLMETIN
976.0	E946.0	E858.7	E950.4	E962.0	E980.4	TOLNAFTATE
976.1	E946.1	E858.7	E950.4	E962.0	E980.4	TOLPROPAMINE
968.0	E938.0	E855.1	E950.4	E962.0	E980.4	TOLSEROL
983.0		E864.0	E950.7	E962.1	E980.6	TOLUENE DIISOCYANATE
983.0		E864.0	E950.7	E962.1	E980.6	TOLUIDINE
987.8		E869.8	E952.8	E962.2	E982.8	TOLUIDINE VAPOR
982.0		E862.4	E950.9	E962.1	E980.9	TOLUOL (LIQUID) (VAPOR)
983.0		E864.0	E950.7	E962.1	E980.6	TOLYLENE-2 4 DIISOCYANATE
972.1	E942.1	E858.3	E950.4	E962.0	E980.4	TONICS CARDIAC
976.6	E946.6	E858.7	E950.4	E962.0	E980.4	TOPICAL AGENTS ANTI-INFECTIVES AND OTHER DRUGS AND PREPARATIONS FOR EAR NOSE AND THROAT
976.1	E946.1	E858.7	E950.4	E962.0	E980.4	TOPICAL AGENTS ANTIPRURITICS
976.7	E946.7	E858.7	E950.4	E962.0	E980.4	TOPICAL AGENTS DENTAL DRUGS TOPICALLY APPLIED
976.3	E946.3	E858.7	E950.4	E962.0	E980.4	TOPICAL AGENTS EMOLLIENTS DEMULCENTS AND PROTECTANTS
976.5	E946.5	E858.7	E950.4	E962.0	E980.4	TOPICAL AGENTS EYE ANTI-INFECTIVES AND OTHER EYE DRUGS
976.5	E946.5	E858.7	E950.4	E962.0	E980.4	TOPICAL AGENTS IDOXURIDINE
976.4	E946.4	E858.7	E950.4	E962.0	E980.4	TOPICAL AGENTS KERATOLYTICS KERATOPLASTICS OTHER HAIR TREATMENT DRUGS AND PREPARATIONS
976.0	E946.0	E858.7	E950.4	E962.0	E980.4	TOPICAL AGENTS LOCAL ANTI-INFECTIVES AND ANTI-INFLAMMATORY DRUGS

POISON	THERA-PEUTIC	ACCIDENT	SUICIDE	ASSAULT	UNDETER-MINED	SUBSTANCE
976.2	E946.2	E858.7	E950.4	E962.0	E980.4	TOPICAL AGENTS LOCAL ASTRINGENTS AND LOCAL DETERGENTS
976.9	E946.9	E858.7	E950.4	E962.0	E980.4	TOPICAL AGENTS NOS AGENT PRIMARILY AFFECTING SKIN AND MUCOUS MEMBRANE
976.8	E946.8	E858.7	E950.4	E962.0	E980.4	TOPICAL AGENTS SPERMICIDES (VAGINAL CONTRACEPTIVES)
982.0		E862.4	E950.9	E962.1	E980.9	TOULENE (LIQUID) (VAPOR)
989.2		E863.0	E950.6	E962.1	E980.7	TOXAPHENE (DUST) (SPRAY)
978.8	E948.8	E858.8	E950.4	E962.0	E980.4	TOXOIDS NEC
981		E862.1	E950.9	E962.1	E980.9	TRACTOR FUEL NEC
973.3	E943.3	E858.4	E950.4	E962.0	E980.4	TRAGACANTH
971.2	E941.2	E855.5	E950.4	E962.0	E980.4	TRAMAZOLINE
969.5	E939.5	E853.9	E950.3	E962.0	E980.3	TRANQUILIZERS
969.4	E939.4	E853.2	E950.3	E962.0	E980.3	TRANQUILIZERS BENZODIAZEPINE-BASED
969.2	E939.2	E853.1	E950.3	E962.0	E980.3	TRANQUILIZERS BUTYROPHENONE-BASED
969.3	E939.3	E853.8	E950.3	E962.0	E980.3	TRANQUILIZERS MAJOR
969.3	E939.3	E853.8	E950.3	E962.0	E980.3	TRANQUILIZERS MAJOR OTHER ANTIPSYCHOTICS NEUROLEPTICS
969.1	E939.1	E853.0	E950.3	E962.0	E980.3	TRANQUILIZERS PHENOTHIAZINE-BASED
969.5	E939.5	E853.8	E950.3	E962.0	E980.3	TRANQUILIZERS SPECIFIED NEC
961.9	E931.9	E857	E950.4	E962.0	E980.4	TRANTOIN
969.4	E939.4	E853.2	E950.3	E962.0	E980.3	TRANXENE
969.0	E939.0	E854.0	E950.3	E962.0	E980.3	TRANYLCYPROMINE (SULFATE)
975.1	E945.1	E858.6	E950.4	E962.0	E980.4	TRASENTINE
974.5	E944.5	E858.5	E950.4	E962.0	E980.4	TRAVERT
961.8	E931.8	E857	E950.4	E962.0	E980.4	TRECATOR
976.8	E946.8	E858.7	E950.4	E962.0	E980.4	TRETINOIN
976.0	E946.0	E858.7	E950.4	E962.0	E980.4	TRIACETIN
960.3	E930.3	E856	E950.4	E962.0	E980.4	TRIACETYLOLEANDO-MYCIN
962.0	E932.0	E858.0	E950.4	E962.0	E980.4	TRIAMCINOLONE
976.6	E946.6	E858.7	E950.4	E962.0	E980.4	TRIAMCINOLONE ENT AGENT
976.5	E946.5	E858.7	E950.4	E962.0	E980.4	TRIAMCINOLONE OPHTHALMIC PREPARATION
976.0	E946.0	E858.7	E950.4	E962.0	E980.4	TRIAMCINOLONE TOPICAL NEC
974.4	E944.4	E858.5	E950.4	E962.0	E980.4	TRIAMTERENE
963.1	E933.1	E858.1	E950.4	E962.0	E980.4	TRIAZIQUONE
967.3	E937.3	E852.2	E950.2	E962.0	E980.2	TRIBROMACETALDEHYDE
968.2	E938.2	E855.1	E950.4	E962.0	E980.4	TRIBROMOETHANOL
967.3	E937.3	E852.2	E950.2	E962.0	E980.2	TRIBROMOMETHANE
983.1		E864.1	E950.7	E962.1	E980.6	TRICHLOROACETIC ACID
976.4	E946.4	E858.7	E950.4	E962.0	E980.4	TRICHLOROACETIC ACID MEDICINAL (KERATOLYTIC)
982.3		E862.4	E950.9	E962.1	E980.9	TRICHLORETHANE
974.3	E944.3	E858.5	E950.4	E962.0	E980.4	TRICHLORMETHIAZIDE
989.2		E863.0	E950.6	E962.1	E980.7	TRICHLOROPHENOXYACETIC ACID (2 4 5-T)
963.1	E933.1	E858.1	E950.4	E962.0	E980.4	TRICHLOROTRIETHYLAMINE
967.1	E937.1	E852.0	E950.2	E962.0	E980.2	TRICHLOROETHANOL
967.1	E937.1	E852.0	E950.2	E962.0	E980.2	TRICHLOROETHYL PHOSPHATE
982.3		E862.4	E950.9	E962.1	E980.9	TRICHLOROETHYLENE (LIQUID) (VAPOR)
968.2	E938.2	E855.1	E950.4	E962.0	E980.4	TRICHLOROETHYLENE ANESTHETIC (GAS)
987.4		E869.2	E952.8	E962.2	E982.8	TRICHLOROFLUORO-METHANE NEC
961.5	E931.5	E857	E950.4	E962.0	E980.4	TRICHOMONACIDES NEC
960.1	E930.1	E856	E950.4	E962.0	E980.4	TRICHOMYCIN
967.1	E937.1	E852.0	E950.2	E962.0	E980.2	TRICLOFOS
989.89		E866.8	E950.9	E962.1	E980.9	TRICRESYL PHOSPHATE
982.8		E862.4	E950.9	E962.1	E980.9	TRICRESYL PHOSPHATE SOLVENT
966.4	E936.4	E855.0	E950.4	E962.0	E980.4	TRICYCLAMOL
969.0	E939.0	E854.0	E950.3	E962.0	E980.3	TRICYCLIC
976.0	E946.0	E858.7	E950.4	E962.0	E980.4	TRIDESILON
971.1	E941.1	E855.4	E950.4	E962.0	E980.4	TRIDIHEXETHYL
966.0	E936.0	E855.0	E950.4	E962.0	E980.4	TRIDIONE
983.2		E861.0	E950.7	E962.1	E980.6	TRIETHANOLAMINE DETERGENT
983.2		E864.2	E950.7	E962.1	E980.6	TRIETHANOLAMINE NEC
972.4	E942.4	E858.3	E950.4	E962.0	E980.4	TRIETHANOLAMINE NEC TRINITRATE
963.1	E933.1	E858.1	E950.4	E962.0	E980.4	TRIETHANOMELAMINE
963.1	E933.1	E858.1	E950.4	E962.0	E980.4	TRIETHYLENE MELAMINE
963.1	E933.1	E858.1	E950.4	E962.0	E980.4	TRIETHYLENE-PHOSPHORAMIDE
963.1	E933.1	E858.1	E950.4	E962.0	E980.4	TRIETHYLENEPHOS-PHORAMIDE
969.1	E939.1	E853.0	E950.3	E962.0	E980.3	TRIFLUOPERAZINE
969.2	E939.2	E853.1	E950.3	E962.0	E980.3	TRIFLUPERIDOL
969.1	E939.1	E853.0	E950.3	E962.0	E980.3	TRIFLUPROMAZINE

POISON	THERA-PEUTIC	ACCIDENT	SUICIDE	ASSAULT	UNDETER-MINED	SUBSTANCE
971.1	E941.1	E855.4	E950.4	E962.0	E980.4	TRIHEXYPHENIDYL
962.7	E932.7	E858.0	E950.4	E962.0	E980.4	TRIIODOTHYRONINE
968.2	E938.2	E855.1	E950.4	E962.0	E980.4	TRILENE
972.4	E942.4	E858.3	E950.4	E962.0	E980.4	TRIMETAZIDINE
966.0	E936.0	E855.0	E950.4	E962.0	E980.4	TRIMETHADIONE
972.3	E942.3	E858.3	E950.4	E962.0	E980.4	TRIMETHAPHAN
972.3	E942.3	E858.3	E950.4	E962.0	E980.4	TRIMETHIDINIUM
963.0	E933.0	E858.1	E950.4	E962.0	E980.4	TRIMETHOBENZAMIDE
980.8		E860.8	E950.9	E962.1	E980.9	TRIMETHYLCARBINOL
976.3	E946.3	E858.7	E950.4	E962.0	E980.4	TRIMETHYLPSORALEN
963.0	E933.0	E858.1	E950.4	E962.0	E980.4	TRIMETON
969.0	E939.0	E854.0	E950.3	E962.0	E980.3	TRIMIPRAMINE
963.1	E933.1	E858.1	E950.4	E962.0	E980.4	TRIMUSTINE
972.4	E942.4	E858.3	E950.4	E962.0	E980.4	TRINITRIN
983.0		E864.0	E950.7	E962.1	E980.6	TRINITROPHENOL
989.89		E866.8	E950.9	E962.1	E980.9	TRINITROTOLUENE
987.8		E869.8	E952.8	E962.2	E982.8	TRINITROTOLUENE FUMES
967.8	E937.8	E852.8	E950.2	E962.0	E980.2	TRIONAL
0						TRIOXIDE OF ARSENIC SEE ARSENIC
976.3	E946.3	E858.7	E950.4	E962.0	E980.4	TRIOXSALEN
963.0	E933.0	E858.1	E950.4	E962.0	E980.4	TRIPELENNAMINE
969.2	E939.2	E853.1	E950.3	E962.0	E980.3	TRIPERIDOL
963.0	E933.0	E858.1	E950.4	E962.0	E980.4	TRIPROLIDINE
976.3	E946.3	E858.7	E950.4	E962.0	E980.4	TRISORALEN
960.3	E930.3	E856	E950.4	E962.0	E980.4	TROLEANDOMYCIN
972.4	E942.4	E858.3	E950.4	E962.0	E980.4	TROLNITRATE (PHOSPHATE)
963.3	E933.3	E858.1	E950.4	E962.0	E980.4	TROMETAMOL
963.3	E933.3	E858.1	E950.4	E962.0	E980.4	TROMETHAMINE
968.5	E938.5	E855.2	E950.4	E962.0	E980.4	TRONOTHANE
971.1	E941.1	E855.4	E950.4	E962.0	E980.4	TROPICAMIDE
966.0	E936.0	E855.0	E950.4	E962.0	E980.4	TROXIDONE
961.1	E931.1	E857	E950.4	E962.0	E980.4	TRYPARSAMIDE
963.4	E933.4	E858.1	E950.4	E962.0	E980.4	TRYPSIN
969.0	E939.0	E854.0	E950.3	E962.0	E980.3	TRYPTIZOL
971.2	E941.2	E855.5	E950.4	E962.0	E980.4	TUAMINOHEPTANE
977.8	E947.8	E858.8	E950.4	E962.0	E980.4	TUBERCULIN (OLD)
975.2	E945.2	E858.6	E950.4	E962.0	E980.4	TUBOCURARE
975.2	E945.2	E858.6	E950.4	E962.0	E980.4	TUBOCURARINE
969.6	E939.6	E854.1	E950.3	E962.0	E980.3	TURKISH GREEN
982.8		E862.4	E950.9	E962.1	E980.9	TURPENTINE (SPIRITS OF) (LIQUID) (VAPOR)
969.5	E939.5	E853.8	E950.3	E962.0	E980.3	TYBAMATE
975.5	E945.5	E858.6	E950.4	E962.0	E980.4	TYLOXAPOL
971.2	E941.2	E855.5	E950.4	E962.0	E980.4	TYMAZOLINE
978.1	E948.1	E858.8	E950.4	E962.0	E980.4	TYPHOID VACCINE
979.2	E949.2	E858.8	E950.4	E962.0	E980.4	TYPHUS VACCINE
976.0	E946.0	E858.7	E950.4	E962.0	E980.4	TYROTHRICIN
976.6	E946.6	E858.7	E950.4	E962.0	E980.4	TYROTHRICIN ENT AGENT
976.5	E946.5	E858.7	E950.4	E962.0	E980.4	TYROTHRICIN OPHTHALMIC PREPARATION
976.0	E946.0	E858.7	E950.4	E962.0	E980.4	UNDECENOIC ACID
976.0	E946.0	E858.7	E950.4	E962.0	E980.4	UNDECYLENIC ACID
976.3	E946.3	E858.7	E950.4	E962.0	E980.4	UNNA'S BOOT
963.1	E933.1	E858.1	E950.4	E962.0	E980.4	URACIL MUSTARD
963.1	E933.1	E858.1	E950.4	E962.0	E980.4	URAMUSTINE
975.2	E945.2	E858.6	E950.4	E962.0	E980.4	URARI
974.4	E944.4	E858.5	E950.4	E962.0	E980.4	UREA
976.8	E946.8	E858.7	E950.4	E962.0	E980.4	UREA TOPICAL
963.1	E933.1	E858.1	E950.4	E962.0	E980.4	URETHAN(E) (ANTINEOPLASTIC)
0						URGINEA (MARITIMA) (SCILLA) SEE SQUILL
974.7	E944.7	E858.5	E950.4	E962.0	E980.4	URIC ACID METABOLISMAGENTS NEC
964.4	E934.4	E858.2	E950.4	E962.0	E980.4	UROKINASE
977.8	E947.8	E858.8	E950.4	E962.0	E980.4	UROKON
961.9	E931.9	E857	E950.4	E962.0	E980.4	UROTROPIN
988.2		E865.4	E950.9	E962.1	E980.9	URTICA
0						UTILITY GAS SEE GAS UTILITY
978.6	E948.6	E858.8	E950.4	E962.0	E980.4	VACCINE (WITH DIPHTHERIA TOXOID) (WITH TETANUS TOXOID)
978.0	E948.0	E858.8	E950.4	E962.0	E980.4	VACCINE BCG
978.2	E948.2	E858.8	E950.4	E962.0	E980.4	VACCINE CHOLERA
978.5	E948.5	E858.8	E950.4	E962.0	E980.4	VACCINE DIPHTHERIA
979.6	E949.6	E858.8	E950.4	E962.0	E980.4	VACCINE INFLUENZA
979.4	E949.4	E858.8	E950.4	E962.0	E980.4	VACCINE MEASLES

POISON	THERA-PEUTIC	ACCIDENT	SUICIDE	ASSAULT	UNDETER-MINED	SUBSTANCE
978.8	E948.8	E858.8	E950.4	E962.0	E980.4	VACCINE MENINGOCOCCAL
978.9	E948.9	E858.8	E950.4	E962.0	E980.4	VACCINE MIXED BACTERIAL VACCINES EXCEPT COMBINATIONS WITH A PERTUSSIS COMPONENT
979.7	E949.7	E858.8	E950.4	E962.0	E980.4	VACCINE MIXED VIRAL-RICKETTSIAL AND BACTERIAL VACCINES EXCEPT COMBINATIONS WITH PERTUSSIS COMP
979.6	E949.6	E858.8	E950.4	E962.0	E980.4	VACCINE MUMPS
979.9	E949.9	E858.8	E950.4	E962.0	E980.4	VACCINE NEC
978.8	E948.8	E858.8	E950.4	E962.0	E980.4	VACCINE OTHER AND NOS BACTERIAL VACCINES
979.9	E949.9	E858.8	E950.4	E962.0	E980.4	VACCINE OTHER AND NOS VACCINES AND BIOLOGICAL SUBSTANCES
978.1	E948.1	E858.8	E950.4	E962.0	E980.4	VACCINE PARATYPHOID
978.6	E948.6	E858.8	E950.4	E962.0	E980.4	VACCINE PERTUSSIS INCLUDING COMBINATIONS WITH A PERTUSSIS COMPONENT
978.3	E948.3	E858.8	E950.4	E962.0	E980.4	VACCINE PLAGUE
979.5	E949.5	E858.8	E950.4	E962.0	E980.4	VACCINE POLIOMYELITIS
979.5	E949.5	E858.8	E950.4	E962.0	E980.4	VACCINE POLIOVIRUS
979.1	E949.1	E858.8	E950.4	E962.0	E980.4	VACCINE RABIES
979.9	E949.6	E858.8	E950.4	E962.0	E980.4	VACCINE RESPIRATORY SYNCYTIAL VIRUS
979.6	E949.6	E858.8	E950.4	E962.0	E980.4	VACCINE RICKETTSIAL NEC
979.6	E949.6	E858.8	E950.4	E962.0	E980.4	VACCINE ROTAVIRUS
979.4	E949.4	E858.8	E950.4	E962.0	E980.4	VACCINE RUBELLA VIRUS
979.0	E949.0	E858.8	E950.4	E962.0	E980.4	VACCINE SMALLPOX
978.4	E948.4	E858.8	E950.4	E962.0	E980.4	VACCINE TETANUS
978.1	E948.1	E858.8	E950.4	E962.0	E980.4	VACCINE TYPHOID AND PARATYPHOID
979.2	E949.2	E858.8	E950.4	E962.0	E980.4	VACCINE TYPHUS
979.6	E949.6	E858.8	E950.4	E962.0	E980.4	VACCINE VIRAL NEC
979.3	E949.3	E858.8	E950.4	E962.0	E980.4	VACCINE YELLOW FEVER
964.6	E934.6	E858.2	E950.4	E962.0	E980.4	VACCINIA IMMUNE GLOBULIN (HUMAN)
976.8	E946.8	E858.7	E950.4	E962.0	E980.4	VAGINAL CONTRACEPTIVES
971.1	E941.1	E855.4	E950.4	E962.0	E980.4	VALETHAMATE
976.0	E946.0	E858.7	E950.4	E962.0	E980.4	VALISONE
969.4	E939.4	E853.2	E950.3	E962.0	E980.3	VALIUM
967.8	E937.8	E852.8	E950.2	E962.0	E980.2	VALMID
985.8		E866.4	E950.9	E962.1	E980.9	VANADIUM
960.8	E930.8	E856	E950.4	E962.0	E980.4	VANCOMYCIN
987.9		E869.9	E952.9	E962.2	E982.9	VAPOR UNSPECIFIED
986		E868.8	E952.1	E962.2	E982.1	VAPOR KILN (CARBON MONOXIDE)
0						VAPOR LEAD SEE LEAD
987.8		E869.8	E952.8	E962.2	E982.8	VAPOR SPECIFIED SOURCE NEC
964.4	E934.4	E858.2	E950.4	E962.0	E980.4	VARIDASE
989.89		E861.6	E950.9	E962.1	E980.9	VARNISH
982.8		E862.9	E950.9	E962.1	E980.9	VARNISH CLEANER
976.3	E946.3	E858.7	E950.4	E962.0	E980.4	VASELINE
972.5	E942.5	E858.3	E950.4	E962.0	E980.4	VASODILAN
972.4	E942.4	E858.3	E950.4	E962.0	E980.4	VASODILATORS CORONARY
972.5	E942.5	E858.3	E950.4	E962.0	E980.4	VASODILATORS NEC
962.5	E932.5	E858.0	E950.4	E962.0	E980.4	VASOPRESSIN
962.5	E932.5	E858.0	E950.4	E962.0	E980.4	VASOPRESSOR DRUGS
989.5		E905.9	E950.9	E962.1	E980.9	VENOM NOS
989.5		E905.5	E950.9	E962.1	E980.9	VENOM ARTHROPOD NEC
989.5		E905.3	E950.9	E962.1	E980.9	VENOM BEE
989.5		E905.4	E950.9	E962.1	E980.9	VENOM CENTIPEDE
989.5		E905.3	E950.9	E962.1	E980.9	VENOM HORNET
989.5		E905.0	E950.9	E962.1	E980.9	VENOM LIZARD
989.5		E905.6	E950.9	E962.1	E980.9	VENOM MARINE ANIMALS OR PLANTS
989.5		E905.4	E950.9	E962.1	E980.9	VENOM MILLIPEDE (TROPICAL)
989.5		E905.7	E950.9	E962.1	E980.9	VENOM PLANT NEC
989.5		E905.6	E950.9	E962.1	E980.9	VENOM PLANT NEC MARINE
989.5		E905.2	E950.9	E962.1	E980.9	VENOM SCORPION
989.5		E905.0	E950.9	E962.1	E980.9	VENOM SNAKE
989.5		E905.8	E950.9	E962.1	E980.9	VENOM SPECIFIED NEC
989.5		E905.1	E950.9	E962.1	E980.9	VENOM SPIDER
989.5		E905.9	E950.9	E962.1	E980.9	VENOM VENOMOUS (BITE) (STING)
989.5		E905.3	E950.9	E962.1	E980.9	VENOM WASP
967.0	E937.0	E851	E950.1	E962.0	E980.1	VERAMON
988.2		E865.4	E950.9	E962.1	E980.9	VERATRUM ALBUM
972.6	E942.6	E858.3	E950.4	E962.0	E980.4	VERATRUM ALKALOIDS
988.2		E865.4	E950.9	E962.1	E980.9	VERATRUM VIRIDE
985.8		E866.4	E950.9	E962.1	E980.9	VERDIGRIS
967.0	E937.0	E851	E950.1	E962.0	E980.1	VERONAL

POISON	THERA-PEUTIC	ACCIDENT	SUICIDE	ASSAULT	UNDETER-MINED	SUBSTANCE
961.6	E931.6	E857	E950.4	E962.0	E980.4	VEROXIL
965.7	E935.7	E850.7	E950.0	E962.0	E980.0	VERSIDYNE
972.5	E942.5	E858.3	E950.4	E962.0	E980.4	VIAGRA
985.1		E866.3	E950.8	E962.1	E980.8	VIENNA GREEN
985.1		E863.4	E950.6	E962.1	E980.7	VIENNA GREEN INSECTICIDE
989.89		E866.8	E950.9	E962.1	E980.9	VIENNA RED
977.4	E947.4	E858.8	E950.4	E962.0	E980.4	VIENNA RED PHARMACEUTICAL DYE
967.0	E937.0	E851	E950.1	E962.0	E980.1	VINBARBITAL
963.1	E933.1	E858.1	E950.4	E962.0	E980.4	VINBLASTINE
963.1	E933.1	E858.1	E950.4	E962.0	E980.4	VINCRISTINE
968.2	E938.2	E855.1	E950.4	E962.0	E980.4	VINESTHENE VINETHENE
967.0	E937.0	E851	E950.1	E962.0	E980.1	VINYL BITAL
968.2	E938.2	E855.1	E950.4	E962.0	E980.4	VINYL ETHER
961.3	E931.3	E857	E950.4	E962.0	E980.4	VIOFORM
976.0	E946.0	E858.7	E950.4	E962.0	E980.4	VIOFORM TOPICAL
960.6	E930.6	E856	E950.4	E962.0	E980.4	VIOMYCIN
963.5	E933.5	E858.1	E950.4	E962.0	E980.4	VIOSTEROL
989.5		E905.0	E950.9	E962.1	E980.9	VIPER (VENOM)
961.6	E931.6	E857	E950.4	E962.0	E980.4	VIPRYNIUM (EMBONATE)
979.7	E949.7	E858.8	E950.4	E962.0	E980.4	VIRAL WITH BACTERIAL COMPONENT VACCINE
978.6	E948.6	E858.8	E950.4	E962.0	E980.4	VIRAL WITH PERTUSSIS COMPONENT VACCINE
979.7	E949.7	E858.8	E950.4	E962.0	E980.4	VIRAL WITH RICKETTSIAL COMPONENT VACCINE
961.7	E931.7	E857	E950.4	E962.0	E980.4	VIRUGON
976.5	E946.5	E858.7	E950.4	E962.0	E980.4	VISINE
963.5	E933.5	E858.1	E950.4	E962.0	E980.4	VITAMIN D
964.3	E934.3	E858.2	E950.4	E962.0	E980.4	VITAMIN K (PHYTONADIONE)
964.1	E934.1	E858.2	E950.4	E962.0	E980.4	VITAMINS HEMATOPOIETIC
963.5	E933.5	E858.1	E950.4	E962.0	E980.4	VITAMINS NEC
964.1	E934.1	E858.2	E950.4	E962.0	E980.4	VITAMINS NEC B12
964.1	E934.1	E858.2	E950.4	E962.0	E980.4	VITAMINS NEC HEMA-TOPOIETIC
976.4	E946.4	E858.7	E950.4	E962.0	E980.4	VLEMINCKX'S SOLUTION
964.2	E934.2	E858.2	E950.4	E962.0	E980.4	WARFARIN (POTASSIUM) (SODIUM)
989.4		E863.7	E950.6	E962.1	E980.7	WARFARIN RODENTICIDE
989.5		E905.3	E950.9	E962.1	E980.9	WASP (STING)
974.5	E944.5	E858.5	E950.4	E962.0	E980.4	WATER BALANCE AGENTS NEC
987.1		E868.1	E951.8	E962.2	E981.8	WATER GAS
988.2		E865.4	E950.9	E962.1	E980.9	WATER HEMLOCK
989.5		E905.0	E950.9	E962.1	E980.9	WATER MOCCASIN (VENOM)
981		E862.3	E950.9	E962.1	E980.9	WAX (PARAFFIN) (PETROLEUM)
989.89		E861.2	E950.9	E962.1	E980.9	WAX AUTOMOBILE
981		E862.0	E950.9	E962.1	E980.9	WAX FLOOR
989.4		E863.5	E950.6	E962.1	E980.7	WEED KILLERS NEC
967.1	E937.1	E852.0	E950.2	E962.0	E980.2	WELLDORM
988.2		E865.4	E950.9	E962.1	E980.9	WHITE HELLEBORE
976.4	E946.4	E858.7	E950.4	E962.0	E980.4	WHITE LOTION (KERATOLYTIC)
981		E862.0	E950.9	E962.1	E980.9	WHITE SPIRIT
989.89		E861.6	E950.9	E962.1	E980.9	WHITEWASHES
964.7	E934.7	E858.2	E950.4	E962.0	E980.4	WHOLE BLOOD
988.2		E865.4	E950.9	E962.1	E980.9	WILD BLACK CHERRY
988.2		E865.4	E950.9	E962.1	E980.9	WILD POISONOUS PLANTS NEC
989.89		E861.3	E950.9	E962.1	E980.9	WINDOW CLEANING FLUID
976.3	E946.3	E858.7	E950.4	E962.0	E980.4	WINTERGREEN (OIL)
976.2	E946.2	E858.7	E950.4	E962.0	E980.4	WITCH HAZEL
980.1		E860.2	E950.9	E962.1	E980.9	WOOD ALCOHOL
980.1		E860.2	E950.9	E962.1	E980.9	WOOD SPIRIT
975.2	E945.2	E858.6	E950.4	E962.0	E980.4	WOORALI
961.6	E931.6	E857	E950.4	E962.0	E980.4	WORMSEED AMERICAN
974.1	E944.1	E858.5	E950.4	E962.0	E980.4	XANTHINE DIURETICS
960.0	E930.0	E856	E950.4	E962.0	E980.4	XANTHOCILLIN
976.3	E946.3	E858.7	E950.4	E962.0	E980.4	XANTHOTOXIN
964.2	E934.2	E858.2	E950.4	E962.0	E980.4	XIGRIS
982.0		E862.4	E950.9	E962.1	E980.9	XYLENE (LIQUID) (VAPOR)
968.5	E938.5	E855.2	E950.4	E962.0	E980.4	XYLOCAINE (INFILTRATION) (TOPICAL)
968.6	E938.6	E855.2	E950.4	E962.0	E980.4	XYLOCAINE NERVE BLOCK (PERIPHERAL) (PLEXUS)
968.7	E938.7	E855.2	E950.4	E962.0	E980.4	XYLOCAINE SPINAL
982.0		E862.4	E950.9	E962.1	E980.9	XYLOL (LIQUID) (VAPOR)
971.2	E941.2	E855.5	E950.4	E962.0	E980.4	XYLOMETAZOLINE
979.3	E949.3	E858.8	E950.4	E962.0	E980.4	YELLOW FEVER VACCINE
988.2		E865.4	E950.9	E962.1	E980.9	YELLOW JASMINE
988.2		E865.4	E950.9	E962.1	E980.9	YEW
965.7	E935.7	E850.7	E950.0	E962.0	E980.0	ZACTANE

POISON	THERA-PEUTIC	ACCIDENT	SUICIDE	ASSAULT	UNDETER-MINED	SUBSTANCE
974.3	E944.3	E858.5	E950.4	E962.0	E980.4	ZAROXOLYN
976.5	E946.5	E858.7	E950.4	E962.0	E980.4	ZEPHIRAN OPHTHALMIC PREPARATION
976.0	E946.0	E858.7	E950.4	E962.0	E980.4	ZEPHIRAN (TOPICAL)
980.1		E860.2	E950.9	E962.1	E980.9	ZERONE
985.8		E866.4	E950.9	E962.1	E980.9	ZINC (COMPOUNDS) (FUMES) (SALTS) (VAPOR) NEC
976.0	E946.0	E858.7	E950.4	E962.0	E980.4	ZINC ANTI-INFECTIVES
972.7	E942.7	E858.3	E950.4	E962.0	E980.4	ZINC ANTIVARICOSE
976.0	E946.0	E858.7	E950.4	E962.0	E980.4	ZINC BACITRACIN
976.2	E946.2	E858.7	E950.4	E962.0	E980.4	ZINC CHLORIDE
976.3	E946.3	E858.7	E950.4	E962.0	E980.4	ZINC GELATIN
976.3	E946.3	E858.7	E950.4	E962.0	E980.4	ZINC OXIDE
976.0	E946.0	E858.7	E950.4	E962.0	E980.4	ZINC PEROXIDE
985.8		E863.4	E950.6	E962.1	E980.7	ZINC PESTICIDES
985.8		E863.7	E950.6	E962.1	E980.7	ZINC PHOSPHIDE (RODENTICIDE)
972.7	E942.7	E866.4	E950.9	E962.1	E980.9	ZINC SALTS
976.3	E946.3	E858.7	E950.4	E962.0	E980.4	ZINC STEARATE
972.7	E942.7	E858.3	E950.4	E962.0	E980.4	ZINC SULFATE (ANTIVARICOSE)
976.5	E946.5	E858.7	E950.4	E962.0	E980.4	ZINC SULFATE OPHTHALMIC SOLUTION
976.0	E946.0	E858.7	E950.4	E962.0	E980.4	ZINC UNDECYLENATE
976.0	E946.0	E858.7	E950.4	E962.0	E980.4	ZINC SULFATE TOPICAL NEC
964.2	E934.2	E858.2	E950.4	E962.0	E980.4	ZOVANT
968.0	E938.0	E855.1	E950.4	E962.0	E980.4	ZOXAZOLAMINE
988.2		E865.4	E950.9	E962.1	E980.9	ZYGADENUS (VENENOSUS)

APPENDIX C

Numerical Reference

001.# Cholera
- 001.0 Due to Vibrio cholerae
- 001.1 Due to Vibrio cholerae el tor
- 001.9 Cholera, unspecified

002.# Typhoid and paratyphoid fevers
- 002.0 Typhoid fever
- 002.1 Paratyphoid fever A
- 002.2 Paratyphoid fever B
- 002.3 Paratyphoid fever C
- 002.9 Paratyphoid fever, unspecified

003.#(#) Other salmonella infections
- 003.0 Salmonella gastroenteritis
- 003.1 Salmonella septicemia
- **003.2#** Localized salmonella infections
  - 003.20 Localized salmonella infection, unspecified
  - 003.21 Salmonella meningitis
  - 003.22 Salmonella pneumonia
  - 003.23 Salmonella arthritis
  - 003.24 Salmonella osteomyelitis
  - 003.29 Other
- 003.8 Other specified salmonella infections
- 003.9 Salmonella infection, unspecified

004.# Shigellosis
- 004.0 Shigella dysenteriae
- 004.1 Shigella flexneri
- 004.2 Shigella boydii
- 004.3 Shigella sonnei
- 004.8 Other specified shigella infections
- 004.9 Shigellosis, unspecified

005.#(#) Other food poisoning (bacterial)
- 005.0 Staphylococcal food poisoning
- 005.1 Botulism food poisoning
- 005.2 Food poisoning due to Clostridium perfringens
- 005.3 Food poisoning due to other Clostridia
- 005.4 Food poisoning due to Vibrio parahaemolyticus
- **005.8#** Other bacterial food poisoning
  - 005.81 Food poisoning due to Vibro vulnificus
  - 005.89 Other bacterial food poisoning
- 005.9 Food poisoning, unspecified

006.# Amebiasis
- 006.0 Acute amebic dysentery without abscess
- 006.1 Chronic intestinal amebiasis without abscess
- 006.2 Amebic nondysenteric colitis
- 006.3 Amebic liver abscess
- 006.4 Amebic lung abscess
- 006.5 Amebic brain abscess
- 006.6 Amebic skin ulceration
- 006.8 Amebic infection of other sites
- 006.9 Amebiasis, unspecified

007.# Other protozoal intestinal diseases
- 007.0 Balantidiasis
- 007.1 Giardiasis
- 007.2 Coccidiosis
- 007.3 Intestinal trichomoniasis
- 007.4 Cryptosporidiosis
- 007.5 Cyclosporiasis
- 007.8 Other specified protozoal intestinal diseases
- 007.9 Unspecified protozoal intestinal disease

008.#(#) Intestinal infections due to other organisms
- **008.0#** Escherichia coli [E. coli]
  - 008.00 E. coli, unspecified
  - 008.01 Enteropathogenic E. coli
  - 008.02 Enterotoxigenic E. coli
  - 008.03 Enteroinvasive E. coli
  - 008.04 Enterohemorrhagic E. coli
  - 008.09 Other intestinal E. coli infections
- 008.1 Arizona group of paracolon bacilli
- 008.2 Aerobacter aerogenes
- 008.3 Proteus (mirabilis) (morganii)
- **008.4#** Other specified bacteria
  - 008.41 Staphylococcus
  - 008.42 Pseudomonas
  - 008.43 Campylobacter
  - 008.44 Yersinia enterocolitica
  - 008.45 Clostridium difficile
  - 008.46 Other anaerobes
  - 008.47 Other gram-negative bacteria
  - 008.49 Other
- 008.5 Bacterial enteritis, unspecified
- **008.6#** Enteritis due to specified virus
  - 008.61 Rotavirus
  - 008.62 Adenovirus
  - 008.63 Norwalk virus
  - 008.64 Other small round viruses
  - 008.65 Calcivirus
  - 008.66 Astrovirus
  - 008.67 Enterovirus NEC
  - 008.69 Other viral enteritis
- 008.8 Other organism, not elsewhere classified

009.# Ill-defined intestinal infections
- 009.0 Infectious colitis, enteritis, and gastroenteritis
- 009.1 Colitis, enteritis, and gastroenteritis of presumed infectious origin
- 009.2 Infectious diarrhea
- 009.3 Diarrhea of presumed infectious origin

010.## Primary tuberculous infection
- **010.0#** Primary tuberculous infection
- **010.1#** Tuberculous pleurisy in primary progressive tuberculosis
- **010.8#** Other primary progressive tuberculosis
- **010.9#** Primary tuberculous infection, unspecified

5th Digit: 010
- **0 Unspecified**
- **1 Bacteriological or histological examination not done**
- **2 Bacteriological or histological examination unknown (at present)**
- **3 Tubercle bacilli found (in sputum) by microscopy**
- **4 Tubercle bacilli not found (in sputum) by microscopy, but found by bacterial culture**
- **5 Tubercle bacilli not found by bacteriological examination, but tuberculosis confirmed histologically**
- **6 Tubercle bacilli not found by bacteriological or histological examination, but tuberculosis confirmed by other methods**

011.## Pulmonary tuberculosis
- 011.0# Tuberculosis of lung, infiltrative
- 011.1# Tuberculosis of lung, nodular
- 011.2# Tuberculosis of lung with cavitation
- 011.3# Tuberculosis of bronchus
- 011.4# Tuberculous fibrosis of lung
- 011.5# Tuberculous bronchiectasis
- 011.6# Tuberculous pneumonia
- 011.7# Tuberculous pneumothorax
- 011.8# Other specified pulmonary tuberculosis
- 011.9# Pulmonary tuberculosis, unspecified

012.## Other respiratory tuberculosis
- 012.0# Tuberculous pleurisy
- 012.1# Tuberculosis of intrathoracic lymph nodes
- 012.2# Isolated tracheal or bronchial tuberculosis
- 012.3# Tuberculous laryngitis
- 012.8# Other specified respiratory tuberculosis

013.## Tuberculosis of meninges and central nervous system
- 013.0# Tuberculous meningitis
- 013.1# Tuberculoma of meninges
- 013.2# Tuberculoma of brain
- 013.3# Tuberculous abscess of brain
- 013.4# Tuberculoma of spinal cord
- 013.5# Tuberculous abscess of spinal cord
- 013.6# Tuberculous encephalitis or myelitis
- 013.8# Other specified tuberculosis of central nervous system
- 013.9# Unspecified tuberculosis of central nervous system

014.## Tuberculosis of intestines, peritoneum, and mesenteric glands
- 014.0# Tuberculous peritonitis
- 014.8# Other

015.## Tuberculosis of bones and joints
- 015.0# Vertebral Column
- 015.1# Hip
- 015.2# Knee
- 015.5# Limb bones
- 015.6# Mastoid
- 015.7# Other specified bone
- 015.8# Other specified joint
- 015.9# Tuberculosis of unspecified bones and joints

016.## Tuberculosis of genitourinary system
- 016.0# Kidney
- 016.1# Bladder
- 016.2# Ureter
- 016.3# Other urinary organs
- 016.4# Epididymis
- 016.5# Other male genital organs
- 016.6# Tuberculous oophoritis and salpingitis
- 016.7# Other female genital organs
- 016.9# Genitourinary tuberculosis, unspecified

017.## Tuberculosis of other organs
- 017.0# Skin and subcutaneous cellular tissue
- 017.1# Erythema nodosum with hypersensitivity reaction in tuberculosis
- 017.2# Peripheral lymph nodes
- 017.3# Eye

017.## *(continued)*
- 017.4# Ear
- 017.5# Thyroid gland
- 017.6# Adrenal glands
- 017.7# Spleen
- 017.8# Esophagus
- 017.9# Other specified organs

018.## Miliary tuberculosis
- 018.0# Acute miliary tuberculosis
- 018.8# Other specified miliary tuberculosis
- 018.9# Miliary tuberculosis, unspecified

5th Digit: 011-018
- **0 Unspecified**
- **1 Bacteriological or histological examination not done**
- **2 Bacteriological or histological examination unknown (at present)**
- **3 Tubercle bacilli found (in sputum) by microscopy**
- **4 Tubercle bacilli not found (in sputum) by microscopy, but found by bacterial culture**
- **5 Tubercle bacilli not found by bacteriological examination, but tuberculosis confirmed histologically**
- **6 Tubercle bacilli not found by bacteriological or histological examination, but tuberculosis confirmed by other methods**

020.# Plague
- 020.0 Bubonic
- 020.1 Cellulocutaneous
- 020.2 Septicemic
- 020.3 Primary pneumonic
- 020.4 Secondary pneumonic
- 020.5 Pneumonic, unspecified
- 020.8 Other specified types of plague
- 020.9 Plague, unspecified

021.# Tularemia
- 021.0 Ulceroglandular Tularemia
- 021.1 Enteric tularemia
- 021.2 Pulmonary tularemia
- 021.3 Oculoglandular tularemia
- 021.8 Other specified tularemia
- 021.9 Unspecified tularemia

022.# Anthrax
- 022.0 Cutaneous anthrax
- 022.1 Pulmonary anthrax
- 022.2 Gastrointestinal anthrax
- 022.3 Anthrax septicemia
- 022.8 Other specified manifestations of anthrax
- 022.9 Anthrax, unspecified

023.# Brucellosis
- 023.0 Brucella melitensis
- 023.1 Brucella abortus
- 023.2 Brucella suis
- 023.3 Brucella canis
- 023.8 Other brucellosis
- 023.9 Brucellosis, unspecified

024 Glanders

025 Melioidosis

026.# Rat-bite fever
- 026.0 Spirillary fever
- 026.1 Streptobacillary fever
- 026.9 Unspecified rat-bite fever

027.# Other zoonotic bacterial diseases
- 027.0 Listeriosis
- 027.1 Erysipelothrix infection
- 027.2 Pasteurellosis
- 027.8 Other specified zoonotic bacterial diseases
- 027.9 Unspecified zoonotic bacterial disease

030.# Leprosy
- 030.0 Lepromatous [type L]
- 030.1 Tuberculoid [type T]
- 030.2 Indeterminate [group I]
- 030.3 Borderline [group B]
- 030.8 Other specified leprosy
- 030.9 Leprosy, unspecified

031.# Diseases due to other mycobacteria
- 031.0 Pulmonary infection by mycobacterium
- 031.1 Cutaneous
- 031.2 Disseminated
- 031.8 Other specified mycobacterial diseases
- 031.9 Unspecified diseases due to mycobacteria

032.#(#) Diphtheria
- 032.0 Faucial diphtheria
- 032.1 Nasopharyngeal diphtheria
- 032.2 Anterior nasal diphtheria
- 032.3 Laryngeal diphtheria
- **032.8#** Other specified diphtheria
  - 032.81 Conjunctival diphtheria
  - 032.82 Diphtheritic myocarditis
  - 032.83 Diphtheritic peritonitis
  - 032.84 Diphtheritic cystitis
  - 032.85 Cutaneous diphtheria
  - 032.89 Other
- 032.9 Diphtheria, unspecified

033.# Whooping cough
- 033.0 Bordetella pertussis [B. pertussis]
- 033.1 Bordetella parapertussis [B. parapertussis]
- 033.8 Whooping cough due to other specified organism
- 033.9 Whooping cough, unspecified organism

034.# Streptococcal sore throat and scarlet fever
- 034.0 Streptococcal sore throat
- 034.1 Scarlet fever

035 Erysipelas

036.#(#) Meningococcal infection
- 036.0 Meningococcal meningitis
- 036.1 Meningococcal encephalitis
- 036.2 Meningococcemia
- 036.3 Waterhouse-Friderichsen syndrome
- **036.4#** Meningococcal carditis
  - 036.40 Meningococcal carditis, unspecified
  - 036.41 Meningococcal pericarditis
  - 036.42 Meningococcal endocarditis
  - 036.43 Meningococcal myocarditis

036.#(#) ***(continued)***
- **036.8#** Other specified meningococcal infections
  - 036.81 Meningococcal optic neuritis
  - 036.82 Meningococcal arthropathy
  - 036.89 Other
- 036.9 Meningococcal infection, unspecified

037 Tetanus

038.#(#) Septicemia
- 038.0 Streptococcal septicemia
- **038.1#** Staphylococcal septicemia
  - 038.10 Staphylococcal septicemia, unspecified
  - 038.11 Staphylococcus aureus septicemia
  - 038.19 Other staphylococcal septicemia
- 038.2 Pneumococcal septicemia
- 038.3 Septicemia due to anaerobes
- **038.4#** Septicemia, gram-negative organisms NEC
  - 038.40 Gram-negative organism, unspecified
  - 038.41 Hemophilus influenzae [H. Influenzae]
  - 038.42 Escherichia coli [E. coli]
  - 038.43 Pseudomonas
  - 038.44 Serratia
  - 038.49 Other
- 038.8 Other specified septicemias
- 038.9 Unspecified septicemia

039.# Actinomycotic infections
- 039.0 Cutaneous
- 039.1 Pulmonary
- 039.2 Abdominal
- 039.3 Cervicofacial
- 039.4 Madura foot
- 039.8 Of other specified sites
- 039.9 Of unspecified site

040.#(#) Other bacterial diseases
- 040.0 Gas gangrene
- 040.1 Rhinoscleroma
- 040.2 Whipple's disease
- 040.3 Necrobacillosis
- **040.4#** Other specified botulism
  - 040.41 Infant botulism
  - 040.42 Wound botulism
- **040.8#** Other specified bacterial diseases
  - 040.81 Tropical pyomyositis
  - 040.82 Toxic Shock Syndrome
  - 040.89 Other

041.#(#) Bacterial infection in conditions classified elsewhere and of unspecified site
- **041.0#** Streptococcus
  - 041.00 Streptococcus, unspecified
  - 041.01 Group A
  - 041.02 Group B
  - 041.03 Group C
  - 041.04 Group D [Enterococcus]
  - 041.05 Group G
  - 041.09 Other Streptococcus
- **041.1#** Staphylococcus
  - 041.10 Staphylococcus, unspecified
  - 041.11 Staphylococcus aureus
  - 041.19 Other Staphylococcus
- 041.2 Pneumococcus
- 041.3 Friedländer's bacillus
- 041.4 Escherichia coli [E.coli]
- 041.5 Hemophilus influenzae [H. influenzae]
- 041.6 Proteus (mirabilis) (morganii)
- 041.7 Pseudomonas

041.#(#) ***(continued)***
- **041.8#** Other specified bacterial infections
  - 041.81 Mycoplasma
  - 041.82 Bacteroides fragilis
  - 041.83 Clostridium perfringens
  - 041.84 Other anaerobes
  - 041.85 Other gram-negative organisms
  - 041.86 Helicobacter pylori (H. pylori)
  - 041.89 Other specified bacteria
- 041.9 Bacterial infection, unspecified

042 Human immunodeficiency virus [HIV] disease

045.## Acute poliomyelitis
- **045.0#** Acute paralytic poliomyelitis specified as bulbar
- **045.1#** Acute poliomyelitis with other paralysis
- **045.2#** Acute nonparalytic poliomyelitis
- **045.9#** Acute poliomyelitis, unspecified

5th Digit: 045
- **0 Poliovirus, unspecified type**
- **1 Poliovirus type I**
- **2 Poliovirus type II**
- **3 Poliovirus type III**

046.# Slow virus infection of central nervous system
- 046.0 Kuru
- 046.1 Jakob-Creutzfeldt disease
- 046.2 Subacute sclerosing panencephalitis
- 046.3 Progressive multifocal leukoencephalopathy
- 046.8 Other specified slow virus infection of central nervous system
- 046.9 Unspecified slow virus infection of central nervous system

047.# Meningitis due to enterovirus
- 047.0 Coxsackie virus
- 047.1 ECHO virus
- 047.8 Other specified viral meningitis
- 047.9 Unspecified viral meningitis

048 Other enterovirus diseases of central nervous system

049.# Other non-arthropod-borne viral diseases of central nervous system
- 049.0 Lymphocytic choriomeningitis
- 049.1 Meningitis due to adenovirus
- 049.8 Other specified non-arthropod-borne viral diseases of central nervous system
- 049.9 Unspecified non-arthropod-borne viral diseases of central nervous system

050.# Smallpox
- 050.0 Variola major
- 050.1 Alastrim
- 050.2 Modified smallpox
- 050.9 Smallpox, unspecified

051.# Cowpox and paravaccinia
- 051.0 Cowpox
- 051.1 Pseudocowpox
- 051.2 Contagious pustular dermatitis
- 051.9 Paravaccinia, unspecified

052.# Chickenpox
- 052.0 Postvaricella encephalitis
- 052.1 Varicella (hemorrhagic) pneumonitis
- 052.2 Postvaricella myelitis
- 052.7 With other specified complications
- 052.8 With unspecified complication
- 052.9 Varicella without mention of complication

053.#(#) Herpes zoster
- 053.0 With meningitis
- **053.1#** With other nervous system complications
  - 053.10 With unspecified nervous system complication
  - 053.11 Geniculate herpes zoster
  - 053.12 Postherpetic trigeminal neuralgia
  - 053.13 Postherpetic polyneuropathy
  - 053.14 Myelitis
  - 053.19 Other
- **053.2#** With ophthalmic complications
  - 053.20 Herpes zoster dermatitis of eyelid
  - 053.21 Herpes zoster keratoconjunctivitis
  - 053.22 Herpes zoster iridocyclitis
  - 053.29 Other
- **053.7#** With other specified complications
  - 053.71 Otitis externa due to herpes zoster
  - 053.79 Other
- 053.8 With unspecified complication
- 053.9 Herpes zoster without mention of complication

054.#(#) Herpes simplex
- 054.0 Eczema herpeticum
- **054.1#** Genital herpes
  - 054.10 Genital herpes, unspecified
  - 054.11 Herpetic vulvovaginitis
  - 054.12 Herpetic ulceration of vulva
  - 054.13 Herpetic infection of penis
  - 054.19 Other
- 054.2 Herpetic gingivostomatitis
- 054.3 Herpetic meningoencephalitis
- **054.4#** With ophthalmic complications
  - 054.40 With unspecified ophthalmic complication
  - 054.41 Herpes simplex dermatitis of eyelid
  - 054.42 Dendritic keratitis
  - 054.43 Herpes simplex disciform keratitis
  - 054.44 Herpes simplex iridocyclitis
  - 054.49 Other
- 054.5 Herpetic septicemia
- 054.6 Herpetic whitlow
- **054.7#** With other specified complications
  - 054.71 Visceral herpes simplex
  - 054.72 Herpes simplex meningitis
  - 054.73 Herpes simplex otitis externa
  - 054.74 Herpes simplex myelitis
  - 054.79 Other
- 054.8 With unspecified complication
- 054.9 Herpes simplex without mention of complication

055.#(#) Measles
- 055.0 Postmeasles encephalitis
- 055.1 Postmeasles pneumonia
- 055.2 Postmeasles otitis media
- **055.7#** With other specified complications
  - 055.71 Measles keratoconjunctivitis
  - 055.79 Other
- 055.8 With unspecified complication
- 055.9 Measles without mention of complication

NUMERICAL REFERENCE

056.#(#) Rubella
056.0# With neurological complications
056.00 With unspecified neurological complication
056.01 Encephalomyelitis due to rubella
056.09 Other
056.7# With other specified complications
056.71 Arthritis due to rubella
056.79 Other
056.8 With unspecified complications
056.9 Rubella without mention of complication

057.# Other viral exanthemata
057.0 Erythema infectiosum [fifth disease]
057.8 Other specified viral exanthemata
057.9 Viral exanthem, unspecified

058.# Other human herpesvirus
058.1# Roseola infantum
058.10 Roseola infantum, unspecified
058.11 Roseola infantum due to human herpesvirus 6
058.12 Roseola infantum due to human herpesvirus 7
058.2# Other human herpesvirus encephalitis
058.21 Human herpesvirus 6 encephalitis
058.29 Other human herpesvirus encephalitis
058.8# Other human herpesvirus infections
058.81 Human herpesvirus 6 infrection
058.82 Human herpesvirus 7 infection
058.89 Other human herpesvirus infection

060.# Yellow fever
060.0 Sylvatic
060.1 Urban
060.9 Yellow fever, unspecified

061 Dengue

062.# Mosquito-borne viral encephalitis
062.0 Japanese encephalitis
062.1 Western equine encephalitis
062.2 Eastern equine encephalitis
062.3 St. Louis encephalitis
062.4 Australian encephalitis
062.5 California virus encephalitis
062.8 Other specified mosquito-borne viral encephalitis
062.9 Mosquito-borne viral encephalitis, unspecified

063.# Tick-borne viral encephalitis
063.0 Russian spring-summer [taiga] encephalitis
063.1 Louping ill
063.2 Central European encephalitis
063.8 Other specified tick-borne viral encephalitis
063.9 Tick-borne viral encephalitis, unspecified

064 Viral encephalitis transmitted by other and unspecified arthropods

065.# Arthropod-borne hemorrhagic fever
065.0 Crimean hemorrhagic fever [CHF Congo virus]
065.1 Omsk hemorrhagic fever
065.2 Kyasanur Forest disease
065.3 Other tick-borne hemorrhagic fever
065.4 Mosquito-borne hemorrhagic fever
065.8 Other specified arthropod-borne hemorrhagic fever
065.9 Arthropod-borne hemorrhagic fever, unspecified

066.#(#) Other arthropod-borne viral diseases
066.0 Phlebotomus fever
066.1 Tick-borne fever
066.2 Venezuelan equine fever
066.3 Other mosquito-borne fever
066.4# West Nile fever
066.40 West Nile fever unspecified
066.41 West Nile fever with encephalitis
066.42 West Nile fever with other neurologic manifestation
066.49 West Nile fever with other complications
066.8 Other specified arthropod-borne viral diseases
066.9 Arthropod-borne viral disease, unspecified

070.#(#) Viral hepatitis
070.0 Viral hepatitis A with hepatic coma
070.1 Viral hepatitis A without mention of hepatic coma
070.2# Viral hepatitis B with hepatic coma
070.3# Viral hepatitis B without mention of hepatic coma
5th Digit: 070.2-070.3
0 Acute or unspecified, without mention of hepatitis delta
1 Acute or unspecified, with hepatitis delta
2 Chronic, without mention of hepatitis delta
3 Chronic, with hepatitis delta
070.4# Other specified viral hepatitis with hepatic coma
070.5# Other specified viral hepatitis without mention of hepatic coma
5th Digit: 070.4-070.5
1 Acute hepatitis C
2 Hepatitis delta without mention of active hepatitis B disease
3 Hepatitis E
4 Chronic hepatitis C
9 Other specified viral hepatitis
070.6 Unspecified viral hepatitis with hepatic coma
070.7# Unspecified viral hepatits C
070.70 Unspecified viral hepatitis C without hepatic coma
070.71 Unspecified viral hepatitis C with hepatic coma
070.9 Unspecified viral hepatitis without mention of hepatic coma

071 Rabies

072.#(#) Mumps
072.0 Mumps orchitis
072.1 Mumps meningitis
072.2 Mumps encephalitis
072.3 Mumps pancreatitis
072.7# Mumps with other specified complications
072.71 Mumps hepatitis
072.72 Mumps polyneuropathy
072.79 Other
072.8 Mumps with unspecified complication
072.9 Mumps without mention of complication

073.# Ornithosis
073.0 With pneumonia
073.7 With other specified complications
073.8 With unspecified complication
073.9 Ornithosis, unspecified

074.#(#) Specific diseases due to Coxsackie virus
074.0 Herpangina
074.1 Epidemic pleurodynia
074.2# Coxsackie carditis
074.20 Coxsackie carditis, unspecified
074.21 Coxsackie pericarditis
074.22 Coxsackie endocarditis
074.23 Coxsackie myocarditis
074.3 Hand, foot, and mouth disease
074.8 Other specified diseases due to Coxsackie virus

075 Infectious mononucleosis

076.# Trachoma
076.0 Initial stage
076.1 Active stage
076.9 Trachoma, unspecified

077.#(#) Other diseases of conjunctiva due to viruses and Chlamydiae
077.0 Inclusion conjunctivitis
077.1 Epidemic keratoconjunctivitis
077.2 Pharyngoconjunctival fever
077.3 Other adenoviral conjunctivitis
077.4 Epidemic hemorrhagic conjunctivitis
077.8 Other viral conjunctivitis
077.9# Unspecified diseases of conjunctiva due to viruses and Chlamydiae
077.98 Due to Chlamydiae
077.99 Due to viruses

078.#(#) Other diseases due to viruses and Chlamydiae
078.0 Molluscum contagiosum
078.1# Viral warts
078.10 Viral warts, unspecified
078.11 Condyloma acuminatum
078.19 Other specified viral warts
078.2 Sweating fever
078.3 Cat-scratch disease
078.4 Foot and mouth disease
078.5 Cytomegaloviral disease
078.6 Hemorrhagic nephrosonephritis
078.7 Arenaviral hemorrhagic fever
078.8# Other specified diseases due to viruses and Chlamydiae
078.81 Epidemic vertigo
078.82 Epidemic vomiting syndrome
078.88 Other specified diseases due to Chlamydiae
078.89 Other specified diseases due to viruses

079.#(#) Viral and chlamydial infection in conditions classified elsewhere and of unspecified site
079.0 Adenovirus
079.1 ECHO virus
079.2 Coxsackie virus
079.3 Rhinovirus
079.4 Human papillomavirus
079.5# Retrovirus
079.50 Retrovirus, unspecified
079.51 Human T-cell lymphotrophic virus, type I [HTLV-I]
079.52 Human T-cell lymphotrophic virus, type II [HTLV-II]
079.53 Human immunodeficiency virus, type 2 [HIV-2]
079.59 Other specified retrovirus
079.6 Respiratory syncytial virus (RSV)
079.8# Other specified viral and chlamydial infections
079.81 Hantavirus
079.82 SARS-associated coronavirus
079.83 Parvovirus B19
079.88 Other specified chlamydial infection
079.89 Other specified viral infection
079.9# Unspecified viral and chlamydial infections
079.98 Unspecified chlamydial infection
079.99 Unspecified viral infection

080 Louse-borne [epidemic] typhus

081.# Other typhus
081.0 Murine [endemic] typhus
081.1 Brill's disease
081.2 Scrub typhus
081.9 Typhus, unspecified

082.#(#) Tick-borne rickettsioses
082.0 Spotted fevers
082.1 Boutonneuse fever
082.2 North Asian tick fever
082.3 Queensland tick typhus
082.4# Ehrlichiosis
082.40 Ehrlichiosis, unspecified
082.41 Ehrlichiosis chaffeensis (E. chaffeensis)
082.49 Other ehrlichiosis
082.8 Other specified tick-borne rickettsioses
082.9 Tick-borne rickettsiosis, unspecified

083.# Other rickettsioses
083.0 Q fever
083.1 Trench fever
083.2 Rickettsialpox
083.8 Other specified rickettsioses
083.9 Rickettsiosis, unspecified

084.# Malaria
084.0 Falciparum malaria [malignant tertian]
084.1 Vivax malaria [benign tertian]
084.2 Quartan malaria
084.3 Ovale malaria
084.4 Other malaria
084.5 Mixed malaria
084.6 Malaria, unspecified
084.7 Induced malaria
084.8 Blackwater fever
084.9 Other pernicious complications of malaria

085.# Leishmaniasis
085.0 Visceral [kala-azar]
085.1 Cutaneous, urban
085.2 Cutaneous, Asian desert
085.3 Cutaneous, Ethiopian
085.4 Cutaneous, American
085.5 Mucocutaneous (American)
085.9 Leishmaniasis, unspecified

086.# Trypanosomiasis
086.0 Chagas' disease with heart involvement
086.1 Chagas' disease with other organ involvement
086.2 Chagas' disease without mention of organ involvement
086.3 Gambian trypanosomiasis
086.4 Rhodesian trypanosomiasis
086.5 African trypanosomiasis, unspecified
086.9 Trypanosomiasis, unspecified

087.# Relapsing fever
087.0 Louse-borne
087.1 Tick-borne
087.9 Relapsing fever, unspecified

NUMERICAL REFERENCE

088.#(#) Other arthropod-borne diseases
088.0 Bartonellosis
088.8# Other specified arthropod-borne diseases
088.81 Lyme disease
088.82 Babesiosis
088.89 Other
088.9 Arthropod-borne disease, unspecified

090.#(#) Congenital syphilis
090.0 Early congenital syphilis, symptomatic
090.1 Early congenital syphilis, latent
090.2 Early congenital syphilis, unspecified
090.3 Syphilitic interstitial keratitis
090.4# Juvenile neurosyphilis
090.40 Juvenile neurosyphilis, unspecified
090.41 Congenital syphilitic encephalitis
090.42 Congenital syphilitic meningitis
090.49 Other
090.5 Other late congenital syphilis, symptomatic
090.6 Late congenital syphilis, latent
090.7 Late congenital syphilis, unspecified
090.9 Congenital syphilis, unspecified

091.#(#) Early syphilis, symptomatic
091.0 Genital syphilis (primary)
091.1 Primary anal syphilis
091.2 Other primary syphilis
091.3 Secondary syphilis of skin or mucous membranes
091.4 Adenopathy due to secondary syphilis
091.5# Uveitis due to secondary syphilis
091.50 Syphilitic uveitis, unspecified
091.51 Syphilitic chorioretinitis (secondary)
091.52 Syphilitic iridocyclitis (secondary)
091.6# Secondary syphilis of viscera and bone
091.61 Secondary syphilitic periostitis
091.62 Secondary syphilitic hepatitis
091.69 Other viscera
091.7 Secondary syphilis, relapse
091.8# Other forms of secondary syphilis
091.81 Acute syphilitic meningitis (secondary)
091.82 Syphilitic alopecia
091.89 Other
091.9 Unspecified secondary syphilis

092.# Early syphilis, latent
092.0 Early syphilis, latent, serological relapse after treatment
092.9 Early syphilis, latent, unspecified

093.#(#) Cardiovascular syphilis
093.0 Aneurysm of aorta, specified as syphilitic
093.1 Syphilitic aortitis
093.2# Syphilitic endocarditis
093.20 Valve, unspecified
093.21 Mitral valve
093.22 Aortic valve
093.23 Tricuspid valve
093.24 Pulmonary valve
093.8# Other specified cardiovascular syphilis
093.81 Syphilitic pericarditis
093.82 Syphilitic myocarditis
093.89 Other
093.9 Cardiovascular syphilis, unspecified

094.#(#) Neurosyphilis
094.0 Tabes dorsalis
094.1 General paresis
094.2 Syphilitic meningitis
094.3 Asymptomatic neurosyphilis

094.#(#) ***(continued)***
094.8# Other specified neurosyphilis
094.81 Syphilitic encephalitis
094.82 Syphilitic Parkinsonism
094.83 Syphilitic disseminated retinochoroiditis
094.84 Syphilitic optic atrophy
094.85 Syphilitic retrobulbar neuritis
094.86 Syphilitic acoustic neuritis
094.87 Syphilitic ruptured cerebral aneurysm
094.89 Other
094.9 Neurosyphilis, unspecified

095.# Other forms of late syphilis, with symptoms
095.0 Syphilitic episcleritis
095.1 Syphilis of lung
095.2 Syphilitic peritonitis
095.3 Syphilis of liver
095.4 Syphilis of kidney
095.5 Syphilis of bone
095.6 Syphilis of muscle
095.7 Syphilis of synovium, tendon, and bursa
095.8 Other specified forms of late symptomatic syphilis
095.9 Late symptomatic syphilis, unspecified

096 Late syphilis, latent

097.# Other and unspecified syphilis
097.0 Late syphilis, unspecified
097.1 Latent syphilis, unspecified
097.9 Syphilis, unspecified

098.#(#) Gonococcal infections
098.0 Acute, of lower genitourinary tract
098.1# Acute, of upper genitourinary tract
098.10 Gonococcal infection (acute) NOS
098.11 Gonococcal cystitis (acute)
098.12 Gonococcal prostatitis (acute)
098.13 Gonococcal epididymo-orchitis (acute)
098.14 Gonococcal seminal vesiculitis (acute)
098.15 Gonococcal cervicitis (acute)
098.16 Gonococcal endometritis (acute)
098.17 Gonococcal salpingitis, specified as acute
098.19 Other
098.2 Chronic, of lower genitourinary tract
098.3# Chronic, of upper genitourinary tract
098.30 Chronic gonococcal infection NOS
098.31 Gonococcal cystitis, chronic
098.32 Gonococcal prostatitis, chronic
098.33 Gonococcal epididymo-orchitis, chronic
098.34 Gonococcal seminal vesiculitis, chronic
098.35 Gonococcal cervicitis chronic
098.36 Gonococcal endometritis, chronic
098.37 Gonococcal salpingitis (chronic)
098.39 Other
098.4# Gonococcal infection of eye
098.40 Gonococcal conjunctivitis (Neonatorum)
098.41 Gonococcal iridocyclitis
098.42 Gonococcal endophthalmia
098.43 Gonococcal keratitis
098.49 Other
098.5# Gonococcal infection of joint
098.50 Gonococcal arthritis
098.51 Gonococcal synovitis and tenosynovitis
098.52 Gonococcal bursitis
098.53 Gonococcal spondylitis
098.59 Other gonococcal rheumatism
098.6 Gonococcal infection of pharynx
098.7 Gonococcal infection of anus and rectum

098.#(#) ***(continued)***
098.8# Gonococcal infection of other specified sites
098.81 Gonococcal keratosis
098.82 Gonococcal meningitis
098.83 Gonococcal pericarditis
098.84 Gonococcal endocarditis
098.85 Other gonococcal heart disease
098.86 Gonococcal peritonitis
098.89 Other gonococcemia

099.#(#) Other venereal diseases
099.0 Chancroid
099.1 Lymphogranuloma venereum
099.2 Granuloma inguinale
099.3 Reiter's disease
099.4# Other nongonococcal urethritis [NGU]
099.40 Unspecified
099.41 Chlamydia trachomatis
099.49 Other specified organism
099.5# Other venereal diseases due to Chlamydia trachomatis
099.50 Unspecified site
099.51 Pharynx
099.52 Anus and rectum
099.53 Lower genitourinary sites
099.54 Other genitourinary sites
099.55 Unspecified genitourinary site
099.56 Peritoneum
099.59 Other specified site
099.8 Other specified venereal diseases
099.9 Venereal disease, unspecified

100.#(#) Leptospirosis
100.0 Leptospirosis icterohemorrhagica
100.8# Other specified leptospiral infections
100.81 Leptospiral meningitis (aseptic)
100.89 Other
100.9 Leptospirosis, unspecified

101 Vincent's angina

102.# Yaws
102.0 Initial lesions
102.1 Multiple papillomata and wet crab yaws
102.2 Other early skin lesions
102.3 Hyperkeratosis
102.4 Gummata and ulcers
102.5 Gangosa
102.6 Bone and joint lesions
102.7 Other manifestations
102.8 Latent yaws
102.9 Yaws, unspecified

103.# Pinta
103.0 Primary lesions
103.1 Intermediate lesions
103.2 Late lesions
103.3 Mixed lesions
103.9 Pinta, unspecified

104.# Other spirochetal infection
104.0 Nonvenereal endemic syphilis
104.8 Other specified spirochetal infections
104.9 Spirochetal infection, unspecified

110.# Dermatophytosis
110.0 Of scalp and beard
110.1 Of nail
110.2 Of hand
110.3 Of groin and perianal area
110.4 Of foot
110.5 Of the body

110.# ***(continued)***
110.6 Deep seated dermatophytosis
110.8 Of other specified sites
110.9 Of unspecified site

111.# Dermatomycosis, other and unspecified
111.0 Pityriasis versicolor
111.1 Tinea nigra
111.2 Tinea blanca
111.3 Black piedra
111.8 Other specified dermatomycoses
111.9 Dermatomycosis, unspecified

112.#(#) Candidiasis
112.0 Of mouth
112.1 Of vulva and vagina
112.2 Of other urogenital sites
112.3 Of skin and nails
112.4 Of lung
112.5 Disseminated
112.8# Of other specified sites
112.81 Candidal endocarditis
112.82 Candidal otitis externa
112.83 Candidal meningitis
112.84 Candidal esophagitis
112.85 Candidal enteritis
112.89 Other
112.9 Of unspecified site

114.# Coccidioidomycosis
114.0 Primary coccidioidomycosis
114.1 Primary extrapulmonary coccidioidomycosis
114.2 Coccidioidal meningitis
114.3 Other forms of progressive coccidioidomycosis
114.4 Chronic pulmonary coccidioidomycosis
114.5 Pulmonary coccidioidomycosis, unspecified
114.9 Coccidioidomycosis, unspecified

115.## Histoplasmosis
115.0# Infection by Histoplasma capsulatum
115.1# Infection by Histoplasma duboisii
115.9# Histoplasmosis, unspecified
5th Digit: 115
0 Without mention of manifestation
1 Meningitis
2 Retinitis
3 Pericarditis
4 Endocarditis
5 Pneumonia
9 Other

116.# Blastomycotic infection
116.0 Blastomycosis
116.1 Paracoccidioidomycosis
116.2 Lobomycosis

117.# Other mycoses
117.0 Rhinosporidiosis
117.1 Sporotrichosis
117.2 Chromoblastomycosis
117.3 Aspergillosis
117.4 Mycotic mycetomas
117.5 Cryptococcosis
117.6 Allescheriosis [Petriellidosis]
117.7 Zygomycosis [Phycomycosis or Mucormycosis]
117.8 Infection by dematiacious fungi
117.9 Other and unspecified mycoses

118 Opportunistic mycoses

120.# Schistosomiasis [bilharziasis]
120.0 Schistosoma haematobium
120.1 Schistosoma mansoni
120.2 Schistosoma japonicum
120.3 Cutaneous
120.8 Other specified schistosomiasis
120.9 Schistosomiasis, unspecified

121.# Other trematode infections
121.0 Opisthorchiasis
121.1 Clonorchiasis
121.2 Paragonimiasis
121.3 Fascioliasis
121.4 Fasciolopsiasis
121.5 Metagonimiasis
121.6 Heterophyiasis
121.8 Other specified trematode infections
121.9 Trematode infection, unspecified

122.# Echinococcosis
122.0 Echinococcus granulosus infection of liver
122.1 Echinococcus granulosus infection of lung
122.2 Echinococcus granulosus infection of thyroid
122.3 Echinococcus granulosus infection, other
122.4 Echinococcus granulosus infection, unspecified
122.5 Echinococcus multilocularis infection of liver
122.6 Echinococcus multilocularis infection, other
122.7 Echinococcus multilocularis infection, unspecified
122.8 Echinococcosis, unspecified, of liver
122.9 Echinococcosis, other and unspecified

123.# Other cestode infection
123.0 Taenia solium infection, intestinal form
123.1 Cysticercosis
123.2 Taenia saginata infection
123.3 Taeniasis, unspecified
123.4 Diphyllobothriasis, intestinal
123.5 Sparganosis [larval diphyllobothriasis]
123.6 Hymenolepiasis
123.8 Other specified cestode infection
123.9 Cestode infection, unspecified

124 Trichinosis

125.# Filarial infection and dracontiasis
125.0 Bancroftian filariasis
125.1 Malayan filariasis
125.2 Loiasis
125.3 Onchocerciasis
125.4 Dipetalonemiasis
125.5 Mansonella ozzardi infection
125.6 Other specified filariasis
125.7 Dracontiasis
125.9 Unspecified filariasis

126.# Ancylostomiasis and necatoriasis
126.0 Ancylostoma duodenale
126.1 Necator americanus
126.2 Ancylostoma braziliense
126.3 Ancylostoma ceylanicum
126.8 Other specified Ancylostoma
126.9 Ancylostomiasis and necatoriasis, unspecified

127.# Other intestinal helminthiases
127.0 Ascariasis
127.1 Anisakiasis
127.2 Strongyloidiasis
127.3 Trichuriasis
127.4 Enterobiasis
127.5 Capillariasis
127.6 Trichostrongyliasis
127.7 Other specified intestinal helminthiasis
127.8 Mixed intestinal helminthiasis
127.9 Intestinal helminthiasis, unspecified

128.# Other and unspecified helminthiases
128.0 Toxocariasis
128.1 Gnathostomiasis
128.8 Other specified helminthiasis
128.9 Helminth infection, unspecified

129 Intestinal parasitism, unspecified

130.# Toxoplasmosis
130.0 Meningoencephalitis due to toxoplasmosis
130.1 Conjunctivitis due to toxoplasmosis
130.2 Chorioretinitis due to toxoplasmosis
130.3 Myocarditis due to toxoplasmosis
130.4 Pneumonitis due to toxoplasmosis
130.5 Hepatitis due to toxoplasmosis
130.7 Toxoplasmosis of other specified sites
130.8 Multisystemic disseminated toxoplasmosis
130.9 Toxoplasmosis, unspecified

131.#(#) Trichomoniasis
131.0# Urogenital trichomoniasis
131.00 Urogenital trichomoniasis, unspecified
131.01 Trichomonal vulvovaginitis
131.02 Trichomonal urethritis
131.03 Trichomonal prostatitis
131.09 Other
131.8 Other specified sites
131.9 Trichomoniasis, unspecified

132.# Pediculosis and phthirus infestation
132.0 Pediculus capitis [head louse]
132.1 Pediculus corporis [body louse]
132.2 Phthirus pubis [pubic louse]
132.3 Mixed infestation
132.9 Pediculosis, unspecified

133.# Acariasis
133.0 Scabies
133.8 Other acariasis
133.9 Acariasis, unspecified

134.# Other infestation
134.0 Myiasis
134.1 Other arthropod infestation
134.2 Hirudiniasis
134.8 Other specified infestations
134.9 Infestation, unspecified

135 Sarcoidosis

136.# Other and unspecified infectious and parasitic diseases
136.0 Ainhum
136.1 Behçet's syndrome
136.2 Specific infections by free-living amebae

136.# ***(continued)***
136.3 Pneumocystosis
136.4 Psorospermiasis
136.5 Sarcosporidiosis
136.8 Other specified infectious and parasitic diseases
136.9 Unspecified infectious and parasitic diseases

137.# Late effects of tuberculosis
137.0 Late effects of respiratory or unspecified tuberculosis
137.1 Late effects of central nervous system tuberculosis
137.2 Late effects of genitourinary tuberculosis
137.3 Late effects of tuberculosis of bones and joints
137.4 Late effects of tuberculosis of other specified organs

138 Late effects of acute poliomyelitis

139.# Late effects of other infectious and parasitic diseases
139.0 Late effects of viral encephalitis
139.1 Late effects of trachoma
139.8 Late effects of other and unspecified infectious and parasitic diseases

140.# Malignant neoplasm of lip
140.0 Upper lip, vermilion border
140.1 Lower lip, vermilion border
140.3 Upper lip, inner aspect
140.4 Lower lip, inner aspect
140.5 Lip, unspecified, inner aspect
140.6 Commissure of lip
140.8 Other sites of lip
140.9 Lip, unspecified, vermilion border

141.# Malignant neoplasm of tongue
141.0 Base of tongue
141.1 Dorsal surface of tongue
141.2 Tip and lateral border of tongue
141.3 Ventral surface of tongue
141.4 Anterior two-thirds of tongue, part unspecified
141.5 Junctional zone
141.6 Lingual tonsil
141.8 Other sites of tongue
141.9 Tongue, unspecified

142.# Malignant neoplasm of major salivary glands
142.0 Parotid gland
142.1 Submandibular gland
142.2 Sublingual gland
142.8 Other major salivary glands
142.9 Salivary gland, unspecified

143.# Malignant neoplasm of gum
143.0 Upper gum
143.1 Lower gum
143.8 Other sites of gum
143.9 Gum, unspecified

144.# Malignant neoplasm of floor of mouth
144.0 Anterior portion
144.1 Lateral portion
144.8 Other sites of floor of mouth
144.9 Floor of mouth, part unspecified

145.# Malignant neoplasm of other and unspecified parts of mouth
145.0 Cheek mucosa
145.1 Vestibule of mouth
145.2 Hard palate
145.3 Soft palate
145.4 Uvula
145.5 Palate, unspecified
145.6 Retromolar area
145.8 Other specified parts of mouth
145.9 Mouth, unspecified

146.# Malignant neoplasm of oropharynx
146.0 Tonsil
146.1 Tonsillar fossa
146.2 Tonsillar pillars (anterior) (posterior)
146.3 Vallecula
146.4 Anterior aspect of epiglottis
146.5 Junctional region
146.6 Lateral wall of oropharynx
146.7 Posterior wall of oropharynx
146.8 Other specified sites of oropharynx
146.9 Oropharynx, unspecified

147.# Malignant neoplasm of nasopharynx
147.0 Superior wall
147.1 Posterior wall
147.2 Lateral wall
147.3 Anterior wall
147.8 Other specified sites of nasopharynx
147.9 Nasopharynx, unspecified

148.# Malignant neoplasm of hypopharynx
148.0 Postcricoid region
148.1 Pyriform sinus
148.2 Aryepiglottic fold, hypopharyngeal aspect
148.3 Posterior hypopharyngeal wall
148.8 Other specified sites of hypopharynx
148.9 Hypopharynx, unspecified

149.# Malignant neoplasm of other and ill-defined sites within the lip, oral cavity, and pharynx
149.0 Pharynx, unspecified
149.1 Waldeyer's ring
149.8 Other
149.9 Ill-defined

150.# Malignant neoplasm of esophagus
150.0 Cervical esophagus
150.1 Thoracic esophagus
150.2 Abdominal esophagus
150.3 Upper third of esophagus
150.4 Middle third of esophagus
150.5 Lower third of esophagus
150.8 Other specified part
150.9 Esophagus, unspecified

151.# Malignant neoplasm of stomach
151.0 Cardia
151.1 Pylorus
151.2 Pyloric antrum
151.3 Fundus of stomach
151.4 Body of stomach
151.5 Lesser curvature, unspecified
151.6 Greater curvature, unspecified
151.8 Other specified sites of stomach
151.9 Stomach, unspecified

152.# Malignant neoplasm of small intestine, including duodenum

152.0 Duodenum
152.1 Jejunum
152.2 Ileum
152.3 Meckel's diverticulum
152.8 Other specified sites of small intestine
152.9 Small intestine, unspecified

153.# Malignant neoplasm of colon

153.0 Hepatic flexure
153.1 Transverse colon
153.2 Descending colon
153.3 Sigmoid colon
153.4 Cecum
153.5 Appendix
153.6 Ascending colon
153.7 Splenic flexure
153.8 Other specified sites of large intestine
153.9 Colon, unspecified

154.# Malignant neoplasm of rectum, rectosigmoid junction, and anus

154.0 Rectosigmoid junction
154.1 Rectum
154.2 Anal canal
154.3 Anus, unspecified
154.8 Other

155.# Malignant neoplasm of liver and intrahepatic bile ducts

155.0 Liver, primary
155.1 Intrahepatic bile ducts
155.2 Liver, not specified as primary or secondary

156.# Malignant neoplasm of gallbladder and extrahepatic bile ducts

156.0 Gallbladder
156.1 Extrahepatic bile ducts
156.2 Ampulla of Vater
156.8 Other specified sites of gallbladder and extrahepatic bile ducts
156.9 Biliary tract, part unspecified

157.# Malignant neoplasm of pancreas

157.0 Head of pancreas
157.1 Body of pancreas
157.2 Tail of pancreas
157.3 Pancreatic duct
157.4 Islets of Langerhans
157.8 Other specified sites of pancreas
157.9 Pancreas, part unspecified

158.# Malignant neoplasm of retroperitoneum and peritoneum

158.0 Retroperitoneum
158.8 Specified parts of peritoneum
158.9 Peritoneum, unspecified

159.# Malignant neoplasm of other and ill-defined sites within the digestive organs and peritoneum

159.0 Intestinal tract, part unspecified
159.1 Spleen, not elsewhere classified
159.8 Other sites of digestive system and intra-abdominal organs
159.9 Ill-defined

160.# Malignant neoplasm of nasal cavities, middle ear, and accessory sinuses

160.0 Nasal cavities
160.1 Auditory tube, middle ear, and mastoid air cells
160.2 Maxillary sinus
160.3 Ethmoidal sinus
160.4 Frontal sinus
160.5 Sphenoidal sinus
160.8 Other
160.9 Accessory sinus, unspecified

161.# Malignant neoplasm of larynx

161.0 Glottis
161.1 Supraglottis
161.2 Subglottis
161.3 Laryngeal cartilages
161.8 Other specified sites of larynx
161.9 Larynx, unspecified

162.# Malignant neoplasm of trachea, bronchus, and lung

162.0 Trachea
162.2 Main bronchus
162.3 Upper lobe, bronchus or lung
162.4 Middle lobe, bronchus or lung
162.5 Lower lobe, bronchus or lung
162.8 Other parts of bronchus or lung
162.9 Bronchus and lung, unspecified

163.# Malignant neoplasm of pleura

163.0 Parietal pleura
163.1 Visceral pleura
163.8 Other specified sites of pleura
163.9 Pleura, unspecified

164.# Malignant neoplasm of thymus, heart, and mediastinum

164.0 Thymus
164.1 Heart
164.2 Anterior mediastinum
164.3 Posterior mediastinum
164.8 Other
164.9 Mediastinum, part unspecified

165.# Malignant neoplasm of other and ill-defined sites within the respiratory system and intrathoracic organs

165.0 Upper respiratory tract, part unspecified
165.8 Other
165.9 Ill-defined sites within the respiratory system

170.# Malignant neoplasm of bone and articular cartilage

170.0 Bones of skull and face, except mandible
170.1 Mandible
170.2 Vertebral column, excluding sacrum and coccyx
170.3 Ribs, sternum, and clavicle
170.4 Scapula and long bones of upper limb
170.5 Short bones of upper limb
170.6 Pelvic bones, sacrum, and coccyx
170.7 Long bones of lower limb
170.8 Short bones of lower limb
170.9 Bone and articular cartilage, site unspecified

171.# Malignant neoplasm of connective and other soft tissue

- 171.0 Head, face, and neck
- 171.2 Upper limb, including shoulder
- 171.3 Lower limb, including hip
- 171.4 Thorax
- 171.5 Abdomen
- 171.6 Pelvis
- 171.7 Trunk, unspecified
- 171.8 Other specified sites of connective and other soft tissue
- 171.9 Connective and other soft tissue, site unspecified

172.# Malignant melanoma of skin

- 172.0 Lip
- 172.1 Eyelid, including canthus
- 172.2 Ear and external auditory canal
- 172.3 Other and unspecified parts of face
- 172.4 Scalp and neck
- 172.5 Trunk, except scrotum
- 172.6 Upper limb, including shoulder
- 172.7 Lower limb, including hip
- 172.8 Other specified sites of skin
- 172.9 Melanoma of skin, site unspecified

173.# Other malignant neoplasm of skin

- 173.0 Skin of lip
- 173.1 Eyelid, including canthus
- 173.2 Skin of ear and external auditory canal
- 173.3 Skin of other and unspecified parts of face
- 173.4 Scalp and skin of neck
- 173.5 Skin of trunk, except scrotum
- 173.6 Skin of upper limb, including shoulder
- 173.7 Skin of lower limb, including hip
- 173.8 Other specified sites of skin
- 173.9 Skin, site unspecified

174.# Malignant neoplasm of female breast

- 174.0 Nipple and areola
- 174.1 Central portion
- 174.2 Upper-inner quadrant
- 174.3 Lower-inner quadrant
- 174.4 Upper-outer quadrant
- 174.5 Lower-outer quadrant
- 174.6 Axillary tail
- 174.8 Other specified sites of female breast
- 174.9 Breast (female), unspecified

175.# Malignant neoplasm of male breast

- 175.0 Nipple and areola
- 175.9 Other and unspecified sites of male breast

176.# Kaposi's sarcoma

- 176.0 Skin
- 176.1 Soft tissue
- 176.2 Palate
- 176.3 Gastrointestinal sites
- 176.4 Lung
- 176.5 Lymph nodes
- 176.8 Other specified sites
- 176.9 Unspecified

179 Malignant neoplasm of uterus, part unspecified

180.# Malignant neoplasm of cervix uteri

- 180.0 Endocervix
- 180.1 Exocervix
- 180.8 Other specified sites of cervix
- 180.9 Cervix uteri, unspecified

181 Malignant neoplasm of placenta

182.# Malignant neoplasm of body of uterus

- 182.0 Corpus uteri, except isthmus
- 182.1 Isthmus
- 182.8 Other specified sites of body of uterus

183.# Malignant neoplasm of ovary and other uterine adnexa

- 183.0 Ovary
- 183.2 Fallopian tube
- 183.3 Broad ligament
- 183.4 Parametrium
- 183.5 Round ligament
- 183.8 Other specified sites of uterine adnexa
- 183.9 Uterine adnexa, unspecified

184.# Malignant neoplasm of other and unspecified female genital organs

- 184.0 Vagina
- 184.1 Labia majora
- 184.2 Labia minora
- 184.3 Clitoris
- 184.4 Vulva, unspecified
- 184.8 Other specified sites of female genital organs
- 184.9 Female genital organ, site unspecified

185 Malignant neoplasm of prostate

186.# Malignant neoplasm of testis

- 186.0 Undescended testis
- 186.9 Other and unspecified testis

187.# Malignant neoplasm of penis and other male genital organs

- 187.1 Prepuce
- 187.2 Glans penis
- 187.3 Body of penis
- 187.4 Penis, part unspecified
- 187.5 Epididymis
- 187.6 Spermatic cord
- 187.7 Scrotum
- 187.8 Other specified sites of male genital organs
- 187.9 Male genital organ, site unspecified

188.# Malignant neoplasm of bladder

- 188.0 Trigone of urinary bladder
- 188.1 Dome of urinary bladder
- 188.2 Lateral wall of urinary bladder
- 188.3 Anterior wall of urinary bladder
- 188.4 Posterior wall of urinary bladder
- 188.5 Bladder neck
- 188.6 Ureteric orifice
- 188.7 Urachus
- 188.8 Other specified sites of bladder
- 188.9 Bladder, part unspecified

189.# Malignant neoplasm of kidney and other and unspecified urinary organs

- 189.0 Kidney, except pelvis
- 189.1 Renal pelvis
- 189.2 Ureter

189.# ***(continued)***
- 189.3 Urethra
- 189.4 Paraurethral glands
- 189.8 Other specified sites of urinary organs
- 189.9 Urinary organ, site unspecified

190.# Malignant neoplasm of eye
- 190.0 Eyeball, except conjunctiva, cornea, retina, and choroid
- 190.1 Orbit
- 190.2 Lacrimal gland
- 190.3 Conjunctiva
- 190.4 Cornea
- 190.5 Retina
- 190.6 Choroid
- 190.7 Lacrimal duct
- 190.8 Other specified sites of eye
- 190.9 Eye, part unspecified

191.# Malignant neoplasm of brain
- 191.0 Cerebrum, except lobes and ventricles
- 191.1 Frontal lobe
- 191.2 Temporal lobe
- 191.3 Parietal lobe
- 191.4 Occipital lobe
- 191.5 Ventricles
- 191.6 Cerebellum NOS
- 191.7 Brain stem
- 191.8 Other parts of brain
- 191.9 Brain, unspecified

192.# Malignant neoplasm of other and unspecified parts of nervous system
- 192.0 Cranial nerves
- 192.1 Cerebral meninges
- 192.2 Spinal cord
- 192.3 Spinal meninges
- 192.8 Other specified sites of nervous system
- 192.9 Nervous system, part unspecified

193 Malignant neoplasm of thyroid gland

194.# Malignant neoplasm of other endocrine glands and related structures
- 194.0 Adrenal gland
- 194.1 Parathyroid gland
- 194.3 Pituitary gland and craniopharyngeal duct
- 194.4 Pineal gland
- 194.5 Carotid body
- 194.6 Aortic body and other paraganglia
- 194.8 Other
- 194.9 Endocrine gland, site unspecified

195.# Malignant neoplasm of other and ill-defined sites
- 195.0 Head, face, and neck
- 195.1 Thorax
- 195.2 Abdomen
- 195.3 Pelvis
- 195.4 Upper limb
- 195.5 Lower limb
- 195.8 Other specified sites

196.# Secondary and unspecified malignant neoplasm of lymph nodes
- 196.0 Lymph nodes of head, face, and neck
- 196.1 Intrathoracic lymph nodes
- 196.2 Intra-abdominal lymph nodes
- 196.3 Lymph nodes of axilla and upper limb

196.# ***(continued)***
- 196.5 Lymph nodes of inguinal region and lower limb
- 196.6 Intrapelvic lymph nodes
- 196.8 Lymph nodes of multiple sites
- 196.9 Site unspecified

197.# Secondary malignant neoplasm of respiratory and digestive systems
- 197.0 Lung
- 197.1 Mediastinum
- 197.2 Pleura
- 197.3 Other respiratory organs
- 197.4 Small intestine, including duodenum
- 197.5 Large intestine and rectum
- 197.6 Retroperitoneum and peritoneum
- 197.7 Liver, specified as secondary
- 197.8 Other digestive organs and spleen

198.#(#) Secondary malignant neoplasm of other specified sites
- 198.0 Kidney
- 198.1 Other urinary organs
- 198.2 Skin
- 198.3 Brain and spinal cord
- 198.4 Other parts of nervous system
- 198.5 Bone and bone marrow
- 198.6 Ovary
- 198.7 Adrenal gland
- **198.8#** Other specified sites
  - 198.81 Breast
  - 198.82 Genital organs
  - 198.89 Other

199.# Malignant neoplasm without specification of site
- 199.0 Disseminated
- 199.1 Other

200.## Lymphosarcoma and reticulosarcoma and other specified malignant tumors or lymphatic tissue
- **200.0#** Reticulosarcoma
- **200.1#** Lymphosarcoma
- **200.2#** Burkitt's tumor or lymphoma
- **200.3#** Marginal zone lymphoma
- **200.4#** Mantle cell lymphoma
- **200.5#** Primary central nervous system lymphoma
- **200.6#** Anaplastic large cell lymphoma
- **200.7#** Large cell lymphoma
- **200.8#** Other named variants

201.## Hodgkin's disease
- **201.0#** Hodgkin's paragranuloma
- **201.1#** Hodgkin's granuloma
- **201.2#** Hodgkin's sarcoma
- **201.4#** Lymphocytic-histiocytic predominance
- **201.5#** Nodular sclerosis
- **201.6#** Mixed cellularity
- **201.7#** Lymphocytic depletion
- **201.9#** Hodgkin's disease, unspecified

5th Digit: 200-201
- **0 Unspecified site,**
- **1 Lymph nodes of head, face, and neck**
- **2 Intrathoracic lymph nodes**
- **3 Intra-abdominal lymph nodes**
- **4 Lymph nodes of axilla and upper limb**
- **5 Lymph nodes of inguinal region and lower limb**
- **6 Intrapelvic lymph nodes**
- **7 Spleen**
- **8 Lymph nodes of multiple sites**

NUMERICAL REFERENCE

202.## Other malignant neoplasms of lymphoid and histiocytic tissue
- **202.0#** Nodular lymphoma
- **202.1#** Mycosis fungoides
- **202.2#** Sézary's disease
- **202.3#** Malignant histiocytosis
- **202.4#** Leukemic reticuloendotheliosis
- **202.5#** Letterer-Siwe disease
- **202.6#** Malignant mast cell tumors
- **202.7#** Peripheral T-cell lymphoma
- **202.8#** Other lymphomas
- **202.9#** Other and unspecified malignant neoplasms of lymphoid and histiocytic tissue

5th Digit: 202
- **0 Unspecified site,**
- **1 Lymph nodes of head, face, and neck**
- **2 Intrathoracic lymph nodes**
- **3 Intra-abdominal lymph nodes**
- **4 Lymph nodes of axilla and upper limb**
- **5 Lymph nodes of inguinal region and lower limb**
- **6 Intrapelvic lymph nodes**
- **7 Spleen**
- **8 Lymph nodes of multiple sites**

203.## Multiple myeloma and immunoproliferative neoplasms
- **203.0#** Multiple myeloma
- **203.1#** Plasma cell leukemia
- **203.8#** Other immunoproliferative neoplasms

204.## Lymphoid leukemia
- **204.0#** Acute
- **204.1#** Chronic
- **204.2#** Subacute
- **204.8#** Other lymphoid leukemia
- **204.9#** Unspecified lymphoid leukemia

205.## Myeloid leukemia
- **205.0#** Acute
- **205.1#** Chronic
- **205.2#** Subacute
- **205.3#** Myeloid sarcoma
- **205.8#** Other myeloid leukemia
- **205.9#** Unspecified myeloid leukemia

206.## Monocytic leukemia
- **206.0#** Acute
- **206.1#** Chronic
- **206.2#** Subacute
- **206.8#** Other monocytic leukemia
- **206.9#** Unspecified monocytic leukemia

207.## Other specified leukemia
- **207.0#** Acute erythremia and erythroleukemia
- **207.1#** Chronic erythremia
- **207.2#** Megakaryocytic leukemia
- **207.8#** Other specified leukemia

208.## Leukemia of unspecified cell type
- **208.0#** Acute
- **208.1#** Chronic
- **208.2#** Subacute
- **208.8#** Other leukemia of unspecified cell type
- **208.9#** Unspecified leukemia

5th Digit: 203-208
- **0 Without mention of remission**
- **1 In remission**

210.# Benign neoplasm of lip, oral cavity, and pharynx
- 210.0 Lip
- 210.1 Tongue
- 210.2 Major salivary glands
- 210.3 Floor of mouth
- 210.4 Other and unspecified parts of mouth
- 210.5 Tonsil
- 210.6 Other parts of oropharynx
- 210.7 Nasopharynx
- 210.8 Hypopharynx
- 210.9 Pharynx, unspecified

211.# Benign neoplasm of other parts of digestive system
- 211.0 Esophagus
- 211.1 Stomach
- 211.2 Duodenum, jejunum, and ileum
- 211.3 Colon
- 211.4 Rectum and anal canal
- 211.5 Liver and biliary passages
- 211.6 Pancreas, except islets of Langerhans
- 211.7 Islets of Langerhans
- 211.8 Retroperitoneum and peritoneum
- 211.9 Other and unspecified site

212.# Benign neoplasm of respiratory and intrathoracic organs
- 212.0 Nasal cavities, middle ear, and accessory sinuses
- 212.1 Larynx
- 212.2 Trachea
- 212.3 Bronchus and lung
- 212.4 Pleura
- 212.5 Mediastinum
- 212.6 Thymus
- 212.7 Heart
- 212.8 Other specified sites
- 212.9 Site unspecified

213.# Benign neoplasm of bone and articular cartilage
- 213.0 Bones of skull and face
- 213.1 Lower jaw bone
- 213.2 Vertebral column, excluding sacrum and coccyx
- 213.3 Ribs, sternum, and clavicle
- 213.4 Scapula and long bones of upper limb
- 213.5 Short bones of upper limb
- 213.6 Pelvic bones, sacrum, and coccyx
- 213.7 Long bones of lower limb
- 213.8 Short bones of lower limb
- 213.9 Bone and articular cartilage, site unspecified

214.# Lipoma
- 214.0 Skin and subcutaneous tissue of face
- 214.1 Other skin and subcutaneous tissue
- 214.2 Intrathoracic organs
- 214.3 Intra-abdominal organs
- 214.4 Spermatic cord
- 214.8 Other specified sites
- 214.9 Lipoma, unspecified site

215.# Other benign neoplasm of connective and other soft tissue
- 215.0 Head, face, and neck
- 215.2 Upper limb, including shoulder
- 215.3 Lower limb, including hip
- 215.4 Thorax
- 215.5 Abdomen

NUMERICAL REFERENCE

215.# *(continued)*
215.6 Pelvis
215.7 Trunk, unspecified
215.8 Other specified sites
215.9 Site unspecified

216.# Benign neoplasm of skin
216.0 Skin of lip
216.1 Eyelid, including canthus
216.2 Ear and external auditory canal
216.3 Skin of other and unspecified parts of face
216.4 Scalp and skin of neck
216.5 Skin of trunk, except scrotum
216.6 Skin of upper limb, including shoulder
216.7 Skin of lower limb, including hip
216.8 Other specified sites of skin
216.9 Skin, site unspecified

217 Benign neoplasm of breast

218.# Uterine leiomyoma
218.0 Submucous leiomyoma of uterus
218.1 Intramural leiomyoma of uterus
218.2 Subserous leiomyoma of uterus
218.9 Leiomyoma of uterus, unspecified

219.# Other benign neoplasm of uterus
219.0 Cervix uteri
219.1 Corpus uteri
219.8 Other specified parts of uterus
219.9 Uterus, part unspecified

220 Benign neoplasm of ovary

221.# Benign neoplasm of other female genital organs
221.0 Fallopian tube and uterine ligaments
221.1 Vagina
221.2 Vulva
221.8 Other specified sites of female genital organs
221.9 Female genital organ, site unspecified

222.# Benign neoplasm of male genital organs
222.0 Testis
222.1 Penis
222.2 Prostate
222.3 Epididymis
222.4 Scrotum
222.8 Other specified sites of male genital organs
222.9 Male genital organ, site unspecified

223.#(#) Benign neoplasm of kidney and other urinary organs
223.0 Kidney, except pelvis
223.1 Renal pelvis
223.2 Ureter
223.3 Bladder
223.8# Other specified sites of urinary organs
223.81 Urethra
223.89 Other
223.9 Urinary organ, site unspecified

224.# Benign neoplasm of eye
224.0 Eyeball, except conjunctiva, cornea, retina, and choroid
224.1 Orbit
224.2 Lacrimal gland

224.# *(continued)*
224.3 Conjunctiva
224.4 Cornea
224.5 Retina
224.6 Choroid
224.7 Lacrimal duct
224.8 Other specified parts of eye
224.9 Eye, part unspecified

225.# Benign neoplasm of brain and other parts of nervous system
225.0 Brain
225.1 Cranial nerves
225.2 Cerebral meninges
225.3 Spinal cord
225.4 Spinal meninges
225.8 Other specified sites of nervous system
225.9 Nervous system, part unspecified

226 Benign neoplasm of thyroid glands

227.# Benign neoplasm of other endocrine glands and related structures
227.0 Adrenal gland
227.1 Parathyroid gland
227.3 Pituitary gland and craniopharyngeal duct
227.4 Pineal gland
227.5 Carotid body
227.6 Aortic body and other paraganglia
227.8 Other
227.9 Endocrine gland, site unspecified

228.#(#) Hemangioma and lymphangioma, any site
228.0# Hemangioma, any site
228.00 Of unspecified site
228.01 Of skin and subcutaneous tissue
228.02 Of intracranial structures
228.03 Of retina
228.04 Of intra-abdominal structures
228.09 Of other sites
228.1 Lymphangioma, any site

229.# Benign neoplasm of other and unspecified sites
229.0 Lymph nodes
229.8 Other specified sites
229.9 Site unspecified

230.# Carcinoma in situ of digestive organs
230.0 Lip, oral cavity, and pharynx
230.1 Esophagus
230.2 Stomach
230.3 Colon
230.4 Rectum
230.5 Anal canal
230.6 Anus, unspecified
230.7 Other and unspecified parts of intestine
230.8 Liver and biliary system
230.9 Other and unspecified digestive organs

231.# Carcinoma in situ of respiratory system
231.0 Larynx
231.1 Trachea
231.2 Bronchus and lung
231.8 Other specified parts of respiratory system
231.9 Respiratory system, part unspecified

232.# Carcinoma in situ of skin
232.0 Skin of lip
232.1 Eyelid, including canthus
232.2 Ear and external auditory canal
232.3 Skin of other and unspecified parts of face
232.4 Scalp and skin of neck
232.5 Skin of trunk, except scrotum
232.6 Skin of upper limb, including shoulder
232.7 Skin of lower limb, including hip
232.8 Other specified sites of skin
232.9 Skin, site unspecified

233.# Carcinoma in situ of breast and genitourinary system
233.0 Breast
233.1 Cervix uteri
233.2 Other and unspecified parts of uterus
233.3# Other and unspecified female genital organs
233.30 Unspecified female genital organ
233.31 Vagina
233.32 Vulva
233.39 Other female genital organ
233.4 Prostate
233.5 Penis
233.6 Other and unspecified male genital organs
233.7 Bladder
233.9 Other and unspecified urinary organs

234.# Carcinoma in situ of other and unspecified sites
234.0 Eye
234.8 Other specified sites
234.9 Site unspecified

235.# Neoplasm of uncertain behavior of digestive and respiratory systems
235.0 Major salivary glands
235.1 Lip, oral cavity, and pharynx
235.2 Stomach, intestines, and rectum
235.3 Liver and biliary passages
235.4 Retroperitoneum and peritoneum
235.5 Other and unspecified digestive organs
235.6 Larynx
235.7 Trachea, bronchus, and lung
235.8 Pleura, thymus, and mediastinum
235.9 Other and unspecified respiratory organs

236.#(#) Neoplasm of uncertain behavior of genitourinary organs
236.0 Uterus
236.1 Placenta
236.2 Ovary
236.3 Other and unspecified female genital organs
236.4 Testis
236.5 Prostate
236.6 Other and unspecified male genital organs
236.7 Bladder
236.9# Other and unspecified urinary organs
236.90 Urinary organ, unspecified
236.91 Kidney and ureter
236.99 Other

237.#(#) Neoplasm of uncertain behavior of endocrine glands and nervous system
237.0 Pituitary gland and craniopharyngeal duct
237.1 Pineal gland
237.2 Adrenal gland
237.3 Paraganglia
237.4 Other and unspecified endocrine glands
237.5 Brain and spinal cord

237.#(#) ***(continued)***
237.6 Meninges
237.7# Neurofibromatosis
237.70 Neurofibromatosis, unspecified
237.71 Neurofibromatosis, type 1
237.72 Neurofibromatosis, type 2
237.9 Other and unspecified parts of nervous system

238.#(#) Neoplasm of uncertain behavior of other and unspecified sites and tissues
238.0 Bone and articular cartilage
238.1 Connective and other soft tissue
238.2 Skin
238.3 Breast
238.4 Polycythemia vera
238.5 Histiocytic and mast cells
238.6 Plasma cells
238.7# Other lymphatic and hematopoietic tissues
238.71 Essential thrombocythemia
238.72 Low grade myelodysplastic syndrome lesions
238.73 High grade myelodysplastic syndrome lesions
238.74 Myelodysplastic syndrome with 5q deletion
238.75 Myelodysplastic syndrome, unspecified
238.76 Myelogibrosis with myeloid metaplasia
238.79 Other lymphatic and hematopoietic tissues
238.8 Other specified sites
238.9 Site unspecified

239.# Neoplasms of unspecified nature
239.0 Digestive system
239.1 Respiratory system
239.2 Bone, soft tissue, and skin
239.3 Breast
239.4 Bladder
239.5 Other genitourinary organs
239.6 Brain
239.7 Endocrine glands and other nervous system
239.8 Other specified sites
239.9 Site unspecified

240.# Simple and unspecified goiter
240.0 Goiter, specified as simple
240.9 Goiter, unspecified

241.# Nontoxic nodular goiter
241.0 Nontoxic uninodular goiter
241.1 Nontoxic multinodular goiter
241.9 Unspecified nontoxic nodular goiter

242.## Thyrotoxicosis with or without goiter
242.0# Toxic diffuse goiter
242.1# Toxic uninodular goiter
242.2# Toxic multinodular goiter
242.3# Toxic nodular goiter, unspecified
242.4# Thyrotoxicosis from ectopic thyroid nodule
242.8# Thyrotoxicosis of other specified origin
242.9# Thyrotoxicosis without mention of goiter or other cause

5th Digit: 242
0 Without mention of thyrotoxic crisis or storm
1 With mention of thyrotoxic crisis or storm

243 Congenital hypothyroidism

NUMERICAL REFERENCE

244.# Acquired hypothyroidism
- 244.0 Postsurgical hypothyroidism
- 244.1 Other postablative hypothyroidism
- 244.2 Iodine hypothyroidism
- 244.3 Other iatrogenic hypothyroidism
- 244.8 Other specified acquired hypothyroidism
- 244.9 Unspecified hypothyroidism

245.# Thyroiditis
- 245.0 Acute thyroiditis
- 245.1 Subacute thyroiditis
- 245.2 Chronic lymphocytic thyroiditis
- 245.3 Chronic fibrous thyroiditis
- 245.4 Iatrogenic thyroiditis
- 245.8 Other and unspecified chronic thyroiditis
- 245.9 Thyroiditis, unspecified

246.# Other disorders of thyroid
- 246.0 Disorders of thyrocalcitonin secretion
- 246.1 Dyshormonogenic goiter
- 246.2 Cyst of thyroid
- 246.3 Hemorrhage and infarction of thyroid
- 246.8 Other specified disorders of thyroid
- 246.9 Unspecified disorder of thyroid

250.## Diabetes mellitus
- **250.0#** Diabetes mellitus without mention of complication
- **250.1#** Diabetes with ketoacidosis
- **250.2#** Diabetes with hyperosmolarity
- **250.3#** Diabetes with other coma
- **250.4#** Diabetes with renal manifestations
- **250.5#** Diabetes with ophthalmic manifestations
- **250.6#** Diabetes with neurological manifestations
- **250.7#** Diabetes with peripheral circulatory disorders
- **250.8#** Diabetes with other specified manifestations
- **250.9#** Diabetes with unspecified complication

5th Digit: 250
- **0 Type II or unspecified type, not stated as uncontrolled**
- **1 Type I [juvenile type], not stated as uncontrolled**
- **2 Type II or unspecified type, uncontrolled**
- **3 Type I [insulin dependent type] [IDDM] [juvenile type], uncontrolled**

251.# Other disorders of pancreatic internal secretion
- 251.0 Hypoglycemic coma
- 251.1 Other specified hypoglycemia
- 251.2 Hypoglycemia, unspecified
- 251.3 Postsurgical hypoinsulinemia
- 251.4 Abnormality of secretion of glucagon
- 251.5 Abnormality of secretion of gastrin
- 251.8 Other specified disorders of pancreatic internal secretion
- 251.9 Unspecified disorder of pancreatic internal secretion

252.#(#) Disorders of parathyroid gland
- 252.0 Hyperparathyroidism
  - 252.00 Hyperparathyroidism, unspecified
  - 252.01 Primary hyperparathyroidism
  - 252.02 Secondary hyperparathyroidism, non-renal
  - 252.08 Other hyperparathyroidism
- 252.1 Hypoparathyroidism
- 252.8 Other specified disorders of parathyroid gland
- 252.9 Unspecified disorder of parathyroid gland

253.# Disorders of the pituitary gland and hypothalamic control
- 253.0 Acromegaly and gigantism
- 253.1 Other and NOS anterior pituitary hyperfunction
- 253.2 Panhypopituitarism
- 253.3 Pituitary dwarfism
- 253.4 Other anterior pituitary disorders
- 253.5 Diabetes insipidus
- 253.6 Other disorders of neurohypophysis
- 253.7 Iatrogenic pituitary disorders
- 253.8 Other disorders of the pituitary and other syndromes of diencephalohypophyseal origin
- 253.9 Unspecified

254.# Diseases of thymus gland
- 254.0 Persistent hyperplasia of thymus
- 254.1 Abscess of thymus
- 254.8 Other specified diseases of thymus gland
- 254.9 Unspecified disease of thymus gland

255.#(#) Disorders of adrenal glands
- 255.0 Cushing's syndrome
- **255.1#** Hyperaldosteronism
  - 255.10 Hyperaldosteronism unspecified
  - 255.11 Glucocorticoid-remediable aldosteronism
  - 255.12 Conn's syndrome
  - 255.13 Bartter's syndrome
  - 255.14 Other secondary aldosteronism
- 255.2 Adrenogenital disorders
- 255.3 Other corticoadrenal overactivity
- **255.4#** Corticoadrenal insufficiency
  - 255.41 Glucoccorticoid deficiency
  - 255.42 Mineralocorticoid deficiency
- 255.5 Other adrenal hypofunction
- 255.6 Medulloadrenal hyperfunction
- 255.8 Other specified disorders of adrenal glands
- 255.9 Unspecified disorder of adrenal glands

256.#(#) Ovarian dysfunction
- 256.0 Hyperestrogenism
- 256.1 Other ovarian hyperfunction
- 256.2 Postablative ovarian failure
- **256.3#** Other ovarian failure
  - 256.31 Premature menopause
  - 256.39 Other ovarian failure
- 256.4 Polycystic ovaries
- 256.8 Other ovarian dysfunction
- 256.9 Unspecified ovarian dysfunction

257.# Testicular dysfunction
- 257.0 Testicular hyperfunction
- 257.1 Postablative testicular hypofunction
- 257.2 Other testicular hypofunction
- 257.8 Other testicular dysfunction
- 257.9 Unspecified testicular dysfunction

258.# Polyglandular dysfunction and related disorders
- **258.0#** Polyglandular activity in multiple endocrine adenomatosis
  - 258.01 Multiple endocrine neoplasia [MEN] type I
  - 258.02 Multiple endocrine neoplasia [MEN] type IIA
  - 258.03 Multiple endocrine neoplasia [MEN] type IIB
- 258.1 Other combinations of endocrine dysfunction
- 258.8 Other specified polyglandular dysfunction
- 258.9 Polyglandular dysfunction, unspecified

259.# Other endocrine disorders
- 259.0 Delay in sexual development and Puberty, NEC
- 259.1 Precocious sexual development and puberty, not elsewhere classified
- 259.2 Carcinoid syndrome
- 259.3 Ectopic hormone secretion, not elsewhere classified
- 259.4 Dwarfism, not elsewhere classified
- 259.5 Androgen insensitivity syndrome
- 259.8 Other specified endocrine disorders
- 259.9 Unspecified endocrine disorder

260 Kwashiorkor

261 Nutritional marasmus

262 Other severe protein-calorie malnutrition

263.# Other and unspecified protein-calorie malnutrition
- 263.0 Malnutrition of moderate degree
- 263.1 Malnutrition of mild degree
- 263.2 Arrested development following protein-calorie malnutrition
- 263.8 Other protein-calorie malnutrition
- 263.9 Unspecified protein-calorie malnutrition

264.# Vitamin A deficiency
- 264.0 With conjunctival xerosis
- 264.1 With conjunctival xerosis and Bitot's spot
- 264.2 With corneal xerosis
- 264.3 With corneal ulceration and xerosis
- 264.4 With keratomalacia
- 264.5 With night blindness
- 264.6 With xerophthalmic scars of cornea
- 264.7 Other ocular manifestations of vitamin A deficiency
- 264.8 Other manifestations of vitamin A deficiency
- 264.9 Unspecified vitamin A deficiency

265.# Thiamine and niacin deficiency states
- 265.0 Beriberi
- 265.1 Other and unspecified manifestations of thiamine deficiency
- 265.2 Pellagra

266.# Deficiency of B-complex components
- 266.0 Ariboflavinosis
- 266.1 Vitamin B6 deficiency
- 266.2 Other B-complex deficiencies
- 266.9 Unspecified vitamin B deficiency

267 Ascorbic acid deficiency

268.# Vitamin D deficiency
- 268.0 Rickets, active
- 268.1 Rickets, late effect
- 268.2 Osteomalacia, unspecified
- 268.9 Unspecified vitamin D deficiency

269.# Other nutritional deficiencies
- 269.0 Deficiency of vitamin K
- 269.1 Deficiency of other vitamins
- 269.2 Unspecified vitamin deficiency
- 269.3 Mineral deficiency, not elsewhere classified
- 269.8 Other nutritional deficiency
- 269.9 Unspecified nutritional deficiency

270.# Disorders of amino-acid transport and metabolism
- 270.0 Disturbances of amino-acid transport
- 270.1 Phenylketonuria [PKU]
- 270.2 Other disturbances of aromatic amino-acid metabolism
- 270.3 Disturbances of branched-chain amino-acid metabolism
- 270.4 Disturbances of sulphur-bearing amino-acid metabolism
- 270.5 Disturbances of histidine metabolism
- 270.7 Other disturbances of straight-chain amino-acid metabolism
- 270.8 Other specified disorders of amino-acid metabolism
- 270.9 Unspecified disorder of amino-acid metabolism

271.# Disorders of carbohydrate transport and metabolism
- 271.0 Glycogenosis
- 271.1 Galactosemia
- 271.2 Hereditary fructose intolerance
- 271.3 Intestinal disaccharidase deficiencies and disaccharide malabsorption
- 271.4 Renal glycosuria
- 271.8 Other specified disorders of carbohydrate transport and metabolism
- 271.9 Unspecified disorder of carbohydrate transport and metabolism

272.# Disorders of lipoid metabolism
- 272.0 Pure hypercholesterolemia
- 272.1 Pure hyperglyceridemia
- 272.2 Mixed hyperlipidemia
- 272.3 Hyperchylomicronemia
- 272.4 Other and unspecified hyperlipidemia
- 272.5 Lipoprotein deficiencies
- 272.6 Lipodystrophy
- 272.7 Lipidoses
- 272.8 Other disorders of lipoid metabolism
- 272.9 Unspecified disorder of lipoid metabolism

273.# Disorders of plasma protein metabolism
- 273.0 Polyclonal hypergammaglobulinemia
- 273.1 Monoclonal paraproteinemia
- 273.2 Other paraproteinemias
- 273.3 Macroglobulinemia
- 273.4 Alpha-1 antitrypsin deficiency
- 273.8 Other disorders of plasma protein metabolism
- 273.9 Unspecified disorder of plasma protein metabolism

274.#(#) Gout
- 274.0 Gouty arthropathy
- **274.1#** Gouty nephropathy
  - 274.10 Gouty nephropathy, unspecified
  - 274.11 Uric acid nephrolithiasis
  - 274.19 Other
- **274.8#** Gout with other specified manifestations
  - 274.81 Gouty tophi of ear
  - 274.82 Gouty tophi of other sites
  - 274.89 Other
- 274.9 Gout, unspecified

275.#(#) Disorders of mineral metabolism
- 275.0 Disorders of iron metabolism
- 275.1 Disorders of copper metabolism
- 275.2 Disorders of magnesium metabolism
- 275.3 Disorders of phosphorus metabolism

NUMERICAL REFERENCE

275.#(#) *(continued)*
275.4# Disorders of calcium metabolism
275.40 Unspecified disorder of calcium metabolism
275.41 Hypocalcemia
275.42 Hypercalcemia
275.49 Other disorders of calcium metabolism
275.8 Other specified disorders of mineral metabolism
275.9 Unspecified disorder of mineral metabolism

276.# Disorders of fluid, electrolyte, and acid-base balance
276.0 Hyperosmolality and/or hypernatremia
276.1 Hyposmolality and/or hyponatremia
276.2 Acidosis
276.3 Alkalosis
276.4 Mixed acid-base balance disorder
276.5# Volume depletion
276.50 Unspecified
276.51 Dehydration
276.52 Hypovolemia
276.6 Fluid overload
276.7 Hyperpotassemia
276.8 Hypopotassemia
276.9 Electrolyte and fluid disorders not elsewhere classified

277.#(#) Other and unspecified disorders of metabolism
277.0# Cystic fibrosis
277.00 Without mention of meconium ileus
277.01 With meconium ileus
277.02 With pulmonary manifestations
277.03 With gastrointestinal manifestations
277.09 With other manifestations
277.1 Disorders of porphyrin metabolism
277.2 Other disorders of purine and pyrimidine metabolism
277.3# Amyloidosis
277.30 Unspecified
277.31 Familial Mediterranean fever
277.39 Other
277.4 Disorders of bilirubin excretion
277.5 Mucopolysaccharidosis
277.6 Other deficiencies of circulating enzymes
277.7 Dysmetabolic syndrome X
277.8# Other specified disorders of metabolism
277.81 Primary carnitine deficiency
277.82 Carnitine deficiency due to inborn errors of metabolism
277.83 Iatrogenic carnitine deficiency
277.84 Other secondary carnitine deficiency
277.85 Disorders of fatty acid oxidation
277.86 Peroxisomal disorders
277.87 Disorders of mitochondrial metabolism
277.89 Other specified disorders of metabolism
277.9 Unspecified disorder of metabolism

278.#(#) Obesity and other hyperalimentation
278.0# Overweight and obesity
278.00 Obesity, unspecified
278.01 Morbid obesity
278.02 Overweight
278.1 Localized adiposity
278.2 Hypervitaminosis A
278.3 Hypercarotinemia
278.4 Hypervitaminosis D
278.8 Other hyperalimentation

279.#(#) Disorders involving the immune mechanism
279.0# Deficiency of humoral immunity
279.00 Hypogammaglobulinemia, unspecified
279.01 Selective IgA immunodeficiency
279.02 Selective IgM immunodeficiency
279.03 Other selective immunoglobulin deficiencies
279.04 Congenital hypogammaglobulinemia
279.05 Immunodeficiency with increased IgM
279.06 Common variable immunodeficiency
279.09 Other
279.1# Deficiency of cell-mediated immunity
279.10 Immunodeficiency with predominant T-cell defect, unspecified
279.11 DiGeorge's syndrome
279.12 Wiskott-Aldrich syndrome
279.13 Nezelof's syndrome
279.19 Other
279.2 Combined immunity deficiency
279.3 Unspecified immunity deficiency
279.4 Autoimmune disease, not elsewhere classified
279.8 Other specified disorders involving the immune mechanism
279.9 Unspecified disorder of immune mechanism

280.# Iron deficiency anemias
280.0 Secondary to blood loss (chronic)
280.1 Secondary to inadequate dietary iron intake
280.8 Other specified iron deficiency anemias
280.9 Iron deficiency anemia, unspecified.

281.# Other deficiency anemias
281.0 Pernicious anemia
281.1 Other vitamin B12 deficiency anemia
281.2 Folate-deficiency anemia
281.3 Other specified megaloblastic anemias, not elsewhere classified
281.4 Protein-deficiency anemia
281.8 Anemia associated with other specified nutritional deficiency
281.9 Unspecified deficiency anemia

282.#(#) Hereditary hemolytic anemias
282.0 Hereditary spherocytosis
282.1 Hereditary elliptocytosis
282.2 Anemias due to disorders of glutathione metabolism
282.3 Other hemolytic anemias due to enzyme deficiency
282.4# Thalassemias
282.41 Sickle cell thalassemia without crisis
282.42 Sickle cell thalassemia with crisis
282.49 Other thalassemia
282.5 Sickle-cell trait
282.6# Sickle-cell disease
282.60 Sickle-cell disease, unspecified
282.61 Hb-SS disease without crisis
282.62 Hb-SS disease with crisis
282.63 Sickle-cell/Hb-C disease without crisis
282.64 Sickle cell/Hb-C disease with crisis
282.68 Other sickle cell disease without crisis
282.69 Other sickle cell disease with crisis
282.7 Other hemoglobinopathies
282.8 Other specified hereditary hemolytic anemias
282.9 Hereditary hemolytic anemia, unspecified

283.#(#) Acquired hemolytic anemias
283.0 Autoimmune hemolytic anemias
283.1# Non-autoimmune hemolytic anemias
283.10 Non-autoimmune hemolytic anemia, NOS
283.11 Hemolytic-uremic syndrome
283.19 Other non-autoimmune hemolytic anemias
283.2 Hemoglobinuria due to hemolysis from external causes
283.9 Acquired hemolytic anemia, unspecified

284.#(#) Aplastic anemia and other bone marrow failure syndromes
284.0# Constitutional aplastic anemia
284.01 Constitutional red blood cell aplasia
284.09 Other
284.1 Pancytopenia
284.2 Myelophthisis
284.8# Other specified aplastic anemias
284.81 Red cell aplasia (acquired) (adult) (with thymoma)
284.89 Other specified aplastic anemias
284.9 Aplastic anemia, unspecified

285.#(#) Other and unspecified anemias
285.0 Sideroblastic anemia
285.1 Acute posthemorrhagic anemia
285.2# Anemia of chronic disease
285.21 Anemia of chronic kidney disease
285.22 Anemia of neoplastic disease
285.29 Anemia of other chronic disease
285.8 Other specified anemias
285.9 Anemia, unspecified

286.# Coagulation defects
286.0 Congenital factor VIII disorder
286.1 Congenital factor IX disorder
286.2 Congenital factor XI deficiency
286.3 Congenital deficiency of other clotting factors
286.4 von Willebrand's disease
286.5 Hemorrhagic disorder due to intrinsic circulating anticoagulants
286.6 Defibrination syndrome
286.7 Acquired coagulation factor deficiency
286.9 Other and unspecified coagulation defects

287.# Purpura and other hemorrhagic conditions
287.0 Allergic purpura
287.1 Qualitative platelet defects
287.2 Other nonthrombocytopenic purpuras
287.3# Primary thrombocytopenia
287.30 Unspecified
287.31 Immune thrombocytopenic purpura
287.32 Evan's syndrome
287.33 Congenital and hereditary thrombocytopenia
287.39 Other
287.4 Secondary thrombocytopenia
287.5 Thrombocytopenia, unspecified
287.8 Other specified hemorrhagic conditions
287.9 Unspecified hemorrhagic conditions

288.#(#) Diseases of white blood cells
288.0# Neutropenia
288.00 Unspecified
288.01 Congenital
288.02 Cyclic
288.03 Drug induced
288.04 Due to infection
288.09 Other

288.#(#) *(continued)*
288.1 Functional disorders of polymorphonuclear neutrophils
288.2 Genetic anomalies of leukocytes
288.3 Eosinophilia
288.4 Hemophagocytic syndromes
288.5# Decreased white blood cell count
288.50 Leukocytopenia, unspecified
288.51 Lymphocytopenia
288.59 Other
288.6# Elevated white blood cell count
288.60 Leukocytosis, unspecified
288.61 Lymphocytosis (symptomatic)
288.62 Leukemoid reaction
288.63 Monocytosis (symptomatic)
288.64 Plasmacytosis
288.65 Basophilia
288.66 Bandemia
288.69 Other
288.8 Other specified disease of white blood cells
288.9 Unspecified disease of white blood cells

289.#(#) Other diseases of blood and blood-forming organs
289.0 Polycythemia, secondary
289.1 Chronic lymphadenitis
289.2 Nonspecific mesenteric lymphadenitis
289.3 Lymphadenitis, unspecified, except mesenteric
289.4 Hypersplenism
289.5# Other diseases of spleen
289.50 Disease of spleen, unspecified
289.51 Chronic congestive splenomegaly
289.52 Splenic sequestration
289.53 Neutropenia splenomegaly
289.59 Other
289.6 Familial polycythemia
289.7 Methemoglobinemia
289.8# Other specified diseases of blood and blood-forming organs
289.81 Primary hypercoagulable state
289.82 Secondary hypercoagulable state
289.83 Myelofibrosis
289.89 Other specified diseases of blood and blood-forming organs
289.9 Diseases of blood and blood-forming organs, NOS

290.#(#) Dementias
290.0 Senile dementia, uncomplicated
290.1# Presenile dementia
290.10 Presenile dementia, uncomplicated
290.11 Presenile dementia with delirium
290.12 Presenile dementia with delusional features
290.13 Presenile dementia with depressive features
290.2# Senile dementia with delusional or depressive features
290.20 Senile dementia with delusional features
290.21 Senile dementia with depressive features
290.3 Senile dementia with delirium
290.4# Vascular dementia
290.40 Vascular dementia, uncomplicated
290.41 Vascular dementia, with delirium
290.42 Vascular dementia, with delusions
290.43 Vascular dementia, with depressed mood
290.8 Other specified senile psychotic condition
290.9 Unspecified senile psychotic condition

291.#(#) Alcohol-induced mental disorders
291.0 Alcohol withdrawal delirium
291.1 Alcohol-induced persisting amnestic disorder
291.2 Alcohol-induced persisting dementia
291.3 Alcohol-induced psychotic disorder withhallucinations
291.4 Idiosyncratic alcohol intoxication
291.5 Alcohol-induced psychotic disorder withdelusions
291.8# Other specified alcohol-induced mental disorders
291.81 Alcohol withdrawal
291.82 Alcohol induced sleep disorders
291.89 Other
291.9 Unspecified alcohol-induced mental disorders

292.#(#) Drug-induced mental disorders
292.0 Drug withdrawal
292.1# Drug-induced psychotic disorders
292.11 Drug-induced psychotic disorder withdelusions
292.12 Drug-induced psychotic disorder withhallucinations
292.2 Pathological drug intoxication
292.8# Other specified drug-induced mental disorders
292.81 Drug-induced delirium
292.82 Drug-induced persisting dementia
292.83 Drug-induced persisting amnestic disorder
292.84 Drug-induced mood disorder
292.85 Drug-induced sleep disorder
292.89 Other
292.9 Unspecified drug-induced mental disorder

293.#(#) Transient mental disorder due to conditions classified elsewhere
293.0 Delirium due to conditions classified elsewhere
293.1 Subacute delirium
293.8# Other specified transient mental disorders dueto conditions classified elsewhere
293.81 Psychotic disorder with delusions in conditions classified elsewhere
293.82 Psychotic disorder with hallucinations in conditions classified elsewhere
293.83 Mood disorder in conditions classified elsewhere
293.84 Anxiety disorder in conditions classified elsewhere
293.89 Other
293.9 Unspecified transient mental disorder in conditions classified elsewhere

294.#(#) Persistent mental disorders due to conditions classified elsewhere
294.0 Amnestic disorder in conditions classified elsewhere
294.1# Dementia in conditions classified elsewhere
294.10 Dementia in conditions classified elsewhere without behavioral disturbance
294.11 Dementia in conditions classified elsewhere with behavioral disturbance
294.8 Other persistent mental disorders due to conditions classified elsewhere
294.9 Unspecified persistent mental disorders due to conditions classified elsewhere

295.## Schizophrenic disorders
295.0# Simple type
295.1# Disorganized type
295.2# Catatonic type
295.3# Paranoid type
295.4# Schizophreniform disorder
295.5# Latent schizophrenia
295.6# Residual type
295.7# Schizoaffective disorder
295.8# Other specified types of schizophrenia
295.9# Unspecified schizophrenia
5th Digit: 295
0 Unspecified
1 Subchronic
2 Chronic
3 Subchronic with acute exacerbation
4 Chronic with acute exacerbation
5 In remission

296.#(#) Episodic mood disorders
296.0# Bipolar I disorder, single manic episode
296.1# Manic disorder, recurrent episode
296.2# Major depressive disorder, single episode
296.3# Major depressive disorder, recurrent episode
296.4# Bipolar I disorder, most recent episode (or current) manic
296.5# Bipolar I disorder, most recent episode (or current) depressed
296.6# Bipolar I disorder, most recent episode (or current) mixed
5th Digit: 296.0-296.6
0 Unspecified
1 Mild
2 Moderate
3 Severe, without mention of psychotic behavior
4 Severe, specified as with psychotic behavior
5 In partial or unspecified remission
6 In full remission
296.7 Bipolar I disorder, most recent episode (or current) unspecified
296.8# Other and unspecified, bipolar disorders
296.80 Bipolar disorder, unspecified
296.81 Atypical manic disorder
296.82 Atypical depressive disorder
296.89 Other
296.9# Other and unspecified episodic mood disorder
296.90 Unspecified episodic mood disorder
296.99 Other specified episodic mood disorder

297.# Delusional disorders
297.0 Paranoid state, simple
297.1 Delusional disorder
297.2 Paraphrenia
297.3 Shared psychotic disorder
297.8 Other specified paranoid states
297.9 Unspecified paranoid state

298.# Other nonorganic psychoses
298.0 Depressive type psychosis
298.1 Excitative type psychosis
298.2 Reactive confusion
298.3 Acute paranoid reaction
298.4 Psychogenic paranoid psychosis
298.8 Other and unspecified reactive psychosis
298.9 Unspecified psychosis

299.## **Pervasive developmental disorders**
- **299.0#** Autism disorder
- **299.1#** Childhood disintegrative disorder
- **299.8#** Other specified pervasive developmental disorders
- **299.9#** Unspecified pervasive developmental disorders

5th Digit: 299
- **0** **Current or active state**
- **1** **Residual state**

300.#(#) **Anxiety, dissociative and somatoform disorders**
- **300.0#** Anxiety states
  - 300.00 Anxiety state, unspecified
  - 300.01 Panic disorder without agoraphobia
  - 300.02 Generalized anxiety disorder
  - 300.09 Other
- **300.1#** Dissociatvie, covversion and factitious disorders
  - 300.10 Hysteria, unspecified
  - 300.11 Conversion disorder
  - 300.12 Dissociative amnesia
  - 300.13 Dissociative fugue
  - 300.14 Dissociative identity disorder
  - 300.15 Dissociative disorder or reaction, unspecified
  - 300.16 Factitious disorder with predominantly psychological signs and symptoms
  - 300.19 Other and unspecified factitious illness
- **300.2#** Phobic disorders
  - 300.20 Phobia, unspecified
  - 300.21 Agoraphobia with panic disorder
  - 300.22 Agoraphobia without mention of panic attacks
  - 300.23 Social phobia
  - 300.29 Other isolated or specific phobias
- 300.3 Obsessive-compulsive disorders
- 300.4 Dysthymic disorder
- 300.5 Neurasthenia
- 300.6 Depersonalization disorder
- 300.7 Hypochondriasis
- **300.8#** Somatoform disorders
  - 300.81 Somatization disorder
  - 300.82 Undifferentiated somatoform disorder
  - 300.89 Other somatoform disorders
- 300.9 Unspecified nonpsychotic mental disorder

301.#(#) **Personality disorders**
- 301.0 Paranoid personality disorder
- **301.1#** Affective personality disorder
  - 301.10 Affective personality disorder, unspecified
  - 301.11 Chronic hypomanic personality disorder
  - 301.12 Chronic depressive personality disorder
  - 301.13 Cyclothymic disorder
- **301.2#** Schizoid personality disorder
  - 301.20 Schizoid personality disorder, NOS
  - 301.21 Introverted personality
  - 301.22 Schizotypal personality disorder
- 301.3 Explosive personality disorder
- 301.4 Obsessive-compulsive personality disorder
- **301.5#** Histrionic personality disorder
  - 301.50 Histrionic personality disorder, unspecified
  - 301.51 Chronic factitious illness with physical symptoms
  - 301.59 Other histrionic personality disorder
- 301.6 Dependent personality disorder
- 301.7 Antisocial personality disorder
- **301.8#** Other personality disorders
  - 301.81 Narcissistic personality disorder
  - 301.82 Avoidant personality disorder
  - 301.83 Borderline personality disorder
  - 301.84 Passive-aggressive personality
  - 301.89 Other

301.#(#) ***(continued)***
- 301.9 Unspecified personality disorder

302.#(#) **Sexual and gender identity disorders**
- 302.0 Ego-dystonic sexual orientation
- 302.1 Zoophilia
- 302.2 Pedophilia
- 302.3 Transvestic fetishism
- 302.4 Exhibitionism
- **302.5#** Trans-sexualism
  - 302.50 With unspecified sexual history
  - 302.51 With asexual history
  - 302.52 With homosexual history
  - 302.53 With heterosexual history
- 302.6 Gender identity disorder in children
- **302.7#** Psychosexual dysfunction
  - 302.70 Psychosexual dysfunction, unspecified
  - 302.71 Hypoactive sexual desire disorder
  - 302.72 With inhibited sexual excitement
  - 302.73 Female orgasmic disorder
  - 302.74 Male orgasic disorder
  - 302.75 Premature ejaculation
  - 302.76 Dyspareunia, psychogenic
  - 302.79 With other specified psychosexual dysfunctions
- **302.8#** Other specified psychosexual disorders
  - 302.81 Fetishism
  - 302.82 Voyeurism
  - 302.83 Sexual masochism
  - 302.84 Sexual sadism
  - 302.85 Gender identity disorder in adolescents or adults
  - 302.89 Other
- 302.9 Unspecified psychosexual disorder

303.## **Alcohol dependence syndrome**
- **303.0#** Acute alcoholic intoxication
- **303.9#** Other and unspecified alcohol dependence

304.## **Drug dependence**
- **304.0#** Opioid type dependence
- **304.1#** Sedative hypnotic or anziolytic dependence
- **304.2#** Cocaine dependence
- **304.3#** Cannabis dependence
- **304.4#** Amphetamine and other psychostimulant dependence
- **304.5#** Hallucinogen dependence
- **304.6#** Other specified drug dependence
- **304.7#** Combinations of opioid type drug with any other
- **304.8#** Combinations of drug dependence excluding opioid type drug
- **304.9#** Unspecified drug dependence

305.#(#) **Nondependent abuse of drugs**
- **305.0#** Alcohol abuse
- 305.1 Tobacco use disorder
- **305.2#** Cannabis abuse
- **305.3#** Hallucinogen abuse
- **305.4#** Sedative, hypnotic or anxiolytic abuse
- **305.5#** Opioid abuse
- **305.6#** Cocaine abuse
- **305.7#** Amphetamine or related acting sympathomimetic abuse
- **305.8#** Antidepressant type abuse
- **305.9#** Other, mixed, or unspecified drug abuse

5th Digit: 303, 304, 305.0, 305.2-305.9
- **0** **Unspecified**
- **1** **Continuous**
- **2** **Episodic**
- **3** **In remission**

306.#(#) Physiological malfunction arising from mental factors
306.0 Musculoskeletal
306.1 Respiratory
306.2 Cardiovascular
306.3 Skin
306.4 Gastrointestinal
306.5# Genitourinary
306.50 Psychogenic genitourinary malfunction, unspecified
306.51 Psychogenic vaginismus
306.52 Psychogenic dysmenorrhea
306.53 Psychogenic dysuria
306.59 Other
306.6 Endocrine
306.7 Organs of special sense
306.8 Other specified psychophysiological
306.9 Unspecified psychophysiological malfunction

307.#(#) Special symptoms or syndromes, not elsewhere classified
307.0 Stuttering
307.1 Anorexia nervosa
307.2# Tics
307.20 Tic disorder, unspecified
307.21 Transient tic disorder
307.22 Chronic motor or vocal tic disorder
307.23 Tourette's disorder
307.3 Stereotypic movement disorder
307.4# Specific disorders of sleep of nonorganic origin
307.40 Nonorganic sleep disorder, unspecified
307.41 Transient disorder of initiating or maintaining sleep
307.42 Persistent disorder of initiating or maintaining sleep
307.43 Transient disorder of initiating or maintaining wakefulness
307.44 Persistent disorder of initiating or maintaining wakefulness
307.45 Circadian rhythm sleep disorder
307.46 Sleep arousal disorder
307.47 Other dysfunctions of sleep stages or arousal from sleep
307.48 Repetitive intrusions of sleep
307.49 Other
307.5# Other and unspecified disorders of eating
307.50 Eating disorder, unspecified
307.51 Bulimia nervosa
307.52 Pica
307.53 Rumination disorder
307.54 Psychogenic vomiting
307.59 Other
307.6 Enuresis
307.7 Encopresis
307.8# Pain disorders related to psychological factors
307.80 Psychogenic pain, site unspecified
307.81 Tension headache
307.89 Other
307.9 Other and unspecified special symptoms or syndromes, not elsewhere classified

308.# Acute reaction to stress
308.0 Predominant disturbance of emotions
308.1 Predominant disturbance of consciousness
308.2 Predominant psychomotor disturbance
308.3 Other acute reactions to stress
308.4 Mixed disorders as reaction to stress
308.9 Unspecified acute reaction to stress

309.#(#) Adjustment reaction
309.0 Adjustment disorder with depressed mood
309.1 Prolonged depressive reaction
309.2# With predominant disturbance of other emotions
309.21 Separation anxiety disorder
309.22 Emancipation disorder of adolescence and early adult life
309.23 Specific academic or work inhibition
309.24 Adjustment disorder with anxiety
309.28 Adjustment disorder with mixed anxiety and depressed mood
309.29 Other
309.3 Adjustment disorder with disturbance of conduct
309.4 Adjustment disorder with mixed disturbance of emotions and conduct
309.8# Other specified adjustment reactions
309.81 Posttraumatic stress disorder
309.82 Adjustment reaction with physical symptoms
309.83 Adjustment reaction with withdrawal
309.89 Other
309.9 Unspecified adjustment reaction

310.# Specific nonpsychotic mental disorders due to brain damage
310.0 Frontal lobe syndrome
310.1 Personality change due to conditions classified elsewhere
310.2 Postconcussion syndrome
310.8 Other specified nonpsychotic mental disorders following organic brain damage
310.9 Unspecified nonpsychotic mental disorder following organic brain damage

311 Depressive disorder, not elsewhere classified

312.#(#) Disturbance of conduct, not elsewhere classified
312.0# Undersocialized conduct disorder, aggressive type
312.1# Undersocialized conduct disorder, unaggressive type
312.2# Socialized conduct disorder
5th Digit: 312.0-312.2
0 Unspecified
1 Mild
2 Moderate
3 Severe
312.3# Disorders of impulse control, not elsewhere classified
312.30 Impulse control disorder, unspecified
312.31 Pathological gambling
312.32 Kleptomania
312.33 Pyromania
312.34 Intermittent explosive disorder
312.35 Isolated explosive disorder
312.39 Other
312.4 Mixed disturbance of conduct and emotions
312.8# Other specified disturbances of conduct, not elsewhere classified
312.81 Conduct disorder, childhood onset type
312.82 Conduct disorder, adolescent onset type
312.89 Other conduct disorder
312.9 Unspecified disturbance of conduct

313.#(#) Disturbance of emotions specific to childhood and adolescence
- 313.0 Overanxious disorder
- 313.1 Misery and unhappiness disorder
- **313.2#** Sensitivity, shyness, and social withdrawal disorder
  - 313.21 Shyness disorder of childhood
  - 313.22 Introverted disorder of childhood
  - 313.23 Selective mutism
- 313.3 Relationship problems
- **313.8#** Other or mixed emotional disturbances of childhood or adolescence
  - 313.81 Oppositional defiant disorder
  - 313.82 Identity disorder
  - 313.83 Academic underachievement disorder
  - 313.89 Other
- 313.9 Unspecified emotional disturbance of childhood or adolescence

314.#(#) Hyperkinetic syndrome of childhood
- **314.0#** Attention deficit disorder
  - 314.00 Without mention of hyperactivity
  - 314.01 With hyperactivity
- 314.1 Hyperkinesis with developmental delay
- 314.2 Hyperkinetic conduct disorder
- 314.8 Other specified manifestations of hyperkinetic syndrome
- 314.9 Unspecified hyperkinetic syndrome

315.#(#) Specific delays in development
- **315.0#** Specific reading disorder
  - 315.00 Reading disorder, unspecified
  - 315.01 Alexia
  - 315.02 Developmental dyslexia
  - 315.09 Other
- 315.1 Mathematics disorder
- 315.2 Other specific learning difficulties
- **315.3#** Developmental speech or language disorder
  - 315.31 Expressive language disorder
  - 315.32 Mixed receptive-expressive language disorder
  - 315.34 Speech and language developmental delay due to hearing loss
  - 315.39 Other
- 315.4 Developmental coordination disorder
- 315.5 Mixed development disorder
- 315.8 Other specified delays in development
- 315.9 Unspecified delay in development

316 Psychic factors associated with diseases classified elsewhere

317 Mild mental retardation

318.# Other specified mental retardation
- 318.0 Moderate mental retardation
- 318.1 Severe mental retardation
- 318.2 Profound mental retardation

319 Unspecified mental retardation

320.#(#) Bacterial meningitis
- 320.0 Hemophilus meningitis
- 320.1 Pneumococcal meningitis
- 320.2 Streptococcal meningitis
- 320.3 Staphylococcal meningitis
- 320.7 Meningitis in other bacterial diseases classified elsewhere

320.#(#) *(continued)*
- **320.8#** Meningitis due to other specified bacteria
  - 320.81 Anaerobic meningitis
  - 320.82 Meningitis due to gram-negative bacteria, not elsewhere classified
  - 320.89 Meningitis due to other specified bacteria
- 320.9 Meningitis due to unspecified bacterium

321.# Meningitis due to other organisms
- 321.0 Cryptococcal meningitis
- 321.1 Meningitis in other fungal diseases
- 321.2 Meningitis due to viruses not elsewhere classified
- 321.3 Meningitis due to trypanosomiasis
- 321.4 Meningitis in sarcoidosis
- 321.8 Meningitis due to other nonbacterial organisms classified elsewhere

322.# Meningitis of unspecified cause
- 322.0 Nonpyogenic meningitis
- 322.1 Eosinophilic meningitis
- 322.2 Chronic meningitis
- 322.9 Meningitis, unspecified

323.#(#) Encephalitis, myelitis, and encephalomyelitis
- **323.0#** Encephalitis, myelitis, and encephalomyelitis in viral diseases classified elsewhere
  - 323.01 Encephalitis and encephalomyelitis in viral diseases classifier elsewhere
  - 323.02 Myelitis in viral diseases classified elsewhere
- 323.1 Encephalitis, myelitis, and encephalomyelitis in rickettsial diseases classified elsewhere
- 323.2 Encephalitis, myelitis, and encephalomyelitis in protozoal diseases classified elsewhere
- **323.4#** Other encephalitis, myelitis, and encephalomyelitis due to infection classified elsewhere
  - 323.41 Other encephalitis and encephalomyelitis due to infection classified elsewhere
  - 323.42 Myelitis due to infection classified elsewhere
- **323.5#** Encephalitis, myelitis, and encephalomyelitis following immunization procedures
  - 323.51 Encephalitisand encephalomyelitis following immunization procedures
  - 323.52 Myelitis following immunization procedures
- **323.6#** Postinfectious encephalitis, myelitis, and encephalomyelitis
  - 323.61 Infectious acute disseminated encephalomyelitis (ADEM)
  - 323.62 Other postinfectious encephalitis and encephalomyelitis
  - 323.63 Postinfectious myelitis
- **323.7#** Toxic encephalitis, myelitis, and encephalomyelitis
  - 323.71 Toxic encephalitis and encephalomyelitis
  - 323.72 Toxic myelitis
- **323.8#** Other causes of encephalitis, myelitis, and encephalomyelitis
  - 323.81 Other causes of encephalitis and encephalomyelitis
  - 323.82 Other causes of myelitis
- 323.9 Unspecified cause of encephalitis, myelitis, and encephalomyelitis

324.# Intracranial and intraspinal abscess
- 324.0 Intracranial abscess
- 324.1 Intraspinal abscess
- 324.9 Of unspecified site

325 **Phlebitis and thrombophlebitis of intracranial venous sinuses**

326 **Late effects of intracranial abscess or pyogenic infection**

327 **Organic sleep disorders**
- **327.0#** Organic disorders of initiating and maintaining sleep
  - 327.00 Unspecified
  - 327.01 Due to medical condition classified elsewhere
  - 327.02 Due to mental disorder
  - 327.09 Other
- **327.1#** Organic disorder of excessive somnolence
  - 327.10 Unspecified
  - 327.11 Idiopathic hypersomnia with long sleep time
  - 327.12 Idiopathic hypersomnia without long sleep time
  - 327.13 Recurrent hypersomnia
  - 327.14 Hypersomnia due to medical condition elsewhere classified
  - 327.15 Hypersomnia due to mental disorder
  - 327.19 Other
- **327.2#** Organic sleep apnea
  - 327.20 Unspecified
  - 327.21 Primary central sleep apnea
  - 327.22 High altitude periodic breathing
  - 327.23 Obstructive sleep apnea (adult) (pediatric)
  - 327.24 Idiopathic sleep related nonobstructive alveolar hypoventilation
  - 327.25 Congenital central alveolar hypoventilation syndrome
  - 327.26 Sleep related hypoventilation/hypoxemia in conditions classifiable elsewhere
  - 327.27 Central sleep apnea in condition classified elsewhere
  - 327.29 Other
- **327.3#** Circadian rhythm sleep disorder
  - 327.30 Unspecified
  - 327.31 Delayed sleep phase type
  - 327.32 Advanced sleep phase type
  - 327.33 Irregular sleep-wake type
  - 327.34 Free-running type
  - 327.35 Jet lag type
  - 327.36 Shift work type
  - 327.37 In conditions classified elsewhere
  - 327.39 Other
- **327.4#** Organic parasomnia
  - 327.40 Unspecified
  - 327.41 confusional arousals
  - 327.42 REM sleep behavior disorder
  - 327.43 Recurrent isolated sleep paralysis
  - 327.44 Parasomnia in conditions classified elsewhere
  - 327.49 Other
- **327.5#** Organic sleep related movement disorders
  - 327.51 Periodic limb movement disorder
  - 327.52 Sleep related leg cramps
  - 327.53 Sleep related bruxism
  - 327.59 Other organic sleep related movement disorders
- 327.8 Other organic sleep disorders

330.# **Cerebral degenerations usually manifest in childhood**
- 330.0 Leukodystrophy
- 330.1 Cerebral lipidoses
- 330.2 Cerebral degeneration in generalized lipidoses

330.# ***(continued)***
- 330.3 Cerebral degeneration of childhood in other diseases classified elsewhere
- 330.8 Other specified cerebral degenerations in childhood
- 330.9 Unspecified cerebral degeneration in childhood

331.#(#) **Other cerebral degenerations**
- 331.0 Alzheimer's disease
- **331.1#** Frontotemporal dementia
  - 331.11 Pick's disease
  - 331.19 Other frontotemporal dementia
- 331.2 Senile degeneration of brain
- 331.3 Communicating hydrocephalus
- 331.4 Obstructive hydrocephalus
- 331.5 Idiopathic normal pressure hydrocephalus
- 331.7 Cerebral degeneration in diseases classified elsewhere
- **331.8#** Other cerebral degeneration
  - 331.81 Reye's syndrome
  - 331.82 Dementia with Lewy bodies
  - 331.83 Mild cognitive impairment, so stated
  - 331.89 Other
- 331.9 Cerebral degeneration, unspecified

332.# **Parkinson's disease**
- 332.0 Paralysis agitans
- 332.1 Secondary Parkinsonism

333.#(#) **Other extrapyramidal disease and abnormal movement disorders**
- 333.0 Other degenerative diseases of the basal ganglia
- 333.1 Essential and other specified forms of tremor
- 333.2 Myoclonus
- 333.3 Tics of organic origin
- 333.4 Huntington's chorea
- 333.5 Other choreas
- 333.6 Genetic torsion dystonia
- **333.7#** Acquired torsion dystonia
  - 333.71 Athetoid cerebral palsy
  - 333.72 Acute dystonia due to drugs
  - 333.79 Other acquired torsion dystonia
- **333.8#** Fragments of torsion dystonia
  - 333.81 Blepharospasm
  - 333.82 Orofacial dyskinesia
  - 333.83 Spasmodic torticollis
  - 333.84 Organic writers' cramp
  - 333.85 Subacute dyskinesia due to drugs
  - 333.89 Other
- **333.9#** Other and unspecified extrapyramidal diseases and abnormal movement disorders
  - 333.90 Unspecified extrapyramidal disease and abnormal movement disorder
  - 333.91 Stiff-man syndrome
  - 333.92 Neuroleptic malignant syndrome
  - 333.93 Benign shuddering attacks
  - 333.94 Restless leg syndrome (RLS)
  - 333.99 Other

334.# **Spinocerebellar disease**
- 334.0 Friedreich's ataxia
- 334.1 Hereditary spastic paraplegia
- 334.2 Primary cerebellar degeneration
- 334.3 Other cerebellar ataxia
- 334.4 Cerebellar ataxia in diseases classified elsewhere
- 334.8 Other spinocerebellar diseases
- 334.9 Spinocerebellar disease, unspecified

335.#(#) Anterior horn cell disease
335.0 Werdnig-Hoffmann disease
335.1# Spinal muscular atrophy
335.10 Spinal muscular atrophy, unspecified
335.11 Kugelberg-Welander disease
335.19 Other
335.2# Motor neuron disease
335.20 Amyotrophic lateral sclerosis
335.21 Progressive muscular atrophy
335.22 Progressive bulbar palsy
335.23 Pseudobulbar palsy
335.24 Primary lateral sclerosis
335.29 Other
335.8 Other anterior horn cell diseases
335.9 Anterior horn cell disease, unspecified

336.# Other diseases of spinal cord
336.0 Syringomyelia and syringobulbia
336.1 Vascular myelopathies
336.2 Subacute combined degeneration of spinal cord in diseases classified elsewhere
336.3 Myelopathy in other diseases classified elsewhere
336.8 Other myelopathy
336.9 Unspecified disease of spinal cord

337.#(#) Disorders of the autonomic nervous system
337.0 Idiopathic peripheral autonomic neuropathy
337.1 Peripheral autonomic neuropathy in disorders classified elsewhere
337.2# Reflex sympathetic dystrophy
337.20 Reflex sympathetic dystrophy, unspecified
337.21 Reflex sympathetic dystrophy, upper limb
337.22 Reflex sympathetic dystrophy, lower limb
337.29 Reflex sympathetic dystrophy, other specified site
337.3 Autonomic dysreflexia
337.9 Unspecified disorder of autonomic nervous system

338.#(#) Pain, not elsewhere classified
338.0 Central pain syndrome
338.1# Acute pain
338.11 Acute pain due to trauma
338.12 Acute post-thoracotomy pain
338.18 Other acute postoperative pain
338.19 Other acute pain
338.2# Chronic pain
338.21 Chronic pain due to trauma
338.22 Chronic post-thoracotomy pain
338.28 Other chronic postoperative pain
338.29 Other chronic pain
338.3 Neoplasm related pain (acute) (chronic)
338.4 Chroic pain syndrome

340 Multiple sclerosis

341.#(#) Other demyelinating diseases of central nervous system
341.0 Neuromyelitis optica
341.1 Schilder's disease
341.2# Acute (tansverse) myelitis
341.20 Acute (tansverse) myelitis NOS
341.21 Acute (tansverse) myelitis in conditions classified elsewhere
341.22 Idiopathic transverse myelitis
341.8 Other demyelinating diseases of central nervous system
341.9 Demyelinating disease of central nervous system, unspecified

342.## Hemiplegia and hemiparesis
342.0# Flaccid hemiplegia
342.1# Spastic hemiplegia
342.8# Other specified hemiplegia
342.9# Hemiplegia, unspecified
5th Digits: 342
0 Affecting unspecified side
1 Affecting dominant side
2 Affecting nondominant side

343.# Infantile cerebral palsy
343.0 Diplegic
343.1 Hemiplegic
343.2 Quadriplegic
343.3 Monoplegic
343.4 Infantile hemiplegia
343.8 Other specified infantile cerebral palsy
343.9 Infantile cerebral palsy, unspecified

344.#(#) Other paralytic syndromes
344.0# Quadriplegia and quadriparesis
344.00 Quadriplegia, unspecified
344.01 C_1-C_4, complete
344.02 C_1-C_4, incomplete
344.03 C_5-C_7, complete
344.04 C_5-C_7, incomplete
344.09 Other
344.1 Paraplegia
344.2 Diplegia of upper limbs
344.3# Monoplegia of lower limb
344.4# Monoplegia of upper limb
5th Digit: 344.3-344.4
0 Affecting unspecified side
1 Affecting dominant side
2 Affecting nondominant side
344.5 Unspecified monoplegia
344.6# Cauda equina syndrome
344.60 Without mention of neurogenic bladder
344.61 With neurogenic bladder
344.8# Other specified paralytic syndromes
344.81 Locked-in state
344.89 Other specified paralytic syndrome
344.9 Paralysis, unspecified

345.#(#) Epilepsy and recurrent seizures
345.0# Generalized nonconvulsive epilepsy
345.1# Generalized convulsive epilepsy
345.2 Petit mal status
345.3 Grand mal status
345.4# Localization-related (focal) (partial) epilepsy and epileptic syndromes with complex partial seizures
345.5# Localization-related (focal) (partial) epilepsy and epileptic syndromes with simple partial seizures
345.6# Infantile spasms
345.7# Epilepsia partialis continua
345.8# Other forms of epilepsy and recurrent seizures
345.9# Epilepsy, unspecified
5th Digit: 345.0, 1, 4-9
0 Without mention of intractable migraine
1 With intractable migraine

NUMERICAL REFERENCE

346.## Migraine
- **346.0#** Classical migraine
- **346.1#** Common migraine
- **346.2#** Variants of migraine
- **346.8#** Other forms of migraine
- **346.9#** Migraine, unspecified

5th Digit: 346
- **0 Without mention of intractable migraine**
- **1 With intractable migraine**

347.## Cataplexy and narcolepsy
- **347.0#** Narcolepsy
  - 347.00 Without cataplexy
  - 347.01 with cataplexy
- **347.1#** Narcolepsy in conditions classified elsewhere
  - 347.10 Without cataplexy
  - 347.11 with cataplexy

348.#(#) Other conditions of brain
- 348.0 Cerebral cysts
- 348.1 Anoxic brain damage
- 348.2 Benign intracranial hypertension
- **348.3#** Encephalopathy not elsewhere classified
  - 348.30 Encephalopathy unspecified
  - 348.31 Metabolic encephalopathy
  - 348.39 Other encephalopathy
- 348.4 Compression of brain
- 348.5 Cerebral edema
- 348.8 Other conditions of brain
- 348.9 Unspecified condition of brain

349.#(#) Other and unspecified disorders of the nervous system
- 349.0 Reaction to spinal or lumbar puncture
- 349.1 Nervous system complications from surgically implanted device
- 349.2 Disorders of meninges, not elsewhere classified
- **349.8#** Other specified disorders of nervous system
  - 349.81 Cerebrospinal fluid rhinorrhea
  - 349.82 Toxic encephalopathy
  - 349.89 Other
- 349.9 Unspecified disorders of nervous system

350.# Trigeminal nerve disorders
- 350.1 Trigeminal neuralgia
- 350.2 Atypical face pain
- 350.8 Other specified trigeminal nerve disorders
- 350.9 Trigeminal nerve disorder, unspecified

351.# Facial nerve disorders
- 351.0 Bell's palsy
- 351.1 Geniculate ganglionitis
- 351.8 Other facial nerve disorders
- 351.9 Facial nerve disorder, unspecified

352.# Disorders of other cranial nerves
- 352.0 Disorders of olfactory [1st] nerve
- 352.1 Glossopharyngeal neuralgia
- 352.2 Other disorders of glossopharyngeal [9th] nerve
- 352.3 Disorders of pneumogastric [10th] nerve
- 352.4 Disorders of accessory [11th] nerve
- 352.5 Disorders of hypoglossal [12th] nerve
- 352.6 Multiple cranial nerve palsies
- 352.9 Unspecified disorder of cranial nerves

353.# Nerve root and plexus disorders
- 353.0 Brachial plexus lesions
- 353.1 Lumbosacral plexus lesions
- 353.2 Cervical root lesions, not elsewhere classified
- 353.3 Thoracic root lesions, not elsewhere classified
- 353.4 Lumbosacral root lesions, not elsewhere classified
- 353.5 Neuralgic amyotrophy
- 353.6 Phantom limb (syndrome)
- 353.8 Other nerve root and plexus disorders
- 353.9 Unspecified nerve root and plexus disorder

354.# Mononeuritis of upper limb and mononeuritis multiplex
- 354.0 Carpal tunnel syndrome
- 354.1 Other lesion of median nerve
- 354.2 Lesion of ulnar nerve
- 354.3 Lesion of radial nerve
- 354.4 Causalgia of upper limb
- 354.5 Mononeuritis multiplex
- 354.8 Other mononeuritis of upper limb
- 354.9 Mononeuritis of upper limb, unspecified

355.#(#) Mononeuritis of lower limb
- 355.0 Lesion of sciatic nerve
- 355.1 Meralgia paresthetica
- 355.2 Other lesion of femoral nerve
- 355.3 Lesion of lateral popliteal nerve
- 355.4 Lesion of medial popliteal nerve
- 355.5 Tarsal tunnel syndrome
- 355.6 Lesion of plantar nerve
- **355.7#** Other mononeuritis of lower limb
  - 355.71 Causalgia of lower limb
  - 355.79 Other mononeuritis of lower limb
- 355.8 Mononeuritis of lower limb, unspecified
- 355.9 Mononeuritis of unspecified site

356.# Hereditary and idiopathic peripheral neuropathy
- 356.0 Hereditary peripheral neuropathy
- 356.1 Peroneal muscular atrophy
- 356.2 Hereditary sensory neuropathy
- 356.3 Refsum's disease
- 356.4 Idiopathic progressive polyneuropathy
- 356.8 Other specified idiopathic peripheral neuropathy
- 356.9 Unspecified

357.#(#) Inflammatory and toxic neuropathy
- 357.0 Acute infective polyneuritis
- 357.1 Polyneuropathy in collagen vascular disease
- 357.2 Polyneuropathy in diabetes
- 357.3 Polyneuropathy in malignant disease
- 357.4 Polyneuropathy in other diseases classified elsewhere
- 357.5 Alcoholic polyneuropathy
- 357.6 Polyneuropathy due to drugs
- 357.7 Polyneuropathy due to other toxic agents
- **357.8#** Other
  - 357.81 Chronic inflammatory demyelinating polyneuritis
  - 357.82 Critical illness polyneuropathy
  - 357.89 Other inflammatory and toxic neuropathy
- 357.9 Unspecified

358.#(#) Myoneural disorders
- **358.0#** Myasthenia gravis
  - 358.00 Myasthenia gravis without (acute) exacerbation
  - 358.01 Myasthenia gravis with (acute) exacerbation
- 358.1 Myasthenic syndromes in diseases classified elsewhere
- 358.2 Toxic myoneural disorders
- 358.8 Other specified myoneural disorders
- 358.9 Myoneural disorders, unspecified

359.#(#) Muscular dystrophies and other myopathies
- 359.0 Congenital hereditary muscular dystrophy
- 359.1 Hereditary progressive muscular dystrophy
- **359.2#** Myotonic disorders
  - 359.21 Myotonic muscular dystrophy
  - 359.22 Myotonic congenita
  - 359.23 Myotonic chondrodystrophy
  - 359.24 Drug induced myotonia
  - 359.29 Other specified myotonic disorder
- 359.3 Periodic paralysis
- 359.4 Toxic myopathy
- 359.5 Myopathy in endocrine diseases classified elsewhere
- 359.6 Symptomatic inflammatory myopathy in diseases classified elsewhere
- **359.8#** Other myopathies
  - 359.81 Critical illness myopathy
  - 359.89 Other myopathies
- 359.9 Myopathy, unspecified

360.#(#) Disorders of the globe
- **360.0#** Purulent endophthalmitis
  - 360.00 Purulent endophthalmitis, unspecified
  - 360.01 Acute endophthalmitis
  - 360.02 Panophthalmitis
  - 360.03 Chronic endophthalmitis
  - 360.04 Vitreous abscess
- **360.1#** Other endophthalmitis
  - 360.11 Sympathetic uveitis
  - 360.12 Panuveitis
  - 360.13 Parasitic endophthalmitis NOS
  - 360.14 Ophthalmia nodosa
  - 360.19 Other
- **360.2#** Degenerative disorders of globe
  - 360.20 Degenerative disorder of globe, unspecified
  - 360.21 Progressive high (degenerative) myopia
  - 360.23 Siderosis
  - 360.24 Other metallosis
  - 360.29 Other
- **360.3#** Hypotony of eye
  - 360.30 Hypotony, unspecified
  - 360.31 Primary hypotony
  - 360.32 Ocular fistula causing hypotony
  - 360.33 Hypotony associated with other ocular disorders
  - 360.34 Flat anterior chamber
- **360.4#** Degenerated conditions of globe
  - 360.40 Degenerated globe or eye, unspecified
  - 360.41 Blind hypotensive eye
  - 360.42 Blind hypertensive eye
  - 360.43 Hemophthalmos, except current injury
  - 360.44 Leucocoria
- **360.5#** Retained (old) intraocular foreign body, magnetic
  - 360.50 Foreign body, magnetic, intraocular, unspecified
  - 360.51 Foreign body, magnetic, in anterior chamber

360.#(#) (continued)
- ***360.5# (continued)***
  - 360.52 Foreign body, magnetic, in iris or ciliary body
  - 360.53 Foreign body, magnetic, in lens
  - 360.54 Foreign body, magnetic, in vitreous
  - 360.55 Foreign body, magnetic, in posterior wall
  - 360.59 Foreign body, magnetic, in other or multiple sites
- **360.6#** Retained (old) intraocular foreign body, nonmagnetic
  - 360.60 Foreign body, intraocular, unspecified
  - 360.61 Foreign body in anterior chamber
  - 360.62 Foreign body in iris or ciliary body
  - 360.63 Foreign body in lens
  - 360.64 Foreign body in vitreous
  - 360.65 Foreign body in posterior wall
  - 360.69 Foreign body in other or multiple sites
- **360.8#** Other disorders of globe
  - 360.81 Luxation of globe
  - 360.89 Other
- 360.9 Unspecified disorder of globe

361.#(#) Retinal detachments and defects
- **361.0#** Retinal detachment with retinal defect
  - 361.00 Retinal detachment with retinal defect, unspecified
  - 361.01 Recent detachment, partial, with single defect
  - 361.02 Recent detachment, partial, with multiple defects
  - 361.03 Recent detachment, partial, with giant tear
  - 361.04 Recent detachment, partial, with retinal dialysis
  - 361.05 Recent detachment, total or subtotal
  - 361.06 Old detachment, partial
  - 361.07 Old detachment, total or subtotal
- **361.1#** Retinoschisis and retinal cysts
  - 361.10 Retinoschisis, unspecified
  - 361.11 Flat retinoschisis
  - 361.12 Bullous retinoschisis
  - 361.13 Primary retinal cysts
  - 361.14 Secondary retinal cysts
  - 361.19 Other
- 361.2 Serous retinal detachment
- **361.3#** Retinal defects without detachment
  - 361.30 Retinal defect, unspecified
  - 361.31 Round hole of retina without detachment
  - 361.32 Horseshoe tear of retina without detachment
  - 361.33 Multiple defects of retina without detachment
- **361.8#** Other forms of retinal detachment
  - 361.81 Traction detachment of retina
  - 361.89 Other
- 361.9 Unspecified retinal detachment

362.#(#) Other retinal disorders
- **362.0#** Diabetic retinopathy
  - 362.01 Background diabetic retinopathy
  - 362.02 Proliferative diabetic retinopathy
  - 362.03 Nonproliferative diabetic retinopathy NOS
  - 362.04 Mild nonproliferative diabetic retinopathy
  - 362.05 Moderate nonproliferative diabetic retinopathy
  - 362.06 Severe nonproliferative diabetic retinopathy
  - 362.07 Diabetic macular edema
- **362.1#** Other background retinopathy and retinal vascular changes
  - 362.10 Background retinopathy, unspecified
  - 362.11 Hypertensive retinopathy

NUMERICAL REFERENCE

362.#(#) ***(continued)***

362.1# ***(continued)***

362.12 Exudative retinopathy
362.13 Changes in vascular appearance
362.14 Retinal microaneurysms NOS
362.15 Retinal telangiectasia
362.16 Retinal neovascularization NOS
362.17 Other intraretinal microvascular abnormalities
362.18 Retinal vasculitis

362.2# Other proliferative retinopathy

362.21 Retrolental fibroplasia
362.29 Other nondiabetic proliferative retinopathy

362.3# Retinal vascular occlusion

362.30 Retinal vascular occlusion, unspecified
362.31 Central retinal artery occlusion
362.32 Arterial branch occlusion
362.33 Partial arterial occlusion
362.34 Transient arterial occlusion
362.35 Central retinal vein occlusion
362.36 Venous tributary (branch) occlusion
362.37 Venous engorgement

362.4# Separation of retinal layers

362.40 Retinal layer separation, unspecified
362.41 Central serous retinopathy
362.42 Serous detachment of retinal pigment epithelium
362.43 Hemorrhagic detachment of retinal pigment epithelium

362.5# Degeneration of macula and posterior pole

362.50 Macular degeneration (senile), unspecified
362.51 Nonexudative senile macular degeneration
362.52 Exudative senile macular degeneration
362.53 Cystoid macular degeneration
362.54 Macular cyst, hole, or pseudohole
362.55 Toxic maculopathy
362.56 Macular puckering
362.57 Drusen (degenerative)

362.6# Peripheral retinal degenerations

362.60 Peripheral retinal degeneration, unspecified
362.61 Paving stone degeneration
362.62 Microcystoid degeneration
362.63 Lattice degeneration
362.64 Senile reticular degeneration
362.65 Secondary pigmentary degeneration
362.66 Secondary vitreoretinal degenerations

362.7# Hereditary retinal dystrophies

362.70 Hereditary retinal dystrophy, unspecified
362.71 Retinal dystrophy in systemic or cerebroretinal lipidoses
362.72 Retinal dystrophy in other systemic disorders and syndromes
362.73 Vitreoretinal dystrophies
362.74 Pigmentary retinal dystrophy
362.75 Other dystrophies primarily involving the sensory retina
362.76 Dystrophies primarily involving the retinal pigment epithelium
362.77 Dystrophies primarily involving Bruch's membrane

362.8# Other retinal disorders

362.81 Retinal hemorrhage
362.82 Retinal exudates and deposits
362.83 Retinal edema
362.84 Retinal ischemia
362.85 Retinal nerve fiber bundle defects
362.89 Other retinal disorders

362.9 Unspecified retinal disorder

363.#(#) Chorioretinal inflammations, scars, and other disorders of choroid

363.0# Focal chorioretinitis and focal retinochoroiditis

363.00 Focal chorioretinitis, unspecified
363.01 Focal choroiditis and chorioretinitis, Juxtapapillary
363.03 Focal choroiditis and chorioretinitis of other posterior pole
363.04 Focal choroiditis and chorioretinitis, peripheral
363.05 Focal retinitis and retinochoroiditis, juxtapapillary
363.06 Focal retinitis and retinochoroiditis, macular or paramacular
363.07 Focal retinitis and retinochoroiditis of other posterior pole
363.08 Focal retinitis and retinochoroiditis, peripheral

363.1# Disseminated chorioretinitis and disseminated retinochoroiditis

363.10 Disseminated chorioretinitis, unspecified
363.11 Disseminated choroiditis and chorioretinitis, posterior pole
363.12 Disseminated choroiditis and chorioretinitis, peripheral
363.13 Disseminated choroiditis and chorioretinitis, generalized
363.14 Disseminated retinitis and retinochoroiditis, metastatic
363.15 Disseminated retinitis and retinochoroiditis, pigment epitheliopathy

363.2# Other and unspecified forms of chorioretinitis and retinochoroiditis

363.20 Chorioretinitis, unspecified
363.21 Pars planitis
363.22 Harada's disease

363.3# Chorioretinal scars

363.30 Chorioretinal scar, unspecified
363.31 Solar retinopathy
363.32 Other macular scars
363.33 Other scars of posterior pole
363.34 Peripheral scars
363.35 Disseminated scars

363.4# Choroidal degenerations

363.40 Choroidal degeneration, unspecified
363.41 Senile atrophy of choroid
363.42 Diffuse secondary atrophy of choroid
363.43 Angioid streaks of choroid

363.5# Hereditary choroidal dystrophies

363.50 Hereditary choroidal dystrophy or atrophy, unspecified
363.51 Circumpapillary dystrophy of choroid, partial
363.52 Circumpapillary dystrophy of choroid, total
363.53 Central dystrophy of choroid, partial
363.54 Central choroidal atrophy, total
363.55 Choroideremia
363.56 Other diffuse or generalized dystrophy, partial
363.57 Other diffuse or generalized dystrophy, total

363.6# Choroidal hemorrhage and rupture

363.61 Choroidal hemorrhage, unspecified
363.62 Expulsive choroidal hemorrhage
363.63 Choroidal rupture

363.7# Choroidal detachment

363.70 Choroidal detachment, unspecified
363.71 Serous choroidal detachment
363.72 Hemorrhagic choroidal detachment

363.#(#) ***(continued)***
363.8 Other disorders of choroid
363.9 Unspecified disorder of choroid

364.#(#) Disorders of iris and ciliary body
364.0# Acute and subacute iridocyclitis
364.00 Acute and subacute iridocyclitis, NOS
364.01 Primary iridocyclitis
364.02 Recurrent iridocyclitis
364.03 Secondary iridocyclitis, infectious
364.04 Secondary iridocyclitis, noninfectious
364.05 Hypopyon
364.1# Chronic iridocyclitis
364.10 Chronic iridocyclitis, unspecified
364.11 Chronic iridocyclitis in diseases classified elsewhere
364.2# Certain types of iridocyclitis
364.21 Fuchs' heterochromic cyclitis
364.22 Glaucomatocyclitic crises
364.23 Lens-induced iridocyclitis
364.24 Vogt-Koyanagi syndrome
364.3 Unspecified iridocyclitis
364.4# Vascular disorders of iris and ciliary body
364.41 Hyphema
364.42 Rubeosis iridis
364.5# Degenerations of iris and ciliary body
364.51 Essential or progressive iris atrophy
364.52 Iridoschisis
364.53 Pigmentary iris degeneration
364.54 Degeneration of pupillary margin
364.55 Miotic cysts of pupillary margin
364.56 Degenerative changes of chamber angle
364.57 Degenerative changes of ciliary body
364.59 Other iris atrophy
364.6# Cysts of iris, ciliary body, and anterior chamber
364.60 Idiopathic cysts
364.61 Implantation cysts
364.62 Exudative cysts of iris or anterior chamber
364.63 Primary cyst of pars plana
364.64 Exudative cyst of pars plana
364.7# Adhesions and disruptions iris and ciliary body
364.70 Adhesions of iris, unspecified
364.71 Posterior synechiae
364.72 Anterior synechiae
364.73 Goniosynechiae
364.74 Pupillary membranes
364.75 Pupillary abnormalities
364.76 Iridodialysis
364.77 Recession of chamber angle
364.8# Other disorders of iris and ciliary body
364.81 Floppy iris syndrome
364.89 Other disorders of the iris and ciliary body
364.9 Unspecified disorder of iris and ciliary body

365.#(#) Glaucoma
365.0# Borderline glaucoma [glaucoma suspect]
365.00 Preglaucoma, unspecified
365.01 Open angle with borderline findings
365.02 Anatomical narrow angle
365.03 Steroid responders
365.04 Ocular hypertension
365.1# Open-angle glaucoma
365.10 Open-angle glaucoma, unspecified
365.11 Primary open angle glaucoma
365.12 Low tension glaucoma
365.13 Pigmentary glaucoma
365.14 Glaucoma of childhood
365.15 Residual stage of open angle glaucoma

365.#(#) ***(continued)***
365.2# Primary angle-closure glaucoma
365.20 Primary angle-closure glaucoma, unspecified
365.21 Intermittent angle-closure glaucoma
365.22 Acute angle-closure glaucoma
365.23 Chronic angle-closure glaucoma
365.24 Residual stage of angle-closure glaucoma
365.3# Corticosteroid-induced glaucoma
365.31 Glaucomatous stage
365.32 Residual stage
365.4# Glaucoma associated with congenital anomalies, dystrophies, and systemic syndromes
365.41 Glaucoma associated with chamber angle anomalies
365.42 Glaucoma associated with anomalies of iris
365.43 Glaucoma associated with other anterior segment anomalies
365.44 Glaucoma associated with systemic syndromes
365.5# Glaucoma associated with disorders of the lens
365.51 Phacolytic glaucoma
365.52 Pseudoexfoliation glaucoma
365.59 Glaucoma associated with other lens disorders
365.6# Glaucoma associated with other ocular disorders
365.60 Glaucoma associated with unspecified ocular disorder
365.61 Glaucoma associated with pupillary block
365.62 Glaucoma associated with ocular inflammations
365.63 Glaucoma associated with vascular disorders
365.64 Glaucoma associated with tumors or cysts
365.65 Glaucoma associated with ocular trauma
365.8# Other specified forms of glaucoma
365.81 Hypersecretion glaucoma
365.82 Glaucoma with increased episcleral venous pressure
365.83 Aqueous misdirection
365.89 Other specified glaucoma
365.9 Unspecified glaucoma

366.#(#) Cataract
366.0# Infantile, juvenile, and presenile cataract
366.00 Nonsenile cataract, unspecified
366.01 Anterior subcapsular polar cataract
366.02 Posterior subcapsular polar cataract
366.03 Cortical, lamellar, or zonular cataract
366.04 Nuclear cataract
366.09 Other and combined forms of nonsenile cataract
366.1# Senile Cataract
366.10 Senile cataract, unspecified
366.11 Pseudoexfoliation of lens capsule
366.12 Incipient cataract
366.13 Anterior subcapsular polar senile cataract
366.14 Posterior subcapsular polar senile cataract
366.15 Cortical senile cataract
366.16 Nuclear sclerosis
366.17 Total or mature cataract
366.18 Hypermature cataract
366.19 Other and combined forms of senile cataract
366.2# Traumatic cataract
366.20 Traumatic cataract, unspecified
366.21 Localized traumatic opacities
366.22 Total traumatic cataract
366.23 Partially resolved traumatic cataract

366.#(#) ***(continued)***

366.3# Cataract secondary to ocular disorders
- 366.30 Cataracta complicata, unspecified
- 366.31 Glaucomatous flecks (subcapsular)
- 366.32 Cataract in inflammatory disorders
- 366.33 Cataract with neovascularization
- 366.34 Cataract in degenerative disorders

366.4# Cataract associated with other disorders
- 366.41 Diabetic cataract
- 366.42 Tetanic cataract
- 366.43 Myotonic cataract
- 366.44 Cataract associated with other syndromes
- 366.45 Toxic cataract
- 366.46 Cataract associated with radiation and other physical influences

366.5# After-cataract
- 366.50 After-cataract, unspecified
- 366.51 Soemmering's ring
- 366.52 Other after-cataract, not obscuring vision
- 366.53 After-cataract, obscuring vision

366.8 Other cataract

366.9 Unspecified cataract

367.#(#) Disorders of refraction and accommodation

367.0 Hypermetropia

367.1 Myopia

367.2# Astigmatism
- 367.20 Astigmatism, unspecified
- 367.21 Regular astigmatism
- 367.22 Irregular astigmatism

367.3# Anisometropia and aniseikonia
- 367.31 Anisometropia
- 367.32 Aniseikonia

367.4 Presbyopia

367.5# Disorders of accommodation
- 367.51 Paresis of accommodation
- 367.52 Total or complete internal ophthalmoplegia
- 367.53 Spasm of accommodation

367.8# Other disorders of refraction and accommodation
- 367.81 Transient refractive change
- 367.89 Other

367.9 Unspecified disorder of refraction and accommodation

368.#(#) Visual disturbances

368.0# Amblyopia ex anopsia
- 368.00 Amblyopia, unspecified
- 368.01 Strabismic amblyopia
- 368.02 Deprivation amblyopia
- 368.03 Refractive amblyopia

368.1# Subjective visual disturbances
- 368.10 Subjective visual disturbance, unspecified
- 368.11 Sudden visual loss
- 368.12 Transient visual loss
- 368.13 Visual discomfort
- 368.14 Visual distortions of shape and size
- 368.15 Other visual distortions and entoptic phenomena
- 368.16 Psychophysical visual disturbances

368.2 Diplopia

368.3# Other disorders of binocular vision
- 368.30 Binocular vision disorder, unspecified
- 368.31 Suppression of binocular vision
- 368.32 Simultaneous visual perception without fusion
- 368.33 Fusion with defective stereopsis
- 368.34 Abnormal retinal correspondence

368.#(#) ***(continued)***

368.4# Visual field defects
- 368.40 Visual field defect, unspecified
- 368.41 Scotoma involving central area
- 368.42 Scotoma of blind spot area
- 368.43 Sector or arcuate defects
- 368.44 Other localized visual field defect
- 368.45 Generalized contraction or constriction
- 368.46 Homonymous bilateral field defects
- 368.47 Heteronymous bilateral field defects

368.5# Color vision deficiencies
- 368.51 Protan defect
- 368.52 Deutan defect
- 368.53 Tritan defect
- 368.54 Achromatopsia
- 368.55 Acquired color vision deficiencies
- 368.59 Other color vision deficiencies

368.6# Night blindness
- 368.60 Night blindness, unspecified
- 368.61 Congenital night blindness
- 368.62 Acquired night blindness
- 368.63 Abnormal dark adaptation curve
- 368.69 Other night blindness

368.8 Other specified visual disturbances

368.9 Unspecified visual disturbance

369.#(#) Blindness and low vision

369.0# Profound impairment, both eyes
- 369.00 Impairment level not further specified
- 369.01 Better eye: total impairment; lesser eye: total impairment
- 369.02 Better eye: near-total impairment; lesser eye: not further specified
- 369.03 Better eye: near-total impairment; lesser eye: total impairment
- 369.04 Better eye: near-total impairment; lesser eye: near-total impairment
- 369.05 Better eye: profound impairment; lesser eye: not further specified
- 369.06 Better eye: profound impairment; lesser eye: total impairment
- 369.07 Better eye: profound impairment; lesser eye: near-total impairment
- 369.08 Better eye: profound impairment; lesser eye: profound impairment

369.1# Moderate or severe impairment, better eye, profound impairment lesser eye
- 369.10 Impairment level not further specified
- 369.11 Better eye: severe impairment; lesser eye: blind, not further specified
- 369.12 Better eye: severe impairment; lesser eye: total impairment
- 369.13 Better eye: severe impairment; lesser eye: near-total impairment
- 369.14 Better eye: severe impairment; lesser eye: profound impairment
- 369.15 Better eye: moderate impairment; lesser eye: blind, not further specified
- 369.16 Better eye: moderate impairment; lesser eye: total impairment
- 369.17 Better eye: moderate impairment; lesser eye: near-total impairment
- 369.18 Better eye: moderate impairment; lesser eye: profound impairment

369.2# Moderate or severe impairment, both eyes
- 369.20 Impairment level not further specified
- 369.21 Better eye: severe impairment; lesser eye: not further specified

369.#(#) *(continued)*

369.2(#) (continued)

369.22 Better eye: severe impairment; lesser eye: severe impairment

369.23 Better eye: moderate impairment; lesser eye: not further specified

369.24 Better eye: moderate impairment; lesser eye: severe impairment

369.25 Better eye: moderate impairment; lesser eye: moderate impairment

369.3 Unqualified visual loss, both eyes

369.4 Legal blindness, as defined in U.S.A.

369.6# Profound impairment, one eye

369.60 Impairment level not further specified

369.61 One eye: total impairment; other eye: not specified

369.62 One eye: total impairment; other eye: near-normal vision

369.63 One eye: total impairment; other eye: normal vision

369.64 One eye: near-total impairment; other eye: not specified

369.65 One eye: near-total impairment; other eye: near-normal vision

369.66 One eye: near-total impairment; other eye: normal vision

369.67 One eye: profound impairment; other eye: not specified

369.68 One eye: profound impairment; other eye: near-normal vision

369.69 One eye: profound impairment; other eye: normal vision

369.7# Moderate or severe impairment, one eye

369.70 Impairment level not further specified

369.71 One eye: severe impairment; other eye: not specified

369.72 One eye: severe impairment; other eye: near-normal vision

369.73 One eye: severe impairment; other eye: normal vision

369.74 One eye: moderate impairment; other eye: not specified

369.75 One eye: moderate impairment; other eye: near-normal vision

369.76 One eye: moderate impairment; other eye: normal vision

369.8 Unqualified visual loss, one eye

369.9 Unspecified visual loss

370.#(#) Keratitis

370.0# Corneal ulcer

370.00 Corneal ulcer, unspecified

370.01 Marginal corneal ulcer

370.02 Ring corneal ulcer

370.03 Central corneal ulcer

370.04 Hypopyon ulcer

370.05 Mycotic corneal ulcer

370.06 Perforated corneal ulcer

370.07 Mooren's ulcer

370.2# Superficial keratitis without conjunctivitis

370.20 Superficial keratitis, unspecified

370.21 Punctate keratitis

370.22 Macular keratitis

370.23 Filamentary keratitis

370.24 Photokeratitis

370.3# Certain types of keratoconjunctivitis

370.31 Phlyctenular keratoconjunctivitis

370.32 Limbar and corneal involvement in vernal conjunctivitis

370.33 Keratoconjunctivitis sicca, not specified as Sjögren's

370.#(#) *(continued)*

370.3# (continued)

370.34 Exposure keratoconjunctivitis

370.35 Neurotrophic keratoconjunctivitis

370.4# Other and unspecified keratoconjunctivitis

370.40 Keratoconjunctivitis, unspecified

370.44 Keratitis or keratoconjunctivitis in exanthema

370.49 Other

370.5# Interstitial and deep keratitis

370.50 Interstitial keratitis, unspecified

370.52 Diffuse interstitial keratitis

370.54 Sclerosing keratitis

370.55 Corneal abscess

370.59 Other

370.6# Corneal neovascularization

370.60 Corneal neovascularization, unspecified

370.61 Localized vascularization of cornea

370.62 Pannus (corneal)

370.63 Deep vascularization of cornea

370.64 Ghost vessels (corneal)

370.8 Other forms of keratitis

370.9 Unspecified keratitis

371.#(#) Corneal opacity and other disorders of cornea

371.0# Corneal scars and opacities

371.00 Corneal opacity, unspecified

371.01 Minor opacity of cornea

371.02 Peripheral opacity of cornea

371.03 Central opacity of cornea

371.04 Adherent leucoma

371.05 Phthisical cornea

371.1# Corneal pigmentations and deposits

371.10 Corneal deposit, unspecified

371.11 Anterior pigmentations

371.12 Stromal pigmentations

371.13 Posterior pigmentations

371.14 Kayser-Fleischer ring

371.15 Other deposits associated with metabolic disorders

371.16 Argentous deposits

371.2# Corneal edema

371.20 Corneal edema, unspecified

371.21 Idiopathic corneal edema

371.22 Secondary corneal edema

371.23 Bullous keratopathy

371.24 Corneal edema due to wearing of contact lenses

371.3# Changes of corneal membranes

371.30 Corneal membrane change, unspecified

371.31 Folds and rupture of Bowman's membrane

371.32 Folds in Descemet's membrane

371.33 Rupture in Descemet's membrane

371.4# Corneal degenerations

371.40 Corneal degeneration, unspecified

371.41 Senile corneal changes

371.42 Recurrent erosion of cornea

371.43 Band-shaped keratopathy

371.44 Other calcerous degenerations of cornea

371.45 Keratomalacia NOS

371.46 Nodular degeneration of cornea

371.48 Peripheral degenerations of cornea

371.49 Other

371.5# Hereditary corneal dystrophies

371.50 Corneal dystrophy, unspecified

371.51 Juvenile epithelial corneal dystrophy

371.52 Other anterior corneal dystrophies

371.53 Granular corneal dystrophy

371.54 Lattice corneal dystrophy

371.55 Macular corneal dystrophy

371.56 Other stromal corneal dystrophies

371.#(#) *(continued)*
- **371.5(#)** (continued)
  - 371.57 Endothelial corneal dystrophy
  - 371.58 Other posterior corneal dystrophies
- **371.6#** Keratoconus
  - 371.60 Keratoconus, unspecified
  - 371.61 Keratoconus, stable condition
  - 371.62 Keratoconus, acute hydrops
- **371.7#** Other corneal deformities
  - 371.70 Corneal deformity, unspecified
  - 371.71 Corneal ectasia
  - 371.72 Descemetocele
  - 371.73 Corneal staphyloma
- **371.8#** Other corneal disorders
  - 371.81 Corneal anesthesia and hypoesthesia
  - 371.82 Corneal disorder due to contact lens
  - 371.89 Other
- 371.9 Unspecified corneal disorder

372.#(#) Disorders of conjunctiva
- **372.0#** Acute conjunctivitis
  - 372.00 Acute conjunctivitis, unspecified
  - 372.01 Serous conjunctivitis, except viral
  - 372.02 Acute follicular conjunctivitis
  - 372.03 Other mucopurulent conjunctivitis
  - 372.04 Pseudomembranous conjunctivitis
  - 372.05 Acute atopic conjunctivitis
- **372.1#** Chronic conjunctivitis
  - 372.10 Chronic conjunctivitis, unspecified
  - 372.11 Simple chronic conjunctivitis
  - 372.12 Chronic follicular conjunctivitis
  - 372.13 Vernal conjunctivitis
  - 372.14 Other chronic allergic conjunctivitis
  - 372.15 Parasitic conjunctivitis
- **372.2#** Blepharoconjunctivitis
  - 372.20 Blepharoconjunctivitis, unspecified
  - 372.21 Angular blepharoconjunctivitis
  - 372.22 Contact blepharoconjunctivitis
- **372.3#** Other and unspecified conjunctivitis
  - 372.30 Conjunctivitis, unspecified
  - 372.31 Rosacea conjunctivitis
  - 372.33 Conjunctivitis in mucocutaneous disease
  - 372.39 Other
- **372.4#** Pterygium
  - 372.40 Pterygium, unspecified
  - 372.41 Peripheral pterygium, stationary
  - 372.42 Peripheral pterygium, progressive
  - 372.43 Central pterygium
  - 372.44 Double pterygium
  - 372.45 Recurrent pterygium
- **372.5#** Conjunctival degenerations and deposits
  - 372.50 Conjunctival degeneration, unspecified
  - 372.51 Pinguecula
  - 372.52 Pseudopterygium
  - 372.53 Conjunctival xerosis
  - 372.54 Conjunctival concretions
  - 372.55 Conjunctival pigmentations
  - 372.56 Conjunctival deposits
- **372.6#** Conjunctival scars
  - 372.61 Granuloma of conjunctiva
  - 372.62 Localized adhesions and strands of conjunctiva
  - 372.63 Symblepharon
  - 372.64 Scarring of conjunctiva
- **372.7#** Conjunctival vascular disorders and cysts
  - 372.71 Hyperemia of conjunctiva
  - 372.72 Conjunctival hemorrhage
  - 372.73 Conjunctival edema
  - 372.74 Vascular abnormalities of conjunctiva
  - 372.75 Conjunctival cysts

372.#(#) *(continued)*
- **372.8#** Other disorders of conjunctiva
  - 372.81 Conjunctivochalasis
  - 372.89 Other disorders of conjunctiva
- 372.9 Unspecified disorder of conjunctiva

373.#(#) Inflammation of eyelids
- **373.0#** Blepharitis
  - 373.00 Blepharitis, unspecified
  - 373.01 Ulcerative blepharitis
  - 373.02 Squamous blepharitis
- **373.1#** Hordeolum and other deep inflammation of eyelid
  - 373.11 Hordeolum externum
  - 373.12 Hordeolum internum
  - 373.13 Abscess of eyelid
- 373.2 Chalazion
- **373.3#** Noninfectious dermatoses of eyelid
  - 373.31 Eczematous dermatitis of eyelid
  - 373.32 Contact and allergic dermatitis of eyelid
  - 373.33 Xeroderma of eyelid
  - 373.34 Discoid lupus erythematosus of eyelid
- 373.4 Infective dermatitis of eyelid of types resulting in deformity
- 373.5 Other infective dermatitis of eyelid
- 373.6 Parasitic infestation of eyelid
- 373.8 Other inflammations of eyelids
- 373.9 Unspecified inflammation of eyelid

374.#(#) Other disorders of eyelids
- **374.0#** Entropion and trichiasis of eyelid
  - 374.00 Entropion, unspecified
  - 374.01 Senile entropion
  - 374.02 Mechanical entropion
  - 374.03 Spastic entropion
  - 374.04 Cicatricial entropion
  - 374.05 Trichiasis without entropion
- **374.1#** Ectropion
  - 374.10 Ectropion, unspecified
  - 374.11 Senile ectropion
  - 374.12 Mechanical ectropion
  - 374.13 Spastic ectropion
  - 374.14 Cicatricial ectropion
- **374.2#** Lagophthalmos
  - 374.20 Lagophthalmos, unspecified
  - 374.21 Paralytic lagophthalmos
  - 374.22 Mechanical lagophthalmos
  - 374.23 Cicatricial lagophthalmos
- **374.3#** Ptosis of eyelid
  - 374.30 Ptosis of eyelid, unspecified
  - 374.31 Paralytic ptosis
  - 374.32 Myogenic ptosis
  - 374.33 Mechanical ptosis
  - 374.34 Blepharochalasis
- **374.4#** Other disorders affecting eyelid function
  - 374.41 Lid retraction or lag
  - 374.43 Abnormal innervation syndrome
  - 374.44 Sensory disorders
  - 374.45 Other sensorimotor disorders
  - 374.46 Blepharophimosis
- **374.5#** Degenerative disorders eyelidand periocular area
  - 374.50 Degenerative disorder of eyelid, NOS
  - 374.51 Xanthelasma
  - 374.52 Hyperpigmentation of eyelid
  - 374.53 Hypopigmentation of eyelid
  - 374.54 Hypertrichosis of eyelid
  - 374.55 Hypotrichosis of eyelid
  - 374.56 Other degenerative disorders of skin affecting eyelid

374.#(#) *(continued)*

374.8# Other disorders of eyelid
- 374.81 Hemorrhage of eyelid
- 374.82 Edema of eyelid
- 374.83 Elephantiasis of eyelid
- 374.84 Cysts of eyelids
- 374.85 Vascular anomalies of eyelid
- 374.86 Retained foreign body of eyelid
- 374.87 Dermatochalasis
- 374.89 Other disorders of eyelid

374.9 Unspecified disorder of eyelid

375.#(#) Disorders of lacrimal system

375.0# Dacryoadenitis
- 375.00 Dacryoadenitis, unspecified
- 375.01 Acute dacryoadenitis
- 375.02 Chronic dacryoadenitis
- 375.03 Chronic enlargement of lacrimal gland

375.1# Other disorders of lacrimal gland
- 375.11 Dacryops
- 375.12 Other lacrimal cysts and cystic degeneration
- 375.13 Primary lacrimal atrophy
- 375.14 Secondary lacrimal atrophy
- 375.15 Tear film insufficiency, unspecified
- 375.16 Dislocation of lacrimal gland

375.2# Epiphora
- 375.20 Epiphora, unspecified as to cause
- 375.21 Epiphora due to excess lacrimation
- 375.22 Epiphora due to insufficient drainage

375.3# Acute and unspecified inflammation of lacrimal passages
- 375.30 Dacryocystitis, unspecified
- 375.31 Acute canaliculitis, lacrimal
- 375.32 Acute dacryocystitis
- 375.33 Phlegmonous dacryocystitis

375.4# Chronic inflammation of lacrimal passages
- 375.41 Chronic canaliculitis
- 375.42 Chronic dacryocystitis
- 375.43 Lacrimal mucocele

375.5# Stenosis and insufficiency of lacrimal passages
- 375.51 Eversion of lacrimal punctum
- 375.52 Stenosis of lacrimal punctum
- 375.53 Stenosis of lacrimal canaliculi
- 375.54 Stenosis of lacrimal sac
- 375.55 Obstruction of nasolacrimal duct, neonatal
- 375.56 Stenosis of nasolacrimal duct, acquired
- 375.57 Dacryolith

375.6# Other changes of lacrimal passages
- 375.61 Lacrimal fistula
- 375.69 Other

375.8# Other disorders of lacrimal system
- 375.81 Granuloma of lacrimal passages
- 375.89 Other

375.9 Unspecified disorder of lacrimal system

376.#(#) Disorders of the orbit

376.0# Acute inflammation of orbit
- 376.00 Acute inflammation of orbit, unspecified
- 376.01 Orbital cellulitis
- 376.02 Orbital periostitis
- 376.03 Orbital osteomyelitis
- 376.04 Tenonitis

376.1# Chronic inflammatory disorders of orbit
- 376.10 Chronic inflammation of orbit, unspecified
- 376.11 Orbital granuloma
- 376.12 Orbital myositis
- 376.13 Parasitic infestation of orbit

376.2# Endocrine exophthalmos
- 376.21 Thyrotoxic exophthalmos
- 376.22 Exophthalmic ophthalmoplegia

376.#(#) *(continued)*

376.3# Other exophthalmic conditions
- 376.30 Exophthalmos, unspecified
- 376.31 Constant exophthalmos
- 376.32 Orbital hemorrhage
- 376.33 Orbital edema or congestion
- 376.34 Intermittent exophthalmos
- 376.35 Pulsating exophthalmos
- 376.36 Lateral displacement of globe

376.4# Deformity of orbit
- 376.40 Deformity of orbit, unspecified
- 376.41 Hypertelorism of orbit
- 376.42 Exostosis of orbit
- 376.43 Local deformities due to bone disease
- 376.44 Orbital deformities associated with craniofacial deformities
- 376.45 Atrophy of orbit
- 376.46 Enlargement of orbit
- 376.47 Deformity due to trauma or surgery

376.5# Enophthalmos
- 376.50 Enophthalmos, unspecified as to cause
- 376.51 Enophthalmos due to atrophy of orbital tissue
- 376.52 Enophthalmos due to trauma or surgery

376.6 Retained (old) foreign body following penetrating wound of orbit

376.8# Other orbital disorders
- 376.81 Orbital cysts
- 376.82 Myopathy of extraocular muscles
- 376.89 Other

376.9 Unspecified disorder of orbit

377.#(#) Disorders of optic nerve and visual pathways

377.0# Papilledema
- 377.00 Papilledema, unspecified
- 377.01 Papilledema associated with increased intracranial pressure
- 377.02 Papilledema associated with decreased ocular pressure
- 377.03 Papilledema associated with retinal disorder
- 377.04 Foster-Kennedy syndrome

377.1# Optic atrophy
- 377.10 Optic atrophy, unspecified
- 377.11 Primary optic atrophy
- 377.12 Postinflammatory optic atrophy
- 377.13 Optic atrophy associated with retinal dystrophies
- 377.14 Glaucomatous atrophy (cupping) of optic disc
- 377.15 Partial optic atrophy
- 377.16 Hereditary optic atrophy

377.2# Other disorders of optic disc
- 377.21 Drusen of optic disc
- 377.22 Crater-like holes of optic disc
- 377.23 Coloboma of optic disc
- 377.24 Pseudopapilledema

377.3# Optic neuritis
- 377.30 Optic neuritis, unspecified
- 377.31 Optic papillitis
- 377.32 Retrobulbar neuritis (acute)
- 377.33 Nutritional optic neuropathy
- 377.34 Toxic optic neuropathy
- 377.39 Other

377.4# Other disorders of optic nerve
- 377.41 Ischemic optic neuropathy
- 377.42 Hemorrhage in optic nerve sheaths
- 377.43 Optic nerve hypoplasia
- 377.49 Other

377.#(#) *(continued)*
377.5# Disorders of optic chiasm
377.51 Associated with pituitary neoplasms and disorders
377.52 Associated with other neoplasms
377.53 Associated with vascular disorders
377.54 Associated with inflammatory disorders
377.6# Disorders of other visual pathways
377.61 Associated with neoplasms
377.62 Associated with vascular disorders
377.63 Associated with inflammatory disorders
377.7# Disorders of visual cortex
377.71 Associated with neoplasms
377.72 Associated with vascular disorders
377.73 Associated with inflammatory disorders
377.75 Cortical blindness
377.9 Unspecified disorder of optic nerve and visual pathways

378.#(#) Strabismus and other disorders of binocular eye movements
378.0# Esotropia
378.1# Exotropia
5th Digit: 378.0-378.1
0 Unspecified
1 Monocular
2 Monocular with A pattern
3 Monocular with V pattern
4 Monocular with other noncomitancies
5 Alternating
6 Alternating with A pattern
7 Alternating with V pattern
8 Alternating with other noncomitancies
378.2# Intermittent heterotropia
378.20 Intermittent heterotropia, unspecified
378.21 Intermittent esotropia, monocular
378.22 Intermittent esotropia, alternating
378.23 Intermittent exotropia, monocular
378.24 Intermittent exotropia, alternating
378.3# Other and unspecified heterotropia
378.30 Heterotropia, unspecified
378.31 Hypertropia
378.32 Hypotropia
378.33 Cyclotropia
378.34 Monofixation syndrome
378.35 Accommodative component in esotropia
378.4# Heterophoria
378.40 Heterophoria, unspecified
378.41 Esophoria
378.42 Exophoria
378.43 Vertical heterophoria
378.44 Cyclophoria
378.45 Alternating hyperphoria
378.5# Paralytic strabismus
378.50 Paralytic strabismus, unspecified
378.51 Third or oculomotor nerve palsy, partial
378.52 Third or oculomotor nerve palsy, total
378.53 Fourth or trochlear nerve palsy
378.54 Sixth or abducens nerve palsy
378.55 External ophthalmoplegia
378.56 Total ophthalmoplegia
378.6# Mechanical strabismus
378.60 Mechanical strabismus, unspecified
378.61 Brown's (tendon) sheath syndrome
378.62 Mechanical strabismus from other musculofascial disorders
378.63 Limited duction associated with other conditions

378.#(#) *(continued)*
378.7# Other specified strabismus
378.71 Duane's syndrome
378.72 Progressive external ophthalmoplegia
378.73 Strabismus in other neuromuscular disorders
378.8# Other disorders of binocular eye movements
378.81 Palsy of conjugate gaze
378.82 Spasm of conjugate gaze
378.83 Convergence insufficiency or palsy
378.84 Convergence excess or spasm
378.85 Anomalies of divergence
378.86 Internuclear ophthalmoplegia
378.87 Other dissociated deviation of eye movements
378.9 Unspecified disorder of eye movements

379.#(#) Other disorders of eye
379.0# Scleritis and episcleritis
379.00 Scleritis, unspecified
379.01 Episcleritis periodica fugax
379.02 Nodular episcleritis
379.03 Anterior scleritis
379.04 Scleromalacia perforans
379.05 Scleritis with corneal involvement
379.06 Brawny scleritis
379.07 Posterior scleritis
379.09 Other
379.1# Other disorders of sclera
379.11 Scleral ectasia
379.12 Staphyloma posticum
379.13 Equatorial staphyloma
379.14 Anterior staphyloma, localized
379.15 Ring staphyloma
379.16 Other degenerative disorders of sclera
379.19 Other
379.2# Disorders of vitreous body
379.21 Vitreous degeneration
379.22 Crystalline deposits in vitreous
379.23 Vitreous hemorrhage
379.24 Other vitreous opacities
379.25 Vitreous membranes and strands
379.26 Vitreous prolapse
379.29 Other disorders of vitreous
379.3# Aphakia and other disorders of lens
379.31 Aphakia
379.32 Subluxation of lens
379.33 Anterior dislocation of lens
379.34 Posterior dislocation of lens
379.39 Other disorders of lens
379.4# Anomalies of pupillary function
379.40 Abnormal pupillary function, unspecified
379.41 Anisocoria
379.42 Miosis (persistent), not due to miotics
379.43 Mydriasis (persistent), not due to mydriatics
379.45 Argyll Robertson pupil, atypical
379.46 Tonic pupillary reaction
379.49 Other
379.5# Nystagmus and other irregular eye movements
379.50 Nystagmus, unspecified
379.51 Congenital nystagmus
379.52 Latent nystagmus
379.53 Visual deprivation nystagmus
379.54 Nystagmus associated with disorders of the vestibular system
379.55 Dissociated nystagmus
379.56 Other forms of nystagmus
379.57 Deficiencies of saccadic eye movements

379.#(#) *(continued)*

379.5(#) (continued)

379.58 Deficiencies of smooth pursuit movements
379.59 Other irregularities of eye movements

379.6# Inflammation (infection) of postprocedural bleb
379.60 Inflammation (infection) of postprocedural bleb unspecified
379.61 Inflammation (infection) of postprocedural bleb stage 1
379.62 Inflammation (infection) of postprocedural bleb stage 2
379.63 Inflammation (infection) of postprocedural bleb stage 3

379.8 Other specified disorders of eye and adnexa

379.9# Unspecified disorder of eye and adnexa
379.90 Disorder of eye, unspecified
379.91 Pain in or around eye
379.92 Swelling or mass of eye
379.93 Redness or discharge of eye
379.99 Other ill-defined disorders of eye

380.#(#) Disorders of external ear

380.0# Perichondritis and chondritis of pinna
380.00 Perichondritis of pinna, unspecified
380.01 Acute perichondritis of pinna
380.02 Chronic perichondritis of pinna
380.03 Chondritis of pinna

380.1# Infective otitis externa
380.10 Infective otitis externa, unspecified
380.11 Acute infection of pinna
380.12 Acute swimmers' ear
380.13 Other acute infections of external ear
380.14 Malignant otitis externa
380.15 Chronic mycotic otitis externa
380.16 Other chronic infective otitis externa

380.2# Other otitis externa
380.21 Cholesteatoma of external ear
380.22 Other acute otitis externa
380.23 Other chronic otitis externa

380.3# Noninfectious disorders of pinna
380.30 Disorder of pinna, unspecified
380.31 Hematoma of auricle or pinna
380.32 Acquired deformities of auricle or pinna
380.39 Other

380.4 Impacted cerumen

380.5# Acquired stenosis of external ear canal
380.50 Acquired stenosis of external ear canal, unspecified as to cause
380.51 Secondary to trauma
380.52 Secondary to surgery
380.53 Secondary to inflammation

380.8# Other disorders of external ear
380.81 Exostosis of external ear canal
380.89 Other

380.9 Unspecified disorder of external ear

381.#(#) Nonsuppurative otitis media and Eustachian tube disorders

381.0# Acute nonsuppurative otitis media
381.00 Acute nonsuppurative otitis media, NOS
381.01 Acute serous otitis media
381.02 Acute mucoid otitis media
381.03 Acute sanguinous otitis media
381.04 Acute allergic serous otitis media
381.05 Acute allergic mucoid otitis media
381.06 Acute allergic sanguinous otitis media

381.1# Chronic serous otitis media
381.10 Chronic serous otitis media, simple or unspecified
381.19 Other

381.#(#) *(continued)*

381.2# Chronic mucoid otitis media
381.20 Chronic mucoid otitis media, simple or unspecified
381.29 Other

381.3 Other and unspecified chronic nonsuppurative otitis media

381.4 Nonsuppurative otitis media, not specified as acute or chronic

381.5# Eustachian salpingitis
381.50 Eustachian salpingitis, unspecified
381.51 Acute Eustachian salpingitis
381.52 Chronic Eustachian salpingitis

381.6# Obstruction of Eustachian tube
381.60 Obstruction of Eustachian tube, unspecified
381.61 Osseous obstruction of Eustachian tube
381.62 Intrinsic cartilagenous obstruction of Eustachian tube
381.63 Extrinsic cartilagenous obstruction of Eustachian tube

381.7 Patulous Eustachian tube

381.8# Other disorders of Eustachian tube
381.81 Dysfunction of Eustachian tube
381.89 Other

381.9 Unspecified Eustachian tube disorder

382.#(#) Suppurative and unspecified otitis media

382.0# Acute suppurative otitis media
382.00 Acute suppurative otitis media without spontaneous rupture of ear drum
382.01 Acute suppurative otitis media with spontaneous rupture of ear drum
382.02 Acute suppurative otitis media in diseases classified elsewhere

382.1 Chronic tubotympanic suppurative otitis media
382.2 Chronic atticoantral suppurative otitis media
382.3 Unspecified chronic suppurative otitis media
382.4 Unspecified suppurative otitis media
382.9 Unspecified otitis media

383.#(#) Mastoiditis and related conditions

383.0# Acute mastoiditis
383.00 Acute mastoiditis without complications
383.01 Subperiosteal abscess of mastoid
383.02 Acute mastoiditis with other complications

383.1 Chronic mastoiditis

383.2# Petrositis
383.20 Petrositis, unspecified
383.21 Acute petrositis
383.22 Chronic petrositis

383.3# Complications following mastoidectomy
383.30 Postmastoidectomy complication, unspecified
383.31 Mucosal cyst of postmastoidectomy cavity
383.32 Recurrent cholesteatoma of postmastoidectomy cavity
383.33 Granulations of postmastoidectomy cavity

383.8# Other disorders of mastoid
383.81 Postauricular fistula
383.89 Other

383.9 Unspecified mastoiditis

384.#(#) Other disorders of tympanic membrane

384.0# Acute myringitis without mention of otitis media
384.00 Acute myringitis, unspecified
384.01 Bullous myringitis
384.09 Other

384.1 Chronic myringitis without mention of otitis media

384.#(#) ***(continued)***

384.2# Perforation of tympanic membrane
384.20 Perforation of tympanic membrane, NOS
384.21 Central perforation of tympanic membrane
384.22 Attic perforation of tympanic membrane
384.23 Other marginal perforation of tympanic membrane
384.24 Multiple perforations of tympanic membrane
384.25 Total perforation of tympanic membrane
384.8# Other specified disorders of tympanic membrane
384.81 Atrophic flaccid tympanic membrane
384.82 Atrophic nonflaccid tympanic membrane
384.9 Unspecified disorder of tympanic membrane

385.#(#) Other disorders of middle ear and mastoid

385.0# Tympanosclerosis
385.00 Tympanosclerosis, unspecified as to involvement
385.01 Tympanosclerosis involving tympanic membrane only
385.02 Tympanosclerosis involving tympanic membrane and ear ossicles
385.03 Tympanosclerosis involving tympanic membrane, ear ossicles, and middle ear
385.09 Tympanosclerosis involving other combination of structures
385.1# Adhesive middle ear disease
385.10 Adhesive middle ear disease, unspecified as to involvement
385.11 Adhesions of drum head to incus
385.12 Adhesions of drum head to stapes
385.13 Adhesions of drum head to promontorium
385.19 Other adhesions and combinations
385.2# Other acquired abnormality of ear ossicles
385.21 Impaired mobility of malleus
385.22 Impaired mobility of other ear ossicles
385.23 Discontinuity or dislocation of ear ossicles
385.24 Partial loss or necrosis of ear ossicles
385.3# Cholesteatoma of middle ear and mastoid
385.30 Cholesteatoma, unspecified
385.31 Cholesteatoma of attic
385.32 Cholesteatoma of middle ear
385.33 Cholesteatoma of middle ear and mastoid
385.35 Diffuse cholesteatosis
385.8# Other disorders of middle ear and mastoid
385.82 Cholesterin granuloma
385.83 Retained foreign body of middle ear
385.89 Other
385.9 Unspecified disorder of middle ear and mastoid

386.#(#) Vertiginous syndromes and other disorders of vestibular system

386.0# Méniére's disease
386.00 Méniére's disease, unspecified
386.01 Active Méniére's disease
386.02 Active Méniére's disease, cochlear
386.03 Active Méniére's disease, vestibular
386.04 Inactive Méniére's disease
386.1# Other and unspecified peripheral vertigo
386.10 Peripheral vertigo, unspecified
386.11 Benign paroxysmal positional vertigo
386.12 Vestibular neuronitis
386.19 Other
386.2 Vertigo of central origin

386.#(#) ***(continued)***

386.3# Labyrinthitis
386.30 Labyrinthitis, unspecified
386.31 Serous labyrinthitis
386.32 Circumscribed labyrinthitis
386.33 Suppurative labyrinthitis
386.34 Toxic labyrinthitis
386.35 Viral labyrinthitis
386.4# Labyrinthine fistula
386.40 Labyrinthine fistula, unspecified
386.41 Round window fistula
386.42 Oval window fistula
386.43 Semicircular canal fistula
386.48 Labyrinthine fistula of combined sites
386.5# Labyrinthine dysfunction
386.50 Labyrinthine dysfunction, unspecified
386.51 Hyperactive labyrinth, unilateral
386.52 Hyperactive labyrinth, bilateral
386.53 Hypoactive labyrinth, unilateral
386.54 Hypoactive labyrinth, bilateral
386.55 Loss of labyrinthine reactivity, unilateral
386.56 Loss of labyrinthine reactivity, bilateral
386.58 Other forms and combinations
386.8 Other disorders of labyrinth
386.9 Unspecified vertiginous syndromes and labyrinthine disorders

387.# Otosclerosis

387.0 Otosclerosis involving oval window, nonobliterative
387.1 Otosclerosis involving oval window, obliterative
387.2 Cochlear otosclerosis
387.8 Other otosclerosis
387.9 Otosclerosis, unspecified

388.#(#) Other disorders of ear

388.0# Degenerative and vascular disorders of ear
388.00 Degenerative and vascular disorders, unspecified
388.01 Presbyacusis
388.02 Transient ischemic deafness
388.1# Noise effects on inner ear
388.10 Noise effects on inner ear, unspecified
388.11 Acoustic trauma (explosive) to ear
388.12 Noise-induced hearing loss
388.2 Sudden hearing loss, unspecified
388.3# Tinnitus
388.30 Tinnitus, unspecified
388.31 Subjective tinnitus
388.32 Objective tinnitus
388.4# Other abnormal auditory perception
388.40 Abnormal auditory perception, unspecified
388.41 Diplacusis
388.42 Hyperacusis
388.43 Impairment of auditory discrimination
388.44 Recruitment
388.45 Acquired auditory processing disorder
388.5 Disorders of acoustic nerve
388.6# Otorrhea
388.60 Otorrhea, unspecified
388.61 Cerebrospinal fluid otorrhea
388.69 Other
388.7# Otalgia
388.70 Otalgia, unspecified
388.71 Otogenic pain
388.72 Referred pain
388.8 Other disorders of ear
388.9 Unspecified disorder of ear

389.#(#) Hearing loss
- **389.0#** Conductive hearing loss
  - 389.00 Conductive hearing loss, unspecified
  - 389.01 Conductive hearing loss, external ear
  - 389.02 Conductive hearing loss, tympanic membrane
  - 389.03 Conductive hearing loss, middle ear
  - 389.04 Conductive hearing loss, inner ear
  - 389.05 Conductive hearing loss, unilateral
  - 389.06 Conductive hearing loss, bilateral
  - 389.08 Conductive hearing loss of combined types
- **389.1#** Sensorineural hearing loss
  - 389.10 Sensorineural hearing loss, unspecified
  - 389.11 Sensory hearing loss, bilateral
  - 389.12 Neural hearing loss, bilateral
  - 389.13 Neural hearing loss, unilateral
  - 389.14 Central hearing loss
  - 389.15 Sensorineural hearing loss, unilateral
  - 389.16 Sensorineural hearing loss, asymmetrical
  - 389.17 Sensory hearing loss, unilateral
  - 389.18 Sensorineural hearing loss, bilateral
- **389.2#** Mixed conductive and sensorineural hearing loss
  - 389.20 Mixed hearing loss, unspecified
  - 389.21 Mixed hearing loss, unilateral
  - 389.22 Mixed hearing loss, bilateral
- 389.7 Deaf, nonspeaking, not elsewhere classifiable
- 389.8 Other specified forms of hearing loss
- 389.9 Unspecified hearing loss

390 Rheumatic fever without mention of heart involvement

391.# Rheumatic fever with heart involvement
- 391.0 Acute rheumatic pericarditis
- 391.1 Acute rheumatic endocarditis
- 391.2 Acute rheumatic myocarditis
- 391.8 Other acute rheumatic heart disease
- 391.9 Acute rheumatic heart disease, unspecified

392.# Rheumatic chorea
- 392.0 With heart involvement
- 392.9 Without mention of heart involvement

393 Chronic rheumatic pericarditis

394.# Diseases of mitral valve
- 394.0 Mitral stenosis
- 394.1 Rheumatic mitral insufficiency
- 394.2 Mitral stenosis with insufficiency
- 394.9 Other and unspecified mitral valve diseases

395.# Diseases of aortic valve
- 395.0 Rheumatic aortic stenosis
- 395.1 Rheumatic aortic insufficiency
- 395.2 Rheumatic aortic stenosis with insufficiency
- 395.9 Other and unspecified rheumatic aortic diseases

396.# Diseases of mitral and aortic valves
- 396.0 Mitral valve stenosis and aortic valve stenosis
- 396.1 Mitral valve stenosis and aortic valve insufficiency
- 396.2 Mitral valve insufficiency and aortic valve stenosis
- 396.3 Mitral valve insufficiency and aortic valve insufficiency
- 396.8 Multiple involvement of mitral and aortic valves
- 396.9 Mitral and aortic valve diseases, unspecified

397.# Diseases of other endocardial structures
- 397.0 Diseases of tricuspid valve
- 397.1 Rheumatic diseases of pulmonary valve
- 397.9 Rheumatic diseases of endocardium, valve unspecified

398.#(#) Other rheumatic heart disease
- 398.0 Rheumatic myocarditis
- **398.9#** Other and unspecified rheumatic heart diseases
  - 398.90 Rheumatic heart disease, unspecified
  - 398.91 Rheumatic heart failure (congestive)
  - 398.99 Other

401.# Essential hypertension
- 401.0 Malignant
- 401.1 Benign
- 401.9 Unspecified

402.## Hypertensive heart disease
- **402.0#** Malignant
- **402.1#** Benign
- **402.9#** Unspecified

5th Digit 402
- **0 Without heart failure**
- **1 With heart failure**

403.## Hypertensive chronic kidney disease
- **403.0#** Malignant
- **403.1#** Benign
- **403.9#** Unspecified

5th Digit: 403
- **0 With chronic kidney disease stage I through stage IV, or unspecified**
- **1 With chronic kidney disease stage V or end stage renal disease**

404.## Hypertensive heart and chronic kidney disease
- **404.0#** Malignant
- **404.1#** Benign
- **404.9#** Unspecified

5th digit: 404
- **0 Without heart failure and with chronic kdney disease stage I through stage IV, or unspecified**
- **1 With heart failure and with chronic kidney disease stage I through stage IV or unspecified**
- **2 Without heart failure and with chronic kidney disease stage V or end stage renal disease**
- **3 With heart failure and chronic kidney disease stage V or end stage renal disease**

405.## Secondary hypertension
- **405.0#** Malignant
- **405.1#** Benign
- **405.9#** Unspecified

5th Digit: 405
- **1 Renovascular**
- **9 Other**

410.## Acute myocardial infarction
- **410.0#** Of anterolateral wall
- **410.1#** Of other anterior wall
- **410.2#** Of inferolateral wall

5th Digit: 410
- **0 Episode of care unspecified**
- **1 Initial episode of care**
- **2 Subsequent episode of care**

410.## ***(continued)***
410.3# Of inferoposterior wall
410.4# Of other inferior wall
410.5# Of other lateral wall
410.6# True posterior wall infarction
410.7# Subendocardial infarction
410.8# Of other specified sites
410.9# Unspecified site
5th Digit: 410
0 Episode of care unspecified
1 Initial episode of care
2 Subsequent episode of care

411.#(#) Other acute and subacute forms of ischemic heart disease
411.0 Postmyocardial infarction syndrome
411.1 Intermediate coronary syndrome
411.8# Other
411.81 Acute coronary occlusion without myocardial infarction
411.89 Other
412 Old myocardial infarction

413.# Angina pectoris
413.0 Angina decubitus
413.1 Prinzmetal angina
413.9 Other and unspecified angina pectoris

414.#(#) Other forms of chronic ischemic heart disease
414.0# Coronary atherosclerosis
414.00 Of unspecified type of vessel, native or graft
414.01 Of native coronary artery
414.02 Of autologous biological bypass graft
414.03 Of nonautologous biological bypass graft
414.04 Of artery bypass graft
414.05 Of unspecified type of bypass graft
414.06 Of native coronary artery of transplanted heart
414.07 Of bypass graft (artery) (vein) of transplanted heart
414.1# Aneurysm and dissection of heart
414.10 Aneurysm of heart (wall)
414.11 Aneurysm of coronary vessels
414.12 Dissection of coronary artery
414.19 Other aneurysm of heart
414.2 Chronic total occlusion of coronary artery
414.8 Other specified forms of chronic ischemic heart disease
414.9 Chronic ischemic heart disease, unspecified

415.#(#) Acute pulmonary heart disease
415.0 Acute cor pulmonale
415.1# Pulmonary embolism and infarction
415.11 Iatrogenic pulmonary embolism and infarction
415.12 Septic pulmonary embolism
415.19 Other pulmonary embolism and infarction
416.# Chronic pulmonary heart disease
416.0 Primary pulmonary hypertension
416.1 Kyphoscoliotic heart disease
416.8 Other chronic pulmonary heart diseases
416.9 Chronic pulmonary heart disease, unspecified

417.# Other diseases of pulmonary circulation
417.0 Arteriovenous fistula of pulmonary vessels
417.1 Aneurysm of pulmonary artery

417.## ***(continued)***
417.8 Other specified diseases of pulmonary circulation
417.9 Unspecified disease of pulmonary circulation

420.#(#) Acute pericarditis
420.0 Acute pericarditis in diseases classified elsewhere
420.9# Other and unspecified acute pericarditis
420.90 Acute pericarditis, unspecified
420.91 Acute idiopathic pericarditis
420.99 Other

421.# Acute and subacute endocarditis
421.0 Acute and subacute bacterial endocarditis
421.1 Acute and subacute infective endocarditis in diseases classified elsewhere
421.9 Acute endocarditis, unspecified

422.#(#) Acute myocarditis
422.0 Acute myocarditis in diseases classified elsewhere
422.9# Other and unspecified acute myocarditis
422.90 Acute myocarditis, unspecified
422.91 Idiopathic myocarditis
422.92 Septic myocarditis
422.93 Toxic myocarditis
422.99 Other

423.# Other diseases of pericardium
423.0 Hemopericardium
423.1 Adhesive pericarditis
423.2 Constrictive pericarditis
423.3 Cardiac tamponade
423.8 Other specified diseases of pericardium
423.9 Unspecified disease of pericardium

424.#(#) Other diseases of endocardium
424.0 Mitral valve disorders
424.1 Aortic valve disorders
424.2 Tricuspid valve disorders, specified as nonrheumatic
424.3 Pulmonary valve disorders
424.9# Endocarditis, valve unspecified
424.90 Endocarditis, valve unspecified, casuse NOS
424.91 Endocarditis in diseases classified elsewhere
424.99 Other

425.# Cardiomyopathy
425.0 Endomyocardial fibrosis
425.1 Hypertrophic obstructive cardiomyopathy
425.2 Obscure cardiomyopathy of Africa
425.3 Endocardial fibroelastosis
425.4 Other primary cardiomyopathies
425.5 Alcoholic cardiomyopathy
425.7 Nutritional and metabolic cardiomyopathy
425.8 Cardiomyopathy in other diseases classified elsewhere
425.9 Secondary cardiomyopathy, unspecified

426.#(#) Conduction disorders
426.0 Atrioventricular block, complete
426.1# Atrioventricular block, other and unspecified
426.10 Atrioventricular block, unspecified
426.11 First degree atrioventricular block
426.12 Mobitz (type) II atrioventricular block
426.13 Other second degree atrioventricular block

NUMERICAL REFERENCE

426.#(#) ***(continued)***
426.2 Left bundle branch hemiblock
426.3 Other left bundle branch block
426.4 Right bundle branch block
426.5# Bundle branch block, other and unspecified
426.50 Bundle branch block, unspecified
426.51 Right bundle branch block and left posterior fascicular block
426.52 Right bundle branch block and left anterior fascicular block
426.53 Other bilateral bundle branch block
426.54 Trifascicular block
426.6 Other heart block
426.7 Anomalous atrioventricular excitation
426.8# Other specified conduction disorders
426.81 Lown-Ganong-Levine syndrome
426.82 Long QT syndrome
426.89 Other
426.9 Conduction disorder, unspecified

427.#(#) Cardiac dysrhythmias
427.0 Paroxysmal supraventricular tachycardia
427.1 Paroxysmal ventricular tachycardia
427.2 Paroxysmal tachycardia, unspecified
427.3# Atrial fibrillation and flutter
427.31 Atrial fibrillation
427.32 Atrial flutter
427.4# Ventricular fibrillation and flutter
427.41 Ventricular fibrillation
427.42 Ventricular flutter
427.5 Cardiac arrest
427.6# Premature beats
427.60 Premature beats, unspecified
427.61 Supraventricular premature beats
427.69 Other
427.8# Other specified cardiac dysrhythmias
427.81 Sinoatrial node dysfunction
427.89 Other
427.9 Cardiac dysrhythmia, unspecified

428.#(#) Heart failure
428.0 Congestive heart failure, unspecified
428.1 Left heart failure
428.2# Systolic heart failure
428.3# Diastolic heart failure
428.4# Systolic and Diastolic heart failure
5th digit: 428.2-4
0 Unspecified
1 Acute
2 Chronic
3 Acute and chronic
428.9 Heart failure, unspecified

429.#(#) Ill-defined descriptions and complications of heart disease
429.0 Myocarditis, unspecified
429.1 Myocardial degeneration
429.2 Cardiovascular disease, unspecified
429.3 Cardiomegaly
429.4 Functional disturbances following cardiac surgery
429.5 Rupture of chordae tendineae
429.6 Rupture of papillary muscle
429.7# Certain sequelae of myocardial infarction, NEC
429.71 Acquired cardiac septal defect
429.79 Other
429.8# Other ill-defined heart diseases
429.81 Other disorders of papillary muscle
429.82 Hyperkinetic heart disease
429.83 Takotsubo syndrome
429.89 Other
429.9 Heart disease, unspecified

430 Subarachnoid hemorrhage

431 Intracerebral hemorrhage

432.# Other and unspecified intracranial hemorrhage
432.0 Nontraumatic extradural hemorrhage
432.1 Subdural hemorrhage
432.9 Unspecified intracranial hemorrhage

433.## Occlusion and stenosis of precerebral arteries
433.0# Basilar artery
433.1# Carotid artery
433.2# Vertebral artery
433.3# Multiple and bilateral
433.8# Other specified precerebral artery
433.9# Unspecified precerebral artery
5th Digit: 433
0 Without mention of cerebral infarction
1 With cerebral infarction

434.## Occlusion of cerebral arteries
434.0# Cerebral thrombosis
434.1# Cerebral embolism
434.9# Cerebral artery occlusion, unspecified
5th Digit: 434
0 Without mention of cerebral infarction
1 With cerebral infarction

435.# Transient cerebral ischemia
435.0 Basilar artery syndrome
435.1 Vertebral artery syndrome
435.2 Subclavian steal syndrome
435.3 Vertebrobasilar artery syndrome
435.8 Other specified transient cerebral ischemias
435.9 Unspecified transient cerebral ischemia

436 Acute, but ill-defined, cerebrovascular disease

437.# Other and ill-defined cerebrovascular disease
437.0 Cerebral atherosclerosis
437.1 Other generalized ischemic cerebrovascular disease
437.2 Hypertensive encephalopathy
437.3 Cerebral aneurysm, nonruptured
437.4 Cerebral arteritis
437.5 Moyamoya disease
437.6 Nonpyogenic thrombosis of intracranial venous sinus
437.7 Transient global amnesia
437.8 Other
437.9 Unspecified

438.#(#) Late effects of cerebrovascular disease
438.0 Cognitive deficits
438.1# Speech and language deficits
438.10 Speech and language deficit, unspecified
438.11 Aphasia
438.12 Dysphasia
438.19 Other speech and language deficits
438.2# Hemiplegia/hemiparesis
438.3# Monoplegia of upper limb
438.4# Monoplegia of lower limb
5th Digit: 438.2-4
0 Affecting unspecified side
1 Affecting dominant side
2 Affecting nondominant side
438.5# Other paralytic syndrome
438.50 Affecting unspecified side
438.51 Affecting dominant side

NUMERICAL REFERENCE

438.#(#) ***(continued)***
438.5# **(continued)**
438.52 Affecting nondominant side
438.53 Bilateral
438.6 Alterations of sensations
438.7 Disturbances of vision
438.8# Other late effects of cerebrovascular disease
438.81 Apraxia
438.82 Dysphagia
438.83 Facial weakness
438.84 Ataxia
438.85 Vertigo
438.89 Other late effects of cerebrovascular disease
438.9 Unspecified late effects of cerebrovascular disease

440.#(#) Atherosclerosis
440.0 Of aorta
440.1 Of renal artery
440.2# Of native arteries of the extremities
440.20 Atherosclerosis of the extremities, unspecified
440.21 Atherosclerosis of the extremities with intermittent claudication
440.22 Atherosclerosis of the extremities with rest pain
440.23 Atherosclerosis of the extremities with ulceration
440.24 Atherosclerosis of the extremities with gangrene
440.29 Other
440.3# Of bypass graft of the extremities
440.30 Of unspecified graft
440.31 Of autologous vein bypass graft
440.32 Of nonautologous vein bypass graft
440.4 Chronic total occlusion of artery of the extremity
440.8 Of other specified arteries
440.9 Generalized and unspecified atherosclerosis

441.#(#) Aortic aneurysm and dissection
441.0# Dissection of aorta
441.00 Unspecified site
441.01 Thoraci
441.02 Abdominal
441.03 Thoracoabdominal
441.1 Thoracic aneurysm, ruptured
441.2 Thoracic aneurysm without mention of rupture
441.3 Abdominal aneurysm, ruptured
441.4 Abdominal aneurysm without mention of rupture
441.5 Aortic aneurysm of unspecified site, ruptured
441.6 Thoracoabdominal aneurysm, ruptured
441.7 Thoracoabdominal aneurysm, without mention of rupture
441.9 Aortic aneurysm of unspecified site without mention of rupture

442.#(#) Other aneurysm
442.0 Of artery of upper extremity
442.1 Of renal artery
442.2 Of iliac artery
442.3 Of artery of lower extremity
442.8# Of other specified artery
442.81 Artery of neck
442.82 Subclavian artery
442.83 Splenic artery
442.84 Other visceral artery
442.89 Other artery
442.9 Of unspecified site

443.#(#) Other peripheral vascular disease
443.0 Raynaud's syndrome
443.1 Thromboangiitis obliterans [Buerger's disease]
443.2# Other arterial dissection
443.21 of carotid artery
443.22 of iliac artery
443.23 of renal artery
443.24 of vertebral artery
443.29 of other artery
443.8# Other specified peripheral vascular diseases
443.81 Peripheral angiopathy in diseases classified elsewhere
443.82 Erythromelalgia
443.89 Other
443.9 Peripheral vascular disease, unspecified

444.#(#) Arterial embolism and thrombosis
444.0 Of abdominal aorta
444.1 Of thoracic aorta
444.2# Of arteries of the extremities
444.21 Upper extremity
444.22 Lower extremity
444.8# Of other specified artery
444.81 Iliac artery
444.89 Other
444.9 Of unspecified artery

445.## Atheroembolism
445.0# Of extremities
445.01 Upper extremity
445.02 Lover extremity
445.8# Other site
445.81 Kidney
445.89 Other site

446.#(#) Polyarteritis nodosa and allied conditions
446.0 Polyarteritis nodosa
446.1 Acute febrile mucocutaneous lymph node syndrome [MCLS]
446.2# Hypersensitivity angiitis
446.20 Hypersensitivity angiitis, unspecified
446.21 Goodpasture's syndrome
446.29 Other specified hypersensitivity angiitis
446.3 Lethal midline granuloma
446.4 Wegener's granulomatosis
446.5 Giant cell arteritis
446.6 Thrombotic microangiopathy
446.7 Takayasu's disease

447.# Other disorders of arteries and arterioles
447.0 Arteriovenous fistula, acquired
447.1 Stricture of artery
447.2 Rupture of artery
447.3 Hyperplasia of renal artery
447.4 Celiac artery compression syndrome
447.5 Necrosis of artery
447.6 Arteritis, unspecified
447.8 Other specified disorders of arteries and arterioles
447.9 Unspecified disorders of arteries and arterioles

448.# Disease of capillaries
448.0 Hereditary hemorrhagic telangiectasia
448.1 Nevus, non-neoplastic
448.9 Other and unspecified capillary diseases

449 Septic arterial embolism

451.#(#) Phlebitis and thrombophlebitis
- 451.0 Of superficial vessels of lower extremities
- **451.1#** Of deep vessels of lower extremities
  - 451.11 Femoral vein (deep) (superficial)
  - 451.19 Other
- 451.2 Of lower extremities, unspecified
- **451.8#** Of other sites
  - 451.81 Iliac vein
  - 451.82 Of superficial veins of upper extremities
  - 451.83 Of deep veins of upper extremities
  - 451.84 Of upper extremities, unspecified
  - 451.89 Other veins
- 451.9 Of unspecified site

452 Portal vein thrombosis

453.#(#) Other venous embolism and thrombosis
- 453.0 Budd-Chiari syndrome
- 453.1 Thrombophlebitis migrans
- 453.2 Of vena cava
- 453.3 Of renal vein
- **453.4#** Venous embolism and thrombosis of deep vessels of lower extremity
  - 453.40 Venous embolism and thrombosis of deep vessels of lower extremity
  - 453.41 Venous embolism and thrombosis of deep vessels of proximal lower extremity
  - 453.42 Venous embolism and thrombosis of deep vessels of distal lower extremity
- 453.8 Of other specified veins
- 453.9 Of unspecified site

454.# Varicose veins of lower extremities
- 454.0 With ulcer
- 454.1 With inflammation
- 454.2 With ulcer and inflammation
- 454.8 With other complication
- 454.9 Asymptomatic varicose veins

455.# Hemorrhoids
- 455.0 Internal hemorrhoids without mention of complication
- 455.1 Internal thrombosed hemorrhoids
- 455.2 Internal hemorrhoids with other complication
- 455.3 External hemorrhoids without complication
- 455.4 External thrombosed hemorrhoids
- 455.5 External hemorrhoids with other complication
- 455.6 Hemorrhoids without complication, NOS
- 455.7 Unspecified thrombosed hemorrhoids
- 455.8 Unspecified hemorrhoids with other complication
- 455.9 Residual hemorrhoidal skin tags

456.#(#) Varicose veins of other sites
- 456.0 Esophageal varices with bleeding
- 456.1 Esophageal varices without mention of bleeding
- **456.2#** Esophageal varices in diseases classified elsewhere
  - 456.20 With bleeding
  - 456.21 Without mention of bleeding
- 456.3 Sublingual varices
- 456.4 Scrotal varices
- 456.5 Pelvic varices
- 456.6 Vulval varices
- 456.8 Varices of other sites

457.# Noninfectious disorders of lymphatic channels
- 457.0 Postmastectomy lymphedema syndrome
- 457.1 Other lymphedema
- 457.2 Lymphangitis

457.# ***(continued)***
- 457.8 Noninfectious disorders of lymphatic channels, other
- 457.9 Unspecified noninfectious disorder of lymphatic channels

458.#(#) Hypotension
- 458.0 Orthostatic hypotension
- 458.1 Chronic hypotension
- **458.2#** Iatrogenic hypotension
  - 458.21 Hypotension of hemodialysis
  - 458.29 Other iatrogenic hypotension
- 458.8 Other specified hypotension
- 458.9 Hypotension, unspecified

459.#(#) Other disorders of circulatory system
- 459.0 Hemorrhage, unspecified
- **459.1#** Postphlebitic syndrome
  - 459.10 without complication
  - 459.11 with ulcer
  - 459.12 with inflammation
  - 459.13 with ulcer and inflammation
  - 459.19 with other complications
- 459.2 Compression of vein
- **459.3# Chronic venous hypertension (idiopathic)**
  - 459.30 without complication
  - 459.31 with ulcer
  - 459.32 with inflammation
  - 459.33 with ulcer and inflammation
  - 459.39 with other complications
- **459.8#** Other specified disorders of circulatory system
  - 459.81 Venous (peripheral) insufficiency, unspecified
  - 459.89 Other
- 459.9 Unspecified circulatory system disorder

460 Acute nasopharyngitis [common cold]

461.# Acute sinusitis
- 461.0 Maxillary
- 461.1 Frontal
- 461.2 Ethmoidal
- 461.3 Sphenoidal
- 461.8 Other acute sinusitis
- 461.9 Acute sinusitis, unspecified

462 Acute pharyngitis

463 Acute tonsillitis

464.#(#) Acute laryngitis and tracheitis
- **464.0#** Acute laryngitis
- **464.1#** Acute tracheitis
- **464.2#** Acute laryngotracheitis
- **464.3#** Acute epiglottitis
  - **5th Digit: 464.0-464.3**
    - **0 Without mention of obstruction**
    - **1 With obstruction**
- 464.4 Croup
- **464.5#** Supraglottitis unspecified
  - **5th Digit: 464.5**
    - **0 Without mention of obstruction**
    - **1 With obstruction**

465.# Acute upper respiratory infections of multiple or unspecified sites
- 465.0 Acute laryngopharyngitis
- 465.8 Other multiple sites
- 465.9 Unspecified site

NUMERICAL REFERENCE

466.#(#) Acute bronchitis and bronchiolitis
466.0 Acute bronchitis
466.1# Acute bronchiolitis
466.11 Acute bronchiolitis due to respiratory syncytial virus (RSV)
466.19 Acute bronchiolitis due to other infectious organisms

470 Deviated nasal septum

471.# Nasal polyps
471.0 Polyp of nasal cavity
471.1 Polypoid sinus degeneration
471.8 Other polyp of sinus
471.9 Unspecified nasal polyp

472.# Chronic pharyngitis and nasopharyngitis
472.0 Chronic rhinitis
472.1 Chronic pharyngitis
472.2 Chronic nasopharyngitis

473.# Chronic sinusitis
473.0 Maxillary
473.1 Frontal
473.2 Ethmoidal
473.3 Sphenoidal
473.8 Other chronic sinusitis
473.9 Unspecified sinusitis (chronic)

474.#(#) Chronic disease of tonsils and adenoids
474.0# Chronic tonsillitis and adenoiditis
474.00 Chronic tonsillitis
474.01 Chronic adenoiditis
474.02 Chronic tonsillitis and adenoiditis
474.1# Hypertrophy of tonsils and adenoids
474.10 Tonsils with adenoids
474.11 Tonsils alone
474.12 Adenoids alone
474.2 Adenoid vegetations
474.8 Other chronic disease of tonsils and adenoids
474.9 Unspecified chronic disease of tonsils and adenoids

475 Peritonsillar abscess

476.# Chronic laryngitis and laryngotracheitis
476.0 Chronic laryngitis
476.1 Chronic laryngotracheitis

477.# Allergic rhinitis
477.0 Due to pollen
477.1 Due to food
477.2 Due to animal (cat) (dog) hair and dander
477.8 Due to other allergen
477.9 Cause unspecified

478.#(#) Other diseases of upper respiratory tract
478.0 Hypertrophy of nasal turbinates
478.1# Other diseases of nasal cavity and sinuses
478.11 Nasal mucositis (ulcerative)
478.19 Other diseases of nasal cavity and sinuses
478.2# Other diseases of pharynx, NEC
478.20 Unspecified disease of pharynx
478.21 Cellulitis of pharynx or nasopharynx
478.22 Parapharyngeal abscess
478.24 Retropharyngeal abscess
478.25 Edema of pharynx or nasopharynx

478.#(#) ***(continued)***
478.2# (continued)
478.26 Cyst of pharynx or nasopharynx
478.29 Other
478.3# Paralysis of vocal cords or larynx
478.30 Paralysis, unspecified
478.31 Unilateral, partial
478.32 Unilateral, complete
478.33 Bilateral, partial
478.34 Bilateral, complete
478.4 Polyp of vocal cord or larynx
478.5 Other diseases of vocal cords
478.6 Edema of larynx
478.7# Other diseases of larynx, NEC
478.70 Unspecified disease of larynx
478.71 Cellulitis and perichondritis of larynx
478.74 Stenosis of larynx
478.75 Laryngeal spasm
478.79 Other
478.8 Upper respiratory tract hypersensitivity reaction, site unspecified
478.9 Other and unspecified diseases of upper respiratory tract

480.# Viral pneumonia
480.0 Pneumonia due to adenovirus
480.1 Pneumonia due to respiratory syncytial virus
480.2 Pneumonia due to parainfluenza virus
480.3 Pneumonia due to SARS-associated coronavirus
480.8 Pneumonia due to other virus not elsewhere classified
480.9 Viral pneumonia, unspecified

481 Pneumococcal pneumonia [streptococcus pneumoniae pneumonia]

482.#(#) Other bacterial pneumonia
482.0 Pneumonia due to Klebsiella pneumoniae
482.1 Pneumonia due to Pseudomonas
482.2 Pneumonia due to Hemophilus influenzae (H. influenzae)
482.3# Pneumonia due to Streptococcus
482.30 Streptococcus, unspecified
482.31 Group A
482.32 Group B
482.39 Other Streptococcus
482.4# Pneumonia due to Staphylococcus
482.40 Pneumonia due to Staphylococcus, NOS
482.41 Pneumonia due to Staphylococcus aureus
482.49 Other Staphylococcus pneumonia
482.8# Pneumonia due to other specified bacteria
482.81 Anaerobes
482.82 Escherichia coli [E. coli]
482.83 Other gram-negative bacteria
482.84 Legionnaires' disease
482.89 Other specified bacteria
482.9 Bacterial pneumonia unspecified

483.# Pneumonia due to other specified organism
483.0 Mycoplasma pneumoniae
483.1 Chlamydia
483.8 Other specified organism

484.# Pneumonia in infectious diseases classified elsewhere
484.1 Pneumonia in cytomegalic inclusion disease
484.3 Pneumonia in whooping cough

NUMERICAL REFERENCE

484.# ***(continued)***
484.5 Pneumonia in anthrax
484.6 Pneumonia in aspergillosis
484.7 Pneumonia in other systemic mycoses
484.8 Pneumonia in other infectious diseases classified elsewhere

485 Bronchopneumonia, organism unspecified

486 Pneumonia, organism unspecified

487.# Influenza
487.0 With pneumonia
487.1 With other respiratory manifestations
487.8 With other manifestations

488 Influenza due to identified avian influenza virus

490 Bronchitis, not specified as acute or chronic

491.#(#) Chronic bronchitis
491.0 Simple chronic bronchitis
491.1 Mucopurulent chronic bronchitis
491.2# Obstructive chronic bronchitis
491.20 Without exacerbation
491.21 With (acute) exacerbation
491.22 With acute bronchitis
491.8 Other chronic bronchitis
491.9 Unspecified chronic bronchitis

492.# Emphysema
492.0 Emphysematous bleb
492.8 Other emphysema

493.## Asthma
493.0# Extrinsic asthma
493.1# Intrinsic asthma
493.2# Chronic obstructive asthma
5th Digit: 493
0 Unspecified
1 With status asthmaticus
2 With (acute) exacerbation
493.8# Other forms of Asthma
493.81 Exercise induced bronchospasm
493.82 Cough variant asthma
493.9# Asthma, unspecified
5th Digit: 493
0 Unspecified
1 With status asthmaticus
2 With (acute) exacerbation

494.# Bronchiectasis
494.0 Bronchiectasis without acute exacerbation
494.1 Bronchiectasis with acute exacerbation

495.# Extrinsic allergic alveolitis
495.0 Farmers' lung
495.1 Bagassosis
495.2 Bird-fanciers' lung
495.3 Suberosis
495.4 Malt workers' lung
495.5 Mushroom workers' lung
495.6 Maple bark-strippers' lung
495.7 "Ventilation" pneumonitis
495.8 Other specified allergic alveolitis and pneumonitis
495.9 Unspecified allergic alveolitis and pneumonitis

496 Chronic airway obstruction, not elsewhere classified

500 Coal workers' pneumoconiosis

501 Asbestosis

502 Pneumoconiosis due to other silica or silicates

503 Pneumoconiosis due to other inorganic dust

504 Pneumonopathy due to inhalation of other dust

505 Pneumoconiosis, unspecified

506.# Respiratory conditions due to chemical fumes and vapors
506.0 Bronchitis and pneumonitis due to fumes and vapors
506.1 Acute pulmonary edema due to fumes and vapors
506.2 Upper respiratory inflammation due to fumes and vapors
506.3 Other acute and subacute respiratory conditions due to fumes and vapors
506.4 Chronic respiratory conditions due to fumes and vapors
506.9 Unspecified respiratory conditions due to fumes and vapors

507.# Pneumonitis due to solids and liquids
507.0 Due to inhalation of food or vomitus
507.1 Due to inhalation of oils and essences
507.8 Due to other solids and liquids

508.# Respiratory conditions due to other and unspecified external agents
508.0 Acute pulmonary manifestations due to radiation
508.1 Chronic and other pulmonary manifestations due to radiation
508.8 Respiratory conditions due to other specified external agents
508.9 Respiratory conditions due to unspecified external agent

510.# Empyema
510.0 With fistula
510.9 Without mention of fistula

511.# Pleurisy
511.0 Without mention of effusion or current tuberculosis
511.1 With effusion, with mention of a bacterial cause other than tuberculosis
511.8 Other specified forms of effusion, except tuberculous
511.9 Unspecified pleural effusion

512.# Pneumothorax
512.0 Spontaneous tension pneumothorax
512.1 Iatrogenic pneumothorax
512.8 Other spontaneous pneumothorax

513.# Abscess of lung and mediastinum
513.0 Abscess of lung
513.1 Abscess of mediastinum

514 Pulmonary congestion and hypostasis

515 Postinflammatory pulmonary fibrosis

516.# Other alveolar and parietoalveolar pneumonopathy
- 516.0 Pulmonary alveolar proteinosis
- 516.1 Idiopathic pulmonary hemosiderosis
- 516.2 Pulmonary alveolar microlithiasis
- 516.3 Idiopathic fibrosing alveolitis
- 516.8 Other specified alveolar and parietoalveolar pneumonopathies
- 516.9 Unspecified alveolar and parietoalveolar pneumonopathy

517.# Lung involvement in conditions classified elsewhere
- 517.1 Rheumatic pneumonia
- 517.2 Lung involvement in systemic sclerosis
- 517.3 Acute chest syndrome
- 517.8 Lung involvement in other diseases classified elsewhere

518.#(#) Other diseases of lung
- 518.0 Pulmonary collapse
- 518.1 Interstitial emphysema
- 518.2 Compensatory emphysema
- 518.3 Pulmonary eosinophilia
- 518.4 Acute edema of lung, unspecified
- 518.5 Pulmonary insufficiency following trauma and surgery
- 518.6 Allergic bronchopulmonary aspergillosis
- 518.7 Transfusion related acute lung injury (TRALI)
- **518.8#** Other diseases of lung
  - 518.81 Acute respiratory failure
  - 518.82 Other pulmonary insufficiency, NEC
  - 518.83 Chronic respiratory failure
  - 518.84 Acute and chronic respiratory failure
  - 518.89 Other diseases of lung, NEC

519.#(#) Other diseases of respiratory system
- **519.0#** Tracheostomy complications
  - 519.00 Tracheostomy complication, unspecified
  - 519.01 Infection of tracheostomy
  - 519.02 Mechanical complication of tracheostomy
  - 519.09 Other tracheostomy complications
- **519.1#** Other diseases of trachea and bronchus, NEC
  - 519.11 Acute bronchospasm
  - 519.19 Other diseases of trachea and bronchus
- 519.2 Mediastinitis
- 519.3 Other diseases of mediastinum, not elsewhere classified
- 519.4 Disorders of diaphragm
- 519.8 Other diseases of respiratory system, not elsewhere classified
- 519.9 Unspecified disease of respiratory system

520.# Disorders of tooth development and eruption
- 520.0 Anodontia
- 520.1 Supernumerary teeth
- 520.2 Abnormalities of size and form
- 520.3 Mottled teeth
- 520.4 Disturbances of tooth formation
- 520.5 Hereditary disturbances in tooth structure, not elsewhere classified
- 520.6 Disturbances in tooth eruption
- 520.7 Teething syndrome
- 520.8 Other specified disorders of tooth development and eruption
- 520.9 Unspecified disorder of tooth development and eruption

521.#(#) Diseases of hard tissues of teeth
- **521.0#** Dental caries
  - 521.00 Dental caries, unspecified
  - 521.01 Dental caries limited to enamel
  - 521.02 Dental caries extending into dentine
  - 521.03 Dental caries extending into pulp
  - 521.04 Arrested dental caries
  - 521.05 Odontoclasia
  - 521.06 Dental caries pit and fissure
  - 521.07 Dental caries smooth surface
  - 521.08 Dental caries root surface
  - 521.09 Other dental caries
- **521.1#** Excessive attrition (approximal wear) (occlusal wear)
  - 521.10 Excessive attrition, unspecified
  - 521.11 Excessive attrition, limited to enamel
  - 521.12 Excessive attrition, extending into dentine
  - 521.13 Excessive attrition, extending into pulp
  - 521.14 Excessive attrition, localized
  - 521.15 Excessive attrition, generalized
- **521.2#** Abrasion
  - 521.20 Abrasion, unspecified
  - 521.21 Abrasion, limited to enamel
  - 521.22 Abrasion, extending into dentine
  - 521.23 Abrasion, extending into pulp
  - 521.24 Abrasion, localized
  - 521.25 Abrasion, generalized
- **521.3#** Erosion
  - 521.30 Erosion, unspecified
  - 521.31 Erosion, limited to enamel
  - 521.32 Erosion, extending into dentine
  - 521.33 Erosion, extending into pulp
  - 521.34 Erosion, localized
  - 521.35 Erosion, generalized
- **521.4#** Pathological resorption
  - 521.40 Pathological resorption, unspecified
  - 521.41 Pathological resorption, internal
  - 521.42 Pathological resorption, external
  - 521.49 Other Pathological resorption
- 521.5 Hypercementosis
- 521.6 Ankylosis of teeth
- 521.7 Intrinsic posteruptive color changes
- **521.8#** Other specified diseases of hard tissues of teeth
  - 521.81 Cracked tooth
  - 521.89 Other specified diseases of hard tissues of teeth
- 521.9 Unspecified disease of hard tissues of teeth

522.# Diseases of pulp and periapical tissues
- 522.0 Pulpitis
- 522.1 Necrosis of the pulp
- 522.2 Pulp degeneration
- 522.3 Abnormal hard tissue formation in pulp
- 522.4 Acute apical periodontitis of pulpal origin
- 522.5 Periapical abscess without sinus
- 522.6 Chronic apical periodontitis
- 522.7 Periapical abscess with sinus
- 522.8 Radicular cyst
- 522.9 Other and unspecified diseases of pulp and periapical tissues

523.#(#) Gingival and periodontal disease
- **523.0#** Acute gingivitis
  - 523.00 Plaque induced
  - 523.01 Non-plaque induced
- **523.1#** Chronic gingivitis
  - 523.10 Plaque induced
  - 523.11 Non-plaque induced

523.#(#) ***(continued)***
523.2# Gingival recession
523.20 Gingival recession, unspecified
523.21 Gingival recession, minimal
523.22 Gingival recession, moderate
523.23 Gingival recession, severe
523.24 Gingival recession, localized
523.25 Gingival recession,, generalized
523.3# Aggressive and acute periodontitis
523.30 Aggressive periodontitis, unspecified
523.31 Aggressive periodontitis, localized
523.32 Aggressive periodontitis, generalized
523.33 Acute periodontitis
523.4# Chronic periodontitis
523.40 Chronic periodontitis, unspecified
523.41 Chronic periodontitis, localized
523.42 Chronic periodontitis, generalized
523.5 Periodontosis
523.6 Accretions on teeth
523.8 Other specified periodontal diseases
523.9 Unspecified gingival and periodontal disease

524.#(#) Dentofacial anomalies, including malocclusion
524.0# Major anomalies of jaw size
524.00 Unspecified anomaly
524.01 Maxillary hyperplasia
524.02 Mandibular hyperplasia
524.03 Maxillary hypoplasia
524.04 Mandibular hypoplasia
524.05 Macrogenia
524.06 Microgenia
524.07 Excessive tuberosity of jaw
524.09 Other specified anomaly
524.1# Anomalies of relationship of jaw to cranial base
524.10 Unspecified anomaly
524.11 Maxillary asymmetry
524.12 Other jaw asymmetry
524.19 Other specified anomaly
524.2# Anomalies of dental arch relationship
524.20 Unspecified anomaly of dental arch relationship
524.21 Malocclusion, Angle's class I
524.22 Malocclusion, Angle's class II
524.23 Malocclusion, Angle's class III
524.24 Open anterior occlusal relationship
524.25 Open posterior occlusal relationship
524.26 Excessive horizontal overlap
524.27 Reverse articulation
524.28 Anomalies of interarch distance
524.29 Other anomalies of dental arch relationship
524.3# Anomalies of tooth position of fuly erupted teeth
524.30 Unspecified anomaly of tooth position
524.31 Crowding of teeth
524.32 Excessive spacing of teeth
524.33 Horizontal displacement of teeth
524.34 Vertical displacement of teeth
524.35 Rotation of tooth/teeth
524.36 Insufficient interocclusal distance of teeth (ridge)
524.37 Excessive interocclusal distance of teeth
524.39 Other anomalies of tooth position
524.4 Malocclusion, unspecified
524.5# Dentofacial functional abnormalities
524.50 Dentofacial functional abnormality, unspecified
524.51 Abnormal jaw closure
524.52 Limited mandibular range of motion
524.53 Deviation in opening and closing of the mandible
524.54 Insufficient anterior guidance

524.#(#) ***(continued)***
524.5(#) (continued)
524.55 Centric occlusion maximum intercuspation discrepancy
524.56 Non-working side interference
524.57 Lack of posterior occlusal support
524.59 Other dentofacial functional abnormalities
524.6# Temporomandibular joint disorders
524.60 Temporomandibular joint disorders, NOS
524.61 Adhesions and ankylosis (bony or fibrous)
524.62 Arthralgia of temporomandibular joint
524.63 Articular disc disorder (reducing or nonreducing)
524.64 Temporomandibular joint sounds on opening and/or closing the jaw
524.69 Other specified temporomandibular joint disorders
524.7# Dental alveolar anomalies
524.70 Unspecified alveolar anomaly
524.71 Alveolar maxillary hyperplasia
524.72 Alveolar mandibular hyperplasia
524.73 Alveolar maxillary hypoplasia
524.74 Alveolar mandibular hypoplasia
524.75 Vertical displacement of alveolus and teeth
524.76 Occlusal plane deviation
524.79 Other specified alveolar anomaly
524.8# Other specified dentofacial anomalies
524.81 Anterior soft tissue impingement
524.82 Posterior soft tissue impingement
524.89 Other specified dentofacial anomalies
524.9 Unspecified dentofacial anomalies

525.#(#) Other diseases and conditions of the teeth and supporting structures
525.0 Exfoliation of teeth due to systemic causes
525.1# Loss of teeth due to trauma, extraction, or local periodontal disease
525.10 Acquired absence of teeth, unspecified
525.11 Loss of teeth due to trauma
525.12 Loss of teeth due to periodontal disease
525.13 Loss of teeth due to caries
525.19 Other loss of teeth
525.2# Atrophy of edentulous alveolar ridge
525.20 Unspecified atrophy of edentulous alveolar ridge
525.21 Minimal atrophy of the mandible
525.22 Moderate atrophy of the mandible
525.23 Severe atrophy of the mandible
525.24 Minimal atrophy of the maxilla
525.25 Moderate atrophy of the maxilla
525.26 Severe atrophy of the maxilla
525.3 Retained dental root
525.4# Complete endentulism
525.40 Unspecified
525.41 Class I
525.42 Class II
525.43 Class III
525.44 Class IV
525.5# Partial endentulism
525.50 Unspecified
525.51 Class I
525.52 Class II
525.53 Class III
525.54 Class IV
525.6# Unsatisfactory restoration of tooth
525.60 Unspecified
525.61 Open restoration margins
525.62 Unrepairable overhanging of dental restorative materials
525.63 Fractured dental restorative material without loss of material

525.#(#) *(continued)*

525.6(#) (continued)

525.64 Fractured dental restorative material with loss of material
525.65 Contour of existing restoration of tooth biologically incompatible with oral health
525.66 Allergy to existing dental restorative material
525.67 Poor anesthetics of existing restoration
525.69 Other unsatisfactory restoration of existing tooth

525.7# Endosseous dental implant failure
525.71 Osseointegration failure of dental implant
525.72 Post-osseointegration biological failure of dental implant
525.73 Post-osseointegration mechanical failure of dental implant
525.79 Other endosseous dental implant failure

525.8 Other specified disorders of the teeth and supporting structures
525.9 Unspecified disorder of the teeth and supporting structures

526.#(#) Diseases of the jaws

526.0 Dental caries
526.1 Fissural cysts of jaw
526.2 Other cysts of jaws
526.3 Central giant cell (reparative) granuloma
526.4 Inflammatory conditions
526.5 Alveolitis of jaw

526.6# Diseases of the jaws
526.61 Perforation of root canal space
526.62 Endodontic overfill
526.63 Endodontic underfill
526.69 Other periradicular pathology associated with previous endodontic treatment

526.8# Other specified diseases of the jaws
526.81 Exostosis of jaw
526.89 Other

526.9 Unspecified disease of the jaws

527.# Diseases of the salivary glands

527.0 Atrophy
527.1 Hypertrophy
527.2 Sialoadenitis
527.3 Abscess
527.4 Fistula
527.5 Sialolithiasis
527.6 Mucocele
527.7 Disturbance of salivary secretion
527.8 Other specified diseases of the salivary glands
527.9 Unspecified disease of the salivary glands

528.#(#) Diseases of the oral soft tissues, excluding lesions specific for gingiva and tongue

528.0# Stomatitis and mucositis (ulcerative)
528.00 Unspecified
528.01 Musositis (ulcerative) due to antineoplastic therapy
528.02 Mucositis (ulcerative) due to other drugs
528.09 Other

528.1 Cancrum oris
528.2 Oral aphthae
528.3 Cellulitis and abscess
528.4 Cysts
528.5 Diseases of lips
528.6 Leukoplakia of oral mucosa, including tongue

528.#(#) ***(continued)***

528.7# Other disturbances of oral epithelium, including tongue
528.71 Minimal keratinized residual ridge mucosa
528.72 Excessive keratinized residual ridge mucosa
528.79 Other disturbances of oral epithelium, including tongue

528.8 Oral submucosal fibrosis, including of tongue
528.9 Other and unspecified diseases of the oral soft tissues

529.# Diseases and other conditions of the tongue

529.0 Glossitis
529.1 Geographic tongue
529.2 Median rhomboid glossitis
529.3 Hypertrophy of tongue papillae
529.4 Atrophy of tongue papillae
529.5 Plicated tongue
529.6 Glossodynia
529.8 Other specified conditions of the tongue
529.9 Unspecified condition of the tongue

530.#(#) Diseases of esophagus

530.0 Achalasia and cardiospasm

530.1# Esophagitis
530.10 Esophagitis NOS
530.11 Reflux esophagitis
530.12 Acute esophagitis
530.19 Other esophagitis

530.2# Ulcer of esophagus
530.20 Ulcer of esophagus without bleeding
530.21 Ulcer of esophagus with bleeding

530.3 Stricture and stenosis of esophagus
530.4 Perforation of esophagus
530.5 Dyskinesia of esophagus
530.6 Diverticulum of esophagus, acquired
530.7 Gastroesophageal laceration-hemorrhage syndrome

530.8# Other specified disorders of esophagus
530.81 Esophageal reflux
530.82 Esophageal hemorrhage
530.83 Esophageal leukoplakia
530.84 Tracheoesophageal fistula
530.85 Barrett's esophagus
530.86 Infection of esophagostomy
530.87 Mechanical complication of esophagostomy
530.89 Other

530.9 Unspecified disorder of esophagus

531.## Gastric ulcer

531.0# Acute with hemorrhage
531.1# Acute with perforation
531.2# Acute with hemorrhage and perforation
531.3# Acute without mention of hemorrhage or perforation
531.4# Chronic or unspecified with hemorrhage
531.5# Chronic or unspecified with perforation
531.6# Chronic or unspecified with hemorrhage and perforation
531.7# Chronic without mention of hemorrhage or perforation
531.9# Unspecified as acute or chronic, without hemorrhage or perforation

5th Digit: 531
0 Without mention of obstruction
1 With obstruction

NUMERICAL REFERENCE

532.## Duodenal ulcer
- **532.0#** Acute with hemorrhage
- **532.1#** Acute with perforation
- **532.2#** Acute with hemorrhage and perforation
- **532.3#** Acute without mention of hemorrhage or perforation
- **532.4#** Chronic or unspecified with hemorrhage
- **532.5#** Chronic or unspecified with perforation
- **532.6#** Chronic or unspecified with hemorrhage and perforation
- **532.7#** Chronic without mention of hemorrhage or perforation
- **532.9#** Unspecified as acute or chronic, without hemorrhage or perforation

533.## Peptic ulcer, site unspecified
- **533.0#** Acute with hemorrhage
- **533.1#** Acute with perforation
- **533.2#** Acute with hemorrhage and perforation
- **533.3#** Acute without mention of hemorrhage and perforation
- **533.4#** Chronic or unspecified with hemorrhage
- **533.5#** Chronic or unspecified with perforation
- **533.6#** Chronic or unspecified with hemorrhage and perforation
- **533.7#** Chronic without mention of hemorrhage or perforation
- **533.9#** Unspecified as acute or chronic, without mention of hemorrhage or perforation

534.## Gastrojejunal ulcer
- **534.0#** Acute with hemorrhage
- **534.1#** Acute with perforation
- **534.2#** Acute with hemorrhage and perforation
- **534.3#** Acute without mention of hemorrhage or perforation
- **534.4#** Chronic or unspecified with hemorrhage
- **534.5#** Chronic or unspecified with perforation
- **534.6#** Chronic or unspecified with hemorrhage and perforation
- **534.7#** Chronic without mention of hemorrhage or perforation
- **534.9#** Unspecified as acute or chronic, without mention of hemorrhage or perforation

535.## Gastritis and duodenitis
- **535.0#** Acute gastritis
- **535.1#** Atrophic gastritis
- **535.2#** Gastric mucosal hypertrophy
- **535.3#** Alcoholic gastritis
- **535.4#** Other specified gastritis
- **535.5#** Unspecified gastritis and gastroduodenitis
- **535.6#** Duodenitis

5th Digit: 532-535
- **0 Without mention of obstruction**
- **1 With obstruction**

536.#(#) Disorders of function of stomach
- 536.0 Achlorhydria
- 536.1 Acute dilatation of stomach
- 536.2 Persistent vomiting
- 536.3 Gastroparesis, Gastroparalysis
- **536.4#** Gastrostomy complications
  - 536.40 Gastrostomy complication, unspecified
  - 536.41 Infection of gastrostomy
  - 536.42 Mechanical complication of gastrostomy
  - 536.49 Other gastrostomy complications
- 536.8 Dyspepsia and other specified disorders of function of stomach
- 536.9 Unspecified functional disorder of stomach

537.#(#) Other disorders of stomach and duodenum
- 537.0 Acquired hypertrophic pyloric stenosis
- 537.1 Gastric diverticulum
- 537.2 Chronic duodenal ileus
- 537.3 Other obstruction of duodenum
- 537.4 Fistula of stomach or duodenum
- 537.5 Gastroptosis
- 537.6 Hourglass stricture or stenosis of stomach
- **537.8#** Other disorders of stomach and duodenum
  - 537.81 Pylorospasm
  - 537.82 Angiodysplasia of stomach and duodenum without mention of hemorrhage
  - 537.83 Angiodysplasia of stomach and duodenum with hemorrhage
  - 537.84 Dieulafoy lesion (hemorrhagic) of stomach and duodenum
  - 537.89 Other
- 537.9 Unspecified disorder of stomach and duodenum

538 Gastrointestinal mucositis (ulcerative)

540.# Acute appendicitis
- 540.0 With generalized peritonitis
- 540.1 With peritoneal abscess
- 540.9 Without mention of peritonitis

541 Appendicitis, unqualified

542 Other appendicitis

543.# Other diseases of appendix
- 543.0 Hyperplasia of appendix (lymphoid)
- 543.9 Other and unspecified diseases of appendix

550.## Inguinal hernia
- **550.0#** Inguinal hernia, with gangrene
- **550.1#** Inguinal hernia, with obstruction, without mention of gangrene
- **550.9#** Inguinal hernia, without mention of obstruction or gangrene

5th Digit: 550
- **0 Unilateral or unspecified (not specified as recurrent)**
- **1 Unilateral or unspecified, recurrent**
- **2 Bilateral (not specified as recurrent) bilateral NOS**
- **3 Bilateral, recurrent**

551.#(#) Other hernia of abdominal cavity, with gangrene
- **551.0#** Femoral hernia with gangrene
  - 551.00 Unilateral or unspecified (not specified as recurrent)
  - 551.01 Unilateral or unspecified, recurrent
  - 551.02 Bilateral (not specified as recurrent)
  - 551.03 Bilateral, recurrent
- 551.1 Umbilical hernia with gangrene
- **551.2#** Ventral hernia with gangrene
  - 551.20 Ventral, unspecified, with gangrene
  - 551.21 Incisional, with gangrene
  - 551.29 Other
- 551.3 Diaphragmatic hernia with gangrene
- 551.8 Hernia of other specified sites, with gangrene
- 551.9 Hernia of unspecified site, with gangrene

552.#(#) Other hernia of abdominal cavity, with obstruction, but without mention of gangrene
- **552.0#** Femoral hernia with obstruction
  - 552.00 Unilateral or unspecified (not specified as recurrent)
  - 552.01 Unilateral or unspecified, recurrent

552.#(#) *(continued)*
552.0(#) (continued)
552.02 Bilateral (not specified as recurrent)
552.03 Bilateral, recurrent
552.1 Umbilical hernia with obstruction
552.2# Ventral hernia with obstruction
552.20 Ventral, unspecified, with obstruction
552.21 Incisional, with obstruction
552.29 Other
552.3 Diaphragmatic hernia with obstruction
552.8 Hernia of other specified sites, with obstruction
552.9 Hernia of unspecified site, with obstruction

553.#(#) Other hernia of abdominal cavity without mention of obstruction or gangrene
553.0# Femoral hernia
553.00 Unilateral or unspecified (not specified as recurrent)
553.01 Unilateral or unspecified, recurrent
553.02 Bilateral (not specified as recurrent)
553.03 Bilateral, recurrent
553.1 Umbilical hernia
553.2# Ventral hernia
553.20 Ventral, unspecified
553.21 Incisional
553.29 Other
553.3 Diaphragmatic hernia
553.8 Hernia of other specified sites
553.9 Hernia of unspecified site

555.# Regional enteritis
555.0 Small intestine
555.1 Large intestine
555.2 Small intestine with large intestine
555.9 Unspecified site

556.# Ulcerative colitis
556.0 Ulcerative (chronic) enterocolitis
556.1 Ulcerative (chronic) ileocolitis
556.2 Ulcerative (chronic) proctitis
556.3 Ulcerative (chronic) proctosigmoiditis
556.4 Pseudopolyposis of colon
556.5 Left-sided ulcerative (chronic) colitis
556.6 Universal ulcerative (chronic) colitis
556.8 Other ulcerative colitis
556.9 Ulcerative colitis, unspecified

557.# Vascular insufficiency of intestine
557.0 Acute vascular insufficiency of intestine
557.1 Chronic vascular insufficiency of intestine
557.9 Unspecified vascular insufficiency of intestine

558.# Other noninfectious gastroenteritis and colitis
558.1 Gastroenteritis and colitis due to radiation
558.2 Toxic gastroenteritis and colitis
558.3 Allergic gastroenteritis and colitis
558.9 Other and unspecified noninfectious gastroenteritis and colitis

560.#(#) Intestinal obstruction without mention of hernia
560.0 Intussusception
560.1 Paralytic ileus
560.2 Volvulus
560.3# Impaction of intestine
560.30 Impaction of intestine, unspecified
560.31 Gallstone ileus
560.39 Other

560.#(#) ***(continued)***
560.8# Other specified intestinal obstruction
560.81 Intestinal or peritoneal adhesions with obstruction (postoperative) (postinfection)
560.89 Other
560.9 Unspecified intestinal obstruction

562.#(#) Diverticula of intestine
562.0# Small intestine
562.00 Diverticulosis of small intestine (without mention of hemorrhage)
562.01 Diverticulitis of small intestine (without mention of hemorrhage)
562.02 Diverticulosis of small intestine with hemorrhage
562.03 Diverticulitis of small intestine with hemorrhage
562.1# Colon
562.10 Diverticulosis of colon (without mention of hemorrhage)
562.11 Diverticulitis of colon (without mention of hemorrhage)
562.12 Diverticulosis of colon with hemorrhage
562.13 Diverticulitis of colon with hemorrhage

564.#(#) Functional digestive disorders, not elsewhere classified
564.0(#) Constipation
564.00 Constipation, unspecified
564.01 Slow transit constipation
564.02 Outlet dysfunction constipation
564.09 Other constipation
564.1 Irritable bowel syndrome
564.2 Postgastric surgery syndromes
564.3 Vomiting following gastrointestinal surgery
564.4 Other postoperative functional disorders
564.5 Functional diarrhea
564.6 Anal spasm
564.7 Megacolon, other than Hirschsprung's
564.8# Other specified functional disorders of intestine
564.81 Neurogenic bowel
564.89 Other functional disorders of intestine
564.9 Unspecified functional disorder of intestine

565.# Anal fissure and fistula
565.0 Anal fissure
565.1 Anal fistula

566 Abscess of anal and rectal regions

567.#(#) Peritonitis and retroeritoneal infections
567.0 Peritonitis in infectious diseases classified elsewhere
567.1 Pneumococcal peritonitis
567.2# Other suppurative peritonitis
567.21 Peritonitis (acute) generalized
567.22 Peritoneal abscess
567.23 Spontaneous bacterial peritonitis
567.29 Other
567.3# Retroperitoneal infections
567.31 Psoas muscle abscess
567.38 Other retroperitoneal abscess
567.39 Other retroperitoneal infections
567.8# Other specified peritonitis
567.81 choleperitonitis
567.82 sclerosing mesenteritis
567.89 other specified peritonitis
567.9 Unspecified peritonitis

NUMERICAL REFERENCE

568.#(#) Other disorders of peritoneum
- 568.0 Peritoneal adhesions (postoperative) (postinfection)
- **568.8#** Other specified disorders of peritoneum
  - 568.81 Hemoperitoneum (nontraumatic)
  - 568.82 Peritoneal effusion (chronic)
  - 568.89 Other
- 568.9 Unspecified disorder of peritoneum

569.#(#) Other disorders of intestine
- 569.0 Anal and rectal polyp
- 569.1 Rectal prolapse
- 569.2 Stenosis of rectum and anus
- 569.3 Hemorrhage of rectum and anus
- **569.4#** Other specified disorders of rectum and anus
  - 569.41 Ulcer of anus and rectum
  - 569.42 Anal or rectal pain
  - 569.43 Anal sphincter tear (healed) (old)
  - 569.49 Other
- 569.5 Abscess of intestine
- **569.6#** Colostomy and enterostomy complications
  - 569.60 Colostomy and enterostomy complication, NOS
  - 569.61 Infection of colostomy and enterostomy
  - 569.62 Mechanical complication of colostomy and enterostomy
  - 569.69 Other complication
- **569.8.#** Other specified disorders of intestine
  - 569.81 Fistula of intestine, except rectum and anus
  - 569.82 Ulceration of intestine
  - 569.83 Perforation of intestine
  - 569.84 Angiodysplasia of intestine (without mention of hemorrhage)
  - 569.85 Angiodysplasia intestine with hemorrhage
  - 569.86 Dieulafoy lesion (hemorrhagic) or intestine
  - 569.89 Other
- 569.9 Unspecified disorder of intestine

570 Acute and subacute necrosis of liver

571.#(#) Chronic liver disease and cirrhosis
- 571.0 Alcoholic fatty liver
- 571.1 Acute alcoholic hepatitis
- 571.2 Alcoholic cirrhosis of liver
- 571.3 Alcoholic liver damage, unspecified
- **571.4#** Chronic hepatitis
  - 571.40 Chronic hepatitis, unspecified
  - 571.41 Chronic persistent hepatitis
  - 571.49 Other
- 571.5 Cirrhosis of liver without mention of alcohol
- 571.6 Biliary cirrhosis
- 571.8 Other chronic nonalcoholic liver disease
- 571.9 Chronic liver disease NOS without mention of alcohol

572.# Liver abscess and sequelae of chronic liver disease
- 572.0 Abscess of liver
- 572.1 Portal pyemia
- 572.2 Hepatic coma
- 572.3 Portal hypertension
- 572.4 Hepatorenal syndrome
- 572.8 Other sequelae of chronic liver disease

573.# Other disorders of liver
- 573.0 Chronic passive congestion of liver
- 573.1 Hepatitis in viral diseases classified elsewhere
- 573.2 Hepatitis in other infectious diseases classified elsewhere
- 573.3 Hepatitis, unspecified

573.# ***(continued)***
- 573.4 Hepatic infarction
- 573.8 Other specified disorders of liver
- 573.9 Unspecified disorder of liver

574.## Cholelithiasis
- **574.0#** Calculus of gallbladder with acute cholecystitis
- **574.1#** Calculus of gallbladder with other cholecystitis
- **574.2#** Calculus of gallbladder without mention of cholecystitis
- **574.3#** Calculus of bile duct with acute cholecystitis
- **574.4#** Calculus of bile duct with other cholecystitis
- **574.5#** Calculus of bile duct without mention of cholecystitis
- **574.6#** Calculus of gallbladder and bile duct with acute cholecystitis
- **574.7#** Calculus of gallbladder and bile duct with other cholecystitis
- **574.8#** Calculus of gallbladder and bile duct with acute and chronic cholecystitis
- **574.9#** Calculus of gallbladder and bile duct without cholecystitis

5th Digit: 574
- **0 Without mention of obstruction**
- **1 With obstruction**

575.#(#) Other disorders of gallbladder
- 575.0 Acute cholecystitis
- **575.1#** Other cholecystitis
  - 575.10 Cholecystitis, unspecified
  - 575.11 Chronic cholecystitis
  - 575.12 Acute and chronic cholecystitis
- 575.2 Obstruction of gallbladder
- 575.3 Hydrops of gallbladder
- 575.4 Perforation of gallbladder
- 575.5 Fistula of gallbladder
- 575.6 Cholesterolosis of gallbladder
- 575.8 Other specified disorders of gallbladder
- 575.9 Unspecified disorder of gallbladder

576.# Other disorders of biliary tract
- 576.0 Postcholecystectomy syndrome
- 576.1 Cholangitis
- 576.2 Obstruction of bile duct
- 576.3 Perforation of bile duct
- 576.4 Fistula of bile duct
- 576.5 Spasm of sphincter of Oddi
- 576.8 Other specified disorders of biliary tract
- 576.9 Unspecified disorder of biliary tract

577.# Diseases of pancreas
- 577.0 Acute pancreatitis
- 577.1 Chronic pancreatitis
- 577.2 Cyst and pseudocyst of pancreas
- 577.8 Other specified diseases of pancreas
- 577.9 Unspecified disease of pancreas

578.# Gastrointestinal hemorrhage
- 578.0 Hematemesis
- 578.1 Blood in stool
- 578.9 Hemorrhage of gastrointestinal tract, NOS

579.# Intestinal malabsorption
- 579.0 Celiac disease
- 579.1 Tropical sprue
- 579.2 Blind loop syndrome
- 579.3 Postsurgical nonabsorption, NOS and NEC
- 579.4 Pancreatic steatorrhea
- 579.8 Other specified intestinal malabsorption
- 579.9 Unspecified intestinal malabsorption

580.#(#) Acute glomerulonephritis
- 580.0 Lesion of proliferative glomerulonephritis
- 580.4 Lesion of rapidly progressive glomerulonephritis
- **580.8#** Pathological lesion in kidney NEC
  - 580.81 Acute glomerulonephritis in diseases classified elsewhere
  - 580.89 Other
- 580.9 Acute glomerulonephritis with pathological lesion in kidney, NOS

581.#(#) Nephrotic syndrome
- 581.0 With lesion of proliferative glomerulonephritis
- 581.1 With lesion of membranous glomerulonephritis
- 581.2 With lesion of membranoproliferative glomerulonephritis
- 581.3 With lesion of minimal change glomerulonephritis
- **581.8#** Pathological lesion in kidney, NEC
  - 581.81 Nephrotic syndrome in diseases classified elsewhere
  - 581.89 Other
- 581.9 Nephrotic syndrome with unspecified pathological lesion in kidney

582.#(#) Chronic glomerulonephritis
- 582.0 With lesion of proliferative glomerulonephritis
- 582.1 With lesion of membranous glomerulonephritis
- 582.2 With lesion of membranoproliferative glomerulonephritis
- 582.4 With lesion of rapidly progressive glomerulonephritis
- **582.8#** With other specified pathological lesion in kidney
  - 582.81 Chronic glomerulonephritis in diseases classified elsewhere
  - 582.89 Other
- 582.9 Chronic glomerulonephritis with unspecified pathological lesion in kidney

583.#(#) Nephritis and nephropathy, not specified as acute or chronic
- 583.0 With lesion of proliferative glomerulonephritis
- 583.1 With lesion of membranous glomerulonephritis
- 583.2 With lesion of membranoproliferative glomerulonephritis
- 583.4 With lesion of rapidly progressive glomerulonephritis
- 583.6 With lesion of renal cortical necrosis
- 583.7 With lesion of renal medullary necrosis
- **583.8#** With other specified pathological lesion in kidney
  - 583.81 Nephritis and nephropathy, not specified as acute or chronic, in diseases classified elsewhere
  - 583.89 Other
- 583.9 With unspecified pathological lesion in kidney

584.# Acute renal failure
- 584.5 With lesion of tubular necrosis
- 584.6 With lesion of renal cortical necrosis
- 584.7 With lesion of renal medullary [papillary] necrosis
- 584.8 Pathological lesion in kidney, NEC
- 584.9 Acute renal failure, unspecified

585.# Chronic kidney disease (CKD)
- 585.1 Stage I
- 585.2 Stage II (mild)
- 585.3 Stage III (moderate)

585.# *(continued)*
- 585.4 Stage IV (severe)
- 585.5 Stage V
- 585.6 End stage renal disease
- 585.9 Unspecified

586 Renal failure, unspecified

587 Renal sclerosis, unspecified

588.#(#) Disorders resulting from impaired renal function
- 588.0 Renal osteodystrophy
- 588.1 Nephrogenic diabetes insipidus
- **588.8#** Other specified disorders resulting from impaired renal function
  - 588.81 Secondary hyperparathyroidism (of renal origin)
  - 588.89 Other specified disorders resulting from impaired renal function
- 588.9 Disorder resulting from impaired renal function, NOS

589.# Small kidney of unknown cause
- 589.0 Unilateral small kidney
- 589.1 Bilateral small kidneys
- 589.9 Small kidney, unspecified

590.#(#) Infections of kidney
- **590.0#** Chronic pyelonephritis
  - 590.00 Without lesion of renal medullary necrosis
  - 590.01 With lesion of renal medullary necrosis
- **590.1#** Acute pyelonephritis
  - 590.10 Without lesion of renal medullary necrosis
  - 590.11 With lesion of renal medullary necrosis
- 590.2 Renal and perinephric abscess
- 590.3 Pyeloureteritis cystica
- **590.8#** Other pyelonephritis or pyonephrosis, NOS
  - 590.80 Pyelonephritis, unspecified
  - 590.81 Pyelitis or pyelonephritis in diseases classified elsewhere
- 590.9 Infection of kidney, unspecified

591 Hydronephrosis

592.# Calculus of kidney and ureter
- 592.0 Calculus of kidney
- 592.1 Calculus of ureter
- 592.9 Urinary calculus, unspecified

593.#(#) Other disorders of kidney and ureter
- 593.0 Nephroptosis
- 593.1 Hypertrophy of kidney
- 593.2 Cyst of kidney, acquired
- 593.3 Stricture or kinking of ureter
- 593.4 Other ureteric obstruction
- 593.5 Hydroureter
- 593.6 Postural proteinuria
- **593.7#** Vesicoureteral reflux
  - 593.70 Unspecified or without reflux nephropathy
  - 593.71 With reflux nephropathy, unilateral
  - 593.72 With reflux nephropathy, bilateral
  - 593.73 With reflux nephropathy NOS
- **593.8#** Other specified disorders of kidney and ureter
  - 593.81 Vascular disorders of kidney
  - 593.82 Ureteral fistula
  - 593.89 Other
- 593.9 Unspecified disorder of kidney and ureter

594.# Calculus of lower urinary tract
594.0 Calculus in diverticulum of bladder
594.1 Other calculus in bladder
594.2 Calculus in urethra
594.8 Other lower urinary tract calculus
594.9 Calculus of lower urinary tract, unspecified

595.#(#) Cystitis
595.0 Acute cystitis
595.1 Chronic interstitial cystitis
595.2 Other chronic cystitis
595.3 Trigonitis
595.4 Cystitis in diseases classified elsewhere
595.8# Other specified types of cystitis
595.81 Cystitis cystica
595.82 Irradiation cystitis
595.89 Other
595.9 Cystitis, unspecified

596.#(#) Other disorders of bladder
596.0 Bladder neck obstruction
596.1 Intestinovesical fistula
596.2 Vesical fistula, not elsewhere classified
596.3 Diverticulum of bladder
596.4 Atony of bladder
596.5# Other functional disorders of bladder
596.51 Hypertonicity of bladder
596.52 Low bladder compliance
596.53 Paralysis of bladder
596.54 Neurogenic bladder NOS
596.55 Detrusor sphincter dyssynergia
596.59 Other functional disorder of bladder
596.6 Rupture of bladder, nontraumatic
596.7 Hemorrhage into bladder wall
596.8 Other specified disorders of bladder
596.9 Unspecified disorder of bladder

597.#(#) Urethritis, not sexually transmitted, and urethral syndrome
597.0 Urethral abscess
597.8# Other urethritis
597.80 Urethritis, unspecified
597.81 Urethral syndrome NOS
597.89 Other

598.#(#) Urethral stricture
598.0# Urethral stricture due to infection
598.00 Due to unspecified infection
598.01 Due to infective diseases classified elsewhere
598.1 Traumatic urethral stricture
598.2 Postoperative urethral stricture
598.8 Other specified causes of urethral stricture
598.9 Urethral stricture, unspecified

599.#(#) Other disorders of urethra and urinary tract
599.0 Urinary tract infection, site not specified
599.1 Urethral fistula
599.2 Urethral diverticulum
599.3 Urethral caruncle
599.4 Urethral false passage
599.5 Prolapsed urethral mucosa
599.6# Urinary obstruction
599.60 Unspecified
599.69 Not elsewhere classified
599.7 Hematuria
599.8# Other specified disorders urethra/urinary tract
599.81 Urethral hypermobility
599.82 Intrinsic (urethral) sphincter deficiency [ISD]

599.#(#) ***(continued)***
599.9# ***(continued)***
599.83 Urethral instability
599.84 Other specified disorders of urethra
599.89 Other specified disorders of urinary tract
599.9 Unspecified disorder of urethra and urinary tract

600.#(#) Hyperplasia of prostate
600.0# Hypertrophy (benign) of prostate
600.00 Hypertrophy (benign) of prostate without urinary obstruction and other lower urinary tract symptoms (LUTS)
600.01 Hypertrophy (benign) of prostate with urinary obstruction and other lower urinary tract symptoms (LUTS)
600.1# Nodular prostate
600.10 Nodular prostate without urinary obstruction
600.11 Nodular prostate with urinary obstruction
600.2# Benign localized hyperplasia of prostate
600.20 Benign localized hyperplasia of prostate without urinary obstruction and other lower urinary tract symptoms (LUTS)
600.21 Benign localized hyperplasia of prostate with urinary obstruction and other lower urinary tract symptoms (LUTS)
600.3 Cyst of prostate
600.9# Hyperplasia of prostate, unspecified
600.90 Hyperplasia of prostate, unspecified, without urinary obstruction and other lower urinary tract symptoms (LUTS)
600.91 Hyperplasia of prostate, unspecified, with urinary obstruction and other lower urinary tract symptoms (LUTS)

601.# Inflammatory diseases of prostate
601.0 Acute prostatitis
601.1 Chronic prostatitis
601.2 Abscess of prostate
601.3 Prostatocystitis
601.4 Prostatitis in diseases classified elsewhere
601.8 Other specified inflammatory diseases prostate
601.9 Prostatitis, unspecified

602.# Other disorders of prostate
602.0 Calculus of prostate
602.1 Congestion or hemorrhage of prostate
602.2 Atrophy of prostate
602.3 Dysplasia of prostate
602.8 Other specified disorders of prostate
602.9 Unspecified disorder of prostate

603.# Hydrocele
603.0 Encysted hydrocele
603.1 Infected hydrocele
603.8 Other specified types of hydrocele
603.9 Hydrocele, unspecified

604.#(#) Orchitis and epididymitis
604.0 Orchitis, epididymitis, and epididymo-orchitis, with abscess
604.9# Other orchitis, epididymitis, and epididymo-orchitis, without mention of abscess
604.90 Orchitis and epididymitis, unspecified
604.91 Orchitis and epididymitis in diseases classified elsewhere
604.99 Other

605 Redundant prepuce and phimosis

606.# Infertility, male
- 606.0 Azoospermia
- 606.1 Oligospermia
- 606.8 Infertility due to extratesticular causes
- 606.9 Male infertility, unspecified

607.#(#) Disorders of penis
- 607.0 Leukoplakia of penis
- 607.1 Balanoposthitis
- 607.2 Other inflammatory disorders of penis
- 607.3 Priapism
- **607.8#** Other specified disorders of penis
  - 607.81 Balanitis xerotica obliterans
  - 607.82 Vascular disorders of penis
  - 607.83 Edema of penis
  - 607.84 Impotence of organic origin
  - 607.85 Peyronie's disease
  - 607.89 Other
- 607.9 Unspecified disorder of penis

608.#(#) Other disorders of male genital organs
- 608.0 Seminal vesiculitis
- 608.1 Spermatocele
- **608.2#** Torsion of testis
  - 608.20 Unspecified
  - 608.21 Extravaginal torsion of spermatic cord
  - 608.22 Intravaginal torsion of spermatic cord
  - 605.23 Torsion of appendix testis
  - 608.24 Torsion of appendix epididymis
- 608.3 Atrophy of testis
- 608.4 Other inflammatory disorders of male genital organs
- **608.8#** Other specified disorders of male genital organs
  - 608.81 Disorders of male genital organs in diseases classified elsewhere
  - 608.82 Hematospermia
  - 608.83 Vascular disorders
  - 608.84 Chylocele of tunica vaginalis
  - 608.85 Stricture
  - 608.86 Edema
  - 608.87 Retrograde ejaculation
  - 608.89 Other
- 608.9 Unspecified disorder of male genital organs

610.# Benign mammary dysplasias
- 610.0 Solitary cyst of breast
- 610.1 Diffuse cystic mastopathy
- 610.2 Fibroadenosis of breast
- 610.3 Fibrosclerosis of breast
- 610.4 Mammary duct ectasia
- 610.8 Other specified benign mammary dysplasias
- 610.9 Benign mammary dysplasia, unspecified

611.#(#) Other disorders of breast
- 611.0 Inflammatory disease of breast
- 611.1 Hypertrophy of breast
- 611.2 Fissure of nipple
- 611.3 Fat necrosis of breast
- 611.4 Atrophy of breast
- 611.5 Galactocele
- 611.6 Galactorrhea not associated with childbirth
- **611.7#** Signs and symptoms in breast
  - 611.71 Mastodynia
  - 611.72 Lump or mass in breast
  - 611.79 Other
- 611.8 Other specified disorders of breast
- 611.9 Unspecified breast disorder

614.# Inflammatory disease of ovary, fallopian tube, pelvic cellular tissue, and peritoneum
- 614.0 Acute salpingitis and oophoritis
- 614.1 Chronic salpingitis and oophoritis
- 614.2 Salpingitis and oophoritis not specified as acute, subacute, or chronic
- 614.3 Acute parametritis and pelvic cellulitis
- 614.4 Chronic or NOS parametritis and pelvic cellulitis
- 614.5 Acute or unspecified pelvic peritonitis, female
- 614.6 Pelvic peritoneal adhesions, female (postoperative) (postinfection)
- 614.7 Other chronic pelvic peritonitis, female
- 614.8 Inflammatory disease of female pelvic organs and tissues, NEC
- 614.9 Inflammatory disease of female pelvic organs and tissues, NOS

615.# Inflammatory diseases of uterus, except cervix
- 615.0 Acute
- 615.1 Chronic
- 615.9 Unspecified inflammatory disease of uterus

616.#(#) Inflammatory disease of cervix, vagina, and vulva
- 616.0 Cervicitis and endocervicitis
- **616.1#** Vaginitis and vulvovaginitis
  - 616.10 Vaginitis and vulvovaginitis, unspecified
  - 616.11 Vaginitis and vulvovaginitis in diseases classified elsewhere
- 616.2 Cyst of Bartholin's gland
- 616.3 Abscess of Bartholin's gland
- 616.4 Other abscess of vulva
- **616.5#** Ulceration of vulva
  - 616.50 Ulceration of vulva, unspecified
  - 616.51 Ulceration of vulva in diseases classified elsewhere
- **616.8#** Inflammatory diseases of cervix, vagina, and vulva, NEC
  - 616.81 Mucositis (ulcerative) of cervix, vagina, and vulva
  - 616.89 Other inflammatory diseases of cervix, vagina, and vulva
- 616.9 Inflammatory disease of cervix, vagina, and vulva, NOS

617.# Endometriosis
- 617.0 Endometriosis of uterus
- 617.1 Endometriosis of ovary
- 617.2 Endometriosis of fallopian tube
- 617.3 Endometriosis of pelvic peritoneum
- 617.4 Endometriosis of rectovaginal septum and vagina
- 617.5 Endometriosis of intestine
- 617.6 Endometriosis in scar of skin
- 617.8 Endometriosis of other specified sites
- 617.9 Endometriosis, site unspecified

618.#(#) Genital prolapse
- **618.0#** Prolapse of vaginal walls without mention of uterine prolapse
  - 618.00 Unspecified prolapse of vaginal walls
  - 618.01 Cystocele, midline
  - 618.02 Cystocele, lateral
  - 618.03 Urethrocele
  - 618.04 Rectocele
  - 618.05 Perineocele
  - 618.09 Other prolapse of vaginal walls without mention of uterine prolapse
- 618.1 Uterine prolapse without mention of vaginal wall prolapse

NUMERICAL REFERENCE

618.#(#) ***(continued)***
618.2 Uterovaginal prolapse, incomplete
618.3 Uterovaginal prolapse, complete
618.4 Uterovaginal prolapse, unspecified
618.5 Prolapse of vaginal vault after hysterectomy
618.6 Vaginal enterocele, congenital or acquired
618.7 Old laceration of muscles of pelvic floor
618.8# Other specified genital prolapse
618.81 Incompetence or weakening of pubocervical tissue
618.82 Incompetence or weakening of rectovaginal tissue
618.83 Pelvic muscle wasting
618.84 Cervical stump prolapse
618.89 Other specified genital prolapse
618.9 Unspecified genital prolapse

619.# Fistula involving female genital tract
619.0 Urinary-genital tract fistula, female
619.1 Digestive-genital tract fistula, female
619.2 Genital tract-skin fistula, female
619.8 Other specified fistulas involving female genital tract
619.9 Unspecified fistula involving female genital tract

620.# Noninflammatory disorders of ovary, fallopian tube, and broad ligament
620.0 Follicular cyst of ovary
620.1 Corpus luteum cyst or hematoma
620.2 Other and unspecified ovarian cyst
620.3 Acquired atrophy of ovary and fallopian tube
620.4 Prolapse or hernia of ovary and fallopian tube
620.5 Torsion of ovary, ovarian pedicle, or fallopian tube
620.6 Broad ligament laceration syndrome
620.7 Hematoma of broad ligament
620.8 Other noninflammatory disorders of ovary, fallopian tube, and broad ligament
620.9 Unspecified noninflammatory disorder of ovary, fallopian tube, and broad ligament

621.#(#) Disorders of uterus, not elsewhere classified
621.0 Polyp of corpus uteri
621.1 Chronic subinvolution of uterus
621.2 Hypertrophy of uterus
621.3# Endometrial hyperplasia
621.30 Endometrial hyperplasia, unspecified
621.31 Simple endometrial hyperplasia without atypia
621.32 Complex endometrial hyperplasia without atypia
621.33 Endometrial hyperplasia with atypia
621.4 Hematometra
621.5 Intrauterine synechiae
621.6 Malposition of uterus
621.7 Chronic inversion of uterus
621.8 Other specified disorders of uterus, not elsewhere classified
621.9 Unspecified disorder of uterus

622.#(#) Noninflammatory disorders of cervix
622.0 Erosion and ectropion of cervix
622.1# Dysplasia of cervix (uteri)
622.10 Dysplasia of cervix, unspecified
622.11 Mild dysplasia of cervix
622.12 Moderate dysplasia of cervix
622.2 Leukoplakia of cervix (uteri)
622.3 Old laceration of cervix
622.4 Stricture and stenosis of cervix
622.5 Incompetence of cervix
622.6 Hypertrophic elongation of cervix

622.#(#) ***(continued)***
622.7 Mucous polyp of cervix
622.8 Other specified noninflammatory disorders of cervix
622.9 Unspecified noninflammatory disorder of cervix

623.# Noninflammatory disorders of vagina
623.0 Dysplasia of vagina
623.1 Leukoplakia of vagina
623.2 Stricture or atresia of vagina
623.3 Tight hymenal ring
623.4 Old vaginal laceration
623.5 Leukorrhea, not specified as infective
623.6 Vaginal hematoma
623.7 Polyp of vagina
623.8 Other specified noninflammatory disorders of vagina
623.9 Unspecified noninflammatory disorder of vagina

624.# Noninflammatory disorders of vulva and perineum
624.0# Dystrophy of vulva
624.01 Vulvar intraepithelial neoplasia I [VIN I]
624.02 Vulvar intraepithelial neoplasia II [VIN II]
624.09 Other dystrophy of vulva
624.1 Atrophy of vulva
624.2 Hypertrophy of clitoris
624.3 Hypertrophy of labia
624.4 Old laceration or scarring of vulva
624.5 Hematoma of vulva
624.6 Polyp of labia and vulva
624.8 Other specified noninflammatory disorders of vulva and perineum
624.9 Unspecified noninflammatory disorder of vulva and perineum

625.# Pain and other symptoms associated with female genital organs
625.0 Dyspareunia
625.1 Vaginismus
625.2 Mittelschmerz
625.3 Dysmenorrhea
625.4 Premenstrual tension syndromes
625.5 Pelvic congestion syndrome
625.6 Stress incontinence, female
625.8 Other specified symptoms associated with female genital organs
625.9 Unspecified symptom associated with female genital organs

626.# Disorders of menstruation and other abnormal bleeding from female genital tract
626.0 Absence of menstruation
626.1 Scanty or infrequent menstruation
626.2 Excessive or frequent menstruation
626.3 Puberty bleeding
626.4 Irregular menstrual cycle
626.5 Ovulation bleeding
626.6 Metrorrhagia
626.7 Postcoital bleeding
626.8 Other
626.9 Unspecified

627.# Menopausal and postmenopausal disorders
627.0 Premenopausal menorrhagia
627.1 Postmenopausal bleeding
627.2 Symptomatic menopausal or female climacteric states
627.3 Postmenopausal atrophic vaginitis
627.4 Symptomatic states associated with artificial menopause

627.# *(continued)*
627.8 Other specified menopausal and postmenopausal disorders
627.9 Unspecified menopausal and postmenopausal disorder

628.# Infertility female
628.0 Associated with anovulation
628.1 Of pituitary-hypothalamic origin
628.2 Of tubal origin
628.3 Of uterine origin
628.4 Of cervical or vaginal origin
628.8 Of other specified origin
628.9 Of unspecified origin

629.#(#) Other disorders of female genital organs
629.0 Hematocele, female, not elsewhere classified
629.1 Hydrocele, canal of Nuck
629.2# Female genital mutilation status
629.20 Female genital mutilation status, unspecified
629.21 Female genital mutilation Type I status
629.22 Female genital mutilation Type II status
629.23 Female genital mutilation Type III status
629.29 Female genital mutilation status other
629.8# Other specified disorders of female genital organs
629.81 Habitual aborter without current pregnancy
629.89 Other specified disorders of female genital organs
629.9 Unspecified disorder of female genital organs

630 Hydatidiform mole
631 Other abnormal product of conception
632 Missed abortion

633.# Ectopic pregnancy
633.0 Abdominal pregnancy
633.1 Tubal pregnancy
633.2 Ovarian pregnancy
633.8 Other ectopic pregnancy
633.9 Unspecified ectopic pregnancy
5th Digit: 633
0 Without intrauterine pregnancy
1 With intrauterine pregnancy

634.## Spontaneous abortion
635.## Legally induced abortion
636.## Illegally induced abortion
637.## Unspecified abortion
4th Digit: 634-637
0 Complicated by genital tract and pelvic infection
1 Complicated by delayed or excessive hemorrhage
2 Complicated by damage to pelvic organs and tissues
3 Complicated by renal failure
4 Complicated by metabolic disorder
5 Complicated by shock
6 Complicated by embolism
7 With other specified complications
8 With unspecified complications
9 Without complication
5th Digit: 634-637
0 Unspecified
1 Incomplete
2 Complete

638.# Failed attempted abortion
638.0 Complicated by genital tract and pelvic infection
638.1 Complicated by delayed or excessive hemorrhage
638.2 Complicated by damage to pelvic organs or tissues
638.3 Complicated by renal failure
638.4 Complicated by metabolic disorder
638.5 Complicated by shock
638.6 Complicated by embolism
638.7 With other specified complications
638.8 With unspecified complication
638.9 Without mention of complication

639.# Complications following abortion and ectopic and molar pregnancies
639.0 Genital tract and pelvic infection
639.1 Delayed or excessive hemorrhage
639.2 Damage to pelvic organs and tissues
639.3 Renal failure
639.4 Metabolic disorders
639.5 Shock
639.6 Embolism
639.8 Other specified complications following abortion or ectopic and molar pregnancy
639.9 Unspecified complication following abortion or ectopic and molar pregnancy

640.## Hemorrhage in early pregnancy
640.0# Threatened abortion
640.8# Other specified hemorrhage in early pregnancy
640.9# Unspecified hemorrhage in early pregnancy

641.## Antepartum hemorrhage, abruptio placentae, and placenta previa
641.0# Placenta previa without hemorrhage
641.1# Hemorrhage from placenta previa
641.2# Premature separation of placenta
641.3# Antepartum hemorrhage associated with coagulation defects
641.8# Other antepartum hemorrhage
641.9# Unspecified antepartum hemorrhage
5th Digit: 640.0-640.9, 641.0-641.9
0 Unspecified as to episode of care or not applicable
1 Delivered, with or without mention of antepartum condition
3 Antepartum condition or complication

642.## Hypertension complicating pregnancy, childbirth, and the puerperium
642.0# Benign essential
642.1# Secondary to renal disease,
642.2# Other pre-existing
642.3# Transient hypertension of pregnancy
642.4# Mild or unspecified pre-eclampsia
642.5# Severe pre-eclampsia
5th Digit: 642
0 Unspecified as to episode of care or not applicable
1 Delivered, with or without mention of antepartum condition
2 Delivered, with mention of postpartum complication
3 Antepartum condition or complication
4 Postpartum condition or complication

642.## ***(continued)***

642.6# Eclampsia
642.7# Pre-eclampsia or eclampsia superimposed on pre-existing hypertension
642.9# Unspecified
5th Digit: 642
0 **Unspecified as to episode of care or not applicable**
1 **Delivered, with or without mention of antepartum condition**
2 **Delivered, with mention of postpartum complication**
3 **Antepartum condition or complication**
4 **Postpartum condition or complication**

643.## **Excessive vomiting in pregnancy**
643.0# Mild hyperemesis gravidarum
643.1# Hyperemesis gravidarum with metabolic disturbance
643.2# Late vomiting of pregnancy
643.8# Other vomiting complicating pregnancy
643.9# Unspecified vomiting of pregnancy
5th Digit: 643
0 **Episode of care NOS or not applicable**
1 **Delivered, with or without mention of antepartum condition**
3 **Antepartum condition or complication**

644.## **Early or threatened labor**
644.0# Threatened premature labor
644.1# Other threatened labor
5th Digit: 644.0-644.1
0 **Episode of care NOS or not applicable**
3 **Antepartum condition or complication**
644.2# Early onset of delivery
5th Digit: 644.2
0 **Episode of care NOS or not applicable**
1 **Delivered, with or without mention of antepartum condition**

645.## **Late pregnancy**
645.1# Post term pregnancy
645.2# Prolonged pregnancy

646.## **Other complications of pregnancy, not elsewhere classified**
646.0# Papyraceous fetus
5th Digit: 645.1, 645.2,, 646.0
0 **Episode of care NOS or not applicable**
1 **Delivered, with or without mention of antepartum condition**
3 **Antepartum condition or complication**
646.1# Edema or excessive weight gain in pregnancy, without mention of hypertension
646.2# Renal disease in pregnancy NOS, without mention of hypertension
5th Digit: 646.1-646.2
0 **Episode of care NOS or not applicable**
1 **Delivered, with or without mention of antepartum condition**
2 **Delivered, with mention of postpartum complication**
3 **Antepartum condition or complication**
4 **Postpartum condition or complication**
646.3# Habitual aborter
5th Digit: 646.3
0 **Episode of care NOS or not applicable**
1 **Delivered, with or without mention of antepartum condition**
3 **Antepartum condition or complication**

646.## ***(continued)***

646.4# Peripheral neuritis in pregnancy
646.5# Asymptomatic bacteriuria in pregnancy
646.6# Infections of genitourinary tract in pregnancy
5th Digit: 646.4-646.6
0 **Episode of care NOS or not applicable**
1 **Delivered, with or without mention of antepartum condition**
2 **Delivered, with mention of postpartum complication**
3 **Antepartum condition or complication**
4 **Postpartum condition or complication**
646.7# Liver disorders in pregnancy
5th Digit: 646.7
0 **Episode of care NOS or not applicable**
1 **Delivered, with or without mention of antepartum condition**
3 **Antepartum condition or complication**
646.8# Other specified complications of pregnancy
5th Digit: 646.8
0 **Episode of care NOS or not applicable**
1 **Delivered, with or without mention of antepartum condition**
2 **Delivered, with mention of postpartum complication**
3 **Antepartum condition or complication**
4 **Postpartum condition or complication**

646.9# Unspecified complication of pregnancy
5th Digit: 646.9
0 **Unspecified as to episode of care or not applicable**
1 **Delivered, with or without mention of antepartum condition**
3 **Antepartum condition or complication**

647.## **Infectious and parasitic conditions in the mother classifiable elsewhere, but complicating pregnancy, childbirth, or the puerperium**
647.0# Syphilis
647.1# Gonorrhea
647.2# Other venereal diseases
647.3# Tuberculosis
647.4# Malaria
647.5# Rubella
647.6# Other viral diseases
647.8# Other specified infectious and parasitic diseases
647.9# Unspecified infection or infestation

648.## **Other current conditions in the mother classifiable elsewhere, but complicating pregnancy, childbirth, or the puerperium**
648.0# Diabetes mellitus
648.1# Thyroid dysfunction
648.2# Anemia
648.3# Drug dependence
648.4# Mental disorders
648.5# Congenital cardiovascular disorders
648.6# Other cardiovascular diseases
648.7# Bone and joint disorders of back, pelvis, and lower limbs
5th Digit: 647-648
0 **Episode of care NOS or not applicable**
1 **Delivered, with or without mention of antepartum condition**
2 **Delivered, with mention of postpartum complication**
3 **Antepartum condition or complication**
4 **Postpartum condition or complication**

NUMERICAL REFERENCE

648.## ***(continued)***
- **648.8#** Abnormal glucose tolerance
- **648.9#** Other current conditions classifiable elsewhere

649.## Other conditions or status of the mother complicating pregnancy, childbirth, or the puerperium
- **649.0#** Tobacco use disorder complicating pregnancy, childbirth, or the puerperium
- **649.1#** Obesity complicating pregnancy, childbirth, or the puerperium
- **649.2#** Bariatric surgery status complicating pregnancy, childbirth, or the puerperium
- **649.3#** Coagulation defects complicating pregnancy, childbirth, or the puerperium
- **649.4#** Epilepsy complicating pregnancy, childbirth, or the puerperium
- **649.5#** Spotting complicating pregnancy
- **649.6#** Uterine size date discrepancy

5th Digit: 648-649
- **0 Episode of care NOS or not applicable**
- **1 Delivered, with or without mention of antepartum condition**
- **2 Delivered, with mention of postpartum complication**
- **3 Antepartum condition or complication**
- **4 Postpartum condition or complication**

650 Normal delivery

651.## Multiple gestation
- **651.0#** Twin pregnancy
- **651.1#** Triplet pregnancy
- **651.2#** Quadruplet pregnancy
- **651.3#** Twin pregnancy with fetal loss and retention of one fetus
- **651.4#** Triplet pregnancy with fetal loss and retention of one or more fetus(es)
- **651.5#** Quadruplet pregnancy with fetal loss and retention of one or more fetus(es)
- **651.6#** Other multiple pregnancy with fetal loss and retention of one or more fetus(es)
- **651.7#** Following (elective) fetal reduction
- **651.8#** Other specified multiple gestation
- **651.9#** Unspecified multiple gestation

652.## Malposition and malpresentation of fetus
- **652.0#** Unstable lie
- **652.1#** Breech or other malpresentation successfully converted to cephalic presentation
- **652.2#** Breech presentation without mention of version
- **652.3#** Transverse or oblique presentation
- **652.4#** Face or brow presentation
- **652.5#** High head at term
- **652.6#** Multiple gestation with malpresentation of one fetus or more

5th Digit: 651
- **0 Episode of care NOS or not applicable**
- **1 Delivered, with or without mention of antepartum condition**
- **3 Antepartum condition or complication**

652.## ***(continued)***
- **652.7#** Prolapsed arm
- **652.8#** Other specified malposition or malpresentation
- **652.9#** Unspecified malposition or malpresentation

653.## Disproportion
- **653.0#** Major abnormality of bony pelvis, NOS
- **653.1#** Generally contracted pelvis
- **653.2#** Inlet contraction of pelvis
- **653.3#** Outlet contraction of pelvis
- **653.4#** Fetopelvic disproportion
- **653.5#** Unusually large fetus causing disproportion
- **653.6#** Hydrocephalic fetus causing disproportion
- **653.7#** Other fetal abnormality causing disproportion
- **653.8#** Disproportion of other origin
- **653.9#** Unspecified disproportion

5th Digit: 652-653
- **0 Episode of care NOS or not applicable**
- **1 Delivered, with or without mention of antepartum condition**
- **3 Antepartum condition or complication**

654.## Abnormality of organs and soft tissues of pelvis
- **654.0#** Congenital abnormalities of uterus
- **654.1#** Tumors of body of uterus

5th Digit: 654.0-654.1
- **0 Episode of care NOS or not applicable**
- **1 Delivered, with or without mention of antepartum condition**
- **2 Delivered, with mention of postpartum complication**
- **3 Antepartum condition or complication**
- **4 Postpartum condition or complication**

- **654.2#** Previous cesarean delivery

5th Digit: 654.2
- **0 Episode of care NOS or not applicable**
- **1 Delivered, with or without mention of antepartum condition**
- **3 Antepartum condition or complication**

- **654.3#** Retroverted and incarcerated gravid uterus
- **654.4#** Other abnormalities in shape or position of gravid uterus and of neighboring structures
- **654.5#** Cervical incompetence
- **654.6#** Congenital or acquired abnormality cervix, NEC
- **654.7#** Congenital or acquired abnormality vagina
- **654.8#** Congenital or acquired abnormality vulva
- **654.9#** Other and unspecified

5th Digit: 654.3-654.9
- **0 Episode of care NOS or not applicable**
- **1 Delivered, with or without mention of antepartum condition**
- **2 Delivered, with mention of postpartum complication**
- **3 Antepartum condition or complication**
- **4 Postpartum condition or complication**

655.## Known or suspected fetal abnormality affecting management of mother

655.0# Central nervous system malformation in fetus
655.1# Chromosomal abnormality in fetus
655.2# Hereditary disease in family possibly affecting fetus
655.3# Suspected damage to fetus from viral disease in mother
655.4# Suspected damage to fetus from other disease in the mother
655.5# Suspected damage to fetus from drugs
655.6# Suspected damage to fetus from radiation
655.7# Decreased fetal movements
655.8# Known or suspected fetal abnormality, NEC
655.9# Unspecified

656.## Other fetal and placental problems affecting management of mother

656.0# Fetal-maternal hemorrhage
656.1# Rhesus isoimmunization
656.2# Isoimmunization, blood-group incompatibility NOS and NEC
656.3# Fetal distress
656.4# Intrauterine death
656.5# Poor fetal growth
656.6# Excessive fetal growth
656.7# Other placental conditions
656.8# Other specified fetal and placental problems
656.9# Unspecified fetal and placental problem

657.0# Polyhydramnios

658.## Other problems associated with amniotic cavity and membranes

658.0# Oligohydramnios
658.1# Premature rupture of membranes
658.2# Delayed delivery after spontaneous or unspecified rupture of membranes
658.3# Delayed delivery after artificial rupture of membranes
658.4# Infection of amniotic cavity
658.8# Other
658.9# Unspecified

659.## Other indications for care or intervention related to labor and delivery, not elsewhere classified

659.0# Failed mechanical induction
659.1# Failed medical or unspecified induction
659.2# Maternal pyrexia during labor, unspecified
659.3# Generalized infection during labor
659.4# Grand multiparity
659.5# Elderly primigravida
659.6# Elderly multigravida
659.7# Abnormality in fetal heart rate or rhythm
659.8# Other specified indications for care or intervention related to labor and delivery
659.9# Indication for care or intervention related to labor and delivery, NOS

5th Digit: 655-659

0 Episode of care NOS or not applicable
1 Delivered, with or without mention of antepartum condition
3 Antepartum condition or complication

660.## Obstructed labor

660.0# Obstruction caused by malposition of fetus at onset of labor
660.1# Obstruction by bony pelvis
660.2# Obstruction by abnormal pelvic soft tissues
660.3# Deep transverse arrest and persistent occipitoposterior position
660.4# Shoulder (girdle) dystocia
660.5# Locked twins
660.6# Failed trial of labor, unspecified
660.7# Failed forceps or vacuum extractor, NOS
660.8# Other causes of obstructed labor
660.9# Unspecified obstructed labor

661.## Abnormality of forces of labor

661.0# Primary uterine inertia
661.1# Secondary uterine inertia
661.2# Other and unspecified uterine inertia
661.3# Precipitate labor
661.4# Hypertonic, incoordinate, or prolonged uterine contractions
661.9# Unspecified abnormality of labor

662.## Long labor

662.0# Prolonged first stage
662.1# Prolonged labor, unspecified
662.2# Prolonged second stage
662.3# Delayed delivery of second twin, triplet, etc.

663.## Umbilical cord complications

663.0# Prolapse of cord
663.1# Cord around neck, with compression
663.2# Other and unspecified cord entanglement, with compression
663.3# Other and unspecified cord entanglement, without mention of compression
663.4# Short cord
663.5# Vasa previa
663.6# Vascular lesions of cord
663.8# Other umbilical cord complications
663.9# Unspecified umbilical cord complication

5th Digit: 660-663

0 Unspecified as to episode of care or not applicable
1 Delivered, with or without mention of antepartum condition
3 Antepartum condition or complication

664.## Trauma to perineum and vulva during delivery

664.0# First-degree perineal laceration
664.1# Second-degree perineal laceration
664.2# Third-degree perineal laceration
664.3# Fourth-degree perineal laceration
664.4# Unspecified perineal laceration
664.5# Vulval and perineal hematoma
664.6# Anal sphincter tear complicating delivery, not associated with third-degree perineal laceration
664.8# Trauma to perineum and vulva, NEC
664.9# Unspecified trauma to perineum and vulva

5th Digit: 664

0 Unspecified as to episode of care or not applicable
1 Delivered, with or without mention of antepartum condition
4 Postpartum condition or complication

NUMERICAL REFERENCE

665.## Other obstetrical trauma
665.0# Rupture of uterus before onset of labor
5th Digit: 665.0
0 Unspecified as to episode of care or not applicable
1 Delivered, with or without mention of antepartum condition
3 Antepartum condition or complication
665.1# Rupture of uterus during labor
5th Digit: 665.1
0 Unspecified as to episode of care or not applicable
1 Delivered, with or without mention of antepartum condition
665.2# Inversion of uterus
5th Digit: 665.2
0 Unspecified as to episode of care or not applicable
2 Delivered, with mention of postpartum complication
4 Postpartum condition or complication
665.3# Laceration of cervix
665.4# High vaginal laceration
665.5# Other injury to pelvic organs
665.6# Damage to pelvic joints and ligaments
5th Digit: 665.3-665.6
0 Unspecified as to episode of care or not applicable
1 Delivered, with or without mention of antepartum condition
4 Postpartum condition or complication
665.7# Pelvic hematoma
5th Digit: 665.7
0 Unspecified as to episode of care or not applicable
1 Delivered, with or without mention of antepartum condition
2 Delivered, with mention of postpartum complication
4 Postpartum condition or complication
665.8# Other specified obstetrical trauma
665.9# Unspecified obstetrical trauma
5th Digit: 665.8-665.9
0 Unspecified as to episode of care or not applicable
1 Delivered, with or without mention of antepartum condition
2 Delivered, with mention of postpartum complication
3 Antepartum condition or complication
4 Postpartum condition or complication

666.## Postpartum hemorrhage
666.0# Third-stage hemorrhage
666.1# Other immediate postpartum hemorrhage
666.2# Delayed and secondary postpartum hemorrhage
666.3# Postpartum coagulation defects
5th Digit: 666
0 Unspecified as to episode of care or not applicable
2 Delivered, with mention of postpartum complication
4 Postpartum condition or complication

667.## Retained placenta or membranes without hemorrhage
667.0# Retained placenta without hemorrhage
667.1# Retained portions of placenta or membranes, without hemorrhage
5th Digit: 667
0 Unspecified as to episode of care or not applicable
2 Delivered, with mention of postpartum complication
4 Postpartum condition or complication

668.## Complications of the administration of anesthetic or other sedation in labor and delivery
668.0# Pulmonary complications
668.1# Cardiac complications
668.2# Central nervous system complications
668.8# Other complications of anesthesia or other sedation in labor and delivery
668.9# Unspecified complication of anesthesia and other sedation

669.## Other complications of labor and delivery, not elsewhere classified
669.0# Maternal distress
669.1# Shock during or following labor and delivery
5th Digit: 668-669.2
0 Unspecified as to episode of care or not applicable
1 Delivered, with or without mention of antepartum condition
2 Delivered, with mention of postpartum complication
3 Antepartum condition or complication
4 Postpartum condition or complication

669.2# Maternal hypotension syndrome
669.3# Acute renal failure following labor and delivery
5th Digit: 669.3
0 Unspecified as to episode of care or not applicable
2 Delivered, with mention of postpartum complication
4 Postpartum condition or complication
669.4# Complications obstetrical surgery and procedures, NEC
5th Digit: 669.4
0 Unspecified as to episode of care or not applicable
1 Delivered, with or without mention of antepartum condition
2 Delivered, with mention of postpartum complication
3 Antepartum condition or complication
4 Postpartum condition or complication
669.5# Forceps/vacuum extractor delivery without mention of indication
669.6# Breech extraction, without mention of indication
669.7# Cesarean delivery, without mention of indication
5th Digit: 669.5-669.7
0 Unspecified as to episode of care or not applicable
1 Delivered, with or without mention of antepartum condition

669.## ***(continued)***
669.8# Other complications of labor and delivery
669.9# Unspecified complication of labor and delivery
5th Digit: 669.8-669.9
- **0** **Unspecified as to episode of care or not applicable**
- **1** **Delivered, with or without mention of antepartum condition**
- **2** **Delivered, with mention of postpartum complication**
- **3** **Antepartum condition or complication**
- **4** **Postpartum condition or complication**

670.0# **Major puerperal infection**
5th Digit: 670.0
- **0** **Unspecified as to episode of care or not applicable**
- **2** **Delivered, with mention of postpartum complication**
- **4** **Postpartum condition or complication**

671.## **Venous complications in pregnancy and the puerperium**
671.0# Varicose veins of legs
671.1# Varicose veins of vulva and perineum
671.2# Superficial thrombophlebitis
5th Digit: 671.0-671.2
- **0** **Unspecified as to episode of care or not applicable**
- **1** **Delivered, with or without mention of antepartum condition**
- **2** **Delivered, with mention of postpartum complication**
- **3** **Antepartum condition or complication**
- **4** **Postpartum condition or complication**

671.3# Deep phlebothrombosis, antepartum
5th Digit: 671.3
- **0** **Unspecified as to episode of care or not applicable**
- **1** **Delivered, with or without mention of antepartum condition**
- **3** **Antepartum condition or complication**

671.4# Deep phlebothrombosis, postpartum
5th Digit: 671.4
- **0** **Episode of care or not applicable, NOS**
- **2** **Delivered, with mention of postpartum complication**
- **4** **Postpartum condition or complication**

671.5# Other phlebitis and thrombosis
671.8# Other venous complications
671.9# Unspecified venous complication
5th Digit: 671.5-671.9
- **0** **Unspecified as to episode of care or not applicable**
- **1** **Delivered, with or without mention of antepartum condition**
- **2** **Delivered, with mention of postpartum complication**
- **3** **Antepartum condition or complication**
- **4** **Postpartum condition or complication**

672.0# **Pyrexia of unknown origin during the puerperium**
5th Digit: 672.0
- **0** **Unspecified as to episode of care or not applicable**
- **2** **Delivered, with mention of postpartum complication**
- **4** **Postpartum condition or complication**

673.## **Obstetrical pulmonary embolism**
673.0# Obstetrical air embolism
673.1# Amniotic fluid embolism
673.2# Obstetrical blood-clot embolism
673.3# Obstetrical pyemic and septic embolism
673.8# Other pulmonary embolism

674.## **Other and unspecified complications of the puerperium, NEC**
674.0# Cerebrovascular disorders in the puerperium
5th Digit: 673-674.0
- **0** **Unspecified as to episode of care or not applicable**
- **1** **Delivered, with or without mention of antepartum condition**
- **2** **Delivered, with mention of postpartum complication**
- **3** **Antepartum condition or complication**
- **4** **Postpartum condition or complication**

674.1# Disruption of cesarean wound
674.2# Disruption of perineal wound
674.3# Complications obstetrical surgical wounds NEC
674.4# Placental polyp
5th Digit: 674.1-674.4
- **0** **Unspecified as to episode of care or not applicable**
- **2** **Delivered, with mention of postpartum complication**
- **4** **Postpartum condition or complication**

674.5# Peripartum cardiomyopathy
5th Digit: 674.5
- **0** **Unspecified as to episode of care or not applicable**
- **1** **Delivered, with or without mention of antepartum condition**
- **2** **Delivered, with mention of postpartum complication**
- **3** **Antepartum condition or complication**
- **4** **Postpartum condition or complication**

674.8# Other
674.9# Unspecified
5th Digit: 674.1-674.9
- **0** **Unspecified as to episode of care or not applicable**
- **2** **Delivered, with mention of postpartum complication**
- **4** **Postpartum condition or complication**

675.## Infections of the breast and nipple associated with childbirth
- **675.0#** Infections of nipple
- **675.1#** Abscess of breast
- **675.2#** Nonpurulent mastitis
- **675.8#** Other specified infections of breast and nipple
- **675.9#** Unspecified infection of the breast and nipple

5th Digit: 675
- **0 Unspecified as to episode of care or not applicable**
- **1 Delivered, with or without mention of antepartum condition**
- **2 Delivered, with mention of postpartum complication**
- **3 Antepartum condition or complication**
- **4 Postpartum condition or complication**

676.## Other disorders of the breast associated with childbirth and disorders of lactation
- **676.0#** Retracted nipple
- **676.1#** Cracked nipple
- **676.2#** Engorgement of breasts
- **676.3#** Other and unspecified disorder of breast
- **676.4#** Failure of lactation
- **676.5#** Suppressed lactation
- **676.6#** Galactorrhea
- **676.8#** Other disorders of lactation
- **676.9#** Unspecified disorder of lactation

5th Digit: 676
- **0 Unspecified as to episode of care or not applicable**
- **1 Delivered, with or without mention of antepartum condition**
- **2 Delivered, with mention of postpartum complication**
- **3 Antepartum condition or complication**
- **4 Postpartum condition or complication**

677 Late effect of complication of pregnancy, childbirth, and the puerperium

680.# Carbuncle and furuncle
- 680.0 Face
- 680.1 Neck
- 680.2 Trunk
- 680.3 Upper arm and forearm
- 680.4 Hand
- 680.5 Buttock
- 680.6 Leg, except foot
- 680.7 Foot
- 680.8 Other specified sites
- 680.9 Unspecified site

681.#(#) Cellulitis and abscess of finger and toe
- **681.0#** Finger
  - 681.00 Cellulitis and abscess, unspecified
  - 681.01 Felon
  - 681.02 Onychia and paronychia of finger
- **681.1#** Toe
  - 681.10 Cellulitis and abscess, unspecified
  - 681.11 Onychia and paronychia of toe
- 681.9 Cellulitis and abscess of unspecified digit

682.# Other cellulitis and abscess
- 682.0 Face
- 682.1 Neck
- 682.2 Trunk
- 682.3 Upper arm and forearm
- 682.4 Hand, except fingers and thumb
- 682.5 Buttock
- 682.6 Leg, except foot
- 682.7 Foot, except toes
- 682.8 Other specified sites
- 682.9 Unspecified site

683 Acute lymphadenitis

684 Impetigo

685.# Pilonidal cyst
- 685.0 With abscess
- 685.1 Without mention of abscess

686.#(#) Other local infections of skin and subcutaneous tissue
- **686.0#** Pyoderma
  - 686.00 Pyoderma, unspecified
  - 686.01 Pyoderma gangrenosum
  - 686.09 Other pyoderma
- 686.1 Pyogenic granuloma
- 686.8 Other specified local infections of skin and subcutaneous tissue
- 686.9 Unspecified local infection of skin and subcutaneous tissue

690.#(#) Erythematosquamous dermatosis
- **690.1#** Seborrheic dermatitis
  - 690.10 Seborheic dermatitis, unspecified
  - 690.11 Seborrhea capitis
  - 690.12 Seborrheic infantile dermatitis
  - 690.18 Other seborrheic dermatitis
- 690.8 Other erythematosquamous dermatosis

691.# Atopic dermatitis and related conditions
- 691.0 Diaper or napkin rash
- 691.8 Other atopic dermatitis and related conditions

692.#(#) Contact dermatitis and other eczema
- 692.0 Due to detergents
- 692.1 Due to oils and greases
- 692.2 Due to solvents
- 692.3 Due to drugs and medicines in contact with skin
- 692.4 Due to other chemical products
- 692.5 Due to food in contact with skin
- 692.6 Due to plants [except food]
- **692.7#** Due to solar radiation
  - 692.70 Unspecified dermatitis due to sun
  - 692.71 Sunburn
  - 692.72 Acute dermatitis due to solar radiation
  - 692.73 Actinic reticuloid and actinic granuloma
  - 692.74 Other chronic dermatitis due to solar radiation
  - 692.75 Disseminated superfician actinic porokeratosis (DSAP)
  - 692.76 Sunburn of second degree
  - 692.77 Sunburn of third degree
  - 692.79 Other dermatitis due to solar radiation

692.#(#) ***(continued)***
- **692.8#** Due to other specified agents
  - 692.81 Dermatitis due to cosmetics
  - 692.82 Dermatitis due to other radiation
  - 692.83 Dermatitis due to metals
  - 692.84 Due to animal (cat) (dog) dander
  - 692.89 Other
- 692.9 Unspecified cause

693.# Dermatitis due to substances taken internally
- 693.0 Due to drugs and medicines
- 693.1 Due to food
- 693.8 Due to other specified substances taken internally
- 693.9 Due to unspecified substance taken internally

694.#(#) Bullous dermatoses
- 694.0 Dermatitis herpetiformis
- 694.1 Subcorneal pustular dermatosis
- 694.2 Juvenile dermatitis herpetiformis
- 694.3 Impetigo herpetiformis
- 694.4 Pemphigus
- 694.5 Pemphigoid
- **694.6#** Benign mucous membrane pemphigoid
  - 694.60 Without mention of ocular involvement
  - 694.61 With ocular involvement
- 694.8 Other specified bullous dermatoses
- 694.9 Unspecified bullous dermatoses

695.#(#) Erythematous conditions
- 695.0 Toxic erythema
- 695.1 Erythema multiforme
- 695.2 Erythema nodosum
- 695.3 Rosacea
- 695.4 Lupus erythematosus
- **695.8#** Other specified erythematous conditions
  - 695.81 Ritter's disease
  - 695.89 Other
- 695.9 Unspecified erythematous condition

696.# Psoriasis and similar disorders
- 696.0 Psoriatic arthropathy
- 696.1 Other psoriasis
- 696.2 Parapsoriasis
- 696.3 Pityriasis rosea
- 696.4 Pityriasis rubra pilaris
- 696.5 Other and unspecified pityriasis
- 696.8 Other

697.# Lichen
- 697.0 Lichen planus
- 697.1 Lichen nitidus
- 697.8 Other lichen, not elsewhere classified
- 697.9 Lichen, unspecified

698.# Pruritus and related conditions
- 698.0 Pruritus ani
- 698.1 Pruritus of genital organs
- 698.2 Prurigo
- 698.3 Lichenification and lichen simplex chronicus
- 698.4 Dermatitis factitia [artefacta]
- 698.8 Other specified pruritic conditions
- 698.9 Unspecified pruritic disorder

700 Corns and callosities

701.# Other hypertrophic and atrophic conditions of skin
- 701.0 Circumscribed scleroderma
- 701.1 Keratoderma, acquired
- 701.2 Acquired acanthosis nigricans
- 701.3 Striae atrophicae
- 701.4 Keloid scar
- 701.5 Other abnormal granulation tissue
- 701.8 Other specified hypertrophic and atrophic conditions of skin
- 701.9 Unspecified hypertrophic and atrophic conditions of skin

702.#(#) Other dermatoses
- 702.0 Actinic keratosis
- **702.1#** Seborrheic keratosis
  - 702.11 Inflamed seborrheic keratosis
  - 702.19 Other seborrheic keratosis
- 702.8 Other specified dermatoses

703.# Diseases of nail
- 703.0 Ingrowing nail
- 703.8 Other specified diseases of nail
- 703.9 Unspecified disease of nail

704.#(#) Diseases of hair and hair follicles
- **704.0#** Alopecia
  - 704.00 Alopecia, unspecified
  - 704.01 Alopecia areata
  - 704.02 Telogen effluvium
  - 704.09 Other
- 704.1 Hirsutism
- 704.2 Abnormalities of the hair
- 704.3 Variations in hair color
- 704.8 Other specified diseases of hair and hair follicles
- 704.9 Unspecified disease of hair and hair follicles

705.#(#) Disorders of sweat glands
- 705.0 Anhidrosis
- 705.1 Prickly heat
- **705.2#** Focal hyperhidrosis
  - 705.21 Primary focal hyperhidrosis
  - 705.22 Secondary focal hyperhidrosis
- **705.8#** Other specified disorders of sweat glands
  - 705.81 Dyshidrosis
  - 705.82 Fox-Fordyce disease
  - 705.83 Hidradenitis
  - 705.89 Other
- 705.9 Unspecified disorder of sweat glands

706.# Diseases of sebaceous glands
- 706.0 Acne varioliformis
- 706.1 Other acne
- 706.2 Sebaceous cyst
- 706.3 Seborrhea
- 706.8 Other specified diseases of sebaceous glands
- 706.9 Unspecified disease of sebaceous glands

707.## Chronic ulcer of skin

707.0# Decubitus ulcer

5th Digit: 707.

- **0 Unspecified site**
- **1 Elbow**
- **2 Upper back**
- **3 Lower back**
- **4 Hip**
- **5 Buttock**
- **6 Ankle**
- **7 Heel**
- **9 Other site**

707.1# Ulcer of lower limbs, except decubitus

5th Digit: 707.1

- **0 Lower limb, unspecified**
- **1 Thigh**
- **2 Calf**
- **3 Ankle**
- **4 Of heel and midfoot**
- **5 Other part of foot**
- **9 Other part of lower limb**

707.8 Chronic ulcer of other specified sites
707.9 Chronic ulcer of unspecified site

708.# Urticaria

708.0 Allergic urticaria
708.1 Idiopathic urticaria
708.2 Urticaria due to cold and heat
708.3 Dermatographic urticaria
708.4 Vibratory urticaria
708.5 Cholinergic urticaria
708.8 Other specified urticaria
708.9 Urticaria, unspecified

709.#(#) Other disorders of skin and subcutaneous tissue

709.0# Dyschromia
709.00 Dyschromia, unspecified
709.01 Vitiligo
709.09 Other
709.1 Vascular disorders of skin
709.2 Scar conditions and fibrosis of skin
709.3 Degenerative skin disorders
709.4 Foreign body granuloma of skin and subcutaneous tissue
709.8 Other specified disorders of skin
709.9 Unspecified disorder of skin and subcutaneous tissue

710.# Diffuse diseases of connective tissue

710.0 Systemic lupus erythematosus
710.1 Systemic sclerosis
710.2 Sicca syndrome
710.3 Dermatomyositis
710.4 Polymyositis
710.5 Eosinophilia myalgia syndrome
710.8 Other specified diffuse diseases of connective tissue
710.9 Unspecified diffuse connective tissue disease

711.## Arthropathy associated with infections

711.0# Pyogenic arthritis
711.1# Arthropathy associated with Reiter's disease and nonspecific urethritis
711.2# Arthropathy in Behçet's syndrome
711.3# Postdysenteric arthropathy
711.4# Arthropathy associated with other bacterial diseases
711.5# Arthropathy associated with other viral diseases
711.6# Arthropathy associated with mycoses
711.7# Arthropathy associated with helminthiasis
711.8# Arthropathy associated with other infectious and parasitic diseases
711.9# Unspecified infective arthritis

712.## Crystal arthropathies

712.1# Chondrocalcinosis due to dicalcium phosphate crystals
712.2# Chondrocalcinosis due to pyrophosphate crystals
712.3# Chondrocalcinosis, unspecified
712.8# Other specified crystal arthropathies
712.9# Unspecified crystal arthropathy

5th Digit: 711-712

- **0 Site unspecified**
- **1 Shoulder region**
- **2 Upper arm**
- **3 Forearm**
- **4 Hand**
- **5 Pelvic region and thigh**
- **6 Lower leg**
- **7 Ankle and foot**
- **8 Other specified sites**
- **9 Multiple sites**

713.# Arthropathy associated with other disorders classified elsewhere

713.0 Arthropathy associated with other endocrine and metabolic disorders
713.1 Arthropathy associated with gastrointestinal conditions other than infections
713.2 Arthropathy associated with hematological disorders
713.3 Arthropathy associated with dermatological disorders
713.4 Arthropathy associated with respiratory disorders
713.5 Arthropathy associated with neurological disorders
713.6 Arthropathy associated with hypersensitivity reaction
713.7 Other general diseases with articular involvement
713.8 Arthropathy associated with other conditions classifiable elsewhere

714.#(#) Rheumatoid arthritis and other inflammatory polyarthropathies
714.0 Rheumatoid arthritis
714.1 Felty's syndrome
714.2 Other rheumatoid arthritis with visceral or systemic involvement
714.3# Juvenile chronic polyarthritis
714.30 Polyarticular juvenile rheumatoid arthritis, chronic or unspecified
714.31 Polyarticular juvenile rheumatoid arthritis, acute
714.32 Pauciarticular juvenile rheumatoid arthritis
714.33 Monoarticular juvenile rheumatoid arthritis
714.4 Chronic postrheumatic arthropathy
714.8# Other specified inflammatory polyarthropathies
714.81 Rheumatoid lung
714.89 Other
714.9 Unspecified inflammatory polyarthropathy

715.## Osteoarthrosis and allied disorders
715.0# Osteoarthrosis, generalized
5th Digit: 715.0
0 Site unspecified
4 Hand
9 Multiple sites
715.1# Osteoarthrosis, localized, primary
715.2# Osteoarthrosis, localized, secondary
715.3# Osteoarthrosis, localized, unspecified as to primary or secondary
5th Digit: 715.1-715.3
0 Site unspecified
1 Shoulder region
2 Upper arm
3 Forearm
4 Hand
5 Pelvic region and thigh
6 Lower leg
7 Ankle and foot
8 Other specified sites
715.8# Osteoarthrosis involving, or with mention of more than one site, but not generalized
5th Digit: 715.8
0 Site unspecified
9 Multiple sites
715.9# Osteoarthrosis, generalized or localized NOS
5th Digit: 715.9
0 Site unspecified
1 Shoulder region
2 Upper arm
3 Forearm
4 Hand
5 Pelvic region and thigh
6 Lower leg
7 Ankle and foot
8 Other specified sites

716.## Other and unspecified arthropathies
716.0# Kaschin-Beck disease
716.1# Traumatic arthropathy
716.2# Allergic arthritis
716.3# Climacteric arthritis
716.4# Transient arthropathy
716.5# Unspecified polyarthropathy or polyarthritis
5th Digit: 716.0 -716.5
0 Site unspecified
1 Shoulder region
2 Upper arm
3 Forearm
4 Hand
5 Pelvic region and thigh
6 Lower leg
7 Ankle and foot
8 Other specified sites
9 Multiple sites
716.6# Unspecified monoarthritis
5th Digit: 716.6
0 Site unspecified
1 Shoulder region
2 Upper arm
3 Forearm
4 Hand
5 Pelvic region and thigh
6 Lower leg
7 Ankle and foot
8 Other specified sites
716.8# Other specified arthropathy
716.9# Arthropathy, unspecified
5th Digit: 716.8-716.9
0 Site unspecified
1 Shoulder region
2 Upper arm
3 Forearm
4 Hand
5 Pelvic region and thigh
6 Lower leg
7 Ankle and foot
8 Other specified sites
9 Multiple sites

717.#(#) Internal derangement of knee
717.0 Old bucket handle tear of medial meniscus
717.1 Derangement, anterior horn, medial meniscus
717.2 Derangement, posterior horn, medial meniscus
717.3 Other and unspecified derangement, medial meniscus
717.4# Derangement of lateral meniscus
717.40 Derangement of lateral meniscus, NOS
717.41 Bucket handle tear of lateral meniscus
717.42 Derangement of anterior horn of lateral meniscus
717.43 Derangement of posterior horn of lateral meniscus
717.49 Other
717.5 Derangement of meniscus, NEC
717.6 Loose body in knee
717.7 Chondromalacia of patella

717.#(#) ***(continued)***

717.8# Other internal derangement of knee
- 717.81 Old disruption of lateral collateral ligament
- 717.82 Old disruption of medial collateral ligament
- 717.83 Old disruption of anterior cruciate ligament
- 717.84 Old disruption of posterior cruciate ligament
- 717.85 Old disruption of other ligaments of knee
- 717.89 Other

717.9 Unspecified internal derangement of knee

718.## Other derangement of joint

718.0# Articular cartilage disorder
718.1# Loose body in joint

5th Digit: 718.0-718.1
- 0 **Site unspecified**
- 1 **Shoulder region**
- 2 **Upper arm**
- 3 **Forearm**
- 4 **Hand**
- 5 **Pelvic region and thigh**
- 7 **Ankle and foot**
- 8 **Other specified sites**
- 9 **Multiple sites**

718.2# Pathological dislocation
718.3# Recurrent dislocation of joint
718.4# Contracture of joint
718.5# Ankylosis of joint

5th Digit: 718.2-718.5
- 0 **Site unspecified**
- 1 **Shoulder region**
- 2 **Upper arm**
- 3 **Forearm**
- 4 **Hand**
- 5 **Pelvic region and thigh**
- 6 **Lower leg**
- 7 **Ankle and foot**
- 8 **Other specified sites**
- 9 **Multiple sites**

718.6# Unspecified intrapelvic protrusion of acetabulum

5th Digit: 718.6
- 0 **Site unspecified**
- 5 **Pelvic region and thigh**

718.7# Developmental dislocation of joint
718.8# Other joint derangement, not elsewhere classified

5th Digit: 718.8
- 0 **Site unspecified**
- 1 **Shoulder region**
- 2 **Upper arm**
- 3 **Forearm**
- 4 **Hand**
- 5 **Pelvic region and thigh**
- 6 **Lower leg**
- 7 **Ankle and foot**
- 8 **Other specified sites**
- 9 **Multiple sites**

718.#(#) ***(continued)***

718.9# Unspecified derangement of joint

5th Digit: 718.9
- 0 **Site unspecified**
- 1 **Shoulder region**
- 2 **Upper arm**
- 3 **Forearm**
- 4 **Hand**
- 5 **Pelvic region and thigh**
- 7 **Ankle and foot**
- 8 **Other specified sites**
- 9 **Multiple sites**

719.#(#) Other and unspecified disorders of joint

719.0# Effusion of joint
719.1# Hemarthrosis
719.2# Villonodular synovitis
719.3# Palindromic rheumatism
719.4# Pain in joint
719.5# Stiffness of joint, not elsewhere classified
719.6# Other symptoms referable to joint

5th Digit: 719.0-719.6
- 0 **Site unspecified**
- 1 **Shoulder region**
- 2 **Upper arm**
- 3 **Forearm**
- 4 **Hand**
- 5 **Pelvic region and thigh**
- 6 **Lower leg**
- 7 **Ankle and foot**
- 8 **Other specified sites**
- 9 **Multiple sites**

719.7 Difficulty in walking
719.8# Other specified disorders of joint
719.9# Unspecified disorder of joint

5th Digit: 719.8-719.9
- 0 **Site unspecified**
- 1 **Shoulder region**
- 2 **Upper arm**
- 3 **Forearm**
- 4 **Hand**
- 5 **Pelvic region and thigh**
- 6 **Lower leg**
- 7 **Ankle and foot**
- 8 **Other specified sites**
- 9 **Multiple sites**

720.#(#) Ankylosing spondylitis and other inflammatory spondylopathies

720.0 Ankylosing spondylitis
720.1 Spinal enthesopathy
720.2 Sacroiliitis, not elsewhere classified
720.8# Other inflammatory spondylopathies
- 720.81 Inflammatory spondylopathies in diseases classified elsewhere
- 720.89 Other

720.9 Unspecified inflammatory spondylopathy

721.#(#) Spondylosis and allied disorders

721.0 Cervical spondylosis without myelopathy
721.1 Cervical spondylosis with myelopathy
721.2 Thoracic spondylosis without myelopathy
721.3 Lumbosacral spondylosis without myelopathy

721.#(#) ***(continued)***

721.4# Thoracic or lumbar spondylosis with myelopathy
- 721.41 Thoracic region
- 721.42 Lumbar region

721.5 Kissing spine
721.6 Ankylosing vertebral hyperostosis
721.7 Traumatic spondylopathy
721.8 Other allied disorders of spine
721.9# Spondylosis of unspecified site
- 721.90 Without mention of myelopathy
- 721.91 With myelopathy

722.#(#) Intervertebral disc disorders

722.0 Displacement of cervical intervertebral disc without myelopathy
722.1.# Displacement of thoracic or lumbar intervertebral disc without myelopathy
- 722.10 Lumbar intervertebral disc without myelopathy
- 722.11 Thoracic intervertebral disc without myelopathy

722.2 Displacement of intervertebral disc, site unspecified, without myelopathy
722.3# Schmorl's nodes
- 722.30 Unspecified region
- 722.31 Thoracic region
- 722.32 Lumbar region
- 722.39 Other

722.4 Degeneration of cervical intervertebral disc
722.5# Degeneration of thoracic or lumbar intervertebral disc
- 722.51 Thoracic or thoracolumbar intervertebral disc
- 722.52 Lumbar or lumbosacral intervertebral disc

722.6 Degeneration of intervertebral disc, site NOS
722.7# Intervertebral disc disorder with myelopathy
722.8# Postlaminectomy syndrome
722.9# Other and unspecified disc disorder

5th Digit: 722.7-722.9
- **0 Unspecified region**
- **1 Cervical region**
- **2 Thoracic region**
- **3 Lumbar region**

723.# Other disorders of cervical region

723.0 Spinal stenosis of cervical region
723.1 Cervicalgia
723.2 Cervicocranial syndrome
723.3 Cervicobrachial syndrome (diffuse)
723.4 Brachia neuritis or radiculitis NOS
723.5 Torticollis, unspecified
723.6 Panniculitis specified as affecting neck
723.7 Ossification of posterior longitudinal ligament in cervical region
723.8 Other syndromes affecting cervical region
723.9 Unspecified musculoskeletal disorders and symptoms referable to neck

724.#(#) Other and unspecified disorders of back

724.0# Spinal stenosis, other than cervical
- 724.00 Spinal stenosis, unspecified region
- 724.01 Thoracic region
- 724.02 Lumbar region
- 724.09 Other

724.1 Pain in thoracic spine
724.2 Lumbago
724.3 Sciatia
724.4 Thoracic or lumbosacral neuritis or radiculitis, NOS

724.#(#) ***(continued)***

724.5 Backache, unspecified
724.6 Disorders of sacrum
724.7# Disorders of coccyx
- 724.70 Unspecified disorder of coccyx
- 724.71 Hypermobility of coccyx
- 724.79 Other

724.8 Other symptoms referable to back
724.9 Other unspecified back disorders

725 Polymyalgia rheumatica

726.#(#) Peripheral enthesopathies and allied syndromes

726.0 Adhesive capsulitis of shoulder
726.1# Rotator cuff syndrome of shoulder and allied disorders
- 726.10 Disorders of bursae and tendons in shoulder region, unspecified
- 726.11 Calcifying tendinitis of shoulder
- 726.12 Bicipital tenosynovitis
- 726.19 Other specified disorders

726.2 Other affections of shoulder region, not elsewhere classified
726.3# Enthesopathy of elbow region
- 726.30 Enthesopathy of elbow, unspecified
- 726.31 Medial epicondylitis
- 726.32 Lateral epicondylitis
- 726.33 Olecranon bursitis
- 726.39 Other

726.4 Enthesopathy of wrist and carpus
726.5 Enthesopathy of hip region
726.6# Enthesopathy of knee
- 726.60 Enthesopathy of knee, unspecified
- 726.61 Pes anserinus tendinitis or bursitis
- 726.62 Tibial collateral ligament bursitis
- 726.63 Fibular collateral ligament bursitis
- 726.64 Patellar tendinitis
- 726.65 Prepatellar bursitis
- 726.69 Other

726.7# Enthesopathy of ankle and tarsus
- 726.70 Enthesopathy of ankle and tarsus, unspecified
- 726.71 Achilles bursitis or tendinitis
- 726.72 Tibialis tendinitis
- 726.73 Calcaneal spur
- 726.79 Other

726.8 Other peripheral enthesopathies
726.9# Unspecified enthesopathy
- 726.90 Enthesopathy of unspecified site
- 726.91 Exostosis of unspecified site

727.#(#) Other disorders of synovium, tendon, and bursa

727.0# Synovitis and tenosynovitis
- 727.00 Synovitis and tenosynovitis, unspecified
- 727.01 Synovitis and tenosynovitis in diseases classified elsewhere
- 727.02 Giant cell tumor of tendon sheath
- 727.03 Trigger finger (acquired)
- 727.04 Radial styloid tenosynovitis
- 727.05 Other tenosynovitis or hand and wrist
- 727.06 Tenosynovitis of foot and ankle
- 727.09 Other

727.1 Bunion
727.2 Specific bursitides often of occupational origin
727.3 Other bursitis

727.#(#) ***(continued)***

727.4# Ganglion and cyst of synovium, tendon, and bursa
- 727.40 Synovial cyst, unspecified
- 727.41 Ganglion of joint
- 727.42 Ganglion of tendon sheath
- 727.43 Ganglion, unspecified
- 727.49 Other

727.5# Rupture of synovium
- 727.50 Rupture of synovium, unspecified
- 727.51 Synovial cyst of popliteal space
- 727.59 Other

727.6# Rupture of tendon, nontraumatic
- 727.60 Nontraumatic rupture of unspecified tendon
- 727.61 Complete rupture of rotator cuff
- 727.62 Tendons of biceps (long head)
- 727.63 Extensor tendons of hand and wrist
- 727.64 Flexor tendons of hand and wrist
- 727.65 Quadriceps tendon
- 727.66 Patellar tendon
- 727.67 Achilles tendon
- 727.68 Other tendons of foot and ankle
- 727.69 Other

727.8# Other disorders of synovium, tendon, and bursa
- 727.81 Contracture of tendon (sheath)
- 727.82 Calcium deposits in tendon and bursa
- 727.83 Plica syndrome
- 727.89 Other

727.9 Unspecified disorder of synovium, tendon, and bursa

728.#(#) Disorders of muscle, ligament, and fascia

728.0 Infective myositis

728.1# Muscular calcification and ossification
- 728.10 Calcification and ossification, unspecified
- 728.11 Progressive myositis ossificans
- 728.12 Traumatic myositis ossificans
- 728.13 Postoperative heterotopic calcification
- 728.19 Other

728.2 Muscular wasting and disuse atrophy, not elsewhere classified

728.3 Other specific muscle disorders

728.4 Laxity of ligament

728.5 Hypermobility syndrome

728.6 Contracture of palmar fascia

728.7# Other fibromatoses
- 728.71 Plantar fascial fibromatosis
- 728.79 Other

728.8# Other disorders of muscle, ligament, and fascia
- 728.81 Interstitial myositis
- 728.82 Foreign body granuloma of muscle
- 728.83 Rupture of muscle, nontraumatic
- 728.84 Diastasis of muscle
- 728.85 Spasm of muscle
- 728.86 Necrotizing fasciitis
- 728.87 Muscle weakness
- 728.88 Rhabdomyolysis
- 728.89 Other

728.9 Unspecified disorder of muscle, ligament, and fascia

729.#(#) Other disorders of soft tissues

729.0 Rheumatism, unspecified and fibrositis

729.1 Mylagia and myositis, unspecified

729.2 Neuralgia, neuritis, and radiculitis,unspecified

729.#(#) ***(continued)***

729.3# Panniculitis, unspecified
- 729.30 Panniculitis, unspecified site
- 729.31 Hypertrophy of fat pad, knee
- 729.39 Other site

729.4 Fasciitis, unspecified

729.5 Pain in limb

729.6 Residual foreign body in soft tissue

729.7# Nontraumatic compartment syndrome
- 729.71 Upper extremity
- 729.72 Lower extremity
- 729.73 abdomen
- 729.79 other sites

729.8# Other musculoskeletal symptoms referable to limbs
- 729.81 Swelling of limb
- 729.82 Cramp
- 729.89 Other

729.9 Other and unspecified disorders of soft tissue

730.## Osteomyelitis, periostitis, and other infections involving bone

730.0# Acute osteomyelitis

730.1# Chronic osteomyelitis

730.2# Unspecified osteomyelitis

730.3# Periostitis without mention of ostemyelitis

730.7# Osteopathy resulting from poliomyelitis

730.8# Other infections involving bone in disease classified elsewhere

730.9# Unspecified infection of bone

5th Digit: 730
- **0 Site unspecified**
- **1 Shoulder region**
- **2 Upper arm**
- **3 Forearm**
- **4 Hand**
- **5 Pelvic region and thigh**
- **6 Lower leg**
- **7 Ankle and foot**
- **8 Other specified sites**
- **9 Multiple sites**

731.# Osteitis deformans and osteopathies associated with other disorders classified elsewhere

731.0 Osteitis deformans without mention of bone tumor

731.1 Osteitis deformans in diseases classified elsewhere

731.2 Hypertrophic pulmonary osteoarthropathy

731.3 Major ossecous defects

731.8 Other bone involvement in diseases classified elsewhere

732.# Osteochondropathies

732.0 Juvenile osteochondrosis of spine

732.1 Juvenile osteochondrosis of hip and pelvis

732.2 Nontraumatic slipped upper femoral epiphysis

732.3 Juvenile osteochondrosis of upper extremity

732.4 Juvenile osteochondrosis of lower extremity, excluding foot

732.5 Juvenile osteochondrosis of foot

732.6 Other juvenile osteochondrosis

732.7 Osteochondritis dissecans

732.8 Other specified forms of osteochondropathy

732.9 Unspecified osteochondropathy

733.#(#) Other disorders of bone and cartilage
- **733.0#** Osteoporosis
  - 733.00 Osteoporosis, unspecified
  - 733.01 Senile osteoporosis
  - 733.02 Idiopathic osteoporosis
  - 733.03 Disuse osteoporosis
  - 733.09 Other
- **733.1#** Pathologic fracture
  - 733.10 Pathologic fracture, unspecified site
  - 733.11 Pathologic fracture of humerus
  - 733.12 Pathologic fracture of distal radius and ulna
  - 733.13 Pathologic fracture of vertebrae
  - 733.14 Pathologic fracture of neck of femur
  - 733.15 Pathologic fracture femur NEC
  - 733.16 Pathologic fracture of tibia and fibula
  - 733.19 Pathologic fracture NEC
- **733.2#** Cyst of bone
  - 733.20 Cyst of bone (localized), unspecified
  - 733.21 Solitary bone cyst
  - 733.22 Aneurysmal bone cyst
  - 733.29 Other
- 733.3 Hyperostosis of skull
- **733.4#** Aseptic necrosis of bone
  - 733.40 Aseptic necrosis of bone, site unspecified
  - 733.41 Head of humerus
  - 733.42 Head and neck of femur
  - 733.43 Medial femoral condyle
  - 733.45 Jaw
  - 733.44 Talus
  - 733.49 Other
- 733.5 Osteitis condensans
- 733.6 Tietze's disease
- 733.7 Algoneurodystrophy
- **733.8#** Malunion and nonunion of fracture
  - 733.81 Malunion of fracture
  - 733.82 Nonunion of fracture
- **733.9#** Other and unspecified disorders of bone and cartilage
  - 733.90 Disorder of bone and cartilage, NOS
  - 733.91 Arrest of bone development or growth
  - 733.92 Chondromalacia
  - 733.93 Stress fracture of tibia or fibula
  - 733.94 Stress fracture of the metatarsals
  - 733.95 Stress fracture of other bone
  - 733.99 Other

734 Flat foot

735.# Acquired deformities of toe
- 735.0 Hallux valgus (acquired)
- 735.1 Hallux varus (acquired)
- 735.2 Hallux rigidus
- 735.3 Hallux malleus
- 735.4 Other hammer toe (acquired)
- 735.5 Claw toe (acquired)
- 735.8 Other acquired deformities of toe
- 735.9 Unspecified acquired deformity of toe

736.#(#) Other acquired deformities of limbs
- **736.0#** Acquired deformities of forearm, except fingers
  - 736.00 Unspecified deformity
  - 736.01 Cubitus valgus (acquired)
  - 736.02 Cubitus varus (acquired)
  - 736.03 Valgus deformity of wrist(acquired)
  - 736.04 Varus deformity of wrist (acquired)
  - 736.05 Wrist drop (acquired)
  - 736.06 Claw hand (acquired)
  - 736.07 Club hand (acquired)
  - 736.09 Other
- 736.1 Mallet finger

736.#(#) ***(continued)***
- **736.2#** Other acquired deformities of finger
  - 736.20 Unspecified deformity
  - 736.21 Boutonniere deformity
  - 736.22 Swan-neck deformity
  - 736.29 Other
- **736.3#** Acquired deformities of hip
  - 736.30 Unspecified deformity
  - 736.31 Coxa valga (acquired)
  - 736.32 Coxa vara (acquired)
  - 736.39 Other
- **736.4#** Genu valgum or varum (acquired)
  - 736.41 Genu valgum (acquired)
  - 736.42 Genu varum (acquired)
- 736.5 Genu recurvatum (acquired)
- 736.6 Other acquired deformities of knee
- **736.7#** Other acquired deformities of ankle and foot
  - 736.70 Deformity of ankle and foot, acquired NOS
  - 736.71 Acquired equinovarus deformity
  - 736.72 Equinus deformity of foot, acquired
  - 736.73 Cavus deformity of foot
  - 736.74 Claw foot, acquired
  - 736.75 Cavovarus deformity of foot, acquired
  - 736.76 Other calcaneus deformity
  - 736.79 Other
- **736.8#** Acquired deformities of other parts of limbs
  - 736.81 Unequal leg length (acquired)
  - 736.89 Other
- 736.9 Acquired deformity of limb, site unspecified

737.#(#) Curvature of spine
- 737.0 Adolescent postural kyphosis
- **737.1#** Kyphosis (acquired)
  - 737.10 Kyphosis (acquired) (postural)
  - 737.11 Kyphosis due to radiation
  - 737.12 Kyphosis, postlaminectomy
  - 737.19 Other
- **737.2#** Lordosis (acquired)
  - 737.20 Lordosis (acquired) (postural)
  - 737.21 Lordosis, postlaminectomy
  - 737.22 Other postsurgical lordosis
  - 737.29 Other
- **737.3#** Kyphoscoliosis and scoliosis
  - 737.30 Scoliosis [and kyphoscoliosis], idiopathic
  - 737.31 Resolving infantile idiopathic scoliosis
  - 737.32 Progressive infantile idiopathic scoliosis
  - 737.33 Scoliosis due to radiation
  - 737.34 Thoracogenic scoliosis
  - 737.39 Other
- **737.4#** Curvature of spine associated with other conditions
  - 737.40 Curvature of spine, unspecified
  - 737.41 Kyphosis
  - 737.42 Lordosis
  - 737.43 Scoliosis
- 737.8 Other curvatures of spine
- 737.9 Unspecified curvature of spine

738.#(#) Other acquired deformity
- 738.0 Acquired deformity of nose
- **738.1#** Other acquired deformity of head
  - 738.10 Unspecified deformity
  - 738.11 Zygomatic hyperplasia
  - 738.12 Zygomatic hypoplasia
  - 738.19 Other specified deformity
- 738.2 Acquired deformity of neck
- 738.3 Acquired deformity of chest and rib
- 738.4 Acquired spondylolisthesis
- 738.5 Other acquired deformity of back or spine
- 738.6 Acquired deformity of pelvis

738.#(#) ***(continued)***

738.7 Cauliflower ear
738.8 Acquired deformity of other specified site
738.9 Acquired deformity of unspecified site

739.# Nonallopathic lesions, not elsewhere classified

739.0 Head region
739.1 Cervical region
739.2 Thoracic region
739.3 Lumbar region
739.4 Sacral region
739.5 Pelvic region
739.6 Lower extremities
739.7 Upper extremities
739.8 Rib cage
739.9 Abdomen and other

740.# Anencephalus and similar anomalies

740.0 Anencephalus
740.1 Craniorachischisis
740.2 Iniencephaly

741.## Spina bifida

741.0# With hydrocephalus
741.9# Without mention of hydrocephalus

5th Digit: 741

0 Unspecified region
1 Cervical region
2 Dorsal (thoracic) region
3 Lumbar region

742.#(#) Other congenital anomalies of nervous system

742.0 Encephalocele
742.1 Microcephalus
742.2 Reduction deformities of brain
742.3 Congenital hydrocephalus
742.4 Other specified anomalies of brain
742.5# Other specified anomalies of spinal cord
742.51 Diastematomyelia
742.53 Hydromyelia
742.59 Other
742.8 Other specified anomalies of nervous system
742.9 Unspecified anomaly of brain, spinal cord, and nervous system

743.#(#) Congenital anomalies of eye

743.0# Anophthalmos
743.00 Clinical anophthalmos, unspecified
743.03 Cystic eyeball, congenital
743.06 Cryptophthalmos
743.1# Microphthalmos
743.10 Microphthalmos, unspecified
743.11 Simple microphthalmos
743.12 Microphthalmos associated with other anomalies of eye and adnexa
743.2# Buphthalmos
743.20 Buphthalmos, unspecified
743.21 Simple buphthalmos
743.22 Buphthalmos associated with other ocular anomalies
743.3# Congenital cataract and lens anomalies
743.30 Congenital cataract, unspecified
743.31 Capsular and subcapsular cataract
743.32 Cortical and zonular cataract
743.33 Nuclear cataract
743.34 Total and subtotal cataract, congenital
743.35 Congenital aphakia
743.36 Anomalies of lens shape
743.37 Congenital ectopic lens
743.39 Other

743.#(#) ***(continued)***

743.4# Coloboma and other anomalies of anterior segment
743.41 Anomalies of corneal size and shape
743.42 Corneal opacities, interfering with vision, congenital
743.43 Other corneal opacities, congenital
743.44 Specified anomalies of anterior chamber, chamber angle, and related structures
743.45 Aniridia
743.46 Other specified anomalies of iris and ciliary body
743.47 Specified anomalies of sclera
743.48 Multiple and combined anomalies of anterior segment
743.49 Other
743.5# Congenital anomalies of posterior segment
743.51 Vitreous anomalies
743.52 Fundus coloboma
743.53 Chorioretinal degeneration, congenital
743.54 Congenital folds and cysts of posterior segment
743.55 Congenital macular changes
743.56 Other retinal changes, congenital
743.57 Specified anomalies of optic disc
743.58 Vascular anomalies
743.59 Other
743.6# Congenital anomalies of eyelids, lacrimal system, and orbit
743.61 Congenital ptosis
743.62 Congenital deformities of eyelids
743.63 Congenital anomalies of eyelid NEC
743.64 Specified congenital anomalies of lacrimal gland
743.65 Specified congenital anomalies of lacrimal passages
743.66 Specified congenital anomalies of orbit
743.69 Other
743.8 Other specified anomalies of eye
743.9 Unspecified anomaly of eye

744.#(#) Congenital anomalies of ear, face, and neck

744.0# Anomalies of ear causing impairment of hearing
744.00 Unspecified anomaly of ear with impairment of hearing
744.01 Absence of external ear
744.02 Other anomalies of external ear with impairment of hearing
744.03 Anomaly of middle ear, except ossicles
744.04 Anomalies of ear ossicles
744.05 Anomalies of inner ear
744.09 Other
744.1 Accessory auricle
744.2# Other specified anomalies of ear
744.21 Absence of ear lobe, congenital
744.22 Macrotia
744.23 Microtia
744.24 Specified anomalies of Eustachian tube
744.29 Other
744.3 Unspecified anomaly of ear
744.4# Branchial cleft cyst or fistula; preauricular sinus
744.41 Branchial cleft sinus or fistula
744.42 Branchial cleft cyst
744.43 Cervical auricle
744.46 Preauricular sinus or fistula
744.47 Preauricular cyst
744.49 Other

744.#(#) ***(continued)***
- 744.5 Webbing of neck
- **744.8#** Other specified anomalies of face and neck
  - 744.81 Macrocheilia
  - 744.82 Microcheilia
  - 744.83 Macrostomia
  - 744.84 Microstomia
  - 744.89 Other
- 744.9 Unspecified anomalies of face and neck

745.#(#) Bulbus cordis anomalies and anomalies of cardiac septal closure
- 745.0 Common truncus
- **745.1#** Transposition of great vessels
  - 745.10 Complete transposition of great vessels
  - 745.11 Double outlet right ventricle
  - 745.12 Corrected transposition of great vessels
  - 745.19 Other
- 745.2 Tetralogy of Fallot
- 745.3 Common ventricle
- 745.4 Ventricular septal defect
- 745.5 Ostium secundum type atrial septal defect
- **745.6#** Endocardial cushion defects
  - 745.60 Endocardial cushion defect, unspecified type
  - 745.61 Ostium primum defect
  - 745.69 Other
- 745.7 Cor biloculare
- 745.8 Other
- 745.9 Unspecified defect of septal closure

746.#(#) Other congenital anomalies of heart
- **746.0#** Anomalies of pulmonary valve
  - 746.00 Pulmonary valve anomaly, unspecified
  - 746.01 Atresia, congenital
  - 746.02 Stenosis, congenital
  - 746.09 Other
- 746.1 Tricuspid atresia and stenosis, congenital
- 746.2 Ebstein's anomaly
- 746.3 Congenital stenosis of aortic valve
- 746.4 Congenital insufficiency of aortic valve
- 746.5 Congenital mitral stenosis
- 746.6 Congenital mitral insufficiency
- 746.7 Hypoplastic left heart syndrome
- **746.8#** Other specified anomalies of heart
  - 746.81 Subaortic stenosis
  - 746.82 Cor triatriatum
  - 746.83 Infundibular pulmonic stenosis
  - 746.84 Obstructive anomalies of heart, NEC
  - 746.85 Coronary artery anomaly
  - 746.86 Congenital heart block
  - 746.87 Malposition of heart and cardiac apex
  - 746.89 Other
- 746.9 Unspecified anomaly of heart

747.#(#) Other congenital anomalies of circulatory system
- 747.0 Patent ductus arteriosus
- **747.1#** Coarctation of aorta
  - 747.10 Coarctation of aorta (preductal) (postductal)
  - 747.11 Interruption of aortic arch
- **747.2#** Other anomalies of aorta
  - 747.20 Anomaly of aorta, unspecified
  - 747.21 Anomalies of aortic arch
  - 747.22 Atresia and stenosis of aorta
  - 747.29 Other
- 747.3 Anomalies of pulmonary artery

747.#(#) ***(continued)***
- **747.4#** Anomalies of great veins
  - 747.40 Anomaly of great veins, unspecified
  - 747.41 Total anomalous pulmonary venous connection
  - 747.42 Partial anomalous pulmonary venous connection
  - 747.49 Other anomalies of great veins
- 747.5 Absence or hypoplasia of umbilical artery
- **747.6#** Other anomalies of peripheral vascular system
  - 747.60 Anomaly of the peripheral vascular system, unspecified site
  - 747.61 Gastrointestinal vessel anomaly
  - 747.62 Renal vessel anomaly
  - 747.63 Upper limb vessel anomaly
  - 747.64 Lower limb vessel anomaly
  - 747.69 Anomalies peripheral vascular system NEC
- **747.8#** Other specified anomalies of circulatory system
  - 747.81 Anomalies of cerebrovascular system
  - 747.82 Spinal vessel anomaly
  - 747.83 Persistent fetal circulation
  - 747.89 Other
- 747.9 Unspecified anomaly of circulatory system

748.#(#) Congenital anomalies of respiratory system
- 748.0 Choanal atresia
- 748.1 Other anomalies of nose
- 748.2 Web of larynx
- 748.3 Other anomalies of larynx, trachea, and bronchus
- 748.4 Congenital cystic lung
- 748.5 Agenesis, hypoplasia, and dysplasia of lung
- **748.6#** Other anomalies of lung
  - 748.60 Anomaly of lung, unspecified
  - 748.61 Congenital bronchiectasis
  - 748.69 Other
- 748.8 Other specified anomalies of respiratory system
- 748.9 Unspecified anomaly of respiratory system

749.#(#) Cleft palate and cleft lip
- **749.0#** Cleft palate
- **749.1#** Cleft lip

  5th Digit: 749.0-749.1
  - **0 Unspecified**
  - **1 Unilateral, complete**
  - **2 Unilateral, incomplete**
  - **3 Bilateral, complete**
  - **4 Bilateral, incomplete**
- **749.2#** Cleft palate with cleft lip
  - 749.20 Cleft palate with cleft lip, unspecified
  - 749.21 Unilateral, complete
  - 749.22 Unilateral, incomplete
  - 749.23 Bilateral, complete
  - 749.24 Bilateral, incomplete
  - 749.25 Other combinations

750.#(#) Other congenital anomalies of upper alimentary tract
- 750.0 Tongue tie
- **750.1#** Other anomalies of tongue
  - 750.10 Anomaly of tongue, unspecified
  - 750.11 Aglossia
  - 750.12 Congenital adhesions of tongue
  - 750.13 Fissure of tongue
  - 750.15 Macroglossia
  - 750.16 Microglossia
  - 750.19 Other

750.#(#) ***(continued)***

750.2# Other specified anomalies of mouth and pharynx
750.21 Absence of salivary gland
750.22 Accessory salivary gland
750.23 Atresia, salivary gland
750.24 Congenital fistula of salivary gland
750.25 Congenital fistula of lip
750.26 Other specified anomalies of mouth
750.27 Diverticulum of pharynx
750.29 Other specified anomalies of pharynx
750.3 Tracheoesophageal fistula, esophageal atresia and stenosis
750.4 Other specified anomalies of esophagus
750.5 Congenital hypertrophic pyloric stenosis
750.6 Congenital hiatus hernia
750.7 Other specified anomalies of stomach
750.8 Anomalies of upper alimentary tract, NEC
750.9 Unspecified anomaly of upper alimentary tract

751.#(#) Other congenital anomalies of digestive system

751.0 Meckel's diverticulum
751.1 Atresia and stenosis of small intestine
751.2 Atresia and stenosis of large intestine, rectum, and anal canal
751.3 Hirschsprung's disease and other congenital functional disorders of colon
751.4 Anomalies of intestinal fixation
751.5 Other anomalies of intestine
751.6# Anomalies of gallbladder, bile ducts, and liver
751.60 Unspecified anomaly of gallbladder, bile ducts, and liver
751.61 Biliary atresia
751.62 Congenital cystic disease of liver
751.69 Other anomalies of gallbladder, bile ducts, and liver
751.7 Anomalies of pancreas
751.8 Other specified anomalies of digestive system
751.9 Unspecified anomaly of digestive system

752.#(#) Congenital anomalies of genital organs

752.0 Anomalies of ovaries
752.1# Anomalies of fallopian tubes and broad ligaments
752.10 Unspecified anomaly of fallopian tubes and broad ligaments
752.11 Embryonic cyst of fallopian tubes and broad ligaments
752.19 Other
752.2 Doubling of uterus
752.3 Other anomalies of uterus
752.4# Anomalies of cervix, vagina, and external female genitalia
752.40 Unspecified anomaly of cervix, vagina, and external female genitalia
752.41 Embryonic cyst of cervix, vagina, and external female genitalia
752.42 Imperforate hymen
752.49 Other anomalies of cervix, vagina, and external female genitalia
752.5# Undescended and retractile testicle
752.51 Undescended testis
752.52 Retractile testis

752.#(#) ***(continued)***

752.6# Hypospadias and epispadias and other penile anomalies
752.61 Hypospadias
752.62 Epispadias
752.63 Congenital chordee
752.64 Micropenis
752.65 Hidden penis
752.69 Other penile anomalies
752.7 Indeterminate sex and pseudohermaphroditism
752.8# Other specified anomalies of genital organs
752.81 Scrotal transposition
752.89 Other specified anomalies of genital organs
752.9 Unspecified anomaly of genital organs

753.#(#) Congenital anomalies of urinary system

753.0 Renal agenesis and dysgenesis
753.1# Cystic kidney disease
753.10 Cystic kidney disease, unspecified
753.11 Congenital single renal cyst
753.12 Polycystic kidney, unspecified type
753.13 Polycystic kidney, autosomal dominant
753.14 Polycystic kidney, autosomal recessive
753.15 Renal dysplasia
753.16 Medullary cystic kidney
753.17 Medullary sponge kidney
753.19 Other specified cystic kidney disease
753.2# Obstructive defects of renal pelvis and ureter
753.20 Unspecified obstructive defect of renal pelvis and ureter
753.21 Congenital obstruction of ureteropelvic junction
753.22 Congenital obstruction of ureterovesical junction
753.23 Congenital ureterocele
753.29 Other
753.3 Other specified anomalies of kidney
753.4 Other specified anomalies of ureter
753.5 Exstrophy of urinary bladder
753.6 Atresia and stenosis of urethra and bladder neck
753.7 Anomalies of urachus
753.8 Anomalies of bladder and urethra, NEC
753.9 Unspecified anomaly of urinary system

754.#(#) Certain congenital musculoskeletal deformities

754.0 Of skull, face, and jaw
754.1 Of sternocleidomastoid muscle
754.2 Of spine
754.3# Congenital dislocation of hip
754.30 Congenital dislocation of hip, unilateral
754.31 Congenital dislocation of hip, bilateral
754.32 Congenital subluxation of hip, unilateral
754.33 Congenital subluxation of hip, bilateral
754.35 Congenital dislocation of one hip with subluxation of other hip
754.4# Congenital genu recurvatum and bowing of long bones of leg
754.40 Genu recurvatum
754.41 Congenital dislocation of knee (with genu recurvatum)
754.42 Congenital bowing of femur
754.43 Congenital bowing of tibia and fibula
754.44 Congenital bowing long bones of leg NOS

NUMERICAL REFERENCE

754.#(#) *(continued)*

754.5# Varus deformities of feet
- 754.50 Talipes varus
- 754.51 Talipes equinovarus
- 754.52 Metatarsus primus varus
- 754.53 Metatarsus varus
- 754.59 Other

754.6# Valgus deformities of feet
- 754.60 Talipes valgus
- 754.61 Congenital pes planus
- 754.62 Talipes calcaneovalgus
- 754.69 Other

754.7# Other deformities of feet
- 754.70 Talipes, unspecified
- 754.71 Talipes cavus
- 754.79 Other

754.8# Other specified nonteratogenic anomalies
- 754.81 Pectus excavatum
- 754.82 Pectus carinatum
- 754.89 Other

755.#(#) Other congenital anomalies of limbs

755.0# Polydactyly
- 755.00 Polydactyly, unspecified digits
- 755.01 Of fingers
- 755.02 Of toes

755.1# Syndactyly
- 755.10 Of multiple and unspecified sites
- 755.11 Of fingers without fusion of bone
- 755.12 Of fingers with fusion of bone
- 755.13 Of toes without fusion of bone
- 755.14 Of toes with fusion of bone

755.2# Reduction deformities of upper limb
- 755.20 Reduction deformity of upper limb NOS
- 755.21 Transverse deficiency of upper limb
- 755.22 Longitudinal deficiency of upper limb, NEC
- 755.23 Longitudinal deficiency, combined, involving humerus, radius, and ulna (complete or incomplete)
- 755.24 Longitudinal deficiency, humeral, complete or partial (with or without distal deficiencies, incomplete)
- 755.25 Longitudinal deficiency, radioulnar, complete or partial (with or without distal deficiencies, incomplete)
- 755.26 Longitudinal deficiency, radial, complete or partial (with or without distal deficiencies, incomplete)
- 755.27 Longitudinal deficiency, ulnar, complete or partial (with or without distal deficiencies, incomplete)
- 755.28 Longitudinal deficiency, carpals or metacarpals, complete or partial (with or without phalangeal deficiency)
- 755.29 Longitudinal deficiency, phalanges, complete or partial

755.3# Reduction deformities of lower limb
- 755.30 Reduction deformity of lower limb NOS
- 755.31 Transverse deficiency of lower limb
- 755.32 Longitudinal deficiency lower limb, NEC
- 755.33 Longitudinal deficiency, combined, involving femur, tibia, and fibula (complete or incomplete)
- 755.34 Longitudinal deficiency, femoral, complete or partial (with or without distal deficiencies, incomplete)
- 755.35 Longitudinal deficiency, tibiofibular, complete or partial (with or without distal deficiencies, incomplete)

755.#(#) *(continued)*

755.3(#) *(continued)*
- 755.36 Longitudinal deficiency, tibia, complete or partial (with or without distal deficiencies, incomplete)
- 755.37 Longitudinal deficiency, fibular, complete or partial (with or without distal deficiencies, incomplete)
- 755.38 Longitudinal deficiency, tarsals or metatarsals, complete or partial (with or without phalangeal deficiency)
- 755.39 Longitudinal deficiency, phalanges, complete or partial

755.4 Reduction deformities, unspecified limb

755.5# Other anomalies of upper limb, including shoulder girdle
- 755.50 Unspecified anomaly of upper limb
- 755.51 Congenital deformity of clavicle
- 755.52 Congenital elevation of scapula
- 755.53 Radioulnar synostosis
- 755.54 Madelung's deformity
- 755.55 Acrocephalosyndactyly
- 755.56 Accessory carpal bones
- 755.57 Macrodactylia (fingers)
- 755.58 Cleft hand, congenital
- 755.59 Other

755.6# Anomalies of lower limb, including pelvic girdle, NEC
- 755.60 Unspecified anomaly of lower limb
- 755.61 Coxa valga, congenital
- 755.62 Coxa vara, congenital
- 755.63 Other congenital deformity of hip (joint)
- 755.64 Congenital deformity of knee (joint)
- 755.65 Macrodactylia of toes
- 755.66 Other anomalies of toes
- 755.67 Anomalies of foot, NEC
- 755.69 Other

755.8 Other specified anomalies of unspecified limb

755.9 Unspecified anomaly of unspecified limb

756.#(#) Other congenital musculoskeletal anomalies

756.0 Anomalies of skull and face bones

756.1# Anomalies of spine
- 756.10 Anomaly of spine, unspecified
- 756.11 Spondylolysis, lumbosacral region
- 756.12 Spondylolisthesis
- 756.13 Absence of vertebra, congenital
- 756.14 Hemivertebra
- 756.15 Fusion of spine [vertebra], congenital
- 756.16 Klippel-Feil syndrome
- 756.17 Spina bifida occulta
- 756.19 Other

756.2 Cervical rib

756.3 Other anomalies of ribs and sternum

756.4 Chondrodystrophy

756.5# Osteodystrophies
- 756.50 Osteodystrophy, unspecified
- 756.51 Osteogenesis imperfecta
- 756.52 Osteopetrosis
- 756.53 Osteopoikilosis
- 756.54 Polyostotic fibrous dysplasia of bone
- 756.55 Chondroectodermal dysplasia
- 756.56 Multiple epiphyseal dysplasia
- 756.59 Other

756.6 Anomalies of diaphragm

756.7# Anomalies of abdominal wall
- 756.70 Anomaly of abdominal wall, unspecified
- 756.71 Prune belly syndrome
- 756.79 Congenital anomalies of abdominal wall, NEC

756.#(#) ***(continued)***

- **756.8#** Other specified anomalies of muscle, tendon, fascia, and connective tissue
  - 756.81 Absence of muscle and tendon
  - 756.82 Accessory muscle
  - 756.83 Ehlers-Danlos syndrome
  - 756.89 Other
- 756.9 Other and unspecified anomalies of musculoskeletal system

757.#(#) Congenital anomalies of the integument

- 757.0 Hereditary edema of legs
- 757.1 Ichthyosis congenital
- 757.2 Dermatoglyphic anomalies
- **757.3#** Other specified anomalies of skin
  - 757.31 Congenital ectodermal dysplasia
  - 757.32 Vascular hamartomas
  - 757.33 Congenital pigmentary anomalies of skin
  - 757.39 Other
- 757.4 Specified anomalies of hair
- 757.5 Specified anomalies of nails
- 757.6 Specified anomalies of breast
- 757.8 Other specified anomalies of the integument
- 757.9 Unspecified anomaly of the integument

758.#(#) Chromosomal anomalies

- 758.0 Down's syndrome
- 758.1 Patau's syndrome
- 758.2 Edward's syndrome
- **758.3#** Autosomal deletion syndromes
  - 758.31 Cri-du-chat syndrome
  - 758.32 Velo-cardio-facial syndrome
  - 758.33 Other microdeletions
  - 758.39 Other autosomal deletions
- 758.4 Balanced autosomal translocation in normal individual
- 758.5 Other conditions due to autosomal anomalies
- 758.6 Gonadal dysgenesis
- 758.7 Klinefelter's syndrome
- **758.8#** Other conditions due to chromosome anomalies
  - 758.81 Other conditions due to sex chromosome anomalies
  - 758.89 Other
- 758.9 Conditions due to anomaly of unspecified chromosome

759.#(#) Other and unspecified congenital anomalies

- 759.0 Anomalies of spleen
- 759.1 Anomalies of adrenal gland
- 759.2 Anomalies of other endocrine glands
- 759.3 Situs inversus
- 759.4 Conjoined twins
- 759.5 Tuberous sclerosis
- 759.6 Other hamartoses, NEC
- 759.7 Multiple congenital anomalies, so described
- **759.8#** Other specified anomalies
  - 759.81 Prader-Willi syndrome
  - 759.82 Marfan syndrome
  - 759.83 Fragile X syndrome
  - 759.89 Other
- 759.9 Congenital anomaly, unspecified

760.#(#) Fetus or newborn affected by maternal conditions which may be unrelated to present pregnancy

- 760.0 Maternal hypertensive disorders
- 760.1 Maternal renal and urinary tract diseases
- 760.2 Maternal infections
- 760.3 Other chronic maternal circulatory and respiratory diseases
- 760.4 Maternal nutritional disorders
- 760.5 Maternal injury
- 760.6 Surgical operation on mother
- **760.7#** Noxious influences affecting fetus or newborn via placenta or breast milk
  - 760.70 Unspecified noxious substance
  - 760.71 Alcohol
  - 760.72 Narcotics
  - 760.73 Hallucinogenic agents
  - 760.74 Anti-infectives
  - 760.75 Cocaine
  - 760.76 Diethylstilbestrol [DES]
  - 760.77 Anticonvulsants
  - 760.78 Antimetabloic agnets
  - 760.79 Other
- 760.8 Other specified maternal conditions affecting fetus or newborn
- 760.9 Other maternal condition affecting fetus or newborn

761.# Fetus or newborn affected by maternal complications of pregnancy

- 761.0 Incompetent cervix
- 761.1 Premature rupture of membranes
- 761.2 Oligohydramnios
- 761.3 Polyhydramnios
- 761.4 Ectopic pregnancy
- 761.5 Multiple pregnancy
- 761.6 Maternal death
- 761.7 Malpresentation before labor
- 761.8 Other specified maternal complications of pregnancy affecting fetus or newborn
- 761.9 Unspecified maternal complication of pregnancy affecting fetus or newborn

762.# Fetus or newborn affected by complications of placenta, cord, and membranes

- 762.0 Placenta previa
- 762.1 Placental separation and hemorrhage NEC
- 762.2 Other and unspecified morphological and functional abnormalities of placenta
- 762.3 Placental transfusion syndromes
- 762.4 Prolapsed cord
- 762.5 Other compression of umbilical cord
- 762.6 Other and unspecified conditions of umbilical cord
- 762.7 Chorioamnionitis
- 762.8 Other specified abnormalities of chorion and amnion
- 762.9 Unspecified abnormality of chorion and amnion

763.#(#) Fetus or newborn affected by other complications of labor and delivery

- 763.0 Breech delivery and extraction
- 763.1 Other malpresentation, malposition, and disproportion during labor and delivery
- 763.2 Forceps delivery
- 763.3 Delivery by vacuum extractor
- 763.4 Cesarean delivery
- 763.5 Maternal anesthesia and analgesia
- 763.6 Precipitate delivery
- 763.7 Abnormal uterine contractions

763.#(#) ***(continued)***

763.8# Other specified complications of labor and delivery affecting fetus or newborn
- 763.81 Abnormality in fetal heart rate or rhythm before the onset of labor
- 763.82 Abnormality in fetal heart rate or rhythm during labor
- 763.83 Abnormality in fetal heart rate or rhythm, unspecified as to time of onset
- 763.84 Meconium passage during delivery
- 763.89 Other specified complications of labor and delivery affecting fetus or newborn

763.9 Unspecified complication of labor and delivery affecting fetus or newborn

764.## Slow fetal growth and fetal malnutrition

764.0# "Light-for-dates" without mention of fetal malnutrition
764.1# "Light-for-dates" with signs of fetal malnutrition
764.2# Fetal malnutrition without mention of "light-for dates"
764.9# Fetal growth retardation, unspecified

765.## Disorders relating to short gestation and unspecified low birthweight

765.0# Extreme immaturity
765.1# Other preterm infants

5th Digit: 764.0-764.9, 765.0-1
- **0 Unspecified [weight]**
- **1 Less than 500 grams**
- **2 500-749 grams**
- **3 750-999 grams**
- **4 1000-1249 grams**
- **5 1250-1499 grams**
- **6 1500-1749 grams**
- **7 1750-1999 grams**
- **8 2000-2499 grams**
- **9 2500 grams and over**

765.2# Weeks of gestation

5th Digit: 765.2
- **0 Unspecified weeks of gestations**
- **1 Less than 24 weeks of gestation**
- **2 24 completed weeks of gestation**
- **3 25-26 completed weeks of gestation**
- **4 27-28 completed weeks of gestation**
- **5 29-30 completed weeks of gestation**
- **6 31-32 completed weeks of gestation**
- **7 33-34 completed weeks of gestation**
- **8 35-36 completed weeks of gestation**
- **9 37or more completed weeks of gestation**

766.#(#) Disorders relating to long gestation and high birthweight

766.0 Exceptionally large baby
766.1 Other "heavy-for-dates" infants
766.2# Post-term infant, not "heavy-for-dates"
- 766.21 Post-term infant (>40-42 completed weeks)
- 766.22 Prolonged gestation (>42 completed weeks)

767.#(#) Birth trauma

767.0 Subdural and cerebral hemorrhage
767.1# Injuries to scalp
- 767.11 Epicranial subaponeurotic hemorrhage (massive)
- 767.19 Other injuries to the scalp

767.2 Fracture of clavicle
767.3 Other injuries to skeleton
767.4 Injury to spine and spinal cord

767.#(#) ***(continued)***

767.5 Facial nerve injury
767.6 Injury to brachial plexus
767.7 Other cranial and peripheral nerve injuries
767.8 Other specified birth trauma
767.9 Birth trauma, unspecified

768.# Intrauterine hypoxia and birth asphyxia

768.0 Fetal death from asphyxia or anoxia before onset of labor or at unspecified time
768.1 Fetal death from asphyxia or anoxia during labor
768.2 Fetal distress before onset of labor, in liveborn infant
768.3 Fetal distress first noted during labor and delivery, in liveborn infant
768.4 Fetal distress, unspecified as to time of onset, in liveborn infant
768.5 Severe birth asphyxia
768.6 Mild or moderate birth asphyxia
768.7 Hypoxic-ischemic encephalopathy (HIE)
768.9 Unspecified birth asphyxia in liveborn infant

769 Respiratory distress syndrome

770.#(#) Other respiratory conditions of fetus and newborn

770.0 Congenital pneumonia
770.1# Fetal and newborn aspiration
- 770.10 Unspecified
- 770.11 Meconium aspiration without respiratory symptoms
- 770.12 Meconium aspiration with respiratory symptoms
- 770.13 Aspiration of clear amniotic fluid without respiratory symptoms
- 770.14 Aspiration of clear amniotic fluid with respiratory symptoms
- 770.15 Aspiration of blood without respiratory symptoms
- 770.16 Aspiration of blood with respiratory symptoms
- 77017 Other fetal and newborn aspiration without respiratory symptoms
- 770.18 Other fetal and newborn aspiration with respiratory symptoms

770.2 Interstitial emphysema and related conditions
770.3 Pulmonary hemorrhage
770.4 Primary atelectasis
770.5 Other and unspecified atelectasis
770.6 Transitory tachypnea of newborn
770.7 Chronic respiratory disease arising in the perinatal period
770.8# Other respiratory problems after birth
- 770.81 Primary apnea of newborn
- 770.82 Other apnea of newborn
- 770.83 Cyanotic attacks of newborn
- 770.84 Respiratory failure of newborn
- 770.85 Aspiration of postnatal stomach contents without respiratory symptoms
- 770.86 Aspiration postnatal stomach contents with respiratory symptoms
- 770.87 Respiratory arrest of newborn
- 770.88 Hypoxemia of newborn
- 770.89 Other respiratory problems after birth

770.9 Unspecified respiratory condition of fetus and newborn

771.#(#) Infections specific to the perinatal period
771.0 Congenital rubella
771.1 Congenital cytomegalovirus infection
771.2 Other congenital infections
771.3 Tetanus neonatorum
771.4 Omphalitis of the newborn
771.5 Neonatal infective mastitis
771.6 Neonatal conjunctivitis and dacryocystitis
771.7 Neonatal Candida infection
771.8# Other infection specific to the perinatal period
771.81 Septicemia (sepsis) of newborn
771.82 Urinary tract infection of newborn
771.83 Bacteremia of newborn
771.89 Other infections specific to the perinatal period

772.#(#) Fetal and neonatal hemorrhage
772.0 Fetal blood loss
772.1# Intraventricular hemorrhage
772.10 Unspecified sgrade
772.11 Grade I
772.12 Grade II
772.13 Grade III
772.14 Grade IV
772.2 Subarachnoid hemorrhage
772.3 Umbilical hemorrhage after birth
772.4 Gastrointestinal hemorrhage
772.5 Adrenal hemorrhage
772.6 Cutaneous hemorrhage
772.8 Other specified hemorrhage of fetus or newborn
772.9 Unspecified hemorrhage of newborn

773.# Hemolytic disease of fetus or newborn, due to isoimmunization
773.0 Hemolytic disease due to Rh isoimmunization
773.1 Hemolytic disease due to ABO isoimmunization
773.2 Hemolytic disease due to other and unspecified isoimmunization
773.3 Hydrops fetalis due to isoimmunization
773.4 Kernicterus due to isoimmunization
773.5 Late anemia due to isoimmunization

774.#(#) Other perinatal jaundice
774.0 Perinatal jaundice from hereditary hemolytic anemias
774.2 Neonatal jaundice associated with preterm delivery
774.3# Neonatal jaundice due to delayed conjugation from other causes
774.30 Neonatal jaundice due to delayed conjugation, cause unspecified
774.31 Neonatal jaundice due to delayed conjugation in diseases classified elsewhere
774.39 Other
774.4 Perinatal jaundice due to hepatocellular damage
774.5 Perinatal jaundice from other causes
774.6 Unspecified fetal and neonatal jaundice
774.7 Kernicterus not due to isoimmunization

775.#(#) Endocrine and metabolic disturbances specific to the fetus and newborn
775.0 Syndrome of "infant of a diabetic mother"
775.1 Neonatal diabetes mellitus
775.2 Neonatal myasthenia gravis
775.3 Neonatal thyrotoxicosis

775.#(#) ***(continued)***
775.4 Hypocalcemia and hypomagnesemia of newborn
775.5 Other transitory neonatal electrolyte disturbances
775.6 Neonatal hypoglycemia
775.7 Late metabolic acidosis of newborn
775.8# Other neonatal endocrine and metabolic disturbances
775.81 Other acidosis of newborn
775.89 Other neonatal endocrine and metabolic disturbances
775.9 Unspecified endocrine and metabolic disturbances specific to the fetus and newborn

776.# Hematological disorders of fetus and newborn
776.0 Hemorrhagic disease of newborn
776.1 Transient neonatal thrombocytopenia
776.2 Disseminated intravascular coagulation in newborn
776.3 Other transient neonatal disorders of coagulation
776.4 Polycythemia neonatorum
776.5 Congenital anemia
776.6 Anemia of prematurity
776.7 Transient neonatal neutropenia
776.8 Other specified transient hematological disorders
776.9 Unspecified hematological disorder specific to fetus or newborn

777.# Perinatal disorders of digestive system
777.1 Meconium obstruction
777.2 Intestinal obstruction due to inspissated milk
777.3 Hematemesis and melena due to swallowed maternal blood
777.4 Transitory ileus of newborn
777.5 Necrotizing enterocolitis in fetus or newborn
777.6 Perinatal intestinal perforation
777.8 Other specified perinatal disorders of digestive system
777.9 Unspecified perinatal disorder of digestive system

778.# Conditions involving the integument and temperature regulation of fetus and newborn
778.0 Hydrops fetalis not due to isoimmunization
778.1 Sclerema neonatorum
778.2 Cold injury syndrome of newborn
778.3 Other hypothermia of newborn
778.4 Other disturbances of temperature regulation of newborn
778.5 Other and unspecified edema of newborn
778.6 Congenital hydrocele
778.7 Breast engorgement in newborn
778.8 Other specified conditions involving the integument of fetus and newborn
778.9 Condition involving the integument and temperature regulation of fetus and newborn NOS

779.#(#) Other and ill-defined conditions originating in the perinatal period
779.0 Convulsions in newborn
779.1 Other and unspecified cerebral irritability in newborn
779.2 Cerebral depression, coma, and other abnormal cerebral signs
779.3 Feeding problems in newborn
779.4 Drug reactions and intoxications specific to newborn

779.#(#) *(continued)*
779.5 Drug withdrawal syndrome in newborn
779.6 Termination of pregnancy (fetus)
779.7 Periventricular leukomalacia
779.8# Other specified conditions originating in the perinatal period
779.81 Neonatal bradycardia
779.82 Neonatal tachycardia
779.83 Delayed seperation of umbilical cord
779.84 Meconium staining
779.85 Cardiac arrest of newborn
779.89 Other specified conditions originating in the perinatal period
779.9 Unspecified condition originating in the perinatal period

780.#(#) General symptoms
780.0# Alteration of consciousness
780.01 Coma
780.02 Transient alteration of awareness
780.03 Persistent vegetative state
780.09 Other
780.1 Hallucinations
780.2 Syncope and collapse
780.3# Convulsions
780.31 Febrile convulsions (simple), unspecified
780.32 Complex febrile convulsions
780.39 Other convulsions
780.4 Dizziness and giddiness
780.5# Sleep disturbances
780.50 Sleep disturbance, unspecified
780.51 Insomnia with sleep apnea, unspecified
780.52 Insomnia, unspecified
780.53 Hypersomnia with sleep apnea, unspecified
780.54 Hypersomnia, unspecified
780.55 Disruptions of 24 hour sleep wake cycle, unspecified
780.56 Dysfunctions associated with sleep stages or arousal from sleep
780.57 Unspecified sleep apnea
780.58 Sleep related movement disorder, unspecified
780.59 Other
780.6 Fever
780.7# Malaise and fatigue
780.71 Chronic fatigue syndrome
780.79 Other malaise and fatigue
780.8 Generalized hyperhidrosis
780.9# Other general symptoms
780.91 Fussy infant (baby)
780.92 Excessive crying of infant (baby)
780.93 Memory loss
780.94 Early satiety
780.95 Excessive crying of child, adolescent, or adult
780.96 Generalized pain
780.97 Altered mental status
780.99 Other general symptoms

781.#(#) Symptoms involving nervous and musculoskeletal systems
781.0 Abnormal involuntary movements
781.1 Disturbances of sensation of smell and taste
781.2 Abnormality of gait
781.3 Lack of coordination
781.4 Transient paralysis of limb
781.5 Clubbing of fingers
781.6 Meningismus
781.7 Tetany
781.8 Neurologic neglect syndrone

781.#(#) *(continued)*
781.9# Other symptoms involving nervous and musculoskeletal systems
781.91 Loss of height
781.92 Abnormal posture
781.93 Ocular torticollis
781.94 Facial weakness
781.99 Other symptoms involving nervous and musculoskeletal systems

782.#(#) Symptoms involving skin and other integumentary tissue
782.0 Disturbance of skin sensation
782.1 Rash and other nonspecific skin eruption
782.2 Localized superficial swelling, mass, or lump
782.3 Edema
782.4 Jaundice, unspecified, not of newborn
782.5 Cyanosis
782.6# Pallor and flushing
782.61 Pallor
782.62 Flushing
782.7 Spontaneous ecchymoses
782.8 Changes in skin texture
782.9 Other symptoms involving skin and integumentary tissues

783.#(#) Symptoms concerning nutrition, metabolism, and development
783.0 Anorexia
783.1 Abnormal weight gain
783.2# Abnormal loss of weight and underweight
783.21 Loss of weight
783.22 Underweight
783.3 Feeding difficulties and mismanagement
783.4# Lack of expected normal physiological development in childhood
783.40 Lack of normal physiological development, unspecified
783.41 Failure to thrive
783.42 Delayed milestones
783.43 Short stature
783.5 Polydipsia
783.6 Polyphagia
783.7 Adult failure to thrive
783.9 Other symptoms concerning nutrition, metabolism, and development

784.#(#) Symptoms involving head and neck
784.0 Headache
784.1 Throat pain
784.2 Swelling, mass, or lump in head and neck
784.3 Aphasia
784.4# Voice disturbance
784.40 Voice disturbance, unspecified
784.41 Aphonia
784.49 Other
784.5 Other speech disturbance
784.6# Other symbolic dysfunction
784.60 Symbolic dysfunction, unspecified
784.61 Alexia and dyslexia
784.69 Other
784.7 Epistaxis
784.8 Hemorrhage from throat
784.9# Other symptoms involving head and neck
784.91 Postnasal drip
784.99 Other symptoms involving head and neck

785.#(#) Symptoms involving cardiovascular system
785.0 Tachycardia, unspecified
785.1 Palpitations
785.2 Undiagnosed cardiac murmurs

785.#(#) ***(continued)***

785.3 Other abnormal heart sounds
785.4 Gangrene
785.5# Shock without mention of trauma
785.50 Shock, unspecified
785.51 Cardiogenic shock
785.52 Septic shock
785.59 Other
785.6 Enlargement of lymph nodes
785.9 Other symptoms involving cardiovascular system

786.#(#) Symptoms involving respiratory system and other chest symptoms

786.0# Dyspnea and respiratory abnormalities
786.00 Respiratory abnormality, unspecified
786.01 Hyperventilation
786.02 Orthopnea
786.03 Apnea
786.04 Cheyne-Stokes respiration
786.05 Shortness of breath
786.06 Tachypnea
786.07 Wheezing
786.09 Other
786.1 Stridor
786.2 Cough
786.3 Hemoptysis
786.4 Abnormal sputum
786.5# Chest pain
786.50 Chest pain, unspecified
786.51 Precordial pain
786.52 Painful respiration
786.59 Other
786.6 Swelling, mass, or lump in chest
786.7 Abnormal chest sounds
786.8 Hiccough
786.9 Other symptoms involving respiratory system and chest

787.#(#) Symptoms involving digestive system

787.0# Nausea and vomiting
787.01 Nausea with vomiting
787.02 Nausea alone
787.03 Vomiting alone
787.1 Heartburn
787.2# Dysphagia
787.20 Unspecified
787.21 Oral phase
787.22 Oropharyngeal phase
787.23 Pharyngeal phase
787.24 Pharyngoesophageal phase
787.29 Other
787.3 Flatulence, eructation, and gas pain
787.4 Visible peristalsis
787.5 Abnormal bowel sounds
787.6 Incontinence of feces
787.7 Abnormal feces
787.9# Other symptoms involving digestive system
787.91 Diarrhea
787.99 Other

788.#(#) Symptoms involving urinary system

788.0 Renal colic
788.1 Dysuria
788.2# Retention of urine
788.20 Retention of urine, unspecified
788.21 Incomplete bladder emptying
788.29 Other specified retention of urine

788.#(#) ***(continued)***

788.3# Urinary incontinence
788.30 Urinary incontinence, unspecified
788.31 Urge incontinence
788.32 Stress incontinence, male
788.33 Mixed incontinence (female) (male)
788.34 Incontinence without sensory awareness
788.35 Post-void dribbling
788.36 Nocturnal enuresis
788.37 Continuous leakage
788.38 Overflow incontinence
788.39 Other urinary incontinence
788.4# Frequency of urination and polyuria
788.41 Urinary frequency
788.42 Polyuria
788.43 Nocturia
788.5 Oliguria and anuria
788.6# Other abnormality of urination
788.61 Splitting of urinary stream
788.62 Slowing of urinary stream
788.63 Urgency of urination
788.64 Urinary hesitancy
788.65 Straining on urination
788.69 Other
788.7 Urethral discharge
788.8 Extravasation of urine
788.9 Other symptoms involving urinary system

789.#(#) Other symptoms involving abdomen and pelvis

789.0# Abdominal pain
789.1 Hepatomegaly
789.2 Splenomegaly
789.3# Abdominal or pelvic swelling, mass, or lump
789.4# Abdominal rigidity
789.5# Ascites
789.51 Malignant
789.59 Other
789.6# Abdominal tenderness
789.9 Other symptoms involving abdomen and pelvis

5th Digit: 789.0, 789.3, 789.4, 789.6
0 Unspecified site
1 Right upper quadrant
2 Left upper quadrant
3 Right lower quadrant
4 Left lower quadrant
5 Periumbilic
6 Epigastric
7 Generalized
9 Other specified site

790.#(#) Nonspecific findings on examination of blood

790.0# Abnormality of red blood cells
790.01 Precipitous drop in hematocrit
790.09 Other abnormality of red blood cells
790.1 Elevated sedimentation rate
790.2# Abnormal glucose
790.21 Impaired fasting glucose
790.22 Impaired glucose tolerance test (oral)
790.29 Other abnormal glucose
790.3 Excessive blood level of alcohol
790.4 Nonspecific elevation of levels of transaminase or lactic acid dehydrogenase [LDH]
790.5 Nonspecific abnormal serum enzyme levels NEC
790.6 Other abnormal blood chemistry
790.7 Bacteremia
790.8 Viremia, unspecified

790.#(#) ***(continued)***

790.9# Other nonspecific findings, examination of blood
- 790.91 Abnormal arterial blood gases
- 790.92 Abnormal coagulation profile
- 790.93 Elevated prostate specific antigen [PSA]
- 790.94 Euthyroid sick syndrome
- 790.95 Elevated C-reactive protein (CRP)
- 790.99 Other

791.# Nonspecific findings on examination of urine
- 791.0 Proteinuria
- 791.1 Chyluria
- 791.2 Hemoglobinuria
- 791.3 Myoglobinuria
- 791.4 Biliuria
- 791.5 Glycosuria
- 791.6 Acetonuria
- 791.7 Other cells and casts in urine
- 791.9 Other nonspecific findings,examination of urine

792.# Nonspecific abnormal findings, other body substances
- 792.0 Cerebrospinal fluid
- 792.1 Stool contents
- 792.2 Semen
- 792.3 Amniotic fluid
- 792.4 Saliva
- 792.5 Cloudy (hemodialysis)(peritoneal) dialysis substances
- 792.9 Other nonspecific abnormal findings in body substances

793.#(#) Nonspecific abnormal findings on radiological and other examination of body structure
- 793.0 Skull and head
- 793.1 Lung field
- 793.2 Other intrathoracic organ
- 793.3 Biliary tract
- 793.4 Gastrointestinal tract
- 793.5 Genitourinary organs
- 793.6 Abdominal area, including retroperitoneum
- 793.7 Musculoskeletal system

793.8(#) Breast
- 793.80 Abnormal mammogram, unspecified
- 793.81 Mammographic microcalcification
- 793.89 Other abnormal findings on radiological examination of breast

793.9# Other
- 793.91 Image test inconclusive due to excess body fat
- 793.99 Other nonspecific abnormal findings on radiological and other examination of body structure

794.#(#) Nonspecific abnormal results of function studies

794.0# Brain and central nervous system
- 794.00 Abnormal function study, unspecified
- 794.01 Abnormal echoencephalogram
- 794.02 Abnormal electroencephalogram [EEG]
- 794.09 Other

794.1# Peripheral nervous system and special senses
- 794.10 Abnormal response nerve stimulation, NOS
- 794.11 Abnormal retinal function studies
- 794.12 Abnormal electro-oculogram [EOG]
- 794.13 Abnormal visually evoked potential
- 794.14 Abnormal oculomotor studies
- 794.15 Abnormal auditory function studies
- 794.16 Abnormal vestibular function studies
- 794.17 Abnormal electromyogram [EMG]
- 794.19 Other

794.2 Pulmonary

794.#(#) ***(continued)***

794.3# Cardiovascular
- 794.30 Abnormal function study, unspecified
- 794.31 Abnormal electrocardiogram [ECG] [EKG]
- 794.39 Other

- 794.4 Kidney
- 794.5 Thyroid
- 794.6 Other endocrine function study
- 794.7 Basal metabolism
- 794.8 Liver
- 794.9 Other

795.#(#) Other and nonspecific abnormal cystological, histological, immunological and DNA test findings

795.0# Abnormal Papanicolaou smear of cervix and cervical HPV
- 795.00 Abnormal glandular Papanicolaou smear of cervix
- 795.01 Papanicolaou smear of cervix with atypical squamous cells of undertermined significance (ASC-US)
- 795.02 Papanicolaou smear of cervix with atypical squamous cells cannot exclude high grade squamous intraepithelial lesion (ASC-H)
- 795.03 Papanicolaou smear of cervix with low grade squamous intraepithelial lesion (LGSIL)
- 795.04 Papanicolaou smear of cervix with high grade squamous intraepithelial lesion (HGSIL)
- 795.05 Cervical high risk human papillomavirus (HPV) DNA test positive
- 795.06 Papanicolaou smear of cervix with cytologic evidence of malignancy
- 795.08 Unsatisfactory smear
- 795.09 Other abnormal Papanicolaou smear of cervix and cervical HPV

- 795.1 Nonspecific abnormal Papanicolaou smear of other site
- 795.2 Nonspecific abnormal findings on chromosomal analysis

795.3# Nonspecific positive culture findings
- 795.31 For antrhrax
- 795.39 Other

- 795.4 Other nonspecific abnormal histological findings
- 795.5 Nonspecific reaction to tuberculin skin test without active tuberculosis
- 795.6 False positive serological test for syphilis

795.7# Other nonspecific immunological findings
- 795.71 Nonspecific serologic evidence of human immunodeficiency virus [HIV]
- 795.79 Other and unspecified nonspecific immunological findings

795.8# Abnormal tumor markers
- 795.81 Elevated carcinoembryonic antigen [CEA]
- 795.82 Elevated cancer antigen 125 [CA 125]
- 795.89 Other abnormal turmor markers

796.# Other nonspecific abnormal findings
- 796.0 Nonspecific abnormal toxicological findings
- 796.1 Abnormal reflex
- 796.2 Elevated blood pressure reading without diagnosis of hypertension
- 796.3 Nonspecific low blood pressure reading
- 796.4 Other abnormal clinical findings
- 796.5 Abnormal finding on antenatal screening
- 796.6 Abnormal findings on neonatal screening
- 796.9 Other

797 Senility without mention of psychosis

NUMERICAL REFERENCE

798.# Sudden death, cause unknown
- 798.0 Sudden infant death syndrome
- 798.1 Instantaneous death
- 798.2 Death occurring in less than 24 hours from onset of symptoms, not otherwise explained
- 798.9 Unattended death

799.#(#) Other ill-defined and unknown causes of morbidity and mortality
- **799.0#** Asphyxia and hypoxemia
  - 799.01 Asphyxia
  - 799.02 Hypoxemia
- 799.1 Respiratory arrest
- 799.2 Nervousness
- 799.3 Debility, unspecified
- 799.4 Cachexia
- **799.8#** Other ill-defined conditions
  - 799.81 Decreased libido
  - 799.89 Other ill defined conditions
- 799.9 Other unknown and unspecified cause

800.## Fracture of vault of skull

801.## Fracture of base of skull

4th Digit: 800, 801
- **0 Closed without mention of intracranial injury**
- **1 Closed with cerebral laceration and contusion**
- **2 Closed wtih subarachnoid, subdural, and extradural hemorrhage**
- **3 Closed with other and unspecified intracranial hemorrhage**
- **4 Closed with intracranial injury of other and unspecified nature**
- **5 Open without mention of intracranial injury**
- **6 Open with cerebral laceration and contusion**
- **7 Open with subarachnoid, subdural, and extradural hemorrhage**
- **8 Open with other and unspecified intracranial hemorrhage**
- **9 Open with intracranial injury of other and unspecified nature**

5th Digit: 800, 801
- **0 Unspecified state of consciousness**
- **1 With no loss of consciousness**
- **2 With brief [less than one hour] loss of consciousness**
- **3 With moderate [1-24 hours] loss of consciousness**
- **4 With prolonged [more than 24 hours] loss of consciousness and return to pre-existing conscious level**
- **5 With prolonged [more than 24 hours] loss of consciousness, without return to pre-existing conscious level**
- **6 With loss of consciousness NOS**
- **9 With concussion, unspecified**

802.#(#) Fracture of face bones
- 802.0 Nasal bones, closed
- 802.1 Nasal bones, open

802.#(#) ***(continued)***
- **802.2#** Mandible, closed
- **802.3#** Mandible, open

5th Digit: 802.2, 802.3
- **0 Unspecified site**
- **1 Condylar process**
- **2 Subcondylar**
- **3 Coronoid process**
- **4 Ramus, unspecified**
- **5 Angle of jaw**
- **6 Symphysis of body**
- **7 Alveolar border of body**
- **8 Body, other and unspecified**
- **9 Multiple sites**

- 802.4 Malar and maxillary bones, closed
- 802.5 Malar and maxillary bones, open
- 802.6 Orbital floor (blow-out), closed
- 802.7 Orbital floor (blow-out), open
- 802.8 Other facial bones, closed
- 802.9 Other facial bones, open

803.## Other and unqualified skull fractures

804.## Multiple fractures involving skull or face with other bones

4th Digit: 803-804
- **0 Closed without mention of intracranial injury**
- **1 Closed with cerebral laceration and contusion**
- **2 Closed with subarachnoid, subdural, and extradural hemorrhage**
- **3 Closed with other and unspecified intracranial hemorrhage**
- **4 Closed with intracranial injury of other and unspecified nature**
- **5 Open without mention of intracranial injury**
- **6 Open with cerebral laceration and contusion**
- **7 Open with subarachnoid, subdural, and extradural hemorrhage**
- **8 Open with other and unspecified intracranial hemorrhage**
- **9 Open with intracranial injury of other and unspecified nature**

5th Digit: 803, 804
- **0 Unspecified state of consciousness**
- **1 With no loss of consciousness**
- **2 With brief [less than one hour] loss of consciousness**
- **3 With moderate [1-24 hours] loss of consciousness**
- **4 With prolonged [more than 24 hours] loss of consciousness and return to pre-existing conscious level**
- **5 With prolonged [more than 24 hours] loss of consciousness, without return to pre-existing conscious level**
- **6 With loss of consciousness of unspecified duration**
- **9 With concussion, unspecified**

805.#(#) Fracture of vertebral column without mention of spinal cord injury

805.0# Cervical, closed
805.1# Cervical, open

5th Digit: 805.0-805.1

- **0 Cervical vertebra, unspecified level**
- **1 First cervical vertebra**
- **2 Second cervical vertebra**
- **3 Third cervical vertebra**
- **4 Fourth cervical vertebra**
- **5 Fifth cervical vertebra**
- **6 Sixth cervical vertebra**
- **7 Seventh cervical vertebra**
- **8 Multiple cervical vertebrae**

805.2 Dorsal [thoracic], closed
805.3 Dorsal [thoracic], open
805.4 Lumbar, closed
805.5 Lumbar, open
805.6 Sacrum and coccyx, closed
805.7 Sacrum and coccyx, open
805.8 Unspecified, closed
805.9 Unspecified, open

806.#(#) Fracture of vertebral column with spinal cord injury

806.0# Cervical, closed
806.1# Cervical, open

5th Digit: 806.0-806.1

- **0 C_1-C_4 level with unspecified spinal cord injury**
- **1 C_1-C_4 level with complete lesion of cord**
- **2 C_1-C_4 level with anterior cord syndrome**
- **3 C_1-C_4 level with central cord syndrome**
- **4 C_1-C_4 level with other specified spinal cord injury**
- **5 C_5-C_7 level with unspecified spinal cord injury**
- **6 C_5-C_7 level with complete lesion of cord**
- **7 C_5-C_7 level with anterior cord syndrome**
- **8 C_5-C_7 level with central cord syndrome**
- **9 C_5-C_7 level with other specified spinal cord injury**

806.2# Dorsal [thoracic], closed
806.3# Dorsal [thoracic], open

5th Digit: 806.2-806.3

- **0 T_1-T_6 level, spinal cord injury NOS**
- **1 T_1-T_6 level, complete lesion of cord**
- **2 T_1-T_6 level, anterior cord syndrome**
- **3 T_1-T_6 level, central cord syndrome**
- **4 T_1-T_6 level, spinal cord injury other**
- **5 T_7-T_{12} level, spinal cord injury NOS**
- **6 T_7-T_{12} level, complete lesion of cord**
- **7 T_7-T_{12} level, anterior cord syndrome**
- **8 T_7-T_{12} level, central cord syndrome**
- **9 T_7-T_{12} level, spinal cord injury other**

806.4 Lumbar, closed
806.5 Lumbar, open
806.6# Sacrum and coccyx, closed
806.7# Sacrum and coccyx, open

5th Digit: 806.6-806.7

- **0 With unspecified spinal cord injury**
- **1 With complete cauda equina lesion**
- **2 With other cauda equina injury**
- **9 With other spinal cord injury**

806.8 Unspecified, closed
806.9 Unspecified, open

807.#(#) Fracture of rib(s), sternum, larynx, and trachea

807.0# Rib(s), closed
807.1# Rib(s), open

5th Digit: 807.0-807.1

- **0 Rib(s), unspecified**
- **1 One rib**
- **2 Two ribs**
- **3 Three ribs**
- **4 Four ribs**
- **5 Five ribs**
- **6 Six ribs**
- **7 Seven ribs**
- **8 Eight or more ribs**
- **9 Multiple ribs, unspecified**

807.2 Sternum, closed
807.3 Sternum, open
807.4 Flail chest
807.5 Larynx and trachea, closed
807.6 Larynx and trachea, open

808.#(#) Fracture of pelvis

808.0 Acetabulum, closed
808.1 Acetabulum, open
808.2 Pubis, closed
808.3 Pubis, open
808.4# Other specified part, closed
808.5# Other specified part, open

5th Digit: 808.4-808.5

- **1 Ilium**
- **2 Ischium**
- **3 Multiple pelvic fractures with disruption of pelvic circle**
- **9 Other**

808.8 Unspecified, closed
808.9 Unspecified, open

809.# Ill-defined fractures of bones of trunk

809.0 Fracture of bones of trunk, closed
809.1 Fracture of bones of trunk, open

810.## Fracture of clavicle

810.0# Closed
810.1# Open

5th Digit 810

- **0 Unspecified part**
- **1 Sternal end of clavicle**
- **2 Shaft of clavicle**
- **3 Acromial end of clavicle**

811.## Fracture of scapula

811.0# Closed
811.1# Open

5th Digit: 811

- **0 Unspecified part**
- **1 Acromial process**
- **2 Coracoid process**
- **3 Glenoid cavity and neck of scapula**
- **9 Other**

812.## Fracture of humerus

812.0# Upper end, closed
812.1# Upper end, open

5th Digit: 812.0-812.1

- **0 Upper end, unspecified part**
- **1 Surgical neck**
- **2 Anatomical neck**
- **3 Greater tuberosity**
- **9 Other**

NUMERICAL REFERENCE

812.## ***(continued)***
- **812.2#** Shaft or unspecified part, closed
- **812.3#** Shaft or unspecified part, open
  - **5th Digit: 812.2-812.3**
    - **0 Unspecified part of humerus**
    - **1 Shaft of humerus**
- **812.4#** Lower end, closed
- **812.5#** Lower end, open
  - **5th Digit: 812.4-812.5**
    - **0 Lower end, unspecified part**
    - **1 Supracondylar fracture of humerus**
    - **2 Lateral condyle**
    - **3 Medial condyle**
    - **4 Condyle(s), unspecified**
    - **9 Other**

813.## Fracture of radius and ulna
- **813.0#** Upper end, closed
- **813.1#** Upper end, open
  - **5th Digit: 813.0-813.1**
    - **0 Upper end of forearm, unspecified**
    - **1 Olecranon process of ulna**
    - **2 Coronoid process of ulna**
    - **3 Monteggia's fracture**
    - **4 Other and unspecified fractures of proximal end of ulna (alone)**
    - **5 Head of radius**
    - **6 Neck of radius**
    - **7 Other and unspecified fractures of proximal end of radius (alone)**
    - **8 Radius with ulna, upper end [any part]**
- **813.2#** Shaft, closed
- **813.3#** Shaft, open
  - **5th Digit: 813.2-813.3**
    - **0 Shaft, unspecified**
    - **1 Radius (alone)**
    - **2 Ulna (alone)**
    - **3 Radius with ulna**
- **813.4#** Lower end, closed
  - **5th Digit: 813.4**
    - **0 Lower end of forearm, unspecified**
    - **1 Colles' fracture**
    - **2 Other fractures of distal end of radius**
    - **3 Distal end of ulna (alone)**
    - **4 Radius with ulna, lower end**
    - **5 Torus fracture of radius**
- **813.5#** Lower end, open
  - **5th Digit: 813.5**
    - **0 Lower end of forearm, unspecified**
    - **1 Colles' fracture**
    - **2 Other fractures of distal end of radius**
    - **3 Distal end of ulna (alone)**
    - **4 Radius with ulna, lower end**
- **813.8#** Unspecified part, closed
- **813.9#** Unspecified part, open
  - **5th Digit: 813.8-813.9**
    - **0 Forearm, unspecified**
    - **1 Radius (alone)**
    - **2 Ulna (alone)**
    - **3 Radius with ulna**

814.## Fracture of carpal bone(s)
- **814.0#** Closed
- **814.1#** Open
  - **5th Digit: 814**
    - **0 Carpal bone, unspecified**
    - **1 Navicular [scaphoid] of wrist**
    - **2 Lunate [semilunar] bone of wrist**
    - **3 Triquetral [cuneiform] bone of wrist**
    - **4 Pisiform**
    - **5 Trapezium bone [larger multangular]**
    - **6 Trapezoid bone [smaller multangular]**
    - **7 Capitate bone [os magnum]**
    - **8 Hamate [unciform] bone**
    - **9 Other**

815.## Fracture of metacarpal bone(s)
- **815.0#** Closed
- **815.1#** Open
  - **5th Digit: 815**
    - **0 Metacarpal bone(s), site unspecified**
    - **1 Base of thumb [first] metacarpal**
    - **2 Base of other metacarpal bone(s)**
    - **3 Shaft of metacarpal bone(s)**
    - **4 Neck of metacarpal bone(s)**
    - **9 Multiple sites of metacarpus**

816.## Fracture of one or more phalanges of hand
- **816.0#** Closed
- **816.1#** Open
  - **5th Digit: 816**
    - **0 Phalanx or phalanges, unspecified**
    - **1 Middle or proximal phalanx or phalanges**
    - **2 Distal phalanx or phalanges**
    - **3 Multiple sites**

817.# Multiple fractures of hand bones
- 817.0 Closed
- 817.1 Open

818.# Ill-defined fractures of upper limb
- 818.0 Closed
- 818.1 Open

819.# Multiple fractures involving both upper limbs, and upper limb with rib(s) and sternum
- 819.0 Closed
- 819.1 Open

820.#(#) Fracture of neck of femur
- **820.0#** Transcervical fracture, closed
- **820.1#** Transcervical fracture, open
  - **5th Digit: 820.0-820.1**
    - **0 Intracapsular section, unspecified**
    - **1 Epiphysis (separation) (upper)**
    - **2 Midcervical section**
    - **3 Base of neck**
    - **9 Other**
- **820.2#** Pertrochanteric fracture, closed
- **820.3#** Pertrochanteric fracture, open
  - **5th Digit: 820.2-820.3**
    - **0 Trochanteric section, unspecified**
    - **1 Intertrochanteric section**
    - **2 Subtrochanteric section**
- 820.8 Unspecified part of neck of femur, closed
- 820.9 Unspecified part of neck of femur, open

NUMERICAL REFERENCE

821.#(#) Fracture of other and unspecified parts of femur
821.0# Shaft or unspecified part, closed
821.1# Shaft or unspecified part, open
5th Digit: 821.0-821.1
0 Unspecified part of femur
1 Shaft
821.2# Lower end, closed
821.3# Lower end, open
5th Digit: 821.2-821.3
0 Lower end, unspecified part
1 Condyle, femoral
2 Epiphysis, lower (separation)
3 Supracondylar fracture of femur
9 Other

822.# Fracture of patella
822.0 Closed
822.1 Open

823.## Fracture of tibia and fibula
823.0# Upper end, closed
823.1# Upper end, open
823.2# Shaft, closed
823.3# Shaft, open
823.4# Torus
823.8# Unspecified part, closed
823.9# Unspecified part, open
5th Digit: 823
0 Tibia alone
1 Fibula alone
2 Fibula with tibia

824.# Fracture of ankle
824.0 Medial malleolus, closed
824.1 Medial malleolus, open
824.2 Lateral malleolus, closed
824.3 Lateral malleolus, open
824.4 Bimalleolar, closed
824.5 Bimalleolar, open
824.6 Trimalleolar, closed
824.7 Trimalleolar, open
824.8 Unspecified, closed
824.9 Unspecified, open

825.#(#) Fracture of one or more tarsal and metatarsal bones
825.0 Fracture of calcaneus, closed
825.1 Fracture of calcaneus, open
825.2# Fracture of other tarsal and metatarsal bones, closed
825.3# Fracture of other tarsal and metatarsal bones, open
5th Digit: 825.2-825.3
0 Unspecified bone(s) of foot [except toes]
1 Astragalus
2 Navicular [scaphoid], foot
3 Cuboid
4 Cuneiform, foot
5 Metatarsal bone(s)
9 Other

826.# Fracture of one or more phalanges of foot
826.0 Closed
826.1 Open

827.# Other, multiple, and ill-defined fractures of lower limb
827.0 Closed
827.1 Open

828.# Multiple fractures involving both lower limbs, lower with upper limb, and lower limb(s) with rib(s) and sternum
828.0 Closed
828.1 Open

829.# Fracture of unspecified bones
829.0 Unspecified bone, closed
829.1 Unspecified bone, open

830.# Dislocation of jaw
830.0 Closed dislocation
830.1 Open dislocation

831.## Dislocation of shoulder
831.0# Closed dislocation
831.1# Open dislocation
5th Digit: 831
0 Shoulder, unspecified
1 Anterior dislocation of humerus
2 Posterior dislocation of humerus
3 Inferior dislocation of humerus
4 Acromioclavicular (joint)
9 Other

832.## Dislocation of elbow
832.0# Closed dislocation
832.1# Open dislocation
5th Digit: 832
0 Elbow unspecified
1 Anterior dislocation of elbow
2 Posterior dislocation of elbow
3 Medial dislocation of elbow
4 Lateral dislocation of elbow
9 Other

833.## Dislocation of wrist
833.0# Closed dislocation
833.1# Open dislocation
5th Digit: 833
0 Wrist, unspecified part
1 Radioulnar (joint), distal
2 Radiocarpal (joint)
3 Midcarpal (joint)
4 Carpometacarpal (joint)
5 Metacarpal (bone), proximal end
9 Other

834.## Dislocation of finger
834.0# Closed dislocation
834.1# Open dislocation
5th Digit: 834
0 Finger, unspecified part
1 Metacarpophalangeal (joint)
2 Interphalangeal (joint), hand

835.## Dislocation of hip
835.0# Closed dislocation
835.1# Open dislocation
5th Digit: 835
0 Dislocation of hip, unspecified
1 Posterior dislocation
2 Obturator dislocation
3 Other anterior dislocation

836.#(#) Dislocation of knee
836.0 Tear of medial cartilage or meniscus of knee, current
836.1 Tear of lateral cartilage or meniscus of knee, current

NUMERICAL REFERENCE

836.#(#) *(continued)*
836.2 Tear cartilage or meniscus of knee, current other
836.3 Dislocation of patella, closed
836.4 Dislocation of patella, open
836.5# Other dislocation of knee, closed
836.6# Other dislocation of knee, open
5th Digit: 836.5-836.6
0 Dislocation of knee, unspecified
1 Anterior dislocation of tibia, proximal end
2 Posterior dislocation of tibia, proximal end
3 Medial dislocation of tibia, proximal end
4 Lateral dislocation of tibia, proximal end
9 Other

837.# Dislocation of ankle
837.0 Closed dislocation
837.1 Open dislocation

838.## Dislocation of foot
838.0# Closed dislocation
838.1# Open dislocation
5th Digit: 838
0 Foot, unspecified
1 Tarsal (bone), joint unspecified
2 Midtarsal (joint)
3 Tarsometatarsal (joint)
4 Metatarsal (bone), joint unspecified
5 Metatarsophalangeal (joint)
6 Interphalangeal (joint), foot
9 Other

839.#(#) Other, multiple, and ill-defined dislocations
839.0# Cervical vertebra, closed
839.1# Cervical vertebra, open
5th Digit: 839.0-839.1
0 Cervical vertebra, unspecified
1 First cervical vertebra
2 Second cervical vertebra
3 Third cervical vertebra
4 Fourth cervical vertebra
5 Fifth cervical vertebra
6 Sixth cervical vertebra
7 Seventh cervical vertebra
8 Multiple cervical vertebrae
839.2# Thoracic and lumbar vertebra, closed
839.3# Thoracic and lumbar vertebra, open
5th Digit: 839.2-839.3
0 Lumbar vertebra
1 Thoracic vertebra
839.4# Other vertebra, closed
839.5# Other vertebra, open
5th Digit: 839.4-839.5
0 Vertebra, unspecified site
1 Coccyx
2 Sacrum
9 Other
839.6# Other location, closed
839.7# Other location, open
5th Digit: 839.6-839.7
1 Sternum
9 Other
839.8 Multiple and ill-defined, closed
839.9 Multiple and ill-defined, open

840.# Sprains and strains of shoulder and upper arm
840.0 Acromioclavicular (joint) (ligament)
840.1 Coracoclavicular (ligament)
840.2 Coracohumeral (ligament)
840.3 Infraspinatus (muscle) (tendon)
840.4 Rotator cuff (capsule)
840.5 Subscapularis (muscle)
840.6 Supraspinatus (muscle) (tendon)
840.7 Superior glenoid labrum lesion
840.8 Other specified sites of shoulder and upper arm
840.9 Unspecified site of shoulder and upper arm

841.# Sprains and strains of elbow and forearm
841.0 Radial collateral ligament
841.1 Ulnar collateral ligament
841.2 Radiohumeral (joint)
841.3 Ulnohumeral (joint)
841.8 Other specified sites of elbow and forearm
841.9 Unspecified site of elbow and forearm

842.## Sprains and strains of wrist and hand
842.0# Wrist
842.00 Unspecified site
842.01 Carpal (joint)
842.02 Radiocarpal (joint) (ligament)
842.09 Other
842.1# Hand
842.10 Unspecified site
842.11 Carpometacarpal (joint)
842.12 Metacarpophalangeal (joint)
842.13 Interphalangeal (joint)
842.19 Other

843.# Sprains and strains of hip and thigh
843.0 Iliofemoral (ligament)
843.1 Ischiocapsular (ligament)
843.8 Other specified sites of hip and thigh
843.9 Unspecified site of hip and thigh

844.# Sprains and strains of knee and leg
844.0 Lateral collateral ligament of knee
844.1 Medial collateral ligament of knee
844.2 Cruciate ligament of knee
844.3 Tibiofibular (joint) (ligament), superior
844.8 Other specified sites of knee and leg
844.9 Unspecified site of knee and leg

845.## Sprains and strains of ankle and foot
845.0# Ankle
845.00 Unspecified site
845.01 Deltoid (ligament), ankle
845.02 Calcaneofibular (ligament)
845.03 Tibiofibular (ligament), distal
845.09 Other
845.1# Foot
845.10 Unspecified site
845.11 Tarsometatarsal (joint) (ligament)
845.12 Metatarsophalangeal (joint)
845.13 Interphalangeal (joint), toe
845.19 Other

846.# Sprains and strains of sacroiliac region
846.0 Lumbosacral (joint) (ligament)
846.1 Sacroiliac ligament
846.2 Sacrospinatus (ligament)
846.3 Sacrotuberous (ligament)
846.8 Other specified sites of sacroiliac region
846.9 Unspecified site of sacroiliac region

847.# Sprains and strains of other and unspecified parts back

847.0 Neck
847.1 Thoracic
847.2 Lumbar
847.3 Sacrum
847.4 Coccyx
847.9 Unspecified site of back

848.#(#) Other and ill-defined sprains and strains

848.0 Septal cartilage of nose
848.1 Jaw
848.2 Thyroid region
848.3 Ribs
848.4# Sternum
848.40 Unspecified site
848.41 Sternoclavicular (joint) (ligament)
848.42 Chondrosternal (joint)
848.49 Other
848.5 Pelvis
848.8 Other specified sites of sprains and strains
848.9 Unspecified site of sprain and strain

850.# Concussion

850.0 With no loss of consciousness
850.1# With brief loss of consciousness
850.11 With loss of consciousness of 30 minutes or less
850.12 With loss of consciousness of 31 to 59 minutes
850.2 With moderate loss of consciousness
850.3 With prolonged loss of consciousness and return to pre-existing conscious level
850.4 With prolonged loss of consousness, without return to pre-existing conscious level
850.5 With loss of consciousness duration NOS
850.9 Concussion, unspecified

851.## Cerebral laceration and contusion

851.0# Cortex (cerebral) contusion without open intracranial wound
851.1# Cortex (cerebral) contusion with open intracranial wound
851.2# Cortex (cerebral) laceration without open intracranial wound
851.3# Cortex (cerebral) laceration with open intracranial wound
851.4# Cerebellar or brain stem contusion without open intracranial wound
851.5# Cerebellar or brain stem contusion with open intracranial wound
851.6# Cerebellar or brain stem laceration without open intracranial wound

5th Digit: 851

0 Unspecified state of consciousness
1 With no loss of consciousness
2 With brief [less than one hour] loss of consciousness
3 With moderate [1-24 hours] loss of consciousness
4 With prolonged [more than 24 hours] loss of consciousness and return to pre-existing conscious level
5 With prolonged [more than 24 hours] loss of consciousness without return to pre-existing conscious level
6 With loss of consciousness of unspecified duration
9 With concussion, unspecified

851.#(#) *(continued)*

851.7# Cerebellar or brain stem laceration with open intracranial wound
851.8# Other and unspecified cerebral laceration and contusion, without open intracranial wound
851.9# Other and unspecified cerebral laceration and contusion, with open intracranial wound

852.## Subarachnoid, subdural, and extradural hemorrhage, following injury

852.0# Subarachnoid hemorrhage following injury without open intracranial wound
852.1# Subarachnoid hemorrhage following injury with open intracranial wound
852.2# Subdural hemorrhage following injury without open intracranial wound
852.3# Subdural hemorrhage following injury with open intracranial wound
852.4# Extradural hemorrhage following injury without open intracranial wound
852.5# Extradural hemorrhage following injury with open intracranial wound

853.## Other and unspecified Intracranial hemorrhage following injury

853.0# Without open intracranial wound
853.1# With open intracranial wound

854.## Intracranial injury of other and unspecified nature

854.0# Without mention of open intracranial wound
854.1# With open intracranial wound

5th Digit: 851-854

0 Unspecified state of consciousness
1 With no loss of consciousness
2 With brief [less than one hour] loss of consciousness
3 With moderate [1-24 hours] loss of consciousness
4 With prolonged [more than 24 hours] loss of consciousness and return to pre-existing conscious level
5 With prolonged [more than 24 hours] loss of consciousness without return to pre-existing conscious level
6 With loss of consciousness of unspecified duration
9 With concussion, unspecified

860.# Traumatic pneumothorax and hemothorax

860.0 Pneumothorax without mention of open wound into thorax
860.1 Pneumothorax with open wound into thorax
860.2 Hemothorax without mention of open wound into thorax
860.3 Hemothorax with open wound into thorax
860.4 Pneumohemothorax without mention of open wound into thorax
860.5 Pneumohemothorax with open wound into thorax

861.## Injury to heart and lung
- **861.0#** Heart, without mention of open wound into thorax
- **861.1#** Heart, with open wound into thorax

5th Digit: 861.0-861.1
- **0 Unspecified injury**
- **1 Contusion**
- **2 Laceration without penetration of heart chambers**
- **3 Laceration with penetration of heart chambers**

- **861.2#** Lung, without mention of open wound into thorax
- **861.3#** Lung, with open wound into thorax

5th Digit: 861.2-861.3
- **0 Unspecified injury**
- **1 Contusion**
- **2 Laceration**

862.#(#) Injury to other and unspecified intrathoracic organs
- 862.0 Diaphragm, without mention of open wound into cavity
- 862.1 Diaphragm, with open wound into cavity
- **862.2#** Other specified intrathoracic organs, without mention of open wound into cavity
- **862.3#** Other specified intrathoracic organs, with open wound into cavity

5th Digit: 862.2-862.3
- **1 Bronchus**
- **2 Esophagus**
- **9 Other**

- 862.8 Multiple and unspecified intrathoracic organs, without mention of open wound into cavity
- 862.9 Multiple and unspecified intrathoracic organs, with open wound into cavity

863.#(#) Injury to gastrointestinal tract
- 863.0 Stomach, without mention of open wound into cavity
- 863.1 Stomach, with open wound into cavity
- **863.2#** Small intestine, without mention of open wound into cavity
- **863.3#** Small intestine, with open wound into cavity

5th Digit: 863.2-863.3
- **0 Small intestine, unspecified site**
- **1 Duodenum**
- **9 Other**

- **863.4#** Colon or rectum, without mention of open wound into cavity
- **863.5#** Colon or rectum, with open wound into cavity

5th Digit: 863.4-863.5
- **0 Colon, unspecified site**
- **1 Ascending [right] colon**
- **2 Transverse colon**
- **3 Descending [left] colon**
- **4 Sigmoid colon**
- **5 Rectum**
- **6 Multiple sites in colon and rectum**
- **9 Other**

863.#(#) ***(continued)***
- **863.8#** Other and unspecified gastrointestinal sites, without mention of open wound into cavity
- **863.9#** Other and unspecified gastrointestinal sites, with open wound into cavity

5th Digit: 863.8-863.9
- **0 Gastrointestinal tract, unspecified site**
- **1 Pancreas, head**
- **2 Pancreas, body**
- **3 Pancreas, tail**
- **4 Pancreas, multiple and sites NOS**
- **5 Appendix**
- **9 Other**

864.## Injury to liver
- **864.0#** Without mention of open wound into cavity
- **864.1#** With open wound into cavity

5th Digit: 864
- **0 Unspecified injury**
- **1 Hematoma and contusion**
- **2 Laceration, minor**
- **3 Laceration, moderate**
- **4 Laceration, major**
- **5 Laceration, unspecified**
- **9 Other**

865.## Injury to spleen
- **865.0#** Without mention of open wound into cavity
- **865.1#** With open wound into cavity

5th Digit: 865
- **0 Unspecified injury**
- **1 Hematoma without rupture of capsule**
- **2 Capsular tears, without major disruption of parenchyma**
- **3 Laceration extending into parenchyma**
- **4 Massive parenchymal disruption**
- **9 Other**

866.## Injury to kidney
- **866.0#** Without mention of open wound into cavity
- **866.1#** With open wound into cavity

5th Digit: 866
- **0 Unspecified injury**
- **1 Hematoma without rupture of capsule**
- **2 Laceration**
- **3 Complete disruption of kidney parenchyma**

867.# Injury to pelvic organs
- 867.0 Bladder and urethra, without mention of open wound into cavity
- 867.1 Bladder and urethra, with open wound into cavity
- 867.2 Ureter, without mention of open wound into cavity
- 867.3 Ureter, with open wound into cavity
- 867.4 Uterus, without mention of open wound into cavity
- 867.5 Uterus, with open wound into cavity
- 867.6 Other specified pelvic organs, without mention of open wound into cavity
- 867.7 Other specified pelvic organs, with open wound into cavity
- 867.8 Unspecified pelvic organ, without mention of open wound into cavity
- 867.9 Unspecified pelvic organ, with open wound into cavity

868.## **Injury to other intra-abdominal organs**
868.0# Without mention of open wound into cavity
868.1# With open wound into cavity
5th Digit: 868
0 **Unspecified intra-abdominal organ**
1 **Adrenal gland**
2 **Bile duct and gallbladder**
3 **Peritoneum**
4 **Retroperitoneum**
9 **Other and multiple intra-abdominal organs**

869.# **Internal injury to unspecified or ill-defined organs**
869.0 Without mention of open wound into cavity
869.1 With open wound into cavity

870.# **Open wound of ocular adnexa**
870.0 Laceration of skin of eyelid and periocular area
870.1 Laceration of eyelid, full-thickness, not involving lacrimal passages
870.2 Laceration of eyelid involving lacrimal passages
870.3 Penetrating wound of orbit, without mention of foreign body
870.4 Penetrating wound of orbit with foreign body
870.8 Other specified open wounds of ocular adnexa
870.9 Unspecified open wound of ocular adnexa

871.# **Open wound of eyeball**
871.0 Ocular laceration without prolapse of intraocular tissue
871.1 Ocular laceration with prolapse or exposure of intraocular tissue
871.2 Rupture of eye with partial loss of intraocular tissue
871.3 Avulsion of eye
871.4 Unspecified laceration of eye
871.5 Penetration of eyeball, magnetic foreign body
871.6 Penetration of eyeball with (nonmagnetic) foreign body
871.7 Unspecified ocular penetration
871.9 Unspecified open wound of eyeball

872.#(#) **Open wound of ear**
872.0# External ear, without mention of complication
872.1# External ear, complicated
5th Digit: 872.0-872.1
0 **External ear, unspecified site**
1 **Auricle, ear**
2 **Auditory canal**
872.6# Other specified parts of ear, without mention of complication
872.7# Other specified parts of ear, complicated
5th Digit: 872.6-872.7
1 **Ear drum**
2 **Ossicles**
3 **Eustachian tube**
4 **Cochlea**
9 **Other and multiple sites**
872.8 Ear, part unspecified, without mention of complication
872.9 Ear, part unspecified, complicated

873.#(#) **Other open wound of head**
873.0 Scalp, without mention of complication
873.1 Scalp, complicated
873.2# Nose, without mention of complication
873.3# Nose, complicated
5th Digit: 873.2-873.3
0 **Nose, unspecified site**
1 **Nasal septum**
2 **Nasal cavity**
3 **Nasal sinus**
9 **Multiple sites**
873.4# Face, without mention of complication
873.5# Face, complicated
5th Digit: 873.4-873.5
0 **Face, unspecified site**
1 **Cheek**
2 **Forehead**
3 **Lip**
4 **Jaw**
9 **Other and multiple sites**
873.6# Internal structures of mouth, without mention of complication
873.7# Internal structures of mouth, complicated
5th Digit: 873.6-873.7
0 **Mouth, unspecified site**
1 **Buccal mucosa**
2 **Gum (alveolar process)**
3 **Tooth (broken) (fractured) (due to trauma)**
4 **Tongue and floor of mouth**
5 **Palate**
9 **Other and multiple sites**
873.8 Other and unspecified open wound of head without mention of complication
873.9 Other and unspecified open wound of head, complicated

874.#(#) **Open wound of neck**
874.0# Larynx and trachea, without mention of complication
874.1# Larynx and trachea, complicated
5th Digit: 874.0-874.1
0 **Larynx with trachea**
1 **Larynx**
2 **Trachea**
874.2 Thyroid gland, without mention of complication
874.3 Thyroid gland, complicated
874.4 Pharynx, without mention of complication
874.5 Pharynx, complicated
874.8 Other and unspecified parts, without mention of complication
874.9 Other and unspecified parts, complicated

875.# **Open wound of chest (wall)**
875.0 Without mention of complication
875.1 Complicated

876.# **Open wound of back**

877.# **Open wound of buttock**
5th Digit: 876-877
0 **Without mention of complication**
1 **Complicated**

NUMERICAL REFERENCE

878.# Open wound of genital organs (external), including traumatic amputation
- 878.0 Penis, without mention of complication
- 878.1 Penis, complicated
- 878.2 Scrotum and testes, without mention of complication
- 878.3 Scrotum and testes, complicated
- 878.4 Vulva, without mention of complication
- 878.5 Vulva, complicated
- 878.6 Vagina, without mention of complication
- 878.7 Vagina, complicated
- 878.8 Other and unspecified parts, without mention of complication
- 878.9 Other and unspecified parts, complicated

879.# Open wound of other and unspecified sites, except limbs
- 879.0 Breast, without mention of complication
- 879.1 Breast, complicated
- 879.2 Abdominal wall, anterior, without mention of complication
- 879.3 Abdominal wall, anterior, complicated
- 879.4 Abdominal wall, lateral, without mention of complication
- 879.5 Abdominal wall, lateral, complicated
- 879.6 Other and unspecified parts of trunk, without mention of complication
- 879.7 Other and unspecified parts of trunk, complicated
- 879.8 Open wound(s) (multiple) of unspecified site(s) without mention of complication
- 879.9 Open wound(s) (multiple) of unspecified site(s), complicated

880.## Open wound of shoulder and upper arm
- **880.0#** Without mention of complication
- **880.1#** Complicated
- **880.2#** With tendon involvement

5th Digit: 880
- **0 Shoulder region**
- **1 Scapular region**
- **2 Axillary region**
- **3 Upper arm**
- **9 Multiple sites**

881.## Open wound of elbow, forearm, and wrist
- **881.0#** Without mention of complication
- **881.1#** Complicated
- **881.2#** With tendon involvement

5th Digit: 881
- **0 Forearm**
- **1 Elbow**
- **2 Wrist**

882.# Open wound of hand except finger(s) alone

883.# Open wound of finger(s)

4th Digit: 882-883
- **0 Without mention of complication**
- **1 Complicated**
- **2 With tendon involvement**

884.# Multiple and unspecified open wound of upper limb
- 884.0 Without mention of complication
- 884.1 Complicated
- 884.2 With tendon involvement

885.# Traumatic amputation of thumb (complete) (partial)

886.# Traumatic amputation of other finger(s) (complete) (partial)

4th Digit: 885-886
- **0 Without mention of complication**
- **1 Complicated**

887.# Traumatic amputation of arm and hand (complete) (partial)
- 887.0 Unilateral, below elbow, without complication
- 887.1 Unilateral, below elbow, complicated
- 887.2 Unilateral, at or above elbow, without mention of complication
- 887.3 Unilateral, at or above elbow, complicated
- 887.4 Unilateral, level not specified, without mention of complication
- 887.5 Unilateral, level not specified, complicated
- 887.6 Bilateral [any level], without mention of complication
- 887.7 Bilateral [any level], complicated

890.# Open wound of hip and thigh

891.# Open wound of knee, leg [except thigh], and ankle

4th Digit: 890-891
- **0 Without mention of complication**
- **1 Complicated**
- **2 With tendon involvement**

892.# Open wound of foot except toe(s) alone

893.# Open wound of toe(s)

4th Digit: 892-893
- **0 Without mention of complication**
- **1 Complicated**
- **2 With tendon involvement**

894.# Multiple and unspecified open wound of lower limb
- 894.0 Without mention of complication
- 894.1 Complicated
- 894.2 With tendon involvement

895.# Traumatic amputation of toe(s) (complete) (partial)
- 895.0 Without mention of complication
- 895.1 Complicated

896.# Traumatic amputation of foot (complete) (partial)
- 896.0 Unilateral, without mention of complication
- 896.1 Unilateral, complicated
- 896.2 Bilateral, without mention of complication
- 896.3 Bilateral, complicated

897.# Traumatic amputation of leg(s) (complete) (partial)
- 897.0 Unilateral, below knee, without mention of complication
- 897.1 Unilateral, below knee, complicated
- 897.2 Unilateral, at or above knee, without mention of complication
- 897.3 Unilateral, at or above knee, complicated
- 897.4 Unilateral, level not specified, without mention of complication

897.# ***(continued)***
897.5 Unilateral, level not specified, complicated
897.6 Bilateral [any level], without mention of complication
897.7 Bilateral [any level], complicated

900.#(#) Injury to blood vessels of head and neck
900.0# Carotid artery
900.00 Carotid artery, unspecified
900.01 Common carotid artery
900.02 External carotid artery
900.03 Internal carotid artery
900.1 Internal jugular vein
900.8# Other specified blood vessels of head and neck
900.81 External jugular vein
900.82 Multiple blood vessels of head and neck
900.89 Other
900.9 Unspecified blood vessel of head and neck

901.#(#) Injury to blood vessels of thorax
901.0 Thoracic aorta
901.1 Innominate and subclavian arteries
901.2 Superior vena cava
901.3 Innominate and subclavian veins
901.4# Pulmonary blood vessels
901.40 Pulmonary vessel(s), unspecified
901.41 Pulmonary artery
901.42 Pulmonary vein
901.8# Other specified blood vessels of thorax
901.81 Intercostal artery or vein
901.82 Internal mammary artery or vein
901.83 Multiple blood vessels of thorax
901.89 Other
901.9# Unspecified blood vessels of thorax

902.#(#) Injury to blood vessels of abdomen and pelvis
902.0 Abdominal aorta
902.1# Inferior vena cava
902.10 Inferior vena cava, unspecified
902.11 Hepatic veins
902.19 Other
902.2# Celiac and mesenteric arteries
902.20 Celiac and mesenteric arteries, unspecified
902.21 Gastric artery
902.22 Hepatic artery
902.23 Splenic artery
902.24 Other specified branches of celiac axis
902.25 Superior mesenteric artery (trunk)
902.26 Primary branches of superior mesenteric artery
902.27 Inferior mesenteric artery
902.29 Other
902.3# Portal and splenic veins
902.31 Superior mesenteric vein and primary subdivisions
902.32 Inferior mesenteric vein
902.33 Portal vein
902.34 Splenic vein
902.39 Other
902.4# Renal blood vessels
902.40 Renal vessel(s), unspecified
902.41 Renal artery
902.42 Renal vein
902.49 Other

902.#(#) ***(continued)***
902.5# Iliac blood vessels
902.50 Iliac vessel(s), unspecified
902.51 Hypogastric artery
902.52 Hypogastric vein
902.53 Iliac artery
902.54 Iliac vein
902.55 Uterine artery
902.56 Uterine vein
902.59 Other
902.8# Other specified blood vessels of abdomen and pelvis
902.81 Ovarian artery
902.82 Ovarian vein
902.87 Multiple blood vessels of abdomen and pelvis
902.89 Other
902.9 Unspecified blood vessel of abdomen and pelvis

903.#(#) Injury to blood vessels of upper extremity
903.0# Axillary blood vessels
903.00 Axillary vessel(s), unspecified
903.01 Axillary artery
903.02 Axillary vein
903.1 Brachial blood vessels
903.2 Radial blood vessels
903.3 Ulnar blood vessels
903.4 Palmar artery
903.5 Digital blood vessels
903.8 Other specified blood vessels of upper extremity
903.9 Unspecified blood vessel of upper extremity

904.#(#) Injury to blood vessels of lower extremity and unspecified sites
904.0 Common femoral artery
904.1 Superficial femoral artery
904.2 Femoral veins
904.3 Saphenous veins
904.4# Popliteal blood vessels
904.40 Popliteal vessel(s), unspecified
904.41 Popliteal artery
904.42 Popliteal vein
904.5# Tibial blood vessels
904.50 Tibial vessel(s), unspecified
904.51 Anterior tibial artery
904.52 Anterior tibial vein
904.53 Posterior tibial artery
904.54 Posterior tibial vein
904.6 Deep plantar blood vessels
904.7 Other specified blood vessels of lower extremity
904.8 Unspecified blood vessel of lower extremity
904.9 Unspecified site

905.# Late effects of musculoskeletal and connective tissue injuries
905.0 Late effect of fracture of skull and face bones
905.1 Late effect of fracture of spine and trunk without mention of spinal cord lesion
905.2 Late effect of fracture of upper extremities
905.3 Late effect of fracture of neck of femur
905.4 Late effect of fracture of lower extremities
905.5 Late effect of fracture of multiple and unspecified bones

NUMERICAL REFERENCE

905.# ***(continued)***
- 905.6 Late effect of dislocation
- 905.7 Late effect of sprain and strain without mention of tendon injury
- 905.8 Late effect of tendon injury
- 905.9 Late effect of traumatic amputation

906.# Late effects of injuries to skin and subcutaneous tissues
- 906.0 Late effect of open wound of head, neck, and trunk
- 906.1 Late effect of open wound of extremities without mention of tendon injury
- 906.2 Late effect of superficial injury
- 906.3 Late effect of contusion
- 906.4 Late effect of crushing
- 906.5 Late effect of burn of eye, face, head, and neck
- 906.6 Late effect of burn of wrist and hand
- 906.7 Late effect of burn of other extremities
- 906.8 Late effect of burns of other specified sites
- 906.9 Late effect of burn of unspecified site

907.# Late effects of injuries to the nervous system
- 907.0 Late effect of intracranial injury without mention of skull fracture
- 907.1 Late effect of injury to cranial nerve
- 907.2 Late effect of spinal cord injury
- 907.3 Late effect of injury to nerve root(s), spinal plexus(es), and other nerves of trunk
- 907.4 Late effect of injury to peripheral nerve of shoulder girdle and upper limb
- 907.5 Late effect of injury to peripheral nerve of pelvic girdle and lower limb
- 907.9 Late effect of injury to other and unspecified nerve

908.# Late effects of other and unspecified injuries
- 908.0 Late effect of internal injury to chest
- 908.1 Late effect of internal injury to intra-abdominal organs
- 908.2 Late effect of internal injury to other internal organs
- 908.3 Late effect of injury to blood vessel of head, neck, and extremities
- 908.4 Late effect of injury to blood vessel of thorax, abdomen, and pelvis
- 908.5 Late effect of foreign body in orifice
- 908.6 Late effect of certain complications of trauma
- 908.9 Late effect of unspecified injury

909.# Late effects of other and unspecified external causes
- 909.0 Late effect of poisoning due to drug, medicinal or biological substance
- 909.1 Late effect of toxic effects of nonmedical substances
- 909.2 Late effect of radiation
- 909.3 Late effect of complications of surgical and medical care
- 909.4 Late effect of certain other external causes
- 909.5 Late effect of adverse effect of drug, medicinal or biological substance
- 909.9 Late effect of other and unspecified external causes

910.# Superficial injury of face, neck, and scalp except eye

911.# Superficial injury of trunk

912.# Superficial injury of shoulder and upper arm

913.# Superficial injury of elbow, forearm, and wrist

914.# Superficial injury of hand(s) except finger(s) alone

915.# Superficial injury of finger(s)

916.# Superficial injury of hip, thigh, leg, and ankle

917.# Superficial injury of foot and toe(s)
4th Digit: 910-917
- **0 Abrasion or friction burn without mention of infection**
- **1 Abrasion or friction burn, infected**
- **2 Blister without mention of infection**
- **3 Blister, infected**
- **4 Insect bite, nonvenomous, without mention of infection**
- **5 Insect bite, nonvenomous, infected**
- **6 Superficial foreign body (splinter) without major open wound and without mention of infection**
- **7 Superficial foreign body (splinter) without major open wound, infected**
- **8 Other and unspecified superficial injury without mention of infection**
- **9 Other and unspecified superficial injury, infected**

918.# Superficial injury of eye and adnexa
- 918.0 Eyelids and periocular area
- 918.1 Cornea
- 918.2 Conjunctiva
- 918.9 Other and unspecified superficial injuries of eye

919.# Superficial injury of other, multiple, and unspecified sites
- 919.0 Abrasion or friction burn without mention of infection
- 919.1 Abrasion or friction burn, infected
- 919.2 Blister without mention of infection
- 919.3 Blister, infected
- 919.4 Insect bite, nonvenomous, without mention of infection
- 919.5 Insect bite, nonvenomous, infected
- 919.6 Superficial foreign body (splinter) without major open wound and without mention of infection
- 919.7 Superficial foreign body (splinter) without major open wound, infected
- 919.8 Other and unspecified superficial injury without mention of infection
- 919.9 Other and unspecified superficial injury, infected

920 Contusion of face, scalp, and neck except eye(s)

921.# Contusion of eye and adnexa
- 921.0 Black eye, NOS
- 921.1 Contusion of eyelids and periocular area
- 921.2 Contusion of orbital tissues
- 921.3 Contusion of eyeball
- 921.9 Unspecified contusion of eye

922.#(#) Contusion of trunk
- 922.0 Breast
- 922.1 Chest wall
- 922.2 Abdominal wall
- **922.3#** Back
  - 922.31 Back
  - 922.32 Buttock
  - 922.33 Interscapular region
- 922.4 Genital organs
- 922.8 Multiple sites of trunk
- 922.9 Unspecified part

923.#(#) Contusion of upper limb
- **923.0#** Shoulder and upper arm
  - 923.00 Shoulder region
  - 923.01 Scapular region
  - 923.02 Axillary region
  - 923.03 Upper arm
  - 923.09 Multiple sites
- **923.1#** Elbow and forearm
  - 923.10 Forearm
  - 923.11 Elbow
- **923.2#** Wrist and hand(s), except finger(s) alone
  - 923.20 Hand(s)
  - 923.21 Wrist
- 923.3 Finger
- 923.8 Multiple sites of upper limb
- 923.9 Unspecified part of upper limb

924.#(#) Contusion of lower limb and of other and unspecified sites
- **924.0#** Hip and thigh
  - 924.00 Thigh
  - 924.01 Hip
- **924.1#** Knee and lower leg
  - 924.10 Lower leg
  - 924.11 Knee
- **924.2#** Ankle and foot, excluding toe(s)
  - 924.20 Foot
  - 924.21 Ankle
- 924.3 Toe, Toenail
- 924.4 Multiple sites of lower limb
- 924.5 Unspecified part of lower limb
- 924.8 Multiple sites, not elsewhere classified
- 924.9 Unspecified site

925.# Crushing injury of face, scalp, and neck
- 925.1 Crushing injury of face and scalp
- 925.2 Crushing injury of neck

926.#(#) Crushing injury of trunk
- 926.0 External genitalia
- **926.1#** Other specified sites
  - 926.11 Back
  - 926.12 Buttock
  - 926.19 Other
- 926.8 Multiple sites of trunk
- 926.9 Unspecified site

927.#(#) Crushing injury of upper limb
- **927.0#** Shoulder and upper arm
  - 927.00 Shoulder region
  - 927.01 Scapular region
  - 927.02 Axillary region
  - 927.03 Upper arm
  - 927.09 Multiple sites
- **927.1#** Elbow and forearm
  - 927.10 Forearm
  - 927.11 Elbow
- **927.2#** Wrist and hand(s), except finger(s) alone
  - 927.20 Hand(s)
  - 927.21 Wrist
- 927.3 Finger(s)
- 927.8 Multiple sites of upper limb
- 927.9 Unspecified site

928.#(#) Crushing injury of lower limb
- **928.0#** Hip and thigh
  - 928.00 Thigh
  - 928.01 Hip
- **928.1#** Knee and lower leg
  - 928.10 Lower leg
  - 928.11 Knee
- **928.2#** Ankle and foot, excluding toe(s) alone
  - 928.20 Foot
  - 928.21 Ankle
- 928.3 Toe(s)
- 928.8 Multiple sites of lower limb
- 928.9 Unspecified site

929.# Crushing injury of multiple and unspecified sites
- 929.0 Multiple sites, not elsewhere classified
- 929.9 Unspecified site

930.# Foreign body on external eye
- 930.0 Corneal foreign body
- 930.1 Foreign body in conjunctival sac
- 930.2 Foreign body in lacrimal punctum
- 930.8 Other and combined sites
- 930.9 Unspecified site

931 Foreign body in ear

932 Foreign body in nose

933.# Foreign body in pharynx and larynx
- 933.0 Pharynx
- 933.1 Larynx

934.# Foreign body in trachea, bronchus, and lung
- 934.0 Trachea
- 934.1 Main bronchus
- 934.8 Other specified parts
- 934.9 Respiratory tree, unspecified

935.# Foreign body in mouth, esophagus, and stomach
- 935.0 Mouth
- 935.1 Esophagus
- 935.2 Stomach

936 Foreign body in intestine and colon

937 Foreign body in anus and rectum

938 Foreign body in digestive system, unspecified

939.# Foreign body in genitourinary tract
- 939.0 Bladder and urethra
- 939.1 Uterus, any part
- 939.2 Vulva and vagina
- 939.3 Penis
- 939.9 Unspecified site

940.# Burn confined to eye and adnexa
- 940.0 Chemical burn of eyelids and periocular area
- 940.1 Other burns of eyelids and periocular area
- 940.2 Alkaline chemical burn of cornea and conjunctival sac
- 940.3 Acid chemical burn of cornea and conjunctival sac
- 940.4 Other burn of cornea and conjunctival sac
- 940.5 Burn with resulting rupture and destruction of eyeball
- 940.9 Unspecified burn of eye and adnexa

941.## Burn of face, head, and neck
- **941.0#** Unspecified degree
- **941.1#** Erythema [first degree]
- **941.2#** Blisters, epidermal loss [second degree]
- **941.3#** Full-thickness skin loss [third degree NOS]
- **941.4#** Deep necrosis of underlying tissues [deep third degree] without mention of loss of a body part
- **941.5#** Deep necrosis of underlying tissues [deep third degree] with loss of a body part

5th Digit: 941
- **0 Face and head, unspecified site**
- **1 Ear [any part]**
- **2 Eye (with other parts of face, head, and neck)**
- **3 Lip(s)**
- **4 Chin**
- **5 Nose (septum)**
- **6 Scalp [any part]**
- **7 Forehead and cheek**
- **8 Neck**
- **9 Multiple sites [except with eye] of face, head, and neck**

942.## Burn of trunk
- **942.0#** Unspecified degree
- **942.1#** Erythema [first degree]
- **942.2#** Blisters, epidermal loss [second degree]
- **942.3#** Full-thickness skin loss [third degree NOS]
- **942.4#** Deep necrosis of underlying tissues [deep third degree] without mention of loss of a body part
- **942.5#** Deep necrosis of underlying tissues [deep third degree] with loss of a body part

5th Digit: 942
- **0 Trunk, unspecified site**
- **1 Breast**
- **2 Chest wall, excluding breast and nipple**
- **3 Abdominal wall**
- **4 Back [any part]**
- **5 Genitalia**
- **9 Other and multiple sites of trunk**

943.## Burn of upper limb, except wrist and hand
- **943.0#** Unspecified degree
- **943.1#** Erythema [first degree]
- **943.2#** Blisters, epidermal loss [second degree]
- **943.3#** Full-thickness skin loss [third degree NOS]
- **943.4#** Deep necrosis of underlying tissues [deep third degree] without mention of loss of a body part
- **943.5#** Deep necrosis of underlying tissues [deep third degree] with loss of a body part

5th Digit: 943
- **0 Upper limb, unspecified site**
- **1 Forearm**
- **2 Elbow**
- **3 Upper arm**
- **4 Axilla**
- **5 Shoulder**
- **6 Scapular region**
- **9 Multiple sites of upper limb, except wrist and hand**

944.## Burn of wrist(s) and hand(s)
- **944.0#** Unspecified degree
- **944.1#** Erythema [first degree]
- **944.2#** Blisters, epidermal loss [second degree]
- **944.3#** Full-thickness skin loss [third degree NOS]
- **944.4#** Deep necrosis of underlying tissues [deep third degree] without mention of loss of a body part
- **944.5#** Deep necrosis of underlying tissues [deep third degree] with loss of a body part

5th Digit: 944
- **0 Hand, unspecified site**
- **1 Dingle digit [finger (nail)] other than thumb**
- **2 Thumb (nail)**
- **3 Two or more digits, not including thumb**
- **4 Two or more digits including thumb**
- **5 Palm**
- **6 Back of hand**
- **7 Wrist**
- **8 Multiple sites of wrist(s) and hand(s)**

945.## Burn of lower limb(s)
- **945.0#** Unspecified degree
- **945.1#** Erythema [first degree]
- **945.2#** Blisters, epidermal loss [second degree]
- **945.3#** Full-thickness skin loss [third degree NOS]
- **945.4#** Deep necrosis of underlying tissues [deep third degree] without mention of loss of a body part
- **945.5#** Deep necrosis of underlying tissues [deep third degree] with loss of a body part

5th Digit: 945
- **0 Lower limb [leg], unspecified site**
- **1 Toe(s) (nail)**
- **2 Foot**
- **3 Ankle**
- **4 Lower leg**
- **5 Knee**
- **6 Thigh [any part]**
- **9 Multiple sites of lower limb(s)**

946.# Burns of multiple specified sites
- 946.0 Unspecified degree
- 946.1 Erythema [first degree]
- 946.2 Blisters, epidermal loss [second degree]
- 946.3 Full-thickness skin loss [third degree NOS]
- 946.4 Deep necrosis of underlying tissues [deep third degree] without mention of loss of a body part
- 946.5 Deep necrosis of underlying tissues [deep third degree] with loss of a body part

947.# Burn of internal organs
- 947.0 Mouth and pharynx
- 947.1 Larynx, trachea, and lung
- 947.2 Esophagus
- 947.3 Gastrointestinal tract
- 947.4 Vagina and uterus
- 947.8 Other specified sites
- 947.9 Unspecified site

948.## Burns classified according to extent of body surface involved

4th Digit: 948
- **0 Burn [any degree] involving less than 10 percent**
- **1 Burn [any degree] 10-19%**
- **2 Burn [any degree] 20-29%**
- **3 Burn [any degree] 30-39%**
- **4 Burn [any degree] 40-49%**
- **5 Burn [any degree] 50-59%**
- **6 Burn [any degree] 60-69%**
- **7 Burn [any degree] 70-79%**
- **8 Burn [any degree] 80-89%**
- **9 Burn [any degree] 90% or more**

5th Digit: 948
- **0 With third degree less than 10 percent or unspecified**
- **1 With third degree 10-19%**
- **2 With third degree 20-29%**
- **3 With third degree 30-39%**
- **4 With third degree 40-49%**
- **5 With third degree 50-59%**
- **6 With third degree 60-69%**
- **7 With third degree 70-79%**
- **8 With third degree 80-89%**
- **9 With third degree 90% or more of body surface**

949.# Burn, unspecified
- 949.0 Unspecified degree
- 949.1 Erythema [first degree]
- 949.2 Blisters, epidermal loss [second degree]
- 949.3 Full-thickness skin loss [third degree NOS]
- 949.4 Deep necrosis of underlying tissues [deep third degree] without mention of loss of a body part
- 949.5 Deep necrosis of underlying tissues [deep third degree] with loss of a body part

950.# Injury to optic nerve and pathways
- 950.0 Optic nerve injury
- 950.1 Injury to optic chiasm
- 950.2 Injury to optic pathways
- 950.3 Injury to visual cortex
- 950.9 Unspecified

951.# Injury to other cranial nerve(s)
- 951.0 Injury to oculomotor nerve
- 951.1 Injury to trochlear nerve
- 951.2 Injury to trigeminal nerve
- 951.3 Injury to abducens nerve
- 951.4 Injury to facial nerve
- 951.5 Injury to acoustic nerve
- 951.6 Injury to accessory nerve
- 951.7 Injury to hypoglossal nerve
- 951.8 Injury to other specified cranial nerves
- 951.9 Injury to unspecified cranial nerve

952.#(#) Spinal cord injury without evidence of spinal bone injury

952.0# Cervical
- 952.00 C_1-C_4 level with unspecified spinal cord injury
- 952.01 C_1-C_4 level with complete lesion of spinal cord
- 952.02 C_1-C_4 level with anterior cord syndrome
- 952.03 C_1-C_4 level with central cord syndrome
- 952.04 C_1-C_4 level with other specified spinal cord injury
- 952.05 C_5-C_7 level with unspecified spinal cord injury
- 952.06 C_5-C_7 level with complete lesion of spinal cord
- 952.07 C_5-C_7 level with anterior cord syndrome
- 952.08 C_5-C_7 level with central cord syndrome
- 952.09 C_5-C_7 level with other specified spinal cord injury

952.1# Dorsal [thoracic]
- 952.10 T_1-T_6 level with unspecified spinal cord injury
- 952.11 T_1-T_6 level with complete lesion of spinal cord
- 952.12 T_1-T_6 level with anterior cord syndrome
- 952.13 T_1-T_6 level with central cord syndrome
- 952.14 T_1-T_6 level with other specified spinal cord injury
- 952.15 T_7-T_{12} level with unspecified spinal cord injury
- 952.16 T_7-T_{12} level with complete lesion of spinal cord
- 952.17 T_7-T_{12} level with anterior cord syndrome
- 952.18 T_7-T_{12} level with central cord syndrome
- 952.19 T_7-T_{12} level with other specified spinal cord injury

- 952.2 Lumbar
- 952.3 Sacral
- 952.4 Cauda equina
- 952.8 Multiple sites of spinal cord
- 952.9 Unspecified site of spinal cord

953.# Injury to nerve roots and spinal plexus
- 953.0 Cervical root
- 953.1 Dorsal root
- 953.2 Lumbar root
- 953.3 Sacral root
- 953.4 Brachial plexus
- 953.5 Lumbosacral plexus
- 953.8 Multiple sites
- 953.9 Unspecified site

954.# Injury to other nerve(s) of trunk, excluding shoulder and pelvic girdles
- 954.0 Cervical sympathetic
- 954.1 Other sympathetic
- 954.8 Other specified nerve(s) of trunk
- 954.9 Unspecified nerve of trunk

955.# Injury to peripheral nerve(s) of shoulder girdle and upper limb
955.0 Axillary nerve
955.1 Median nerve
955.2 Ulnar nerve
955.3 Radial nerve
955.4 Musculocutaneous nerve
955.5 Cutaneous sensory nerve, upper limb
955.6 Digital nerve
955.7 Other specified nerve(s) of shoulder girdle and upper limb
955.8 Multiple nerves of shoulder girdle and upper limb
955.9 Unspecified nerve of shoulder girdle and upper limb

956.# Injury to peripheral nerve(s) of pelvic girdle and lower limb
956.0 Sciatic nerve
956.1 Femoral nerve
956.2 Posterior tibial nerve
956.3 Peroneal nerve
956.4 Cutaneous sensory nerve, lower limb
956.5 Other specified nerve(s) of pelvic girdle and lower limb
956.8 Multiple nerves of pelvic girdle and lower limb
956.9 Unspecified nerve of pelvic girdle and lower limb

957.# Injury to other and unspecified nerves
957.0 Superficial nerves of head and neck
957.1 Other specified nerve(s)
957.8 Multiple nerves in several parts
957.9 Unspecified site

958.#(#) Certain early complications of trauma
958.0 Air embolism
958.1 Fat embolism
958.2 Secondary and recurrent hemorrhage
958.3 Posttraumatic wound infection, not elsewhere classified
958.4 Traumatic shock
958.5 Traumatic anuria
958.6 Volkmann's ischemic contracture
958.7 Traumatic subcutaneous emphysema
958.8 Other early complications of trauma
958.9# Traumatic compartment syndrome
958.90 Unspecified
958.91 Upper extremity
958.92 Lower extremity
958.93 Abdomen
958.99 Other sites

959.#(#) Injury, other and unspecified
959.0# Head, face and neck
959.01 Head injury, unspecified
959.09 Injury of face and neck
959.1# Trunk
959.11 Chest wall
959.12 Abdomen
959.13 Fracture of corpus cavernosum penis
959.14 Other injury of external genitals
959.19 Other and unspecified sites of trunk
959.2 Shoulder and upper arm
959.3 Elbow, forearm, and wrist
959.4 Hand, except finger
959.5 Finger
959.6 Hip and thigh
959.7 Knee, leg, ankle, and foot

959.#(#) ***(continued)***
959.8 Other specified sites, including multiple
959.9 Unspecified site

960.# Poisoning by antibiotics
960.0 Penicillins
960.1 Antifungal antibiotics
960.2 Chloramphenicol group
960.3 Erythromycin and other macrolides
960.4 Tetracycline group
960.5 Cephalosporin group
960.6 Antimycobacterial antibiotics
960.7 Antineoplastic antibiotics
960.8 Other specified antibiotics
960.9 Unspecified antibiotic

961.# Poisoning by other anti-infectives
961.0 Sulfonamides
961.1 Arsenical anti-infectives
961.2 Heavy metal anti-infectives
961.3 Quinoline and hydroxyquinoline derivatives
961.4 Antimalarials and drugs acting on other blood protozoa
961.5 Other antiprotozoal drugs
961.6 Anthelmintics
961.7 Antiviral drugs
961.8 Other antimycobacterial drugs
961.9 Other and unspecified anti-infectives

962.# Poisoning by hormones and synthetic substitutes
962.0 Adrenal cortical steroids
962.1 Androgens and anabolic congeners
962.2 Ovarian hormones and synthetic substitutes
962.3 Insulins and antidiabetic agents
962.4 Anterior pituitary hormones
962.5 Posterior pituitary hormones
962.6 Parathyroid and parathyroid derivatives
962.7 Thyroid and thyroid derivatives
962.8 Antithyroid agents
962.9 Other and unspecified hormones and synthetic substitutes

963.# Poisoning by primarily systemic agents
963.0 Antiallergic and antiemetic drugs
963.1 Antineoplastic and immunosuppressive drugs
963.2 Acidifying agents
963.3 Alkalizing agents
963.4 Enzymes, not elsewhere classified
963.5 Vitamins, not elsewhere classified
963.8 Other specified systemic agents
963.9 Unspecified systemic agent

964.# Poisoning by agents primarily affecting blood constituents
964.0 Iron and its compounds
964.1 Liver preparations and other antianemic agents
964.2 Anticoagulants
964.3 Vitamin K [phytonadione]
964.4 Fibrinolysis-affecting drugs
964.5 Anticoagulant antagonists and other coagulants
964.6 Gamma globulin
964.7 Natural blood and blood products
964.8 Other specified agents affecting blood constituents
964.9 Unspecified agents affecting blood constituents

965.#(#) Poisoning by analgesics, antipyretics, and antirheumatics
- **965.0#** Opiates and related narcotics
  - 965.00 Opium (alkaloids), unspecified
  - 965.01 Heroin
  - 965.02 Methadone
  - 965.09 Other
- 965.1 Salicylates
- 965.4 Aromatic analgesics, not elsewhere classified
- 965.5 Pyrazole derivatives
- **965.6#** Antirheumatics [antiphlogistics]
  - 965.61 Propionic acid derivatives
  - 965.69 Other antirheumatics
- 965.7 Other non-narcotic analgesics
- 965.8 Other specified analgesics and antipyretics
- 965.9 Unspecified analgesic and antipyretic

966.# Poisoning by anticonvulsants and anti-Parkinsonism drugs
- 966.0 Oxazolidine derivatives
- 966.1 Hydantoin derivatives
- 966.2 Succinimides
- 966.3 Other and unspecified anticonvulsants
- 966.4 Anti-Parkinsonism drugs

967.# Poisoning by sedatives and hypnotics
- 967.0 Barbiturates
- 967.1 Chloral hydrate group
- 967.2 Paraldehyde
- 967.3 Bromine compounds
- 967.4 Methaqualone compounds
- 967.5 Glutethimide group
- 967.6 Mixed sedatives, not elsewhere classified
- 967.8 Other sedatives and hypnotics
- 967.9 Unspecified sedative or hypnotic

968.# Poisoning by other central nervous system depressants and anesthetics
- 968.0 Central nervous system muscle-tone depressants
- 968.1 Halothane
- 968.2 Other gaseous anesthetics
- 968.3 Intravenous anesthetics
- 968.4 Other and unspecified general anesthetics
- 968.5 Surface [topical] and infiltration anesthetics
- 968.6 Peripheral nerve- and plexus-blocking anesthetics
- 968.7 Spinal anesthetics
- 968.9 Other and unspecified local anesthetics

969.# Poisoning by psychotropic agents
- 969.0 Antidepressants
- 969.1 Phenothiazine-based tranquilizers
- 969.2 Butyrophenone-based tranquilizers
- 969.3 Other antipsychotics, neuroleptics, and major tranquilizers
- 969.4 Benzodiazepine-based tranquilizers
- 969.5 Other tranquilizers
- 969.6 Psychodysleptics [hallucinogens]
- 969.7 Psychostimulants
- 969.8 Other specified psychotropic agents
- 969.9 Unspecified psychotropic agent

970.# Poisoning by central nervous system stimulants
- 970.0 Analeptics
- 970.1 Opiate antagonists
- 970.8 Other specified central nervous system stimulants
- 970.9 Unspecified central nervous system stimulant

971.# Poisoning by drugs primarily affecting the autonomic nervous system
- 971.0 Parasympathomimetics [cholinergics]
- 971.1 Parasympatholytics [anticholinergics and antimuscarinics] and spasmolytics
- 971.2 Sympathomimetics [adrenergics]
- 971.3 Sympatholytics [antiadrenergics]
- 971.9 Unspecified drug primarily affecting autonomic nervous system

972.# Poisoning by agents primarily affecting the cardiovascular system
- 972.0 Cardiac rhythm regulators
- 972.1 Cardiotonic glycosides and drugs of similar action
- 972.2 Antilipemic and antiarteriosclerotic drugs
- 972.3 Ganglion-blocking agents
- 972.4 Coronary vasodilators
- 972.5 Other vasodilators
- 972.6 Other antihypertensive agents
- 972.7 Antivaricose drugs, including sclerosing agents
- 972.8 Capillary-active drugs
- 972.9 Other and unspecified agents primarily affecting the cardiovascular system

973.# Poisoning by agents primarily affecting the gastrointestinal system
- 973.0 Antacids and antigastric secretion drugs
- 973.1 Irritant cathartics
- 973.2 Emollient cathartics
- 973.3 Other cathartics, including intestinal atonia drugs
- 973.4 Digestants
- 973.5 Antidiarrheal drugs
- 973.6 Emetics
- 973.8 Other specified agents primarily affecting the gastrointestinal system
- 973.9 Unspecified agent primarily affecting the gastrointestinal system

974.# Poisoning by water, mineral, and uric acid metabolism drugs
- 974.0 Mercurial diuretics
- 974.1 Purine derivative diuretics
- 974.2 Carbonic acid anhydrase inhibitors
- 974.3 Saluretics
- 974.4 Other diuretics
- 974.5 Electrolytic, caloric, and water-balance agents
- 974.6 Other mineral salts, not elsewhere classified
- 974.7 Uric acid metabolism drugs

975.# Poisoning by agents primarily acting on the smooth and skeletal muscles and respiratory system
- 975.0 Oxytocic agents
- 975.1 Smooth muscle relaxants
- 975.2 Skeletal muscle relaxants
- 975.3 Other and unspecified drugs acting on muscles

975.# ***(continued)***

- 975.4 Antitussives
- 975.5 Expectorants
- 975.6 Anti-common cold drugs
- 975.7 Antiasthmatics
- 975.8 Other and unspecified respiratory drugs

976.# Poisoning by agents primarily affecting skin and mucous membrane, ophthalmological, otorhinolaryngological, and dental drugs

- 976.0 Local anti-infectives and anti-inflammatory drugs
- 976.1 Antipruritics
- 976.2 Local astringents and local detergents
- 976.3 Emollients, demulcents, and protectants
- 976.4 Keratolytics, keratoplastics, other hair treatment drugs and preparations
- 976.5 Eye anti-infectives and other eye drugs
- 976.6 Anti-infectives and other drugs and preparations for ear, nose, and throat
- 976.7 Dental drugs topically applied
- 976.8 Other agents primarily affecting skin and mucous membrane
- 976.9 Unspecified agent primarily affecting skin and mucous membrane

977.# Poisoning by other and unspecified drugs and medicinal substances

- 977.0 Dietetics
- 977.1 Lipotropic drugs
- 977.2 Antidotes and chelating agents, not elsewhere classified
- 977.3 Alcohol deterrents
- 977.4 Pharmaceutical excipients
- 977.8 Other specified drugs and medicinal substances
- 977.9 Unspecified drug or medicinal substance

978.# Poisoning by bacterial vaccines

- 978.0 BCG
- 978.1 Typhoid and paratyphoid
- 978.2 Cholera
- 978.3 Plague
- 978.4 Tetanus
- 978.5 Diphtheria
- 978.6 Pertussis vaccine, including combinations with a pertussis component
- 978.8 Other and unspecified bacterial vaccines
- 978.9 Mixed bacterial vaccines, except combinations with a pertussis component

979.# Poisoning by other vaccines and biological substances

- 979.0 Smallpox vaccine
- 979.1 Rabies vaccine
- 979.2 Typhus vaccine
- 979.3 Yellow fever vaccine
- 979.4 Measles vaccine
- 979.5 Poliomyelitis vaccine
- 979.6 Other and unspecified viral and rickettsial vaccines
- 979.7 Mixed viral-rickettsial and bacterial vaccines, except combinations with a pertussis component
- 979.9 Other and unspecified vaccines and biological substances

980.# Toxic effect of alcohol

- 980.0 Ethyl alcohol
- 980.1 Methyl alcohol
- 980.2 Isopropyl alcohol
- 980.3 Fusel oil
- 980.8 Other specified alcohols
- 980.9 Unspecified alcohol

981 Toxic effect of petroleum products

982.# Toxic effect of solvents other than petroleumbased

- 982.0 Benzene and homologues
- 982.1 Carbon tetrachloride
- 982.2 Carbon disulfide
- 982.3 Other chlorinated hydrocarbon solvents
- 982.4 Nitroglycol
- 982.8 Other nonpetroleum-based solvents

983.# Toxic effect of corrosive aromatics, acids, and caustic alkalis

- 983.0 Corrosive aromatics
- 983.1 Acids
- 983.2 Caustic alkalis
- 983.9 Caustic, unspecified

984.# Toxic effect of lead and its compounds (including fumes)

- 984.0 Inorganic lead compounds
- 984.1 Organic lead compounds
- 984.8 Other lead compounds
- 984.9 Unspecified lead compound

985.# Toxic effect of other metals

- 985.0 Mercury and its compounds
- 985.1 Arsenic and its compounds
- 985.2 Manganese and its compounds
- 985.3 Beryllium and its compounds
- 985.4 Antimony and its compounds
- 985.5 Cadmium and its compounds
- 985.6 Chromium
- 985.8 Other specified metals
- 985.9 Unspecified metal

986 Toxic effect of carbon monoxide

987.# Toxic effect of other gases, fumes, or vapors

- 987.0 Liquefied petroleum gases
- 987.1 Other hydrocarbon gas
- 987.2 Nitrogen oxides
- 987.3 Sulfur dioxide
- 987.4 Freon
- 987.5 Lacrimogenic gas
- 987.6 Chlorine gas
- 987.7 Hydrocyanic acid gas
- 987.8 Other specified gases, fumes, or vapors
- 987.9 Unspecified gas, fume, or vapor

988.# Toxic effect of noxious substances eaten as food

- 988.0 Fish and shellfish
- 988.1 Mushrooms
- 988.2 Berries and other plants
- 988.8 Noxious substances eaten as food NEC
- 988.9 Unspecified noxious substance eaten as food

989.#(#) Toxic effect of other substances, chiefly nonmedicinal as to source
989.0 Hydrocyanic acid and cyanides
989.1 Strychnine and salts
989.2 Chlorinated hydrocarbons
989.3 Organophosphate and carbamate
989.4 Other pesticides, not elsewhere classified
989.5 Venom
989.6 Soaps and detergents
989.7 Aflatoxin and other mycotoxin
989.8# Other substances, chiefly nonmedicinal as to source
989.81 Asbestos
989.82 Latex
989.83 Silicone
989.84 Tobacco
989.89 Other
989.9 Unspecified substance, chiefly nonmedicinal as to source

990 Effects of radiation, unspecified

991.# Effects of reduced temperature
991.0 Frostbite of face
991.1 Frostbite of hand
991.2 Frostbite of foot
991.3 Frostbite of other and unspecified sites
991.4 Immersion foot
991.5 Chilblains
991.6 Hypothermia
991.8 Other specified effects of reduced temperature
991.9 Unspecified effect of reduced temperature

992.# Effects of heat and light
992.0 Heat stroke and sunstroke
992.1 Heat syncope
992.2 Heat cramps
992.3 Heat exhaustion, anhydrotic
992.4 Heat exhaustion due to salt depletion
992.5 Heat exhaustion, unspecified
992.6 Heat fatigue, transient
992.7 Heat edema
992.8 Other specified heat effects
992.9 Unspecified

993.# Effects of air pressure
993.0 Barotrauma, otitic
993.1 Barotrauma, sinus
993.2 Other and unspecified effects of high altitude
993.3 Caisson disease
993.4 Effects of air pressure caused by explosion
993.8 Other specified effects of air pressure
993.9 Unspecified effect of air pressure

994.# Effects of other external causes
994.0 Effects of lightning
994.1 Drowning and nonfatal submersion
994.2 Effects of hunger
994.3 Effects of thirst
994.4 Exhaustion due to exposure
994.5 Exhaustion due to excessive exertion
994.6 Motion sickness
994.7 Asphyxiation and strangulation
994.8 Electrocution and nonfatal effects of electric current
994.9 Other effects of external causes

995.#(#) Certain adverse effects not elsewhere classified
995.0 Other anaphylactic shock
995.1 Angioneurotic edema
995.2# Other and unspecified adverse effect of drug, medicinal and biological substance
995.20 Unspecified adverse effect of unspecified drug, medicinal and biological sustance
995.21 Arthus phenomenon
995.22 Uspecified adverse effect of anesthesia
995.23 Unspecified adverse effect of insulin
995.27 Other drug allergy
995.29 Unspecified adverse effect of other drug
995.3 Allergy, unspecified
995.4 Shock due to anesthesia
995.5# Child maltreatment syndrome
995.50 Child abuse, unspecified
995.51 Child emotional/psychological abuse
995.52 Child neglect (nutritional)
995.53 Child sexual abuse
995.54 Child physical abuse
995.55 Shaken infant syndrome
995.59 Other child abuse and neglect
995.6# Anaphylactic shock due to adverse food reaction
995.60 Due to unspecified food
995.61 Due to peanuts
995.62 Due to crustaceans
995.63 Due to fruits and vegetables
995.64 Due to tree nuts and seeds
995.65 Due to fish
995.66 Due to food additives
995.67 Due to milk products
995.68 Due to eggs
995.69 Due to other specified food
995.7 Other adverse food reactions, not elsewhere classified
995.8# Other specified adverse effects, not elsewhere classified
995.80 Adult maltreatment, unspecified
995.81 Adult physical abuse
995.82 Adult emotional/psychological abuse
995.83 Adult sexual abuse
995.84 Adult neglect (nutritional)
995.85 Other adult abuse and neglect
995.86 Malignant hyperthermia
995.89 Other
995.9# Systemic inflammatory response syndrome (SIRS)
995.90 Unspecified
995.91 Sepsis
995.92 Severe sepsis
995.93 Due to non-infectious process without acute organ dysfunction
995.94 Due to non-infectious process with acute organ dysfunction

996.#(#) Complications peculiar to certain specified procedures
996.0# Mechanical complication of cardiac device, implant, and graft
996.00 Unspecified device, implant, and graft
996.01 Due to cardiac pacemaker (electrode)
996.02 Due to heart valve prosthesis
996.03 Due to coronary bypass graft
996.04 Due to automatic implantable cardiac defibrillator
996.09 Other
996.1 Mechanical complication of other vascular device, implant, and graft
996.2 Mechanical complication of nervous system device, implant, and graft

NUMERICAL REFERENCE

996.#(#) ***(continued)***

996.3# Mechanical complication of genitourinary device, implant, and graft
- 996.30 Unspecified device, implant, and graft
- 996.31 Due to urethral [indwelling] catheter
- 996.32 Due to intrauterine contraceptive device
- 996.39 Other

996.4# Mechanical complication of internal orthopedic device, implant, and graft
- 996.40 Unspecified
- 996.41 Mechanical loosening of prosthetic joint
- 996.42 Disolocation of prosthetic joint
- 996.43 Prosthetic joint implant failure
- 996.44 Peri-prosthetic fracture around prosthetic joint
- 996.45 Peri-prosthetic osteolysis
- 996.46 Articular bearing surgace wear of prosthetic joint
- 996.47 Other mechanical complication of prosthetic joint
- 996.49 Other

996.5# Mechanical complication of other specified prosthetic device, implant, and graft
- 996.51 Due to corneal graft
- 996.52 Due to graft of other tissue, not elsewhere classified
- 996.53 Due to ocular lens prosthesis
- 996.54 Due to breast prosthesis
- 996.55 Due to artificial skin graft and decellularized allodermis
- 996.56 Due to peritoneal dialysis catheter
- 996.57 Due to insulin pump
- 996.59 Due to other implant and internal device, not elsewhere classified

996.6# Infection and inflammatory reaction due to internal prosthetic device, implant, and graft
- 996.60 Due to unspecified device, implant and graft
- 996.61 Due to cardiac device, implant and graft
- 996.62 Due to vascular device, implant and graft
- 996.63 Due to nervous system device, implant and graft
- 996.64 Due to indwelling urinary catheter
- 996.65 Due to other genitourinary device, implant and graft
- 996.66 Due to internal joint prosthesis
- 996.67 Due to other internal orthopedic device, implant and graft
- 996.68 Due to peritoneal dialysis catheter
- 996.69 Due to other internal prosthetic device, implant, and graft

996.7# Other complications of internal (biological) (synthetic) prosthetic device, implant, and graft
- 996.70 Due to unspecified device, implant, and graft
- 996.71 Due to heart valve prosthesis
- 996.72 Due to other cardiac device, implant, and graft
- 996.73 Due to renal dialysis device, implant, and graft
- 996.74 Due to vascular device, implant, and graft
- 996.75 Due to nervous system device, implant, and graft
- 996.76 Due to genitourinary device, implant, and graft
- 996.77 Due to internal joint prosthesis

996.#(#) ***(continued)***

996.7# ***(continued)***
- 996.78 Due to other internal orthopedic device, implant, and graft
- 996.79 Due to other internal prosthetic device, implant, and graft

996.8# Complications of transplanted organ
- 996.80 Transplanted organ, unspecified
- 996.81 Kidney
- 996.82 Liver
- 996.83 Heart
- 996.84 Lung
- 996.85 Bone marrow
- 996.86 Pancreas
- 996.87 Intestine
- 996.89 Other specified transplanted organ

996.9# Complications of reattached extremity or body part
- 996.90 Unspecified extremity
- 996.91 Forearm
- 996.92 Hand
- 996.93 Finger(s)
- 996.94 Upper extremity, other and unspecified
- 996.95 Foot and toe(s)
- 996.96 Lower extremity, other and unspecified
- 996.99 Other specified body part

997.#(#) Complications affecting specified body systems, not elsewhere classified

997.0# Nervous system complications
- 997.00 Nervous system complication, NOS
- 997.01 Central nervous system complication
- 997.02 Iatrogenic cerebrovascular infarction or hemorrhage
- 997.09 Other nervous system complications

997.1 Cardiac complications

997.2 Peripheral vascular complications

997.3 Respiratory complications

997.4 Digestive system complications

997.5 Urinary complications

997.6# Amputation stump complication
- 997.60 Unspecified complication
- 997.61 Neuroma of amputation stump
- 997.62 Infection (chronic)
- 997.69 NEC

997.7# Vascular complications of other vessels
- 997.71 Vascular complications of mesenteric artery
- 997.72 Vascular complications of renal artery
- 997.79 Vascular complications of other vessels

997.9# Complications affecting other specified body systems, not elsewhere classified
- 997.91 Hypertension
- 997.99 Other

998.#(#) Other complications of procedures, NEC

998.0 Postoperative shock

998.1# Hemorrhage or hematoma or seroma complicating a procedure
- 998.11 Hemorrhage complicating a procedure
- 998.12 Hematoma complicating a procedure
- 998.13 Seroma complicating a procedure

998.2 Accidental puncture or laceration during a procedure

998.3# Disruption of operation wound
- 998.31 Internal
- 998.32 External

998.4 Foreign body accidentally left during a procedure

998.#(#) ***(continued)***

998.5# Postoperative infection
998.51 Infected postoperative seroma
998.59 Other postoperative infection
998.6 Persistent postoperative fistula
998.7 Acute reaction to foreign substance accidentally left during a procedure
998.8# Other specified complications of procedures, not elsewhere classified
998.81 Emphysema (subcutaneous) (surgical) resulting from a procedure
998.82 Cataract fragments in eye following cataract surgery
998.83 Non-healing surgical wound
998.89 Other specified complications
998.9 Unspecified complication of procedure, not elsewhere classified

999.# Complications of medical care, not elsewhere classified

999.0 Generalized vaccinia
999.1 Air embolism
999.2 Other vascular complications
999.3# Other infection
999.31 Infection due to central venous catheter
999.39 Infection following other infusion, injection, transfusion, or vaccination
999.4 Anaphylactic shock due to serum
999.5 Other serum reaction
999.6 ABO incompatibility reaction
999.7 Rh incompatibility reaction
999.8 Other transfusion reaction
999.9 Other and unspecified complications of medical care, not elsewhere classified

V01.#(#) Contact with or exposure to communicable diseases

V01.0 Cholera
V01.1 Tuberculosis
V01.2 Poliomyelitis
V01.3 Smallpox
V01.4 Rubella
V01.5 Rabies
V01.6 Venereal diseases
V01.7# Other viral diseases
V01.71 Varicella
V01.79 Other viral diseases
V01.8# Other communicable diseases
V01.81 Anthrax
V01.82 SARS –associated coronavirus
V01.83 Escherichia coli (E. coli)
V01.84 Meningococcus
V01.89 Other
V01.9 Unspecified communicable disease

V02.#(#) Carrier or suspected carrier of infectious diseases

V02.0 Cholera
V02.1 Typhoid
V02.2 Amebiasis
V02.3 Other gastrointestinal pathogens
V02.4 Diphtheria
V02.5# Other specified bacterial diseases
V02.51 Group B streptococcus
V02.52 Other streptococcus
V02.59 Other specified bacterial diseases
V02.6# Viral hepatitis
V02.60 Viral hepatitis carrier, unspecified
V02.61 Hepatitis B carrier
V02.62 Hepatitis C carrier
V02.69 Other viral hepatitis carrier

V02.#(#) ***(continued)***

V02.7 Gonorrhea
V02.8 Other venereal diseases
V02.9 Other specified infectious organism

V03.#(#) Need for prophylactic vaccination and inoculation against bacterial diseases

V03.0 Cholera alone
V03.1 Typhoid-paratyphoid alone [TAB]
V03.2 Tuberculosis [BCG]
V03.3 Plague
V03.4 Tularemia
V03.5 Diphtheria alone
V03.6 Pertussis alone
V03.7 Tetanus toxoid alone
V03.8# Other specified vaccinations against single bacterial diseases
V03.81 Hemophilus influenza, type B [Hib]
V03.82 Streptococcus pneumoniae
V03.89 Other specified vaccination
V03.9 Unspecified single bacterial disease

V04.#(#) Need for prophylactic vaccination and inoculation against certain diseases

V04.0 Poliomyelitis
V04.1 Smallpox
V04.2 Measles alone
V04.3 Rubella alone
V04.4 Yellow fever
V04.5 Rabies
V04.6 Mumps alone
V04.7 Common cold
V04.8# Other viral diseases
V04.81 Influenza
V04.82 Respiratory syncytial virus (RSV)
V04.89 Other viral diseases

V05.# Need for prophylactic vaccination and inoculation against single diseases

V05.0 Arthropod-borne viral encephalitis
V05.1 Other arthropod-borne viral diseases
V05.2 Leishmaniasis
V05.3 Viral hepatitis
V05.4 Varicella
V05.8 Other specified disease
V05.9 Unspecified single disease

V06.# Need for prophylactic vaccination and inoculation against combinations of diseases

V06.0 Cholera with typhoid-paratyphoid [cholera + TAB]
V06.1 Diphtheria-tetanus-pertussis, combined [DTP] [DTaP]
V06.2 Diphtheria-tetanus-pertussis with typhoid-paratyphoid [DTP + TAB]
V06.3 Diphtheria-tetanus-pertussis with poliomyelitis [DTP+polio]
V06.4 Measles-mumps-rubella [MMR]
V06.5 Tetanus-diphtheria [Td] [DT]
V06.6 Streptococcus pneumoniae [pneumococcus] and influenza
V06.8 Other combinations
V06.9 Unspecified combined vaccine

V07.#(#) Need for isolation and other prophylactic measures

V07.0 Isolation
V07.1 Desensitization to allergens
V07.2 Prophylactic immunotherapy

V07.#(#) ***(continued)***

V07.3# Other prophylactic chemotherapy
V07.31 Prophylactic fluoride administration
V07.39 Other prophylactic chemotherapy
V07.4 Hormone replacement therapy (postmenopausal)
V07.8 Other specified prophylactic measure
V07.9 Unspecified prophylactic measure

V08 Asymptomatic human immunodeficiency virus [HIV] infection status

V09.#(#) Infection with drug-resistant microorganisms

V09.0 Infection with microorganisms resistant to penicillins
V09.1 Infection with microorganisms resistant to cephalosporins and other B-lactam antibiotics
V09.2 Infection with microorganisms resistant to macrolides
V09.3 Infection with microorganisms resistant to tetracyclines
V09.4 Infection with microorganisms resistant to aminoglycosides
V09.5# Infection with microorganisms resistant to quinolones and fluoroquinolones
V09.50 Without mention of resistance to multiple quinolones and fluoroquinoles
V09.51 With resistance to multiple quinolones and fluoroquinoles
V09.6 Infection with microorganisms resistant to sulfonamides
V09.7# Infection with microorganisms resistant to other specified antimycobacterial agents
V09.70 Without mention of resistance to multiple antimycobacterial agents
V09.71 With resistance to multiple antimycobacterial agents
V09.8# Infection with microorganisms resistant to other specified drugs
V09.9# Infection with drug-resistant microorganisms, unspecified

5th Digit: V09.8-V09.9
0 Without mention of resistance to multiple drugs
1 With resistance to multiple drugs

V10.#(#) Personal history of malignant neoplasm

V10.0# Gastrointestinal tract
V10.00 Gastrointestinal tract, unspecified
V10.01 Tongue
V10.02 Other and unspecified oral cavity and pharynx
V10.03 Esophagus
V10.04 Stomach
V10.05 Large intestine
V10.06 Rectum, rectosigmoid junction, and anus
V10.07 Liver
V10.09 Other
V10.1# Trachea, bronchus, and lung
V10.11 Bronchus and lung
V10.12 Trachea
V10.2# Other respiratory and intrathoracic organs
V10.20 Respiratory organ, unspecified
V10.21 Larynx
V10.22 Nasal cavities, middle ear, and accessory sinuses
V10.29 Other

V10.#(#) ***(continued)***

V10.3 Breast
V10.4# Genital organs
V10.40 Female genital organ, unspecified
V10.41 Cervix uteri
V10.42 Other parts of uterus
V10.43 Ovary
V10.44 Other female genital organs
V10.45 Male genital organ, unspecified
V10.46 Prostate
V10.47 Testis
V10.48 Epididymis
V10.49 Other male genital organs
V10.5# Urinary organs
V10.50 Urinary organ, unspecified
V10.51 Bladder
V10.52 Kidney
V10.53 Renal pelvis
V10.59 Other
V10.6# Leukemia
V10.60 Leukemia, unspecified
V10.61 Lymphoid leukemia
V10.62 Myeloid leukemia
V10.63 Monocytic leukemia
V10.69 Other
V10.7# Other lymphatic and hematopoietic neoplasms
V10.71 Lymphosarcoma and reticulosarcoma
V10.72 Hodgkin's disease
V10.79 Other
V10.8# Personal history of malignant neoplasm of other sites
V10.81 Bone
V10.82 Malignant melanoma of skin
V10.83 Other malignant neoplasm of skin
V10.84 Eye
V10.85 Brain
V10.86 Other parts of nervous system
V10.87 Thyroid
V10.88 Other endocrine glands and related structures
V10.89 Other
V10.9 Unspecified personal history of malignant neoplasm

V11.# Personal history of mental disorder

V11.0 Schizophrenia
V11.1 Affective disorders
V11.2 Neurosis
V11.3 Alcoholism
V11.8 Other mental disorders
V11.9 Unspecified mental disorder

V12.#(#) Personal history of certain other diseases

V12.0# Infectious and parasitic diseases
V12.00 Unspecified infectious and parasitic disease
V12.01 Tuberculosis
V12.02 Poliomyelitis
V12.03 Malaria
V12.09 Other
V12.1 Nutritional deficiency
V12.2 Endocrine, metabolic, and immunity disorders
V12.3 Diseases of blood and blood-forming organs

V12.#(#) *(continued)*

V12.4# Disorders of nervous system and sense organs
- V12.40 Unspecified disorder of nervous system and sense organs
- V12.41 Benign neoplasm of the brain
- V12.42 Infections of central nervous system
- V12.49 Other disorders of nervous system and sense organs

V12.5# Diseases of circulatory system
- V12.50 Unspecified circulatory disease
- V12.51 Venous thrombosis and embolism
- V12.52 Thrombophlebitis
- V12.53 Sudden cardiac arrest
- V12.54 Transient ischemic attack (TIA), and cerebral infarction without residual deficits
- V12.59 Other

V12.6# Diseases of respiratory system
- V12.60 Unspecified
- V12.61 Pneumonia (recurrent)
- V12.69 Other

V12.7# Diseases of digestive system
- V12.70 Unspecified digestive disease
- V12.71 Peptic ulcer disease
- V12.72 Colonic polyps
- V12.79 Other

V13.#(#) Personal history of other diseases

V13.0# Disorders of urinary system
- V13.00 Unspecified urinary disorder
- V13.01 Urinary calculi
- V13.02 Urinary (tract) infection
- V13.03 Nephrotic syndrome
- V13.09 Other

V13.1 Trophoblastic disease

V13.2# Other genital system and obstetric disorders
- V13.21 Personal history of pre-term labor
- V13.22 Personal history or cervical dysplasia
- V13.29 Other

V13.3 Diseases of skin and subcutaneous tissue
V13.4 Arthritis
V13.5 Other musculoskeletal disorders

V13.6# Congenital malformations
- V13.61 Hypospadias
- V13.69 Other congenital malformations

V13.7 Perinatal problems
V13.8 Other specified diseases
V13.9 Unspecified disease

V14.# Personal history of allergy to medicinal agents

V14.0 Penicillin
V14.1 Other antibiotic agent
V14.2 Sulfonamides
V14.3 Other anti-infective agent
V14.4 Anesthetic agent
V14.5 Narcotic agent
V14.6 Analgesic agent
V14.7 Serum or vaccine
V14.8 Other specified medicinal agents
V14.9 Unspecified medicinal agent

V15.#(#) Other personal history presenting hazards to health

V15.0# Allergy, other than to medicinal agents
- V15.01 Allergy to peanuts
- V15.02 Allergy to milk products
- V15.03 Allergy to eggs
- V15.04 Allergy to seafood
- V15.05 Allergy to other foods
- V15.06 Allergy to insects
- V15.07 Allergy to latex
- V15.08 Allergy to radiographic dye
- V15.09 Allergy other than medicinal agents

V15.#(#) *(continued)*

V15.1 Surgery to heart and great vessels
V15.2 Surgery to other major organs
V15.3 Irradiation

V15.4# Psychological trauma
- V15.41 History of physical abuse
- V15.42 History of emotional abuse
- V15.49 Other

V15.5 Injury
V15.6 Poisoning
V15.7 Contraception

V15.8# Other specified personal history presenting hazards to health
- V15.81 Noncompliance with medical treatment
- V15.82 History of tobacco use
- V15.84 Exposure to asbestos
- V15.85 Exposure to potentially hazardous body fluids
- V15.86 Exposure to lead
- V15.87 History of extracorporeal membrane oxygenation [ECMO]
- V15.88 History of fall
- V15.89 Other

V15.9 Unspecified personal history presenting hazards to health

V16.#(#) Family history of malignant neoplasm

V16.0 Gastrointestinal tract
V16.1 Trachea, bronchus, and lung
V16.2 Other respiratory and intrathoracic organs
V16.3 Breast

V16.4# Genital organs
- V16.40 Genital organ, unspecified
- V16.41 Ovary
- V16.42 Prostate
- V16.43 Testis
- V16.49 Other

V16.5# Urinary organs
- V16.51 Kidney
- V16.52 Bladder
- V16.59 Other

V16.6 Leukemia
V16.7 Other lymphatic and hematopoietic neoplasms
V16.8 Other specified malignant neoplasm
V16.9 Unspecified malignant neoplasm

V17.#(#) Family history of certain chronic disabling diseases

V17.0 Psychiatric condition
V17.1 Stroke (cerebrovascular)
V17.2 Other neurological diseases
V17.3 Ischemic heart disease

V17.4# Other cardiovascular diseases
- V17.41 Sudden cardiac death (SCD)
- V17.49 Other cardiovascular disease

V17.5 Asthma
V17.6 Other chronic respiratory conditions
V17.7 Arthritis

V17.8# Other musculoskeletal diseases
- V17.81 Osteoporosis
- V17.82 Other

V18.#(#) Family history of certain other specific conditions

V18.0 Diabetes mellitus

V18.1# Other endocrine and metabolic diseases
- V18.11 Multiple endocrine neoplasia [MEN\ syndrome
- V18.19 Other endocrine and metabolic diseases

V18.2 Anemia
V18.3 Other blood disorders
V18.4 Mental retardation

V18.#(#) ***(continued)***
- **V18.5#** Digestive disorders
  - V18.51 Colonic polyps
  - V18.59 Other digestive disorder
- **V18.6#** Kidney diseases
  - V18.61 Polycystic kidney
  - V18.69 Other kidney diseases
- V18.7 Other genitourinary diseases
- V18.8 Infectious and parasitic diseases
- V18.9 Genetic disease carrier

V19.# Family history of other conditions
- V19.0 Blindness or visual loss
- V19.1 Other eye disorders
- V19.2 Deafness or hearing loss
- V19.3 Other ear disorders
- V19.4 Skin conditions
- V19.5 Congenital anomalies
- V19.6 Allergic disorders
- V19.7 Consanguinity
- V19.8 Other condition

V20.# Health supervision of infant or child
- V20.0 Foundling
- V20.1 Other healthy infant or child receiving care
- V20.2 Routine infant or child health check

V21.# Constitutional states in development
- V21.0 Period of rapid growth in childhood
- V21.1 Puberty
- V21.2 Other adolescence
- **V21.3#** Low birth weight status
  - V21.30 NOS
  - V21.31 less than 500 grams
  - V21.32 500-999 grams
  - V21.33 1000-1499 grams
  - V21.34 1500-1599 grams
  - V21.35 2000-2500 grams
- V21.8 Other specified constitutional states in development
- V21.9 Unspecified constitutional state in development

V22.# Normal pregnancy
- V22.0 Supervision of normal first pregnancy
- V22.1 Supervision of other normal pregnancy
- V22.2 Pregnant state, incidental

V23.#(#) Supervision of high-risk pregnancy
- V23.0 Pregnancy with history of infertility
- V23.1 Pregnancy with history of trophoblastic disease
- V23.2 Pregnancy with history of abortion
- V23.3 Grand multiparity
- **V23.4#** Pregnancy with other poor obstetric history
  - V23.41 Hisotry of pre-term labor
  - V23.49 other poor obstetric history
- V23.5 Pregnancy with other poor reproductive history
- V23.7 Insufficient prenatal care
- **V23.8#** Other high-risk pregnancy
  - V23.81 Elderly primigravida
  - V23.82 Elderly multigravida
  - V23.83 Young primigravida
  - V23.84 Young multigravida
  - V23.89 Other high-risk pregnancy
- V23.9 Unspecified high-risk pregnancy

V24.# Postpartum care and examination
- V24.0 Immediately after delivery
- V24.1 Lactating mother
- V24.2 Routine postpartum follow-up

V25.#(#) Encounter for contraceptive management
- **V25.0#** General counseling and advice
  - V25.01 Prescription of oral contraceptives
  - V25.02 Initiation of other contraceptive measures
  - V25.03 Emergency contraceptive counseling and prescription
  - V25.04 Counseling and instruction in natural family planning to avoid pregnancy
  - V25.09 Other
- V25.1 Insertion of intrauterine contraceptive device
- V25.2 Sterilization
- V25.3 Menstrual extraction
- **V25.4#** Surveillance of previously prescribed contraceptive methods
  - V25.40 Contraceptive surveillance, unspecified
  - V25.41 Contraceptive pill
  - V25.42 Intrauterine contraceptive device
  - V25.43 Implantable subdermal contraceptive
  - V25.49 Other contraceptive method
- V25.5 Insertion of implantable subdermal contraceptive
- V25.8 Other specified contraceptive management
- V25.9 Unspecified contraceptive management

V26.#(#) Procreative management
- V26.0 Tuboplasty or vasoplasty after previous sterilization
- V26.1 Artificial insemination
- **V26.2#** Investigation and testing
  - V26.21 Fertility testing
  - V26.22 Aftercare following sterilization reversal
  - V26.29 Other investigation and testing of female
- **V26.3#** Genetic counseling and testing
  - V26.31 Testing of female for genetic disease carrier status
  - V26.32 Other genetic testing of female
  - V26.33 Genetic counseling
  - V26.34 Testing of male for genetic disease carrier status
  - V26.35 Encounter for testing of male partner of habitual aborter
  - V26.39 Other genetic testing of male
- **V26.4#** General counseling and advice
  - V26.41 Procreative counseling and advice using natural family planning
  - V26.49 Other procreative management counseling and advice
- **V26.5#** Sterilization status
  - V26.51 Tubal ligation status
  - V26.52 Vasectomy status
- **V26.8#** Other specified procreative management
  - V26.81 Encounter for assisted reproductive fertility
  - V26.89 Other specified procreative management
- V26.9 Unspecified procreative management

V27.# Outcome of delivery
- V27.0 Single liveborn
- V27.1 Single stillborn
- V27.2 Twins, both liveborn
- V27.3 Twins, one liveborn and one stillborn
- V27.4 Twins, both stillborn
- V27.5 Other multiple birth, all liveborn
- V27.6 Other multiple birth, some liveborn
- V27.7 Other multiple birth, all stillborn
- V27.9 Unspecified outcome of delivery

V28.# Encounter for antenatal screening
- V28.0 Screening for chromosomal anomalies by amniocentesis
- V28.1 Screening for raised alpha-fetoprotein levels in amniotic fluid
- V28.2 Other screening based on amniocentesis
- V28.3 Screening for malformation using ultrasonics
- V28.4 Screening for fetal growth retardation using ultrasonics
- V28.5 Screening for isoimmunization
- V28.6 Screening for Streptococcus B
- V28.8 Other specified antenatal screening
- V28.9 Unspecified antenatal screening

V29.# Observation and evaluation of newborns for suspected condition not found
- V29.0 Observation for suspected infectious condition
- V29.1 Observation for suspected neurological condition
- V29.2 Observation for suspected respiratory condition
- V29.3 Observation for suspected genetic or metabolic condition
- V29.8 Observation for other specified suspected condition
- V29.9 Observation for unspecified suspected condition

V30.#(#) Single liveborn

V31.#(#) Twin, mate liveborn

V32.#(#) Twin, mate stillborn

V33.#(#) Twin, unspecified

V34.#(#) Other multiple, mates all liveborn

V35.#(#) Other multiple, mates all stillborn

V36.#(#) Other multiple, mates live- and stillborn

V37.#(#) Other multiple, unspecified

V39.#(#) Unspecified

4th Digit: V30-V39
- **0 Born in hospital**
- **1 Born before admission to hospital**
- **2 Born outside hospital and not hospitalized**

5th Digit: V30.0, V31.0, V32.0, V33.0, V34.0, V35.0, V36.0, V37.0, V38.0, V39.0
- **0 Delivered without mention of cesarean delivery**
- **1 Delivered by cesarean delivery**

V40.# Mental and behavioral problems
- V40.0 Problems with learning
- V40.1 Problems with communication [includidng speech]
- V40.2 Other mental problems
- V40.3 Other behavioral problems
- V40.9 Unspecified mental or behavioral problem

V41.# Problems with special senses and other special functions
- V41.0 Problems with sight
- V41.1 Other eye problems
- V41.2 Problems with hearing

V41.# *(continued)*
- V41.3 Other ear problems
- V41.4 Problems with voice production
- V41.5 Problems with smell and taste
- V41.6 Problems with swallowing and mastication
- V41.7 Problems with sexual function
- V41.8 Other problems with special functions
- V41.9 Unspecified problem with special functions

V42.#(#) Organ or tissue replaced by transplant
- V42.0 Kidney
- V42.1 Heart
- V42.2 Heart valve
- V42.3 Skin
- V42.4 Bone
- V42.5 Cornea
- V42.6 Lung
- V42.7 Liver
- **V42.8#** Other specified organ or tissue
  - V42.81 Bone marrow
  - V42.82 Peripheral stem cells
  - V42.83 Pancreas
  - V42.84 Intestines
  - V42.89 Other
- V42.9 Unspecified organ or tissue

V43.#(#) Organ or tissue replaced by other means
- V43.0 Eye globe
- V43.1 Lens
- **V43.2#** Heart
  - V43.21 Heart assist device
  - V43.22 Fully implantable artificial heart
- V43.3 Heart valve
- V43.4 Blood vessel
- V43.5 Bladder
- **V43.6#** Joint
  - V43.60 Unspecified joint
  - V43.61 Shoulder
  - V43.62 Elbow
  - V43.63 Wrist
  - V43.64 Hip
  - V43.65 Knee
  - V43.66 Ankle
  - V43.69 Other
- V43.7 Limb
- **V43.8#** Other organ or tissue
  - V43.81 Larynx
  - V43.82 Breast
  - V43.83 Artificial skin
  - V43.89 Other

V44.#(#) Artificial opening status
- V44.0 Tracheostomy
- V44.1 Gastrostomy
- V44.2 Ileostomy
- V44.3 Colostomy
- V44.4 Other artificial opening of gastrointestinal tract
- **V44.5#** Cystostomy
  - V44.50 Cystostomy, unspecified
  - V44.51 Cutaneous-vesicostomy
  - V44.52 Appendico-vesicostomy
  - V44.59 Other cystostomy
- V44.6 Other artificial opening of urinary tract
- V44.7 Artificial vagina
- V44.8 Other artificial opening status
- V44.9 Unspecified artificial opening status

V45.#(#) Other postsurgical states
- **V45.0#** Cardiac device in situ
  - V45.00 Unspecified cardiac device
  - V45.01 Cardiac pacemaker

V45.#(#) ***(continued)***

V45.0(#) (continued)

V45.02 Automatic implantable cardiac defibrillator
V45.09 Other specified cardiac device

V45.1 Renal dialysis status
V45.2 Presence of cerebrospinal fluid drainage device
V45.3 Intestinal bypass or anastomosis status
V45.4 Arthrodesis status

V45.5# Presence of contraceptive device

V45.51 Intrauterine contraceptive device
V45.52 Subdermal contraceptive implant
V45.59 Other

V45.6# States following surgery of eye and adnexa

V45.61 Cataract extraction status
V45.69 Other states following surgery of eye and adnexa

V45.7# Acquired absence of organ

V45.71 Acquired absence of breast
V45.72 Acquired absence of intestine
V45.73 Acquired absence of kidney
V45.74 Other parts of urinary tract
V45.75 Stomach
V45.76 Lung
V45.77 Genital organs
V45.78 Eye
V45.79 Other acquired absence of organ

V45.8# Other postprocedural status

V45.81 Aortocoronary bypass status
V45.82 Percutaneous transluminal coronary angioplasty status
V45.83 Breast implant removal status
V45.84 Dental restoration status
V45.85 Insulin pump
V45.86 Bariatric surgery status
V45.89 Other

V46.# Other dependence on machines

V46.0 Aspirator

V46.1# Respirator [Ventilator]

V46.11 Dependence on respirator, status
V46.12 Encounter for respirator dependence dring power failure
V46.13 Encounter for weaning from respirator [ventilator]
V46.14 Mechanical complication of respirator [ventilator]

V46.2 Supplemental oxygen
V46.8 Other enabling machines
V46.9 Unspecified machine dependence

V47.# Other problems with internal organs

V47.0 Deficiencies of internal organs
V47.1 Mechanical and motor problems, internal organs
V47.2 Other cardiorespiratory problems
V47.3 Other digestive problems
V47.4 Other urinary problems
V47.5 Other genital problems
V47.9 Unspecified

V48.# Problems with head, neck, and trunk

V48.0 Deficiencies of head
V48.1 Deficiencies of neck and trunk
V48.2 Mechanical and motor problems with head
V48.3 Mechanical and motor problems, neck and trunk
V48.4 Sensory problem with head
V48.5 Sensory problem with neck and trunk
V48.6 Disfigurements of head
V48.7 Disfigurements of neck and trunk

V48.#(#) ***(continued)***

V48.8 Other problems with head, neck, and trunk
V48.9 Unspecified problem with head, neck, or trunk

V49.#(#) Problems with limbs and other problems

V49.0 Deficiencies of limbs
V49.1 Mechanical problems with limbs
V49.2 Motor problems with limbs
V49.3 Sensory problems with limbs
V49.4 Disfigurements of limbs
V49.5 Other problems of limbs

V49.6# Upper limb amputation status

V49.60 Unspecified level
V49.61 Thumb
V49.62 Other finger(s)
V49.63 Hand
V49.64 Wrist
V49.65 Below elbow
V49.66 Above elbow
V49.67 Shoulder

V49.7# Lower limb amputation status

V49.70 Unspecified level
V49.71 Great toe
V49.72 Other toe(s)
V49.73 Foot
V49.74 Ankle
V49.75 Below knee
V49.76 Above knee
V49.77 Hip

V49.8# Other specified conditions influencing health status

V49.81 Asymptomatic postmenopausal status (age-related) (natural)
V49.82 Dental sealant status
V49.83 Awaiting organ transplant status
V49.84 Bed confinement status
V49.85 Dual sensory impairment
V49.89 Other specified conditions influencing health status

V49.9 Unspecified

V50.#(#) Elective surgery for purposes other than remedying health states

V50.0 Hair transplant
V50.1 Other plastic surgery for unacceptable cosmetic appearance
V50.2 Routine or ritual circumcision
V50.3 Ear piercing

V50.4# Prophylactic organ removal

V50.41 Breast
V50.42 Ovary
V50.49 Other

V50.8 Other
V50.9 Unspecified

V51 Aftercare involving the use of plastic surgery

V52.# Fitting and adjustment of prosthetic device and implant

V52.0 Artificial arm (complete) (partial)
V52.1 Artificial leg (complete) (partial)
V52.2 Artificial eye
V52.3 Dental prosthetic device
V52.4 Breast prosthesis and implant
V52.8 Other specified prosthetic device
V52.9 Unspecified prosthetic device

V53.#(#) Fitting and adjustment of other device
V53.0# Devices related to nervous system and special senses
V53.01 Fitting and adjustment of cerebral ventricle (communicating) shunt
V53.02 Neuropacemaker (brain) (peripheral nerve) (spinal cord)
V53.09 Fitting and adjustment of other devices related to nervous system and special senses
V53.1 Spectacles and contact lenses
V53.2 Hearing aid
V53.3# Cardiac device
V53.31 Cardiac pacemaker
V53.32 Automatic implantable cardiac defibrillator
V53.39 Other cardiac device
V53.4 Orthodontic devices
V53.5 Other intestinal appliance
V53.6 Urinary devices
V53.7 Orthopedic devices
V53.8 Wheelchair
V53.9# Other and unspecified device
V53.90 Unspecified device
V53.91 Fitting and adjustment of insulin pump
V53.99 Other device

V54.#(#) Other orthopedic aftercare
V54.0# Aftercare involving internal fixation device
V54.01 Aftercare for removal of internal fixation device
V54.02 Aftercare for legnthening/adjustment of growth rod
V54.09 Other aftercare involving internal fixation device
V54.1# Aftercare for healing traumatic fracture
V54.2# Aftercare for healing pathologic fracture
5th Digit: V54.1- V54.2
0 Arm unspecified
1 Upper arm
2 Lower arm
3 Hip
4 Leg unspecified
5 Upper leg
6 Lower leg
7 Vertebrae
9 Other bone
V54.8# Other orthopedic aftercare
V54.81 Following joint replacement
V54.89 Other
V54.9 Unspecified orthopedic aftercare

V55.# Attention to artificial openings
V55.0 Tracheostomy
V55.1 Gastrostomy
V55.2 Ileostomy
V55.3 Colostomy
V55.4 Other artificial opening of digestive tract
V55.5 Cystostomy
V55.6 Other artificial opening of urinary tract
V55.7 Artificial vagina
V55.8 Other specified artificial opening
V55.9 Unspecified artificial opening

V56.#(#) Encounter for dialysis and dialysis catheter care
V56.0 Extracorporeal dialysis
V56.1 Fitting and adjustment of extracorporeal dialysis catheter
V56.2 Fitting and adjustment of peritoneal dialysis catheter

V56.#(#) *(continued)*
V56.3# Encounter for adequacy testing for dialysis
V56.31 Encounter for adequacy testing for hemodialysis
V56.32 Encounter for adequacy testing for peritoneal dialysis
V56.8 Other dialysis

V57.#(#) Care involving use of rehabilitation procedures
V57.0 Breathing exercises
V57.1 Other physical therapy
V57.2# Occupational therapy and vocational rehabilitation
V57.21 Encounter for occupational therapy
V57.22 Encounter for vocational therapy
V57.3 Speech therapy
V57.4 Orthoptic training
V57.8# Other specified rehabilitation procedure
V57.81 Orthotic training
V57.89 Other
V57.9 Unspecified rehabilitation procedure

V58.#(#) Encounter for other and unspecified procedures and aftercare
V58.0 Radiotherapy
V58.1# Encounter for antineoplastic chemotherapy and immunotherapy
V58.11 Chemotherapy
V58.12 Immunotherapy
V58.2 Blood transfusion, without reported diagnosis
V58.3# Attention to dressings and sutures
V58.30 Encounter for change or removal of nonsurgical wound dressing
V58.31 Encounter for change or removal of surgical wound dressing
V58.32 Encounter for removal of sutures
V58.4# Other aftercare following surgery
V58.41 Encounter for planned post-operative wound closure
V58.42 For neoplasm
V58.43 For injury and trauma
V58.44 Aftercare following organ transplant
V58.49 Other specified aftercare following surgery
V58.5 Orthodontics
V58.6# Long-term (current) drug use
V58.61 Long-term (current) use of anticoagulants
V58.62 Long-term (current) use of antibiotics
V58.63 Long-term (current) use of antiplatelets/antithrombotics
V58.64 Long-term (current) use of non-steroidal anti-inflammatories (NSAID)
V58.65 Long term (current) use of steroids
V58.66 Long-term (current) use of aspirin
V58.67 Long-term (current) use of insulin
V58.69 Long-term (current) use of other medications
V58.7# Aftercare following surgery to specified body systems, NEC
V58.71 Sense organs, NEC
V58.72 Nervous Systems, NEC
V58.73 Circulatory systems, NEC
V58.74 Respiratory systems NEC
V58.75 Teeth, oral cavity and digestive system, NEC
V58.76 Genitourinary system NEC
V58.77 Skin and subcutaneous tissue NEC
V58,78 Musculoskeletal system NEC
V58.8# Other specified procedures and aftercare
V58.81 Fitting and adjustment of vascular catheter
V58.82 Fitting and adjustment of non-vascular catheter NEC

V58.#(#) ***(continued)***
V58.8(#) (continued)
V58.83 Encounter for therapeutic drug monitoring
V58.89 Other specified aftercare
V58.9 Unspecified aftercare

V59.#(#) Donors
V59.0# Blood
V59.01 Whole blood
V59.02 Stem cells
V59.09 Other
V59.1 Skin
V59.2 Bone
V59.3 Bone marrow
V59.4 Kidney
V59.5 Cornea
V59.6 Liver
V59.7# Egg (oocyte) (ovum)
V59.70 Donor, unspecified
V59.71 Donor, under age 35, anonymous recipent
V59.72 Donor, under age 35, designated recipient
V59.73 Donor, age 35 and over, anonymous recipent
V59.74 Donor, age 35 and over, designated recipent
V59.8 Other specified organ or tissue
V59.9 Unspecified organ or tissue

V60.# Housing, household, and economic circumstances
V60.0 Lack of housing
V60.1 Inadequate housing
V60.2 Inadequate material resources
V60.3 Person living alone
V60.4 No other household member able to render care
V60.5 Holiday relief care
V60.6 Person living in residential institution
V60.8 Other specified housing or economic circumstances
V60.9 Unspecified housing or economic circumstance

V61.#(#) Other family circumstances
V61.0 Family disruption
V61.1# Counseling for marital and partner problems
V61.10 Counseling for marital and partner problems, unspecified
V61.11 Counseling for victim of spousal and partner abuse
V61.12 Counseling for perpetrator of spousal and partner abuse
V61.2# Parent-child problems
V61.20 Counseling for parent-child problem, unspecified
V61.21 Counseling for victim of child abuse
V61.22 Counseling for perpetrator of parental child abuse
V61.29 Other
V61.3 Problems with aged parents or in-laws
V61.4# Health problems within family
V61.41 Alcoholism in family
V61.49 Other
V61.5 Multiparity
V61.6 Illegitimacy or illegitimate pregnancy
V61.7 Other unwanted pregnancy
V61.8 Other specified family circumstances
V61.9 Unspecified family circumstance

V62.#(#) Other psychosocial circumstances
V62.0 Unemployment
V62.1 Adverse effects of work environment
V62.2 Other occupational circumstances or maladjustment
V62.3 Educational circumstances
V62.4 Social maladjustment
V62.5 Legal circumstances
V62.6 Refusal of treatment for reasons of religion or conscience
V62.8# Other psychological or physical stress, NEC
V62.81 Interpersonal problems, not elsewhere classified
V62.82 Bereavement, uncomplicated
V62.83 Counseling for perpetrator of physical/sexual abuse
V62.84 Suicidal ideation
V62.89 Other
V62.9 Unspecified psychosocial circumstance

V63.# Unavailability of other medical facilities for care
V63.0 Residence remote from hospital or other health care facility
V63.1 Medical services in home not available
V63.2 Person awaiting admission to adequate facility elsewhere
V63.8 Other specified reasons for unavailability of medical facilities
V63.9 Unspecified reason for unavailability of medical facilities

V64.#(#) Persons encountering health services for specific procedures, not carried out
V64.0# Vaccination not carried out
V64.00 Unspecified reason
V64.01 Due to acute illness
V64.02 Due to chronic illness or condition
V64.03 Due to immune compromised state
V64.04 Due to allergy to vaccine or component
V64.05 Due to caregiver refusal
V64.06 Due to patient refusal
V64.07 Due to religious reasons
V64.08 Due to patient having disease being vaccinated against
V64.09 Other reason
V64.1 Surgical or other procedure not carried out because of contraindication
V64.2 Surgical or other procedure not carried out because of patient's decision
V64.3 Procedure not carried out for other reasons
V64.4# Closed surgical procedure converted to open procedure
V64.41 Laparoscopic surgical procedure converted to open procedure
V64.42 Thoracoscopic surgical procedure converted to open procedure
V64.43 Arthroscopic surgical procedure converted to open procedure

V65.#(#) Other persons seeking consultation without complaint or sickness
V65.0 Healthy person accompanying sick person
V65.1# Person consulting on behalf of another person
V65.11 Pediatric pre-birth visit for expectant mother
V65.19 Other person consulting on behalf of another person
V65.2 Person feigning illness
V65.3 Dietary surveillance and counseling

V65.#(#) ***(continued)***

V65.4# Other counseling, not elsewhere classified
- V65.40 Counseling NOS
- V65.41 Exercise counseling
- V65.42 Counseling on substance use and abuse
- V65.43 Counseling on injury prevention
- V65.44 Human immunodeficiency virus [HIV] counseling
- V65.45 Counseling on other sexually transmitted diseases
- V65.46 Encounter for insulin pump training
- V65.49 Other specified counseling

V65.5 Person with feared complaint in whom no diagnosis was made
V65.8 Other reasons for seeking consultation
V65.9 Unspecified reason for consultation

V66.# Convalescence and palliative care

V66.0 Following surgery
V66.1 Following radiotherapy
V66.2 Following chemotherapy
V66.3 Following psychotherapy and other treatment for mental disorder
V66.4 Following treatment of fracture
V66.5 Following other treatment
V66.6 Following combined treatment
V66.7 Encounter for palliative care
V66.9 Unspecified convalescence

V67.#(#) Follow-up examination

V67.0# Following surgery
- V67.00 Following surgery, unspecified
- V67.01 Follow-up vaginal pap smear
- V67.09 Following other surgery

V67.1 Following radiotherapy
V67.2 Following chemotherapy
V67.3 Following psychotherapy and other treatment for mental disorder
V67.4 Following treatment of healed fracture
V67.5# Following other treatment
- V67.51 Following completed treatment with high-risk medication, not elsewhere classified
- V67.59 Other

V67.6 Following combined treatment
V67.9 Unspecified follow-up examination

V68.#(#) Encounters for administrative purposes

V68.0# Issue of medical certificates
- V68.01 Disability examination
- V68.09 Other issue of medical certificates

V68.1 Issue of repeat prescriptions
V68.2 Request for expert evidence
V68.8# Other specified administrative purpose
- V68.81 Referral of patient without examination or treatment
- V68.89 Other

V68.9 Unspecified administrative purpose

V69.# Problems related to lifestyle

V69.0 Lack of physical exercise
V69.1 Inappropriate diet and eating habits
V69.2 High-risk sexual behavior
V69.3 Gambling and betting
V69.4 Lack of adequate sleep
V69.5 Behavioral insomnia of childhood
V69.8 Other problems related to lifestyle
V69.9 Problem related to lifestyle, unspecified

V70.# General medical examination

V70.0 Routine general medical examination at a health care facility
V70.1 General psychiatric examination, requested by the authority
V70.2 General psychiatric examination, other and unspecified
V70.3 Other medical examination for administrative purposes
V70.4 Examination for medicolegal reasons
V70.5 Health examination of defined subpopulations
V70.6 Health examination in population surveys
V70.7 Examination for normal comparison or control in clinical research
V70.8 Other specified general medical examinations
V70.9 Unspecified general medical examination

V71.#(#) Observation and evaluation for suspected conditions not found

V71.0# Observation for suspected mental condition
- V71.01 Adult antisocial behavior
- V71.02 Childhood or adolescent antisocial behavior
- V71.09 Other suspected mental condition

V71.1 Observation for suspected malignant neoplasm
V71.2 Observation for suspected tuberculosis
V71.3 Observation following accident at work
V71.4 Observation following other accident
V71.5 Observation following alleged rape or seduction
V71.6 Observation following other inflicted injury
V71.7 Observation for suspected cardiovascular disease
V71.8# Observation for other specified suspected conditions
- V71.81 Abuse and neglect
- V71.82 Anthrax
- V71.83 Other biological agent
- V71.89 Other specified suspected conditions

V71.9 Observation for unspecified suspected condition

V72.#(#) Special investigations and examinations

V72.0 Examination of eyes and vision
V72.1# Examination of ears and hearing
- V72.11 Encounter for hearing examination following failed hearing exam
- V72.12 Encounter for hearing conservation and treatment
- V72.19 Other examination of ears and hearing

V72.2 Dental examination
V72.3# Gynecological examination
- V72.31 Routine gynecological examination
- V72.32 Encounter for Papanicolaou cervical smear to confirm findings of recent normal smear following initial abnormal smear

V72.4# Pregnancy examination or test
- V72.40 Pregnancy unconfirmed
- V72.41 Negative result
- V72.42 Positive result

V72.5 Radiological examination, not elsewhere classified
V72.6 Laboratory examination
V72.7 Diagnostic skin and sensitization tests
V72.8# Other specified examinations
- V72.81 Preoperative cardiovascular examination
- V72.82 Preoperative respiratory examination
- V72.83 Other specified preoperative examination

V72.#(#) ***(continued)***

V72.8# ***(continued)***

V72.84 Preoperative examination, unspecified
V72.85 Other specified examination
V72.86 Encounter for blood typing

V72.9 Unspecified examination

V73.#(#) Special screening examination for viral and chlamydial diseases

V73.0 Poliomyelitis
V73.1 Smallpox
V73.2 Measles
V73.3 Rubella
V73.4 Yellow fever
V73.5 Other arthropod-borne viral diseases
V73.6 Trachoma
V73.8# Other specified viral and chlamydial diseases
V73.81 Human papilomavirus (HPV)
V73.88 Other specified chlamydial diseases
V73.89 Other specified viral diseases
V73.9# Unspecified viral and chlamydial disease
V73.98 Unspecified chlamydial disease
V73.99 Unspecified viral disease

V74.# Special screening examination for bacterial and spirochetal diseases

V74.0 Cholera
V74.1 Pulmonary tuberculosis
V74.2 Leprosy [Hansen's disease]
V74.3 Diphtheria
V74.4 Bacterial conjunctivitis
V74.5 Venereal disease
V74.6 Yaws
V74.8 Other specified bacterial and spirochetal diseases
V74.9 Unspecified bacterial and spirochetal disease

V75.# Special screening examination for other infectious diseases

V75.0 Rickettsial diseases
V75.1 Malaria
V75.2 Leishmaniasis
V75.3 Trypanosomiasis
V75.4 Mycotic infections
V75.5 Schistosomiasis
V75.6 Filariasis
V75.7 Intestinal helminthiasis
V75.8 Other specified parasitic infections
V75.9 Unspecified infectious disease

V76.#(#) Special screening for malignant neoplasms

V76.0 Respiratory organs
V76.1# Breast
V76.10 Breast screening, unspecified
V76.11 Screening mammogram for high-risk patient
V76.12 Other screening mammogram
V76.19 Other screening breast examination
V76.2 Cervix
V76.3 Bladder
V76.4# Other sites
V76.41 Rectum
V76.42 Oral cavity
V76.43 Skin
V76.44 Prostate
V76.45 Testis
V76.46 Ovary
V76.47 Vagina
V76.49 Other sites

V76.#(#) ***(continued)***

V76.5# Intestine
V76.50 Intestine
V76.51 Colon
V76.52 Small Intestine
V76.8# Other neoplasm
V76.81 Nervous system
V76.89 Other neoplasm
V76.9 Unspecified

V77.#(#) Special screening for endocrine, nutritional, metabolic, and immunity disorders

V77.0 Thyroid disorders
V77.1 Diabetes mellitus
V77.2 Malnutrition
V77.3 Phenylketonuria [PKU]
V77.4 Galactosemia
V77.5 Gout
V77.6 Cystic fibrosis
V77.7 Other inborn errors of metabolism
V77.8 Obesity
V77.9# Other and unspecified endocrine, nutritional, metabolic, and immunity disorders
V77.91 Screening for lipoid disorders
V77.99 Other and unspecified endocrine, nutritional, metabolic and immunity disorders

V78.# Special screening for disorders of blood and blood-forming organs

V78.0 Iron deficiency anemia
V78.1 Other and unspecified deficiency anemia
V78.2 Sickle-cell disease or trait
V78.3 Other hemoglobinopathies
V78.8 Other disorders of blood and blood-forming organs
V78.9 Unspecified disorder of blood and blood-forming organs

V79.# Special screening for mental disorders and developmental handicaps

V79.0 Depression
V79.1 Alcoholism
V79.2 Mental retardation
V79.3 Developmental handicaps in early childhood
V79.8 Other specified mental disorders and developmental handicaps
V79.9 Unspecified mental disorder and developmental handicap

V80.# Special screening for neurological, eye, and ear diseases

V80.0 Neurological conditions
V80.1 Glaucoma
V80.2 Other eye conditions
V80.3 Ear diseases

V81.# Special screening for cardiovascular, respiratory, and genitourinary diseases

V81.0 Ischemic heart disease
V81.1 Hypertension
V81.2 Other and unspecified cardiovascular conditions
V81.3 Chronic bronchitis and emphysema
V81.4 Other and unspecified respiratory conditions
V81.5 Nephropathy
V81.6 Other and unspecified genitourinary conditions

V82.#(#)/ Special screening for other conditions
- V82.0 Skin conditions
- V82.1 Rheumatoid arthritis
- V82.2 Other rheumatic disorders
- V82.3 Congenital dislocation of hip
- V82.4 Maternal postnatal screening for chromosomal anomalies
- V82.5 Chemical poisoning and other contamination
- V82.6 Multiphasic screening
- **V82.7#** Genetic screening
  - V82.71 Screening for genetic disease carrier status
  - V82.79 Other genetic screening
- **V82.8#** Other specified conditions
  - V82.81 Osteoporosis
  - V82.89 Other specified conditions
- V82.9 Unspecified condition

V83.## Genetic carrier status
- **V83.0#** Hemophilia A carrier
  - V83.01 Asymptomatic hemophilia A carrier
  - V83.02 Symptomatic hemophilia A carrier
- **V83.8#** Other genetic carrier status
  - V83.81 Cystic fibrosis gene carrier
  - V83.89 Other genetic carrier status

V84.#(#) Genetic susceptibility to disease
- V84.0#Genetic susceptibility to malignant neoplasm
  - V84.01 Beast
  - V84.02 Ovary
  - V84.03 Prostate
  - V84.04 Endometrium
  - V84.09 Other Malignant neoplasm
- **V84.8#** Genetic susceptibility to other disease
  - V84.81 Genetic susceptibility to multiple endocrine neoplasia [MEN]
  - V84.89 Genetic susceptibility to other disease

V85.#(#) Body mass index [BMI]
- V85.0 Body mass index less than, 19, adult
- V85.1 Body mass index between 19-24, adult
- **V85.2(#)** Body mass index between 25-29, adult
  - V85.20 25.0-25.9
  - V85.21 26.0-26.9
  - V85.22 27.0-27.9
  - V85.23 28.0-28.9
  - V85.24 29.0-29.9
- **V85.3(#)** Body mass index between 30-39,adult
  - V85.30 30.0-30.9
  - V85.31 31.0-31.9
  - V85.32 32.0-32.9
  - V85.33 33.0-33.9
  - V85.34 34.0-34.9
  - V85.35 35.0-35.9
  - V85.36 36.0-36.9
  - V85.37 37.0-37.9
  - V85.38 38.0-38.9
  - V85.39 39.0-39.9
- V85.4 Body mass index 40 and over, adult
- **V85.5#** Body Mass Index, pediatric
  - V85.51 Body Mass Index, pediatric, less than 5th percentile for age
  - V85.52 Body Mass Index, pediatric, 5th percentile to less that 85th percentile for age
  - V85.53 Body Mass Index, pediatric, 85th percentile to less that 95th percentile for age
  - V85.54 Body Mass Index, pediatric, greater than or equal to 95th percentile for age

V86.# Estrogen receptor status
- V86.0 Estrogen receptor positive status [ER+]
- V86.1 Estrogen receptor negative status [ER-]

NUMERICAL REFERENCE

APPENDIX D
CODING GUIDELINES

This section of coding guidelines is not intended to be a comprehensive tutorial on ICD-9 coding. This compilation of guidelines covers many of the basic principles of outpatient coding, including many of the topics most frequently requested on the Unicor Medical coding hotline and in our monthly newsletter. The information presented is based on official government and industry publications. We have made every attempt to assure that the information is accurate; however, no warranty or guarantee is given that this information is error-free and we accept no responsibility or liability should an error occur.

GUIDELINES

ETHICAL STANDARDS OF CODING

In this era of payment based on diagnostic and procedural coding, the professional ethics of health information continue to be challenged. The following standards for ethical coding were developed by the American Health Information Management Association (AHIMA) Council on Coding and Classification and approved by the AHIMA Board of Directors.

I. Diagnoses that are present on admission or diagnoses and procedures that occur during the current encounter are to be abstracted after a thorough review of the entire medical record. Those diagnoses not applicable to the current encounter should not be abstracted.

II. For inpatient settings, the selection of the principal diagnosis and principal procedure, along with other diagnoses and procedures, must meet the definitions of the Uniform Hospital Discharge Data Set (UHDDS). *

III. Assessment must be made of the documentation in the chart to ensure that it is adequate and appropriate to support the diagnoses and procedures selected to be abstracted.

IV. Medical record coders should use their skills, their knowledge of ICD-9-CM and CPT, and any available resources to select diagnostic and procedural codes.

V. Medical record coders should not change codes or narratives of codes so that the meanings are misrepresented. Nor should diagnoses or procedures be included or excluded because the payment will be affected. Statistical clinical data is an important result of coding, and maintaining a quality database should be a conscientious goal.

VI. Physicians should be consulted for clarification when they enter conflicting or ambiguous documentation in the chart.

VII. The medical record coder is a member of the healthcare team and, as such, should assist physicians who are unfamiliar with ICD-9-CM, CPT, or DRG methodology by suggesting resequencing or inclusion of diagnoses or procedures when needed to most accurately reflect the occurrence of events during the encounter.

VIII. The medical record coder is expected to strive for the optimal payment to which the facility is legally entitled, but it is unethical and illegal to maximize payment by means that contradict regulatory guidelines.

Reprinted with permission from the American Health Information Management Association (AHIMA).

(* Note that for outpatient settings, the reason for the encounter is coded first. If the major work or effort is directed at another diagnosis, however, that diagnosis may become primary.)

UNDERSTANDING WHAT YOU CODE

"Understand what you are coding" is one of the most fundamental rules of coding. This rule does not mean you should be able to diagnose patients or practice medicine, but you need to have a basic understanding of the diagnoses that you are coding. All too frequently the diagnosis the physician has written cannot be found exactly in the code book.

In these cases, it is essential to have access to reference books that can help you get on track and provide terminology that you may use to find the code. For starters, invest in a comprehensive medical dictionary, The Merck Manual, and a good anatomy and physiology textbook. Make sure you also keep up to date on your reference books, always using the current edition. Make sure you have a current ICD-9 book! The terminology for code descriptions changes from year to year.

Remember that as a coder, your job is to accurately reflect what occurred in the encounter and show through coding the reasons for any procedure and the complexity of any evaluation and management. This requires that you have some basic understanding of the patient's situation along with knowledge of basic coding rules.

Understanding what you are coding is especially important now that you are required to match your ICD-9 codes with your procedure codes. If you do not understand the medical problem, test, exam, or treatment, you will not know which diagnosis corresponds to each procedure. Your reference books and your growing base of knowledge will prove invaluable resources.

DOCUMENTATION

When the physician does not provide enough information for the coder, the coder cannot provide enough information for the carrier. The physician must clearly and carefully document all diagnoses in detail so the coder can translate the information into specific and accurate codes reflecting as much detail and precision as the documentation and the ICD-9 system allows. Here are some responsibilities the physician has in order for the coder to be able to assign the correct codes:

Write legibly. Illegible handwriting holds up the coding/billing process.

Describe the patient's condition using terminology which includes specific diagnoses as well as symptoms, problems, or reasons for the encounter.

Remember you are submitting code numbers, not narrative descriptions. Somewhere in the patient documentation there must be specific and explicit information about what diagnoses were treated and what services were provided. Be clear and detailed, noting the site, type, cause, etc. that specifies the exact diagnosis. This is the information the coder must use to accurately translate the documentation into code numbers.

You must document all conditions or problems existing at the time of the visit that impact the treatment or management of the patient. The coder needs all this information in order to adequately convey the patient encounter to the carrier and to justify the services provided.

You must clearly denote which diagnosis or diagnoses are related to which procedure or procedures. The coder is required to link at least one diagnosis to each service billed for, and he or she needs some supporting documentation in order to correctly do this.

MEDICAL NECESSITY

Medical necessity is a determination that items or services furnished, or to be furnished, by any health care provider (for which third party payment may be made) are reasonable and medically necessary for the treatment provided for an illness or injury, for the improvement of function of a malformed body member, or for prevention of an illness. Remember that medical necessity is determined by the diagnoses you submit. Procedure codes may determine the amount being charged, but ICD-9 diagnoses provide the information that determines whether or not payment will be made.

For years, CMS has warned physicians to be specific and file correctly—this means document records fully, be unfailingly accurate with code assignments, use the correct number of digits, correctly link your diagnosis code to the correct procedure code, and make sure you adequately show medical necessity with your diagnoses. Failure to follow these steps can result in lowered reimbursement, claims rejection, and possible civil or criminal prosecution.

CORRECT CODE VERSUS PAYABLE CODE

As health care data is used for more and more purposes, the demand for accuracy and quality continues to increase. Of course, one of the major purposes to providers is reimbursement.

Sometimes it is true that the correct code (the code that most accurately describes the patient encounter) is not necessarily a payable code (a code that a carrier will reimburse the physician for). It is the coder's job to assign the correct code on the patient's record; hopefully, the correct code will also be a payable code. But the assignment must be based on what is correct, not what is payable.

If you submit a bill with an incorrect code, not only can the physician see repercussions (such as downcoding, rejection, inaccurate practice profile, and long-term audit risk), but the patient can, too.

The appropriate course of action is for physicians and coders to work together to correctly document and code each patient encounter. For each encounter, concentrate on choosing the correct code, not just the first similar code you come across, and not necessarily the code you know is payable.

BASIC CODING RULES

Outpatient coders: Code first the diagnosis, condition, problem, or other reason for the encounter that is shown in the medical record to be chiefly responsible for the services provided. Then code any additional diagnoses and co-existing conditions.

Inpatient coders: Follow UHDDS guidelines on selecting the principal diagnosis.

Code all current conditions and only current conditions that affect the treatment of the patient. Do not code conditions that have previously been treated and no longer exist, even if reference was made to their previous existence in the current record. (An exception to this would be in the case of late effects of previous injury or illness, or appropriate V-codes for history, family history or status codes.)

If a patient has a chronic disease, it can be coded on an ongoing basis as long as the patient is receiving treatment for the condition or it is a complicating factor that contributes to the complexity of the medical decision-making by the physician.

For physician billing, do not code diagnoses documented as suspected, probable, possible, or rule out as if they are established. If the physician does not document a definite diagnosis at the conclusion of a patient visit, you may code the chief complaint as the reason for the encounter.

Be sure to review the chart to get the details you need (cause, site, type, etc.) to assign the exact code. Don't hesitate to refer to a medical dictionary or a medical terminology book to verify the meanings or synonyms if necessary.

Be sure to check the accuracy of information such as patient's age and sex. You do not need this information to find the right codes, but it never hurts to make sure that you are not giving an obstetric code to one of your male patients or some other scenario that will almost assuredly be rejected by a carrier.

AVOID CODING FROM CONDENSED DIAGNOSIS LISTS

Code directly from the medical record. Don't rely solely on a diagnosis list from a superbill. For every diagnosis on the superbill, hundreds, sometimes thousands, are not on there. A condensed list cannot possibly contain the specificity required for accurate coding. Arthritis, for example, can be coded hundreds of different ways. By always coding with the appropriate acuity and specificity you will avoid setting a profile that causes either your treatment protocol or your billing practices to be questioned.

"RULE OUT", "PROBABLE", "POSSIBLE", "SUSPECTED", OR "VERSUS" CONDITIONS

When coding in an outpatient setting, conditions indicated by the terms "rule out", "probable", "possible", "suspected", or "versus" should never be coded as though they exist. Though allowed in inpatient settings, (with some caveats on certain diseases such as epilepsy and AIDS), coding of these "rule out" conditions is never allowed in the outpatient setting. Assigning a code to these unconfirmed conditions permanently affixes these diagnoses to the patient's medical history with potentially serious medicolegal consequences for the physician and patient. Imagine the consequences of an insurance coverage denial for a "pre-existing" condition that was erroneously coded from a "rule out" statement.

ULTIMATE SPECIFICITY

Always code to ultimate specificity, using all the digits available for the code. Use as many digits in the code as there are digits offered. If you can use five digits, use five. If there are only four digits possible for a code, use all four. Only use three digits if there are no fourth or fifth digit options. Take the code to as many digits as are available.

Remember that each digit helps to specify the diagnosis further and explain to the carrier what the patient's condition is. The claim will not be processed by most carriers if it is not at ultimate specificity.

MULTIPLE CODING

The basic rule of multiple coding is to be sure to fully code the patient's underlying problem(s) that were addressed, along with any complications or conditions that contribute to their medical complexity.

Some examples of this would be fluid overload in a patient with CHF, pneumonia in a patient with COPD, influenza in a patient with asthma, fracture in a diabetic patient, a shunt/catheter infection in a dialysis patient in chronic renal failure, an open wound in a diabetic patient, a urinary tract infection in a patient who is pregnant, arm weakness in a patient with hypertension, or chest tightness in a patient who had previously suffered a myocardial infarction.

Multiple coding is also required for certain conditions when a single code does not fully identify the condition being coded. For instance, you need both 250.5# and 362.01 to correctly code diabetic retinopathy. The 250.5# shows the diabetes with ophthalmic manifestation, and the 362.01 shows the background retinopathy due to diabetes. As is customary in multiple coding, the underlying disease or the condition that the manisfestation is "due to" is coded first, (250.5# in this case).

Use multiple coding whenever applicable. Generally, though, you should not code symptoms of a diagnosed disease or a disorder. For example, if a patient presents with abdominal pain and through the course of the encounter is found to have appendicitis, you would code only the appendicitis.

Multiple coding is divided into three categories: multiple coding for multiple concurrent diagnoses ("due to" , "with" or "secondary to"), mandatory multiple coding, and discretionary multiple coding.

Multiple coding for multiple concurrent diagnoses
The phrase "due to" indicates a cause and effect relationship between the two diagnoses. You should code both the cause and the effect. For example, if a patient was diagnosed with urinary incontinence due to BPH, you would code both the urinary retention and the BPH.

600.00 BPH
788.3# urinary retention

When "with" is used in a diagnosis it means that both conditions are present together, so you should use a code for each condition.

Note that the exception to using multiple codes for multiple concurrent diagnoses is the case in which there is one ICD-9 code that incorporates each of the conditions under one description. One example is 540.1, the code for abscess of the peritoneum with appendicitis. When a combination code exists for a condition with its manifestation/etiology, no additional code is required.

Mandatory multiple coding
There are certain codes that will not stand alone. Both the underlying condition (etiology) and the specific manifestation must be coded, with the underlying disease sequenced first. For example, a diagnosis of diabetic gangrene requires a code for the diabetes (the underlying disease) as well as a code for the gangrene.

250.7# diabetes
785.4 gangrene

GUIDELINES

Discretionary multiple coding
This type of multiple coding is indicated by the phrase "use additional code". An additional code should be used if the physician documents information that further describes the diagnosis. Every essential part of a diagnosis should be coded in order to fully describe a patient encounter.

An example of discretionary multiple coding would be a diagnosis of acute peritonitis caused by staphylococcus aureus. The correct coding for this disease would include two codes, one for peritonitis and one for the bacterial organism.

567.21 peritonitis acute
041.11 staphylococcus aureus

COMBINATION CODES

A combination code is a single code used to classify one of three things:

1. Two diagnoses at once, such as chronic cholecystitis with choledocholelithiasis, 574.40.

2. A diagnosis with an associated secondary process or manifestation, such as peritoneal abscess with appendicitis, 540.1.

3. An associated complication, such as arteriosclerotic gangrene of the extremities, 440.24.

You should assign a combination code only when the code fully identifies both conditions involved. If only one complication is present, do not use the combination code.

"UNSPECIFIED" (NOS) CODES

The "not otherwise specified" (NOS) or "unspecified" descriptions are used when the information in the record is not as specific as the information in the code book. For example, if the diagnosis provided is "osteoporosis", you must choose the NOS code for osteoporosis, 733.00, because you have not been given enough information to correctly choose from the more specific listings for osteoporosis.

Be careful when choosing an NOS code. If possible, follow up with the physician or get more information from the patient's chart so that you can specify the diagnosis more. Carriers are reluctant to accept and/or pay for NOS codes, but if an NOS code is your only option based on the documentation that you have, you must use it.

"NOT ELSEWHERE CLASSIFIED" (NEC) CODES

"Not elsewhere classified" (NEC) codes or "other specified" codes are used when the description given for the diagnosis is more specific than the descriptions for the codes in ICD-9. When a code does not exist for a definitive diagnosis, assign the "other specified" or "NEC" code in the category most accurately describing the condition. A diagnosis of breast discharge, for example would be coded as other specified disorder of breast, 611.79.

LATE EFFECTS

A late effect is a condition that is related to, but occurs after, an acute illness or injury. Late effects are also called sequelae, residual effects, or residual conditions. There is no set time period that must elapse before a sequelae becomes a late effect. Some residual conditions may appear immediately following injury or illness, such as aphasia following cerebrovascular disease. Others may appear years after the illness or injury, such as contractures from burns. Descriptive statements in the record such as "old", "late", "following", or "due to previous..." may be indicative of late effects that must be coded.

When coding a late effect, you may need multiple codes. Some code categories, such as cerebrovascular disease, have combination codes indicating the late effect diagnosis. In most cases, though, you will need two codes. The first code indicates the residual condition. The second code indicates that the condition is a late effect (codes 905-909).

If there is no appropriate code to indicate a late effect, code only the residual condition.

If the specific residual condition is not identified, such a "residual of traumatic arm amputation", use only the late effect code.

Never use the code for the acute condition when the diagnosis is a late effect of that condition.

Sequence the residual condition first, followed by the late effect code, unless specific instructions for the codes indicate otherwise.

Following are some examples:

Malunion of a femur fracture shortly after initial (acute) treatment:
733.81 Malunion
905.4 Late effect of fracture

Brain damage following cerebral abscess six months earlier:

348.9 brain damage
326 late effect abscess intracranial

ADVERSE REACTIONS TO PROPERLY ADMINISTERED SUBSTANCES

An adverse reaction is defined as a reaction to a correct substance properly administered. Adverse reactions are usually indicated in the diagnostic statement by one of the following terms: accumulative effect, intoxication due to, allergic reaction, idiosyncratic reaction, hypersensitivity, side effects, toxicity, synergistic reaction, or interaction between two drugs.

At least two codes are required to correctly code an adverse reaction. First, code the manifestation or condition caused by the drug—the adverse reaction itself. Second, code the substance or substances that caused the reaction. To code the substance, use the corresponding E-code from the "therapeutic" column of the Table of Drugs and Chemicals in the back of your ICD-9 book.

Sequence the reaction code first, followed by the E-code indicating the substance.

Here are a couple of examples of correctly coded adverse reactions:

The diagnosis is dizziness due to valium taken as prescribed.

780.4 dizziness
E939.4 adverse effect of valium, therapeutic use

When the manifestation of an adverse reaction is not identified, use code 995.2. Then use the E-code for the substance as you normally would. Here's an example:

995.2 adverse reaction to drug
E930.0 penicillin–therapeutic use

POISONINGS

A poisoning is any condition caused by drugs, medicines, or other chemical substances not used in accordance with the physician's instructions. Poisonings are identified in the diagnostic statement by the following terms: intoxication, overdose, poisoning, toxic effect, wrong dosage given in error, wrong dosage taken in error.

Drug interactions are also considered to be poisonings. For example, any condition caused by an interaction between a drug taken with alcohol or between prescribed drugs and nonprescribed drugs (over the counter medications) is considered a poisoning.

Poisonings due to drugs and related substances such as antibiotics, analgesics, and vaccinations are classified to categories 960-979. The table of drugs and chemicals also includes chemical substances that are non-medicinal in categories 980-989. This second category would include substances such as gases, acids, lead materials, and fumes. In both cases, the code you use will identify the type of substance that caused the poisoning.

To code a poisoning, use the table of drugs and chemicals in the back of your ICD-9 book. The substance will be found alphabetically and the corresponding code found in the "poisoning" column. The poison code should be sequenced first. When the manifestation of the poisoning is identified, it is sequenced second.

For example, here are the codes for a coma due to a valium overdose:

969.4 valium poisoning
780.01 coma

The use of E-codes to identify the external cause of the poisoning is the final step to fully coding poisonings. ICD-9 provides the following E-code categories for poisonings:

E850-869 accidental
E950-959 suicide and self-inflicted injury
E962 assault
E980-989 undetermined

Following are the codes for a patient in a coma due to a suicide attempt by valium overdose:

969.4 valium poisoning
780.01 coma
E950.3 suicide attempt-valium

To code a late effect of a poisoning, apply the same rules you would apply for coding late effects of an injury. The code identifying the residual effect is sequenced first, followed by the code for the late effect of the poisoning, and then the E-code for the late effect.

Here are the E-codes for late effects of poisonings:

E929 accidental
E959 self-inflicted
E969 assault
E989 undetermined

Here's an example of those codes in use for the diagnosis anoxic brain damage due to attempted suicide by barbiturate overdose four years ago:

348.1 anoxic brain damage
909.0 late effect poisoning
E959 late effect self-inflicted injury

GUIDELINES

V-CODES

The V-codes in ICD-9 CM are provided to identify health service encounters or contact with health services for reasons other than illness or injury. The following circumstances or problems are the primary reason for assigning V-codes:

1. When a person who is not currently sick encounters health services to act as an organ or tissue donor, because of the need for prophylactic vaccination, to discuss a problem, for counseling, or for health screenings.

2. When a person with known disease or injury (current, chronic or resolving) encounters health services for specific treatment of that disease or injury including aftercare, cast change, chemotherapy, dialysis, gastrostomy care/closure, or radiotherapy.

3. A. A circumstance or problem is present which influences the person's health status but is not a current illness or injury. Examples include alcoholism, family problems (reason for encounter), divorce estrangement (reason for encounter), and stress/unemployment problems (reason for encounter).

B. A circumstance or problem is present (the person may or may not currently be sick) and the V-code is assigned as an additional code to show a personal or family history of certain diseases or show a person with replacement status, such as heart valve (artificial)(prosthesis).

4. Newborn birth status.

Assignments of V-codes is appropriate both in the inpatient and outpatient setting but are particularly useful in coding ambulatory care encounters. V-codes indicate the reason for an encounter (V55.1 gastrostomy closure) and should not be confused with the procedure code that documents what procedure was actually performed.

Sequencing of V-codes may be first or second depending on the circumstances of the encounter.

V-code categories include:

1. Contact/exposure to communicable diseases

2. Need for inoculation and vaccination

3. Status: Indicates that a patient underwent a procedure that may influence future health or treatment.

4. History codes (personal) (family)
There are two types of history codes, personal and family. Personal history codes are valuable additional codes to denote past medical history of conditions that have been treated and for which no treatment is currently being rendered. However, the potential for recurrence is possible and the condition may need monitoring. History codes will usually be sequenced second. History codes may be assigned as additional codes on any record to provide further information regardless of the reason for the visit or whether the condition is still present or in any way alters the treatment provided.

5. Screening codes
Codes for screening exams are not assigned to individual tests administered to a patient to "screen for" a suspected condition. Screening exams are coded only when exams are used to screen for disease in defined population groups. The code does not in itself apply to any particular test or study.

(Remember, the testing of a person to rule out or confirm a suspected condition is usually done because there are some signs or symptoms to suspect a problem. This is a diagnostic exam, not a screening exam. In this case, do not assign a screening code, assign a code for the sign or symptoms.)

6. Observation codes
There are two categories of observation codes in ICD-9-CM. These codes are used only when a person is being observed for a suspected condition that is ruled out. These observation codes should not be used if an injury, illness, or any sign or symptom related to the suspected condition is present. In such cases, assign the diagnosis or symptom code with appropriate E-code.

7. Aftercare codes
Aftercare codes are codes that are used after the initial treatment of the acute disease or injury is completed and the patient requires continued care during the recovery period or care for long-term consequences of the original disease.

For routine visits for the purpose of changing surgical dressings, monitoring, or removing sutures form wounds without mention of complication, use code V58.3, attention to surgical dressings and sutures.

8. Follow-Up codes
V24.# and V67.# are used to explain continuing surveillance following completed treatment of a disease or injury. Follow-up codes denote that the condition has been satisfactorily treated and no longer exist. They are sequenced first and may be used with an additional history code to explain fully the healed condition.

9. Donor codes
V59.# or V59.## are not used for self-donation (autogenous) of tissue or organ, but rather for non-autogenous donation by other living individual who is donating tissue, blood, or other body tissue for person other than self.

10. Counseling codes
Counseling codes are used for counseling of a patient or patient's family member, following illness, injury, or other type of family or social crisis. These codes are used when support is needed to assist the person in coping with their problem. Reference these codes under Counseling.

11. Reproduction and Development V-codes
V-codes for obstetric care are used for the following reasons:
V20.# supervision child infant (healthy) well baby check
V22.# supervision of pregnancy normal
V23.#(#) supervision of pregnancy high risk
V24.# postpartum care
V25.#(#) contraception, contraceptive device/management
V26.#(#) procreative management
V27.# outcome of delivery (code on mother's chart) (inpatient only)
V28.# screening antenatal

12. Liveborn Infants Observation and Outcome
V29.0 – V29.9 observation newborn /infant suspected condition not found (undiagnosed)
V30.0# – V39.9# liveborn infants according to type of birth (code on infant's record) (inpatient only)

13. Examinations Administrative and Routine

14. V-codes miscellaneous
These codes include other health encounters not mentioned as the reason for the encounter and sequence first.

15. V-codes nonspecific
These codes are so nonspecific or redundant that there is little reason for their use in an inpatient setting.

In the outpatient setting, use these codes only when there is insufficient documentation in the chart to select a better diagnosis, and when you have made the physician aware of the lack of documentation. When possible and documentation allows, select any other sign or symptom code as the reason for the encounter rather than the nonspecific V-code.

WHERE CAN I GET CERTIFICATION AS A CODER?

Becoming involved in a professional organization for coders is an ideal way to make contacts, learn more about coding, share problems and solutions, and receive accreditation. Here's a brief rundown of a few professional organizations that you may be interested in joining.

AAPC

The American Academy of Professional Coders is designed to aid healthcare professionals interested in reimbursement and procedural and diagnosis coding.

The AAPC offers an Independent Study Program, which allows participants to work at their own pace as they learn more about CPT coding and reimbursement issues. Through the AAPC, you may earn the certification of Certified Professional Coder (CPC) or Certified Professional Coder-Hospital (CPC-H).

For more information about the AAPC, call 1-800-626-CODE or visit their web site at www.aapc.com.

AHIMA

AHIMA, the American Health Information Management Association, offers membership to anyone who is interested in the knowledge and understanding of health information issues.

AHIMA has various state and local chapters, and several particular sections and societies that deal with a specific area of health information. Members may be certified as Registered Health Information Administrator (RHIA), Registered Health Information Technician (RHIT), or Certified Coding Specialist (CCS).

For information about AHIMA, call 312-787-2672 or e-mail info@ahima.org.

PAHCOM

PAHCOM stands for the Professional Association of Health Care Office Managers. It provides support for managers of small group and solo health care practices.

Local chapters routinely meet to discuss relevant issues and educational programs for their communities. PAHCOM offers accreditation as a Certified Medical Manager (CMM).

For information on PAHCOM, call 1-800-451-9311.

CODE UPDATES

APPENDIX E

NEW – REVISED – INVALID DIAGNOSIS

NEW DIAGNOSIS CODES

040.41 Infant botulism
040.42 Wound botulism
058.10 Roseola infantum, unspecified
058.11 Roseola infantum due to human herpesvirus 6
058.12 Roseola infantum due to human herpesvirus 7
058.21 Human herpesvirus 6 encephalitis
058.29 Other human herpesvirus encephalitis
058.81 Human herpesvirus 6 infection
058.82 Human herpesvirus 7 infection
058.89 Other human herpesvirus infection
079.83 Parvovirus B19
200.30 Marginal zone lymphoma, unspecified site, extranodal and solid organ sites
200.31 Marginal zone lymphoma, lymph nodes of head, face, and neck
200.32 Marginal zone lymphoma, intrathoracic lymph nodes
200.33 Marginal zone lymphoma, intraabdominal lymph nodes
200.34 Marginal zone lymphoma, lymph nodes of axilla and upper limb
200.35 Marginal zone lymphoma, lymph nodes of inguinal region and lower limb
200.36 Marginal zone lymphoma, intrapelvic lymph nodes
200.37 Marginal zone lymphoma, spleen
200.38 Marginal zone lymphoma, lymph nodes of multiple sites
200.40 Mantle cell lymphoma, unspecified site, extranodal and solid organ sites
200.41 Mantle cell lymphoma, lymph nodes of head, face, and neck
200.42 Mantle cell lymphoma, intrathoracic lymph nodes
200.43 Mantle cell lymphoma, intra-abdominal lymph nodes
200.44 Mantle cell lymphoma, lymph nodes of axilla and upper limb
200.45 Mantle cell lymphoma, lymph nodes of inguinal region and lower limb
200.46 Mantle cell lymphoma, intrapelvic lymph nodes
200.47 Mantle cell lymphoma, spleen
200.48 Mantle cell lymphoma, lymph nodes of multiple sites
200.50 Primary central nervous system lymphoma, unspecified site, extranodal and solid organ sites
200.51 Primary central nervous system lymphoma, lymph nodes of head, face, and neck
200.52 Primary central nervous system lymphoma, intrathoracic lymph nodes
200.53 Primary central nervous system lymphoma, intra-abdominal lymph nodes
200.54 Primary central nervous system lymphoma, lymph nodes of axilla and upper limb
200.55 Primary central nervous system lymphoma, lymph nodes of inguinal region and lower limb
200.56 Primary central nervous system lymphoma, intrapelvic lymph nodes
200.57 Primary central nervous system lymphoma, spleen
200.58 Primary central nervous system lymphoma, lymph nodes of multiple sites
200.60 Anaplastic large cell lymphoma, unspecified site, extranodal and solid organ sites
200.61 Anaplastic large cell lymphoma, lymph nodes of head, face, and neck
200.62 Anaplastic large cell lymphoma, intrathoracic lymph nodes
200.63 Anaplastic large cell lymphoma, intra-abdominal lymph nodes
200.64 Anaplastic large cell lymphoma, lymph nodes of axilla and upper limb
200.65 Anaplastic large cell lymphoma, lymph nodes of inguinal region and lower limb

NEW DIAGNOSIS CODES (continued)

200.66 Anaplastic large cell lymphoma, intrapelvic lymph nodes
200.67 Anaplastic large cell lymphoma, spleen
200.68 Anaplastic large cell lymphoma, lymph nodes of multiple sites
200.70 Large cell lymphoma, unspecified site, extranodal and solid organ sites
200.71 Large cell lymphoma, lymph nodes of head, face, and neck
200.72 Large cell lymphoma, intrathoracic lymph nodes
200.73 Large cell lymphoma, intra-abdominal lymph nodes
200.74 Large cell lymphoma, lymph nodes of axilla and upper limb
200.75 Large cell lymphoma, lymph nodes of inguinal region and lower limb
200.76 Large cell lymphoma, intrapelvic lymph nodes
200.77 Large cell lymphoma, spleen
200.78 Large cell lymphoma, lymph nodes of multiple sites
202.70 Peripheral T cell lymphoma, unspecified site, extranodal and solid organ sites
202.71 Peripheral T cell lymphoma, lymph nodes of head, face, and neck
202.72 Peripheral T cell lymphoma, intrathoracic lymph nodes
202.73 Peripheral T cell lymphoma, intra-abdominal lymph nodes
202.74 Peripheral T cell lymphoma, lymph nodes of axilla and upper limb
202.75 Peripheral T cell lymphoma, lymph nodes of inguinal region and lower limb
202.76 Peripheral T cell lymphoma, intrapelvic lymph nodes
202.77 Peripheral T cell lymphoma, spleen
202.78 Peripheral T cell lymphoma, lymph nodes of multiple sites
233.30 Carcinoma in situ, unspecified female genital organ
233.31 Carcinoma in situ,vagina
233.32 Carcinoma in situ,vulva
233.39 Carcinoma in situ, other female genital organ
255.41 Glucocorticoid deficiency
255.42 Mineralocorticoid deficiency
258.01 Multiple endocrine neoplasia [MEN] type I
258.02 Multiple endocrine neoplasia [MEN] type IIA
258.03 Multiple endocrine neoplasia [MEN] type IIB
284.81 Red cell aplasia (acquired)(adult)(with thymoma)
284.89 Other specified aplastic anemias
288.66 Bandemia
315.34 Speech and language developmental delay due to hearing loss
331.5 Idiopathic normal pressure hydrocephalus (INPH)
359.21 Myotonic muscular dystrophy
359.22 Myotonia congenital
359.23 Myotonic chondrodystrophy
359.24 Drug induced myotonia
359.29 Other specified myotonic disorder
364.81 Floppy iris syndrome
364.89 Other disorders of iris and ciliary body
388.45 Acquired auditory processing disorder
389.05 Conductive hearing loss, unilateral
389.06 Conductive hearing loss, bilateral
389.13 Neural hearing loss, unilateral
389.17 Sensory hearing loss, unilateral
389.20 Mixed hearing loss, unspecified
389.21 Mixed hearing loss, unilateral
389.22 Mixed hearing loss, bilateral
414.2 Chronic total occlusion of coronary artery
415.12 Septic pulmonary embolism
423.3 Cardiac tamponade

NEW DIAGNOSIS CODES (continued)

440.4	Chronic total occlusion of artery of the extremities
449	Septic arterial embolism
488	Influenza due to identified avian influenza virus
525.71	Osseointegration failure of dental implant
525.72	Post-osseointegration biological failure of dental implant
525.73	Post-osseointegration mechanical failure of dental implant
525.79	Other endosseous dental implant failure
569.43	Anal sphincter tear (healed) (old)
624.01	Vulvar intraepithelial neoplasia I [VIN I]
624.02	Vulvar intraepithelial neoplasia II [VIN II]
624.09	Other dystrophy of vulva
629.82	Acquired absence of both uterus and cervix
629.83	Acquired absence of uterus, with remaining cervical stump
629.84	Acquired absence of cervix with remaining uterus
664.60	Anal sphincter tear complicating delivery, not associated with third-degree perineal laceration, unspecified as to episode of care or not applicable
664.61	Anal sphincter tear complicating delivery, not associated with third-degree perineal laceration, delivered, with or without mention of antepartum condition
664.64	Anal sphincter tear complicating delivery, not associated with third-degree perineal laceration, postpartum condition or complication
733.45	Aseptic necrosis of bone, jaw
787.20	Dysphagia, unspecified
787.21	Dysphagia, oral phase
787.22	Dysphagia, oropharyngeal phase
787.23	Dysphagia, pharyngeal phase
787.24	Dysphagia, pharyngoesophageal phase
787.29	Other dysphagia
789.51	Malignant ascites
789.59	Other ascites
V12.53	Personal history of sudden cardiac arrest
V12.54	Personal history of transient ischemic attack (TIA), and cerebral infarction without residual deficits
V13.22	Personal history of cervical dysplasia
V16.52	Family history of malignant neoplasm, bladder
V17.40	Family history of cardiovascular diseases,unspecified
V17.41	Family history of sudden cardiac death (SCD)
V17.49	Family history of other cardiovascular diseases
V18.11	Family history of multiple endocrine neoplasia [MEN] syndrome
V18.19	Family history of other endocrine and metabolic diseases
V25.04	Counseling and instruction in natural family planning to avoid pregnancy
V26.41	Procreative counseling and advice using natural family planning
V26.49	Other procreative management, counseling and advice
V26.81	Encounter for assisted reproductive fertility procedure cycle
V26.89	Other specified procreative management
V49.85	Dual sensory impairment
V68.01	Disability examination
V68.09	Other issue of medical certificates
V72.12	Encounter for hearing conservation and treatment
V73.81	Special screening examination, Human papillomavirus (HPV)
V84.81	Genetic susceptibility to multiple endocrine neoplasia [MEN]
V84.89	Genetic susceptibility to other disease

REVISED DIAGNOSIS CODES

005.1	Botulism food poisoning
359.3	Periodic paralysis
389.14	Central hearing loss
389.18	Sensorineural hearing loss, bilateral
389.7	Deaf, nonspeaking, not elsewhere classifiable

DELETED DIAGNOSIS CODES

233.3	Carcinoma in situ,other and unspecified female genital organs
255.4	Corticoadrenal insufficiency
258.0	Polyglandular activity in multiple endocrine adenomatosis
284.8	Other specified aplastic anemias
359.2	Myotonic disorders
364.8	Other disorders of iris and ciliary body
389.2	Mixed conductive and sensorineural hearing loss
624.0	Dystrophy of vulva
787.2	Dysphagia
789.5	Ascites
V17.4	Family history of other cardiovascular diseases
V18.1	Family history of other endocrine and metabolic diseases
V26.4	Procreative management,general counseling and advice
V26.8	Other specified procreative management
V68.0	Issue of medical certificates
V84.8	Genetic susceptibility to other disease

NOTES

NOTES

NOTES

NOTES

NOTES

NOTES

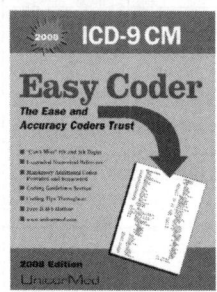

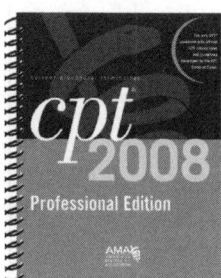

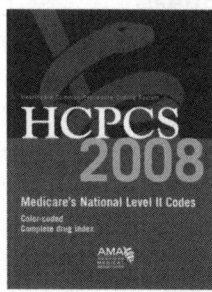

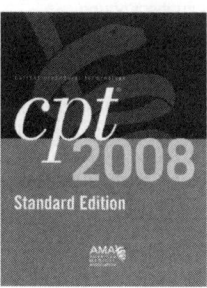

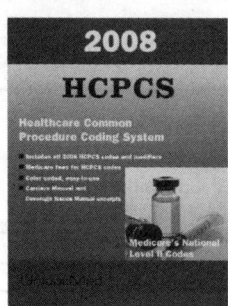

UnicorMed

unifying coding, compliance, and reimbursement

PRODUCTS	PRICE	QTY	TOTAL
2008 ICD-9 Easy Coder *Comprehensive*	$ 62.00		
2008 ICD-9 Easy Coder *Cardiology*	$ 62.00		
2008 ICD-9 Easy Coder *Chiropractic*	$ 62.00		
2008 ICD-9 Easy Coder *Dermatology*	$ 62.00		
2008 ICD-9 Easy Coder *ENT*	$ 62.00		
2008 ICD-9 Easy Coder *Family Practice*	$ 62.00		
2008 ICD-9 Easy Coder *Internal Medicine*	$ 62.00		
2008 ICD-9 Easy Coder *OB/Gyn*	$ 62.00		
2008 ICD-9 Easy Coder *Ophthalmology*	$ 62.00		
2008 ICD-9 Easy Coder *Optometry*	$ 62.00		
2008 ICD-9 Easy Coder *Orthopedics*	$ 62.00		
2008 ICD-9 Easy Coder *Psychiatry*	$ 62.00		
2008 ICD-9 Easy Coder *Urology*	$ 62.00		
2008 ICD-9 Easy Coder *Includ. Volume Three*	$ 72.00		
2008 CPT® Standard – *softbound*	$ 71.95		
2008 CPT® Professional – *spiral*	$ 99.95		
2008 CPT® Changes	$ 65.95		
2008 CPT® Coding Workbook	$ 59.95		
2008 HCPCS UnicorMed– *spiral*	$ 84.95		
2008 HCPCS AMA – *softbound*	$ 94.95		
2008 ICD-9 AMA *spiral*	$ 92.95		
2008 ICD-9 AMA *softbound*	$ 89.95		
2008 ICD-9 AMA *compact*	$ 74.95		
2008 ICD-9 Mag Mutual *spiral*	$ 74.95		
2008 ICD-9 Mag Mutual *softbound*	$ 69.95		
Principles of ICD-9 Coding	$ 69.95		
Principles of CPT® Coding 4th ed	$ 64.95		
Coding with Modifiers	$ 89.95		
2008 Physicians' Fee & Coding Guide, Vol. 1 *spiral*	$169.95		
2008 Physicians' Fee & Coding Guide, Vol. 1 *softbound*	$169.95		
2008 Physicians' Fee & Coding Guide, Vol. 2 – *softbound*	$109.95		
2008 Physicians' Fee & Coding Guide Vol 3 *Indicate specialty*	$129.95		
Practical E/M	$ 84.95		
Netter's Atlas of Human Anatomy for CPT	$ 89.95		
Step by Step Medical Coding	$ 61.95		
Compliance Guide for the Medical Practice	$ 99.95		
HIPAA Plain and Simple	$ 49.95		
Secrets of the Best Run Practices	$ 64.95		
Medical Practice Policies and Procedures	$125.00		
Tech. and Fin. Gde. to EHR Implementation	$ 99.95		

SHIPPING CHARGES
1 item: $ 7.95
2-3 items: $10.95
4-5 items: $14.95
6-7 items: $17.95
8-9 items: $19.95
10+ items: Each additional item, add $2.00

These charges are not valid in HI, AK, PR, or Guam. For delivery outside the Continental US or for rush delivery, please call [800] 825-7421 to arrange the most efficient shipping method.

SUBTOTAL	
SHIPPING CHARGES	
TOTAL	

SHIP TO

Is the ship-to address listed below a commercial or residential address? ☐ commercial ☐ residential

Name__________

Title__________

Company__________

Billing address__________

City, State, ZIP__________

Shipping address__________

City, State, ZIP__________

Phone__________ Fax__________

Email__________

Ok to send product info and promotions via email? ☐ Yes ☐ No

PAYMENT INFORMATION

☐ Check enclosed payable to Unicor Medical

Please charge my: ☐ MC ☐ VISA ☐ AMEX

Name on card__________

Account No__________

Exp. Date__________

Signature__________

☐ P.O. No__________

Signature__________

P.O.s accepted on orders of $300 or more, subject to credit approval.

30-Day Money Back Guarantee: You may return any product within 30 days for a full refund, minus shipping charges. Product should be in resalable condition and in its original shipping package. We do not accept CODs.

TO ORDER | UnicorMed [800] 825-7421 | FAX [800] 305-8030 | WWW.UNICORMED.COM | SALES @UNICORMED.COM
MAIL TO: UnicorMed 4160 CARMICHAEL ROAD MONTGOMERY, AL 36106

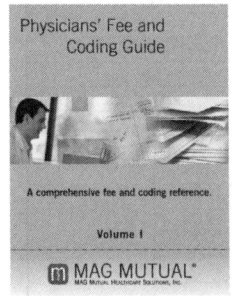

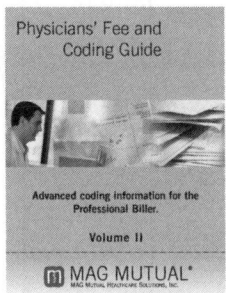

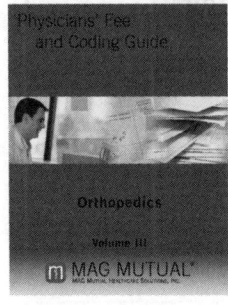